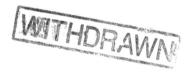

# Critical Care Obstetrics

## Third Edition

# Critical Care Obstetrics

## Third Edition

Edited by

### STEVEN L. CLARK, MD
**Director, Intermountain Health Care Perinatal Centers**
**Professor of Obstetrics and Gynecology**
University of Utah
Salt Lake City, Utah

### DAVID B. COTTON, MD
**Professor, Department of Obstetrics and Gynecology**
Hutzel Hospital/Wayne State University
Detroit, Michigan

### GARY D.V. HANKINS, MD
**Professor and Vice Chairman**
Department of Obstetrics and Gynecology
**Chief, Maternal/Fetal Medicine and Obstetrics**
University of Texas Medical Branch at Galveston
Galveston, Texas

### JEFFREY P. PHELAN, MD
**Co-Director, Maternal-Fetal Medicine**
Pomona Valley Hospital Medical Center
Pomona, California

*b*

**Blackwell**
**Science**

**Blackwell Science**

**Editorial Offices:**
Commerce Place, 350 Main Street, Malden,
Massachusetts 02148, USA
Osney Mead, Oxford OX2 0E1, England
25 John Street, London WC1N 2BL, England
23 Ainslie Place, Edinburgh EH3 6AJ, Scotland
54 University Street, Carlton, Victoria 3053,
Australia

**Other Editorial Offices:**
Blackwell Wissenschafts-Verlag GmbH
    Kurfürstendamm 57, 10707 Berlin, Germany
Zehetnergasse 6, A-1140 Vienna, Austria

**Distributors:**

*USA*
    Blackwell Science, Inc.
    Commerce Place
    350 Main Street
    Malden, Massachusetts 02148
    (Telephone orders: 800-215-1000 or
        617-388-8250; Fax orders: 617-388-8270)

*Australia*
    Blackwell Science Pty., Ltd.
    54 University Street
    Carlton, Victoria 3053
    (Telephone orders: 03-9347-0300;
        Fax orders: 03-9349-3016)

*Canada*
    Copp Clark, Ltd.
    2775 Matheson Blvd. East
    Mississauga, Ontario
    Canada, L4W 4P7
    (Telephone orders: 800-263-4374 or
        905-238-6074)

*Outside North America and Australia*
    Blackwell Science, Ltd.
    ℅ Marston Book Services, Ltd.
    P.O. Box 269, Abingdon
    Oxon OX14 4YN
    England
    (Telephone orders: 44-01235-465500;
        Fax orders 44-01235-465555)

Acquisitions: Joy Denomme
Production: Colophon
Manufacturing: Lisa Flanagan
Typeset by Publication Services/WG, Inc.
Printed and bound by Braun-Brumfield, Inc.
© 1997 by Steven L. Clark, David B. Cotton, Gary D.V. Hankins, and Jeffrey P. Phelan

Printed in the United States of America

97  98  99  00   5  4  3  2  1

**Library of Congress Cataloging-in-Publication Data**

Critical care obstetrics / [edited by] Steven L. Clark . . . [et al.] —3rd ed.
    p.    cm.
    Includes bibliographical references and index.
    ISBN 0-86542-538-8
    1. Pregnancy—Complications. 2. Obstetrical emergencies.
  I. Clark, Steven L.
    [DNLM: 1. Pregnancy Complications—therapy. 2. Critical Care—in pregnancy.    WQ 240 C9339 1997]
RG571.C68   1997
618.3′028—dc21
DNLM/DLC
for Library of Congress

    97-5559
    CIP

To Dr. Richard Paul,
under whose guidance the
discipline of Maternal-Fetal
Medicine was formed, and
who directed the training of a
generation of leaders in the field

# Contents

PART **IV**

Fetal Consideration

# Preface

*Critical Care Obstetrics* was introduced originally in 1987. Since that time, interest in this area has continued to grow, as the complex interactions between pregnancy-induced maternal physiologic changes, the fetus, and critical illness are increasingly appreciated. While many maternal fetal medicine specialists are expanding the scope of their expertise into the domains traditionally reserved for the anesthesiologist and medical intensivist, so, too, the latter specialists are paying increased attention to the unique needs of the critically ill mother and her unborn child. It is against this background that the third edition of *Critical Care Obstetrics* was developed.

This text does not represent a simple update of the second edition; rather, most chapters have been rewritten extensively. We have involved a number of new subspecialist authors, many of them trained and board certified in areas beyond obstetrics or maternal fetal medicine. We also have paid particular attention to an expanded treatment of basic physiologic principles, such as fluid and electrolyte balance, and of procedures such as ventilator management and complex arterial/venous access that are often vital in current intensive care management. We anticipate that the third edition of *Critical Care Obstetrics* will continue to be of assistance to those involved in providing care to these important patients.

SLC
DBC
GDVH
JPP

# List of Contributors

**Manuel Alvarez, MD**
Chairman
Department of Obstetrics, Gynecology, and
  Reproductive Science
Hackensack University Medical Center
Hackensack, New Jersey
Chapter 10

**Peter L. Bailey, MD**
Associate Professor of Anesthesiology
Department of Anesthesiology
University of Utah
Salt Lake City, Utah
Chapter 13

**William H. Barth, Jr., MD**
Chairman, Dept. of OB/GYN
Maternal Fetal Medicine
Wilford Hall Medical Center
San Antonio, Texas
Chapter 17

**Michael A. Belfort, MD**
Associate Professor, Dept. of OB/GYN
Baylor College of Medicine
Houston, Texas
Chapter 35

**James W. Bernasko, MD**
Assistant Clinical Professor
Division of Maternal-Fetal Medicine
Mount Sinai School of Medicine
New York, New York
Chapter 10

**Renee A. Bobrowski, MD**
Assistant Professor
Department of Obstetrics and Gynecology
Indiana University Medical Center
Indianapolis, Indiana
Chapter 2

**Gerald G. Briggs, BPharm**
Careline Pharmacist/Clinical Coordinator
Long Beach Memorial Medical Center, Women's
  Hospital
Long Beach, California
Chapter 37

**Steven L. Clark, MD**
Director, Intermountain Health Care Perinatal
  Centers
Professor of Obstetrics and Gynecology
University of Utah
Salt Lake City, Utah
Chapters 5, 15, 20, 21

**David B. Cotton, MD**
Professor, Department of Obstetrics and
  Gynecology
Hutzel Hospital/Wayne State University
Detroit, Michigan
Chapters 1, 3, 14

**Barbara J. Davey-Sullivan, MD**
Clinical Professor
The Woman's Clinic
Jackson, Mississippi
Chapter 32

**Lowell E. Davis, MD**
Professor
Department of Obstetrics and Gynecology
Oregon Health Sciences University
Portland, Oregon
Chapter 28

**Gary A. Dildy, MD**
Director, Utah Valley Regional Perinatal Center
Associate Professor
Department of Obstetrics and Gynecology
Provo, Utah
Chapter 14

**Donna Dizon-Townson, MD**
Assistant Professor
Department of Obstetrics and Gynecology
University of Utah School of Medicine
Salt Lake City, Utah
Chapter 23

**Thomas J. Garite, MD**
Professor and Chairman
Department of Obstetrics and Gynecology
UCI Women's Health Care
Orange, California
Chapter 37

**Bernard Gonik, MD**
Professor and Associate Chairman
Department of Obstetrics and Gynecology
Wayne State University/Grace Hospital
Detroit, Michigan
Chapters 23, 31

**Cornelia R. Graves, MD**
Assistant Professor
Division of Maternal/Fetal Medicine
Vanderbilt Medical Center
Nashville, Tennessee
Chapter 34

**Gary D.V. Hankins, MD**
Professor and Vice Chairman
Department of Obstetrics and Gynecology
Chief, Maternal/Fetal Medicine and Obstetrics
University of Texas Medical Branch at Galveston
Galveston, Texas
Chapters 6, 18, 29, 33

**David P. Kissinger, MD**
Chairman, Dept. of General Surgery
Wilford Hall Medical Center
San Antonio, Texas
Chapter 7

**Wayne B. Kramer, MD**
Assistant Professor, Maternal-Fetal Medicine
Department of Obstetrics and Gynecology
University of Maryland
Baltimore, Maryland
Chapter 4

**Wesley Lee, MD**
Attending Staff
Department of Obstetrics and Gynecology
William Beaumont Hospital
Royal Oak, Michigan
Associate Professor of Obstetrics and
   Gynecology
Wayne State University
Detroit, Michigan
Chapter 1

**Michael R. Leonardi, MD**
Division of Maternal-Fetal Medicine
Department of Obstetrics and Gynecology
Wilford Hall Medical Center
San Antonio, Texas
Chapter 22

**James N. Martin, Jr., MD**
Professor of Obstetrics and Gynecology
Director of Maternal/Fetal Medicine
University of Mississippi Medical Center
Jackson, Mississippi
Chapters 27, 30, 32

**Julie Martin-Arafch, RN, MSN**
Division of Maternal/Fetal Medicine
Vanderbilt Medical Center
Nashville, Tennessee
Chapter 34

**Brian M. Mason, MD**
Division of Maternal/Fetal Medicine
Department of Obstetrics and Gynecology
University of Tennessee, Memphis
Memphis, Tennessee
Chapter 18

**Kenneth J. Moise, Jr., MD**
Associate Professor
Department of Obstetrics and Gynecology
Director, Division of Maternal/Fetal Medicine
Baylor College of Medicine
Houston, Texas
Chapter 3

**Mary P. O'Day, MD**
Assistant Professor of Maternal/Fetal Medicine
University of Texas Medical Branch at Galveston
Galveston, Texas
Chapter 29

**Jeffrey P. Phelan, MD**
Co-Director, Maternal-Fetal Medicine
Pomona Valley Hospital Medical Center
Pomona, California
Chapters 19, 36

**T. Flint Porter, MD**
Assistant Professor
Department of Obstetrics and Gynecology
University of Utah
Salt Lake City, Utah
Chapter 24

**Brendan S. Ross, MD**
Assistant Professor
Department of Obstetrics and Gynecology
University of Mississippi Medical Center
Jackson, Mississippi
Chapter 30

**Elaine L. Ross, MD**
Assistant Professor
Department of Obstetrics and Gynecology
University of Mississippi Medical Center
Jackson, Mississippi
Chapter 30

**David A. Sacks, MD**
Director, Division of Maternal-Fetal Medicine
Department of Obstetrics and Gynecology
Kaiser Foundation Hospital
Bellflower, California
Clinical Professor
Department of Obstetrics and Gynecology
Los Angeles County-University of Southern
    California Medical Center
Los Angeles, California
Chapter 11

**Andrew J. Satin, MD**
Associate Professor
Department of Obstetrics and Gynecology
Uniformed Services University of the Health
    Sciences
Bethesda, Maryland
Chapter 12

**Gail L. Seiken, MD**
Staff Nephrologist
Walter Reed Medical Center
Washington, D.C.
Chapters 9, 16

**Christopher A. Sullivan, MD**
Director, Maternal/Fetal Medicine
Stamford Hospital
Stamford, Connecticut
Assistant Professor
Obstetrics and Gynecology at New York Medical
    College
Chapter 27

**Mark W. Tomlinson, MD**
Assistant Professor, Maternal-Fetal Medicine
Department of Obstetrics and Gynecology
Wayne State University School of Medicine
Detroit Medical Center/Grace Hospital
Detroit, Michigan
Chapter 31

**James W. Van Hook, MD**
Assistant Professor
Department of Obstetrics and Gynecology
Vice Chief, Maternal/Fetal Medicine
The University of Texas Medical Branch at
    Galveston
Galveston, Texas
Chapters 8, 33

**Karen A. Zempolich, MD**
Fellow in Gynecologic Oncology
USC School of Medicine
Los Angeles, California
Chapter 25

# PART I

# Physiology

CHAPTER *1*

# Pregnancy-Induced Physiologic Alterations

*C*ritical illnesses that compromise the heart and lungs are among the most challenging problems affecting pregnant women. Normal physiologic changes should be considered when evaluating patients for circulatory shock, hypertension, cardiac disease, and pulmonary insufficiency. For example, maternal hemodynamic variables including blood volume, BP, heart rate, stroke volume, cardiac output, and systemic vascular resistance (SVR) may be modified by gestational age, body position, pain, labor, blood loss, and maternal respiratory status. This chapter reviews these relationships and their clinical relevance to the intensive care of obstetric patients.

## Blood Volume

Most plasma volume measurements have been made with Evans blue dye or radioactive isotope bound to serum albumin (McLennon, 1948; Caton, 1951; Hytten, 1963; Lund, 1967). Clapp and co-workers (1988) reported maternal plasma volume to increase by 11% as early as the seventh week of pregnancy. As summarized in Figure 1-1, this increase reaches a plateau at 32 weeks, remaining stable thereafter until delivery (Scott, 1972). Although wide variations are recognized, the increase in plasma volume at term averages approximately 45% to 50%. Placental production of chorionic somatomammotropin, progesterone, and possibly prolactin stimulates maternal eryth-

ropoiesis, but it results in a smaller (20% less) red-cell mass increase (Jepson, 1968; Letsky, 1995). These changes account for the maternal anemia that often occurs despite adequate iron stores (Cavill, 1995). Maximal hemodilution develops by approximately 30 to 32 weeks. Intervillous thrombosis and infarction have been reported to occur during normal pregnancies (Rolschau, 1978). In this regard, Koller (1982) suggests that the hemodilution of pregnancy has a beneficial effect on the uteroplacental circulation by decreasing blood viscosity.

The magnitude of hypervolemia shows considerable variation among different women, despite a tendency for the same plasma volume pattern to be repeated during successive pregnancies (Pritchard, 1965a; Lund, 1967). Increased blood volume is positively correlated to the number of fetuses (Pritchard, 1965a; Rovinsky, 1965). Pritchard (1965a) observed that the overall increase in blood volume for singleton pregnancies was estimated to be 1570 mL, which represented a 48% increase over nonpregnant values. These women received iron supplementation during pregnancy and served as their own postpartum controls. By comparison, twin pregnancies had an average blood volume of 1960 mL (Table 1-1).

Pregnancy should be considered a natural volume-overload state resulting from renal sodium and water retention, with a shift of fluid from the intravascular to the extravascular space. Increased renal glomerular filtration rate and progesterone levels lead to increased urinary sodium

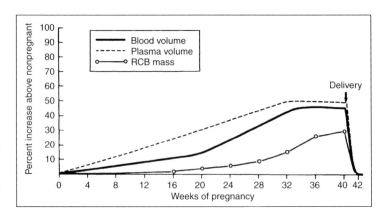

F I G U R E   **1-1**

**Blood volume changes during pregnancy.** (Reproduced by permission from Scott DE. Anemia during pregnancy. Obstet Gynecol Annu 1972;1:219.

excretion (Oparil, 1975). By contrast, sodium-sparing mechanisms must counterbalance these natriuretic effects primarily through increased mineralocorticoid activity. These processes cause an overall accumulation of approximately 500 to 900 mEq of sodium and 6 to 8 liters of total body water in the maternal circulation (Seitchik, 1967; Lindheimer, 1973). Clinicians should remember that a substantial part of maternal weight gain results from not only fetal growth, but also fluid accumulation.

Unlike other arterial vasodilatory states, pregnancy is uniquely associated with increased renal glomerular filtration and filtered sodium load (Schrier, 1991). Enhanced distal tubular sodium delivery opposes the sodium-retaining effects of aldosterone. No known substance, including the prostaglandins, has been shown to exhibit such a profound effect on renal hemodynamics. There-fore, an unknown vasodilator could be responsible as a primary stimulus to volume expansion. This concept is supported by studies demonstrating that systemic vasodilatation occurs prior to blood volume increases during baboon pregnancy (Phippard, 1986). A hypothetical vasodilating substance may also be responsible for the well-described vascular resistance to angiotensin during pregnancy.

Plasma volume changes may be regulated by both the mother and her fetus. For example, increased maternal mineralocorticoid activity results from extra-adrenal conversion of progesterone to deoxycorticosterone (Winkel, 1980). The fetal adrenal gland may regulate maternal plasma volume by controlling the amount of estrogen precursor (dehydroepiandrosterone) reaching the placenta (Longo, 1984). Placental estrogen then triggers increased production of aldosterone through

T A B L E   **1-1**

Blood and red-cell volumes in normal women late in pregnancy and again when not pregnant

|  | Late Pregnant | Nonpregnant | Increase (mL) | Increase (%) |
|---|---|---|---|---|
| *Single Fetus* (n = 50) | | | | |
| Blood volume | 4820 | 3250 | 1570 | 48 |
| RBC volume | 1790 | 1355 | 430 | 32 |
| Hematocrit | 37.0 | 41.7 | — | — |
| *Twins* (n = 30) | | | | |
| Blood volume | 5820 | 3865 | 1960 | 51 |
| RBC volume | 2065 | 1580 | 485 | 31 |
| Hematocrit | 35.5 | 41 | — | — |

Reproduced by permission from Pritchard JA. Changes in the blood volume during pregnancy and delivery. Anesthesiology 1965;26:393.

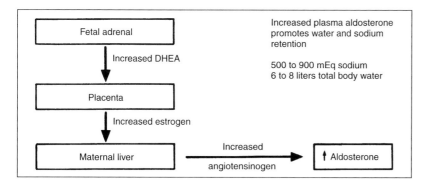

Increased plasma aldosterone promotes water and sodium retention

500 to 900 mEq sodium
6 to 8 liters total body water

F I G U R E   **1-2**

Hypothesis for fetal regulation of maternal plasma volume changes.

the renin-angiotensin system (Fig 1-2). The fetus, however, is not essential for the development of gestational hypervolemia because this has also been described in molar pregnancies (Pritchard, 1965b).

Blood volume changes are related closely to pregnancy outcome, and hypervolemia can act as a protective mechanism against excessive maternal blood loss. For example, eclamptic women do not expand their vascular space to the extent that they demonstrate in subsequent nonhypertensive pregnancies (Table 1-2) (Pritchard, 1984). Patients with this disease are less tolerant of peripartum blood loss when compared with pregnant women who normally expand their blood volume. Clinicians should appreciate that these patients have a contracted, but not underfilled, intravascular compartment.

Maternal blood volume expansion abnormalities also are associated with fetal problems. Salas et al (1993) used Evans blue dye to compare plasma volume between growth-retarded and normal fetuses. Smaller fetuses (n = 30) had significantly less maternal plasma volume (2976 ± 76

mL vs. 3594 ± 103 mL) near term gestation. Growth-retarded pregnancies also had lower maternal levels of aldosterone and vasodilator substances such as prostacyclin and kallikrein.

## Blood Pressure

Blood pressure reflects the heart's ability to maintain adequate cardiac output and perfusion to surrounding tissues. Quantitatively, it is the product of SVR and cardiac output. Maternal BP can be affected by gestational age, measurement technique, and maternal position. Clinicians should consider these factors when evaluating a gravid patient with circulatory abnormalities. For example, a maternal BP reading of 130/84 mm Hg would be normal for term pregnancy but abnormally high for 20 weeks' gestation. Earlier reports suggested that increases of 30 mm Hg systolic or 15 mm Hg diastolic from second trimester values helped to establish maternal hypertension. This concept is no longer valid because many women

T A B L E   **1-2**

Blood volumes in five women

|  | Eclampsia | Nonpregnant | Normal Pregnant |
|---|---|---|---|
| Blood volume (mL) | 3530 | 3035 | 4425 |
| Change (%) | + 16 |  | + 47 |
| Hematocrit (%) | 40.5 | 38.2 | 34.7 |

Measured (chromium 51) during antepartum eclampsia, again when nonpregnant, and finally at comparable time in second pregnancy uncomplicated by hypertension.

Adapted by permission from Pritchard JA, Cunningham FG, Pritchard SA. The Parkland Memorial Hospital protocol for treatment of eclampsia: evaluation of 245 cases. Am J Obstet Gynecol 1984;148:951.

can exhibit these findings during normal pregnancy (Villar, 1989; ACOG, 1996).

Maternal BP decreases by 9% as early as the seventh week of pregnancy (Clapp, 1988). These changes may be due to hormonal and cardiovascular factors. Animal studies indicate that systemic vasodilation and a synchronous fall in arterial pressure occur very early in baboon pregnancy (Phippard, 1986). In fact, the fall in BP was caused entirely by decreased SVR. Cardiac output did not completely compensate for decreased afterload, thereby providing a reasonable explanation for lower mean arterial BP during the first trimester.

Systolic and diastolic BPs decrease during pregnancy until midpregnancy, with gradual recovery to nonpregnant values by term. A longitudinal study of 69 women during normal pregnancy documented the lowest arterial BPs occurring by 28 weeks' gestation (Fig 1-3) (Wilson, 1980). In this series, the lowest BPs were obtained from the maternal left lateral decubitus position. When subjects were moved from the left lateral decubitus to the supine position, mean BP increased by approximately 14 mm Hg (Fig 1-4).

Occasionally, BP measurements also can be influenced by specific measurement techniques. Ginsberg and Duncan (1969) observed a difference between intra-arterial and manual BP measurements during pregnancy. In this series of 70 women, directly measured systolic and diastolic pressures were lower ($-6$ mm Hg and $-15$ mm Hg, respectively), when compared with readings measured indirectly by cuff sphygmomanometry. Kirshon and colleagues (1987) found automated cuff systolic BP to be significantly lower than direct intra-arterial measurements in postpartum patients. No differences were found in the diastolic BP measurements between direct radial and automated measurements.

## Heart Rate

Maternal heart rate increases occur as early as the seventh week of pregnancy. By late pregnancy, maternal heart rate is increased approximately 20% over postpartum values (Wilson, 1980) (Fig 1-5). These increases may be caused by a primary fall in SVR (Duvekot, 1993). Alternatively, hormonal factors may account for these changes. It seems unlikely that human chorionic gonadotropin causes maternal tachycardia, because its nadir by 20 weeks' gestation does not correlate well with the degree of heart rate increases occurring during the second trimester (Glinoer, 1990). This hormone does not cause heart rate increases in women who receive pharmacologic doses of the hormone for infertility. Free thyroxine levels increase by 10 weeks and remain elevated throughout pregnancy (Harada, 1979; Glinoer, 1990); the

FIGURE **1-3**

Sequential changes in average systolic and diastolic BPs, with subjects sitting and standing throughout pregnancy (n = 69 patients with SEMs). Postpartum values drawn on the ordinate are used as a baseline, and dotted lines represent the presumed changes during the first 8 weeks. (Reprinted by permission of the publisher from Wilson M, Morganti AA, Zervodakis I, et al. Blood pressure, the renin-aldosterone system, and sex steroids throughout normal pregnancy. Am J Med 68:97. Copyright 1980 by Excerpta Medica Inc.)

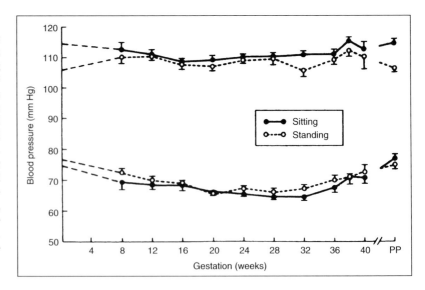

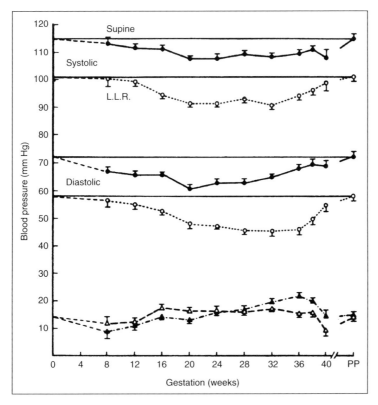

F I G U R E   **1-4**

Sequential changes in BP throughout pregnancy with subjects in the supine and left lateral decubitus positions (n = 69 patients with SEMs). The change in systolic (open triangles) and diastolic (closed triangles) BPs produced by movement from the left lateral decubitus position is illustrated. LLR, left lateral recumbent. (Reprinted by permission of the publisher from Wilson M, Morganti AA, Zervodakis I, et al. Blood pressure, the renin-aldosterone system, and sex steroids throughout normal pregnancy. Am J Med 68:97. Copyright 1980 by Excerpta Medica Inc.)

F I G U R E   **1-5**

Sequential changes in mean heart rate in three positions throughout pregnancy (n = 69 patients with SEMs). (Reprinted by permission of the publisher from Wilson M, Morganti AA, Zervodakis I, et al. Blood pressure, the renin-aldosterone system, and sex steroids throughout normal pregnancy. Am J Med 68:97. Copyright 1980 by Excerpta Medica Inc.)

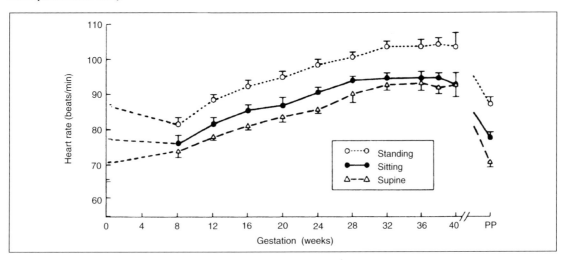

possibility that thyroid hormones are responsible for maternal tachycardia warrants further investigation.

Several conditions, such as fever, pain, blood loss, hyperthyroidism, respiratory insufficiency, and cardiac disease, can lead to increased heart rate. Tachycardia can be particularly important for the critically ill gravida. For example, women with severe mitral stenosis must rely on diastolic ventricular filling to achieve satisfactory cardiac output. Maternal tachycardia can limit severely their capacity for maintaining adequate BP because left ventricular diastolic filling is heart rate–dependent. Consequently, a very fine balance between heart rate and BP exists for these patients. Any exogenous factor leading to increased heart rate can actually cause cardiovascular shock and fetal distress. These patients should be stabilized by controlling maternal tachycardia in addition to conventional diuretic therapy that is based on invasive hemodynamic monitoring.

## Stroke Volume and Cardiac Output

Cardiac output is the product of heart rate and stroke volume. It reflects the overall capacity of the left ventricle for maintaining systemic BP and organ perfusion. Cardiac index is calculated by dividing cardiac output by body surface area. A clinically significant correlation between cardiac output (by Doppler echocardiography or thoracic electrical impedance) and body surface area, however, is not observed during normal pregnancy (van Oppen, 1995). Considering that the widely used DuBois (1916) body surface area nomogram was based on only nine nongravid subjects, the routine use of cardiac index may not be a well-justified practice during pregnancy.

In 1915, Linhard first reported a 50% cardiac output increase during pregnancy by the indirect Fick method. Others have studied maternal cardiac output by invasive catheterization (Hamilton, 1949; Palmer, 1949; Bader, 1955; Clark, 1989), indicator-dye dilution (Walters, 1966; Lees, 1967; Ueland, 1969a,b,c), impedance cardiography (Atkins, 1981a,b), and echocardiography or Doppler technique (Katz, 1978; Laird-Meeter, 1979; Mashini, 1987; Easterling, 1990; van Oppen, 1996). De-

spite controversy about the relative contributions of stroke volume and heart rate, maternal cardiac output increases as early as 10 weeks' gestation and peaks at 30% to 50% over control values by the latter part of the second trimester. This rise, from approximately 4.5 to 6.0 liters/min, is sustained for the remainder of the pregnancy if cardiac output is measured from the lateral decubitus position. Nulliparous women have a higher mean cardiac output than multiparous women (van Oppen, 1996).

Beginning in the late 1940s, right heart catheterization provided a more refined, although invasive, method for studying maternal cardiac output. Hamilton (1949) measured cardiac output in 24 nongravid and 68 normal pregnant women by this technique. Cardiac output in nonpregnant women averaged 4.51 ± 0.38 liters/min as compared with pregnant women with a maximum of 5.73 liters/min at 26 to 29 weeks' gestation. This increase began at approximately 10 to 13 weeks' gestation and eventually returned to nonpregnant levels by term. An early rise in cardiac output with an eventual fall toward nonpregnant levels by term gestation was consistent with the findings from two other cross-sectional right heart catheterization studies performed by Palmer and Walker (1949) and Bader et al (1955), respectively.

Longitudinal studies employing M-mode echocardiography have provided further insight into the relationship of heart rate and stroke volume throughout pregnancy. In a study of 19 pregnant women, Katz and associates (1978) observed progressive stroke volume increases when patients were studied in the lateral decubitus position, although this increase was not significant for supine women. Maternal cardiac output increases ( +59% by the third trimester) were attributable to both heart rate and stroke volume increases. Laird-Meeter et al (1979) also performed M-mode echocardiography in 13 normal pregnant women. The initial cardiac output increase occurring before 20 weeks' gestation was due to maternal tachycardia. After 20 weeks' gestation, stroke volume increased significantly and was associated with reversible myocardial hypertrophy. The researchers hypothesized that the mechanism of cardiac output increase may shift from elevated heart rate early in pregnancy to an elevation in stroke volume after 20 weeks' gestation. Mashini and colleagues (1987) reported yet another longitudinal study of 16 pregnancies. Cardiac output was not elevated prior to 20 weeks' gestation. By the early third trimester, however, it had increased by 32% over postpartum values, primarily due to heart rate but not stroke volume.

Therefore, the major M-mode ultrasound studies of maternal cardiac output report somewhat conflicting results about the relative contributions of heart rate and stroke volume to cardiac output during pregnancy. Some of this confusion may be related to maternal body position, from which these measurements were actually taken. It must be emphasized, however, that these calculations are based on geometric assumptions, which may not be valid during pregnancy. Although M-mode estimations of stroke volume have been correlated satisfactorily with angiographic studies of nongravid subjects, similar validation studies have not been carried out during pregnancy (Pombo, 1971; Murray, 1972).

Doppler ultrasound measurements of maternal volume flow have also been validated against thermodilution techniques (Robson, 1987a,b,c; Easterling, 1987; Lee, 1988). Mabie and colleagues (1994) studied serial maternal hemodynamic changes for 18 gravid women from the left lateral recumbent position. Their Doppler ultrasound measurements were compared with 12-week postpartum values. Cardiac output increased from 6.7 ± 0.9 liters/min at 8 to 11 weeks' gestation to 8.7 ± 1.4 liters/min at 36 to 39 weeks' gestation. Cardiac output increases were due to augmentation of both heart rate (+29%) and stroke volume (+18%). Their results suggested that stroke volume had a greater influence on cardiac output increases than heart rate prior to 20 weeks' gestation (Fig 1-6).

Unfortunately, serial studies of maternal hemodynamic changes are usually compared with measurements from postpartum control subjects. This may create problems because cardiac output is still elevated weeks after delivery (Robson, 1987c; Capeless, 1991). Robson et al (1989a) studied maternal cardiac output and compared their measurements with those of the same subjects

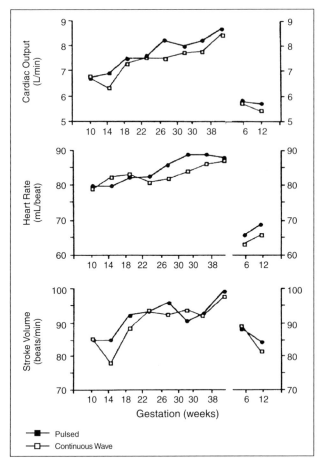

**F I G U R E  1-6**

**Hemodynamic changes during pregnancy and postpartum.** (Reproduced by permission from Mabie W, Ratts TE, Sibai S. A longitudinal study of cardiac output in normal human pregnancy. Am J Obstet Gynecol 1994;170:849.)

prior to pregnancy. Thirteen women were studied by Doppler echocardiography twice before conception and at monthly intervals throughout pregnancy. Heart rate increased significantly by 5 weeks' gestation and continued to do so until stabilizing at 32 weeks (+17% above prepartum values). Stroke volumes increased by 8 weeks of pregnancy, with maximal values (+32% over prepartum values) obtained by 16 to 20 weeks. Overall, cardiac output increased as early as 5 weeks' gestation from 4.88 liters/min to 7.21 liters/min (+48%) by 32 weeks (Fig 1-7).

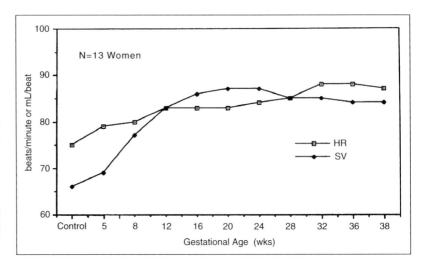

F I G U R E **1-7**
Serial changes in maternal heart rate (HR) and stroke volume (SV) by M-mode and Doppler echocardiography in 13 women. (Adapted by permission from Robson SC, Hunter S, Boys RJ, et al. Serial study of factors influencing changes in cardiac output during human pregnancy. Am J Physiol 1989;256:H1060.)

Maternal cardiac output augmentation may result from increased blood volume, arteriovenous shunting, and/or hormonal mechanisms. Blood volume changes are not directly responsible for increased cardiac output because the latter occurs much earlier than gestational hypervolemia in pregnant baboons (Phippard, 1986) (Fig 1-8). Burwell (1938) has proposed that the increased plasma volume, cardiac output, and heart rate during pregnancy is similar to the hemodynamic changes following the development of an arteriovenous fistula in the uteroplacental circulation. A third hypothesis suggests that left ventricular dilation is caused by hormonal factors and is analogous to decreased venous tone observed with normal pregnancy (McCalden, 1975) or after the administration of oral contraceptives (Wook, 1964). Morton and co-workers (1984) believe that early stroke volume increases are caused by a "shift to the right" of the left ventricular pressure-volume curve (Frank-Starling mechanism). In this regard, high-dose estrogen administration has been shown to increase stroke volume and cardiac output in male transsexuals (Slater, 1986).

Toward this end, a hormonal factor may cause increased cardiac output by triggering a primary fall in systemic vascular tone. Duvekot and colleagues (1993) studied serial echocardiographic, hormonal, and renal electrolyte measurements from 10 pregnant women. They proposed that a primary fall in SVR leads to compensatory tachy-cardia with activation of volume-restoring mechanisms. In this manner, increased stroke volume may be a direct result of "normalized" vascular filling, despite systemic afterload reduction.

## Systemic Vascular Resistance

Systemic vascular resistance is a measure of the impedance to the ejection of blood into the maternal circulation (e.g., afterload). Bader et al (1955) used cardiac catheterization to document the lowest values for SVR (980 dyne·sec·cm$^{-5}$) during the fourteenth to twenty-fourth week of pregnancy. According to their data, SVR rises progressively toward a nonpregnant value of 1240 dyne·sec·cm$^{-5}$ by term gestation. These findings are consistent with subsequent invasive studies (Clark, 1989), which found the mean SVR to be 1210 ± 266 dyne·sec·cm$^{-5}$ during late pregnancy.

When describing the physiologic relationships between pressure and flow, it is customary to measure vascular impedance as a ratio of pressure to flow. The following formula may be used to estimate this value:

$$SVR = \frac{(\text{Mean arterial pressure} - \text{Central venous pressure}) \times 80}{\text{Cardiac output}}$$

Quantitatively, the decreased SVR observed during pregnancy largely reflects decreased mean arterial pressure and increased cardiac output. It

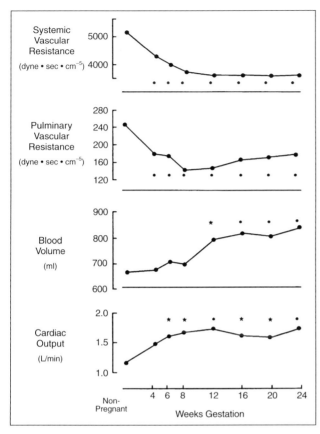

F I G U R E  **1-8**

**Early hemodynamic and humoral profile for pregnant baboons. Significant rises in cardiac output occurred at 4 to 6 weeks of pregnancy and coincided with decreases in pulmonary and systemic vascular resistances. However, significant blood volume increases did not occur until 12 weeks.** *p < .05. (Adapted by permission from Phippard AF, Horvath JS, Glynn EM, et al. Circulatory adaptation to pregnancy—serial studies of haemodynamics, blood volume, renin, and aldosterone in the baboon (*Papio hamadryas*). J Hypertens 1986;4:773.)

is very important to recognize the inverse relationship between cardiac output and SVR.

The uteroplacental circulation is a low-resistance circuit that reduces cardiac afterload. Peripheral arterial vasodilation with relative underfilling of the arterial circulation could account for decreased SVR (Schrier, 1988; 1990; 1991). Arterial vascular underfilling is possible despite overall blood volume expansion because much

of the circulation is contained within the central venous system. As seen in Figure 1-9, pregnancy may cause decreased SVR as the result of an unknown vasodilatory substance. The peripheral arterial vasodilation hypothesis can explain increased cardiac output, water accumulation, and sodium retention as homeostatic mechanisms that maintain maternal arterial blood volume. This is accomplished through activation of arterial baroreceptors, vasopressin stimulation, stimulation of the sympathetic nervous system, and increased mineralocorticoid activity. However, the hypothesis assumes the existence of a potent vasodilatory substance, which remains to be characterized. Recent in vitro work by Seligman and colleagues (1996) have examined the significance of nitrous oxide in the pathogenesis of pregnancy-induced hypertension. Nitrous oxide maintains decreased vascular tone in the uteroplacental circulation. Their study suggests that hypoxia-induced impairment of nitrous oxide production by placental syncytiotrophoblast may lead to uteroplacental insufficiency.

Atrial natriuretic peptide (ANP) is a peptide hormone that is produced within atrial cardiocytes and appears to regulate fluid and electrolyte homeostasis (Brenner, 1990). This substance promotes renal sodium excretion and diuresis in nonpregnant subjects. In vitro studies suggest that ANP has significant vasodilating effects on vascular smooth muscle that has been precontracted with angiotensin II. Several studies have found increased ANP levels during pregnancy, and these findings have raised the possibility that this substance may cause decreased maternal SVR (Cusson, 1985; Thomsen, 1988).

Earlier cross-sectional studies did not simultaneously correlate ANP levels with blood volume and hemodynamic measurements. Thomsen and colleagues (1993) reported a prospective longitudinal study of 40 primigravid women that showed a highly significant decrease of plasma ANP levels during the third trimester. Plasma ANP levels were positively correlated with Doppler ultrasound estimates of peripheral vascular resistance. Their results substantiate the physiologic significance of plasma ANP as a blood volume regulator but suggests that ANP does not function as a significant vasodilator during pregnancy.

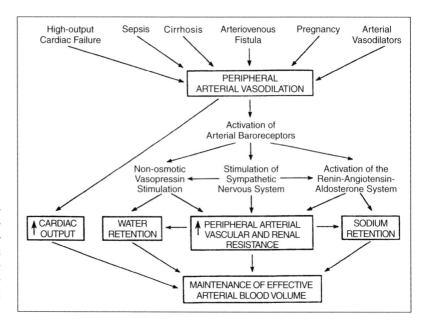

F I G U R E   **1-9**

Unifying hypothesis of renal sodium and water retention initiated by peripheral arterial vasodilation. (Reprinted with permission from The American College of Obstetricians and Gynecologists [Obstetrics and Gynecology, 1991; 77:632].)

## Regional Blood Flow

Significant regional blood flow changes have been documented during pregnancy. Renal blood flow has been shown to increase to approximately 30% over nonpregnant values by midpregnancy (Chesley, 1960; Gabert, 1985). In these studies, increased renal flow remained stable until term gestation, when measurements were taken from the lateral decubitus position. The supine position, however, can decrease renal flow related to aortocaval compression by the gravid uterus (Chesley, 1960; Lindheimer, 1972). The glomerular filtration rate can increase 30% to 50% over control values as a result of elevated renal plasma flow (Schrier, 1988).

In two studies, uterine blood flow increased from approximately 50 mL/min at 10 weeks' gestation to 500 mL/min at term, a figure that represents more than 10% of systemic cardiac output (Metcalfe, 1955; Assali, 1960). This increase in blood flow may be related to hormonal factors, because animal studies have shown a significant decrease in uterine vascular resistance in response to the administration of estrogen and progesterone (Ueland, 1966; Caton, 1974).

Pulmonary hemodynamics have been examined by Doppler echocardiography (Robson, 1991) and by analyzing pulmonary artery acceleration and ejection times (Kitabatake, 1983). In the latter study, mean pulmonary artery pressure was about 14 mm Hg, which was not significantly different from the nongravid state. Pulmonary blood flow increased more than 32% (4.88 liters/min to 7.19 liters/min) by 38 weeks' gestation. A small decrease in pulmonary vascular resistance was noted until 8 weeks without any subsequent significant change thereafter. These findings are consistent with invasive studies suggesting that mean pulmonary artery pressure does not significantly change during pregnancy (Werko, 1954; Bader, 1955). While confirming a lack of change in pulmonary artery pressures, Clark et al (1989) demonstrated a 34% decline in pulmonary vascular resistance in late pregnancy, compared with postpartum values.

Skin perfusion begins to increase slowly in early pregnancy, up to 18 to 20 weeks' gestation, and is followed by a sharp rise between 20 and 30 weeks (Katz, 1980). The increased skin perfusion then remains stable until delivery and is measurable for approximately 1 week postpartum. Earlier studies have documented the increased skin temperature that results from dilatation of dermal capillaries (Burt, 1949; Herbert, 1958). This may serve as a mechanism by which the excessive heat of fetal metabolism is allowed to dissipate via the maternal circulation.

## Effect of Posture on Maternal Hemodynamics

Prior to the 1960s, clinical investigators had not appreciated the effects of maternal postural changes on cardiac output, and their patients were often studied in the supine position. The unique angiographic studies of Bieniarz et al (1966, 1968) indicate that the gravid uterus can block caval blood flow significantly in approximately 90% of women studied in the supine position. Elevated caval pressure resulting from the weight of the gravid uterus predisposes the parturient to increased dependent edema and varicosities of the lower extremities. Significant partial obstruction of the aorta and its ancillary branches has also been shown to result from compression by the gravid uterus in the supine position. Central venous return is reduced in supine gravidas and may result in decreased cardiac output, a sudden drop in BP, bradycardia, and syncope (Fig 1-10) (Kerr, 1968).

These clinical changes were described extensively by Howard et al (1953) and are now commonly referred to as the "supine hypotensive syndrome." Holmes (1960) documented significant supine hypotension in 8.2% of 500 women during late pregnancy. Pregnant women who are symptomatic from this syndrome have poor circulation in the paravertebral vessels (e.g., azygous, lumbar, and paraspinal) that usually serve as an alternate route for blood return from the pelvic organs and the lower extremities back to the heart. The varying degree of collateral circulation that returns blood around the gravid uterus explains the reason why pregnant women respond so differently while in the supine position near term gestation. Kinsella and associates (1994) comprehensively reviewed potential mechanisms for the supine hypotensive syndrome involving vena caval obstruction, aortic compression, and/or neurogenic factors.

Vorys et al (1961) first described the reduction of cardiac output to the heart due to the mechanical effects of the gravid uterus on the vena cava during late pregnancy. A 16% cardiac output reduction from the lateral position was

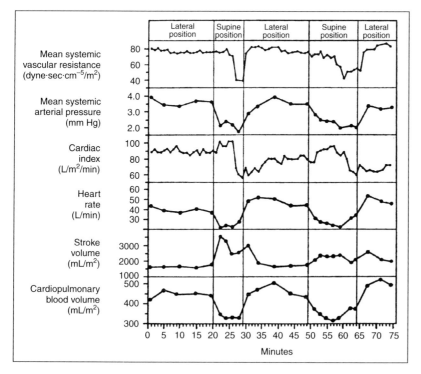

**F I G U R E   1-10**

Serial hemodynamic changes in a gravid woman who experienced the supine hypotensive syndrome. After the patient had been lying supine for 6 minutes, a profound fall in arterial BP was observed. (Reproduced by permission from Kerr MG. Cardiovascular dynamics in pregnancy and labour. Br Med Bull 1968;24:19.)

observed in the dorsal lithotomy position (Table 1-3). Calvin and associates (1988) monitored BP, oxygen saturation, and pulse amplitude in 42 gravid women (mean gestational age, 28 to 42 weeks) in the supine position. As seen in Figure 1-11, four general responses were observed: type A (BP elevation without pulse change, 64%), types B and C (isolated tachycardia or BP decreases, 21%), and type D (supine hypotensive syndrome, 14%). An important finding of this study indicates that significant oxygen desaturation does not normally result from supine hypotension.

The relationship of gestational age on the maternal cardiovascular response to posture was examined by Ueland et al (1969a). Figure 1-12 illustrates serial changes in resting heart rate, stroke volume, and cardiac output for 11 normal gravid women in various positions. Cardiac output was measured by a dye-dilution technique at four different study periods: 20 to 24 weeks, 28 to 32 weeks, 38 to 42 weeks, and 6 to 8 weeks postpartum. Measurements were taken from patients in the sitting, supine, and left lateral decubitus positions. Maternal heart rate was maximal (range, +13% to 20%) by 28 to 32 weeks of pregnancy, especially in the sitting position. Stroke volume increased early, with maximal values by 20 to 24 weeks (range, +21% to 33%), followed by a progressive decline toward term gestation that was quite striking in the supine position. In fact, assumption of the supine position at term led to stroke volume and cardiac output values that

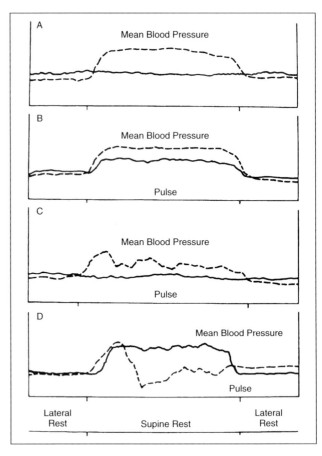

**F I G U R E  1-11**

Four general types of BP (dashed line) and pulse (solid line) responses to supine rest. (A) Type A was experienced by 64% of patients. (B, C) Types B and C were experienced by 21% of patients. (D) Representing the supine hypotensive syndrome, type D occurred in 14% of the women. (Reprinted with permission from The American College of Obstetricians and Gynecologists [Obstetrics and Gynecology, 1988;71:872].)

T A B L E  **1-3**

Cardiac output changes with maternal position (n = 31)

| Late-Trimester Women (sulphobromophthalein dye) | Change from Supine (%) |
| --- | --- |
| Horizontal left side | +14 |
| Trendelenburg left side | +13 |
| Lithotomy | −16 |
| Supine Trendelenburg | −18 |

Reproduced by permission from Vorys N, Ullery JC, Hanusek GE. The cardiac output changes in various positions in pregnancy. Am J Obstet Gynecol 1961;82:1312.

were even below their corresponding postpartum measurements.

Easterling et al (1988) examined by Doppler ultrasound the effects of standing on cardiac output and SVR during early (11.1 ± 1.4 wk) and late (36.7 ± 1.6 wk) pregnancy. Subjects were studied from the recumbent, sitting, and standing positions. Changes from the recumbent to standing position resulted in cardiac output decreases of

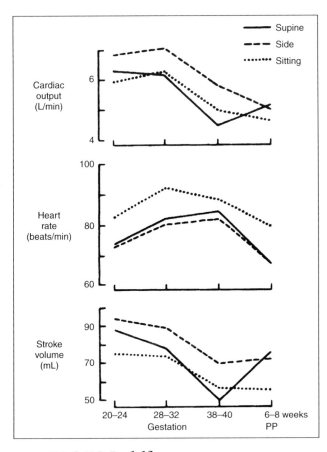

FIGURE **1-12**

Effect of posture on maternal hemodynamics. PP, postpartum. (Reproduced by permission from Ueland K, Metcalfe J. Circulatory changes in pregnancy. Clin Obstet Gynecol 1975;18:41; modified from Ueland K, Novy MJ, Peterson EN, et al. Maternal cardiovascular dynamics. IV. The influence of gestational age on the maternal cardiovascular response to posture and exercise. Am J Obstet Gynecol 1969; 104:856.)

about 1.7 liters/min with compensatory SVR augmentation (Table 1-4). They also observed that SVR increases were blunted during late pregnancy, when compared with nongravid subjects. Smaller SVR decreases may be related to blunted norepinephrine responses during pregnancy (Nisell, 1988; Barron, 1986).

Pulmonary artery catheterization also has been used to examine orthostatic stress during late pregnancy (Clark, 1991). The direct Fick method was used on 10 normal subjects to study cardiac output changes from various positions before and after delivery. Maternal BP was maintained despite varying effects on cardiac output, even during the lowest cardiac output measurement from the sitting position (Table 1-5). The standing position led to decreased cardiac output ($-18\%$) and increased heart rate ($+30\%$). Systemic vascular resistance increases resulting from the standing position were again blunted when compared with the same nongravid subjects (Fig 1-13, Table 1-6). Decreased left ventricular stroke work index ($-22\%$) was attributed to the subject's inability to compensate for decreased stroke volume by heart rate alone as a result of Starling forces.

Decreased left ventricular stroke work index suggested a diminution of intrinsic ventricular function for standing pregnant women. The relationship of these hemodynamic changes to the reported association of the standing position with decreased birth weight, placental infarction, and preterm delivery warrants further investigation (Naeye 1982; Henriksen, 1995). Intrapulmonary shunting ($Q_s/Q_t$) is not influenced by maternal position (Hankins, 1996).

## Antepartum Hemodynamic Values for Late Pregnancy

Cross-sectional cardiac catheterization studies by Bader and colleagues (1955) examined right ventricular, pulmonary arterial, and pulmonary capillary wedge pressures in 46 normal women throughout pregnancy. These parameters were not significantly different from nonpregnant control values.

Clark and colleagues (1989) also examined the maternal circulation by invasive hemodynamic monitoring. Ten primiparous women underwent right heart catheterization during late pregnancy (35 to 38 wk) and again postpartum (11 to 13 wk) to establish normal values for central maternal hemodynamics (Table 1-7). When compared with the postpartum state, late pregnancy was associated with significant increases in the following parameters (measured in the left lateral recumbent position): heart rate ($+17\%$), stroke volume

T A B L E  **1-4**

Net change in hemodynamic parameters from
recumbent to standing positions

| | Nonpregnant | Early Pregnancy | Late Pregnancy | *p*\* |
|---|---|---|---|---|
| MAP (mm Hg) | 7.8 ± 8.3 | 3.7 ± 7.7 | 5.0 ± 11.3 | NS |
| HR (beats/min) | 15.5 ± 9.2 | 25.7 ± 11.8 | 16.7 ± 11.2 | NS |
| CO (liters/min) | −1.8 ± 0.84 | −1.8 ± 0.79 | −1.7 ± 1.2 | NS |
| SV (mL) | −41.1 ± 15.8 | −38.7 ± 13.5 | −30.8 ± 17.5 | NS |
| SVR (dyne·sec·cm$^{-5}$) | 732 ± 363 | 588 ± 246 | 379 ± 214 | .005 |

Data are presented as mean ± SD.

*Determined by analysis of variance.

MAP, mean arterial pressure; HR, heart rate; CO, cardiac output; SV, stroke
volume; SVR, systemic vascular resistance; NS, not significant.

Reprinted with permission from The American College of Obstetricians and
Gynecologists (Obstetrics and Gynecology, 1988;72:550).

(+23%), and cardiac output (+43%). Significant decreases occurred in late pregnancy in SVR (−21%), pulmonary vascular resistance (−34%), serum colloid osmotic pressure (−14%), and the colloid osmotic pressure to pulmonary capillary wedge pressure gradient (−28%). No significant changes were found in the pulmonary capillary wedge or central venous pressures. These women did not exhibit hyperdynamic left ventricular function on the basis of Starling function curves (left ventricular stroke work index ÷ pulmonary capillary wedge pressure).

T A B L E  **1-5**

Hemodynamic alterations in response to position change
late in third trimester of pregnancy

| Hemodynamic Parameter | Position | | | | | |
|---|---|---|---|---|---|---|
| | LL | RL | SUP | SIT | ST | KC |
| MAP (mm Hg) | 90 ± 6 | 90 ± 5 | 90 ± 8 | 90 ± 8 | 91 ± 14 | 95 ± 6 |
| CO (liters/min) | 6.6 ± 1.4 | 6.8 ± 1.3 | 6.0 ± 1.4* | 6.2 ± 2.0 | 5.4 ± 2.0* | 6.9 ± 2.1 |
| P (beats/min) | 82 ± 10 | 87 ± 12 | 84 ± 10 | 91 ± 11 | 107 ± 17* | 93 ± 12 |
| SVR (dyne·cm· sec$^{-5}$) | 1210 ± 266 | 1321 ± 305 | 1437 ± 338 | 1217 ± 254 | 1319 ± 394 | 1223 ± 289 |
| PVR (dyne·cm· sec$^{-5}$) | 76 ± 16 | 81 ± 33 | 101 ± 45 | 102 ± 35 | 117 + 35* | 79 ± 27 |
| PCWP (mm Hg) | 8 ± 2 | 7 ± 1 | 6 ± 3 | 4 ± 4 | 4 ± 2 | 8 ± 3 |
| CVP (mm Hg) | 4 ± 3 | 3 ± 2 | 3 ± 2 | 1 ± 1 | 1 ± 2 | 3 ± 2 |
| LVSWI (g·min·m$^{-2}$) | 43 ± 9 | 42 ± 9 | 40 ± 9 | 44 ± 5 | 34 ± 7* | 47 ± 9 |

*$p < .05$, compared with left lateral position.

CO, cardiac output; P, pulse; SVR, systemic vascular resistance; PVR, pulmonary vascular resistance; PCWP, pulmonary capillary wedge pressure; CVP, central venous pressure; LVSWI, left ventricular stroke work index; LL, left lateral; RL, right lateral; SUP, supine; SIT, sitting; ST, standing; KC, knee-chest.

Reproduced by permission from Clark SL, Cotton DB, Pivarnik JM, et al. Position change and central hemodynamic profile during normal third-trimester pregnancy and postpartum. Am J Obstet Gynecol 1991;164:883.

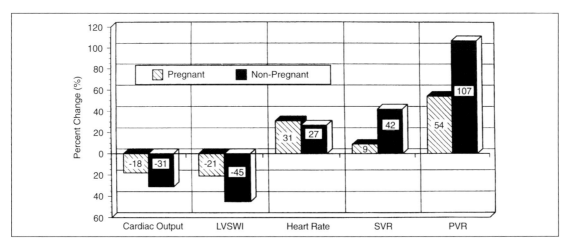

F I G U R E   **1-13**

Position change and hemodynamic parameters during pregnancy and postpartum. Percent changes were documented from maternal standing, as compared with the left lateral position. LVSWI, left ventricular stroke work index; SVR, systemic vascular resistance; PVR, pulmonary vascular resistance. (Adapted by permission from Clark SL, Cotton DB, Pivarnik JM, et al. Position change and central hemodynamic profile during normal third-trimester pregnancy and post partum. Am J Obstet Gynecol 1991;164:883.)

T A B L E   **1-6**

Hemodynamic alterations in response to position change in nonpregnant women

| Hemodynamic Parameter | Position | | |
|---|---|---|---|
| | LL | SUP | ST |
| MAP (mm Hg) | 86 ± 8 | 85 ± 9 | 79 ± 13 |
| CO (liters/min) | 4.2 ± .6 | 4.7 ± 1.0 | 2.9 ± .6* |
| P (beats/min) | 71 ± 10 | 70 ± 14 | 90 ± 19* |
| SVR (dyne·cm·sec$^{-5}$) | 1530 ± 520 | 1598 ± 568 | 2175 ± 709* |
| PVR (dyne·cm·sec$^{-5}$) | 123 ± 38 | 140 ± 87 | 254 ± 167* |
| PCWP (mm Hg) | 6 ± 2 | 8 ± 3 | 3 ± 2 |
| CVP (mm Hg) | 4 ± 3 | 4 ± 3 | 1 ± 2 |
| LVSWI (g·min·m$^{-2}$) | 42 ± 7 | 39 ± 12 | 23 ± 11* |

*$p < .05$, compared with left lateral position.

CO, Cardiac output; P, pulse; SVR, systemic vascular resistance; PVR pulmonary vascular resistance; PCWP, pulmonary capillary wedge pressure; CVP, central venous pressure; LVSWI, left ventricular stroke work index; LL, left lateral; SUP, supine; ST, standing.

Reproduced by permission from Clark SL, Cotton DB, Pivarnik JM, et al. Position change and central hemodynamic profile during normal third-trimester pregnancy and postpartum. Am J Obstet Gynecol 1991;164:883.

T A B L E   1-7

Central hemodynamic changes associated
with late pregnancy (n = 10)

| | Nongravid | Gravid | Change (%) |
|---|---|---|---|
| Mean arterial pressure (mm Hg) | 86 ± 8 | 90 ± 6 | NS |
| Pulmonary capillary wedge pressure (mm Hg) | 6 ± 2 | 8 ± 2 | NS |
| Central venous pressure (mm Hg) | 4 ± 3 | 4 ± 3 | NS |
| Heart rate (beats/min) | 71 ± 10 | 83 ± 10 | +17 |
| Cardiac output (liters/min) | 4.3 ± 0.9 | 6.2 ± 1.0 | +43 |
| Systemic vascular resistance (dyne·sec·cm$^{-5}$) | 1530 ± 520 | 1210 ± 266 | −21 |
| Pulmonary vascular resistance (dyne·sec·cm$^{-5}$) | 119 ± 47 | 78 ± 22 | −34 |
| Serum colloid osmotic pressure (COP: mm Hg) | 20.8 ± 1.0 | 18.0 ± 1.5 | −14 |
| COP-PCWP gradient (mm Hg) | 14.5 ± 2.5 | 10.5 ± 2.7 | −28 |
| Left ventricular stroke work index (g·min·m$^2$) | 41 ± 8 | 48 ± 6 | NS |

Measurements from the left lateral decubitus position are expressed as mean
    ± SD. Significant changes are noted at the $p$ < .05 level, paired two-
    tailed $t$-test. NS, nonsignificant.

Adapted by permission from Clark SL, Cotton DB, Lee W, et al. Central
    hemodynamic assessment of normal term pregnancy. Am J Obstet Gy-
    necol 1989;161:1439.

## Hemodynamic Changes During Labor

Repetitive and forceful uterine contractions can have a significant effect on the cardiovascular system during labor. The quantity of blood expressed by each uterine contraction has been estimated to be approximately 300 to 500 mL (Adams, 1958; Hendricks, 1958). During uterine contractions, angiographic studies suggest that the ball-shaped uterus improves blood flow from pelvic organs and lower extremities back to the heart.

Hendricks and Qulligan (1958) provided the first clinical estimation of cardiac output during labor. Using a modified pulse pressure method for estimating cardiac output, he found that cardiac output increased approximately 31% over the resting state. Additionally, other factors that augmented maternal cardiac output during labor included the Valsalva maneuver during contractions, pain, and anxiety. No consistent relationship between an ineffectual uterine contraction and cardiac output was found. These investigators hypothesized that the increased venous return to the heart during uterine contractions was responsible for a transient bradycardia followed by an increase in cardiac output and compensatory bradycardia.

Others also have investigated hemodynamic changes during labor (Winner, 1966; Ueland, 1969d). Ueland and co-workers (1969b,c) studied the role of posture on maternal hemodynamics. Measurements employing the dye-dilution technique were obtained from catheters inserted into the brachial artery and superior vena cava of 23 pregnant women. When patients moved from the supine to the lateral decubitus position, their cardiac output increased 21.7%, their heart rate decreased 5.6%, and their stroke volume increased 26.5%. Figure 1-14 illustrates the effect of postural changes and uterine contractions on maternal hemodynamics during the first stage of labor. Under these conditions, effective uterine contractions resulted in a 15.3% rise in cardiac output, a 7.6% heart rate decrease, and a 21.5% increase in stroke volume. These hemodynamic changes were of less magnitude in the lateral decubitus position, although cardiac output measurements between contractions were actually higher when patients were on their side.

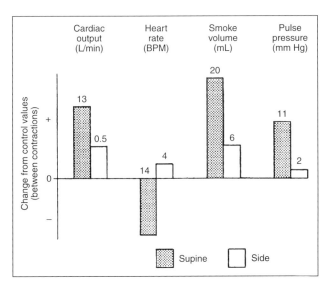

F I G U R E   **1-14**
Effect of posture on the maternal hemodynamic response to uterine contractions in early labor. (Reproduced by permission from Ueland K, Metcalfe J. Circulatory changes in pregnancy. Clin Obstet Gynecol 1975;18:41; modified from Ueland K, Hansen JM. Maternal cardiovascular dynamics. II. Posture and uterine contractions. Am J Obstet Gynecol 1969;103:8.)

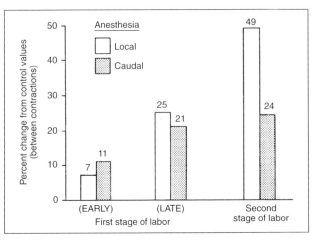

F I G U R E   **1-15**
Changes in cardiac output during local and caudal anesthesia. (Reproduced by permission from Ueland K, Metcalfe J. Circulatory changes in pregnancy. Clin Obstet Gynecol 1975;18:41; modified from Ueland K, Hansen JM. Maternal cardiovascular dynamics. III. Labor and delivery under local and caudal analgesia. Am J Obstet Gynecol 1969;103:8.)

The first stage of labor is associated with progressive increases of cardiac output. Kjeldsen (1979) found cardiac output to increase by 1.10 liters/min in the latent phase of labor, 2.46 liters/min in the accelerating phase, and 2.17 liters/min in the decelerating phase. Ueland and Hansen (1969c) also described an increase in cardiac output between early and late first stages of labor in the supine position. The increase in cardiac output during the first and second stages of labor were not as pronounced when the patient was given caudal anesthesia, compared with local anesthesia (paracervical or pudendal) (Fig 1-15). These investigators concluded that the relative lack of pain and anxiety in patients receiving caudal analgesia may limit the absolute increase in cardiac output encountered at delivery.

Robson and colleagues (1987a) reported the first use of Doppler ultrasound for serial maternal cardiac output measurements during labor. Serial cardiac output values were taken from 15 women in the left semilateral position under me-peridine labor analgesia. Prelabor cardiac output (between contractions) increased from 6.99 liters/min to 7.88 liters/min (+13%) by 8-cm cervical dilation, primarily as a result of stroke volume augmentation. During contractions, there were even further cardiac output increases due to augmentation of both heart rate and stroke volume. The magnitude of these contraction-induced cardiac output changes increased with progression of labor: less than or equal to 3 cm (+17%), 4 to 7 cm (+23%), and greater than or equal to 8 cm (+34%). Lee and co-workers (1989b) also used Doppler and M-mode echocardiography to study parturients with epidural analgesia from the left lateral decubitus position. Cardiac output increases during firm contractions under epidural labor analgesia were similiar to Robson's observations. A 16% increase in stroke volume was associated with an overall 11% cardiac output increase during firm contractions in the first stage of labor. Under epidural anesthesia, however, heart rate was minimally influenced by uterine contractions.

## Labor Analgesia

Cesarean section is sometimes performed to avoid the hemodynamic alterations of labor, but this procedure can lead to a significant amount of apprehension, anxiety, pain, anesthesia, and surgical manipulation, all of which can result in significant cardiovascular responses. Ueland et al (1968; 1970; 1972) studied the influence of analgesia and anesthesia and type of delivery (vaginal or surgical) on the maternal cardiovascular system. As seen in Figure 1-16, the greatest changes in cardiac output occurred during vaginal delivery with the administration of local or caudal anesthesia (Ueland, 1969c). When patients were delivered operatively, the greatest cardiac output changes were seen prior to surgery after the administration of subarachnoid anesthesia (Ueland, 1970, 1972). Although epidural anesthesia with epinephrine resulted in only a 29% decrease in cardiac output prior to surgery, 10 of 12 of these patients required further therapy to treat pro-

FIGURE 1-16
Influence of anesthesia and type of delivery on the maternal cardiovascular system, expressed as percentage change from prelabor (●) and preanesthesia (†) values. Ten of 12 patients (*) required therapy to treat profound hypotension unresponsive to uterine displacement. (Reproduced by permission from Ueland K, Metcalfe J. Circulatory changes in pregnancy. Clin Obstet Gynecol 1975;18:41.)

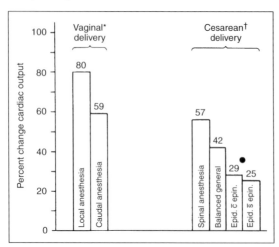

found hypotension that was unresponsive to lateral displacement of the uterus. Balanced anesthesia with thiopental, nitrous oxide, and succinylcholine or epidural anesthesia without epinephrine are associated with smaller hemodynamic fluctuations and thus should be considered for select women with compromised cardiopulmonary reserve (Ueland, 1970, 1972).

James et al (1989) used Doppler ultrasound to examine potential differences in maternal cardiac output prior to cesarean section under regional or general anesthesia. Cardiac output peaked by 37% and 26% of baseline values at 15 and 30 minutes, respectively, after delivery with epidural anesthesia (2% lidocaine; epinephrine 1:200,000; T4–8 sensory level). By comparison, general anesthesia (rapid-sequence thiopental with succinylcholine and nitrous oxide) led to peak cardiac output values of 28% and 17% above baseline at 15 and 30 minutes, respectively, after delivery. This study demonstrated similar patterns of cardiac output augmentation by either anesthetic method and a return by 60 minutes postpartum to preoperative levels that persisted for at least 24 hours after delivery. They concluded that stroke volume increases are primarily responsible for maternal cardiac augmentation during epidural anesthesia. However, both stroke volume and heart rate led to cardiac output increases during general anesthesia.

Hemodynamic stability following regional labor anesthesia has been studied by Doppler echocardiography. Robson and co-workers (1989b) found that the infusion of 800 mL of Ringer's lactate leads to a 12% stroke volume increase and an overall augmentation of cardiac output from 7.01 liters/min to 7.70 liters/min. Epidural anesthesia employing 0.5% bupivacaine did not significantly affect resting maternal heart rate in nonlaboring term gravidas.

## Postpartum Hemodynamics

There is a common misconception that gravidas with cardiac disease are at low risk for compromise following delivery. Significant hemodynamic fluctuations may even occur during the postpartum period. These cardiovascular changes largely reflect the net effect of blood loss at delivery and the body's physiologic compensation to peripartum hemorrhage. Similar to the findings of other investigators (Wilcox, 1959; Newton, 1961) but employing different methodology, Pritchard and colleagues (1962) used chromium-labeled RBCs to quantify blood loss associated with vaginal delivery (505 mL) and cesarean section (1028 mL). They found that normal pregnant women can lose up to 30% of the predelivery blood volume as a result of parturition with little change in postpartum hematocrit.

Ueland (1976) compared intrapartum blood volume and hematocrit changes between vaginal delivery (n = 26) and elective cesarean section (n = 34) (Fig 1-17). The percentage changes in venous hematocrit and blood volume were serially measured in both groups. The average blood loss from vaginal delivery was 610 mL, compared with 1030 mL with cesarean section. Blood volume decreased steadily from 1 hour postpartum until the third day following vaginal delivery, whereas it remained fairly stable in the surgical group. Similar blood volume decreases (−16.2%) were observed in both groups by the third postpartum day. However, differences in hematocrit changes in vaginal (+5.2%) versus cesarean (−5.8%) patients indicated that most of the volume loss by the former was due to postpartum diuresis.

During the first week after delivery, Chesley et al (1959) reported a 2-liter decrease in the sodium space compartment associated with 3 kg of weight loss. This well-known postpartum diuresis usually occurs between the second and fifth day and provides a physiologic mechanism by which increased extracellular fluid accumulated during pregnancy may be dissipated (Cunningham, 1993).

The clinical significance of this phenomenon was demonstrated by Hankins and co-workers (1984), who performed serial invasive hemodynamic measurements from eight eclamptic women. Typically, these patients were found to have initial low biventricular filling pressures, elevated SVR, and hyperdynamic left ventricular function. Three women who did not demonstrate a significant diuresis by 48 to 72 hours postpartum were noted to have elevated pulmonary capillary wedge pressures (mean, 16.7 mm Hg). Their wedge pressures eventually normalized following postpartum diuresis. These investigators suggested that this phenomenon was due to mobilization of extravascular fluid prior to diuresis. Thus, postpartum pulmonary edema may develop in high-risk patients who fail to diurese before mobilization of extravascular fluid.

Significant changes in cardiac output, stroke volume, and heart rate also occur after delivery (Kjeldsen, 1979). Ueland and Hansen (1969c) measured these parameters in 13 patients who received caudal anesthesia and found a 59% and a 71% increase, respectively, in cardiac output and stroke volume by 10 minutes postpartum. By

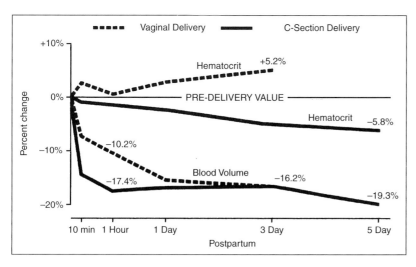

F I G U R E   **1-17**

**Percentage changes in blood volume and venous hematocrit following vaginal delivery or cesarean section.** (Reproduced by permission from Metcalfe J, Ueland K. Heart disease and pregnancy. In: Fowler NO, ed. Cardiac diagnosis and treatment. 3rd ed. Hagerstown, MD: Harper and Row, 1980: 1153–1170.)

1 hour postpartum, cardiac output was elevated 49% above baseline values, which paralleled the 67% increase in stroke volume. At that time, a 15% decrease in heart rate was observed, although no statistically significant changes in BP were noted. The postpartum high cardiac output state probably results from increased venous return to the heart secondary to the following: (1) a shift of blood from the uterus to the intravascular space, (2) the release of caval compression from the gravid uterus, and (3) the mobilization of extravascular fluid into the intravascular compartment.

Robson et al (1987c) used M-mode and Doppler echocardiography to study 15 normal parturients at 38 weeks' gestation and then at 2, 6, 12, and 24 weeks after delivery. Cardiac output fell from a mean of 7.42 liters/min at 38 weeks to 4.96 liters/min at 24 weeks after delivery. This was caused by reductions in both heart rate ($-20\%$) and stroke volume ($-18\%$). By 2 weeks postpartum, there were substantial decreases in left ventricular size and contractility. Left ventricular contractility in the postnatal group was slightly less than age-matched nongravid control subjects by 24 weeks postpartum. Left ventricular mass also was slightly hypertrophied by 24 weeks postpartum. Because the control group's echocardiographic parameters agreed with previously published reports, this suggested a small diminution

in myocardial function long after delivery. This is an interesting finding because patients with peripartum cardiomyopathy usually develop their disease within 5 months of delivery (Lee, 1989a).

## Cardiorespiratory Interactions During Pregnancy

The maternal respiratory system experiences significant mechanical and functional changes during pregnancy. Oxygen consumption and basal metabolic rate are increased 21% and 14%, respectively (Fig 1-18). Other changes include upward displacement of the diaphragm and increased diameter of the thoracic cage. Chest wall compliance and total pulmonary compliance improve after delivery (McGinty, 1938; Farman, 1969).

Cugell and associates (1953) measured lung volume changes throughout pregnancy. In this study of 19 women, no significant alterations in the functional lung profile were seen until the second half of normal pregnancy. At that time, a decrease in both the expiratory reserve volume and residual volume led to a net 18% mean decrease in functional residual capacity. Despite decreasing functional residual capacity from the mechanical effects of the uterus on the diaphragm, there is a mild increase in inspiratory capacity.

F I G U R E   **1-18**

**Percentage changes of minute volume, oxygen uptake, basal metabolism, and the ventilation equivalent for oxygen at monthly intervals throughout pregnancy.** (Reproduced by permission from Prowse CM, Gaensler EA. Respiratory and acid-base changes during pregnancy. Anesthesiology 1965; 26:381.)

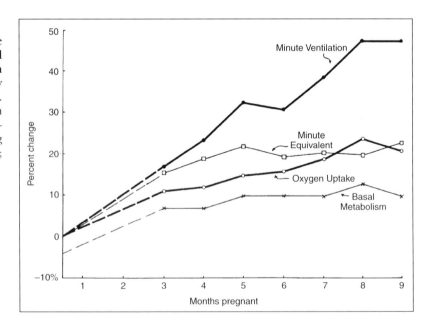

These alterations result in a minimal change for overall total lung capacity. A more recent study agrees with these earlier observations and suggests no significant change in the forced expiratory volume in 1 second as well (Puranik, 1994). Representative maternal lung volumes are summarized in Figure 1-19 (Bonica, 1962).

The relative hyperventilation of pregnancy begins in the first trimester and increases as much as 48% by term gestation (Cugell, 1953; Prowse, 1965). Minute ventilation, however, is a consequence of increased tidal volume, not respiratory rate (Fishburne, 1979). Because hyperventilation has been observed during the luteal phase of the menstrual cycle (Goodland, 1952) and progesterone can induce similar changes in nonpregnant women (Lyons, 1968), it is likely that this phenomenon results from hormonal factors. Although the mechanism of progesterone-induced hyperventilation has not been defined clearly, it has been suggested that this hormone acts as a primary respiratory center stimulant (Skatrud, 1978). Progesterone also may change the sensitivity of the respiratory centers to carbon dioxide.

Maternal blood gas measurements are also altered during pregnancy. Resting arterial carbon dioxide tension is typically below 30 mm Hg (Lu-cius, 1970). Chronic respiratory alkalosis is partially compensated by increased renal bicarbonate excretion into the urine (Lim, 1976). By comparison, first-trimester arterial oxygen tension ranges from 106 to 108 mm Hg and decreases to 101 to 104 mm by late pregnancy (Anderson, 1969; Templeton, 1976). The oxyhemoglobin dissociation curve is also altered during pregnancy due to a rightward shift that results in lower oxygen saturation for a given $Pao_2$ (Kambam, 1983).

Arterial oxygen tension is dependent on maternal body position during term pregnancy. In a study of 23 pregnant women, arterial oxygen tensions were found to be greater than 90 mm Hg in the sitting position (Awe, 1979). Moderate hypoxemia (arterial oxygen tension < 90 mm Hg) occurred in 25% of their supine patients. The supine position also was associated with a much greater likelihood for the alveolar-arterial oxygen tension gradient to be abnormal (> 10 mm Hg) when compared with the upright position. There was, however, significant improvement in this gradient when women shifted from the supine to the sitting position. These results emphasize the clinical importance of maternal body position relative to the interpretation of arterial blood gas measurements.

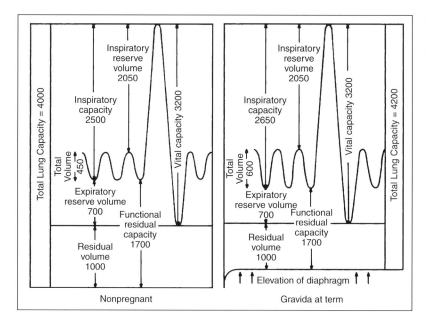

F I G U R E   **1-19**

**Respiratory changes during pregnancy.** (Reproduced by permission from Bonica JJ. Principles and Practice of Obstetrical Analgesia and Anesthesia. Philadelphia: FA Davis, 1962.)

## Cardiorespiratory Signs and Symptoms

Maternal cardiorespiratory changes can lead to signs and symptoms that simulate heart disease during normal pregnancy. Milne and associates (1978) found the incidence of dyspnea to increase from 15% in the first trimester to approximately 50% by 19 weeks and 75% by 31 weeks' gestation. Although the exact mechanism for the dyspnea of pregnancy is not known, Hytten and Leitch (1971) suggested that this symptom may be related to a ventilatory response that is out of proportion for the observed metabolic demand. Maternal dyspnea is probably caused by heightened subjective awareness of increased minute ventilation during pregnancy (Field, 1991).

Easily produced fatigue and decreased exercise tolerance are common during pregnancy. Occasionally, the mechanical effects of the uterus may reduce venous return to the heart, leading to dizziness or even syncope. Increased venous pressure distal to this partial obstruction contributes to the dependent lower-extremity edema commonly seen during pregnancy. A mild amount of pulmonary atelectasis from the enlarging uterus adjacent to the diaphragm occasionally leads to the presence of basilar rales by auscultation.

All of these changes can make the confirmation of maternal heart disease very difficult by history and physical examination alone. In fact, the commonly used New York Heart Classification does not always reliably reflect the severity of cardiac disease during pregnancy. Maternal dyspnea or fatigue actually may confuse physicians who use this subjective classification; in such patients, echocardiography may provide important objective information about heart disease that is not reliably described by physical symptoms.

The physiologic basis of maternal cardiac murmurs also should be understood when trying to evaluate pregnant women. Cutforth and MacDonald (1966) carefully compared auscultatory findings with phonocardiograms in 50 normal primigravid women during pregnancy. As summarized in Figure 1-20, a loud and widely split first heart sound was documented in 88% of these patients from early closure of the mitral valve. The only significant change noted in the second heart sound was a tendency for persistent expiratory splitting. A third heart sound was heard in 84% of women. Systolic ejection murmurs were found in 92% of their subjects. By contrast, only nine patients demonstrated an early soft diastolic murmur (often transient), which was thought to result from increased flow through the atrioventricular valve. The changes in heart sounds and murmurs during pregnancy begin between 12 and 20 weeks' gestation and usually disappear by 1 week postpartum. Occasionally, a benign cervical venous hum or murmur associated with the breast vasculature is also detected.

Echocardiography can also be used to determine the nature of maternal cardiac murmurs. Limacher et al (1985) used pulsed Doppler echocardiography to detect tricuspid regurgitation in 35 of 81 asymptomatic pregnant women with newly diagnosed systolic precordial murmurs. Their study indicates that functional tricuspid regurgitation is common during pregnancy and appears to be related to dilation of the tricuspid annulus. A longitudinal study of 18 women by

**Summarization of cardiac auscultatory findings in 50 pregnant women.** MC, mitral closure; TC, tricuspid closure; $A_2$ and $P_2$, aortic and pulmonary (respectively) closure element of the second sound. (Reproduced by permission from Cutforth R, MacDonald CB. Heart sounds and murmurs during pregnancy. Am Heart J 1966;71:741.)

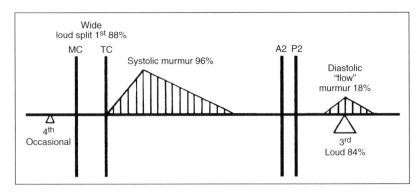

Doppler echocardiography also examined the prevalence of physiologic valvular regurgitation during normal pregnancy (Campos, 1993). Early pregnancy revealed no significant changes from a control group of nongravid women (no aortic or mitral regurgitation; pulmonary, 22.2%; tricuspid, 38.9%). As pregnancy evolved, there was a progressive and significant increase of multivalvular regurgitation, which was maximal at term gestation (mitral, 27.8%; tricuspid, 94.4%; pulmonary, 94.4%). Aortic regurgitation was never detected during any stage of normal pregnancy.

Radiographic changes also occur in normal pregnant women (Fig 1-21). Hollander and Crawford (1943) serially followed 18 pregnant women with chest films (posteroanterior with oblique views) and esophagrams. Aside from the enlargement of the heart, another consistent radiographic change—an indentation of the anterior esophageal wall by the enlarged left atrium—was detected. Turner (1975) reviewed 200 chest films from pregnant women to characterize changes specific to this condition. Aside from cardiac enlargement, there were no specific changes in cardiac contour or pulmonary vascularity when compared with nonpregnant women. It was rec-ommended that the same criteria for interpretation of chest films should be applied to both pregnant and nonpregnant women.

Finally, Hollander and Crawford examined electrocardiographic changes during pregnancy and described the development of a deep Q wave and a negative T wave in lead III. Additionally, the QRS axis changed an average of 15 degrees to the left. Carruth and colleagues (1981) examined 102 pregnant women at Grady Memorial Hospital and found that the pattern of QRS axis change was not predictable for a given individual. Small decreases in the PR and QT intervals occur as a result of maternal tachycardia. Mean electrocardiographic values during pregnancy are summarized in Table 1-8.

## Conclusion

The maternal circulation can be modified by gestational age, body position, pain, labor, and peripartum blood loss. Physiologic adjustment to these factors should be considered while caring for the critically ill obstetric patient. Clinicians

F I G U R E  **1-21**

Example of typical chest radiographic changes during and after pregnancy. (A) The patient at 22 weeks' gestation. (B) The same patient 3 weeks postpartum. Note the increased fullness of the cardiac silhouette, more pronounced breast tissue density, and increased pulmonary vasculature seen during pregnancy. (Courtesy of Dr. L. Leduc.)

**A**

**B**

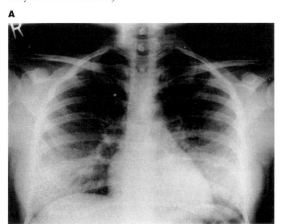
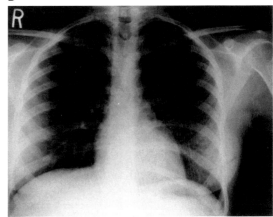

T A B L E    **1-8**

Mean electrocardiogram measurements during normal
pregnancy, delivery, and postpartum in 102 patients

|  | 1TM | 2TM | 3TM | D | PP |
|---|---|---|---|---|---|
| Heart rate (beats/min) | 77 | 79 | 87 | 80 | 66 |
| QT interval (sec) | 0.378 | 0.375 | 0.361 | 0.362 | 0.406 |
| $QT_c$ interval (sec) | 0.424 | 0.427 | 0.431 | 0.414 | 0.423 |
| PR interval (sec) | 0.160 | 0.160 | 0.155 | 0.155 | 0.160 |
| P wave |  |  |  |  |  |
|     Duration (sec) | 0.092 | 0.092 | 0.091 | 0.091 | 0.096 |
|     Amplitude (mm) | 1.9 | 1.9 | 2.0 | 2.0 | 1.9 |
|     Axis (degrees) | 40 | 38 | 38 | 41 | 35 |
| QRS complex |  |  |  |  |  |
|     Duration (sec) | 0.074 | 0.074 | 0.074 | 0.076 | 0.077 |
|     Amplitude (mm) | 11.5 | 11.5 | 12.4 | 12.2 | 11.2 |
|     Axis (degrees) | 49 | 46 | 40 | 44 | 44 |
| T wave |  |  |  |  |  |
|     Duration (sec) | 0.168 | 0.171 | 0.165 | 0.166 | 0.176 |
|     Amplitude (mm) | 3.4 | 3.5 | 3.4 | 3.6 | 3.5 |
|     Axis (degrees) | 27 | 25 | 22 | 33 | 34 |

1TM, 2TM, 3TM, first, second, and third trimesters, respectively; D, 1–3 days
    after delivery (D); PP, 6–8 weeks postpartum (PP).

Reproduced by permission from Carruth JE, Mirvis SB, Brogan DR, et al. The
    electrocardiogram in normal pregnancy. Am Heart J 1981;6:1075.

should appreciate the basic importance of adequate volume replacement, maintenance of BP, and systematic correction of hemodynamic abnormalities that adversely affect cardiac output, oxygenation status, or fetal well-being. Toward this end, the normal adaptation of the patient and her fetus must be well understood before they can be effectively treated in the face of serious medical complications.

**R E F E R E N C E S**

Adams JQ, Alexander AM. Alterations in cardiovascular physiology during labor. Obstet Gynecol 1958;12:542.

American College of Obstetricians and Gynecologists. Hypertension in pregnancy. ACOG Technical Bulletin 219, 1996.

Anderson GJ, James GB, Mathers NP, et al. The maternal oxygen tension and acid-base status during pregnancy. J Obstet Gynaecol Br Cwlth 1969;76:16.

Assali NS, Rauamo L, Peltonen T. Measurement of uterine blood flow and uterine metabolism. VII. Uterine and fetal blood flow and oxygen consumption in early human pregnancy. Am J Obstet Gynecol 1960;79:86.

Atkins AFJ, Watt JM, Milan P, et al. A longitudinal study of cardiovascular dynamics throughout pregnancy. Eur J Obstet Reprod Biol 1981a; 12:215.

Atkins AFJ, Watt JM, Milan P, et al. The influence of posture upon cardiovascular dynamics throughout pregnancy. Eur J Obstet Gynecol Reprod Biol 1981b;12:357.

Awe RJ, Nicotra MB, Newsom TD, et al. Arterial oxygenation and alveolar-arterial gradients in term pregnancy. Obstet Gynecol 1979;53:182.

Bader RA, Bader MG, Rose DJ, et al. Hemodynamics at rest and during exercise in normal pregnancy as studied by cardiac catheterization. J Clin Invest 1955;34:1524.

Barron WM, Mujais SK, Zinaman M, et al. Plasma catecholamine responses to physiologic stimuli in normal human pregnancy. Am J Obstet Gynecol 1986;154:80.

Bieniarz J, Maqueda E, Caldeyro-Barcia R: Compression of aorta by the uterus in late human pregnancy. I. Variations between femoral and brachial artery pressure with changes from hypertension to hypotension. Am J Obstet Gynecol 1966;95:795.

Bieniarz J, Crottogini JJ, Curuchet E, et al. Aortocaval compression by the uterus in late human pregnancy. II. An arteriographic study. Am J Obstet Gynecol 1968;100:203.

Bonica J. Principles and practice of obstetric analgesia and anesthesia. Philadelphia: FA Davis, 1962.

Brenner BM, Ballermann BJ, Gunning ME, Zeidel ML. Diverse biological actions of atrial natriuretic peptide. Physiol Rev 1990;70:665.

Burt CC. Peripheral skin temperature in normal pregnancy. Lancet1949;2:787.

Burwell CS, Strayhorn WD, Flickinger D, et al. Circulation during pregnancy. Arch Intern Med 1938;62:979.

Calvin S, Jones OW, Knieriem K, Weinstein L. Oxygen saturation in the supine hypotensive syndrome. Obstet Gynecol 1988;71:872.

Campos O, Andreade JF, Bocanegra J, et al. Physiologic multivalvular regurgitation during pregnancy: a longitudinal Doppler echocardiographic study. Int J Cardiol 1993;40:265.

Capeless EL, Clapp JF. When do cardiovascular parameters return to their preconception values? Am J Obstet Gynecol 1991;165:883.

Carruth JE, Mirvis SB, Brogan DR, et al. The electrocardiogram in normal pregnancy. Am Heart J 1981;6:1075.

Caton WL, Roby CC, Reid DE, et al. The circulating red cell volume and body hematocrit in normal pregnancy and the puerperium. Am J Obstet Gynecol 1951;61:1207.

Caton D, Abrams RM, Clapp JF, et al. The effect of exogenous progesterone on the rate of blood flow of the uterus of ovariectomized sheep. Q J Exp Physiol 1974;59:225.

Cavill I. Iron and erythropoiesis in normal subjects and in pregnancy. J Perinat Med 1995;23:47.

Chesley LC, Valenti C, Uichano L. Alterations in body fluid compartments and exchangeable sodium in early puerperium. Am J Obstet Gynecol 1959;77:1054.

Chesley LC. Renal functional changes in normal pregnancy. Clin Obstet Gynecol 1960;3:349.

Clapp JF, Seaward BL, Sleamaker RH, et al. Maternal physiologic adaptations to early human pregnancy. Am J Obstet Gynecol 1988;156:1456.

Clark SL, Cotton DB, Lee W, et al. Central hemodynamic assessment of normal term pregnancy. Am J Obstet Gynecol 1989;161:1439.

Clark SL, Cotton DB, Pivarnik JM, et al. Position change and central hemodynamic profile during normal third-trimester pregnancy and post partum. Am J Obstet Gynecol 1991;164:883.

Cugell DW, Frank NR, Gaensler EA, et al. Pulmonary function in pregnancy. I. Serial observations in normal women. Am Rev Tuberc Pulmon Dis 1953;67:568.

Cunningham FG, MacDonald PC, Gant NF, et al. The puerperium. In: Williams Obstetrics. 19th ed. Norwalk, CT: Appleton & Lange, 1993:467.

Cusson JR, Gutkowska J, Rey E, et al. Plasma concentration of atrial natriuretic factor in normal pregnancy. N Engl J Med 1985;313:1230.

Cutforth R, MacDonald CB. Heart sounds and murmurs during pregnancy. Am Heart J 1966;71:741.

Du Bois D, Du Bois EF. A formula to estimate the approximate area if height and weight be known. Arch Intern Med 1916;17:863.

Duvekot JJ, Cheriew EC, Pieters FAA, et al. Early pregnancy changes in hemodynamics and volume homeostasis are consecutive adjustments triggered by a primary fall in systemic vascular tone. Am J Obstet Gynecol 1993;169:1382.

Easterling TR, Watts DH, Schmucker BC, Benedetti TJ. Measurement of cardiac output during pregnancy: validation of Doppler technique and clinical observations in preeclampsia. Obstet Gynecol 1987;69:845.

Easterling TR, Schmucker BC, Benedetti TJ. The hemodynamic effects of orthostatic stress during pregnancy. Obstet Gynecol 1988;72:550.

Easterling TR, Benedetti TJ, Schmucker BC, Millard SP. Maternal hemodynamics in normal and preeclamptic pregnancies: a longitudinal study. Obstet Gynecol 1990;76:1061.

Farman JV, Thorpe ME. Compliance changes during caesarean section. Br J Anaesth 1969;41:999.

Field SK, Bell SG, Cenaiko DF, Whitelaw WA. Relationship between inspiratory effort and breathlessness in pregnancy. J Appl Physiol 1991;71:1897.

Fishburne JI. Physiology and disease of the respiratory system in pregnancy. J Reprod Med 1979;22:177.

Gabert HA, Miller JM. Renal disease during pregnancy. Obstet Gynecol Surv 1985;40:449.

Ginsberg J, Duncan SL. Direct and indirect blood pressure measurement in pregnancy. J Obstet Gynaecol Br Cwlth 1969;76:705.

Glinoer D, De Nayer P, Bourdoux P, et al. Regulation of maternal thyroid during pregnancy. J Clin Endocrinol Metab 1990;71:276.

Goodland RL, Pommerenke WT. Cyclic fluctuations of the alveolar carbon dioxide tension during the normal menstrual cycle. Fertil Steril 1952; 3:394.

Hamilton HGH. The cardiac output in normal pregnancy as determined by the Cournard right heart catheterization technique. J Obstet Gynaecol Br Emp 1949;56:548.

Hankins GDV, Wendel GD, Cunningham FG, et al. Longitudinal evaluation of hemodynamic changes in eclampsia. Am J Obstet Gynecol 1984;150:506.

Hankins GDV, Harvey CJ, Clark SL, et al. The effects of maternal position and cardiac output on intrapulmonary shunt in normal third-trimester pregnancy. Obstet Gynecol 1996;88:327.

Harada A, Hershman JM, Reed AW, et al. Comparison of thyroid stimulators and thyroid hormone concentrations in the sera of pregnant women. J Clin Endocrinol Metab 1979;48:793.

Hendricks ECH, Qulligan EJ. Cardiac output during labor. Am J Obstet Gynecol 1958;76:969.

Henriksen TB, Hedegaard M, Secher NJ, Wilcox AJ. Standing at work and preterm delivery. Br J Obstet Gynaecol 1995;102:198.

Herbert CM, Banner EA, Wakim KG. Variations in the peripheral circulation during pregnancy. Am J Obstet Gynecol 1958;76:742.

Hollander AG, Crawford JH. Roentgenologic and electrocardiographic changes in the normal heart during pregnancy. Am Heart J 1943; 26:364.

Holmes F. Incidence of the supine hypotensive syndrome in late pregnancy. J Obstet Gynaecol Br Emp 1960;67:254.

Howard BK, Goodson JH, Mengert WF. Supine hypotensive syndrome in late pregnancy. Obstet Gynecol 1953;1:371.

Hytten FE, Paintin DB. Increase in plasma volume during normal pregnancy. J Obstet Gynaecol Br Cwlth 1963;70:402.

Hytten FE, Leitch I. The Physiology of Human Pregnancy. 2nd ed. Oxford: Blackwell Scientific, 1971.

James CF, Banner T, Caton D. Cardiac output in women undergoing cesarean section with epidural or general anesthesia. Am J Obstet Gynecol 1989;160:1178.

Jepson JH. Endocrine control of maternal and fetal erythropoiesis. Can Med Assoc J 1968;98:844.

Kambam JR, Handte RE, Brown WR, et al. Effect of pregnancy on oxygen dissociation. Anesthesiology 1983;59:A395.

Katz R, Karliner JS, Resnik R. Effects of a natural volume overload state (pregnancy) on left ventricular performance in normal human subjects. Circulation 1978;58:434.

Katz M, Sokal MM. Skin perfusion in pregnancy. Am J Obstet Gynecol 1980;137:30.

Kerr MG. Cardiovascular dynamics in pregnancy and labour. Br Med Bull 1968;24:19.

Kinsella SM, Lohmann G. Supine hypotensive syndrome. Obstet Gynecol 1994:774.

Kirshon B, Lee W, Cotton DB, et al. Indirect blood pressure monitoring in the obstetric patient. Obstet Gynecol 1987;70:799.

Kitabatake A, Inoue M, Asao M, et al. Noninvasive evaluation of pulmonary hypertension by a pulsed Doppler technique. Circulation 1983; 68:302.

Kjeldsen J. Hemodynamic investigations during labor and delivery. Acta Obstet Gynecol Scand [Suppl] 1979;89:1.

Koller O. The clinical significance of hemodilution during pregnancy. Obstet Gynecol Surv 1982; 37:649.

Laird-Meeter K, van de Ley G, Bom TH, et al. Cardiocirculatory adjustments during pregnancy—an echocardiographic study. Clin Cardiol 1979; 2:328.

Lee W, Rokey R, Cotton DB. Noninvasive maternal stroke volume and cardiac output determinations by pulsed Doppler echocardiography. Am J Obstet Gynecol 1988;158:505.

Lee W, Cotton DB. Peripartum cardiomyopathy: current concepts and clinical management. Clin Obstet Gynecol 1989a;32:54.

Lee W, Rokey R, Cotton DB, Miller JF. Maternal hemodynamic effects of uterine contractions by M-mode and pulsed-Doppler echocardiography. Am J Obstet Gynecol 1989b;161:974.

Lees MM, Taylor SH, Scott DB, et al. A study of cardiac output at rest throughout pregnancy. J Obstet Gynaecol Br Cwlth 1967;74:319.

Letsky EA. Erythropoiesis in pregnancy. J Perinat Med 1995;23:39.

Lim VS, Katz AI, Lindheimer MD. Acid-base regulation in pregnancy. Am J Physiol 1976;231:1764.

Limacher MC, Ware JA, O'Meara ME, et al. Tricuspid regurgitation during pregnancy. Two dimensional and pulsed Doppler echocardiographic observations. Am J Cardiol 1985;55:1059.

Lindheimer MD, Katz AI. Renal function in pregnancy. Obstet Gynecol Annu 1972;1:139.

Lindheimer MD, Katz AI. Sodium and diuretics in pregnancy. N Engl J Med 1973;288:891.

Linhard J. Uber das minutevolumens des herzens bei ruhe und bei muskelarbeit. Pflugers Arch 1915;1612:233.

Longo LD, Hardesty JS. Maternal blood volume: measurement, hypothesis of control, and clinical considerations. Rev Perinatal Med 1984;5:35.

Lucius H, Gahlenbeck H, Kleine HO, et al. Respiratory functions, buffer system, and electrolyte concentrations of blood during human pregnancy. Respir Physiol 1970;9:311.

Lund CJ, Donovan JC. Blood volume during pregnancy. Am J Obstet Gynecol 1967;98:393.

Lyons HA, Huang CT. Therapeutic use of progesterone in alveolar hypoventilation associated with obesity. Am J Med 1968;44:881.

Mabie WC, DiSessa TG, Crocker LG, et al. A longitudinal study of cardiac output in normal pregnancy. Am J Obstet Gynecol 1994;170:849.

Mashini IS, Albazzaz SJ, Fadel HE, et al. Serial noninvasive evaluation of cardiovascular hemodynamics during pregnancy. Am J Obstet Gynecol 1987;156:1208.

McCalden RA. The inhibitory action of oestradiol-17β and progesterone on venous smooth muscle. Br J Pharmacol 1975;53:183.

McGinty AP. The comparative effects of pregnancy and phrenic nerve interruption on the diaphragm and their relation to pulmonary tuberculosis. Am J Obstet Gynecol 1938;35:237.

McLennon CE, Thouin LG. Blood volume in pregnancy. Am J Obstet Gynecol 1948;55:1189.

Metcalfe J, Romney SL, Ramsy LH, et al. Estimation of uterine blood flow in normal human pregnancy at term. J Clin Invest 1955;34:1632.

Milne JA, Howie AD, Pack AL. Dyspnoea during normal pregnancy. Br J Obstet Gynaecol 1978; 85:260.

Morton M, Tsang H, Hohimer R, et al. Left ventricular size, output, and structure during guinea pig pregnancy. Am J Physiol 1984;246:R40.

Murray JA, Johnston W, Reid JM. Echocardiographic determination of left ventricular dimensions, volumes, and performance. Am J Cardiol 1972;30:252.

Naeye RL, Peters EC. Working during pregnancy: effects on the fetus. Pediatrics 1982;69:724.

Newton M, Mosey LM, Egli GE, et al. Blood loss during and immediately after delivery. Obstet Gynecol 1961;17:9.

Nisell H, Lunell N, Linde B. Maternal hemodynamics and impaired fetal growth in pregnancy-induced hypertension. Obstet Gynecol 1988;71:163.

Oparil S, Ehrlich EN, Lindheimer MD. Effect of progesterone on renal sodium handling in man: relation to aldosterone excretion and plasma renin activity. Clin Sci Mol Med 1975;49:139.

Palmer AJ, Walker AHC. The maternal circulation in normal pregnancy. J Obstet Gynaecol Br Emp 1949;56:537.

Phippard AF, Horvath JS, Glynn EM. Circulatory adaptation to pregnancy—serial studies of haemodynamics, blood volume, renin and aldosterone in the baboon (*Papio hamadryas*). J Hypertens 1986;4:773.

Pombo JF, Troy BL, Russell RO. Left ventricular volumes and ejection fraction by echocardiography. Circulation 1971;43:480.

Pritchard JA, Baldwin RM, Dickey JC, Wiggins KM. Blood volume changes in pregnancy and the puerperium. II. Red blood cell loss and changes in apparent blood volume during and following vaginal delivery, cesarean section, and cesarean section plus total hysterectomy. Am J Obstet Gynecol 1962;84:1271.

Pritchard JA. Changes in the blood volume during pregnancy and delivery. Anesthesiology 1965a; 26:393.

Pritchard JA. Blood volume changes in pregnancy and the puerperium. IV. Anemia associated with hydatidiform mole. Am J Obstet Gynecol 1965b;91:621.

Pritchard JA, Cunningham FG, Pritchard SA. The Parkland Memorial Hospital protocol for treatment of eclampsia: evaluation of 245 cases. Am J Obstet Gynecol 1984;148:951.

Prowse CM, Gaensler EA. Respiratory and acid-base changes during pregnancy. Anesthesiology 1965;26:381.

Puranik BM, Kaore SB, Kurhade A, et al. A longitudinal study of pulmonary function tests during pregnancy. Indian J Physiol Pharmacol 1994; 38:129.

Robson SC, Dunlop W, Boys RJ, Hunter S. Cardiac output during labor. Br Med J 1987a;295:1169.

Robson SC, Dunlop W, Moore M, Hunter S. Combined Doppler and echocardiographic measurement of cardiac output: theory and application in pregnancy. Br J Obstet Gynaecol 1987b; 94:1014.

Robson SC, Hunter S, Moore M, Dunlop W. Haemodynamic changes during the puerperium: a Doppler and M-mode echocardiographic study. Br J Obstet Gynaecol 1987c;94:1028.

Robson SC, Hunter S, Boys RJ, Dunlop W. Serial study of factors influencing changes in cardiac output during human pregnancy. Am J Physiol 1989a;256:H1060.

Robson SC, Hunter R, Boys W, et al. Changes in cardiac output during epidural anaesthesia for caesarean section. Anaesthesia 1989b;44:475.

Robson SC, Hunter S, Boys J, Dunlop W. Serial changes in pulmonary haemodynamics during human pregnancy: a non-invasive study using Doppler echocardiography. Clin Sci 1991;80: 113.

Rolschau J. Infarction and intervillous thrombosis in placenta and their association with intrauterine growth retardation. Acta Obstet Gynecol Scand [Suppl] 1978;72:22.

Rovinsky JJ, Jaffin H. Cardiovascular hemodynamics in pregnancy. I. Blood and plasma volumes in multiple pregnancy. Am J Obstet Gynecol 1965;93:1.

Salas SP, Rosso P, Espinoza R, et al. Maternal plasma volume expansion and hormonal changes in women with idiopathic fetal growth retardation. Obstet Gynecol 1993;81:1029.

Schrier RW. Medical progress: pathogenesis of sodium and water retention in high-output and low-output cardiac failure, nephrotic syndrome, cirrhosis, and pregnancy. N Engl J Med 1988;319:1127.

Schrier RW. Body fluid volume regulation in health and disease: a unifying hypothesis. Ann Intern Med 1990;113:155.

Schrier RW, Briner VA. Peripheral arterial vasodilation hypothesis of sodium and water retention in pregnancy: implications for pathogenesis of preeclampsia-eclampsia. Obstet Gynecol 1991; 77:632.

Scott DE. Anemia during pregnancy. Obstet Gynecol Annu 1972;1:219.

Seitchik J. Total body water and total body density of pregnant women. Obstet Gynecol 1967; 29:155.

Seligman SP, Kadner SS, Finlay TH. Relationship between preeclampsia, hypoxia, and production of nitric oxide by the placenta. Am J Obstet Gynecol 1996;174:xxiii. Abstract.

Skatrud JJB, Dempsey JA, Kaiser DG. Ventilatory response to medroxyprogesterone acetate in normal subjects: time course and mechanism. J Appl Physiol 1978;44:939.

Slater AJ, Gude N, Clarke IJ, Walters WA. Haemodynamic changes and left ventricular preformance during high-dose oestrogen administration to male transsexuals. Br J Obstet Gynaecol 1986;93:532.

Templeton A, Kelman GR. Maternal blood-gases, ($P_AO_2$-$P_aO_2$), physiologic shunt, and VD/VT in normal pregnancy. Br J Anaesth 1976;48:1001.

Thomsen JK, Storm TL, Thamsborg G, et al. Increased concentration of circulating atrial natriuretic peptide during normal pregnancy. Eur J Obstet Gynecol Reprod Biol 1988;27:197.

Thomsen JK, Fogh-Anderson N, Jaszczak P, Giese J. Atrial natriuretic peptide (ANP) decrease during normal pregnancy as related to hemodynamic changes and volume regulation. Acta Obstet Gynecol Scand 1993;72:103.

Turner AF. The chest radiograph during pregnancy. Clin Obstet Gynecol 1975;18:65.

Ueland K, Parer JT. Effects of estrogens on the cardiovascular system of the ewe. Am J Obstet Gynecol 1966;96:400.

Ueland K, Gills RE, Hansen JM. Maternal cardiovascular dynamics. I. Cesarean section under subarachnoid block anesthesia. Am J Obstet Gynecol 1968;100:42.

Ueland K, Novy MJ, Peterson EN, et al. Maternal cardiovascular dynamics. IV. The influence of gestational age on the maternal cardiovascular response to posture and exercise. Am J Obstet Gynecol 1969a;104:856.

Ueland K, Hansen JM. Maternal cardiovascular dynamics. II. Posture and uterine contractions. Am J Obstet Gynecol 1969b;103:1.

Ueland K, Hansen JM. Maternal cardiovascular hemodynamics. III. Labor and delivery under local and caudal anesthesia. Am J Obstet Gynecol 1969c;103:8.

Ueland K, Hansen J, Eng M, et al. Maternal cardiovascular hemodynamics. VI. Cesarean section under thiopental, nitrous oxide, and succinylcholine anesthesia. Am J Obstet Gynecol 1970;106:615.

Ueland K, Akamatsu TJ, Eng M, et al. Maternal cardiovascular dynamics. IV. Cesarean section under epidural anesthesia. Am J Obstet Gynecol 1972;114:775.

Ueland K, Metcalfe J. Circulatory changes in pregnancy. Clin Obstet Gynecol 1975;18:41.

Ueland K. Maternal cardiovascular dynamics. VII. Intrapartum blood volume changes. Am J Obstet Gynecol 1976;126:671.

van Oppen AC, van der Tweel I, Duvekot JJ, Bruinse HW. Use of cardiac output in pregnancy: is it justified? Am J Obstet Gynecol 1995;173:923.

van Oppen ACC, van der Tweel I, Alsbach GPJ, et al. A longitudinal study of maternal hemodynamics during normal pregnancy. Obstet Gynecol 1996;88:40.

Villar MA, Sibai BM. Clinical significance of elevated mean arterial pressure in second trimester and threshold increase in systolic and diastolic blood pressure during third trimester. Am J Obstet Gynecol 1989;160:419.

Vorys N, Ullery JC, Hanusek GE. The cardiac output changes in various positions in pregnancy. Am J Obstet Gynecol 1961;82:1312.

Walters WAW, MacGregor WG, Hills M. Cardiac output at rest during pregnancy and the puerperium. Clin Sci 1966;30:1.

Werko L. Pregnancy and heart disease. Acta Obstet Gynecol Scand 1954;33:162.

Wilcox CF, Hunt AR, Owen FA. The measurement of blood lost during cesarean section. Am J Obstet Gynecol 1959;77:772.

Wilson M, Morganti AA, Zervodakis I, et al. Blood pressure, the renin-aldosterone system, and sex steroids throughout normal pregnancy. Am J Med 1980;68:97.

Winkel CA, Milewich L, Parker R, et al. Conversion of plasma progesterone to desoxycorticosterone in men, nonpregnant, and pregnant women, and adrenalectomized subjects. J Clin Invest 1980;66:803.

Winner W, Romney SL. Cardiovascular responses to labor and delivery. Am J Obstet Gynecol 1966;96:1004.

Wook JE, Goodrich SM. Dilation of the veins with pregnancy or with oral contraceptive therapy. Trans Am Clin Climatol Assoc 1964;76:174.

# CHAPTER 2

# Blood Gas Physiology

$\mathcal{A}$bnormalities in acid-base and respiratory homeostasis are common among patients requiring intensive medical support. Critically ill patients frequently require assessment of metabolic and respiratory status as a result of both their illness and our therapeutic interventions. An understanding and clinical application of basic physiologic principles are, therefore, essential to the care of these patients. It is important also that clinicians involved in the care of critically ill gravidas be familiar with the metabolic changes of pregnancy and their effect on arterial blood gas interpretation.

The arterial blood gas provides information regarding acid-base balance, oxygenation, and ventilation. A blood gas should be considered when a patient has significant respiratory symptoms, experiences oxygen desaturation, or as a baseline in the evaluation of preexisting pulmonary disease. In this chapter we focus on fundamental physiology, analytical considerations, effective interpretation of an arterial blood gas, and acid-base disturbances.

## Essential Physiology

### Acid-Base Homeostasis

Normal acid-base balance depends on production, buffering, and excretion of acid. The delicate balance that is crucial for survival is maintained by buffer systems, the lungs and kidneys.

Each day, approximately 15,000 mEq of volatile acids (e.g., carbonic acid) are produced by the metabolism of carbohydrates and fats. These acids are transported to and removed via the lungs as carbon dioxide ($CO_2$) gas. Breakdown of proteins and other substances results in 1.0 to 1.5 mEq/kg/day of nonvolatile or fixed acids (predominantly phosphoric and sulfuric acids) that are removed by the kidney.

Buffers are substances that can absorb or donate protons and thereby resist or reduce changes in $H^+$ ion concentration. Acids produced by cellular metabolism move out of cells and into the extracellular space where buffers absorb the protons. These protons are then transported to the kidney and excreted in urine. The intra- and extracellular buffer systems that maintain homeostasis in the human include the carbonic acid–bicarbonate system, plasma proteins, hemoglobin, and bone.

The carbonic acid–bicarbonate system is the principal extracellular buffer. Its effectiveness is due predominantly to the ability of the lungs to excrete carbon dioxide. In this system, bicarbonate, carbonic acid, and carbon dioxide are related by the equation:

$$CO_2 \quad \leftrightarrow \quad H_2O + CO_2 \quad \leftrightarrow \quad \text{Carbonic}$$

Gaseous phase / Dissolved / anhydrase

↓
LUNG

$$\leftrightarrow \quad H_2CO_3 \quad \leftrightarrow \quad H^+ \quad + \quad HCO_3^-$$

Carbonic acid / Bicarbonate

↓
KIDNEY

Carbon dioxide is produced as an end product of aerobic metabolism and physically dissolves in body fluids. A portion of dissolved carbon dioxide reacts with water to form carbonic acid, which dissociates into bicarbonate and hydrogen ions. The concentration of carbonic acid is normally very low relative to that of dissolved carbon dioxide and $HCO_3^-$. If the $H^+$ ion concentration increases, however, the acid load is buffered by bicarbonate, and additional carbonic acid is formed. The equilibrium of the equation is then driven to the left, and excess acid can be excreted as carbon dioxide gas.

The Henderson-Hasselbalch equation expresses the relationship between the reactants of the carbonic acid–bicarbonate system under conditions of equilibrium:

$$pH = pK + \log \frac{[HCO_3^-]\ (\text{metabolic})}{(s)[P_{CO_2}]\ (\text{respiratory})}$$

As the equation demonstrates, the ratio of $[HCO_3^-]/P_{CO_2}$ determines pH ($H^+$ ion concentration) and not individual or absolute concentrations. This ratio is influenced to a large extent by the function of the kidneys ($HCO_3^-$) and lungs ($P_{CO_2}$). The constant $s$ represents the solubility coefficient of carbon dioxide gas in plasma and relates $P_{CO_2}$ to the concentration of dissolved $CO_2$ and $HCO_3^-$. The value of $s$ is 0.03 mmol/liter/mm Hg at 37°C. The dissociation constant (pK) of blood carbonic acid is equivalent to 6.1 at 37°C.

The lungs are the second component of acid-base regulation. Alveolar ventilation controls $P_{CO_2}$ independent of bicarbonate excretion. When the bicarbonate concentration is altered, respiratory changes attempt to return the ratio of $[HCO_3^-]/P_{CO_2}$ toward the normal 20:1. Thus, in the presence of metabolic acidosis (decreased $HCO_3^-$), ventilation increases, $P_{CO_2}$ is lowered, and the ratio normalizes. In metabolic alkalosis, the opposite occurs as $P_{CO_2}$ rises in response to the primary increase in $HCO_3^-$.

The kidney is the final element of acid-base regulation. The main functions of the renal system are excretion of fixed acids and regulation of plasma bicarbonate levels. Carbonic acid that has been transported to the kidney dissociates into $H^+$ and $HCO_3^-$ in renal tubular cells. Each $H^+$ ion secreted into the tubular lumen is exchanged for sodium, and $HCO_3^-$ is passively reabsorbed into the blood. Essentially all bicarbonate must be reabsorbed by the kidney before acid can be excreted, because the loss of one $HCO_3^-$ is equivalent to the addition of one $H^+$ ion. Mono- and diphasic phosphates and ammonia are urinary buffers that combine with $H^+$ ions in the renal tubules and are excreted. Under normal conditions, the amount of $H^+$ excreted approximates the amount of nonvolatile acids produced.

The buffer systems, the lungs and kidneys, interact to maintain very tight control of the body's acid-base balance. The sequence of responses to a $H^+$ ion load and the time required for each may be summarized:

| Extracellular buffering by $HCO_3^-$ (Immediate) | → | Respiratory buffering $P_{CO_2}$ (Minutes to hours) | → | Renal excretion of $H^+$ (Hours to days) |
|---|---|---|---|---|

In contrast, when $P_{CO_2}$ changes:

| Intracellular buffering (Minutes) | → | Renal excretion of $H^+$ (Hours to days) |
|---|---|---|

Unlike the response to an acid load, no extracellular buffering occurs with a change in $P_{CO_2}$. Since $HCO_3^-$ is not an effective buffer against $H_2CO_3$, the only protection against respiratory acidosis or alkalosis is intracellular buffering (i.e., by hemoglobin) and renal $H^+$ ion excretion.

## Acid-Base Disturbances

Disturbances in acid-base balance are classified according to whether the underlying process results in an abnormal rise or fall in arterial pH. The suffix -osis refers to a pathologic process that causes a gain or loss of acid or base. Thus, *acidosis* describes any condition that leads to a fall in blood pH if the process continues uncorrected. Conversely, *alkalosis* characterizes any process that will cause a rise in pH if unopposed. The terms *acidosis* and *alkalosis* do not require the pH to be abnormal. The suffix -emia refers to the state of the blood, and *acidemia* and *alkalemia* are appropriately used when adult blood pH is abnormally low ($<7.36$) or high ($>7.44$), respectively (Kruse, 1993).

In addition, alterations in acid-base homeostasis are classified based on whether the underlying mechanism is metabolic or respiratory. If the primary abnormality is a net gain or loss of carbon dioxide, this is respiratory acidosis or alkalosis, respectively. Alternatively, a net gain or loss of bicarbonate results in metabolic alkalosis or acidosis, respectively. If only one primary process is present, then the acid-base disturbance is simple, and bicarbonate and $PCO_2$ always deviate in the same direction. A mixed disturbance develops when two or more primary processes are present, and the changes in $HCO_3^-$ and $PCO_2$ are in opposite directions.

The compensatory response attempts to normalize the $[HCO_3^-]/PCO_2$ ratio and maintain pH. Renal and pulmonary function must be adequate for these responses to be effective, and adequate time must be allowed for the complete response. The compensatory response for a primary respiratory abnormality is via the bicarbonate system or acid excretion by the kidney and requires several days for a complete response. Compensation for a metabolic aberration is through ventilation changes and occurs quite rapidly.

Compensatory responses cannot, however, completely return the pH to normal, with the exception of chronic respiratory alkalosis. The more severe the primary disorder, the more difficult it is to return the pH to normal. When the pH is normal but $PCO_2$ and $HCO_3^-$ are abnormal or the expected compensatory responses do not occur, then a second primary disorder exists. The four types of acid-base abnormalities and the compensatory response associated with each are listed in Table 2-1.

## Respiratory and Acid-Base Changes During Pregnancy

A variety of physiologic changes occur during pregnancy, affecting maternal respiratory function and gas exchange. As a result, an arterial blood gas obtained during pregnancy must be interpreted with an understanding of these alterations. Because these changes begin early in gestation and persist into the puerperium, they must be taken into consideration regardless of the stage of pregnancy (MacRae, 1967). In addition, the altitude at which a patient lives will affect arterial blood gas values, and normative data for each individual population should be established (Hankins, 1996a).

T A B L E   **2-1**

Summary of acid-base disorders: the primary disturbance, compensatory response, and expected degree of compensation

| | Primary Disturbance | Compensatory Response | Expected Degree of Compensation |
|---|---|---|---|
| Metabolic acidosis | Decreased $HCO_3^-$ | Decreased $PCO_2$ | $PaCO_2 = [1.5 \times (\text{serum bicarbonate})] + 8$<br>$PaCO_2 = $ last 2 digits of pH |
| Metabolic alkalosis | Increased $HCO_3^-$ | Increased $PCO_2$ | $PaCO_2 = [0.7 \times (\text{serum bicarbonate})] + 20$ |
| Respiratory acidosis | Increased $PCO_2$ | Increased $HCO_3^-$ | Acute: $pH = 0.08 \times (\text{measured } PaCO_2 - 40)/10$<br>Chronic: $pH = 0.03 \times (\text{measured } PaCO_2 - 40)/10$ |
| Respiratory alkalosis | Decreased $PCO_2$ | Decreased $HCO_3^-$ | Acute: $pH = 0.08 \times (40 - \text{measured } PaCO_2)/10$<br>Chronic: $pH = 0.03 \times (40 - \text{measured } PaCO_2)/10$ |

Minute ventilation increases by 30% to 50% during pregnancy (Cruikshank, 1991; Artal, 1986), and alveolar and arterial $P_{CO_2}$ decrease. Normal maternal arterial $P_{CO_2}$ levels range from 26 to 32 mm Hg (Liberatore, 1984; Andersen, 1969; Dayal, 1972). Because the fetus depends on the maternal respiratory system for carbon dioxide excretion, the decreased maternal $P_{CO_2}$ creates a gradient that allows the fetus to offload carbon dioxide. Nevertheless, fetal $P_{CO_2}$ is approximately 10 mm Hg higher than the maternal level when uteroplacental perfusion is normal.

Maternal alveolar oxygen tension increases as alveolar carbon dioxide tension decreases, and arterial $P_{O_2}$ levels rise as high as 106 mm Hg during the first trimester (Andersen, 1969; Templeton, 1976). Airway closing pressures increase with advancing gestation, causing a slight fall in arterial $P_{O_2}$ in the third trimester (101–104 mm Hg) (Pernoll, 1975; Templeton, 1976; Andersen, 1969). The arterial $P_{O_2}$ level, however, is dependent on the altitude at which the patient resides. The mean arterial $P_{O_2}$ for gravidas at sea level ranges from 95 to 102 mm Hg (Awe, 1979; Templeton, 1976), while the average values reported for those living at 1388 m are 87 mm Hg (Hankins, 1996a) and 61 mm Hg at 4200 m (Sobrevilla, 1971). As with carbon dioxide transfer, the fetus depends on the oxygen gradient for continued diffusion across the placenta. Maternal arterial oxygen content, uterine artery perfusion, and maternal hematocrit contribute to fetal oxygenation, and compromise of any of these factors can cause fetal hypoxemia and eventually acidemia (Novy, 1967).

Despite the increased ventilation, maternal arterial pH remains essentially unchanged during pregnancy (Andersen, 1969; Weinberger, 1980). A slightly higher pH value has been noted in women living at a moderate altitude, with a reported mean of 7.46 at 1388 meters above sea level (Hankins, 1996a). Bicarbonate excretion by the kidney is increased during normal pregnancy to compensate for the lowered $P_{CO_2}$, and serum bicarbonate levels are normally 18 to 21 mEq/liter (Andersen, 1969; Dayal, 1972; MacRae, 1967; Lucius, 1970). Thus, the metabolic state of pregnancy is a chronic respiratory alkalosis with a compensatory metabolic acidosis (Table 2-2).

T A B L E   **2-2**

**Arterial blood gas values during pregnancy at mild to moderate altitude**

| Parameter | Normal Range |
|---|---|
| pH | 7.40–7.46 |
| $P_{CO_2}$ | 26–32 mm Hg |
| $P_{O_2}$ | 87–106 mm Hg |
| $HCO_3^-$ | 18–21 mEq/liter |

Normative data should be established for individual populations residing at high altitude.

## Oxygen Delivery and Consumption

All tissues require oxygen for the combustion of organic compounds to fuel cellular metabolism. The cardiopulmonary system serves to deliver a continuous supply of oxygen and other essential substrates to tissues. Oxygen delivery is dependent on oxygenation of blood in the lungs, oxygen carrying capacity of the blood, and cardiac output. Under normal conditions, oxygen delivery ($D_{O_2}$) exceeds oxygen consumption ($V_{O_2}$) by about 75% (Cain, 1983). The amount of oxygen delivered is determined by the cardiac output (CO liters/min) times the arterial oxygen content ($C_{aO_2}$ mL/$O_2$/dL):

$$D_{O_2} = CO \times C_{aO_2} \times 10 \text{ dL/L}$$

Arterial oxygen content ($C_{aO_2}$) is determined by the amount of oxygen that is bound to hemoglobin ($S_{aO_2}$) and by the amount of oxygen that is dissolved in plasma ($P_{aO_2} \times 0.003$):

$$C_{aO_2} = (1.39 \times Hb \times S_{aO_2}) + (P_{aO_2} \times 0.003)$$

It is clear from this formula that the amount of oxygen dissolved in plasma is negligible and, therefore, that arterial oxygen content is dependent largely on hemoglobin concentration and arterial oxygen saturation. Oxygen delivery can be impaired by conditions that affect either cardiac output (flow), arterial oxygen content, or both (Table 2-3). Anemia leads to low arterial oxygen content because of a lack of hemoglobin binding sites for oxygen (Stock, 1986). Carbon monoxide poisoning likewise will decrease oxyhemoglobin because of blockage of binding sites for oxygen. The patient with hypoxemic respiratory failure

T A B L E   **2-3**

Commonly used formulas for assessment of oxygenation

| | Formula | Normal Value |
|---|---|---|
| Estimated alveolar oxygen tension | $Pao_2 = 145 - Paco_2$ | |
| Pulmonary capillary oxygen content | $Cco_2 = (1.39 \times Hb) + (PAo_2)(0.003)$ | |
| Arterial oxygen content | $Cao_2 = (1.39 \times Hb \times Sao_2) + (Pao_2 \times 0.003)$ | 18–21 mL/dL |
| Venous oxygen content | $Cvo_2 = (1.39 \times Hb \times Svo_2) + (Pvo_2 \times 0.003)$ | 15 mL/dL |
| Oxygen delivery | $Do_2 = Cao_2 \times Q_T \times 10\ dL/L$ | 700–1400 mL/min |
| Oxygen consumption | $Vo_2 = Q_T (Cao_2 - Cvo_2)$ $= 13.9\ (Hb)\ (Q_T)\ (Sao_2 - Svo_2)/100$ | 180–280 mL/min |
| Shunt equation | $\dfrac{Qsp}{Qt} = \dfrac{Cco_2 - Cao_2}{Cco_2 - Cvo_2}$ | 3%–8% |
| Estimated shunt | Estimated $Qsp/Qt = \dfrac{Cco_2 - Cao_2}{[Cco_2 - Cao_2] + [Cao_2 - Cvo_2]}$ | |

$Paco_2$, partial pressure of arterial carbon dioxide; $Pao_2$, partial pressure of arterial oxygen; $Pvo_2$, partial pressure of venous oxygen; Hb, hemoglobin, $Sao_2$, arterial oxygen saturation; $Svo_2$, venous oxygen saturation; $Q_T$, cardiac output; $PAo_2$, partial pressure of alveolar oxygen.

will not have sufficient oxygen available to saturate the hemoglobin molecule. Furthermore, it has been demonstrated that desaturated hemoglobin is altered structurally in such a fashion as to have a diminished affinity for oxygen (Bryan-Brown, 1973). It must be kept in mind that the amount of oxygen actually available to tissues also is affected by the affinity of the hemoglobin molecule for oxygen. Thus, the oxyhemoglobin dissociation curve (Fig 2-1) and those conditions that influence the binding of oxygen either negatively or positively must be considered when attempts are made to maximize oxygen delivery (Perutz, 1978). An increase in the plasma pH level, or a decrease in temperature or 2,3 diphosphoglycerate (2,3-DPG) will increase hemoglobin affinity for oxygen, shifting the curve to the left and resulting in diminished tissue oxygenation. If the plasma pH level or temperature falls, or if 2,3-DPG increases, hemoglobin affinity for oxygen will decrease and more oxygen will be available to tissues (Perutz, 1978).

In certain clinical conditions, such as septic shock and adult respiratory distress syndrome, there is maldistribution of flow relative to oxygen demand, leading to diminished delivery and loss

F I G U R E   **2-1**

The oxygen binding curve for human hemoglobin A under physiologic conditions (*dark curve*). The affinity is shifted by changes in pH, diphosphoglycerate concentration, and temperature, as indicated. $P_{50}$ represents the oxygen tension at half saturation. (Reproduced by permission from Bunn HF, Forget BG. Hemoglobin: molecular, genetic, and clinical aspects. Philadelphia: WB Saunders, 1986.)

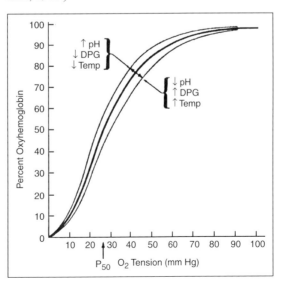

of normal mechanisms of vascular autoregulation, producing regional and microcirculatory imbalances in blood flow (Rackow, 1991). This mismatching of blood flow with metabolic demand causes excessive blood flow to some areas, with relative hypoperfusion of other areas, limiting optimal systemic utilization of oxygen (Rackow, 1991).

The patient with diminished cardiac output secondary to hypovolemia or pump failure is unable to distribute oxygenated blood to tissues. Therapy directed at increasing volume with normal saline, or with blood if the hemoglobin level is less than 10 g/dL, increases oxygen delivery in the hypovolemic patient. The patient with pump failure may benefit from inotropic support and afterload reduction in addition to supplementation of intravascular volume.

## Relationship of Oxygen Delivery to Consumption

Oxygen consumption ($Vo_2$) is the product of the arteriovenous oxygen content difference ($C(a-v)o_2$) and cardiac output. Under normal conditions, oxygen consumption is a direct function of the metabolic rate (Shoemaker, 1989).

$$Vo_2 = C(a-v)o_2 \times CO \times 10 \ dL/L$$

The oxygen extraction ratio (OER) is the fraction of delivered oxygen that actually is consumed:

$$OER = Vo_2/Do_2$$

The normal OER is about 0.25. A rise in the OER is a compensatory mechanism employed when oxygen delivery is inadequate for the level of metabolic activity. A subnormal value suggests flow maldistribution, peripheral diffusion defects, or functional shunting (Shoemaker, 1989). As the supply of oxygen is reduced, the fraction extracted from blood increases and oxygen consumption is maintained. If a severe reduction in oxygen delivery occurs, the limits of oxygen extraction are reached, tissues are unable to sustain aerobic energy production, and consumption decreases. The level of oxygen delivery at which oxygen consumption begins to decrease has been termed the "critical $Do_2$" (Shibutani, 1983). At the critical $Do_2$, tissues begin to use anaerobic glycolysis,

with resultant lactate production and metabolic acidosis (Shibutani, 1983). If this oxygen deprivation continues, irreversible tissue damage and death ensue.

## Oxygen Delivery and Consumption in Pregnancy

The physiologic anemia of pregnancy results in a reduction in the hemoglobin concentration and arterial oxygen content. Oxygen delivery is maintained at or above normal in spite of this because of the 50% increase that occurs in cardiac output. It is important to remember, therefore, that the pregnant woman is more dependent on cardiac output for maintenance of oxygen delivery than is the nonpregnant patient (Barron, 1991). Oxygen consumption increases steadily throughout pregnancy and is greatest at term, reaching an average of 331 mL/min at rest and 1167 mL/min with exercise (Pernoll, 1975). During labor, oxygen consumption increases by 40% to 60%, and cardiac output increases by about 22% (Gemzell, 1957; Ueland, 1969). Because oxygen delivery normally far exceeds consumption, the normal pregnant patient usually is able to maintain adequate delivery of oxygen to herself and her fetus, even during labor. When a pregnant patient has a low oxygen delivery, however, she very quickly can reach the critical $Do_2$, especially during labor, compromising both herself and her fetus. The obstetrician, therefore, must make every effort to optimize oxygen delivery before allowing labor to begin in the compromised patient.

## Blood Gas Analysis

The accuracy of a blood gas determination relies on many factors, including blood collection techniques, specimen transport, and laboratory equipment. Up to 16% of specimens may be improperly handled, diminishing diagnostic utility in a number of cases (Walton, 1981). Factors that can influence blood gas results include excessive heparin in the collection syringe, catheter dead space, air bubbles in the blood sample, time delays to laboratory analysis, as well as other less common causes. This section highlights considerations for obtaining a blood sample and potential sources of error, and briefly describes laboratory methods.

## Sample Collection

The collection syringe typically contains heparin to prevent clotting of the specimen. Excessive heparin in the syringe prior to blood collection, however, can significantly decrease the $P_{CO_2}$ and bicarbonate of the sample. The spurious $P_{CO_2}$ level results in a falsely lowered bicarbonate concentration when calculated using the Henderson-Hasselbalch equation. Although sodium heparin is an acid, pH is minimally affected because whole blood is an adequate buffer. Expelling all heparin except that in the dead space of the syringe and needle and ensuring adequate dilution by obtaining a minimum of 3 mL of blood will help avoid anticoagulant-related errors (Bloom, 1985).

In the intensive care unit setting, an arterial catheter is often placed when frequent blood sampling is anticipated. Dilutional errors occur when a blood sample is contaminated with fluids in the catheter (Ng, 1984). An adequate volume of maintenance fluid or flush solution must be withdrawn from the catheter and discarded prior to obtaining the sample for analysis, but estimating the appropriate amount can be difficult. Although a 2.5-mL discard volume has been suggested, it also has been recommended that each intensive care unit establish its own policy based on individual catheter and connection systems (Al-Ameri, 1986; Kruse, 1993; Bhaskaran, 1988).

Air bubbles in the collection syringe cause time-dependent changes in the arterial blood gas. Air trapped as froth accelerates these changes because of their increased surface area (Biswas, 1982). The degree of change in $P_{O_2}$ depends on the initial $P_{O_2}$ of the sample. Because an air bubble has a $P_{O_2}$ of 150 mm Hg (room air), the bubble will cause a falsely elevated $P_{O_2}$ if the sample $P_{O_2}$ is less than 150 mm Hg. The opposite occurs if the sample has an initial $P_{O_2}$ greater than 150 mm Hg (Mueller, 1982; Kruse, 1993). Oxygen saturation is most significantly affected when the sample $P_{O_2}$ is less than 60 mm Hg because saturation changes rapidly with changes in $P_{O_2}$, as predicted by the oxyhemoglobin dissociation curve. $P_{CO_2}$ in the sample decreases within several minutes of exposure to ambient air (Biswas, 1982; Harsten, 1988).

When a blood sample remains at room temperature following collection, $P_{O_2}$ and pH may decrease while $P_{CO_2}$ increases. Specimens analyzed within 10 to 20 minutes of collection give accurate results even when transported at room temperature (Nanji, 1984; Madiedo, 1980). In most clinical settings, however, the time between sampling and laboratory analysis of the specimen exceeds this limit. Therefore, the syringe should be placed into an ice bath immediately after sample collection. The combination of ice and water provides better cooling of the syringe than ice alone, and a sample may be stored for up to 1 hour without adversely affecting blood gas results (Harsten, 1988).

Several additional factors can influence blood gas results (Urbina, 1993). Insufficient time between an adjustment in fractional inspired oxygen or mechanical ventilator settings and blood gas analysis may not accurately reflect the change. Equilibration is rapid, however, and has been reported to occur as soon as 10 minutes after changing ventilator settings of postoperative cardiac patients (Schuch, 1986). General anesthesia with halothane will falsely elevate $P_{O_2}$ determination because it mimics oxygen during sample analysis (McHugh, 1979; Douglas, 1978; Maekawa, 1980; Dent, 1976). Finally, severe leukocytosis causes a false lowering of $P_{O_2}$ due to consumption by the cells in the collection syringe (Hess, 1979). The effect of the WBCs may be minimized, but not necessarily eliminated, by cooling the sample immediately after it is obtained.

While maternal pH may affect fetal pH as assessed by fetal scalp blood sampling, such changes are generally not of clinical significance, and assessment of maternal pH is not essential to proper clinical evaluation of fetal scalp pH.

## The Blood Gas Analyzer

The blood gas analyzer is designed to simultaneously measure the pH, $P_{O_2}$, and $P_{CO_2}$ of blood.

An aliquot of heparinized blood is injected into a chamber containing one reference and three measuring electrodes. Each measuring electrode is connected to the reference electrode by an Ag/AgCl wire. The electrodes and injected sample are kept at a constant 37°C by a warm water bath or heat exchanger. The accuracy of the measurements depends on routine calibration of equipment, proper sample collection, and constant electrode temperature.

Blood pH and $Pco_2$ are potentiometric determinations, with the potential difference between each electrode and the reference electrode quantitated. The pH electrode detects hydrogen ions, and the electrical potential developed by the electrode varies with the ion $H^+$ activity of the sample. The potential difference between the pH and reference electrode is measured by a voltmeter and converted to the pH. The $Pco_2$ electrode is actually a modified pH electrode. A glass electrode is surrounded with a weak bicarbonate solution and enclosed in a silicone membrane. Carbon dioxide in the sample diffuses through this membrane that is permeable to carbon dioxide but not water and $H^+$ ions. As carbon dioxide diffuses through the membrane, the pH of the bicarbonate solution changes. Thus, the pH measured by the electrode is related to carbon dioxide tension.

The measurement of $Po_2$ is amperometric, because the current generated between an anode and cathode estimates the partial pressure of oxygen. The $Po_2$ electrode surrounds a membrane permeable to oxygen but not other blood constituents. The electrode consists of an anode and a cathode, and constant voltage is maintained between them. Current is produced by an electrolytic process that occurs in the presence of oxygen, and the magnitude of the current is proportional to the partial pressure of oxygen in the sample. As oxygen tension increases, the electrical current generated between the anode and cathode increases.

Bicarbonate concentration as reported on a blood gas result is not directly measured in the blood gas laboratory. Once pH and $Pco_2$ are determined, bicarbonate concentration is calculated using the Henderson-Hasselbalch equation or determined from a nomogram. In contrast, the total serum carbon dioxide ($tCO_2$) content is measured by automated methods and reported with routine serum electrolyte measurements.

Oxygen saturation ($So_2$) is the ratio of oxygenated hemoglobin to total hemoglobin. It can be plotted graphically once $Po_2$ is determined, calculated using an equation that estimates the oxyhemoglobin dissociation curve, or determined spectrophotometrically by a co-oximeter. The latter is the most accurate method because saturation is determined by a direct reading.

## Pulse Oximetry

The oximetry system determines arterial oxygen saturation by measuring the absorption of selected wavelengths of light in pulsatile blood flow (New, 1985). Oxyhemoglobin absorbs much less red and slightly more infrared light than reduced hemoglobin. Oxygen saturation thereby determines the ratio of red to infrared absorption.

Red and infrared light are detected from light-emitting diodes to a photodetector across a pulsatile tissue bed; the absorption of each wavelength of the tissue bed varies cyclically with pulse. The pulse rate, therefore, also is determined. When assessing the accuracy of the arterial saturation measured by the pulse oximeter, correlation of the pulse rate determined by the oximeter and the patient's heart rate is an indication of proper placement of the electrode. The sites usually used for measurement are the nail bed on the finger and the ear lobe. Under ideal circumstances, most oximeters measure saturation ($Spo_2$) to within 2% of $Sao_2$ (New, 1985).

Pulse oximetry is ideal for noninvasive monitoring of the arterial oxygen saturation near the steep portion of the oxygen hemoglobin dissociation curve, namely at a $Pao_2$ less than or equal to 70 mm Hg (Demling, 1993). $Pao_2$ levels greater than or equal to 80 mm Hg result in very small changes in oxygen saturation, namely 97% to 99%. Large changes in the $Pao_2$ from 90 mm Hg to 60 mm Hg can occur without significant change in arterial oxygen saturation. This technique, therefore, is useful as a continuous monitor of the adequacy of blood oxygenation and not as a method to quantitate the level of impaired gas exchange (Huch, 1988).

Poor tissue perfusion, hyperbilirubinemia, and severe anemia may lead to oximetry inconsistencies (Demling, 1993). Carbon monoxide poisoning will lead to an overestimation of the $Pao_2$. With methemoglobin levels greater than 5%, the pulse oximeter no longer accurately predicts oxygen saturation. Methylene blue, the treatment for methemoglobinemia, will also lead to oximetry inaccuracies.

## Mixed Venous Oxygenation

The mixed venous oxygen tension ($Pvo_2$) and mixed venous oxygen saturation ($Svo_2$) are parameters of tissue oxygenation (Shoemaker, 1989). $Pvo_2$ is 40 mm Hg with a saturation of 73%. Saturations less than 60% are abnormally low. These parameters can be measured directly by obtaining a blood sample from the distal port of the pulmonary artery catheter. The $Svo_2$ also can be measured continuously with special pulmonary artery catheters equipped with fiberoptics. Mixed venous oxygenation is a reliable parameter in the patient with hypoxemia or low cardiac output, but findings must be interpreted with caution. When the $Svo_2$ is low, oxygen delivery can be assumed to be low. However, normal or high $Svo_2$ does not guarantee that tissues are well oxygenated. In conditions such as septic shock and adult respiratory distress syndrome, the maldistribution of systemic flow may lead to abnormally high $Svo_2$ in the face of severe tissue hypoxia (Rackow, 1991). The oxygen dissociation curve must be considered when interpreting the $Svo_2$ as an indicator of tissue oxygenation (Bryan-Brown, 1973). Conditions that result in a left shift of the curve cause the venous oxygen saturation to be normal or high, even when the mixed venous oxygen content is low. The $Svo_2$ is useful for monitoring trends in a particular patient, because a significant decrease will occur when oxygen delivery has decreased secondary to hypoxemia or a fall in cardiac output.

## Blood Gas Interpretation

The processes leading to acid-base disturbances are well described, and blood gas analysis may facilitate identification of the cause of a serious illness. Because many critically ill patients have metabolic and respiratory derangements, correct interpretation of a blood gas is fundamental to their care. Misinterpretation, however, can result in treatment delays and inappropriate therapy. Several methods of acid-base interpretation have been devised, including graphic nomograms and step-by-step analysis. Each method is detailed in this section to aid in rapid and correct diagnosis of disturbances in acid-base balance.

Blood gas results are not a substitute for clinical evaluation of a patient, and laboratory values do not necessarily correlate with the degree of clinical compromise. A typical example is the patient with an acute exacerbation of asthma who experiences severe dyspnea and respiratory compromise prior to developing hypercapnea and hypoxemia. Thus, a blood gas is an adjunct to clinical judgment, and decision making should not be based on a single test.

### *Graphic Nomogram*

Nomograms are a graphic display of an equation and have been designed to facilitate identification of simple acid-base disturbances (Goldberg, 1973; Davenport, 1974; Arbus, 1973; Cogan, 1986). Figure 2-2 is an example of a nomogram with arterial blood pH represented on the X-axis, $HCO_3^-$ concentration on the Y-axis, and arterial $Pco_2$ on the regression lines. Nomograms are accurate for simple acid-base disturbances, and a single disorder can be identified by plotting measured blood gas values. When blood gas values fall between labeled areas, a mixed disorder is present and the nomogram does not apply. These complex disorders must then be characterized by quantitative assessment of the expected compensatory changes (see Table 2-1).

## A Systematic Approach to an Acid-Base Abnormality

Several different approaches for blood gas interpretation have been devised (Haber, 1991; Tremper, 1992). A six-step approach modified from Narins and Emmitt provides a simple and reliable method to analyze a blood gas, particularly

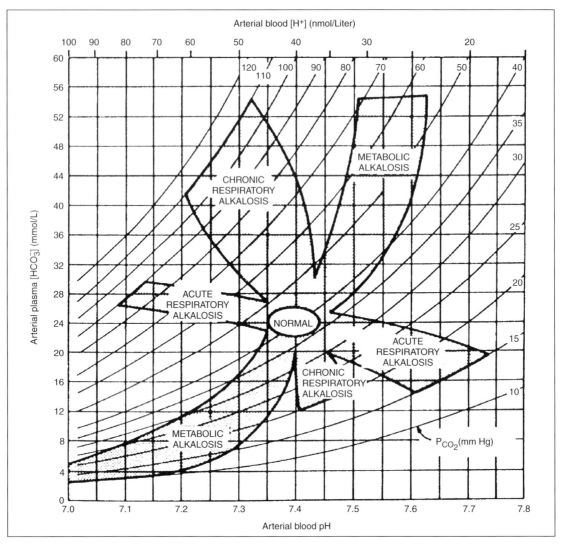

FIGURE   **2-2**

**Nomogram for interpretation of simple acid-base disorders**. (Reproduced by permission from Cogan MJ. In: Brenner BM, Rector FC Jr, eds. The kidney. Philadelphia: WB Saunders, 1986:473.)

when a complicated mixed disorder is present (Narins, 1980; Morganroth, 1990a). This method, adjusted for pregnancy, is as follows (Fig 2-3):

1. Is the patient acidemic or alkalemic? If the arterial blood pH is less than 7.36, the patient is acidemic, while a pH greater than 7.44 defines alkalemia.

2. Is the primary disturbance respiratory or metabolic? The primary alteration associ-

ated with each of the four primary disorders is shown in Table 2-1.

3. If a *respiratory* disturbance is present, is it acute or chronic? The equations listed in Table 2-1 are used to determine the acuteness of the disturbance. The expected change in the pH is calculated and the measured pH is compared with the pH that would be expected based on the patient's $P_{CO_2}$.

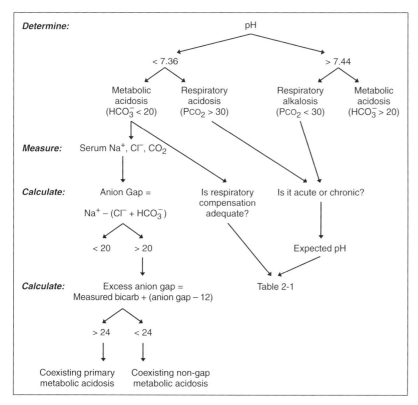

A systematic approach to the interpretation of an arterial blood gas during pregnancy.

4. If a *metabolic acidosis* is present, is the anion gap increased? Metabolic acidosis is classified according to the presence or absence of an anion gap.

5. If a *metabolic* disturbance is present, is the respiratory compensation adequate? The expected $P_{CO_2}$ for a given degree of metabolic acidosis can be predicted by Winter's formula (see Table 2-1), because the relationship between $P_{CO_2}$ and $HCO_3^-$ is linear. Predicting respiratory compensation for metabolic alkalosis, however, is not nearly as consistent as with acidosis.

6. If the patient has an anion gap metabolic acidosis, are additional metabolic disturbances present? The excess anion gap represents bicarbonate concentration before the anion gap acidosis developed. By calculating the excess gap, an otherwise undetected non-anion gap acidosis or metabolic alkalosis may be detected.

## Respiratory Components of the Arterial Blood Gas

**Partial Pressure of Arterial Oxygen $Pa_{O_2}$** The $Pa_{O_2}$ reflects the lung's ability to provide adequate arterial oxygen. Normal arterial oxygen tension during pregnancy ranges from 87 to 106 mm Hg, depending on the altitude at which a patient lives (Hankins, 1996a). Although $Pa_{O_2}$ has been reported to decrease by 25% when samples are obtained from gravidas in the supine position (Awe, 1979), arterial blood gas values recently were shown to be unaffected by a change in maternal position (Hankins, 1996a). Abnormal gas exchange, inadequate ventilation, or both can lead to a fall in $Pa_{O_2}$. Hypoxemia is defined as a $Pa_{O_2}$ below 60 mm Hg or a saturation less than 90%. At this level, the oxygen content of blood is near its maximum for a given hemoglobin concentration, and any additional increase in arterial oxygen tension will increase oxygen content only a small amount.

The amount of oxygen combined with hemoglobin is related to the $Pa_{O_2}$ by the oxyhemoglobin dissociation curve and influenced by a variety of factors (Fig 2-4). The shape of the oxyhemoglobin dissociation curve allows $Pa_{O_2}$ to decrease faster than oxygen saturation until the $Pa_{O_2}$ is approximately 60 mm Hg. A left shift of the curve increases hemoglobin's affinity for oxygen and oxygen content, but decreases release of $O_2$ in peripheral tissues. The fetal or neonatal oxyhemoglobin dissociation curve is shifted to the left as a result of fetal hemoglobin (see Fig 2-4). The increased affinity of hemoglobin for oxygen allows the fetus to extract maximal oxygen from maternal blood. A shift to the right has the opposite effect, with decreased oxygen affinity and content but increased release in the periphery.

F I G U R E  **2-4**

**Maternal and fetal oxyhemoglobin dissociation curves.** (Reproduced by permission from Semin Perinatol 1984;8:168.)

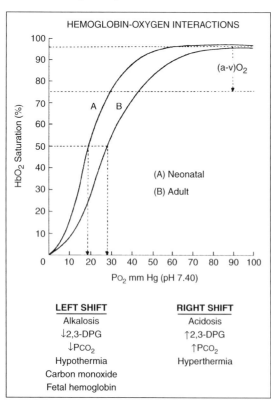

**Assessment of Lung Function** Impairment of lung function can be estimated using an oxygen tension– or oxygen content–based index. Oxygen tension–based indices include (1) expected $Pa_{O_2}$ for a given fraction of inspired oxygen ($Fi_{O_2}$), (2) $Pa_{O_2}/Fi_{O_2}$ ratio, and (3) alveolar-arterial oxygen gradient ($P_{(A-a)}O_2$). These methods are quick and easy to use but have limitations in the critically ill patient (Cane, 1988). The shunt calculation (Qsp/Qt) is an oxygen content–based index and is the most reliable method of determining the extent to which pulmonary disease is contributing to arterial hypoxemia. The need for a pulmonary artery blood sample is a disadvantage, however, because not all patients require invasive monitoring. The estimated shunt calculation (est. Qsp/Qt) is derived from the shunt equation and is the optimal method to estimate lung compromise when a pulmonary artery catheter is not placed.

The expected $Pa_{O_2}$ is an oxygen tension–based calculation and can be estimated quickly by multiplying the actual percentage of inspired oxygen by 6 (Wilson, 1992a). Thus, a patient receiving 50% oxygen has an expected $P_{O_2}$ of (50 × 6) or 300 mm Hg. Alternatively, the $Fi_{O_2}$ (e.g., 0.50 in a patient receiving 50% oxygen) may be multiplied by 500 to estimate the minimum $P_{O_2}$ (Shapiro, 1992). The $Pa_{O_2}/Fi_{O_2}$ ratio has been used to estimate the amount of shunt. The normal ratio is 500 to 600 and correlates with a shunt of 3% to 5%, while a shunt of 20% or more is present when the ratio is less than 200.

Calculation of the alveolar-arterial oxygen gradient is also an oxygen tension calculation. The A-a gradient is most reliable when breathing room air and is normally less than 20. An increased gradient indicates pulmonary dysfunction. A-a gradient values, however, can change unpredictably with changes in $Fi_{O_2}$ and vary with alterations in oxygen saturation and consumption. Thus, the utility of this measurement in critically ill patients has been questioned because these patients often require a high $Fi_{O_2}$ and have unstable oxygenation (Nearman, 1982). Caution is indicated in interpreting the A-a gradient during pregnancy (Awe, 1979).

Oxygen content–based indices include the shunt equation and estimated shunt as derived from the shunt equation (see Table 2-3). The estimated shunt has been shown to be superior to the oxygen tension–based indices described previously (Cane, 1988). The patient is given 100% oxygen for at least 20 minutes prior to determining arterial and venous blood gases and hemoglobin. Because the estimated shunt equation does not require a pulmonary artery blood sample, the C(a-v)$o_2$ difference is assumed to be 3.5 mL/dL. A normal shunt in nonpregnant patients is less than 10%, while a 20% to 29% shunt may be life-threatening in a patient with compromised cardiovascular or neurologic function, and a shunt of 30% and greater usually requires significant cardiopulmonary support.

Intrapulmonary shunt values during normal pregnancy, however, have been reported to be nearly three times above the mean for nonpregnant individuals (Hankins, 1996b). The mean Qs/Qt in normotensive primiparous women at 36 to 38 weeks' gestation ranges from 10% in the knee-chest position to 13% in the standing position and 15% in the lateral position. The increased Qs/Qt can be explained by the physiologic changes of pregnancy as follows. Lung volumes decrease during gestation, and the amount of shunt increases. In addition, pulmonary blood flow increases secondary to increased cardiac output. The combined effect of decreased lung volumes and increased pulmonary flow results in a higher intrapulmonary shunt during pregnancy.

**Oxygenation of Peripheral Tissues** An adequate $Pao_2$ is only the initial step in oxygen transport and it does not guarantee well-oxygenated tissues. The degree of intrapulmonary shunt, oxygen delivery, and oxygen consumption all contribute to adequate tissue oxygenation. Accurate assessment of peripheral oxygenation requires measurement of arterial and venous partial pressures of oxygen, arterial and venous oxygen saturation, hemoglobin, and cardiac output (see Table 2-3).

The amount of oxygen (mL) contained in 100 mL of blood defines oxygen content. Oxygen delivery ($Do_2$) is the volume of oxygen brought to peripheral tissues in 1 minute, and consumption ($Vo_2$) is the volume used by the tissues in 1 minute. Under normal conditions, delivery of oxygen is 3 to 4 times greater than consumption. Oxygen extraction measures the amount of $O_2$ transferred to tissues from 100 mL of blood and can be thought of as $Cao_2 - Cvo_2$. Thus, an oxygen extraction of 3 to 4 mL/dL suggests adequate cardiac reserve to supply additional oxygen if demand increases. Inadequate cardiac reserve is indicated by an oxygen extraction of 5 mL/dL or greater, and tissue extraction must be increased to meet changing metabolic needs (Shapiro, 1995).

Mixed venous oxygen tension ($Pvo_2$) and saturation ($Svo_2$) are measured from pulmonary artery blood. These measurements are better indicators of tissue oxygenation than arterial values because venous blood reflects peripheral tissue extraction. Normal arterial oxygen saturation is 100% and venous saturation is 75%, yielding a normal arteriovenous difference ($Sao_2 - Svo_2$) of 25%. An increased $Svo_2$ (>80%) can occur when oxygen delivery increases, oxygen consumption decreases (or some combination of these two), cardiac output increases, or the pulmonary artery catheter tip is in a pulmonary capillary instead of the artery. A decrease in $Svo_2$ (<50% to 60%) may be due to increased oxygen consumption, decreased cardiac output, or compromised pulmonary function. The venous oxygen saturation may not change at all, however, even with significant cardiovascular changes.

**Partial Pressure of Arterial Carbon Dioxide ($Paco_2$)** The metabolic rate determines the amount of carbon dioxide that enters the blood. Carbon dioxide is then transported to the lung as dissolved carbon dioxide, bicarbonate, and carbamates. It diffuses from blood into alveoli and is removed from the body by ventilation, or the movement of gas into and out of the pulmonary system. Measurement of the arterial partial pressure of carbon dioxide allows assessment of alveolar ventilation in relation to the metabolic rate.

Ventilation ($V_E$) is the amount of gas exhaled in 1 minute and is the sum of alveolar and dead space ventilation ($V_E = V_A + V_{DS}$). Alveolar ventilation ($V_A$) is that portion of the lung that removes carbon dioxide and transfers oxygen to the blood, while dead space ($V_{DS}$) has no respiratory function. As dead space increases, ventilation must increase to maintain adequate alveolar ventilation. Dead space increases with a high ventilation-perfusion ratio (V/Q) (i.e., an acute decrease in cardiac output, acute pulmonary embolism, acute pulmonary hypertension, or adult respiratory distress syndrome) and positive pressure ventilation.

Because $Pa_{CO_2}$ reflects the balance between production and alveolar excretion of $CO_2$, accumulation of carbon dioxide indicates failure of the respiratory system to excrete the products of metabolism. The primary disease process may be respiratory or a process outside the lungs. Extrapulmonary processes that increase metabolism and carbon dioxide production include fever, shivering, seizures, sepsis, or physiologic stress. Parenteral nutrition with glucose providing more than 50% of nonprotein calories also can contribute to high carbon dioxide production.

Recognizing respiratory acid-base imbalance is important because of the need to assist in carbon dioxide elimination. As $V_E$ increases, the work of breathing can cause fatigue and respiratory failure. It is important to recognize that the $Pa_{CO_2}$ may be normal initially but rises as the work of breathing exceeds a patient's functional reserve. Ventilatory failure occurs when the pulmonary system can no longer provide adequate excretion of carbon dioxide. Clinically, this is recognized as tachypnea, tachycardia, intercostal muscle retraction, accessory muscle use, diaphoresis, and paradoxic breathing.

### *Metabolic Component of Arterial Blood Gas (Bicarbonate)*

Measurement of bicarbonate reflects a patient's acid-base status. The bicarbonate concentration reported with a blood gas is calculated using the Henderson-Hasselbalch equation and represents a single ionic species. Total serum carbon dioxide ($tCO_2$) content is measured with serum electrolytes and is the sum of the various forms of carbon dioxide in serum. Bicarbonate is the major contributor to $tCO_2$, and additional forms include dissolved carbon dioxide, carbamates, carbonate, and carbonic acid. The calculated bicarbonate concentration does not include carbonic acid, carbonate, and carbamates.

Frequently, arterial and venous blood samples are obtained simultaneously, making arterial blood gas bicarbonate and venous serum $tCO_2$ measurements available. Venous serum $tCO_2$ content is 2.5 to 3.0 mEq/liter higher than arterial blood gas bicarbonate, because carbon dioxide content is higher in venous than arterial blood and all species of carbon dioxide are included in the determination of $tCO_2$. If the blood sample is arterial, the $tCO_2$ content reported on the electrolyte panel should be 1.5 to 2.0 mEq/liter higher than the calculated bicarbonate. The $tCO_2$ measured directly with serum electrolytes will be higher because it includes the different forms of carbon dioxide. Because both blood gas bicarbonate and electrolyte $tCO_2$ determinations are usually available, the clinical utility of one compared with the other has been a subject of controversy (Kruse, 1989). A recent review, however, concludes that calculated and measured bicarbonate values are close enough in most cases that either is acceptable for clinical use (Kruse, 1995).

## Disorders of Acid-Base Balance

### Metabolic Acidosis

Metabolic acidosis is diagnosed on the basis of a decreased serum bicarbonate and arterial pH. The baseline bicarbonate concentration during pregnancy should, of course, be kept in mind when interpreting bicarbonate concentration. Metabolic acidosis develops when fixed acids accumulate or bicarbonate is lost. Accumulation of fixed acid occurs with overproduction as in diabetic ketoacidosis or lactic acidosis, or with decreased acid excretion as in renal failure. Diarrhea, a small bowel fistula, and renal tubular acidosis can all result in loss of extracellular bicarbonate.

Although the clinical signs associated with metabolic acidosis are not specific, multiple organ systems may be affected. Tachycardia develops with the initial fall in pH, but bradycardia usually predominates as the pH drops below 7.10. Acidosis causes venous constriction and impairs cardiac contractility, increasing venous return while cardiac output decreases. Arteriolar dilation

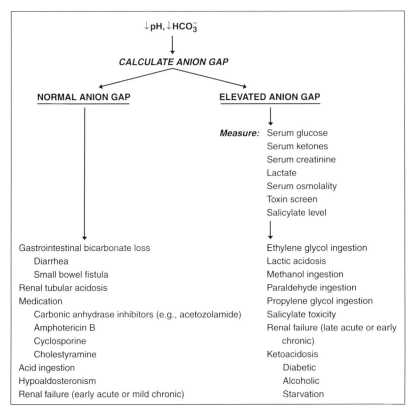

$\downarrow$pH, $\downarrow$HCO$_3^-$

$\downarrow$

*CALCULATE ANION GAP*

**NORMAL ANION GAP**                    **ELEVATED ANION GAP**

$\downarrow$

*Measure:*  Serum glucose
Serum ketones
Serum creatinine
Lactate
Serum osmolality
Toxin screen
Salicylate level

$\downarrow$

| NORMAL ANION GAP | ELEVATED ANION GAP |
|---|---|
| Gastrointestinal bicarbonate loss | Ethylene glycol ingestion |
|   Diarrhea | Lactic acidosis |
|   Small bowel fistula | Methanol ingestion |
| Renal tubular acidosis | Paraldehyde ingestion |
| Medication | Propylene glycol ingestion |
|   Carbonic anhydrase inhibitors (e.g., acetozolamide) | Salicylate toxicity |
|   Amphotericin B | Renal failure (late acute or early |
|   Cyclosporine |   chronic) |
|   Cholestyramine | Ketoacidosis |
| Acid ingestion |   Diabetic |
| Hypoaldosteronism |   Alcoholic |
| Renal failure (early acute or mild chronic) |   Starvation |

F I G U R E  **2-5**

Etiology and evaluation of metabolic acidosis.

occurs at pH less than 7.20. Respiratory rate and tidal volume increase in an attempt to compensate for the acidosis. Maternal acidosis can result in fetal acidosis as H$^+$ ions equilibrate across the placenta, and fetal pH is generally 0.1 pH units less than the maternal pH.

The compensatory response to metabolic acidosis is an increase in ventilation that is stimulated by the fall in the pH. Hyperventilation lowers $P$co$_2$ as the body attempts to return the [HCO$_3^-$]/$P$co$_2$ ratio toward normal. The respiratory response is proportional to the degree of acidosis and allows calculation of the expected $P$co$_2$ for a given bicarbonate level (see Table 2-1). When the measured $P$co$_2$ is higher or lower than expected for the measured serum bicarbonate, a mixed acid-base disorder must be present. This formula is applied ideally once the patient has reached a steady state, when $P$co$_2$ nadirs 12 to 24 hours after the onset of acidosis (Narins, 1980).

The classification of metabolic acidosis as non-anion gap or anion gap acidosis is helpful in determining the pathologic process involved. Once a metabolic acidosis is detected, serum electrolytes should be obtained and the anion gap calculated. Frequently the underlying abnormality can be identified by clinical history and a few additional diagnostic studies (Fig 2-5) (Battle, 1988).

Electroneutrality in the body is maintained because the sum of all anions equals the sum of all cations. Na$^+$, K$^+$, Cl$^-$, and HCO$_3^-$ are the routinely measured serum ions, while Mg$^+$, Ca$^{++}$, proteins (particularly albumin), lactate, HPO$_4^-$, and SO$_4^-$ are the unmeasured ions. Na$^+$ and K$^+$ account for 95% of cations, while HCO$_3^-$ and Cl$^-$ represent 85% of anions (Preuss, 1993). Thus, unmeasured anions are greater than unmeasured cations. The anion gap is the difference between measured plasma cations (Na$^+$) minus measured anions (Cl$^-$, HCO$_3^-$) and is derived:

Total anions = Total cations

Measured anions + Unmeasured anions

  = Measured cations + Unmeasured cations

$([Cl^-] + [tCO_2^-] + $ Unmeasured anions)

  $= ([Na^+] + $ Unmeasured cations)

Unmeasured anions − Unmeasured cations

  $= [Na^+] - ([Cl^-] + [tCO_2^-])$

Anion gap $= [Na^+] - ([Cl^-] + [tCO_2^-])$

A normal anion gap is 8 to 16 mEq/liter. Potassium may be included as a measured cation, although it contributes little to the accuracy or utility of the gap. If $K^+$ is included in the calculation, however, the normal range becomes 12 to 20 mEq/liter (Kruse, 1994).

A change in the gap involves a change in unmeasured cations or anions. An elevated gap is most commonly due to an accumulation of unmeasured anions that include organic acids (i.e., ketoacids or lactic acid) or inorganic acids (i.e., sulfate and phosphate) (Oh, 1977). A decrease in cations (i.e., magnesium and calcium) also will increase the gap, but the serum level is usually life-threatening.

The following example demonstrates use of the anion gap in a patient who had been experiencing dysuria, polyuria, and polydypsia of several days' duration. Initial evaluation of this 19-year-old gravida at 24 weeks' gestation was notable for a serum glucose level of 460 mg/dL and 4+ urinary ketones. Further investigation revealed arterial pH, 7.30; $HCO_3^-$, 14 mEq/liter; serum $Na^+$, 133 mEq/liter; $K^+$, 4.1 mEq/liter; $tCO_2$, 15 mEq/liter; and $Cl^-$, 95 mEq/liter. The anion gap was determined:

Anion gap $= [Na^+] - ([Cl^-] + [tCO_2^-])$

  $= 133$ mEq/liter − (95 mEq/liter
  + 15 mEq/liter)

  $= 133$ mEq/liter − 110 mEq/liter

Anion gap $= 23$ mEq/liter

The elevated anion gap is the result of unmeasured organic anions or ketoacids that have accumulated and decreased serum bicarbonate. As this patient with type I diabetes mellitus receives insulin therapy, the anion gap will normalize, reflecting disappearance of the ketoacids from serum.

The limitations of the anion gap, however, should be recognized. Various factors can lower

the anion gap, but its importance is not so much in the etiology of the decrease as in its ability to mask an elevated gap. Because albumin accounts for the majority of unmeasured anions, the gap decreases as albumin levels fall. For each 1-g decrease in albumin, the gap may be lowered by 2.5 to 3.0 mEq/liter. Decreased serum albumin is the most common cause of a lowered gap, and other less common causes include markedly elevated levels of unmeasured cations ($K^+$, $Mg^+$, and $Ca^{++}$), hyperlipidemia, lithium carbonate intoxication, multiple myeloma, and bromide or iodide intoxication.

Although an elevated anion gap is associated traditionally with metabolic acidosis, it also may occur in the presence of severe metabolic alkalosis. The ionic activity of albumin changes with increasing pH, and protons are released. The net negative charge on each molecule increases, thereby increasing unmeasured anions. Volume contraction leads to hyperproteinemia and augments the anion gap.

If an anion gap acidosis is present, the ratio of the change in the anion gap (the delta gap) to the change in $HCO_3^-$ can be helpful in determining the type of disturbances present:

$$\frac{\Delta \text{ gap}}{\Delta HCO_3^-} = \frac{\text{Anion gap} - 12}{24 - [HCO_3^-]}$$

In simple anion gap metabolic acidosis, the ratio approximates 1.0, because the decrease in bicarbonate equals the increase in anions. The delta gap for the previously described patient with diabetes and ketoacidosis is calculated as follows:

$$\frac{\Delta \text{ gap}}{\Delta HCO_3^-} = \frac{\text{Anion gap} - 12}{24 - [HCO_3^-]} = \frac{23 - 12}{24 - 14} = \frac{11}{10} = 1.1$$

The delta gap is 0 when the acidosis is a pure non-anion gap acidosis. A delta gap of 0.3 to 0.7 is associated with one of two mixed metabolic disorders: (1) a high anion gap acidosis and respiratory alkalosis and (2) a high anion gap with a pre-existing normal or low anion gap. A ratio greater than 1.2 implies a metabolic alkalosis superimposed on a high anion gap acidosis or a mixed high anion gap acidosis and chronic respiratory acidosis. The use of the delta gap is limited, however, by the wide range of normal values for the anion gap and bicarbonate, and its accuracy has been questioned (Salem, 1992).

When a normal anion gap metabolic acidosis is present, the urinary anion gap may be helpful in distinguishing the cause of the acidosis:

Urinary anion gap
$$= ([Urine\ Na^+] + [Urine\ K^+]) - [Urine\ Cl^-]$$

The urinary anion gap is a clinically useful method to estimate urinary ammonium ($NH_4^+$) excretion. Because the amount of $NH_4^+$ excreted in the urine cannot be measured directly, the urinary anion gap helps determine whether the kidney is responding appropriately to a metabolic acidosis (Halperin, 1988). Normally, the urine anion gap is positive or close to zero. A negative gap ($Cl^- > Na^+$ and $K^+$) occurs with gastrointestinal bicarbonate loss, and $NH_4^+$ excretion by the kidney is appropriately increased. In contrast, a positive gap ($Cl^- < Na^+$ and $K^+$) in a patient with acidosis suggests impaired distal urinary acidification with inappropriately low $NH_4^+$ excretion.

A variety of processes can lead to metabolic acidosis, and therapy will depend on the underlying condition. Adequate oxygenation should be ensured and mechanical ventilation instituted for impending respiratory failure. The use of bicarbonate solutions to correct acidosis has been suggested when arterial pH is less than 7.10 or bicarbonate is lower than 5 mEq/liter. Bicarbonate solutions must be administered with caution because an "overshoot" alkalosis can lower seizure threshold, impair oxygen availability to peripheral tissues, and stimulate additional lactate production.

## Metabolic Alkalosis

Metabolic alkalosis is characterized by a rise in serum bicarbonate concentration and an elevated arterial pH. The most impressive clinical effects of metabolic alkalosis are neurologic and include confusion, obtundation, and tetany. Cardiac arrhythmia's, hypotension, hypoventilation, and various metabolic aberrations may accompany these neurologic changes.

Metabolic alkalosis results from a loss of acid or the addition of alkali. The development of metabolic alkalosis occurs in two phases, with the initial addition or generation of $HCO_3^-$ followed by the inability of the kidney to excrete the excess $HCO_3^-$. The two most common causes of metabolic alkalosis are excessive loss of gastric secretions and diuretic administration. Once established, volume contraction, hypercapnea, hypokalemia, glucose loading, and acute hypercalcemia promote $HCO_3^-$ reabsorption by the kidney and sustain the alkalosis.

The degree of respiratory compensation for metabolic alkalosis is more variable than with metabolic acidosis, and formulas to estimate the expected $Paco_2$ have not proven useful (Narins, 1980). Alkalosis tends to cause hypoventilation, but $Paco_2$ rarely exceeds 55 mm Hg (Narins, 1980; Wilson, 1992b). Tissue and RBCs attempt to lower $HCO_3^-$ by exchanging intracellular $H^+$ ions for extracellular $Na^+$ and $K^+$.

Once metabolic alkalosis is diagnosed, determination of urinary chloride concentration can be helpful in determining the etiology (Fig 2-6). Urinary chloride is a more reliable indicator of volume status than is urinary sodium concentration in this group of patients. Sodium is excreted in the urine with bicarbonate to maintain electroneutrality and occurs independent of volume status. Therefore, in patients with volume contraction, low urinary chloride accurately reflects sodium chloride retention by the kidney.

A urinary chloride concentration less than 10 mEq/liter that improves with sodium chloride administration is a chloride-responsive metabolic alkalosis. In contrast, a urine chloride greater than 20 mEq/liter indicates the alkalosis will not improve with saline administration and is called a chloride-resistant alkalosis. Urine chloride levels must be interpreted with caution because levels are falsely elevated when obtained within several hours of diuretic administration.

Treatment of metabolic alkalosis is aimed at eliminating excess bicarbonate and reversing factors responsible for maintaining the alkalosis. If the urinary chloride level indicates a responsive disorder, infusion of sodium chloride will correct the abnormality. Conversely, saline administration will not correct a chloride-resistant disorder

FIGURE 2-6

Etiology and evaluation of metabolic alkalosis.

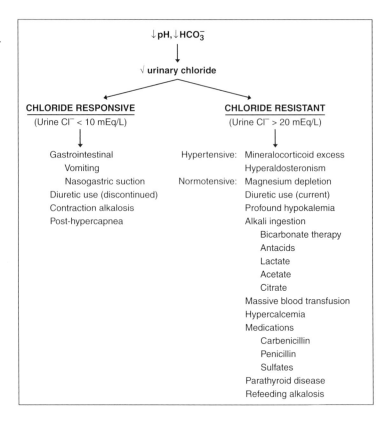

and can be harmful. Treatment of the primary disease will concurrently correct the alkalosis. Although mild alkalemia is generally well tolerated, critically ill surgical patients with a pH > 7.55 have increased mortality (Wilson, 1972; Rimmer, 1987).

## Respiratory Acidosis

Respiratory acidosis is characterized by hypercapnea (a rise in $Pco_2$) and a decreased arterial pH. The development of respiratory acidosis indicates the failure of carbon dioxide excretion to match carbon dioxide production. A variety of disorders can contribute to this acid-base abnormality (Table 2-4). It is important to remember that the normal $Pco_2$ in pregnancy is 30 mm Hg, and normative data for nonpregnant patients do not apply to the gravida.

The clinical manifestations of acute respiratory acidosis are particularly evident in the CNS.

Because carbon dioxide readily penetrates the blood-brain barrier and CSF buffering capacity is not as great as blood, $Pco_2$ elevations quickly decrease the pH of the brain. Thus, neurologic compromise may be more significant with respiratory acidosis than metabolic acidosis (Wilson, 1992b). Acute hypercapnia also decreases cerebral vascular resistance, leading to increased cerebral blood flow and intracranial pressure.

The compensatory response depends on the duration of the respiratory acidosis. In acute respiratory acidosis, the respiratory center is stimulated to increase ventilation. Carbon dioxide is neutralized in erythrocytes by hemoglobin and other buffers, and bicarbonate is generated. An acute disturbance implies that renal compensation is not yet complete. Sustained respiratory acidosis (longer than 6–12 hr) stimulates the kidney to increase acid excretion, but this mechanism usually requires 3 to 5 days for full compensation (Narins, 1994).

T A B L E   **2-4**

Causes of respiratory acidosis

*Airway Obstruction*
Aspiration
Laryngospasm
Severe bronchospasm

*Impaired Ventilation*
Pneumothorax
Hemothorax
Severe pneumonia
Pulmonary edema
Acute respiratory distress syndrome

*Circulatory Collapse*
Massive pulmonary embolism
Cardiac arrest

*CNS Depression*
Medication
    Sedative
    Narcotics
Cerebral infarct, trauma, or encephalopathy
Obesity-hypoventilation syndrome

*Neuromuscular Disease*
Myasthenic crisis
Severe hypokalemia
Guillain-Barré syndrome
Medication

The primary goal in the management of respiratory acidosis is to improve alveolar ventilation and decrease arterial $P_{CO_2}$. Assessment and support of pulmonary function are paramount when a patient has respiratory acidosis. Carbon dioxide accumulates rapidly, and $P_{CO_2}$ rises 2 to 3 mm Hg/min in a patient with apnea. The underlying condition should be corrected rapidly and may include relief of an airway obstruction or pneumothorax, administration of bronchodilator therapy, narcotic reversal, or a diuretic.

Adequate oxygenation is crucial because hypoxemia is more life-threatening than hypercapnia. In the pregnant patient, hypoxemia also compromises the fetus. Uterine perfusion should be optimized and maternal oxygenation ensured because the combination of maternal hypoxemia and uterine artery hypoperfusion profoundly affects the fetus. When a patient cannot maintain adequate ventilation despite aggressive support, endotracheal intubation and mechanical ventilation should be performed without delay.

## Respiratory Alkalosis

Respiratory alkalosis is characterized by hypocapnea (decreased $P_{CO_2}$) and an increased arterial pH. Acute hypocapnea frequently is accompanied by striking clinical symptoms, including paresthesias, circumoral numbness, and confusion. Tachycardia, chest tightness, and decreased cerebral blood flow are some of the prominent cardiovascular effects. Chronic respiratory alkalosis, however, is usually asymptomatic.

Respiratory alkalosis is the result of increased alveolar ventilation (Table 2-5). Hyperventilation can develop from stimulation of brain stem or peripheral chemoreceptors and nociceptive lung receptors. Higher brain centers can override chemoreceptors, and this occurs with involuntary hyperventilation. Respiratory alkalosis is commonly encountered in critically ill patients in

T A B L E   **2-5**

Causes of respiratory alkalosis

*Pulmonary Disease*
Pneumonia
Pulmonary embolism
Pulmonary congestion
Asthma

*Drugs*
Salicylates
Xanthines
Nicotine

*CNS Disorders*
Voluntary hyperventilation
Anxiety
Neurologic disease
    Infection
    Trauma
    Cerebrovascular accident
    Tumor

*Other Causes*
Pregnancy
Pain
Sepsis
Hepatic failure
Iatrogenic mechanical hyperventilation

response to hypoxemia or acidosis, or secondary to CNS dysfunction.

The compensatory response is divided into acute and chronic phases. In acute alkalosis, there is an instantaneous decrease in $H^+$ ion concentration due to tissue and RBC buffer release of $H^+$ ions. If the duration of hypocapnea is greater than a few hours, renal excretion of bicarbonate is increased and acid excretion is decreased. This response requires at least several days to reach a steady state. Chronic respiratory alkalosis is the only acid-base disorder in which the compensatory response can return the pH to normal.

Respiratory alkalosis may be diagnostic of an underlying condition and is usually corrected with treatment of the primary problem. Hypocapnea itself is not life-threatening, but the disease causing the alkalosis may be. The presence of respiratory alkalosis should always raise suspicion for hypoxemia, pulmonary embolism, or sepsis. These conditions, however, can be overlooked if the only concern is correction of the alkalosis. Mechanical ventilation may lead to iatrogenic respiratory alkalosis, and the $P_{CO_2}$ can usually be corrected by lowering the machine-set respiratory rate.

## REFERENCES

Al-Ameri MW, Kruse JA, Carlson RW. Blood sampling from arterial catheters: minimum discard volume to achieve accurate laboratory results. Crit Care Med 1986;14:399.

Andersen GJ, James GB, Mathers NP, et al. The maternal oxygen tension and acid-base status during pregnancy. J Obstet Gynaecol Br Cwlth 1969;76:16.

Arbus GS. An in vivo acid-base nomogram for clinical use. Can Med Assoc J 1973;109:291.

Artal R, Wiswell R, Romem Y, Dorey F. Pulmonary responses to exercise in pregnancy. Am J Obstet Gynecol 1986;154:378.

Awe RJ, Nicotra MB, Newsom TD, Viles R. Arterial oxygenation and alveolar-arterial gradients in term pregnancy. Obstet Gynecol 1979;53:182.

Barron W, Lindheimer M. Medical disorders during pregnancy. 1st ed. St. Louis: Mosby-Year Book, 1991:234.

Battle DC, Hizon M, Cohen E, et al. The use of the urinary anion gap in the diagnosis of hyperchloremic metabolic acidosis. N Engl J Med 1988;318:594.

Bhaskaran NC, Lawler PG. How much blood for a blood gas? Anesthesiology 1988;43:811.

Biswas CK, Ramos JM, Agroyannis B, Kerr DNS. Blood gas analysis: effect of air bubbles in syringe and delay in estimation. Br Med J 1982;284:923.

Bloom SA, Canzanello VJ, Strom JA, Madias NE. Spurious assessment of acid-base status due to dilutional effect of heparin. Am J Med 1985;79:528.

Bryan-Brown CW, Back SM, Malcabalig, et al. Consumable oxygen: oxygen availability in relation to oxyhemoglobin dissociation. Crit Care Med 1973;1:17.

Cain SM. Peripheral uptake and delivery in health and disease. Clin Chest Med 1983;4:139.

Cane RD, Shapiro BA, Templin R, Walther K. Unreliability of oxygen tension-based indices in reflecting intrapulmonary shunting in critically ill patients. Crit Care Med 1988;16:1243.

Cogan MJ. In: Brenner BM, Rector FC Jr, eds. The kidney. 3rd ed. Philadelphia: WB Saunders, 1986:473.

Cruikshank DP, Hays PM. Maternal physiology in pregnancy. In: Gabbe S, Niebyl J, Simpson JL, eds. Obstetrics: normal and problem pregnancies. 2nd ed. New York: Churchill Livingstone, 1991:129.

Davenport HW. Normal acid-base paths. In: The ABC of acid-base chemistry. 6th ed. Chicago: University of Chicago Press, 1974:69.

Dayal P, Murata Y, Takamura H. Antepartum and postpartum acid-base changes in maternal blood in normal and complicated pregnancies. J Obstet Gynaecol Br Cwlth 1972;79:612.

Demling BK, Knox JB. Basic concepts of lung function and dysfunction: oxygenation, ventilation and mechanics. New Horiz 1993;1:362.

Dent JG, Netter KJ. Errors in oxygen tension measurements caused by halothane. Br J Anaesth 1976;48:195.

Douglas IHS, McKenzie PJ, Ledingham IM, Smith G. Effect of halothane on $P_{O_2}$ electrode. Lancet 1978;2:1370.

Gemzell CA, Robbe H, Strom G, et al. Observations on circulatory changes and muscular work in normal labor. Acta Obstet Gynecol Scand 1957;36:75.

Goldberg M, Green SB, Moss ML, et al. Computer-based instruction and diagnosis of acid-base disorders. JAMA 1973;223:269.

Haber RJ. A practical approach to acid-base disorders. West J Med 1991;155:146.

Halperin ML, Richardson RMA, Bear RA, et al. Urine ammonium: the key to the diagnosis of distal renal tubular acidosis. Nephron 1988;50:1.

Hankins GDV, Harvey CJ, Clark SL, Uckan EM. The effects of maternal position and cardiac output on intrapulmonary shunt in normal third-trimester pregnancy. Obstet Gynecol 1996; 88:327.

Hankins GDV, Clark SL, Uckan EM, et al. Third trimester arterial blood gas and acid-base values in normal pregnancy at moderate altitude. Obstet Gynecol 1996;88:347.

Harsten A, Berg B, Inerot S, Muth L. Importance of correct handling of samples for the results of blood gas analysis. Acta Anesthesiol Scand 1988;32:365.

Hess CE, Nichols AB, Hunt WB. Pseudohypoxemia secondary to leukemia and thrombocytopenia. N Engl J Med 1979;301:363.

Huch A, Huch R, Konig V, et al. Limitations of pulse oximetry. Lancet 1988;1:357.

Kruse JA. Acid-base interpretations. Crit Care 1993;14:275.

Kruse JA. Calculation of plasma bicarbonate concentration versus measurement of serum $CO_2$ content. pK′ revisited. Clin Int Care 1995;6:15.

Kruse JA, Hukku P, Carlson RW. Relationship between the apparent dissociation constant of blood carbonic acid and severity of illness. J Lab Clin Med 1989;114:568.

Kruse JA. Use of the anion gap in intensive care and emergency medicine. In: Vincent MJ, ed. Yearbook of intensive care and emergency medicine. New York: Springer, 1994:685–696.

Liberatore SM, Pistelli R, Patalano F, et al. Respiratory function during pregnancy. Respiration 1984;46:145.

Lucius H, Gahlenbeck H, Kleine HO, et al. Respiratory functions, buffer system, and electrolyte concentrations of blood during human pregnancy. Respir Physiol 1970;9:311.

MacRae DJ, Palavradji. Maternal acid-base changes in pregnancy. J Obstet Gynaecol Br Cwlth 1967;74:11.

Madiedo G, Sciacca R, Hause L. Air bubbles and temperature effect on blood gas analysis. J Clin Pathol 1980;33:864.

Maekawa T, Okuda Y, McDowall DG. Effect of low concentrations of halothane on the oxygen electrode. Br J Anaesth 1980;52:585.

McHugh RD, Epstein RM, Longnecker DE. Halothane mimics oxygen in oxygen microelectrodes. Anesthesiology 1979;50:47.

Morganroth ML. An analytic approach to diagnosing acid-base disorders. J Crit Ill 1990;5:138.

Morganroth ML. Six steps to acid-base analysis: clinical applications. J Crit Ill 1990;5:460.

Mueller RG, Lang GE. Blood gas analysis: effect of air bubbles in syringe and delay in estimation. Br Med J 1982;285:1659.

Nanji AA, Whitlow KJ. Is it necessary to transport arterial blood samples on ice for pH and gas analysis? Can Anaesth Soc J 1984;31:568.

Narins RG. Acid-base disorders: definitions and introductory concepts. In: Narins RG, ed. Clinical disorders of fluid and electrolyte metabolism, 5th ed. New York: McGraw-Hill, 1994:755–767.

Narins RG, Emmett M. Simple and mixed acid-base disorders: a practical approach. Medicine 1980;59:161.

Nearman HS, Sampliner JE. Respiratory monitoring. In: Berk JL, Sampliner JE, eds. Handbook of critical care. 3rd ed. Boston: Little Brown, 1982:125–143.

New W. Pulse oximetry. J Clin Monit 1985;1:126.

Ng RH, Dennis RC, Yeston N, et al. Factitious cause of unexpected arterial blood-gas results. N Engl J Med 1984;310:1189.

Novy MJ, Edwards MJ. Respiratory problems in pregnancy. Am J Obstet Gynecol 1967;99:1024.

Oh MS, Carroll HJ. Current concepts: the anion gap. N Engl J Med 1977;297:814.

Pernoll ML, Metcalfe J, Kovach PA, et al. Ventilation during rest and exercise in pregnancy and postpartum. Respir Physiol 1975;25:295.

Perutz MF. Hemoglobin structure and respiratory transport. Sci Ann 1978;239:92.

Preuss HG. Fundamentals of clinical acid-base evaluation. Clin Lab Med 1993;13:103.

Rackow EC, Astiz M. Pathophysiology and treatment of septic shock. JAMA 1991;266:548.

Rimmer JM, Gennari FJ. Metabolic alkalosis. J Intens Care Med 1987;2:137.

Salem MM, Mujais SK. Gaps in the anion gap. Arch Intern Med 1992;152:1625.

Schuch CS, Price JG. Determination of time required for blood gas homeostasis in the intubated, post-open-heart surgery adult following a ventilator change. NTI Res Abs 1986;15:314.

Shapiro BA, Peruzzi WT. Interpretation of blood gases. In: Ayers SM, Grenvik A, Holbrook PR, Shoemaker WC, eds. Textbook of critical care. 3rd ed. Philadelphia: WB Saunders, 1995:278–294.

Shapiro BA, Peruzzi WT. Blood gas analysis. In: Civetta J, Taylor R, Kirby J, eds. Critical care. 2nd ed. Philadelphia: Lippincott, 1992:325–342.

Shibutani K, Komatsu T, Kubal K, et al. Critical levels of oxygen delivery in anesthetical man. Crit Care Med 1983;11:640.

Shoemaker WC, Ayers S, Grenuik A, et al. Textbook of critical care. 2nd ed. Philadelphia: WB Saunders, 1989.

Sobrevilla LA, Cassinelli MT, Carcelen A, et al. Human fetal and maternal oxygen tension and acid-base status during delivery at high altitude. Am J Obstet Gynecol 1971;111:1111.

Stock MC, Shapiro BA, Cane RD. Reliability of $S_vO_2$ in predicting A-$V_{DO_2}$ and the effect of anemia. Crit Care Med 1986;14:402.

Templeton A, Kelman GR. Maternal blood-gases, ($PaO_2$-$PaO_2$), physiological shunt and $V_D/V_T$ in normal pregnancy. Br J Anaesth 1976;48:1001.

Tremper KK, Barker SJ. Blood-gas analysis. In: Hall JB, Schmidt GA, Wood LDH, eds. Principles of critical care. New York: McGraw-Hill, 1992:181–196.

Ueland K, Hansen JM. Maternal cardiovascular hemodynamics: II. Posture and uterine contractions. Am J Obstet Gynecol 1969;103:1.

Urbina LR, Kruse JA. Blood gas analysis and related techniques. In: Carlson RW, Geheb MA, eds. Principles and practice of medical intensive care. Philadelphia: WB Saunders, 1993:235–250.

Walton JR, Shapiro BA, Wine C. Pre-analytic error in arterial blood gas measurement. Respir Care 1981;26:1136.

Weinberger SE, Weiss ST, Cohen WR, et al. Pregnancy and the lung. Am Rev Respir Dis 1980; 121:559.

Wilson RF. Acid-base problems. In: Critical care manual: applied physiology and principles of therapy, 2nd ed. Philadelphia: FA Davis, 1992a:715–756.

Wilson RF. Blood gases: pathophysiology and interpretation. In: Critical care manual: applied physiology and principles of therapy. 2nd ed. Philadelphia: FA Davis, 1992b:389–421.

Wilson RF, Gibson D, Percinel AK, et al. Severe alkalosis in critically ill surgical patients. Arch Surg 1972;105:197.

# CHAPTER 3

# Colloid Oncotic Pressure

*7*he role of plasma colloid osmotic pressure ($COP_p$) in capillary hemodynamics was described first by Starling in 1986. The clinical importance of this parameter was not apparent, however, until the studies of Guyton and Lindsey in 1959. Experimental reduction of plasma proteins in animals resulted in the appearance of pulmonary edema with only minimal increases in left atrial pressure. This finding was attributed to a decrease in the oncotic pressure produced by plasma proteins. With the advent of membrane transducer systems in the late 1960s, measurement of $COP_p$ became a reality (Hansen, 1961; Prather, 1968). Interest in the clinical application of COP followed. Multiple studies have demonstrated the role of $COP_p$ in the development of pulmonary edema in both the pregnant and the nonpregnant state (Cotton, 1985; Benedetti, 1985; Stein, 1974; Weil, 1978).

## Definition

The concept of osmolality is confused frequently with the concept of osmotic pressure. *Osmolality* is an intrinsic property of a fluid. It is an expression of all the dissolved particles (both crystalloid and colloid) in a solution. Osmolality is measured indirectly through the use of a vapor pressure or freezing-point depression. The *osmotic pressure* (also known as the *oncotic pressure*) of a fluid is a relative property and can be demonstrated only when two solutions of differing colloid concentrations are separated by a semipermeable membrane. Those molecules that are unable to pass through the membrane are referred to as *colloids* and are responsible for the oncotic pressure of a solution.

In biologic terms, the semipermeable membrane is the capillary membrane, and the colloid molecules are the various protein molecules of plasma. Plasma is composed of three major proteins: albumin, globulin, and fibrinogen. The plasma concentration of albumin is twice that of the globulin concentration and 15 times that of fibrinogen. Osmotic pressure is related to the number of molecules rather than the size of the molecules; therefore, it becomes apparent that albumin is responsible for up to 75% of the oncotic pressure of plasma. The majority of the remaining oncotic effect is exerted by the globulin fraction, with fibrinogen playing only a minor role. Because the net protein charge of plasma proteins is negative at physiologic pH, positively charged ions (mainly sodium cations) become trapped with the protein molecules in order to maintain electroneutrality across the capillary membrane. This phenomenon is referred to as the *Gibbs-Donnan effect*. The resulting $COP_p$ is approximately 50% greater than would result from the proteins alone (Guyton, 1981). As seen in Figure 3-1, the Gibbs-Donnan effect is not related in a simple linear fashion to the concentration of the colloid. The pressure component resulting

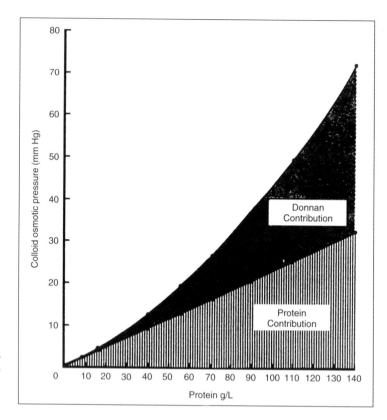

FIGURE   3-1

Relative contributions of proteins and the Gibbs-Donnan effect to plasma colloid osmotic pressure ($COP_p$).

from the Gibbs-Donnan effect is a function of the square of the electrical charge carried by the colloid component.

## Starling's Law and the Lung

The Starling law of the capillary can be expressed by the equation:

$$Q_f = K_f[(P_c - P_i) - R(COP_p - COP_i)]$$

where

$Q_f$  = the total flow of fluid across a capillary membrane

$K_f$  = the fluid filtration coefficient

$P_c$  = the capillary hydrostatic pressure

$P_i$  = the interstitial hydrostatic pressure

$R$  = the reflection coefficient

$COP_p$  = the capillary osmotic pressure of the plasma

$COP_i$  = the osmotic pressure of the interstitial fluid

The fluid filtration coefficient ($K_f$) represents the net amount of fluid crossing the capillary bed for a given imbalance in the Starling forces. This parameter (expressed in mL/min/mm Hg/100 g tissue) is affected by both the conductance of the capillary wall and the ease of fluid movement in the interstitial tissues (Guyton, 1981). The reflection coefficient ($R$) is a measurement of the permeability of a particular capillary bed. A value of 1.0 indicates a membrane impermeable to protein, whereas a value of 0 indicates a situation in which there is total permeability to protein molecules. The average R value for pulmonary capillaries is 0.7 (Wittmers, 1976), with values as low as 0.4 seen in increased permeability states (Taylor, 1981). The predominant force resulting in the movement of fluid out of the vascular space is the capillary hydrostatic pressure ($P_c$), which has been estimated to be on the order of 7 mm Hg in the pulmonary vasculature (Guyton, 1981). The interstitial osmotic pressure ($COP_i$) also results in a net movement of fluid from the vascular space. Although this value has been difficult to quantitate in experimental studies, it is thought to be approximately 16 mm Hg (Guyton, 1981). Interstitial fluid hydrostatic pressure ($P_i$) has been measured by the implantation of capsules in the lungs of dogs and is thought to be approximately a negative 6 mm Hg (Meyer, 1968). The summation of the Starling forces in the lung, therefore, can be represented as follows:

1. Forces affecting fluid movement out of the pulmonary capillary:

   | | |
   |---|---|
   | Capillary hydrostatic pressure | 7 mm Hg |
   | Interstitial fluid colloid osmotic pressure | + 16 mm Hg |
   | Total outward force | 23 mm Hg |

2. Forces affecting fluid movement into the pulmonary capillaries:

   | | |
   |---|---|
   | Plasma colloid osmotic pressure | 25.4 mm Hg |
   | Interstitial hydrostatic pressure | − 6.0 mm Hg |
   | Total inward force | 19.4 mm Hg |

3. Net mean filtration force:

   | | |
   |---|---|
   | Total inward force | 23.0 mm Hg |
   | Total outward force | − 19.4 mm Hg |
   | Net force | 3.6 mm Hg |

The total net filtration pressure at the pulmonary capillary is felt, therefore, to be slightly positive and results in a net movement of fluid into the interstitial spaces (Guyton, 1981). The balance of the Starling forces in the normal lung is illustrated in Figure 3-2A.

Figure 3-2B represents the clinical situation in which an elevated capillary hydrostatic pressure is the primary derangement in the Starling forces that results in pulmonary edema formation. In this example, the capillary hydrostatic pressure is elevated form a normal value of 7 mm Hg to 25 mm Hg. The $COP_p$ is unchanged. The increase in hydrostatic pressure results in a net movement of fluid into the interstitial space. This movement effects an elevation in the tissue hydrostatic pressure and a decrease in the $COP_i$ because of the dilution of interstitial proteins. A common example of this set of circumstances is pulmonary vascular congestion secondary to mitral

stenosis or congestive heart failure. This alteration in pulmonary capillary hydrostatic pressure can be detected by monitoring the pulmonary capillary wedge pressure (PCWP) through the use of a pulmonary artery catheter.

Figure 3-2C depicts the findings in a patient with a fall in the normal $COP_p$ from 25.4 mm Hg to 14.0 mm Hg. The capillary hydrostatic pressure is unchanged. Again, there is net movement of fluid into the interstitial space as a result of the loss of the protective effect of the $COP_p$. Fluid moves into the interstitial spaces of the pulmonary parenchyma; this movement produces an increase in hydrostatic pressure and a decrease in the $COP_i$. A reduction in plasma proteins as a result of dilution secondary to massive crystalloid infusions and severe proteinuria are two common causes of a low $COP_p$. The derangement of the Starling forces can be detected by monitoring the $COP_p$ with an osmometer.

Figure 3-2D illustrates the consequences of an increase in the pulmonary capillary permeability. The COP in the vascular space falls, and the COP of the interstitial space rises as a result of the movement of protein molecules across the capillary membrane. Fluid follows the movement of the colloid molecules, producing a rise in the interstitial hydrostatic pressure. The capillary hydrostatic pressure remains unchanged. Acute respiratory distress syndrome (ARDS) and heroin overdose are examples of situations in which leaky capillaries are noted. With the exception of direct measurements of the osmotic pressure of edema fluid, only experimental methods using radiolabeled proteins are available for detecting the presence of increased pulmonary capillary permeability. Therefore, this is usually a diagnosis of exclusion when the $COP_p$ and PCWP are normal.

Pulmonary lymphatic obstruction, as depicted in Figure 3-2E, is probably not a causative factor in the genesis of acute pulmonary edema in the absence of other factors. Normal protein loss across pulmonary capillary membranes is balanced by lymphatic drainage with subsequent return of proteins to the vascular circulation. However, when interstitial hydrostatic pressure increases as a result of any of the previously mentioned alterations in Starling forces, lymphatic capillaries in the pulmonary interstitium collapse.

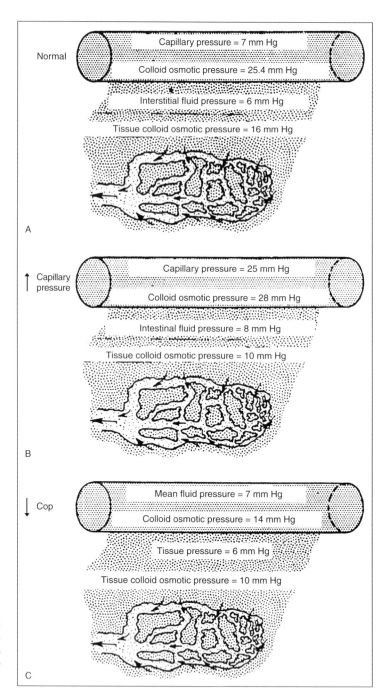

FIGURE **3-2**

(A) Starling forces in the normal lung. (B) Pulmonary edema related to increased capillary hydrostatic pressure. (C) Pulmonary edema related to low $COP_p$.

Interstitial proteins increase as a result of this functional obstruction of the lymphatic, and tissue colloid osmotic pressure becomes elevated. Fluid is drawn from the vascular space, resulting in a further increase in the interstitial hydrostatic pressure and subsequent pulmonary edema. Lymphatics, therefore, play an important role in the prevention of pulmonary edema. Lymph flow has been shown to increase by a factor of 10 when interstitial fluid volume or pressure increases

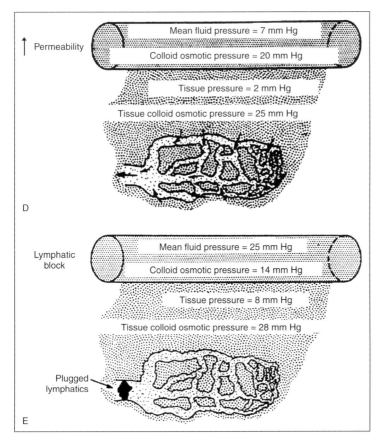

FIGURE **3-2**

(*continued*) (D) Pulmonary edema related to increased capillary permeability. (E) Pulmonary edema related to obstruction of the pulmonary lymphatics. (Modified from Guyton AC. Textbook of medical physiology, 6th ed. Philadelphia: WB Saunders, 1981:377.)

(Parker, 1981). In addition, experiments in animals have revealed that chronic interruption of lymphatic vessels results in a tendency to develop more severe pulmonary edema with a similar stress when compared with animals with intact lymphatic vessels (Uhley, 1962).

## Normal Starling Forces in Pregnancy

Oian and co-workers (1985) measured Starling forces in 10 normal patients in the first trimester of pregnancy and in 10 additional normal women in the third trimester (Fig 3-3). Values for $COP_p$ in early pregnancy (23.2 ± 0.8 mm Hg) were noted to be statistically higher than values obtained in the third trimester (21.1 ± 1.2 mm Hg).

Using wicks sewn into the subcutaneous tissue at the level of the thorax and ankle of pregnant volunteers, these same investigators col-

lected interstitial fluid and were able to quantitate its $COP_i$ (Oian, 1985). Values obtained in the ankle were found to be lower than those in the thorax. In addition, a marked reduction in $COP_i$ was noted when comparing first and third trimester values, a decline that exceeded the fall of $COP_p$ with advancing gestation. The $COP_i$ values in the thorax were 13.1 ± 1.2 mm Hg in the first trimester and 8.4 ± 0.8 mm Hg in the third trimester, while corresponding values for the ankle were 9.6 ± 1.8 mm Hg and 5.5 ± 1.4 mm Hg, respectively. The authors proposed that, as pregnancy progressed, an increase in capillary filtration secondary to elevated capillary hydrostatic pressure initially would lead to a fall in $COP_i$ by simple dilution. To account for the greater decline in $COP_i$ as compared with $COP_p$ with advancing gestation, proteins would have to be removed from the interstitium at an increased rate. The authors proposed that an increase in lymphatic flow would

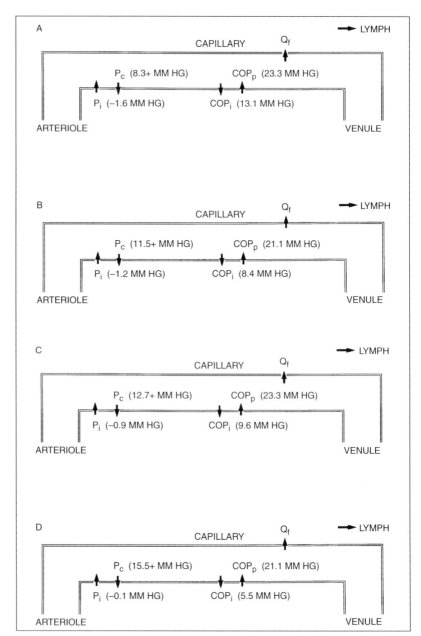

F I G U R E  **3-3**

Starling forces in normal pregnancy. (A) At level of thorax in first trimester. (B) At level of thorax in third trimester. (C) At level of ankle in first trimester. (D) At level of ankle in third trimester. $P_c$, capillary hydrostatic pressure; $P_i$, interstitial hydrostatic pressure; $COP_p$, plasma colloid osmotic pressure; $COP_i$, interstitial colloid osmotic pressure.

effect such a reduction in the protein concentration of the interstitium.

Oian and co-workers (1985) also measured interstitial fluid hydrostatic pressure ($P_i$) by inserting specialized steel cannulas into the subcutaneous tissue of pregnant patients. The $P_i$ was noted to be subatmospheric and to increase with advancing gestational age. The $P_i$ of the thorax was recorded at $-1.6 \pm 0.7$ mm Hg in the first trimester of pregnancy, rising to $-1.2 \pm 0.9$ mm Hg in the third trimester. Likewise, the $P_i$ at the level of the ankle increased from $-0.9 \pm 0.5$ mm Hg to $-0.1 \pm 0.4$ mm Hg when first and third trimester measurements were compared.

Having measured three of the four Starling forces in the pregnant patient, the Norwegian group then calculated capillary hydrostatic pressure ($P_c$) from the Starling equation (Oian, 1987). Their calculations were based on two assumptions. Their first assumption was that flow across the capillary membrane ($Q_f$) was zero. Because this would dictate that lymphatic flow was zero, the authors admitted that their calculated capillary hydrostatic pressures were an underestimation of the true values. Secondly, the authors assumed that the capillary reflection coefficient (R) was 1.0, indicating that capillaries are impermeable to proteins. A significant increase in $P_c$ with advancing gestational age was noted at the level of both the thorax and the ankle. Thoracic $P_c$ was noted to increase from 8.3 ± 1.9 mm Hg in the first trimester to 11.5 ± 2.3 mm Hg in the third trimester. Likewise, ankle $P_c$ increased from 12.7 ± 2.2 mm Hg to 15.5 ± 2.3 mm Hg.

In summary, pregnancy is associated with a moderate fall in $COP_p$ and a rise in $P_c$. Such alterations of these Starling forces would tend to increase fluid filtration from the intravascular compartment to the interstitium. A progressive fall in the COP of the interstitium exerts a protective effect. Despite this mechanism, increasing $P_c$ in late gestation probably overwhelms this mechanism, allowing for increased fluid egress from capillaries. When lymphatic drainage is no longer capable of removing this fluid, edema formation results. Higher $P_c$ in the lower extremity may well explain why edema occurs commonly in the legs of the pregnant patient.

## Measurement and Calculation of $COP_p$

Although the various Starling forces have been measured with experimental techniques, only $COP_p$ can be measured with any degree of practicality. Several commercial devices are available for the determination of $COP_p$. As illustrated in Figure 3-4, a semipermeable membrane usually selectively permeable to proteins exceeding 30,000 particle weight separates two chambers. A sensitive pressure transducer incorporating a Wheatstone bridge is located in the membrane. The chamber below the membrane is the reference chamber, and the one above the membrane

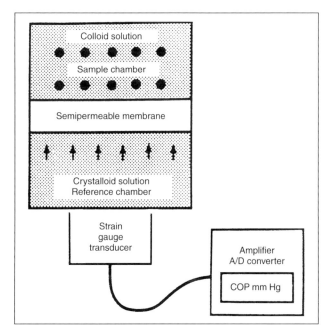

F I G U R E   **3-4**

**Membrane-transducer osmometer used for measuring COP.** (Reproduced by permission from Shoemaker WC, Thompson WL, Holbrook PR. Textbook of critical care. Philadelphia: WB Saunders, 1984: 734.)

is the sample chamber. First, both chambers are filled with isotonic saline, and the device is zeroed. Isotonic saline on both sides of the membrane results in no net fluid movement between the chambers; therefore, no oncotic pressure is created. In addition, daily calibration of various COP values is performed through the use of a water manometer connected to the sample chamber or through the use of a standard solution of known COP value. The sample to be processed is placed in the upper chamber, and the solutions are allowed to equilibrate for a short time, usually 30 to 90 seconds. Saline in the reference chamber is drawn across the semipermeable membrane and into the sample chamber, a result of the presence of colloid protein molecules. The net movement of fluid results in a negative pressure in the reference chamber. After amplification of the electronic signal, a value for the oncotic pressure of the sample is displayed. Several determinations are made, and the results are averaged.

In situations in which an osmometer is not available, $COP_p$ can be calculated after determination of serum albumin or total protein concentration. The $COP_p$ can be calculated from the equation

$$COP_p = 2.1TP + 0.16TP^2 + 0.009TP^3$$

where the $COP_p$ is expressed in millimeters of mercury and TP is the total protein concentration in grams per deciliter (Landis, 1963). Weil et al (1974) reported poor correlation between $COP_p$ and serum albumin and total protein concentrations. However, computerized analysis of serum albumin, total protein, and $COP_p$ in normotensive gravid patients and patients with pregnancy-induced hypertension (PIH) has resulted in two equations for the calculation of $COP_p$ during pregnancy (Nguyen, 1986):

$$COP_p(mm\ Hg) = 5.21 \times Total\ serum\ protein - 11.4$$

and

$$COP_p(mm\ Hg) = 8.1 \times Serum\ albumin - 8.2$$

These two equations are thought to be accurate, with a 10% range of error in 75% and 80% of cases, respectively. Although such calculations are relatively accurate in the healthy patient, variation in pH, BP, and albumin–total protein or globulin–total protein ratios do affect the $COP_p$ in the critically ill patient. Direct measurement of the $COP_p$, therefore, may be preferred if this parameter is to be used in clinical management.

## Normal Values

The $COP_p$ in the fetus appears to increase during intrauterine life and achieves a value of 10 ± 2.3 mm Hg at 40 weeks of gestation (Wu, 1982). Weil and associates (1974) reported that the mean $COP_p$ in healthy ambulatory adult volunteers was 25.4 ± 2.3 mm Hg. A slightly lower $COP_p$ has been noted in female patients when compared with their male counterparts (Morissette, 1983). A downward trend in values is noted with advancing age.

As illustrated in Figure 3-5, maternal $COP_p$ values in normal pregnancy decrease and reach a nadir at approximately 34 to 36 weeks of gestation (Wu, 1983). This trend closely parallels the decrease in maternal serum albumin concentrations (Robertson, 1972). A mean value at term is reported to be 22.4 ± 0.54 mm Hg (Wu, 1983). Oian et al (1985) found hematocrit, serum albumin concentration, and total serum protein concentration to be significantly lower in the third trimester as compared with the first trimester. The authors concluded that reduction of the $COP_p$ in the third trimester was the result of a dilution of plasma proteins secondary to a rise in plasma volume. Because albumin is thought to be the major protein responsible for plasma oncotic pressure, Robertson et al (1972) have proposed that the fall in albumin concentration that occurs in pregnancy is the probable explanation for declining $COP_p$ in the gravid state.

F I G U R E  **3-5**

**Relationship between serum COP and serum albumin during gestation.** (Modified from Robertson EG, Cheyne GA. Plasma biochemistry in relation to oedema of pregnancy. J Obstet Gynaecol Br Cwlth 1972;79:773.)

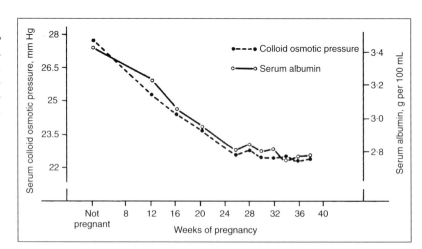

## Technical Variations in $COP_p$

Various collection techniques can affect $COP_p$ (Tables 3-1 and 3-2). For example, prolonged use of a tourniquet when drawing samples from peripheral veins artificially increases $COP_p$ values (Ladegaard-Pedersen, 1967). Venous stasis results in an increase in capillary pressure, movement of fluid into the interstitium, and subsequent elevation of the $COP_p$. Hemolysis is noted to increase values of $COP_p$ by as much as 10% (Ladegaard-Pedersen, 1967). Free hemoglobin molecules released by hemolysis act as colloids. Values obtained from plasma are approximately 0.35 mm Hg higher than those obtained from serum because fibrinogen (not present in serum) does contribute to a small fraction of the total $COP_p$ (Ladegaard-Pedersen, 1967). Most authorities feel that the difference between serum and plasma is sufficiently small that either can be used for COP determinations (Weil, 1974). If plasma is to be used, dried heparin should be employed as an anticoagulant. Amounts exceeding 200 units/mL can elevate COP (Weil, 1974) because the heparin molecule also can act as a colloid. Samples of plasma (but not whole blood) can be refrigerated for up to 1 week without affecting the reliability of $COP_p$ determinations (Ladegaard-Pedersen, 1967).

The COP is noted to decrease by 15% when measured in patients in the supine position for several hours (Ladegaard-Pedersen, 1973). This effect is probably related to the decrease in hydrostatic pressure seen at the capillary level in the reclining position. The reduction in hydrostatic pressure allows fluid to move from the interstitial space into the intravascular space, producing a lower $COP_p$. Increases in the mean systemic arterial BP of 10 mm Hg are noted to increase the value of $COP_p$ by 0.75 mm Hg (Ladegaard-Pedersen, 1973). Elevation of the hydrostatic pressure results in a net movement of fluid into the interstitium, causing a rise in the serum protein concentration. An increase in the $COP_p$ also is noted to be directly proportional to pH because of the Gibbs-Donnan effect (Morissette, 1983).

### TABLE 3-1
Factors associated with increased $COP_p$

Prolonged use of tourniquet prior to drawing sample
Hemolysis of sample
Plasma > serum
Increases in BP
Increases in pH

### TABLE 3-2
Factors associated with decreased $COP_p$

Decreases in BP
Decreases in pH
Supine position
Age
Male > female
Pregnancy
Normotensive pregnancy > PIH
Hypertension
Antepartum > postpartum
Tocolytic therapy
Excessive use of crystalloid fluids
Disease states associated with protein loss: sepsis, peritonitis

## Fluids and $COP_p$

Intravenous (IV) fluids can be divided into crystalloids and colloids. Information on the effect of crystalloids on $COP_p$ is limited to normal saline and lactated Ringer's solution because these fluids are used commonly in the treatment of hypovolemic shock. They contain only cations and anions mixed in various combinations with water. Because the capillary membrane is permeable to such low-molecular-weight molecules as sodium and chloride, the addition of crystalloids to the intravascular compartment would not be expected to elevate $COP_p$. Massive crystalloid resuscitation has been shown to dilute the plasma protein concentration. This dilution results in marked reduction in $COP_p$ (Laks, 1976). Haupt and Rackow (1982) found that 1 liter of normal saline administered to patients in hypovolemic shock caused a 12% decrease in $COP_p$ from baseline levels. Continued use of saline was associated with a further decline in the $COP_p$. Ramanathan et al (1983) noted a decline in $COP_p$ when a 1200-mL volume of lactated Ringer's solution was administered to gravid patients prior to epidural anesthesia. These investigators suggested that the fall in $COP_p$ was related to the decline in total protein and albumin fractions observed after prehydration with crystalloid solutions in this group of patients.

Colloids include products derived from human plasma (albumin and plasma protein fraction) as well as such synthetic products as Hespan (Du Pont Ltd.), Haemacel (Hoechst Ltd., UK), Gelofusine (Consolidated Chemicals Ltd.), Dextraven 10 (Fisons pic), and Gentran 70 (Travenol Laboratories Ltd.). Human serum albumin is available in concentrations of 5% and 25%. The 5% solution is composed of 50 g albumin in 1 liter of normal saline and has a COP of approximately 20 mm Hg, and the 25% solution has a COP of 100 mm Hg (Rackow, 1977a). The fate of exogenous albumin is poorly understood but probably involves elimination at multiple sites, including kidneys, liver, and intestines (Katz, 1964; Tullis, 1977). The effect of albumin has been found to last for approximately 24 hours.

Plasma protein fraction (PPF) is a 5% solution of human albumin and globulins in a buffered electrolyte solution. Albumin comprises the majority of the protein in this solution. For this reason, PPF is expected to have a COP slightly greater than albumin.

Hetastarch (Hespan) is a synthetic colloid consisting of hydroxyethyl-substituted branched-chain polysaccharides with an average molecular weight of 69,000. The COP of hetastarch is 20 mm Hg (Haupt, 1982). Larger particles are degraded by the liver and excreted in the stool and urine (Rothschild, 1955). Low-molecular-weight particles are eliminated from the vascular space by diffusion through systemic capillaries or filtration through the kidneys (Thompson, 1970). The volume-expanding effect of hetastarch has been found to last from 24 to 36 hours.

In vitro analysis comparing the synthetic colloid solutions with 4.5% albumin has revealed that hetastarch showed the least capability for diffusion across capillary membranes (Webb, 1989). This property is probably related to this substance's high-molecular-weight particles. In vivo comparisons of various colloid solutions and their effect on $COP_p$ have revealed that use of 1 liter of hetastarch results in a 36% increase and use of 1 liter of 5% albumin results in an 11% increase (Haupt, 1982). In this study, patients initially given either of these colloids, followed by maintenance crystalloid therapy, had continued elevation of their $COP_p$ for 48 hours. Patients treated with only saline showed depressed $COP_p$ values when compared with baseline levels. The lowered levels continued for up to 5 days (Fig 3-6). Shippy and Shoemaker (1983) compared 500-mL PPF with 25 g of 25% albumin and noted a greater and more sustained elevation in the $COP_p$ with the latter. It appears, therefore, that hetastarch will cause the greatest elevation in the $COP_p$. Lesser degrees of elevation are achieved with PPF, and albumin results in the least elevation of $COP_p$ when compared with other colloids. Colloid therapy increases $COP_p$, whereas crystalloid therapy depresses $COP_p$. However, the clinical superiority of crystalloid versus colloid therapy for resuscitation of patients in shock remains unproven.

## $COP_p$ Values in Pregnancy-Induced Hypertension

Measurements of $COP_p$ at term in patients with PIH have revealed values that are lower than those from a similar group of normotensive patients ($17.9 \pm 0.68$ mm Hg vs. $22 \pm 0.48$ mm Hg) (Nguyen, 1986; Benedetti, 1979). The degree of hypertension, however, does not seem to correlate with the magnitude of reduction in the $COP_p$ (Goodlin, 1982).

Chesley (1978) first proposed that proteinuria was the etiology for decreased $COP_p$ in preeclampsia, but several studies have shed new light on the mechanism for reduced $COP_p$. Bhatia et al (1987) measured fibronectin levels in 12 patients with mild PIH and 20 patients with severe PIH and compared these values with those of a control gravid population. Fibronectin levels in both the mild and severe PIH groups were significantly higher than those in controls ($444 \pm 122$, $401 \pm 102$, and $217 \pm 61$ µg/mL, respectively). Using fibronectin as a sensitive indication of capillary damage, these authors proposed that altered capillary permeability to plasma proteins was

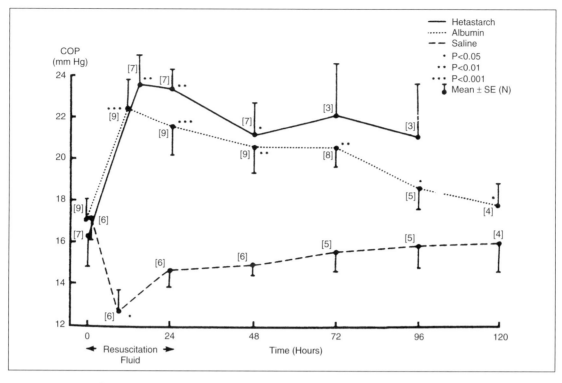

F I G U R E  **3-6**
Changes in $COP_p$ during fluid resuscitation and maintenance on
crystalloid fluid. (Reproduced by permission from Haupt MT, Rackow
EC. Colloid osmotic pressure and fluid resuscitation with hetastarch,
albumin, and saline solutions. Crit Care Med 1982;10:161. Copyright
© 1982, Williams & Wilkins Co, Baltimore.)

the etiology of decreased $COP_p$ in PIH patients.
Statistical analysis revealed that vascular damage
was fourfold more important than proteinuria in
explaining decreased $COP_p$. Parallel research by
Norwegian investigators has confirmed this mechanism. Oian and co-workers (1986) attempted to
correlate 24-hour excretion rates of urine protein
with $COP_p$ in patients with PIH and were unable
to demonstrate a relationship. Using subcutaneous wicks, this group measured $COP_i$ in PIH patients. Patients with severe PIH were noted to
have higher values for interstitial fluid COP at the
level of the thorax and the ankle when compared
with patients with moderate PIH. Such a finding
would suggest that increased microvascular permeability to plasma proteins is the etiology of the
increased $COP_i$ associated with more severe forms
of PIH. The loss of plasma proteins into the inter-

stitium would account for the lower $COP_p$ that
has been reported with PIH. Although these data
would appear conclusive, in a later report, Oian
and Maltau (1987) found that values for $COP_i$ at
the level of the thorax in a group of normal gravid
patients in the third trimester exceeded that of a
group of patients with severe PIH. No explanation for these findings was offered by the authors. It would appear, therefore, that the majority of the experimental evidence indicates that
lowered $COP_p$ in the patient with PIH is the result of loss of serum proteins across capillary
membranes. Urinary protein loss probably also
contributes to lower the $COP_p$ (Fig 3-7).

Magnesium sulfate is used routinely in the
United States in patients with PIH for seizure
prophylaxis. In the majority of institutions, it is
administered IV in association with crystalloid

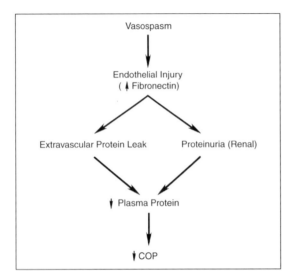

Vasospasm

↓

Endothelial Injury
( ↓ Fibronectin)

Extravascular Protein Leak          Proteinuria (Renal)

↓ Plasma Protein

↓ COP

F I G U R E   **3-7**

Proposed mechanism of lowered $COP_p$ in PIH. (Reproduced by permission from Bhatia RK, Bottoms SF, Saleh AA, et al. Mechanisms for reduced colloid osmotic pressure in preeclampsia. Am J Obstet Gynecol 1987;157:106.)

therapy. Yeast et al (1993) studied the effects of magnesium sulfate on $COP_p$ in 120 patients with PIH maintained on a fluid regimen of 100 mL/hr. $COP_p$ was measured at baseline and every 6 hours thereafter. $COP_p$ tended to fall during the course of therapy, but a significant difference from baseline values was not detected until 44 hours after the initiation of therapy.

## $COP_p$ in the Postpartum Period

When compared with intrapartum values, values of $COP_p$ measured in the first 24 hours postpartum exhibit a significant reduction. Cotton et al (1984) reported a $COP_p$ value of 15.4 ± 2.1 mm Hg postpartum, as compared with a value of 21.0 ± 2.1 mm Hg in the intrapartum period in a group of 72 normal patients at term. The fall in $COP_p$ was not related to the type of anesthesia or mode of delivery.

The nadir of the $COP_p$ appears to occur from 6 to 16 hours after delivery (Gonik, 1985). After 24 hours postpartum, a trend toward recovery of the $COP_p$ to intrapartum levels has been noted (Oian, 1986).

Patients with PIH show a similar decrease in $COP_p$ values in the postpartum period. Benedetti et al (1985) found $COP_p$ values of 17.9 ± 0.68 mm Hg in the postpartum period. This decline in $COP_p$ in the first 24 hours after delivery was noted to be of similar magnitude to the postpartum decline seen in normotensive pregnant patients (Table 3-3). Explanations for the postpartum decrease in $COP_p$ included (1) supine

T A B L E   **3-3**

Normal values for $COP_p$

|  | Variable | COP (mm Hg) (Mean ± SD) |
|---|---|---|
| Condition | Ambulatory | 25.4 ± 2.3 |
|  | Supine | 21.6 ± 3.6 |
| Age (yr) | < 50 | 21.6 ± 4.7 |
|  | 50–70 | 20.7 ± 4.2 |
|  | 70–89 | 19.7 ± 3.7 |
| Sex | Male | 21.6 ± 4.8 |
|  | Female | 19.6 ± 4.2 |
| Normotensive pregnancy | Antepartum (at term) | 22.4 ± 0.5 |
|  | Postpartum (first 24 hr) | 15.4 ± 2.1 |
| Pregnancy-induced hypertension | Antepartum (at term) | 17.9 ± 0.7 |
|  | Postpartum (first 24 hr) | 13.7 ± 0.5 |

positioning during the labor and delivery process, (2) blood loss at delivery, (3) administration of large amounts of crystalloid IV fluids during labor, and (4) mobilization of extravascular fluid to the intravascular space.

Elevations in PCWP have been reported in gravid patients with PIH after endotracheal intubation (Rafferty, 1980). These elevations can persist for up to 8 hours postpartum and therefore coincide with the normal reduction in $COP_p$ after delivery. An increase in the capillary hydrostatic pressure and a reduction in the plasma $COP_p$ represent two derangements in the Starling forces, which could predispose the patient to the development of pulmonary edema.

Gonik and Cotton (1984) compared birthing room patients who received only oral fluids during labor with normal gravid patients who received IV fluids during labor. A greater reduction in the $COP_p$ was noted in patients receiving IV fluid therapy. The authors recommended that careful scrutiny of IV fluid use in labor be undertaken in order to prevent pulmonary edema. Hauch and co-workers (1995) also studied the effect of IV fluids on $COP_p$ in the peripartum period. Thirty women received a 1500-mL bolus of isotonic fluid (Ringer's lactate) prior to the institution of spinal anesthesia for cesarean section. An acute decline in mean $COP_p$ from 23.1 mm Hg to 15.8 mm Hg was noted.

This dramatic fall in $COP_p$ secondary to the use of IV crytalloid fluids might lead to the conclusion that colloids would be preferred. In one study, patients given 5% albumin were noted to have less of a fall in the postpartum $COP_p$ when compared with patients who were administered PlasmaLyte A (Jones, 1986). In addition, the colloid group returned to baseline $COP_p$ levels within 36 hours of delivery; continued reduction in the $COP_p$ was noted in the crystalloid group for 48 hours postpartum.

Although the administration of albumin has been demonstrated to result in less reduction in $COP_p$ after delivery, its routine use is not warranted in the normal parturient. The use of colloid therapy in patients at high risk to subsequently develop pulmonary edema after delivery remains controversial. The administration of large volumes of crystalloid, however, should be avoided in these patients.

## $COP_p$ and Tocolytic Therapy

$COP_p$ is noted to fall slightly when betamimetic therapy is used for tocolysis in the pregnant patient. Nadir values are noted to occur 9 hours after the initiation of IV terbutaline. Long-term betamimetic therapy has been associated with a more dramatic reduction in $COP_p$ values. Goyert and co-workers (1987) studied 15 patients in premature labor who were treated with IV ritodrine. As with administration of terbutaline, $COP_p$ was noted to fall from preinfusion levels of 15.4 ± 2.1 mm Hg to 14.3 ± 1.7 mm Hg after 12 hours of ritodrine infusion. Using serum fibronectin as a sensitive indicator of capillary endothelial damage, no increase in fibronectin levels could be detected before, as compared with during, ritodrine therapy. These investigators concluded that the decreased $COP_p$ associated with ritodrine therapy was not secondary to leakage of serum proteins across damaged capillary membranes but was more likely due to an increase in plasma volume.

Further investigation by Armson et al (1992) supports this concept. Seven patients with preterm labor were treated initially with a 1-liter bolus of normal saline followed by an IV infusion of 125 mL/hr. During infusion with ritodrine, patients retained 54% of administered fluids. This was associated with a change in the mean baseline $COP_p$ from 22.5 mm Hg to a nadir at 8 hours of 19.5 mm Hg. The authors documented a marked rise in arginine vasopressin at 2 hours of therapy and postulated that this was one of the main mechanisms of fluid retention in their study population. Another possible explanation for the fluid retention in the study population was a reported association between betamimetics and elevated plasma renin levels with subsequent antinatriuresis (Grospietsch, 1980). Although Armson et al (1992) did not measure plasma renin activity, urinary fractional excretion of sodium remained less than 1% in all of the studied patients. This would suggest an increased sodium resorption with subsequent fluid retention.

Intravenous magnesium sulfate has gained widespread acceptance as a tocolytic agent. Studies have demonstrated a minimal effect on $COP_p$.

Yeast et al (1993) evaluated serial changes in $COP_p$ in 175 patients receiving magnesium sulfate for premature labor. All patients received a 6-g loading dose followed by a continuous infusion of 3 g/hr. Total oral and IV fluid therapy was limited to 2400 mL in 24 hours. Plasma colloid pressure was noted to fall over the course of therapy, but this decline did not achieve statistical significance until after 56 hours of therapy (Fig 3-8). In a randomized study of 14 patients in premature labor, Armson and co-workers (1992) also noted a decline in $COP_p$ in patients treated with magnesium sulfate, although this fall was not as pronounced as that in the group of patients treated with IV ritodrine. Patients treated with magnesium sulfate retained 22% of administered fluids, as compared with 55% in the ritodrine group. A marked contrast in other measured parameters was noted in those treated with magnesium sulfate compared with ritodrine. Arginine vasopressin levels were unaffected, and fractional excretion of sodium was increased in the magnesium group.

In summary, lower $COP_p$ levels are noted after tocolytic therapy with either betamimetics or magnesium sulfate therapy. This change is more marked with betamimetics due to the fluid retention that occurs secondary to elevated arginine vasopressin and renin activity.

## $COP_p$ and Pyelonephritis

Acute respiratory distress syndrome complicates the clinical course of approximately one in 50 pregnant women admitted for the treatment of pyelonephritis (Cunningham, 1987). Evidence of respiratory failure usually is not apparent until 24 to 48 hours after admission. Although the etiology of this complication is not well understood, increased pulmonary capillary permeability secondary to circulating endotoxins has been proposed as a major etiology. Ridgway and co-workers (1991) studied alterations in $COP_p$ in 17 pregnant women with pyelonephritis. Although no patient developed respiratory compromise, mean oxygen saturation by pulse oximetry decreased significantly by 16 hours after admission. $COP_p$ was markedly decreased from admission values after 24 hours. To investigate whether this

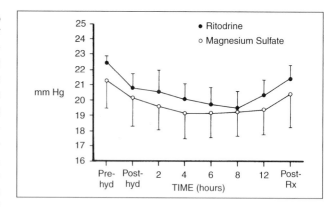

F I G U R E **3-8**

Plasma colloid osmotic pressures at baseline (Prehyd), after infusion of 1 liter of normal saline (Post-hyd), during 12 hours of tocolytic therapy, and 4 hours after cessation of agent (Post-Rx). Open circles, ritodrine; closed circles, magnesium sulfate. (Reproduced by permission from Armson BA, Samuels P, Miller F, et al. Evaluation of maternal fluid dynamics during tocolytic therapy with ritodrine hydrochloride and magnesium sulfate. Am J Obstet Gynecol 1992;167:758.)

decline in $COP_p$ was secondary to protein loss across the pulmonary capillaries or was secondary to the dilutional effect from exogenous fluid therapy, a $COP_p$–total protein ratio was calculated. In the case of loss of osmotically active proteins from the intravascular space, the ratio would be expected to increase over time. If the decline in $COP_p$ were secondary to dilution, the ratio would remain constant. In their series of patients, Ridgway et al (1991) noted no change in the $COP_p$–total protein ratio. It would therefore appear that a dilutional decrease in $COP_p$ in conjunction with an increase in pulmonary capillary permeability contributes to the etiology of pulmonary compromise in a small percentage of pregnant women with pyelonephritis.

## Clinical Application of $COP_p$

### $COP_p$ to Pulmonary Capillary Wedge Pressure Gradient

With the advent of the pulmonary artery catheter in 1970, the measurement of pulmonary capillary hydrostatic pressures became a reality (Swan, 1970). Early clinical and radiographic signs of pulmonary congestion are noted to occur at a PCWP of 18 to 22 mm Hg (McHugh, 1972). Frank pulmonary congestion is noted at a value of 22 to 25 mm Hg (Kostuk, 1973). Subsequently, cases of pulmonary edema have been reported with normal or only slightly elevated levels of PCWP (Stein, 1974). Weil's group (1978) discovered that low $COP_p$ values were commonly found in this subset of patients. They postulated that a decrease in the normal forces keeping fluid in the pulmonary microvasculature ($COP_p$) or an increase in the forces moving fluid out of the pulmonary capillaries (PCWP) could result in the formation of pulmonary edema. Therefore, the concept of a critical $COP_p$-PCWP gradient was proposed. This explanation for the etiology of pulmonary edema is probably an oversimplification of the complex Starling forces in the lung. The other components of the Starling equation are ignored: capillary permeability, interstitial hydrostatic pressure, and $COP_i$. In addition, other protective mechanisms, such as alveolar endothelial permeability, pulmonary lymphatic flow, and surfactant, play vital roles in preventing the accumulation of excess lung water. Because $COP_p$ and capillary hydrostatic pressure are the only two Starling forces that can be measured by current clinical methodology, the $COP_p$-PCWP gradient is probably the closest approximation currently available of the net Starling interactions in the lung.

Rackow et al (1977b) reported that a large percentage of patients with a $COP_p$-PCWP gradient of less than 4 mm Hg were noted to develop pulmonary edema. Decreasing values of this gradient were correlated with increasing severity of pulmonary edema by radiologic analysis (Da Luz, 1975). As demonstrated in Figure 3-9, measurement of the $COP_p$-PCWP gradient during the resolution of pulmonary edema has been associated with normalization of this value (Levine, 1967).

Studies in pregnant patients with PIH have noted that pulmonary edema also may be related to reductions in the $COP_p$-PCWP gradient. Cotton et al (1985) noted a negative $COP_p$-PCWP in five patients with severe PIH and pulmonary edema. Benedetti and co-workers (1985) measured $COP_p$ and hemodynamic parameters in 10

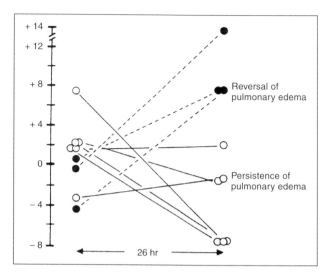

FIGURE 3-9

Changes in $COP_p$-PCWP gradient after treatment with digoxin and furosemide in patients with acute myocardial infarction and pulmonary edema. (Reproduced by permission from Weil MH, Henning RJ, Puri VK. Colloid oncotic pressure: clinical significance. Crit Care Med 1979;7:113. Copyright © 1979, Williams & Wilkins Co, Baltimore.)

patients with severe PIH who developed pulmonary edema in the postpartum period. These authors proposed that in half of the patients, a mild to moderate reduction in $COP_p$ coupled with an elevation in PCWP was the etiology for the pulmonary edema. Increased pulmonary capillary permeability was thought to be the etiology of pulmonary edema in three patients, while left ventricular dysfunction was proposed as the etiology in the remaining two patients in the series. In a second report by Cotton and co-workers (1986), the $COP_p$-PCWP gradient in three patients with severe PIH and pulmonary edema ranged from $-6.8$ mm Hg to $-11.6$ mm Hg.

## The Role of $COP_p$ in Guiding Fluid Therapy in PIH Patients

Several authors have advocated that $COP_p$ determinations should be used to guide fluid therapy in the gravid patient with PIH (Tullis, 1977;

Freund, 1977; Goodlin, 1978). This recommendation has been based on previous data suggesting that $COP_p$ is lower in this disease than in the normotensive pregnancy and that depressed $COP_p$ levels in the postpartum period have been associated with pulmonary edema. Colloids would appear to be the IV fluids of choice to maintain or increase the $COP_p$ in the antepartum period. However, the routine use of colloidal fluids to correct low $COP_p$ and hypovolemia in the PIH patient has generated controversy for years.

In 1977, Assali and Vaughn proposed that the hypovolemia associated with preeclampsia represents a physiologic response to a constricted vascular bed. These authors felt that normalization of intravascular volume would simply increase the work for an already hyperdynamic cardiovascular system. The following year, Goodlin et al (1978) reported that plasma volume expansion with colloids effected reversal of preeclampsia in 10% of cases. Pulmonary edema was said to be a rare complication of such therapy. In 1981, Jouppila et al (1983) provided evidence that cast doubt on the idea that plasma expansion with colloids was beneficial in the treatment of PIH. Using IV xenon-133, these investigators failed to demonstrate an increase in the intervillous pla-

cental blood flow after the infusion of 100 mL of 20% albumin.

Hankins et al (1984) later reported the hemodynamic findings in eight women with eclampsia. Despite fluid restriction prior to delivery, two of the patients exhibited marked elevation of the PCWP to levels associated with pulmonary vascular congestion. Neither patient developed frank pulmonary edema. These authors then plotted the Starling curves of their patients with the 10 patients from Benedetti's series (1980) in which total IV fluids were restricted to 75 to 100 mL/hr of crystalloid solution. The Starling curves of 13 additional patients from two series (Phelan, 1982; Rafferty, 1980) in which the liberal use of crystalloid and colloids was allowed prior to delivery were then presented for comparison (Fig 3-10). The authors concluded that aggressive fluid management resulted in elevations in the normal filling pressures of the left side of the heart and further increased a hyperdynamic cardiac output.

In opposition to the approach by Hankins' group, Kirshon and co-workers (1988) sought to correct the derangement in $COP_p$ with aggressive volume expansion using colloids. Fifteen patients with severe PIH were managed by

FIGURE **3-10**

(A) **Starling curves of eclamptic and severe PIH patients treated with maintenance IV fluids prior to delivery.** (B) **Starling curves of severe PIH patients treated with aggressive crystalloid and colloid therapy prior to delivery.** LVSWI, left ventricular stroke work index. (Reproduced by permission from Hankins GD, Wendel GD, Cunningham FG, Leveno KJ. Longitudinal evaluation of hemodynamic changes in eclampsia. Am J Obstet Gynecol 1984;150:506.)

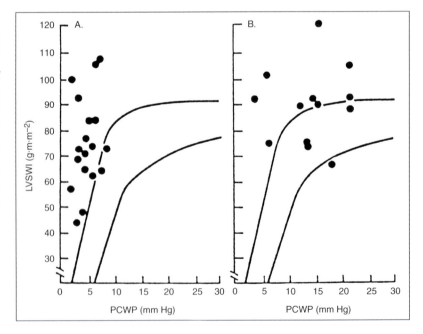

maintaining the $COP_p$ above 17 mm Hg and the PCWP below 15 mm Hg through the use of a 25% albumin infusion. Eleven of the 15 patients required the administration of furosemide in the postpartum period for the treatment of a rising PCWP above 15 mm Hg. Five of the patients were delivered by cesarean section for fetal distress despite optimization of maternal hemodynamic parameters. The authors concluded that $COP_p$ correction was unnecessary unless either a markedly depressed initial value of less than 12 mm Hg or a prolonged negative $COP_p$-PCWP gradient was present.

Yeast and co-workers (1993) have advocated the use of $COP_p$ as a method of monitoring patients with PIH that are at risk for pulmonary edema during treatment with magnesium sulfate. Four of the 120 patients in their study developed pulmonary edema in association with a depressed $COP_p$ ranging from 9.8 mm Hg to 16.6 mm Hg. In three of the four cases, however, the initial $COP_p$ value was not markedly depressed, but serial determinations revealed a marked decline in association with the onset of pulmonary insufficiency. More important, 13 additional patients exhibited $COP_p$ values below 13 mm Hg at some point in their clinical course yet failed to develop pulmonary edema.

It would appear, therefore, that investigative studies do not support the acute correction of a low $COP_p$ in the patient with PIH. In addition, accumulated evidence does not support $COP_p$ as a useful tool to predict the onset of pulmonary edema in these patients.

## $COP_p$ and Acute Respiratory Distress Syndrome

Colloid osmotic pressure has been used to distinguish the leaky-membrane pulmonary edema found in patients with ARDS from other forms of pulmonary edema. Acute respiratory distress syndrome can occur in a variety of conditions associated with pregnancy, including sepsis, preeclampsia (Benedetti, 1985), amniotic fluid embolism, and betamimetic-associated pulmonary edema (Benedetti, 1986). In pulmonary edema related to elevated capillary hydrostatic pressure,

the endobronchial fluid (edema fluid from endotracheal tube suctioning) has a COP of less than 60% of that of simultaneously measured plasma (Weil, 1977). In pulmonary edema secondary to increased permeability of pulmonary capillary membranes, the COP of endobronchial fluid exceeds 75% of that of plasma (Weil, 1977). In more advanced stages, the oncotic pressure of the two determinations may be identical (Weil, 1977).

The role of colloid versus crystalloid therapy is controversial in patients with ARDS. Proponents of colloid therapy argue that increasing $COP_p$ will prevent extravasation of fluid into the interstitium. Those opposed to the use of colloids in ARDS patients maintain that pulmonary interstitial edema is worsened as colloid extravasates into the interstitium, leading to further fluid movement out of the capillary. Despite these theoretical concerns, an investigation using radiolabeled tracers failed to demonstrate a significant increase in the microvascular flux of albumin into pulmonary edema fluid in patients with ARDS (Sibbald, 1983). Appel and Shoemaker (1981) studied the use of various colloids in patients with ARDS and found that optimization of the $COP_p$-PCWP gradient with these solutions improved the cardiorespiratory status. Metildi and co-workers (1984) randomized 46 patients with ARDS to receive either crystalloid or albumin therapy for resuscitation. Although the intrapulmonary shunt did not improve to the same degree in the crystalloid group, as compared with the albumin group, no difference in survival between the two groups was detected. The authors concluded that because colloid therapy did not provide a clear advantage over crystalloids, the latter should be the preferred fluid therapy for the patient with ARDS.

## $COP_p$ and Mortality

Reduced values of $COP_p$ have been associated with increasing mortality rates. Weil and associates (1979) noted a 50% survival rate in 99 patients with myocardial infarction having a $COP_p$ value of 14.1 mm Hg or greater. Lower $COP_p$ values were associated with decreasing survival. Rackow and colleagues (1977b) noted a 100%

mortality rate in a series of 128 patients admitted to a critical care unit with a $COP_p$ of less than 12.5 mm Hg. This relationship between $COP_p$ and mortality is illustrated in Figure 3-11. One investigation, however, has failed to demonstrate improved patient survival when the $COP_p$ is corrected with albumin infusion (Grundmann, 1985).

The finding of a low $COP_p$ may, therefore, indicate a severe disease state, such as sepsis or peritonitis, in which large protein losses are noted to occur. A depressed $COP_p$ may simply be a characteristic of a disease state that ultimately results in the patient's demise. Despite the reported association of low $COP_p$ and mortality in the nongravida patient, no such association has been described in pregnancy.

## Conclusion

The measurement of $COP_p$ *may* be a useful clinical tool in conjunction with the use of hemodynamic monitoring by pulmonary flow-directed catheters in certain critically ill patients. Routine optimization of $COP_p$ in patients with PIH is unwarranted and may lead to complications of fluid overload in the postpartum period. The observation that, even in normal pregnancy, the $COP_p$-PCWP gradient is reduced, compared with the nonpregnant state, suggests that pregnant patients are at increased risk for the development of pulmonary edema, given any further reduction in $COP_p$, elevation of PCWP, or alteration in pulmonary capillary permeability (Clark, 1989).

F I G U R E   **3-11**

$COP_p$ **versus mortality in 128 critically ill patients.** (Reproduced by permission from Rackow EC, Fein IA, Leppo J. Colloid osmotic pressure as a prognostic indicator of pulmonary edema and mortality in the critically ill. Chest 1977;72:712.)

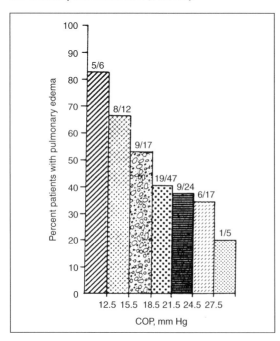

R E F E R E N C E S

Appel PL, Shoemaker WC. Evaluation of fluid therapy in adult respiratory failure. Crit Care Med 1981;9:862.

Armson BA, Samuels P, Miller F, et al. Evaluation of maternal fluid dynamics during tocolytic therapy with ritodrine hydrochloride and magnesium sulfate. Am J Obstet Gynecol 1992; 167:758.

Assali NS, Vaughn DL. Blood volume in preeclampsia: fantasy and reality. Am J Obstet Gynecol 1977;129:355.

Benedetti TJ. Life-threatening complications of betamimetic therapy for preterm labor inhibition. Clin Perinatol 1986;13:84.

Benedetti TJ, Carlson RW. Studies of colloid osmotic pressure in pregnancy-induced hypertension. Am J Obstet Gynecol 1979;135:308.

Benedetti TJ, Cotton DB, Read JC, Miller FC. Hemodynamic observations in severe pre-eclampsia with a flow-directed pulmonary artery catheter. Am J Obstet Gynecol 1980;136:465.

Benedetti TJ, Kates R, Williams V. Hemodynamic observations of severe preeclampsia complicated by pulmonary edema. Am J Obstet Gynecol 1985;152:330.

Bhatia RK, Bottoms SF, Saleh AA, et al. Mechanisms for reduced colloid osmotic pressure in pre-eclampsia. Am J Obstet Gynecol 1987;157:106.

Chesley L. Hypertensive disorders of pregnancy. New York: Appleton-Century-Crofts, 1978:115.

Clark SL, Cotton DB, Lee W, et al. Central hemodynamic assessment of normal term pregnancy. Am J Obstet Gynecol 1989;161:1439.

Cotton DB, Gonik B, Dorman K, Harrist R. Cardiovascular alterations in severe pregnancy-induced hypertension: relationship of central venous pressure to pulmonary capillary wedge pressure. Am J Obstet Gynecol 1985;151:762.

Cotton DB, Gonik B, Spillman T, Dorman KF. Intrapartum to postpartum changes in colloid osmotic pressure. Am J Obstet Gynecol 1984; 149:174.

Cotton DB, Jones MM, Longmire S, et al. Role of intravenous nitroglycerin in the treatment of severe pregnancy-induced hypertension complicated by pulmonary edema. Am J Obstet Gynecol 1986;154:91.

Cunningham FG, Lucas MJ, Hankins GV. Pulmonary injury complicating antepartum pyelonephritis. Am J Obstet Gynecol 1987;156:797.

Da Luz PL, Shubin H, Weil MH, et al. Pulmonary edema related to changes in osmotic and pulmonary artery wedge pressure in patients after acute myocardial infarction. Circulation 1975; 51:350.

Freund U, French W, Carlson RW, et al. Hemodynamic and metabolic studies of a case of toxemia of pregnancy. Am J Obstet Gynecol 1977; 127:206.

Gonik B, Cotton DB. Peripartum colloid osmotic pressure changes: influence of intravenous hydration. Am J Obstet Gynecol 1984;150:99.

Gonik B, Cotton D, Spillman T, et al. Peripartum colloid osmotic changes: effects of controlled fluid management. Am J Obstet Gynecol 1985; 151:812.

Goodlin RC, Cotton DB, Haesslein HC. Severe edema proteinuria-hypertension gestosis. Am J Obstet Gynecol 1978;132:595.

Goodlin R, Kurpershoek C, Haesslein H. Colloid osmotic pressure changes during hypertensive pregnancy. Clin Exp Hypertens 1982;1:49.

Goyert G, Bhatia R, Schubert C, et al: Does intravenous ritodrine therapy cause capillary endothelial damage? Am J Perinatol 1987;4:331.

Grospietsch G, Fenske M, Girndt J, et al. The renin-angiotensin aldosterone system, antidiuretic hormone levels and water balance under tocolytic therapy with Fenoterol and Verapamil. Int J Gynaecol Obstet 1980;17:590.

Grundmann R, Heistermann S. Postoperative albumin infusion therapy based on colloid osmotic pressure. Arch Surg 1985;120:911.

Guyton AC. Textbook of medical physiology. 6th ed. Philadelphia: WB Saunders, 1981:363–382.

Guyton AC, Lindsey AW. Effect of elevated left atrial pressure and decreased plasma protein concentration on the development of pulmonary edema. Circ Res 1959;7:649.

Hankins GD, Wendel GD, Cunningham FG, Leveno KJ. Longitudinal evaluation of hemodynamic changes in eclampsia. Am J Obstet Gynecol 1984;150:506.

Hansen AT. A self-recording electronic osmometer for quick, direct measurement of colloid osmotic pressure in small samples. Acta Physiol Scand 1961;53:197.

Hauch MA, Gaiser RR, Hartwell BL, Datta S. Maternal and fetal colloid osmotic pressure following fluid expansion during cesarean section. Crit Care Med 1995;23:510.

Haupt MT, Rackow EC. Colloid osmotic pressure and fluid resuscitation with hetastarch, albumin, and saline solutions. Crit Care Med 1982;10:159.

Jones MM, Longmire S, Cotton DB, et al. Influence of crystalloid versus colloid infusion on peripartum colloid osmotic pressure changes. Obstet Gynecol 1986;68:659.

Jouppila P, Jouppila R, Koivula A. Albumin infusion does not alter the intervillous blood flow in severe pre-eclampsia. Acta Obstet Gynecol Scand 1983;62:345.

Katz J, Sellers AL, Bonorris G. Effect of nephrectomy on plasma albumin catabolism in experimental nephrosis. J Lab Clin Med 1964;63:680.

Kirshon B, Moise KJ, Cotton DB, et al. Role of volume expansion in severe preeclampsia. Surg Gynecol Obstet 1988;167:367.

Kostuk W, Barr JW, Simon AL, Ross J. Correlations between the chest film and hemodynamics in acute myocardial infarction. Circulation 1973; 48:624.

Ladegaard-Pedersen HJ. Measurement of the colloid osmotic pressure in patients. Scand J Clin Lab Invest 1967;20:79.

Ladegaard-Pedersen HJ. The colloid osmotic pressure in nonoperated surgical patients. Acta Chir Scand 1973;139:135.

Laks H, O'Connor NE, Anderson W, Pilon RN. Crystalloid versus colloid hemodilution in man. Surg Gynecol Obstet 1976;142:506.

Landis EM, Pappenheimer JR. Handbook of physiology. vol 2. Baltimore: Williams and Wilkins, 1963:961.

Levine OR, Mellins RB, Senior RM, Fishman AP. The application of Starling's law of capillary exchange to the lungs. J Clin Invest 1967;46: 934.

McHugh TJ, Forrester JS, Adler L, et al. Pulmonary vascular congestion in acute myocardial infarction: hemodynamic and radiologic correlations. Ann Intern Med 1972;76:29.

Metildi LA, Shackford SR, Virgitio RW, Peters RM. Crystalloid versus colloid fluid resuscitation of patients with severe pulmonary insufficiency. Surg Gynecol Obstet 1984;158:207.

Meyer BJ, Meyer A, Guyton AC. Interstitial fluid pressure. Circ Res 1968;22:263.

Morissette MP. Colloid osmotic pressure: its measurement and clinical value. Can Med Assoc J 1983;116:897.

Nguyen HN, Clark SL, Greenspoon J, et al. Peripartum colloid osmotic pressures: correlation with serum proteins. Obstet Gynecol 1986;68:807.

Oian P, Maltau JM. Calculated capillary hydrostatic pressure in normal pregnancy and preeclampsia. Am J Obstet Gynecol 1987;157:102.

Oian P, Maltau JM, Noddeland H, Fadness HO. Transcapillary fluid balance in preeclampsia. Br J Obstet Gynaecol 1986;93:235.

Oian P, Maltau JM, Noddeland H, Fadness HO. Oedema-preventing mechanisms in subcutaneous tissue of normal pregnant women. Br J Obstet Gynaecol 1985;92:1113.

Parker JC, Parker RE, Granger DN, Taylor AE. Vascular permeability and transvascular fluid and protein transport in the dog lung. Circ Res 1981;48:549.

Phelan JP, Yurth DA. Severe preeclampsia I. Peripartum hemodynamic observations. Am J Obstet Gynecol 1982;144:17.

Prather JW, Gaar KA, Guyton AC. Direct continuous recording of plasma colloid osmotic pressure of whole blood. J Appl Physiol 1968;24:602.

Rackow EC, Fein IA, Leppo J. Colloid osmotic pressure as a prognostic indicator of pulmonary edema and mortality in the critically ill. Chest 1977a;72:712.

Rackow EC, Fein IA, Leppo J. Colloid osmotic pressure as a prognostic indicator of pulmonary edema and mortality in the critically ill. Chest 1977b;72:709.

Rafferty TD, Berkowitz RL. Hemodynamics in patients with severe toxemia during labor and delivery. Am J Obstet Gynecol 1980;138:263.

Ramanathan S, Masih A, Rock I, et al. Maternal and fetal effects of prophylactic hydration with crystalloids or colloids before epidural anesthesia. Anesth Analg 1983;62:673.

Ridgway LE, Martin RW, Hess LW, et al. Acute gestational pyelonephritis: the impact on colloid osmotic pressure, plasma fibronectin, and arterial oxygen saturation. Am J Perinatol 1991;8:222.

Robertson EG, Cheyne GA. Plasma biochemistry in relation to oedema of pregnancy. J Obstet Gynaecol Br Cwlth 1972;79:769.

Rothschild MA, Bauman A, Yalow RS, Berson SA. Tissue distribution of $I^{131}$ labeled human serum albumin following intravenous administration. J Clin Invest 1955;34:1354.

Shippy CR, Shoemaker WC. Hemodynamic and colloid osmotic pressure alterations in the surgical patient. Crit Care Med 1983;11:191.

Sibbald WJ, Dreidger AA, Wells GA, et al. The short-term effects of increasing plasma colloid osmotic pressure in patients with noncardiac pulmonary edema. Surgery 1983;93:620.

Starling EH. On the absorption of fluids from the connective tissue spaces. J Physiol 1896;19:312.

Stein L, Beraud J, Cavanilles J, et al. Pulmonary edema during fluid infusion in the absence of heart failure. JAMA 1974;229:65.

Swan HJ, Ganz W, Forrester J, et al. Catheterization of the heart in man with use of a flow-directed balloon-tipped catheter. N Engl J Med 1970; 283:447.

Taylor AE. Capillary fluid filtration: Starling forces and lymph flow. Circ Res 1981;49:557.

Thompson WL, Fukushima T, Rutherford RB, Walton RP. Intravascular persistence, tissue storage, and excretion of hydroxyethyl starch. Surg Gynecol Obstet 1970;131:965.

Tullis JL. Albumin. I. Background and use. JAMA 1977;237:355.

Uhley HN, Leeds SE, Sampson JJ, Friedman M. Role of pulmonary lymphatics in chronic pulmonary edema. Circ Res 1962;11:966.

Webb AR, Barclay SA, Bennett ED. In vitro colloid osmotic pressure of commonly used plasma expanders and substitutes: a study of the diffusibility of colloid molecules. Intensive Care Med 1989;15:116.

Weil MH, Afifi AA. Experimental and clinical studies on lactate and pyruvate as indicators of the severity of acute circulatory failure. Circulation 1970;41:989.

Weil MH, Carlson RW. Colloid osmotic pressure and pulmonary edema. Chest 1977;72:692.

Weil MH, Henning RJ, Morissette M, Michaels S. Relationship between colloid osmotic pressure and pulmonary artery wedge pressure in patients with acute cardiorespiratory failure. Am J Med 1978;64:643.

Weil MH, Henning RJ, Puri VK. Colloid oncotic pressure: clinical significance. Crit Care Med 1979; 7:113.

Weil MH, Morissette M, Michaels S, et al. Routine plasma colloid osmotic pressure measurements. Crit Care Med 1974;2:229.

Wittmers LE, Bartlett M, Johnson JA. Estimation of capillary permeability coefficient of insulin in various tissues of the rabbit. Microvasc Res 1976;11:67.

Wu PY. Colloid oncotic pressure: current status and clinical applications in neonatal medicine. Clin Perinatol 1982;9:645.

Wu PY, Udani V, Chan L, et al. Colloid osmotic pressure: variations in normal pregnancy. J Perinatol Med 1983;11:193.

Yeast JD, Halberstadt C, Meyer BA, et al. The risk of pulmonary edema and colloid osmotic pressure changes during magnesium sulfate infusion. Am J Obstet Gynecol 1993;169:1566.

# CHAPTER 4

# Fluid and Electrolyte Balance

## Fluid Resuscitation

The infusion of fluid remains a cornerstone of therapy when treating critically ill pregnant women with hypovolemia. An understanding of the distribution and pharmacokinetics of plasma expanders, as well as knowledge of normal fluid exchange, is needed to allow for prompt resuscitation of patients in various forms of shock, as well as to provide maintenance therapy for other critically ill patients. Controversy exists as to the appropriate intravenous (IV) solutions to use in the management of hypovolemic shock. As long as physiologic endpoints are used to guide therapy and adjustments are made based on the individual's needs, side effects associated with inadequate or overaggressive resuscitation can be avoided.

In most types of critical illness, intravascular volume is decreased. Hemorrhagic shock has been shown to deplete the extracellular fluid (ECF) compartment with an increase in intracellular water secondary to cell membrane and sodium-potassium pump dysfunction (Carrico, 1976; Skillman, 1967, 1975, 1976). Surgical patients posttrauma are found to have an expanded ECF, while the intravascular volume is depleted (Shoemaker 1973). Most available studies of fluid balance have been conducted in patients in the nonpregnant state; very little data exist documenting these changes in pregnant women. Whatever the underlying pathology, intravascular volume is decreased in many types of critical illnesses.

Successful resuscitation thus remains dependent on the prompt restoration of intravascular volume.

## Normal Fluid Dynamics

The total body water (TBW) ranges from 45% to 65% of total body weight in the human adult. Total body water is distributed between two major compartments, the intracellular fluid (ICF) space and the ECF space. Two thirds of the TBW resides in the ICF space and one third in the ECF space. The ECF is further subdivided into the interstitial and intravascular spaces in a ratio of 3:1. Regulation of the ICF is mostly achieved by changes in water balance, whereas the changes in plasma volume are related to the regulation of sodium balance. Because water can freely cross most cell membranes, the osmolalities within each compartment are the same. When water is added into one compartment, it distributes evenly throughout the TBW, and the amount of volume added to any given compartment is proportional to its fractional representation of the TBW. Infusion of fluids that are isotonic with plasma are distributed initially within the ECF; however, only one fourth of the infused volume remains in the intravascular space after 30 minutes. Because most fluids are a combination of free water and isotonic fluids, one can predict the space of distribution and thus the volume transfused into each compartment.

During pregnancy, the ECF accumulates 6 to 8 liters of extra fluid, with the plasma volume increasing by 50% (Gallery, 1987). The plasma volume slowly increases during the first 30 weeks of pregnancy and is then maintained at that level until term (Wittaker, 1993). The plasma volume to ECF ratio is also increased in pregnancy (Brown, 1992). Plasma volume is increased by a greater fraction in multiple pregnancies (MacGillivray, 1971; Thomsen, 1993), with the increase being proportional to the number of fetuses (Fullerton, 1965). Reduced plasma volume expansion has been shown to occur in pregnancies complicated by fetal growth retardation (Hytten, 1963; Salas, 1993), hypertensive disorders (Arias, 1965; Brown, 1992; Gallery, 1979; Goodlin, 1981; MacGillivray, 1971; Sibai, 1983), prematurity (Goodlin, 1981; Raiha 1964), oligohydramnios (Goodlin, 1981, 1983), and maternal smoking (Pirani, 1978). In pregnancy-induced hypertension the total ECF is unchanged (Brown, 1989, 1992), supporting an altered distribution of ECF between the two compartments, possibly secondary to the rise in capillary permeability. A similar mechanism may occur in other conditions in which the plama volume is reduced; the clinician needs to be cognizant of this when choosing fluids for resuscitation. Blood volume decreases over the first 24 hours postpartum (Ueland, 1976), with nonpregnant levels reached at 6 to 9 weeks postpartum (Lund, 1967). With intrapartum hemorrhage, ICF can be mobilized to restore the plasma volume (Ueland, 1976).

Red-cell mass is increased by 24% during the course of pregnancy (Thomsen, 1993), resulting in physiologic hemodilution and relative anemia. The decrease in the hematocrit is characterized by a gradual fall until week 30, followed by a gradual rise afterward (Peeters, 1989). This is also associated with a decrease in whole blood viscosity, which may be beneficial for intervillous perfusion (Peeters, 1987). With hemorrhagic shock and mobilization of fluid from the ICF, the hematocrit, and thus oxygen carrying capacity, would be further reduced, requiring replacement with appropriate fluids.

## Crystalloid Solutions

The most commonly employed crystalloid products for fluid resuscitation are 0.9% saline and lactated Ringer's solutions. The contents of normal saline and Ringer's lactate solutions are shown in Table 4-1. These are isotonic solutions that distribute evenly throughout the extracellular space but will not promote intracellular cell shifts. The infusion of hypertonic saline, however, leads to the redistribution of ICF to the extracellular space and will be discussed later in the chapter.

## Isotonic Crystalloids

Isotonic crystalloid solutions are generally readily available, easily stored, nontoxic, and reaction-free. They are an inexpensive form of volume resuscitation. The infusion of large volumes of 0.9% saline and Ringer's lactate is not a problem clinically; when administered in large volumes to patients with traumatic shock, no acidosis is seen

T A B L E   **4-1**

Characteristics of various volume-expanding agents

| Agent | Na$^+$ (mEq/liter) | Cl$^-$ (mEq/liter) | Lactate (mEq/liter ) | Osmolarity (mosm/liter) | Oncotic Pressure (mm Hg) |
|---|---|---|---|---|---|
| Ringer's lactate | 130 | 109 | 28 | 275 | 0 |
| Normal saline | 154 | 154 | 0 | 310 | 0 |
| Hypertonic saline (3%) | 513 | 513 | 0 | 1025 | 0 |
| Albumin (5%) | 130–160 | 130–160 | 0 | 310 | 20 |
| Dextran-70 (6%) | 154 | 154 | 0 | 310 | 60 |
| Hetastarch (6%) | 154 | 154 | 0 | 310 | 30 |

(Lowery, 1971). The excess circulating chloride ion resulting from saline infusion is excreted readily by the kidney. In a similar manner, the lactate load in Ringer's solution does not potentiate the lactacidemia associated with shock (Trudnowski, 1967), nor has it been shown to effect the reliability of blood lactate measurements (Lowery, 1971).

Using the Starling-Landis-Staverman equation for fluid flux across a microvascular wall, one can predict that crystalloids will distribute rapidly between the ICF and ECF. Equilibration within the extracellular space occurs within 20 to 30 minutes after infusion. In healthy nonpregnant adults, approximately 25% of the volume infused remains in the intravascular space after 1 hour. In the critically ill or injured patient, however, only 20% or less of the infusion remains in the circulation after 1 to 2 hours (Carey, 1970; Hauser, 1980). The volemic effects of various crystalloid solutions compared with albumin and whole blood are shown in Table 4-2. At equivalent volumes, crystalloids are less effective than colloids for expansion of the intravascular volume. Two to 12 times the volume of crystalloids are necessary to achieve similar hemodynamic and volemic endpoints (Dawidson, 1981, 1982; Hanshiro, 1967; Hauser, 1980; Moss, 1981; Skillman, 1976). Proponents of crystalloid administration for hemorrhagic shock, however, feel that crystalloid solutions most effectively replace the interstitial deficits that occur (Shires, 1960). Further, the rapid equilibration between the ICF and ECF seen with crystalloid infusion reduces the incidence of pulmonary edema (Virgilio, 1979a,b), whereas exogenous colloid administration promotes the accumulation of interstitial fluid (Lucas, 1988; Siegel, 1970).

## Indications

**Shock** Crystalloids—either normal saline or Ringer's lactate—are used to replenish plasma volume deficits and replace fluid and electrolyte losses from the interstitium (Lowe, 1977; Moss, 1971, 1981; Shoemaker, 1973; Takaori, 1967; Virgilio, 1979). Patients in shock from any cause should receive immediate volume replacement with crystalloid solution during the initial clinical evaluation. Aggressive administration of crystalloid may promptly restore BP and peripheral perfusion. Given in a quantity of 3 to 4 times the amount of blood lost, they can adequately replace an acute loss of up to 20% of the blood volume, although 3 to 5 liters of crystalloid may be required to replace a 1-liter blood loss (Baue, 1967; Siegel, 1970; Singh, 1992; Virgilio, 1979c; Waxman, 1989). After the initial resuscitation with crystalloid, the selection of fluids becomes controversial, especially if microvascular integrity is not preserved (as in sepsis, burns, trauma, and anaphylaxis). Further fluid resuscitation should be guided by continous bedside observation of urine ouput, mental status, heart rate, pulse pressure, respiratory rate, BP, and temperature monitoring, together with serial measurements of hematocrit, serum albumin, platelet count, prothrombin, and partial thromboplastin times. More

T A B L E   **4-2**

Typical volemic effects of various resuscitative fluids
after 1-liter infusion

| Fluid* | ICV (mL) | ECV (mL) | IV (mL) | PV (mL) |
|---|---|---|---|---|
| 0.5% Dextrose/water | 660 | 340 | 255 | 85 |
| Normal saline or lactated Ringer's | − 100 | 1100 | 825 | 275 |
| Sodium chloride | − 2950 | 3950 | 2690 | 990 |
| Albumin | 0 | 1000 | 500 | 500 |
| Whole blood | 0 | 1000 | 0 | 1000 |

*Based on infusion of 1-liter volumes.

IVC, intracellular volume; ECV, extracellular volume; IV, interstitial volume; PV, plasma volume.

Source: Carlson RW, Rattan S, Haupt M. Fluid resuscitation in conditions of increased permeability. Anesth Rev 1990;17(suppl 3):14.

aggressive monitoring is required in patients who remain in shock or fail to respond to the initial resuscitatory efforts and in patients with poor physiologic reserve who are unlikely to tolerate imprecisions in resuscitation efforts.

**Diagnosis of Oliguria**  In critically ill patients, it is often extremely difficult to distinguish volume depletion from congestive heart failure (CHF). Because prerenal hypoperfusion resulting in a urine output of less than 0.5 mL/kg/hr can result in renal failure, it is extremely important to separate the two conditions and treat accordingly. An adequate fluid challenge consists of at least 500 mL of Ringer's lactate or normal saline administered over 5 to 10 minutes. Increasing the patient's IV infusion rate to 200 mL/hr or giving the bolus over 30 minutes or longer will not expand the intravascular volume sufficiently to help differentiate the etiology or treat the volume depletion. If there is no response from the initial fluid challenge, one may repeat it. If no increase in urine output occurs, one is probably not dealing with intravascular depletion, and further fluid management should be guided by invasive monitoring with a pulmonary artery catheter or repetitive echocardiograms. Patients with CHF do not experience a prolonged increase in vascular volume because crystalloid fluids distribute out of the intravascular space rapidly with only a transient increase in intravascular volume.

---

*Side Effects*

Crystalloid solutions are generally nontoxic and free of side effects. However, fluid overload may result in pulmonary, cerebral, myocardial, mesenteric, and skin edema; hypoproteinemia; and altered tissue oxygen tension.

**Pulmonary Edema**  Isotonic crystalloid resuscitation lowers the colloid oncotic pressure (COP) (Haupt, 1982; Waxman, 1989), although it is uncertain whether such alterations in COP actually worsen lung function (Hauser, 1980; Skillman, 1967; Virgilio, 1979a,b). The lung has a variety of mechanisms that act to prevent the development of pulmonary edema. These include increased lymphatic flow, diminished pulmonary intersti-

tial oncotic pressure, and increased interstitial hydrostatic pressure. Together they limit the effect of the lowered COP (Lewis, 1980). In patients with intact microvascular integrity, studies have failed to demonstrate an increase in extravascular lung water after appropriate crystalloid loading (Miller, 1971). Irrespective of the amount of fluid administered, strict attention to physiologic endpoints and oxygenation is essential in order to prevent pulmonary edema.

**Peripheral Edema**  Peripheral edema is a frequent side effect of fluid resuscitation but can be limited by appropriate monitoring of the resuscitatory effort. Excess peripheral edema may result in decreased oxygen tension in the soft tissue, promoting complications such as poor wound healing, skin breakdown, and infection (Hohn, 1976; Kaufman, 1984; Myers, 1967). Despite this, burn patients have shown improvement in survival after massive crystalloid resuscitation (Barone, 1991).

**Myocardial Edema**  Aggressive fluid resuscitation may lead to intravascular overload and increased myocardial water. A 3% to 30% increase in myocardial water has been demonstrated in patients receiving crystalloid resuscitation (Barone, 1991; Lowenstein, 1975; Schupbach, 1978). Although the increased myocardial water may theoretically result in decreased contractility and compliance, reliable clinical evidence of such side effects is lacking.

**Bowel Edema**  Edema of the gastrointestinal system seen with aggressive crystalloid resuscitation may result in ileus and diarrhea, probably secondary to hypoalbuminemia (Granger, 1984). This may be limited by monitoring of the COP and correction of hypo-oncotic states.

**Central Nervous System**  Under normal circumstances, the brain is protected from volume-related injury by the blood-brain barrier and cerebral autoregulation. However, a patient in shock may have a primary or coincidental CNS injury, which may damage either or both of these protective mechanisms. In this situation, the COP and osmotic gradients should be monitored closely to prevent edema.

## Hypertonic Saline

With administration of hypertonic solutions, fluid is recruited from the ICF to the ECF, mainly to the intravascular compartment. This results in plasma volumes in excess of the volume infused (see Table 4-2), with rapid improvement in all hemodynamic profiles. Hypertonic saline provides more rapid resuscitation to normal hemodynamic parameters with less total volume infused than do standard crystalloids (Pascual, 1992). The intravascular benefit lasts for 15 minutes, after which there is redistribution between intravascular and interstitial space. This problem is solved with the addition of a hyperoncotic agent such as 6% dextran.

Hypertonic saline also evokes a vagal pulmonary reflex that leads to selective blood flow restriction to the skeletal muscles and causes visceral and pulmonary precapillary dilation (Nakayama, 1984; Rocha-Silva, 1986; Rothschild, 1957). This results in restoration of normal blood flow to the vital organs and shunting from skeletal muscles. The mechanism by which an increase in cardiac output occurs is unclear. It may be secondary to increased cardiac compliance (Curtis, 1992), a positive inotropic effect, or decreased afterload secondary to the visceral capillary dilation (Nakayama, 1984; Templeton, 1972). In the brain, hypertonic solutions not only improve cerebral blood flow, but also prevent the development of cerebral edema and increased intracranial pressure.

### Indications

Hypertonic saline (3%, 5%, and 7.5%) has been advocated for various forms of circulatory shock (Bitterman, 1987; DeFellipe, 1980; Prough, 1985). Although clinical studies have demonstrated that reduced volumes of hypertonic saline were required for resuscitation, careful monitoring was essential to avoid hyperosmolar and hypernatremic complications (Shackford, 1983). In burn patients resuscitated with hypertonic saline, the volume requirements were reduced by 20% to 25%, with reduced severity of edema when compared with isotonic fluids (Moss, 1981). Experimentally, hypertonic saline has been an efficient volume expander in models of endotoxic shock (Kreimeier, 1991) and may have a future role in resuscitation of patients with septic shock. Because of their association with improved cerebral blood flow and prevention of cerebral edema, such fluids have been shown to be effective in the resuscitation of patients with various types of head injury (Walsh, 1991).

### Side Effects

Hypertonic saline has the potential for causing hypernatremia, hyperchloremia, and hypokalemia. In clinical trails, these side effects generally have not been of clinical significance (Mattox, 1991). When compared with standard crystalloids, there seems to be no added risk for the development of pulmonary edema unless the resuscitatory effort has been overly aggressive. Hypertonic saline given in excessive amounts may result in prolongation of the partial thromboplastin time and interfere with platelet aggregation (Reed, 1991). The addition of dextran to hypertonic saline may compound these problems. Despite theoretical benefits, hypertonic saline is rarely used in obstetrics.

## Colloid Solutions

Colloids are large-molecular-weight substances to which cell membranes are relatively impermeable. They increase the COP (see Chapter 3), resulting in the movement of fluid from the interstitial compartment to the intravascular compartment. Their ability to remain intravascular prolongs their duration of action. The net result is a lower volume of infusate necessary to expand the intravascular space when compared with crystalloid solutions.

### Albumin

Albumin is the colloidal agent against which all others are judged (Tullis, 1977). Albumin is produced in the liver and represents 50% of hepatic protein production (Rothschild, 1972). It contributes to 70% to 80% of the serum COP (Lewis,

1980; Thompson, 1975). A 50% reduction in the serum albumin concentration will lower the COP to one third of normal (Thompson, 1975).

Albumin is a highly water-soluble polypeptide with a molecular weight ranging from 66,300 to 69,000 daltons (Thompson, 1975) and is distributed unevenly between the intravascular (40%) and interstitial (60%) compartments (Thompson, 1975). The normal serum albumin concentration is maintained between 3.5 and 5 g/dL and is affected by albumin secretion, volume of distribution, rate of loss from the intravascular space, and degradation. The albumin level also is well correlated with nutritional status (Grant, 1981). Hypoalbuminemia secondary to diminished production (starvation) or excess loss (hemorrhage) results in a decrease in its degradation and a compensatory increase in its distribution in the interstitial space (Rosenoer, 1980; Rothschild, 1972). In acute injury or stress with depletion of the intravascular compartment, interstitial albumin is mobilized and transported to the intravascular department by lymphatic channels or transcapillary refill (Moss, 1966). Albumin synthesis is stimulated by thyroid hormone (Rothschild, 1958) and cortisol (Rothschild, 1957) and decreased by an elevated COP (Liljedahl, 1968).

The capacity of albumin to bind water is related to the amount of albumin given as well as to the plasma volume deficit (Lamke, 1957a,b). One gram of albumin increases the plasma volume by approximately 18 mL (Granger, 1978; Holcroft, 1974; Lewis, 1980). Albumin is available as a 5% or 25% solution in isotonic saline. Thus, 100 mL of 25% albumin solution increases the intravascular volume by approximately 450 mL over 30 to 60 minutes (Hauser, 1980). With depletion of the ECF, this equilibration is not sufficiently brisk or complete unless supplementation with isotonic fluids is provided as part of the resuscitation regimen (Lewis, 1980). A 500-mL solution of 5% albumin containing 25 g of albumin will increase the intravascular space by 450 mL. In this instance, however, the albumin is administered in conjunction with the fluid to be retained.

Infused albumin has an initial plasma half-life of 16 hours, with 90% of the albumin dose remaining in the plasma 2 hours after administration (Lewis, 1980; Berson, 1957). The albumin equilibrates between the intravascular and interstitial compartments over a 7- to 10-day period (Sterling, 1951), with 75% of the albumin being absent from the plasma in 2 days. In patients with shock, the administration of plasma albumin has been shown to significantly increase the COP for at least 2 days after resuscitation (Haupt, 1982).

## Indications

Albumin is used primarily for the resuscitation of patients with hypovolemic shock. A major goal in the resuscitation of a patient in acute shock is to replace the intravascular volume in order to restore tissue perfusion. In patients with acute blood loss of greater than 30% of blood volume, it probably should be used early in conjunction with a crystalloid infusion to maintain peripheral perfusion. Treatment goals are to maintain a serum albumin of greater than 2.5 g/dL in the acute resuscitatory period. With non-edematous patients, 5% albumin and crystalloid can be used, but with edematous patients, 25% albumin may assist the patient in mobilizing her own interstitial volume. In patients with suspected loss of capillary wall integrity (especially in the lung in patients at risk for the subsequent development of acute respiratory distress syndrome), the use of albumin should be limited, because it crosses the capillary wall and exerts an oncotic influence in the interstitial space. Albumin may be used in patients with burns (Rothschild, 1972) once capillary integrity is restored, approximately 24 hours after the initial event.

## Side Effects

A number of potential adverse effects of albumin have been reported. This agent may accentuate respiratory failure and contribute to the development of pulmonary edema. However, the presence or absence of infection, together with the method of resuscitation and volumes used, affect respiratory function far more than the type of fluid infused (Poole, 1982; Shoemaker, 1981; Virgilio, 1979b,c; Vito, 1974). Albumin may lower the serum ionized calcium concentration, resulting in a negative inotrophic effect on the myocardium (Kovalik, 1981; Lucas, 1978, 1980; Weaver,

1978), and it may impair immune responsiveness. Infusion of albumin results in moderate to transient abnormalities in prothrombin time, partial thromboplastin time, and platelet counts (Coghill, 1981). However, the clinical implications of these defects, if any, are unknown. Albumin-induced anaphylaxis is reported in 0.47% to 1.53% of recipients (Rothschild, 1972). These reactions are short lived and include urticaria, chills, fever, and rarely, hypertension. There is no hepatitis or known risk of acquired immunodeficiency syndrome (AIDS) with the use of albumin.

## Dextran

Dextrans are large glucose polymers that were first introduced into clinical practice in the 1940s. They are produced by the action of the bacterium *Leuconostoc mesenteroides* when grown on sucrose medium. Its original structure is a branched polysaccharide of 200,000 glucose units. Acid hydrolysis and ethanol fractionation of the resulting polysaccharide macromolecule produce a heterogeneous mixture of dextrans with differing molecular weights. These are commercially available as preparations with an average molecular weight of 40,000 daltons (D-40) or 70,000 daltons (D-70).

Dextran molecules are distributed mainly in the ECF within the intravascular compartment. Dextran-70 has an average molecular weight of 70,000, with 90% of the molecules being between 25,000 and 125,000 daltons (Data, 1974). It is available as a 6% solution in normal saline or in 5% dextrose. Dextran-40 has an average molecular weight of 40,000, with 90% of the molecules falling in the range of 10,000 to 80,000 daltons (Data, 1974). It is available as a 10% solution in normal saline or 5% dextrose. The circulating half-life of dextran varies with its particle size (Dawidson, 1981). Sixty percent to 70% of D-40 and 30% to 40% of D-70 are cleared within 12 hours (Arthurson, 1964; Atik, 1969; Thoren, 1981). Dextran-40 is lost from the circulation more rapidly than is D-70 because the former compound contains a larger amount of smaller particles, which are more readily cleared from the circulation. Only 20% of a D-40 dose and 30% of a D-70 dose remains in the circulation up to 24 hours.

Most of the dextran load is excreted by the kidney (Christensen, 1979). Small particles are filtered rapidly, not reabsorbed, and lost in the urine. While in the circulation, smaller particles exert large osmotic activity, whereas larger particles remain in the circulation for longer but have less osmotic activity. The larger fractions are broken down by the reticuloendothelial system to carbon dioxide and water. Thus, D-40 is a more potent plasma expander than D-70 because D-40 has greater colloid osmotic pressure. However, this increase in plasma volume is relatively short lived because D-40 is excreted more rapidly than is D-70.

### Indications

Dextran has been reported to increase survival and improve hemodynamic parameters in patients in shock (Cohn, 1967; Dawidson, 1979, 1980, 1981, 1982; Gelin, 1961; Lamke, 1976a; Risberg, 1981; Shoemaker, 1976; Skillman, 1967; Takaori, 1967; Modig, 1986). When used in hypovolemic patients, dextran is associated with an increase in renal plasma flow and a decrease in plasma antidiuretic hormone (ADH) levels (Thoren, 1981). Infusion of dextran increases the intravascular volume by an amount greater than or equal to the amount infused. The subsequent osmotic diuresis, however, limits the duration of volume expansion. One gram of dextran results in a shift of 20 to 30 mL of water to the intravascular space (Dawidson, 1981; Gruber, 1977; Thoren, 1981). A 500-mL bolus of D-40 results in a 750-mL expansion of the intravascular volume at 1 hour and 1050 mL at 2 hours (Shoemaker, 1976). The degree of intravascular volume expansion is similar and approximately equal to the amount infused 4 to 6 hours after the infusion of either D-40 or D-70 (Thoren, 1981).

Dextran coats endothelial surfaces, reducing interactions with the cellular elements in the blood (Thoren, 1981). Coating of cellular elements and reduction of blood viscosity decrease the sludging and cellular aggregation seen in shock (Cohn, 1967). Platelet function is altered, limiting thrombus formation and activation of the clotting cascade (Aberg, 1979; Lewis, 1966; Weil, 1979). Dextran also has been found to be effective in reducing the incidence of thromboembolic disease (Atik, 1969; Rose, 1979; Sasahara, 1979) and has been used in therapy of ischemic ulceration of the skin, arterial occlusion, frostbite, stroke, and for cell harvesting in plasmapheresis and priming for extracorporeal circulation. The maximum recommended daily dosage of dextran for volume expansion is 20 mL/kg.

### Side Effects

Precipitation of the dextran with cast formation can lead to plugging of the renal tubules and development of dextran-induced renal failure (Chinitz, 1971; Feest, 1976; Mailoux, 1967; Matheson, 1970). This is accentuated by the presence of hypovolemia and preexisting renal dysfunction (Chinitz, 1971). Renal failure in these patients is caused by a combination of decreased renal perfusion pressure, dextran in the tubules, and a continuous stimulus for water reabsorption, conditions all existing following intravascular volume depletion and resuscitation with dextran. Renal failure has been observed only rarely after administration of a larger-molecular-weight D-70; thus, the use of D-40 is not recommended in patients with established or incipient renal failure.

Anaphylactic reactions to dextran occur in approximately 1.0% to 5.3% of the population (Ring, 1977; Thompson, 1975). This is a result of naturally occurring antibodies, which may exist in the general population as a consequence of exposure to dextran in food, as well as the presence of dextran-producing bacteria in the intestine. Symptoms occur within 30 minutes of starting the infusion and include urticaria, rash, nausea, bronchospasm, shock, and occasionally, death.

Dextrans produce a dose-related abnormality in hemostasis by a reduction in platelet adhesion and aggregation (Lewis, 1966; Weiss, 1967). A decrease in serum fibrinogen and other factor levels (Data, 1974) with an increase in the Ivy bleeding time and incisional bleeding (Thompson, 1975; Hess, 1992) are sometimes noted. Dextran inhibits erythrocyte aggregation in vivo (Cohn, 1967).

If blood glucose levels are measured by an acid analysis, which converts dextran to dextrose, a false elevation of the blood glucose levels may be seen. Dextran also may cause false increases of the total protein concentration and can interfere with cross-matching of blood. Other observations include spurious increases in serum bilirubin level and alteration of COP measurements (Guyton, 1971).

In patients receiving D-40, and to a lesser extent D-70, urine volume production cannot serve as a guide to adequacy of intravascular volume replacement because of the osmotic diuresis that occurs immediately upon infusion of dextran.

## Hetastarch

Hetastarch is a synthetic colloid molecule that closely resembles glycogen. It is prepared by incorporating hydroxyethyl ether into the glucose residues of amylopectin (Solanke, 1971). Amylopectin, which is a major component of cornstarch, undergoes rapid hydrolysis in vivo, has a half-life of 20 minutes, and is not clinically useful. Hetastarch is available clinically as a 6% solution in normal saline. The molecular weight of the particles is 480,000 daltons, with 80% of the molecules in the range of 30,000 to 2,400,000 daltons. Hetastarch is metabolized rapidly in the blood by alpha-amylase (Farrow, 1970; Ferber, 1985; Yacobi, 1982), with the rate of degradation dependent on the dose and the degree of glucose hydroxyethylation or substitution (Ferber, 1985; Thompson, 1962; Mischler, 1980).

There is an almost immediate appearance of smaller-molecular-weight particles (molecular weight, 50,000 daltons or less) in the urine after IV infusion of hetastarch (Mischler, 1977). Forty percent of this compound is excreted in the urine after 24 hours, with 46% excreted by 2 days and 64% by 8 days (Puri, 1981; Yacobi, 1982). Bilirubin excretion accounts for less than 1% of total elimination in humans (Ring, 1977). The larger particles are metabolized by the reticuloendothelial system (Metcalf, 1970; Thompson, 1970; Bogan, 1969) and remain in the body for an extended period (Mischler, 1979b; Mischler, 1980). Blood alpha-amylase also degrades larger particles to smaller starch polymers and free glucose. The smaller particles eventually are cleared through the urine and bowel. The amount of glucose thus produced does not cause significant hyperglycemia in a diabetic animal model (Hofer, 1992). The half-life of hetastarch represents a composite of the half-lives of the various-sized particles. Ninety percent of a single infusion of hetastarch is removed from the circulation within 42 days, with a terminal half-life of 17 days (Yacobi, 1982).

## Indications

Hetastarch is an effective long-acting plasma volume-expanding agent that can be used in patients suffering from shock secondary to hemorrhage, trauma, sepsis, and burns. It initially expands plasma volume by an amount equal to or greater than the volume infused (Ballinger, 1966; Kilian, 1975; Lamke, 1976a). The volume expansion seen after the infusion of hetastarch is equal to or greater than that produced by D-70 (Lee, 1968; Metcalf, 1970; Khosropour, 1980) or 5% albumin. The plasma volume remains 70% expanded for 3 hours after the infusion and 40% expanded for 12 hours after the infusion (Metcalf, 1970). At 24 hours after infusion, the plasma volume expansion is approximately 28%, with 38% of the drug actually remaining intravascular (Laks, 1974a). The increase in intravascular volume has been associated with improvement in hemodynamic parameters in critically ill patients (Diehl, 1982; Kirklin, 1984; Puri, 1981; Shatney, 1983). Hetastarch also has been shown to increase the COP to the same degree as albumin (Haupt, 1982; Kirklin, 1984). The maximum recommended daily dose for adults is 1500 mL/70 kg of body weight.

## Side Effects

Starch infusions increase serum amylase levels two- to threefold. Peak levels occur 12 to 24 hours after infusion, with elevated levels present for 3 days or longer (Boon, 1976; Kohler, 1977; Mishler, 1977; Korttila, 1984). No alterations in normal pancreatic function have been noted (Kohler, 1977). Liver dysfunction with ascites secondary to intrahepatic obstuction after hetastarch infusions have been reported (Lucas, 1980).

Hetastarch does not seem to promote histamine release (Lorenz, 1975) or to be immuno-

genic (Maurer, 1968; Ring, 1976). Anaphylactic reactions occur in less than 0.085% of the population, with shock or cardiopulmonary arrest occurring in 0.008% (Ring, 1977). When given in doses below 1500 mL/day, hetastarch has not been associated with clinical bleeding, but minor alterations in laboratory measurements may be seen (Lee, 1968; Muller, 1977). There is a transient decrease in the platelet count, prolonged prothrombin and partial thromboplastin times, acceleration of fibrinolysis, reduced levels of Factor VIII, a decrease in the tensile clot strength and platelet adhesion, and an increased bleeding time (Mattox, 1991; Solanke, 1968; Strauss, 1985; Weatherbee, 1974). Hetastarch-induced disseminated intravascular coagulation (Chang, 1990) and intracranial bleeding in patients with subarachnoid hemorrhage have been documented (Damon, 1987; Cully, 1987).

## Pentastarch

Pentastarch is a hydroxyethyl starch derivative. It has a molecular weight of 264,000 daltons (80% of the molecules in the range of 10,000 to 2,000,000 daltons), with fewer hydroxyethyl groups added per molecule than hetastarch. It has a shorter tissue-retention time when compared with hetastarch, secondary to its lower average molecular weight and fewer hydroxyethyl groups, and it is rapidly excreted by the kidney, with an average half-life of 2.5 hours (Mishler, 1977). Sixty percent of the total infused dose is excreted in the urine within 24 hours, with 4% remaining intravascular and 33% unaccounted for (Mishler, 1979a). When compared with hetastarch, there is a greater volume of expansion per volume infused. A 500-mL infusion of pentastarch results in a 700-mL increase in plasma volume within 30 minutes. This agent is available as a 10% solution in normal saline.

## Indications

Currently, pentastarch is approved only by the Food and Drug Administration as an adjunctive to leukophoresis. Studies have demonstrated its successful use in sepsis, patients with burns, and as a plasma expander in cardiac surgery (London,

1989; Rackow, 1989; Waxman, 1989). In studies using pentastarch as a volume expander, it is given as a 500-mL bolus infusion with a limit of 2000 mL total.

### Side Effects

Pentastarch produces changes similar to those of albumin in the prothrombin time, partial thromboplastin time, coagulation factor activity, and platelet counts (Rackow, 1989; London, 1989; Strauss, 1988; Waxman, 1989).

## Electrolyte Disorders

### Hyponatremia

*Hyponatremia* is defined as a plasma sodium concentration of less than 135 mEq/liter. This usually reflects hypo-osmolarity and is the most common electrolyte disorder. The low plasma osmolality ($P_{osm}$) results in water movement into cells, leading to cellular overhydration, which is responsible for most of the symptoms associated with this disorder.

### Etiology

Hyponatremia occurs secondary to solute loss or water retention. Solute loss occurs in fluid that is isotonic with plasma; therefore, hyponatremia occurs only if these losses are replaced with ingested or administered water. After ingestion of a water load, there is a fall in the $P_{osm}$, resulting in decreased secretion and synthesis of ADH. This leads to decreased water reabsorption in the collecting tubules, the production of dilute urine, and rapid excretion of excess water. When the plasma sodium is less than 135 mEq/liter and/or the $P_{osm}$ is below 275 mosm/kg, ADH secretion generally ceases. A defect in renal water excretion will thus lead to hyponatremia. A reduction in free water excretion is caused by either decreased generation of free water in the loop of Henle and distal tubule or enhanced water permeability of the collecting tubules due to the presence of ADH (Table 4-3). Hyponatremia may occur with normal renal water excretion in primary

| T A B L E 4-3 |
| :--- |
| **Common causes of decreased renal water excretion** |

*Effective Circulating Volume Depletion*
Gastrointestinal losses (vomiting, diarrhea)
Renal losses (diuretics, hypoaldosteronism)
Skin losses (burns)
Edematous states (heart failure, nephrotic syndrome, cirrhosis)

*Renal Failure*

*Administration of Diuretics*

*Syndrome of Inappropriate ADH Secretion*
Drugs (e.g., indomethacin, chlorpropamide, barbiturates)
Tumors
CNS diseases
Pulmonary diseases
Physical and emotional distress
Glucocorticoid deficiency

*Adrenal Insufficiency*

*Hypothyroidism*

polydipsia and in conditions in which there is a resetting of the plasma osmostat, such as in psychosis and malnutrition (Anderson, 1985). Levels of atrial natriuretic peptide (ANP) and aldosterone lead to significant alteration in sodium excretion in twins, as opposed to singleton pregnancy (Thompson, 1994).

Pseudohyponatremia is a reduction in serum sodium concentration with a normal or increased $P_{osm}$. This is commonly due to a measurement error resulting from dilution of the sample (Ladenson, 1981). A low plasma sodium concentration with a normal plasma osmolality need not always indicate the presence of pseudohyponatremia. True hyponatremia may be accompanied by a normal plasma osmolality because of hyperglycemia, azotemia, or after the administration of hypertonic mannitol (Weinberg, 1989).

### Clinical Presentation

Most of the symptoms reflect neurologic dysfunction induced by hypo-osmolarity. The severity of the symptoms correlates with the degree of cerebral overhydration together with the speed at which this occurs, as well as the degree of reduction in the plasma sodium concentration (Arief, 1986; Pollock, 1980). Acute hyponatremia may lead to permanent neurologic damage secondary to cerebral overhydration, as seen with postoperative patients given large quantities of hypotonic fluid. With chronic hyponatremia, symptoms are unusual unless there is a marked reduction in the plasma sodium concentration (Table 4-4). Premenopausal women are at greater risk of developing severe and irreversible neurologic damage than are men.

## Diagnosis

Eliciting a good history and a thorough physical examination will help separate the different etiologies and guide laboratory testing toward the correct diagnosis. Initial laboratory evaluation should include $P_{osm}$, serum electrolytes, BUN, creatinine, urea, urine sodium concentration, and osmolality.

The presence of a low plasma sodium and normal osmolality suggests pseudohyponatremia but does not confirm it. The cause of pseudohyponatremia is investigated by examining the serum (may have a milky appearance in patients with hyperlipidemia), and measurement of the serum lipid profile, plasma proteins, plasma sodium, osmolality, and glucose. A urine osmolality below 100 mosm/kg (sp gr $\leq$ 1.003) is seen with primary polydipsia or a reset osmostat. A urine osmolality greater than 100 mosm/kg is seen in patients with the syndrome of inappropriate ADH (SIADH).

When evaluating hyponatremia associated with hypo-osmolality, one needs to distinguish between SIADH, effective circulating volume depletion, adrenal insufficiency, and hypothyroidism. Urinary sodium excretion is less than 25 mEq/ liter in hypovolemic states and greater than 40 mEq/liter in SIADH, reset osmostat, renal disease, and adrenal insufficiency. A BUN less than 10 mg/dL (Decaux, 1980), a serum creatinine of less than 1 mg/dL, and a serum urate of less than 4.0 mg/dL (Beck, 1979) are all suggestive of normal circulating volume.

## Treatment

In the treatment of hyponatremia, the plasma sodium concentration should be raised at a safe rate while treating the underlying cause. Treatment involves the administration of sodium to volume-depleted patients and restriction of water intake in normovolemic and edematous patients. Water is removed in hyponatremic states with normal or increased body sodium content. Vigorous therapy with hypertonic saline is required with acute hyponatremia (developing over 1–3 days) when symptoms are present or the sodium concentration is less than 110 mEq/liter.

Overly rapid correction of hyponatremia can be harmful, leading to central demyelinating lesions (central pontine myelinolysis). This is characterized by paraparesis or quadriparesis, dysarthria, dysphagia, coma, and less commonly, seizures. It is best diagnosed by magnetic resonance imaging, but it may not be detected radiologically for 4 weeks (Sterns, 1990). The risk of central pontine myelinolysis is lower in patients with acute hyponatremia who have cerebral edema. To minimize this complication, chronic hyponatremia should be corrected at a speed of less than 0.5 mEq/liter/hr (Sterns, 1986). The degree of correction over the first day ($< 12$ mEq/liter), however, seems to be more important than the rate at which it is infused (Soupart, 1992). Rapid correction at a rate of 1.5 to 2.0 mEq/liter/hr (for 3–4 hours) should be restricted to only those patients with acute symptomatic hyponatremia. With concomitant hypokalemia, replacement potassium may raise the plasma sodium at close to the maximum rate (Kamel, 1993); therefore, the appropriate treatment is 0.45% sodium chloride containing 40 mEq of potassium in each liter.

For rapid replacement of sodium depletion in patients with symptomatic hypo-osmolality, the IV administration of sodium as hypertonic saline

T A B L E    **4-4**

Neurologic symptoms associated with an acute reduction in plasma sodium

| Plasma Sodium Level (mEq/liter) | Symptoms |
| --- | --- |
| 120–125 | Nausea, malaise |
| 115–120 | Headache, lethargy, obtundation |
| < 115 | Seizures, coma |

will effectively correct the hypo-osmolality. The sodium needed to raise the sodium concentration to a chosen level is approximated to 0.5 × lean body weight (kg) × (Na), where Na is the desired serum sodium minus the actual serum sodium. Sodium may be administered as a 3% or 5% sodium chloride solution.

With hyponatremia secondary to excess water accumulation, the water may be removed rapidly by administration of IV furosemide together with hypertonic saline. Furosemide results in the loss of water and sodium, but the latter is given back as hypertonic saline, with the net result being a loss of water only (Hartman, 1973). In extreme cases, peritoneal dialysis or hemodialysis may be required. The usual adult starting dose of furosemide for this purpose is 40 mg IV. The same dose can be repeated at 2- to 4-hour intervals while hypertonic saline is being given. Potassium supplements are usually needed with this therapy.

Chronic hyponatremia may be treated by water restriction or by an increase in renal water excretion. Water restriction may be difficult to achieve in patients with heart failure. In these and similar patients, administration of a loop diuretic such as furosemide, in conjunction with an angiotensin-converting enzyme inhibitor (Packer, 1984), is effective.

## Hypernatremia

*Hypernatremia* is defined as an increased sodium concentration in plasma water. Because sodium is an effective osmole, it represents hyperosmolality. The increased $P_{osm}$ results in water moving extracellularly with cellular dehydration occurring. However, the extracellular volume in hypernatremia may be normal, decreased, or increased (Oh, 1992).

### *Etiology*

Hypernatremia represents water loss, sodium retention, or a combination of both (Table 4-5). Loss of water is due to either increased loss or reduced intake, and gain of sodium is due to either increased intake or reduced renal excretion. The cause of hypernatremia is often iatrogenic (e.g., from hypertonic saline infusion or

T A B L E    **4-5**

Common causes of hypernatremia

*Water Loss*
Insensible loss: burns, respiratory infections, exercise
Gastrointestinal loss: gastroenteritis, malabsorption syndromes, osmotic diarrhea
Renal loss: central diabetes insidious (Sheehan's syndrome, cardiopulmonary arrest), nephrogenic diabetes insipidus (pregnancy, X-linked recessive, sickle-cell disease, renal failure, drugs [lithium, diuresis with mannitol, or glucose])

*Decreased Water Intake*
Hypothalamic disorders
Loss of consciousness
Limited access to water or inability to drink it

*Sodium Retention*
Increased intake of sodium or administration of hypertonic solutions

accidental entry into maternal circulation during abortion with hypertonic saline). The body maintains the $P_{osm}$ in the range of 280 to 290 mosm/kg by release of ADH and stimulation of thirst via hypothalamic receptors. Free water is lost from the skin, the respiratory tract, and in dilute urine. Thus, hypernatremia will occur in this situation only if the individual is unable to ask for water (Robertson, 1984). Dilute urine may result from decreased secretion of ADH (central diabetes insipidus [CDI]) (Leaf, 1979) or end-organ resistance (nephrogenic diabetes insipidus [NDI]) (Culpepper, 1983). Reduced renal sodium excretion leading to sodium gain and hypernatremia is most commonly observed in patients who are water-depleted.

### *Clinical Presentation*

The symptoms are primarily neurologic. The earliest findings are lethargy, weakness, and irritability. These may progress to seizures, coma, and death (Arieff, 1976; Ross, 1969). It is often difficult to discern whether the symptoms are secondary to neurologic disease or hypernatremia. Patients also may exhibit signs of volume expansion or volume depletion. With diabetes insipidus, the patient may complain of nocturia, polyuria, and polydipsia.

## Diagnosis

Hypernatremia usually occurs in patients with altered mental status; therefore, obtaining a good history is difficult. Physical examination should help to evaluate the volume status of the patient as well as demonstrate any focal neurologic abnormalities. The urine sp gr of less than 1.010 usually indicates diabetes insipidus. Administration of ADH in this situation will differentiate CDI (increased sp gr with decreased urine volume) from NDI (no change) (Miller, 1970). An sp gr greater than 1.023 is often seen with excessive insensible or gastrointestinal water losses, primary hypodipsia, and excessive administration of hypertonic fluids. Urine volume should be recorded, because volumes in excess of 5 liters/day are seen only with lithium toxicity, primary polydipsia, hypercalcemia, CDI, and congenital NDI. A water restriction test may be the only way to differentiate the etiologies of CDI and NDI.

## Management

Hypernatremia is treated by either the addition of water or removal of sodium, the choice of which depends on the status of the body sodium and water content. If water depletion is the cause of hypernatremia, water is added. If sodium excess is the cause, sodium needs to be removed. Rapid correction of hypernatremia can cause cerebral edema, seizures, permanent neurologic damage, and death (Pollock, 1980). The plasma sodium content should be lowered slowly to normal unless the patient has symptomatic hypernatremia.

Hypernatremia is generally secondary to water loss; therefore, calculation of the water deficit is essential. The water deficit can be estimated from the following equation:

Water deficit = Body weight (kg) $\times$ 0.55 $\times$ Na/Na$_b$

where Na$_b$ is the desired serum sodium level and Na is the difference between the desired and observed serum sodium. This relationship allows calculation of the volume of fluid replacement necessary to reduce the sodium to the desired level. In acute symptomatic hypernatremia, serum sodium may be reduced by 6 to 8 mEq/liter in the first 3 to 4 hours, but thereafter the rate of decline should not exceed 0.5 mEq/liter/hr. As with hyponatremia, chronic hypernatremia usually does not cause CNS symptoms and therefore does not require rapid correction. As with hyponatremia, a safe rate of correction is 0.7 mEq/liter/hr or 12 mEq/liter/day (Blum, 1986). The type of fluid administered to correct losses depends on the patient's clinical state. Dextrose in water (either orally or IV) can be given in patients with pure water loss. If sodium depletion is also present, such as in vomiting and diarrhea, 0.25 N saline is recommended. In hypotensive patients, normal saline should be used until tissue perfusion has been corrected; thereafter, a more dilute saline solution should be used.

In patients with excess sodium, the restoration of normal volume usually initiates natriuresis, but if natriuresis does not occur promptly, sodium may be removed with diuretics. Furosemide with a 5% dextrose solution can be used in this situation, but care must be taken not to allow serum sodium concentration to decline too rapidly. Furosemide can be administered at a dose of up to 60 mg IV every 2 to 4 hours. Patients with renal failure can be treated with dialysis.

Central diabetes insipidus is treated with the administration of exogenous ADH. Desmopressin (dDAVP) can be administered as a nasal spray, subcutaneously, or IV (Robinson, 1976). Desmopressin is usually used as a 0.2-mL nasal spray once or twice a day, which is then titrated to ensure an adequate urine output. Acute CDI can be treated with injectable dDAVP administered subcutaneously or IV at a rate of 2 to 4 µg daily in two to three divided doses. Although ADH is the treatment of choice, other drugs can be given to lower the urine output. Thiazide diuretics can be given in a dose of 12.5 to 25.0 mg once or twice daily. They work by increasing weight loss, which then reduces urine output. With this therapy, the patient should be placed on a low-sodium diet. The addition of amiloride will help restrict thiazide-induced hypokalemia (Knoers, 1990). Chlorpropamide is an oral hypoglycemic agent that will enhance the action of ADH and thus can also be combined with ADH. The usual dose is 125 to 250 mg/day. Both clofibrate and carbamazapine have been used effectively to decrease urine output in partial CDI.

Nephrogenic diabetes insipidus will not respond to ADH, dDAVP, or drugs that depend on ADH for their action. Patients should be treated with a thiazide diuretic combined with a low-sodium, low-protein diet. Subjects with primary hypodipsia should be educated to drink on schedule. Stimulation of the thirst center with chlorpropamide has met with some success in these patients (Bode, 1971).

## Hypokalemia

The average adult contains about 3500 mEq potassium (Brown, 1986; Smith, 1985). Potassium is a predominantly intracellular ion, with less than 2% extracellular. Plasma potassium (K) is thus a poor indicator of total potassium; however, it is the plasma concentrations that usually reflect the total body stores of potassium and that are of real importance when guiding therapy. Hypokalemia is usually the result of potassium depletion, but it also may occur without depletion if there is a shift into cells, as occurs in alkalotic states. *Hypokalemia* is defined as a serum potassium concentration below 3.5 mEq/liter.

### *Etiology*

Hypokalemia can be classified according to three basic mechanisms: redistribution within the body, reduced potassium intake, or increased loss from the body (Table 4-6). Potassium is continuously lost from the cell down a concentration gradient. This loss is opposed by the sodium pump at the surface, which pumps sodium out of the cell in exchange for potassium and hydrogen ions. The activity of the sodium pump is increased by metabolic alkalosis and glucose and insulin (Scribner, 1956). Alkalosis also increases potassium secretion in the distal tubules of the kidneys, probably because of competition between potassium and hydrogen ions for receptor sites.

Increased loss from the body is due to either renal or gastrointestinal losses. There are numerous causes of renal loss, but the two most constant factors are increased sodium delivery to the distal nephron and increased mineralocorticoid activity. Increased sodium delivery occurs with chronic diuretic therapy and primary hyperaldo-

T A B L E   **4-6**
Causes of hypokalemia

***Redistribution Within the Body***
Glucose and insulin therapy
Acute alkalosis or correction of acute acidosis
$B_2$ agonists
Familial periodic paralysis
Barium poisoning

***Reduced Intake***
Chronic starvation

***Increased Loss***
Gastrointestinal loss
    Prolonged vomiting or nasogastric suction
    Diarrhea or intestinal fistula
Renal loss
    Primary hypoaldosteronism
    Secondary hypoaldosteronism (renal artery stenosis, diuretic therapy, malignant hypertension)
    Cushing's syndrome and steroid therapy
    Carbenoxolone
    Licorice-containing substances
    Renal tubular acidosis
    Acute myelocytic and monocytic leukemia
    Magnesium deficiency

steronism. Hypomagnesemia probably causes hypokalemia by increasing aldosterone production, but the mechanism is unclear (Francisco, 1981). Gastrointestinal losses include vomiting and nasogastric suction. The hypokalemia caused is not only due to direct loss of potassium from the stomach but is also attributable to the renal bicarbonate wasting that occurs with metabolic alkalosis.

### *Clinical Presentation*

Muscle weakness, hypotonia, and mental status changes may occur when the serum potassium is below 2.5 mEq/liter. ECG changes occur 50% of the time with hypokalemia (Flakeb, 1986) and involve a decrease in T-wave amplitude and the development of prominent U waves. Hypokalemia does not produce serious arrhythmias but can potentiate arrhythmias due to digitalis toxicity (Flakeb, 1986).

### *Diagnosis*

After obtaining a history and physical examination, serum and urine electrolytes plus serum calcium and magnesium should be obtained. The urine potassium will help differentiate renal from extrarenal losses. A urine potassium below 30 mEq/liter signifies extrarenal losses, seen commonly in patients with diarrhea or redistribution within the body (see Table 4-6). A urine potassium of greater than 30 mEq/liter is seen with renal losses. In this situation, a serum bicarbonate will help separate renal tubular acidosis (<24 mEq/liter) from other causes. A urine chloride less than 10 mEq/liter is seen with vomiting, nasogastric suctioning, and overventilation. A level greater than 10 mEq/liter is seen with diuretic and steroid therapy.

## Management

Hypokalemia is treated either by the administration of potassium or by preventing the renal loss of potassium. Once the potassium falls below 3.5 mEq/liter, there is already a 200-mEq deficit in potassium; therefore, any additional decrease in potassium is significant regardless of the magnitude (Marino, 1991c).

If the serum potassium level is below 2.5 mEq/liter, clinical symptoms or ECG changes are generally present, and one should initiate IV therapy. While it is theoretically useful to estimate the potassium deficit prior to initiating therapy, such calculations are of limited value because they can vary considerably secondary to transcellular shifts. As a rough estimate, a serum potassium of 3.0 mEq/liter is associated with a potassium deficit of 350 mEq, and a potassium level of 2.0 mEq/liter with a deficit of 700 mEq. The recommended IV replacement dose is 0.7 mEq/kg lean body weight over 1 to 2 hours (Smith, 1985). In obese patients, 30 mEq/m$^2$ body surface area is administered. The dose should not increase the serum potassium by more than 1.0 to 1.5 mEq/liter unless an acidosis is present. In life-threatening situations, a rate in excess of 100 mEq/hr may be needed (Smith, 1985). If aggressive replacement therapy does not correct the serum potassium, magnesium depletion should be considered and the magnesium then replaced.

With an underlying metabolic alkalosis, one should use potassium chloride for replacement of hypokalemia. The chloride salt is necessary to correct the alkalosis, which otherwise would result in the administered potassium being lost in the urine. When rapidly replacing potassium chloride, glucose-containing solutions should not be used because they will stimulate release of insulin, which will drive potassium into the cells. Potassium at concentrations exceeding 40 mEq/liter may produce pain at the infusion site and may lead to sclerosis of smaller vessels; thus, it is advisable to split the dosage and administer each portion via a separate peripheral vein. One should avoid central venous infusion of potassium at high concentrations because this can produce life-threatening cardiotoxicity.

Renal loss of potassium is prevented either by treating its cause or by the administration of potassium-sparing diuretics. Spironolactone (25–150 mg twice a day), triamterine (50–100 mg twice a day) or amiloride (5–20 mg/day) is effective in reducing potassium loss. Amiloride should be administered with food to avoid gastric irritation. Mild potassium loss can be replaced orally in the form of potassium chloride or $KPO_4$.

## Hyperkalemia

Hyperkalemia is defined as a serum potassium greater than 5.5 mEq/liter. Because of its potential for producing dysrhythmias, hyperkalemia should be managed far more aggressively than hypokalemia. *Pseudohyperkalemia* is defined as an increase in potassium concentration only in the local blood vessel or in vitro and has no physiologic consequences. Hemolysis during venipuncture, thrombocytosis (greater than 1 million/$\mu$L), and severe leukocytosis (over 50,000) cause pseudohyperkalemia. Pseudohypokalemia should always be investigated immediately, with careful attention paid to avoiding cell trauma during blood collection. Both thrombocytosis and leukocytosis release potassium from the platelets and WBC during blood clotting (Hartman, 1958; Robertson, 1984). Suspected pseudohyperkalemia should be investigated by obtaining simultaneous serum potassium specimens from clotted and unclotted specimens. The potassium in the clotted sample should be 0.3 mEq/liter higher than in the unclotted specimen.

## Etiology

The causes of hyperkalemia can be classified according to three basic mechanisms: redistribution within the body, increased potassium intake, or reduced renal potassium excretion (Table 4-7). Severe tissue injury leads to direct release of potassium due to disruption of cell membranes. Rhabdomyolysis and hemolysis cause hyperkalemia only when causing renal failure. Metabolic acidosis results in increased potassium shift across membranes, with reduced renal excretion of potassium. This can increase the serum potassium by up to 1 mEq/liter (Smith, 1985). Hyperkalemia is less predictable with organic causes of acidosis, such as diabetic and lactic acidosis, when compared with the inorganic causes of acidosis (Oster, 1978). Respiratory acidosis does not often produce hyperkalemia. Digitalis toxicity leads to disruption of the membrane sodium-potassium pump, which normally keeps potassium intracellular (Bismuth, 1973).

Diminished renal potassium excretion is due to either renal failure, reduced aldosterone or aldosterone responsiveness, or reduced distal delivery of sodium. Renal failure usually does not cause hyperkalemia until the glomerular filtration rate is below 10 mL/min or urine output is

T A B L E   4-7
### Causes of hyperkalemia

***Redistribution Within the Body***
Severe tissue damage (e.g., myonecrosis)
Insulin deficiency
Metabolic acidosis
Digitalis toxicity
Severe acute starvation
Hypoxia

***Increased Potassium Intake***
Overenthusiastic potassium therapy
Failure to stop therapy when depletion corrected

***Reduced Renal Excretion of Potassium***
Adrenal insufficiency
Drugs
   Angiotensin-converting enzyme inhibitors
   Potassium-sparing diuretics
   Nonsteroidal antiinflammatory agents
   Heparin
Renal glomerular failure

less than 1 liter/day (Williams, 1988). Deficiency of aldosterone may be due to an absence of hormone, such as occurs in Addison's disease, or may be part of a selective process, such as occurs in hyporeninemic hypoaldosteronism, which is the most common cause of chronic hyperkalemia (Phelps, 1980). Heparin in a small dose can reversibly inhibit aldosterone synthesis causing hypokalemia. Angiotensin-converting enzyme inhibitors, potassium-sparing diuretics, and nonsteroidal antiinflammatory agents limit the supply of renin or angiotensin II, resulting in decreased aldosterone and hyperkalemia. Severe dehydration may result in the delivery of sodium to the distal nephron being markedly reduced with the development of hyperkalemia (Oh, 1982).

## Clinical Presentation

Skeletal muscle and cardiac conduction abnormalities are the dominant features of clinical hyperkalemia. Neuromuscular weakness may occur, with severe flaccid quadriplegia being reported (Villabona, 1987). Electrocardiogram changes begin when the serum potassium reaches 6.0 mEq/liter and are always abnormal when a serum level of 8.0 mEq/liter is reached (Williams, 1988). The earliest changes are tall, narrow T waves on precordial leads V2–4. The T wave in hyperkalemia has a narrow base, which helps to separate it from other causes of tall T waves. As the serum potassium level increases, the P-wave amplitude decreases with lengthening of the PR interval until the P waves disappear. The QRS complex may be prolonged, resulting in ventricular asystole. Occasionally, gastrointestinal symptoms occur.

## Diagnosis

After obtaining a history and physical examination, serum and urine electrolytes plus serum calcium and magnesium should be obtained. The urine potassium will help differentiate renal from extrarenal losses. A urine potassium above 30 mEq/liter suggests a transcellular potassium shift; below this level, reduced renal excretion is suggested.

## Management

Therapy always should be initiated when the serum potassium exceeds 6.0 mEq/liter, irrespective of ECG findings, because ventricular tachycardia can appear without premonitory ECG signs (Smith, 1985). Therapy should be monitored by frequent serum potassium level sampling and ECG. The plan is to acutely manage the hyperkalemia and then achieve and maintain a normal serum level (Table 4-8).

Calcium gluconate is recommended in patients with ECG changes. This agent directly antagonizes the action of potassium and increases the membrane threshold. These effects last only 20 to 30 minutes; therefore, other forms of therapy need to be instituted during this period. In patients not responding to calcium, an insulin-glucose infusion will promote potassium shift into cells, decreasing the serum potassium by 1 mEq after 1 to 2 hours.

Removal of potassium may be accomplished by several routes: through the gastrointestinal tract with a potassium exchange resin given orally or by enema; through the kidney by diuretics, mineralocorticoids, and increased salt intake; or by hemodialysis or peritoneal dialysis. A potassium exchange resin, sodium polystyrene sulfonate (Kayexalate), is more effective when it is given with agents that cause osmotic diarrhea, such as sorbitol or mannitol. One tablespoon of Kayexalate mixed with 100 mL of 10% sorbitol or mannitol can be given by mouth 2 to 4 times a day. A shift of potassium into cells can be accomplished with glucose and insulin or by increasing the blood pH with sodium bicarbonate. Specific

$\beta_2$ agonists such as salbutamol have shown striking efficacy in driving potassium into cells by stimulating the sodium-potassium–dependent adenosine triphosphatase (ATPase). Reduced intake of potassium is an additional measure to be added to any of the methods discussed for the long-term management of hyperkalemia.

## Hypocalcemia

Calcium ($Ca^{2+}$) is the most abundant electrolyte in the human body, 99% of which is in the skeleton. It is involved with all cellular activities involving movement. Calcium is separated into three fractions within blood. Forty percent to 50% circulates bound to protein (albumin accounts for 80% of this binding), 10% is chelated with other ions, and the remainder is the ionized fraction. It is this fraction that is thought to be physiologically active and homeostatically regulated. The normal serum range for the ionized fraction is between 1.1 and 1.3 mM/liter (Marino, 1991a).

The total serum calcium levels may not accurately reflect ionized calcium level. Alterations in the patient's serum albumin concentration can influence the protein-bound fraction, leading to an incorrect assessment of the ionized calcium level. One should always measure the serum albumin level simultaneously and use a correction factor that increases the total calcium by 0.8 mg/dL for each 1-mg/dL decrease in albumin (Kassirer, 1989). For best accuracy, one should measure the ionized calcium directly. In pregnancy, the serum albumin concentrations drop with an increase in ionized calcium activity. The ionized

T A B L E   **4-8**

Management of hyperkalemia

---

***Acute Management***

| | |
|---|---|
| Calcium gluconate | 10 mL (10% solution) IV over 3 minutes; repeat in 5 minutes if no response |
| Insulin-glucose infusion | 10 units regular insulin in 500 mL of 20% dextrose and infuse over 1 hour |
| Sodium bicarbonate | 1–2 ampules (44–88 mEq) over 5 to 10 minutes |
| Furosemide | 40 mg IV, up to 200 mg IV over 2–3 minutes |
| Dialysis | |

***Chronic Management***

| | |
|---|---|
| Kayexalate | Oral: 30 g in 50 mL of 20% sorbitol |
| | Rectal: 50 g in 200 mL of 20% sorbitol retention enema |

calcium level also is influenced by blood pH. Acidosis leads to decreased binding of calcium to the serum proteins with an increase in the ionized calcium level. Alkalosis has the opposite effect. Free fatty acids (FFAs) increase calcium binding to albumin. Serum levels of FFAs are often increased during critical illness as a result of illness-induced elevations in plasma concentrations of epinephrine, glucagon, growth hormone, and corticotrophin, as well as decreases in serum insulin concentrations. Anticoagulants bind calcium in the blood sample and so should be avoided. Hypernatremia decreases calcium binding to serum proteins, whereas hyponatremia has the opposite effect (Zaloga, 1985a). The serum ionized calcium value in patients on hemodialysis may be altered depending on the calcium concentration of the dialysate (Heinrich 1984; Maynard, 1986; Zaloga, 1986).

## Etiology

The most common causes of hypocalcemia include both metabolic and respiratory alkalosis, sepsis, magnesium depletion, and renal failure (Table 4-9). Magnesium deficiency is common in critically ill patients and also may cause hypocalcemia (Anast, 1976; Zaloga, 1987c). Magnesium reduces serum calcium by inhibiting parathyroid hormone (PTH) secretion, reduces the end-organ response to PTH, and causes vitamin D resistance

T A B L E    **4-9**
**Common causes of hypocalcemia**

Acid-base disorders
    Respiratory and metabolic alkalosis
Shock
Renal failure
Malabsorption syndromes
Magnesium depletion
Hypoparathyroidism
    Surgically produced
    Idiopathic
Pancreatitis
Massive blood transfusion
Fat embolism syndrome
Drugs
    Heparin, aminoglycosides, cis-platinum, phenytoin, phenobarbital, and loop diuretics

(Benabe, 1987; Medalle, 1976; Miravet, 1980; Rude, 1976). One cannot correct a calcium deficiency until the magnesium deficit has been corrected.

Sepsis can lead to hypocalcemia, presumably as a result of calcium efflux across a disrupted microcirculation (Zaloga, 1987a). This effect may be linked to an underlying respiratory alkalosis; this combination confers a poor prognosis. Hypocalcemia commonly is seen in patients with acute pancreatitis and also is associated with a poor prognosis (Zaloga, 1985b). Renal failure leads to phosphorous retention, which may cause hypocalcemia as a result of calcium precipitation, inhibition of bone resorption, and suppression of renal 1-hydroxylation of vitamin D (Chernow, 1981; Zaloga, 1990b). Thus, the treatment of hypocalcemia in this setting is to lower the serum $PO_4$ level. Citrated blood (massive blood transfusion), albumin, and radiocontrast dyes are the most common chelators that cause hypocalcemia in critically ill patients. Primary hypoparathyroidism is seen rarely, whereas secondary hypoparathyroidism after neck surgery is a common cause of hypocalcemia (Nagant, 1978).

## Clinical Presentation

Hypocalcemia may present with a variety of clinical signs and symptoms. The most common manifestations are caused by increased neuronal irritability and decreased cardiac contractility (Zaloga, 1985a,b). Neuronal symptoms include seizures, weakness, muscle spasm, paresthesias, tetany, and Chvostek's and Trousseau's signs. Neither Chvostek's nor Trousseau's signs are sensitive or specific (Zaloga, 1985a). Cardiovascular manifestations include hypotension, cardiac insufficiency, bradycardia, arrhythmias, left ventricular failure, and cardiac arrest. Electrocardiogram findings include Q-T and S-T interval prolongation and T-wave inversion. Other clinical findings include anxiety, irritability, confusion, brittle nails, dry scaly skin, and brittle hair.

## Diagnosis

A complete history and physical examination are required. Serum electrolyte, calcium (total and ionized), magnesium, $PO_4$, and albumin levels should be obtained, and renal function should be evaluated. Measurement of thyroid hormone and thyroid-stimulating hormone (TSH) should be obtained if suggested by the history and physical examination, and an ECG should be evaluated.

### Treatment

All patients with an ionized calcium concentration below 0.8 mM/liter should receive treatment. Life-threatening arrhythmias can develop when the ionized calcium level approaches 0.5 to 0.65 mM/liter. Acute symptomatic hypocalcemia is a medical emergency that necessitates IV calcium therapy (Table 4-10). With acute symptoms, a calcium bolus can be given at an initial dose of 100 to 200 mg IV over 10 minutes, followed by a continuous infusion of 1 to 2 mg/kg/hr. This will raise the serum total calcium by 1 mg/dL, with levels returning to baseline by 30 minutes after injection. Intravenous calcium preparations are irritating to veins and should be diluted (10-mL vial in 100 mL of D5W and warmed to body temperature). If IV access is not available, calcium gluceptate may be given intramuscularly (IM) (Haynes, 1985).

Anticonvulsant drugs, sedation, and paralysis may help eliminate signs of neuronal irritability. Once the serum calcium is in the low normal range, oral replacement with enteral calcium is recommended.

### Hypercalcemia

Hypercalcemia occurs uncommonly and is usually asymptomatic. It (ionized calcium > 1.3 mM/liter) occurs when calcium enters the vascular space faster than it can be excreted or sequestered.

T A B L E    **4-10**

**Calcium preparations**

| Parenteral | Rate |
| --- | --- |
| Calcium gluconate | 1.0 mL/min |
| Calcium chloride | 0.5 mL/min |

| Oral | Contents |
| --- | --- |
| Calcium carbonate | 500 mg calcium |
| Calcium gluconate | 500 mg calcium |

### Etiology

The most common cause of hypercalcemia in an intensive care setting is malignancy, while primary hyperparathyroidism is the most common cause in the general population (Table 4-11). Ten percent to 20% of patients with malignancy develop hypercalcemia because of direct tumor osteolysis of bone and secretion of humoral substances that stimulate bone resorption (Benabe, 1987; Mundy, 1989).

### Clinical Presentation

General features such as constipation, anorexia, nausea, and vomiting are common. The cardiovascular effects of hypercalcemia include hypertension and arrhythmias with Q-T shortening seen on ECG. Hypercalcemia can lead to nephrocalcinosis, nephrolithiasis, and renal tubular dysfunction. The predominant neuromuscular manifestations are weakness, atrophy, and hyporeflexia. Personality changes, memory impairment, psychosis, disorientation, coma, seizures, and EEG abnormalities also may occur in some patients.

### Diagnosis

A complete history and physical examination should be obtained. Serum electrolyte, total and ionized calcium, magnesium, $PO_4$, and albumin

T A B L E    **4-11**

**Common causes of hypercalcemia**

Malignancy
Hyperparathyroidism
Chronic renal failure
Recovery from acute renal failure
Immobilization
Calcium administration
Hypocalciuric hypercalcemia
Granulomatous disease
  Sarcoidosis
  Tuberculosis
Hyperthyroidism
AIDS
Drug-induced
  Lithium, theophylline, thiazides, and vitamin D or A

levels should be obtained. Measurement of thyroid hormone, TSH, and PTH should be obtained if needed, and the ECG should be evaluated. Renal function should be assessed. A 24-hour urine collection for $Ca^{2+}$ and creatinine determinations helps to separate hypocalciuric from hypercalciuric syndromes.

## Treatment

A serum calcium of 13 mg/dL or higher needs to be treated. Acute therapy is required in the obtunded or comatose patient (Table 4-12). Hypercalcemia leads to hyperuricemia with concomitant volume depletion and further elevation in the serum calcium level. Aggressive volume replacement will often lead to correction of serum calcium by expansion of intravascular volume, which dilutes the calcium concentration in the blood and promotes renal flow (Baker, 1992; Hosking, 1981). Renal calcium excretion can be enhanced with the use of saline and loop diuretics. Furosemide can be given in doses of 40 to 100 mg every 2 hours and adjusted to maintain a urine output of 200 to 300 mL/hr. Urine output needs to be closely monitored, and all urinary losses should be replaced with saline.

Calcium may be acutely lowered by agents that inhibit bone resorption (Silva, 1973). Synthetic salmon-calcitonin has the greatest potency and can return serum calcium levels to normal in 2 to 3 hours (Roswell, 1987). Normal dosage is 4 units/kg IM or two doses subcutaneously 12 hours apart. It is useful in treating patients with CHF or renal failure in whom large quantities of saline are contraindicated. Mithramycin is an antineoplastic agent that also inhibits bone resorption. It is administered as a 25-μg/kg dose given IV or as a 6-hour infusion. This dose can be repeated in 2 days. The response takes from 24 to 36 hours to appear (Roswell, 1987).

Chelators such as phosphates also can be used in the management of hypercalcemic emergencies. They bind and precipitate $Ca^{2+}$, inhibit bone resorption, and decrease renal activation of vitamin D. Intravenous phosphates should not be given in doses exceeding 50 mM over 6 to 8 hours. The serum $Ca^{2+}$ may fall from 1 to 6 mg/dL, depending on the dose of $PO_4$ administered. This effect is usually seen within 6 to 24 hours. When administered rectally or orally (500–1000 mg every 6 hours), several days are required for maximum effect. Calcium channel blockers such as verapamil can be used in patients with life-threatening effects on the cardiovascular system (Zaloga, 1987b). Hemodialysis is indicated when all other measures have failed (Cardella, 1979; Roswell, 1987).

## Hypomagnesemia

Magnesium ($Mg^{2+}$) is the second most abundant intracellular cation in the body. It is a cofactor for all enzyme reactions involved in the splitting of high-energy adenosine triphosphate bonds required for the activity of phosphatases. Such enzymes are essential and provide energy for the sodium-potassium ATPase pump, proton pump, calcium ATPase pump, neurochemical transmission, muscle contraction, glucose-fat-protein metabolism, oxidative phosphorylation, and DNA synthesis (Quamme, 1987; Salem, 1991; Zaloga,

T A B L E   **4-12**

**Acute management of hypercalcemia**

| Agent | Dose | Comments |
|---|---|---|
| Furosemide and saline | 40–100 mg IV q 2 hr | Need to maintain urine output at 200–300 mL/hr |
| Calcitonin | 4 units/kg IM or SQ q 12 hr | Nausea and vomiting |
| Mithramycin | 25 μg/kg IV q 2 days | Nausea and vomiting |
| Phosphates | 25–50 mM/6–8 hrs IV | Monitor electrolytes, replace urine output |
| Verapamil | 5–10 mg IV | |
| Nifedipine | 10–20 mg sublingually | |
| Hemodialysis | | Use when all other management fails |

1990a). Mg is also required for the activity of adenylate cyclase.

Magnesium is not distributed uniformly within the body. Less than 1% of total body magnesium is found in the serum, with 50% to 60% found in the skeleton and 20% in muscle (Quamme, 1987). Serum levels, thus, may not reflect true intracellular stores accurately and may be normal in the face of magnesium depletion or excess (Reinhart, 1988; Zaloga, 1990a). In the blood, there are three fractions: an ionized fraction (55%), which is physiologically active and homeostatically regulated; a protein-bound fraction (30%); and a chelated fraction (15%).

Magnesium depletion is one of the most common electrolyte abnormalities in hospitalized patients. The normal magnesium concentration is between 1.7 and 2.4 mg/dL (1.4–2.0 mEq/liter); however, a normal reading should not deter one from considering hypomagnesemia in the presence of a suggestive clinical presentation (Marino, 1991b).

### Etiology

Increased renal losses secondary to the use of diuretics and aminoglycosides constitute the most common cause of magnesium loss in a hospital setting (Table 4-13). Diuretics such as furosemide and ethacrynic acid and aminoglycosides inhibit magnesium reabsorption in the loop of Henle and also block absorption at this site, leading to increased urinary losses (Ryan, 1987). Up to 30% of patients receiving aminoglycosides will develop hypomagnesemia (Elin, 1988).

Hypomagnesemia can result from internal redistribution of magnesium. Following the administration of glucose or amino acids, magnesium shifts into cells (Berkelhammer, 1985; Brauthbar, 1987). A similar effect is seen with increased catecholamine levels, correction of acidosis, and hungry bone syndromes. Lower gastrointestinal tract secretions are rich in magnesium; thus, severe diarrhea leads to hypomagnesemia.

### Clinical Presentation

The signs and symptoms of hypomagnesemia are very similar to those of hypocalcemia and hy-

T A B L E    4-13

Common causes of hypomagnesemia

Drug-induced
  Diuretics (furosemide, thiazides, mannitol)
  Aminoglycosides
  Neoplastic agents (cis-platinum, carbenicillin,
    cyclosporine)
  Amphotericin B
  Digoxin
  Thyroid hormone
  Insulin
Malabsorption, laxative abuse, fistulas
Malnutrition
Hyperalimentation and prolonged IV therapy
Renal losses
  Glomerulonephritis, interstitial nephritis
  Tubular disorders
Hyperthyroidism
Diabetic ketoacidosis
Pregnancy and lactation
Sepsis
Hypothermia
Burns
Blood transfusion (citrate)

pokalemia, and it is not entirely clear whether hypomagnesemia alone is responsible for these symptoms (Kingston, 1986; Zaloga, 1989). Most symptomatic patients have levels below 1.0 mg/dL. Cardiovascular symptoms include hypertension, heart failure, arrhythmias, increased risk for digitalis toxicity, and decreased pressor response (Abraham, 1987; Berkelhammer, 1985; Brauthbar, 1987; Burch, 1977; Iseri, 1975; Rasmussen, 1986). The ECG may demonstrate a prolonged P-R and Q-T interval with S-T depression. Tall, peaked T waves occur early and slowly broaden with decreased amplitude together with the development of a widened QRS interval as the magnesium level falls. As with hypocalcemia, there is increased neuronal irritability with weakness, muscle spasms, tremors, seizures, tetany, confusion, psychosis, and coma. Patients also complain of anorexia, nausea, and abdominal cramps.

### Diagnosis

Following a complete history, physical examination, and ECG, serum electrolyte, calcium, magnesium, and $PO_4$ levels are obtained. A 24-hour urine magnesium measurement is helpful in separating renal from nonrenal causes. An increased urinary magnesium level suggests increased renal loss of magnesium as the etiology of hypomagnesemia.

### Treatment

Patients with life-threatening arrhythmias, acute symptomatic hypomagnesemia, or severe hypomagnesemia are best treated with IV magnesium sulfate (Cronin, 1983; Flink, 1969; Heath, 1980; Rude, 1981; Salem, 1991; Zaloga, 1990a). A 2-g bolus of magnesium sulfate is administered IV over 1 to 2 minutes, followed by a continuous infusion at a rate of 2 g/hr. After a few hours, this can be reduced to a 0.5- to 1.0-g/hr maintenance infusion. Magnesium chloride is used in patients with concurrent hypocalcemia, because sulfate can bind calcium and worsen the hypocalcemia. During magnesium replacement, one should monitor the serum levels of magnesium, calcium, potassium, and creatinine. Blood pressure, respiratory status, and neurologic status (mental alertness, deep tendon reflexes) should be assessed periodically. As magnesium sulfate is renally excreted, its dose should be reduced in patients with renal insufficiency.

With moderate magnesium deficiency, 50 to 100 mEq magnesium sulfate per day (600–1200 mg elemental magnesium) can be administered in patients without renal insufficiency. Mild asymptomatic magnesium deficiency can also be replaced with diet alone. It can take up to 3 to 5 days to replace intracellular stores.

Magnesium is important for the maintenance of normal potassium metabolism (Whang, 1985; Zaloga, 1990a). Magnesium deficiency can lead to renal potassium wasting, resulting in a cellular potassium deficiency. Magnesium levels must, therefore, be adequate prior to successful correction of potassium deficiency.

## Hypermagnesemia

Hypermagnesemia, like hypomagnesemia, is difficult to detect because of the unreliability of serum levels in predicting clinical symptoms. Hypermagnesemia (serum magnesium >3 mg/dL or 2.4 mEq/liter or 1.2 mmol/liter) occurs in up to 10% of hospitalized patients (Iseri, 1975), most commonly secondary to iatrogenic causes (Mordes, 1977; Rude, 1981; Stewart, 1980; Zaloga, 1990a).

### Etiology

The most common cause of hypermagnesemia is renal failure, usually in combination with excess magnesium ingestion. The most common source of excess magnesium ingestion is magnesium-containing antacids and cathartics. Other causes include diabetic ketoacidosis, pheochromocytoma, hypothyroidism, Addison's disease, lithium intoxication, and magnesium sulfate therapy for preeclampsia and preterm labor.

### Clinical Presentation

Hypermagnesemia can lead to neuromuscular blockade and depress skeletal muscle function. Conduction through the cardiac conducting system is slowed, with ECG changes noted at a serum concentration as low as 5 mEq/liter and heart block seen at 7.5 mEq/liter (Reinhart, 1988). Hypotension is seen at levels between 3.0 and 5.0 mEq/liter and is common at higher levels (Reinhart, 1988). Loss of deep tendon reflexes occurs at a serum concentration of 10 mEq/liter, with respiratory paralysis and general anesthesia occurring at a serum concentration of 15 mEq/liter. Cardiac arrest occurs at a serum concentration of greater than 25 mEq/liter.

### Diagnosis

A complete history, physical examination, ECG, and serum electrolyte, calcium, magnesium, and $PO_4$ levels should be obtained.

### Treatment

Intravenous calcium gluconate (10 mL of 10% solution over 3 minutes) is effective in reversing the physiologic effects of hypermagnesemia (Fassler, 1985). If this fails, hemodialysis is the recommended therapy. In patients who can tolerate fluid therapy, aggressive infusion of IV saline with furosemide may be effective in increasing renal magnesium losses. All agents containing magnesium should be discontinued.

## REFERENCES

Aberg M, Hedner V, Bergentz S. Effect of dextran on factor VIII and platelet function. Ann Surg 1979; 189:243–247.

Abraham AS, Rosenmann D, Kramer M, et al. Magnesium in the prevention of lethal arrhythmias in acute myocardial infarction. Arch Intern Med 1987;147:753.

Anast CS, Winnacker JL, Forte LR, Burns TW. Impaired release of parathyroid hormone in magnesium deficiency. J Clin Endocrinol Metab 1976;42:707.

Anderson RJ, Chung H-M, Kluge R, Schrier RW. Hyponatremia: a prospective analysis of its epidemiology and pathogenetic role of vasopressin. Ann Intern Med 1985;102:164.

Arias F. Expansion of intravascular volume and fetal outcome in patients with chronic hypertension and pregnancy. Am J Obstet Gynecol 1965; 123:610.

Arieff AI. Hyponatremia, convulsions, respiratory arrest, and permanent brain damage after elective surgery in healthy women. N Engl J Med 1986;314:1529.

Arieff AI, Guisado R. Effects on the central nervous system of hypernatremic and hyponatremic states. Kidney Int 1976;10:104.

Arthurson G, Granath K, Thoren L, Wallenius G. The renal excretion of LMW dextran. Acta Clin Scand 1964;127:543–551.

Atik M. Dextran-40 and dextran-70, a review. Arch Surg 1967;94:664–672.

Atik M. The uses of dextran in surgery: a current evaluation. Surgery 1969;65:548–562.

Baker JR, Wray HL. Early management of hypercalcemic crisis: case report and literature review. Milit Med 1982;147:756.

Ballinger WF. Preliminary report on the use of hydroxyethyl starch solution in man. J Surg Res 1966;6:180–183.

Barone JE, Snyder AB. Treatment strategies in shock: use of oxygen transport measurements. Heart Lung 1991;20:81.

Baue AE, Tragus ET, Wolfson SK. Hemodynamic and metabolic effects of Ringer's lactate solution in hemorrhagic shock. Ann Surg 1967; 166:29–38.

Beck LH. Hypouricemia in the syndrome of inappropriate secretion of antidiuretic hormone. N Engl J Med 1979;301:528.

Benabe JE, Martinez-Maldonado R. Disorders of calcium metabolism. In: Maxwell MH, Kleeman CR, Narins RG, eds. Clinical disorders of fluid and electrolyte metabolism. 4th ed. New York: McGraw-Hill, 1987:758.

Berkelhammer C, Bear RA. A clinical approach to common electrolyte problems: hypomagnesemia. Can Med Assoc J 1985;132:360.

Berson SA, Yalow RS. Distribution and metabolism of I131 labeled proteins in man. Fed Proc 1957; 16:13S–18S.

Bismuth C, Gaultier M, Conso F, et al. Hyperkalemia in acute digitalis poisoning: prognostic significance and therapeutic implications. Clin Toxicol 1973;6:153.

Bitterman H, Triolo J, Lefer A. Use of hypertonic saline in the treatment of hemorrhagic shock. Circ Shock 1987;21:271.

Blum D, Brasseur D, Kahn A, Brachet E. Safe oral rehydration of hypertonic dehydration. J Pediatr Gastroenterol Nutr 1986;5:232.

Bode HH, Harley BM, Crawford JD. Restoration of normal drinking behavior by chlorpropamide in patients with hypodipsia and diabetes insipidus. Am J Med 1971;51:304.

Bogan RK, Gale GR, Walton RP. Fate of 14C-label hydroxyethyl starch in animals. Toxicol Appl Pharmacol 1969;15:206–211.

Boon JC, Jesch F, Ring J, et al. Intravascular persistence of hydroxyethyl starch in man. Eur Surg Res 1976;8:497–503.

Brauthbar N, Massry SG. Hypomagnesemia and hypermagnesemia. In: Maxwell MH, Kleeman CR, Narins RG, eds. Clinical disorders of fluid and electrolyte metabolism. 4th ed. New York: McGraw-Hill, 1987:831.

Brown MA, Zammit VC, Lowe SA. Capillary permeability and extracellular fluid volumes in pregnancy-induced hypertension. Clin Sci 1989;77:599.

Brown MA, Zammitt VC, Mitar DM. Extracellular fluid volumes in pregnancy-induced hypertension. J Hypertension 1992;10:61–68.

Brown RS. Extrarenal potassium homeostasis. Kidney Int 1986;30:116–127.

Burch GE, Giles TD. The importance of magnesium deficiency in cardiovascular disease. Am Heart J 1977;94:649.

Cardella CJ, Birkin BL, Rapoport A. Role of dialysis in the treatment of severe hypercalcemia: report of two cases successfully treated with hemodialysis and review of the literature. Clin Nephrol 1979;12:285.

Carey JS, Scharschmidt BF, Culliford AT. Hemodynamic effectiveness of colloid and electrolyte solutions for replacement of simulated operative blood loss. Surg Gynecol Obstet 1970; 131:679–686.

Carrico CJ, Canizaro PC, Shires GT. Fluid resuscitation following injury; rational for the use of balanced salt solutions. Crit Care Med 1976;4:46–54.

Chang JC, Gross HM, Jang NS. Disseminated intravascular coagulation due to intravenous administration of hetastarch. Am J Med Sci 1990; 300:301–303.

Chernow B, Rainey TG, Georges L, O'Brian JT. Iatrogenic hyperphosphatemia: a metabolic consideration in critical care medicine. Crit Care Med 1981;9:772.

Chinitz JL. Pathophysiology and prevention of dextran-40 induced anuria. J Lab Clin Med 1971;77:76–87.

Christensen EI, Moundsback AB. Effects of dextran on lysosomal ultrastructure and protein digestion in renal proximal tubule. Kidney Int 1979;16:301–311.

Coghill TH, Moore EE, Dunn EI. Coagulation changes after albumin resuscitation. Crit Care Med 1981;9:22–26.

Cohn JN, Luria MH, Daddario RC. Studies in clinical shock and hypotension. V. Hemodynamic effects of dextran. Circulation 1967;35:316–326.

Cronin RE, Knochel JP. Magnesium deficiency. Adv Intern Med 1983;28:509.

Cully MD, Larson CP, Silverberg GD. Hetastarch coagulopathy in a neurosurgical patient. Anesthesiology 1987;66:706–707.

Culpepper R, Hebert SC, Andreoli TE. Nephrogenic diabetes insipidus. In: Stanbury JB, Frederickson DS, Goldstein JL, et al, eds. The metabolic basis of inherited disease. 5th ed. New York: McGraw-Hill, 1983:1877–1884.

Curtis SE, Cain SM. Systemic and regional $O_2$ delivery and uptake in bled dogs given hypertonic saline, whole blood, or dextran. Am J Physiol 1992;262:H778–H786.

Damon L, Adams M, Striker RB, et al. Intracranial bleeding during treatment with hydroxyethyl starch. N Engl J Med 1987;317:364–365.

Data JL, Nies AS. Dextran 40. Ann Intern Med 1974;81:500–504.

Dawidson I, Eriksson B. Statistical evaluations of plasma substitutes based on 10 variables. Crit Care Med 1982;10:653–657.

Dawidson I, Eriksson B, Gelin LE. Oxygen consumption and recovery from surgical shock in rats: a comparison on the efficacy of different plasma substitutes. Crit Care Med 1979;7:460–465.

Dawidson I, Gelin LE, Haglind E. Plasma volume, intravascular protein content, hemodynamic and oxygen transport changes during intestinal shock in dogs. Comparison of relative effectiveness of various plasma expanders. Crit Care Med 1980;8:73–80.

Dawidson I, Gelin LE, Hedman L. Hemodilution and recovery from experimental intestinal shock in rats: a comparison of the efficacy of three colloids and one electrolyte solution. Crit Care Med 1981;9:42–46.

Decaux G, Genette F, Mockel J. Hypouremia in the syndrome of inappropriate secretion of antidiuretic hormone. Ann Intern Med 1980;93:716.

DeFelippe J, Timoner J, Velasco IT, et al. Treatment of refractory hypovolemic shock by 7.5% sodium chloride injections. Lancet 1980;2:1002.

Diehl JT, Lester JL, Cosgrove DM. Clinical comparison of hetastarch and albumin in postoperative cardiac patients. Ann Thorac Surg 1982;34:674–679.

Elin RJ. Magnesium metabolism in health and disease. DM 1988;34:173.

Farrow SP, Hall M, Ricketts CR. Changes in the molecular composition of circulating hydroxyethyl starch. Br J Pharmacol 1970;38:725–730.

Fassler CA, Rodriguez RM, Badesch DB, et al. Magnesium toxicity as a cause of hypotension and hypoventilation. Arch Intern Med 1985; 14:1604.

Feest TG. Low molecular weight dextran: a continuing cause of acute renal failure. Br Med J 1976;2:1300.

Ferber HP, Nitsch E, Forster H. Studies on hydroxyethyl starch. Part II: changes of the molecular weight distribution for hydroxyethyl starch types 450/0.7, 450/0.3, 300/0.4, 200/0.7, 200/0.5, 200/0.3, 200/0.1 after infusion in serum and urine of volunteers. Arzneimittelforsch, 1985; 35:615–622.

Flakeb G, Villarread D, Chapman D. Is hypokalemia a cause of ventricular arrhythmias? J Crit Illness 1986;1:66.

Flink EB. Therapy of magnesium deficiency. Ann NY Acad Sci 1969;162:901.

Francisco LL, Sawin LL, DiBona GF. Mechanism of negative potassium balance in the magnesium deficient rat. Proc Soc Exp Biol Med 1981; 168:382.

Fullerton WT, Hytten FE, Klopper AL, et al. A case of quadruplet pregnancy. J Obstet Gynaecol Br Cmwlth 1965;72:791.

Gallery EDM, Hunyor SN, Gyory AZ. Plasma volume contraction: a significant factor in both pregnancy-associated hypertension (preeclampsia) and chronic hypertension in pregnancy. Q J Med 1979;48:593.

Gallery EDM, Brown MA. Volume homeostasis in normal and hypertensive human pregnancy. Clin Obstet Gynecol 1987;1:835.

Gelin LE, Solvell L, Zederfeldt B. Plasma volume expanding effect of low viscous dextran and macrodex. Acta Chir Scand 1961;122:309–322.

Goodlin RC, Quaife MA, Dirksen JW. The significance, diagnosis, and treatment of maternal hypovolemia as associated with fetal/maternal illness. Semin Perinatol 1981;5:163.

Goodlin RC, Anderson JC, Gallagher TE. Relationship between amniotic fluid volume and maternal plasma volume expansion. Am J Obstet Gynecol 1983;146:505.

Granger DN, Gabel JC, Drahe RE, et al. Physiologic basis for the clinical use of albumin solutions. Surg Gynecol Obstet 1978;146:97–104.

Granger DW, Udrich M, Parks DA, et al. Transcapillary exchange during intestinal fluid absorption. In: Sheppard AP, Granger DW, eds. Physiology of the intestinal circulation. New York: Raven, 1984:107.

Grant JP, Custer PB, Thurlow J. Current techniques of nutritional assessment. Surg Clin North Am, 1981;61:437–463.

Gruber VF, Messmer K. Colloids for blood volume support. Prog Surg 1977;15:49–76.

Guyton AC. Textbook of medical physiology. 4th ed. Philadelphia: WB Saunders, 1971:247–251.

Hanshiro PK, Weil MH. Anaphylactic shock in man. Arch Intern Med 1967;119:129.

Hartman D, Rossier B, Zohlman R, et al. Rapid correction of hyponatremia in the syndrome of appropriate secretion of antidiuretic hormone. Ann Intern Med 1973;78:870.

Hartman RC, Auditore JC, Jackson DP. Studies in thrombocytosis. I. Hyperkalemia due to release of potassium from platelets during coagulation. J Clin Invest 1958;37:699.

Haupt MT, Rackow EC. Colloid osmotic pressure and fluid resuscitation with hetastarch, albumin and saline solutions. Crit Care Med 1982; 10:159–162.

Hauser CJ, Shoemaker WC, Turpin I. Oxygen transport responses to colloids and crystalloids in critically ill surgical patients. Surg Gynecol Obstet 1980;150:811–816.

Haynes RC, Murad F. Agents affecting calcification: calcium, parathyroid hormone, calcitonin, vitamin D, and other compounds. In: Gilman AG, Goodman LS, Rall TW, Murad F, eds. The pharmacological basis of therapeutics. New York: Macmillan, 1985:1517.

Heath DA. The emergency management of disorders of calcium and magnesium. Clin Endocrinol Metab 1980;9:487.

Henrich WL, Hunt JM, Nixon JV. Increased ionized calcium and left ventricular contractility during hemodialysis. N Engl J Med 1984;310:19.

Hess J, Dubick MA, Summary JJ, et al. The effects of 7.5% NaCl/6% dextran-70 on coagulation and platelet aggregation in humans. J Trauma 1992; 32:40–44.

Hofer RE, Lanier WL. Effect of hydroxyethyl starch solutions on blood glucose concentrations in diabetic and nondiabetic rats. Crit Care Med 1992;20:211–215.

Hohn DC, Makay RD, Holliday B, et al. The effect of oxygen tension on microbicidal function of leukocytes in wounds and in vitro. Surg Forum 1976;27:18.

Holcroft JW, Trunkey DD. Extravascular lung water following hemorrhagic shock in the baboon: comparison between resuscitation with Ringer's lactate and plasmanate. Ann Surg 1974; 180:408–417.

Hosking DJ, Cowley A, Bucknall CA. Rehydration in the treatment of severe hypercalcemia. Q J Med 1981;22:473.

Hytten FE, Paintin DB. Increase in plasma volume during normal pregnancy. J Obstet Gynaecol Br Cmwlth, 1973;70:402.

Iseri LT, Freed J, Bures AR. Magnesium deficiency and cardiac disorders. Am J Med 1975;58:837.

Kamel KS, Bear RA. Treatment of hyponatremia: a quantitative analysis. Am J Kidney Dis 1993; 21:439.

Kassirer JP, Hricik DE, Cohen JJ. Repairing body fluids. Philadelphia: WB Saunders, 1989:73.

Kaufman BS, Rackow EC, Falk JL. The relationship between oxygen delivery and consumption during fluid resuscitation of hypovolemic and septic shock. Chest 1984;85:336.

Khosropour R, Lackner F, Steinbereithnerk J, et al. Comparison of the effect of pre- and intraoperative administration of medium molecular weight hydroxyethyl starch (HES 200/0.5) and dextran 40 (60) in vascular surgery. Anaesthesist 1980;29:616–622.

Kilian J, Spilker D, Borst R. Effect of 6% hydroxyethyl starch, 4.5% dextran 60 and 5.5% oxypolygelatine on blood volume and circulation in human volunteers. Anaesthesist 1975;24: 193–197.

Kingston ME, Al-Siba'i MB, Skooge WC. Clinical manifestations of hypomagnesemia. Crit Care Med 1986;14:950.

Kirklin JK, Lell WA, Kouchoukos NT. Hydroxyethyl starch vs. albumin for colloid infusion following cardiopulmonary bypass in patients undergoing myocardial revascularization. Ann Thorac Surg 1984;37:40–46.

Knoers N, Monnens LAH. Amiloride-hydrochlorothiazide versus indomethacin-hydrochlorothiazide in the treatment of nephrogenic diabetes insipidus. J Pediatr 1990;117:499.

Kohler H, Kirch W, Horstmann HJ. Hydroxyethyl starch-induced macroamylasemia. Int J Clin Pharmacol 1977;15:428–431.

Korttila K, Grohn P, Gordin A, et al. Effect of hydroxyethyl starch and dextran on plasma volume and blood hemostasis and coagulation. J Clin Pharmacol 1984;24:273–282.

Kovalik SG, Ledgerwood AM, Lucas CE. The cardiac effect of altered calcium homeostasis after albumin resuscitation. J Trauma 1981;21:275–279.

Kreimeier U, Frey L, Dentz J, et al. Hypertonic saline dextran resuscitation during the initial phase of acute endotoxemia: effect on regional blood flow. Crit Care Med 1991;19:801–809.

Ladenson JK, Apple FS, Koch DD. Misleading hyponatremia due to hyperlipemia: a method-dependent error. Ann Intern Med 1981;95:707.

Laks H, Pilon RN, Anderson W, et al. Acute normovolemic hemodilution with crystalloid vs colloid replacement. Surg Forum 1974a;25:21–22.

Laks H, Pilon RN, Klovekorn WP. Acute hemodilution: its effects on hemodynamics and oxygen transport in anesthetized man. Ann Surg 1974b;180:103–109.

Laks H, Pilon RN, Anderson W, et al. Intraoperative prebleeding in man: effect of colloid hemodilution on blood volume, lung water, hemodynamics and oxygen transport. Surgery 1975; 78:130–137.

Lamke LO, Liljedahl SO. Plasma volume changes after infusion of various plasma expanders. Resuscitation 1976a;5:93–102.

Lamke LO, Liljedahl SO. Plasma volume expansion after infusion of 5%, 20%, and 25% albumin solutions in patients. Resuscitation 1976b;5:85–92.

Leaf A. Neurogenic diabetes insipidus. Kidney Int 1979;15:572.

Lee WH, Cooper N, Weidner MG. Clinical evaluation of a new plasma expander: hydroxyethyl starch. J Trauma 1968;8:381–393.

Lewis JH, Szetol LF, Beyer WL. Severe hemodilution with hydroxyethyl starch and dextrans. Arch Surg 1966;93:941–950.

Lewis RT. Albumin: role and discriminative use in surgery. Can J Surg 1980;23:322–328.

Liljedahl SO, Rieger A. Blood volume and plasma protein. IV. Importance of thoracic-duct lymph in restitution of plasma volume and plasma proteins after bleeding and immediate substitution in the splenectomized dog. Acta Chir Scand 1968;379(suppl):39–51.

Linas SL, Berl T, Robertson GL, et al. Role of vasopressin in the impaired water excretion of glucocorticoid deficiency. Kidney Int 1980;18:58.

London MJ, Ho JS, Triedman JK, et al. A randomized clinical trial of 10% pentastarch (low molecular weight hydroxyethyl starch) versus 5% albumin for plasma volume expansion after cardiac operations. J Thorac Cardiovasc Surg 1989;97:785–797.

Lorenz W, Dolniche A, Freund M. Plasma histamine levels in man following infusion of hydroxyethyl starch: a contribution to the question of allergic or anaphylactoid reactions following administration of a new plasma substitute. Anaesthesist 1975;24:228–230.

Lowe RJ, Moss GS, Jilek J, et al. Crystalloid vs. colloid in the etiology of pulmonary failure after trauma: a randomized trial in man. Surgery 1977;81:676–683.

Lowenstein E, Cooper JD, Erdman AF III, et al. Lung and heart water accumulation produced by hemodilution. Bibl Haematologica 1975;41:190.

Lowery BD, Cloutier CT, Carey LC. Electrolyte solutions in resuscitation in human hemorrhagic shock. Surg Gynecol Obstet 1971;133:273–284.

Lucas CE, Ledgerwood AM, Higgins RF. Impaired pulmonary function after albumin resuscitation from shock. J Trauma 1980;20:446–451.

Lucas CE, Weaver D, Higgins RF. Effects of albumin vs. nonalbumin resuscitation on plasma volume and renal excretory function. J Trauma 1978;18:564–570.

Lucas CE, Denis R, Ledgerwood AM, et al. The effects of hespan on serum and lymphatic albumin, globulin and coagulant protein. Ann Surg 1988;207:416.

Lund CJ, Donovan JC. Blood volume during pregnancy. Significance of plasma and red cell volumes. Am J Obstet Gynaecol 1967;98:393.

MacGillivray I, Campbell D, Duffus GM. Maternal metabolic response to twin pregnancy in primigravidae. J Obstet Gynaecol Br Cmwlth, 1971;78:530.

Mailoux L, Swartz CD, Capizzi R, et al. Acute renal failure after administration of LMW dextran. N Engl J Med 1967;277:1113–1118.

Marino P. Calcium and phosphorous. In: Marino P, ed. The ICU book. Philadelphia: Lea & Febiger, 1991a:499.

Marino P. Magnesium: the hidden ion. In: Marino P, ed. The ICU book. Philadelphia: Lea & Febiger, 1991b:489.

Marino P. Potassium. In: Marino P, ed. The ICU book. Philadelphia: Lea & Febiger, 1991c:478.

Matheson NA, Diomi P. Renal failure after the administration of dextran-40. Surg Gynecol Obstet 1970;131:661–668.

Mattox KL, Maningas PA, Moore EE, et al. Prehospital hypertonic saline/dextran infusion for posttraumatic hypotension. Ann Surg 1991;213:482–491.

Maurer PH, Berardinelli B. Immunologic studies with hydroxyethyl starch (HES). Transfusion 1968;8:265–268.

Maynard JC, Cruz C, Kleerekoper M, Levin NW. Blood pressure response to changes in serum ionized calcium during hemodialysis. Ann Intern Med 1986;104:358.

Medalle R, Waterhouse C, Hahn TJ. Vitamin D resistance in magnesium deficiency. Am J Clin Nutr 1976;29:854.

Metcalf W, Papadopoulos A, Turfaro R, et al. A clinical physiologic study of hydroxyethyl starch. Surg Gynecol Obstet 1970;131:255–267.

Miller M, Kalkos T, Moses AM, et al. Recognition of partial defects in antidiuretic hormone secretion. Ann Intern Med 1970;73:721.

Miller RD, Robbins TO, Tong MJ, et al. Coagulation defects associated with massive blood transfusions. Ann Surg 1971;174:794.

Miravet L, Ayigbede O, Carre M, et al. Lack of vitamin D action on serum calcium in magnesium deficient rats. In: Catin M, Seelig MS, eds. Magnesium in health and disease. New York: SP Medical Scientific, 1980:281.

Mishler JM, Borberg H, Emerson PM. Hydroxyethyl starch, an agent for hypovolemic shock treatment. II. Urinary excretion in normal volunteers following three consecutive daily infusions. Br J Pharmacol 1977;4:591–595.

Mishler JM, Hester JP, Heustis DW, et al. Dosage and scheduling regimens for erythrocyte-sedimenting macromolecules. J Clin Apheresis 1983;1:130–143.

Mishler JM, Parry ES, Sutherland BA, et al. A clinical study of low molecular weight hydroxyethyl starch, a new plasma expander. Br J Clin Pharmacol 1979a;7:619–622.

Mishler JM, Ricketts CR, Parkhouse EJ. Changes in molecular composition of circulating hydroxyethyl starch following consecutive daily infusions in man. Br J Clin Pharmacol 1979b;7: 505–509.

Mishler JM, Ricketts CR, Parkhouse EJ. Post transfusion survival of hydroxyethyl starch 450/0.7 in man: a long term study. J Clin Pathol 1980; 33:155–159.

Modig J. Effectiveness of dextran 70 vs. Ringer's lactate in traumatic shock and adult respiratory distress syndrome. Crit Care Med 1986;14:454–457.

Mordes JP, Wacker WE. Excess magnesium. Pharmacol Rev 1977;29:273.

Moss GS, Proctor JH, Homer LD. A comparison of asanguineous fluids and whole blood in the treatment of hemorrhagic shock. Surg Gynecol Obstet 1966;129:1247–1257.

Moss GS, Lower RJ, Jilek J, et al. Colloid of crystalloid in the resuscitation of hemorrhagic shock. A controlled clinical trial. Surgery 1981;89:434–438.

Moss GS, Siegel DC, Cochin A, et al. Effects of saline and colloid solutions on pulmonary function in hemorrhagic shock. Surg Gynecol Obstet 1971;133:53–58.

Muller N, Popov-Cenic S, Kladetzky RG. The effect of hydroxyethyl starch on the intra- and post-operative behavior of haemostasis. Bibl Anat 1977;16:460–462.

Mundy GR. Calcium homeostasis: hypercalcemia and hypocalcemia. London: Martin Dunitz 1989:1.

Myers MB, Cherry G, Heimberger S, et al. Effect of edema and external pressure on wound healing. Arch Surg 1967;94:218.

Nagant De Deuxchaisnes C, Krane SM. Hypoparathyroidism. In: Avioli LV, Krane SM, eds. Metabolic bone disease. vol 2. Orlando, FL: Academic, 1978:217.

Nakayama S, Sibley C, Gunther RA, et al. Small volume resuscitation and hypertonic saline (2400 mOsm/liter) during hemorrhagic shock. Cir Shock 1984;13:149–159.

Oh MS, Carroll HJ. Hypernatremia. 3rd ed. In: Hurst JW, ed. Medicine for the practicing physician. Boston: Butterworth-Heinemann, 1992:1293.

Oh MS. Selective hypoaldosteronism. Resident Staff Phys 1982;28:46S.

Oster JR, Perez GO, Vaamonde CA. Relationship between blood pH and phosphorus during acute metabolic acidosis. Am J Physiol 1978;235: F345.

Packer M, Medina N, Yushnak M. Correction of dilutional hyponatremia in severe chronic heart failure by converting-enzyme inhibition. Ann Intern Med 1984;100:777.

Pascual JMS, Watson JC, Runyon AE, et al. Resuscitation of intraoperative hypovolemia: a comparison of normal saline and hyperosmotic/hyperoncotic solutions in swine. Crit Care Med 1992;20:200–210.

Peeters LLH, Buchan PC. Blood viscosity in perinatology. Rev Perinatol Med 1989;6:53.

Peeters LLH, Verkeste CM, Saxena PR, et al. Relationship between maternal hemodynamics and hematocrit and hemodynamic effects of isovolemic hemodilution and hemoconcentration. I. The awake late-pregnancy guinea pig. Pediatr Res 1987;21:584.

Phelps KR, Lieberman RL, Oh MS, et al. The syndrome of hyporeninemic hypoaldosteronism. Metabolism 1980;29:185.

Pirani BBK, MacGillivray I. Smoking during pregnancy. Its effect on maternal metabolism and fetoplacental function. Obstet Gynecol 1978;52:257.

Pollock AS, Arieff AL. Abnormalities of cell volume regulation and their functional consequences. Am J Physiol 1980;239:F195.

Poole GV, Meredith JW, Pernell T, et al. Comparison of colloids and crystalloids in resuscitation from hemorrhagic shock. Surg Gynecol Obstet 1982;154:577–586.

Prough DS, Johnson JC, Poole GV Jr, et al. Effects on intracranial pressure of resuscitation from hemorrhagic shock with hypertonic saline versus lactated Ringer's solution. Crit Care Med 1985;13:407.

Puri VK, Paidipaty B, White L. Hydroxyethyl starch for resuscitation of patients with hypovolemia in shock. Crit Care Med 1981;9:833–837.

Quamme GA, Dirks KJ. Magnesium metabolism. In: Maxwell MH, Kleeman CR, Narins RG, eds. Clinical disorders of fluid and electrolyte metabolism. 4th ed. New York: McGraw-Hill 1987:297.

Rackow EC, Mecher C, Astiz ME, et al. Effects of pentastarch and albumin infusion on cardiorespiratory function and coagulation in patients with severe sepsis and systemic hypoperfusion. Crit Care Med 1989;17:394–398.

Raiha CE. Prematurity, perinatal mortality, and maternal heart volume. Guy's Hosp Rep 1964;113:96.

Rasmussen HS, McNair P, Norregard P, et al. Intravenous magnesium in acute myocardial infarction. Lancet 1986;1:234.

Reed RL, Johnston TD, Chen Y, Fischer RP. Hypertonic saline alters plasma clotting times and platelet aggregation. J Trauma 1991;31:8–14.

Reinhart RA. Magnesium metabolism. A review with special reference to the relationship between intracellular content and serum levels. Arch Intern Med 1988;148:2415.

Ring J, Messmer K. Incidence and severity of anaphylactoid reactions to colloid volume substitutes. Lancet 1977;1:466–469.

Ring J, Siefert J, Messmer K. Anaphylactoid reactions due to hydroxyethyl starch infusion. Eur Surg Res 1976;8:389–399.

Risberg B, Miller E, Hughes J. Comparison of the pulmonary effects of rapid infusion of a crystalloid and a colloid solution. Acta Chir Scand 1981;147:613–618.

Robertson GL. Abnormalities of thirst regulation. Kidney Int 1984;25:460.

Robinson AG. DDAVP in the treatment of central diabetes insipidus. N Engl J Med 1976;294:320.

Rocha-Silva M, Negraes GA, Soares AM, et al. Hypertonic resuscitation from severe hemorrhagic shock: patterns of regional circulation. Circ Shock 1986;19:165–175.

Rose SD. Prophylaxis of thromboembolic disease. Med Clin North Am 1979;63:1205–1224.

Rosenoer VM, Skillman JJ, Hastings PR. Albumin synthesis and nitrogen balance in postoperative patients. Surgery 1980;87:305–312.

Ross EJ, Christie SBM. Hypernatremia. Medicine 1969;48:441.

Roswell RH. Severe hypercalcemia: Causes and specific therapy. J Crit Illness 1987;2:14.

Rothschild MA, Oratz M, Schreiber SS. Albumin synthesis. N Engl J Med 1972;286:748–756, 816–820.

Rothschild MA, Schreiber SS, Oratz M, et al. The effects of adrenocortical hormones on albumin metabolism studies with albumin-I131. J Clin Invest 1958;37:1229–1235.

Rothschild MA, Bauman A, Yalow RS, et al. The effect of large doses of desiccated thyroid on the distribution and metabolism of albumin-I131 in euthyroid subjects. J Clin Invest 1957;36:422–428.

Rude RK, Oldham SB, Singer FR. Functional hypoparathyroidism and parathyroid hormone end-organ resistance in human magnesium deficiency. Clin Endocrinol 1976;5:209.

Rude RK, Singer FR. Magnesium deficiency and excess. Annu Rev Med 1981;32:245.

Ryan MP. Diuretics and potassium/magnesium depletion. Am J Med 1987;82:38.

Salas SP, Rosso P, Espinoza R, et al. Maternal plasma volume expansion and hormonal changes in women with idiopathic fetal growth retardation. Obstet Gynecol 1993;81:1029.

Salem M, Munoz R, Chernow B. Hypomagnesemia in critical illness. A common and clinically important problem. Crit Care Clin 1991;7:225.

Sasahara AA, Sharma GV, Parisi AF. New developments in the detection and prevention of venous thromboembolism. Am J Cardiol 1979; 43:1214–1224.

Schupbach P, Pappova E, Schilt W, et al. Perfusate oncotic pressure during cardiopulmonary bypass. Vox Sang 1978;35:332.

Scribner BH, Burnell JM. Interpretation of serum potassium concentration. Metabolism 1956; 5:468.

Shackford SR, Sisc JM, Fridlund PH, et al. Hypertonic sodium lactate versus lactated Ringer's solution for intravenous fluid therapy in operations of the abdominal aorta. Surgery 1983; 94:41.

Shatney CH, Deapiha K, Militello PR, et al. Efficacy of hetastarch in the resuscitation of patients with multisystem trauma and shock. Arch Surg 1983;118:804–809.

Shires GT, Braun FT, Canizaro PC, et al. Distributional changes in extracellular fluid during acute hemorrhagic shock. Surg Forum 1960;11:115.

Shoemaker WC. Comparison of the relative effectiveness of whole blood transfusions and various types of fluid therapy in resuscitation. Crit Care Med 1976;4:71–78.

Shoemaker WC, Bryan-Brown CW, Quigley L. Body fluid shifts in depletion and post-stress states and their correction with adequate nutrition. Surg Gynecol Obstet 1973;136:371–374.

Shoemaker WC, Schluchter M, Hopkins JA. Comparison of the relative effectiveness of colloids and crystalloids in emergency resuscitation. Am J Cardiol 1981;142:73–84.

Sibai BM, Anderson GD, Spinnato JA, et al. Plasma volume findings in patients with mild pregnancy-induced hypertension. Am J Obstet Gynecol 1983;147:16.

Siegel SC, Moss GS, Cochin A. Pulmonary changes following treatment for hemorrhagic shock: saline vs. colloid infusion. Surg Forum 1970; 921:17–19.

Silva OL, Becker KL. Salmon calcitonin in the treatment of hypercalcemia. Arch Intern Med 1973;132:337.

Singh G, Chaudry KI, Chaudry IH. Crystalloid is as effective as blood in resuscitation of hemorrhagic shock. Ann Surg 1992;215:377–382.

Skillman JJ, Hassan AK, Moore FD. Plasma protein kinetics of the early transcapillary refill after hemorrhage in man. Surg Gynecol Obstet 1967;125:983–996.

Skillman JJ, Restall DS, Salzman EW. Randomized trial of albumin vs. electrolyte solutions during abdominal aortic operations. Surgery 1975; 78:291–303.

Skillman JJ, Rosenoer VM, Smith PC. Improved albumin synthesis in postoperative patients by amino acid infusion. N Engl J Med 1976; 295:1037–1040.

Smith JD, Bia MJ, DeFronzo RA. Clinical disorders of potassium metabolism. In: Arieff AI, DeFronzo RA, eds. Fluid, electrolyte and acid-base disorders. New York: Churchill Livingstone, 1985:413.

Solanke TF. Clinical trial of 6% hydroxyethyl starch (a new plasma expander). Br Med J 1968;3:783–785.

Solanke TF, Khwaja MS, Madojemu EI. Plasma volume studies with four different plasma volume expanders. J Surg Res 1971;11:140–143.

Soupart A, Penninckx R, Stenuit A, et al. Treatment of chronic hyponatremia in rats by intravenous saline: comparison of rate versus magnitude of correction. Kidney Int 1992;41:1667.

Sterling K. The turnover rate of serum albumin in man as measured by I-131 tagged albumin. J Clin Invest 1951;30:1228–1237.

Sterns RH, Riggs JE, Schochet SS Jr. Osmotic demyelinating syndrome following correction of hyponatremia. N Engl J Med 1986;314:1535.

Sterns RH. The treatment of hyponatremia: first, do no harm. Am J Med 1990;88:557.

Stewart AF, Horst R, Deftos LJ, et al. Biochemical evaluation of patients with cancer-associated hypercalcemia: evidence for humoral and non-humoral groups. N Engl J Med 1980;303:1377.

Strauss RG, Stansfield C, Henriksen RA, Vilaahaauer PJ. Pentastarch may cause fewer effects on coagulation than hetastarch. Transfusion 1988; 28:257–260.

Strauss RG, Stump DC, Henriksen RA. Hydroxyethyl starch accentuates von Willebrand's disease. Transfusion 1985;25:235–237.

Takaori M, Safer P. Acute severe hemodilution with lactated Ringer's solution. Arch Surg 1967; 94:67–73.

Templeton GH, Mitchell JH, Wildenthal K. Influence of hyperosmolarity on left ventricular stiffness. Am J Physiol 1972;222:1406–1411.

Thompson JK, Fogh-Andersen N, Jaszczak P. Atrial natriuretic peptide, blood volume, aldosterone, and sodium excretion during twin pregnancy. Acta Obstet Gynecol Scand 1994;73:14.

Thompson WL, Britton JJ, Walton RP. Persistence of starch derivatives and dextran when infused after hemorrhage. Pharmacol Exp Ther 1962; 136:125–132.

Thompson WL, Fukushima T, Rutherford RB, et al. Intravascular persistence, tissue storage, and excretion of hydroxyethyl starch. Surg Gynecol Obstet 1970;131:965–972.

Thompson WL. Rational use of albumin and plasma substitutes. Johns Hopkins Med J 1975;136: 220–225.

Thomsen JK, Fogh-Andersen N, Jaszczak P, et al. Atrial natriuretic peptide decrease during normal pregnancy as related to hemodynamic changes and volume regulation. Acta Obstet Gynecol Scand 1993;72:103.

Thoren L. The dextrans-clinical data. Joint WHO/ IABS symposium on the standardization of albumin plasma substitutes and plasmapheresis, Geneva 1980. Dev Biol Stand 1981;48:157–167.

Trudnowski RJ, Goel SB, Lam FT, et al. Effect of Ringer's lactate solution and sodium bicarbonate on surgical acidosis. Surg Gynecol Obstet 1967;125:807–814.

Tullis JL. Albumin. I. Background and use. JAMA 1977;237:355–360.

Ueland K. Maternal cardiovascular dynamics. VII. Intrapartum blood volume changes. Am J Obstet Gynecol 1976;126:671.

Villabona C, Rodriguez P, Joven J. Potassium disturbances as a cause of metabolic neuromyopathy. Intensive Care Med 1987;13:208.

Virgilio RW. Crystalloid vs. colloid resuscitation [reply to letter to editor]. Surgery 1979a;86:515.

Virgilio RW, Rice CL, Smith DE. Crystalloid vs colloid resuscitation: is one better? A randomized clinical study. Surgery 1979b;85:129–139.

Virgilio RW, Smith DE, Zarino DK. Balanced electrolyte solutions: experimental and clinical studies. Crit Care Med 1979c;7:98–106.

Vito L, Dennis RC, Weisel RD. Sepsis presenting as acute respiratory insufficiency. Surg Gynecol Obstet 1974;138:896–900.

Walsh JC, Zhuamg J, Shackford SR. A comparison of hypertonic to isotonic fluid in the resuscitation of brain injury and hemorrhagic shock. J Surg Res 1991;50:284–292.

Waxman K, Honess R, Tominaga G, et al. Hemodynamic and oxygen transport effects of pentastarch in burn resuscitation. Ann Surg 1989;209:341–345.

Weatherbee L, Spencer HH, Knopp CT. Coagulation studies after the transfusion of hydroxyethyl starch protected frozen blood in primates. Transfusion 1974;14:109–115.

Weaver DW, Ledgerwood AM, Lucas CE. Pulmonary effects of albumin resuscitation for severe hypovolemic shock. Arch Surg 1978;113:387–392.

Weil MH, Hennin RJ, Puri VK. Colloid oncotic pressure: clinical significance. Crit Care Med 1979;7:113–116.

Weinberg LS. Pseudohyponatremia: a reappraisal. Am J Med 1989;86:315.

Weiss HJ. The effect of clinical dextran on platelet aggregation, adhesion and ADP release in man:

in vivo and in vitro studies. J Lab Clin Med 1967;69:37–46.

Whang R, Flink EB, Cyckner T, et al. Magnesium depletion as a cause of refractory potassium repletion. Arch Intern Med 1985;145:1686.

Williams ME, Rosa RM. Hyperkalemia: disorders of internal and external potassium balance. J Intensive Care Med 1988;3:52.

Wittaker PG, Lind T. The intravascular mass of albumin during human pregnancy: A serial study in normal and diabetic women. Br J Obstet Gynaecol 1993;100:587.

Yacobi A, Stoll RG, Sum CY, et al. Pharmacokinetics on hydroxyethyl starch in normal subjects. J Clin Pharmacol 1982;22:206–212.

Zaloga GP, Chernow B. Calcium metabolism. Clin Crit Care Med 1985a;5.

Zaloga GP, Chernow B. Stress-induced changes in calcium metabolism. Semin Respir Med 1985b; 7:56.

Zaloga GP, Chernow B. Hypercalcemia in critical illness. JAMA 1986;256:1924.

Zaloga GP, Chernow B. The multifactorial basis for hypocalcemia during sepsis. Studies of the parathyroid hormone–vitamin D axis. Ann Intern Med 1987a;107:36.

Zaloga GP, Malcolm DS, Holaday J, Chernow B. Verapamil reverses calcium cardiotoxicity. Ann Emerg Med 1987b;16:637.

Zaloga GP, Wilkens R, Tourville J, et al. A simple method for determining physiologically active calcium and magnesium concentrations in critically ill patients. Crit Care Med 1987;15:813.

Zaloga GP. Interpretation of the serum magnesium level. Chest 1989;95:257.

Zaloga GP, Roberts JE. Magnesium disorders. Probl Crit Care 1990a;4:425.

Zaloga GP. Phosphate disorders. Probl Crit Care 1990b;4:416.

# PART II

# Instrumentation and Procedures

# CHAPTER 5

# Pulmonary Artery Catheterization

Since its introduction into clinical medicine over 2 decades ago, the pulmonary artery catheter has come to play an indispensable role in the management of critically ill patients in a number of specialties, including obstetrics (Swan, 1970; Clark, 1988, 1985; European Society, 1991). Several prospective trials demonstrate the benefits of pulmonary artery catheterization in select critically ill patients. These include a reduction in operative morbidity and mortality in certain complicated surgical patients and a significant decrease in death rate in patients in shock in whom catheter-obtained parameters lead to changes in therapy (Mimoz, 1994; Sola, 1993). In one study, management recommendations changed as a direct result of knowledge obtained by pulmonary artery catheter placement in 56% of patients admitted to an intensive care unit (Coles, 1993). In patients with major burn injuries, survival is predicted by early response to pulmonary artery catheter-guided resuscitation (Schiller, 1995). This technique, however, is not without its critics; in a nonrandomized observational study, Califf (1996) demonstrated increased mortality and cost associated with pulmonary artery catheterization, and suggested that a randomized trial aimed at better patient selection is needed. This chapter provides an overview of placement techniques and complications; indications for the use of this diagnostic tool in the obstetric patient are examined in more detail in the ensuing chapters.

## Catheter Placement

The procedure for catheter placement involves two phases. The initial phase in pulmonary artery catheterization is establishing venous access with a large-bore sheath. Access is most commonly obtained via the internal jugular or subclavian veins; however, under certain circumstances (e.g., where access to the neck or thoracic region is difficult or in a patient with a coagulopathy where bleeding from a major artery could be hazardous), peripheral veins—including cephalic or femoral—can be used (Findling, 1994). Insertion of the introducer sheath via the right internal jugular vein is described here.

## Insertion of the Sheath

To catheterize the internal jugular vein, the patient is placed supine with the head turned to the left in a mild Trendelenburg position. The landmark for insertion is the junction of the clavicular and sternal heads of the sternocleidomastoid muscle. When this junction is indistinct, its identification can be facilitated by having the patient raise her head slightly. When the landmark has been identified, 1% lidocaine is infiltrated into the skin and superficial subcutaneous tissue.

The internal jugular vein is entered first with a *finder needle*, consisting of a 21-gauge needle on a 10-mL syringe. The skin is punctured at the junction of the two clavicular heads, and the needle is directed with constant aspiration toward the ipsilateral nipple at an angle approximately 30 degrees superior to the plane of the skin. Free flow of venous blood confirms the position of the internal jugular vein. Next, the needle is withdrawn and the vein once again entered with a 16-gauge needle and syringe. Then a guidewire is placed through the needle and into the jugular vein. This placement is perhaps the most crucial part of the entire procedure, and it is vital that the guidewire pass freely without any resistance whatsoever. Free passage confirms entrance into the vein.

Next, the needle is removed and the guidewire left in place. The incision is widened with a scalpel, and the introducer sheath–vein dilator apparatus is introduced over the guidewire. During introduction of the introducer sheath–vein dilator, it is crucial that the proximal tip of the guidewire be visible at all times, to avoid inadvertent loss of the guidewire into the central venous system. The introducer sheath–vein dilator apparatus is advanced with a slight turning motion along the guidewire. In general, the point of entry into the vein is felt clearly by a sudden decrease in resistance. The sheath apparatus then is advanced to the hilt. The conscious patient is instructed to hold her breath to prevent negative intrathoracic pressure and inadvertent air embolism, and the guidewire and trocar are quickly removed and the sheath left in place.

Occasionally, portable real-time sonography may be helpful in guiding central venous cannulation (Lee, 1989; Sherer, 1993).

Most current introducer systems contain an accessory port, which attaches to the proximal end of the introducer sheath and includes a one-way valve that prevents air introduction into the central venous system during removal of the guidewire and trocar. To keep the line open, the sheath then is infused with a crystalloid solution containing 1 unit of heparin per milliliter and secured in place with suture.

## Insertion of the Catheter

Phase two involves the actual placement of the pulmonary artery catheter (Fig 5-1). Careful attention must be paid to maintaining sterile technique as the catheter is removed from the package. The distal and proximal ports are flushed to assure patency. The balloon then is tested with 1 mL of air. When the catheter has been attached to the physiologic monitor and the air completely flushed from the system, minute movements in the catheter tip should produce corresponding oscillations on the monitor. The catheter tip is introduced through the sheath and advanced approximately 20 cm. At this point, the balloon is inflated and the catheter advanced through the introducer sheath into the central venous system. Occasionally, portable real-time sonography

F I G U R E    **5-1**

**The pulmonary artery catheter.** (Reproduced by permission from American Edwards Laboratories.)

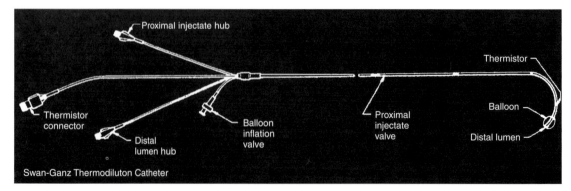

may be helpful in guiding central venous cannulation (Sherer, 1993).

## Waveforms and Catheter Placement

Once within the superior vena cava, the balloon on the tip of the catheter will advance with the flow of blood into the heart. Characteristic waveforms and pressure observed are detailed in Figure 5-2. Entrance into the right ventricle is signaled by a high spiking waveform with diastolic pressures near zero. This is the time of maximum potential complications during the catheter place-

ment, because most arrhythmias occur as the catheter tip impinges on the interventricular septum. For this reason, the catheter must be advanced rapidly through the right ventricle and into the pulmonary artery. If premature ventricular contractions occur during this process and the catheter does not advance promptly out of the right ventricle, the balloon should be deflated and the catheter withdrawn to the right atrium.

As soon as the catheter enters the pulmonary artery, the waveform has two notable characteristics. First, and most important, is the rise in diastolic pressure from that seen in the right ventricle. Second, a notching of the peak systolic waveform often is seen and represents closure of

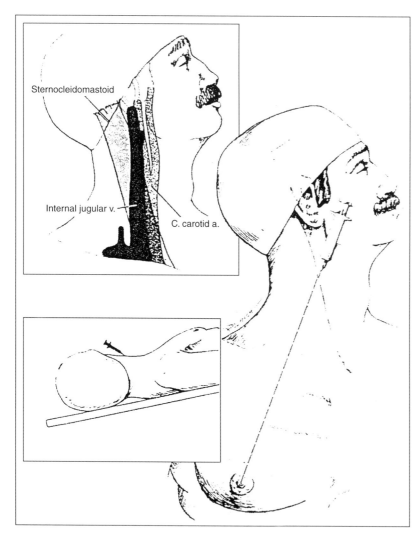

Sternocleidomastoid

Internal jugular v.

C. carotid a.

the pulmonic valve. After entrance into the pulmonary artery has been confirmed (in most pregnant women, this occurs between 40 and 45 cm of catheter length), the catheter is advanced farther until the tip reaches a point within the pulmonary vasculature where the balloon diameter exceeds that of the corresponding pulmonary arterial branch. At this point, a wedge tracing is observed. If the balloon is deflated, the tracing should return to a pulmonary artery pattern.

Following catheter placement, it is essential that health-care personnel skilled in the interpretation of these waveforms continuously monitor the waveforms for evidence of catheter migration (spontaneous advancement), which may lead to pulmonary infarction. This may be manifest by the appearance of a spontaneous "wedge" tracing at the distal port, rather than the pulmonary artery waveform, which should be continuously manifest on the display monitor. Alternately, the appearance of a pulmonary artery waveform in the central venous pressure port will alert the attendant to distal catheter migration and the need for adjustment (Santora, 1991). Komadina et al described disturbingly high interobserver variability in the interpretation of waveform tracings, although agreement on numerical wedge pressure readings was high (Komadina, 1991). In a similar manner, Iberti et al reported a wide variation in the understanding of pulmonary artery catheter waveforms and techniques among critical care nurses using this device (Iberti, 1994). It would appear that graphic recording at end expiration is the most reliable means of measuring hemodynamic pressures (Johnson, 1995). Clearly, continuous training and credentialing programs are essential for health-care providers utilizing these techniques.

Caution also is advised during pulmonary artery catheter removal; techniques to avoid complications have been reviewed by Wadas (1994).

## Cardiac Output Determination

Once in place, cardiac output is obtained with the use of a cardiac output computer connected to a terminal on the pulmonary artery catheter. This instrument derives cardiac output from thermodilution curves created by the injection of cold or room-temperature saline into the proximal central venous port of the catheter. The resultant flow-related temperature changes detected at the distal thermistor are converted into cardiac output by the computer and correlate well in pregnant women with those obtained by the more precise, but clinically cumbersome, oxygen extraction (Fick) technique (Clark, 1989). Nevertheless, it should be emphasized that cardiac output determinations are of most value in following trends in individual patients; caution is advised in relying on absolute cardiac output values, and sound clinical judgment is essential in data interpretation (Vender, 1993). One study suggests that the thermodilution technique may overestimate cardiac output, especially with very low values (Jensen, 1995). In addition, meticulous attention must be paid to technique if reliable information regarding cardiac output is to be obtained. The exact injectate temperature must be known, the proximal injectate port must have advanced beyond the introducer sheath, and the introducer sheath sidearm must be closed (Boyd, 1994). If the central venous port line becomes nonfunctional, room-temperature thermodilution cardiac outputs can be used with saline injection into the sideport, with the understanding that a slight overestimation of cardiac output will occur (Pesola, 1993). Additional issues that effect the validity of cardiac output measurements include the rate of injection, the timing of injection during the respiratory cycle, the position of the patient, and the presence of other, concurrent infusions (Sommers, 1993). Recently, techniques have been evaluated for continuous cardiac output measurement, both by thermodilution and with the use of a special flow-directed Doppler pulmonary artery catheter (Segal, 1991; Mihaljevic, 1994).

With appropriate modification of technique, right ventricular ejection fraction measurements also may be obtained with the pulmonary artery catheter (Cockroft, 1993; Safcsak, 1994). Specially designed fiberoptic catheters allow continuous assessment of mixed venous oxygen saturation in critically ill surgical and nonsurgical patients. Newer techniques for continuous thermodilution measurement compare well with conventional methods (Inomata, 1994; Lefrant, 1995).

## Complications

Most complications actually seen in patients undergoing pulmonary artery catheterization are a result of obtaining central venous access. Such events include pneumothorax and insertion site infection and occur in 1% to 5% of patients undergoing this procedure (Scott, 1988; Patel, 1986). Potential complications of pulmonary artery catheterization per se include air embolism, thromboembolism, pulmonary infarction, catheter-related sepsis, direct trauma to the heart or pulmonary artery, postganglionic Horner's syndrome, and catheter entrapment (Soding, 1994; Bernardin, 1994; Yellin, 1991; Manager, 1993; Lanigan, 1991; Vaswani, 1991). Such complications occur in 1% or less of patients. More recently, a pressure release balloon has been described to limit overinflation and potentially reduce the risk of vessel rupture (Sheuede, 1994). Arrhythmias, consisting of transient premature ventricular contractions, occur during catheter insertion in 30% to 50% of patients and are generally of no clinical consequence.

The remaining complications can be minimized or eliminated by careful attention to proper insertion maintenance and removal techniques (Wadas, 1994). In patients with right-to-left shunts, the use of this catheter is hazardous; when its placement is deemed mandatory, the use of carbon dioxide instead of air for ballon inflation may minimize the risk of systemic air embolism (Moorthy, 1991). A Food and Drug Administration task force has summarized recommendations regarding methods to minimize complications of central venous catheterization procedures (U.S. Food and Drug Administration, 1989).

Numerous studies have documented the frequent discrepancy between measurements of pulmonary capillary wedge pressure and central venous pressure (Benedetti, 1980; Cotton, 1985; Clark, 1988). In such circumstances, clinical use of the central venous pressure would be misleading. For these reasons, in a modern perinatal intensive care unit, central venous monitoring is seldom, if ever, indicated. Where proper equipment and personnel exist, the vast amount of additional information obtainable by pulmonary artery catheterization far outweighs the slight potential increase in risk attributable to catheter placement and pulmonary artery catheterization is nearly always preferable.

## Noninvasive Techniques

Despite the small risks associated with properly managed pulmonary artery catheterization, the search continues for noninvasive methods of central hemodynamic assessment of the critically ill patient. Such techniques generally focus on sonographic or bioimpedance techniques to estimate cardiac output, and have been described in both pregnant and nonpregnant patients (Clark, 1994; Belfort, 1991, 1996; Easterling, 1987; Weiss, 1995). In addition, investigation continues into techniques to allow noninvasive central pressure determination (Ensing, 1994). These techniques appear to be useful in a research setting or in patients requiring only a single evaluation of hemodynamics in order to classify their disease and initiate appropriate therapy. Invasive techniques, however, remain the mainstay of long-term management of complex, critically ill obstetric patients.

**REFERENCES**

Belfort MA, Rokey R, Saade GR, et al. Rapid echocardiographic assessment of left and right heart hemodynamics in critically ill obstetric patients. Am J Obstet Gynecol 1991;171:884.

Belfort MA, Mares A, Saade G, et al. A re-evaluation of the indications for pulmonary artery catheters in obstetrics: the role of 2-D echocardiography and Doppler ultrasound. Am J Obstet Gynecol 1996;174:331.

Benedetti TJ, Cotton DB, Read JC, et al. Hemodynamic observations in severe preeclampsia with a flow-directed pulmonary artery catheter. Am J Obstet Gynecol 1980;136:465.

Bernardin G, Milhaud D, Roger PM, et al. Swan-Ganz catheter related pulmonary valve infective endocarditis: a case report. Intensive Care Med 1994;20:142.

Boyd O, Mackay CJ, Newman P, et al. Effects of insertion depth and use of the sidearm of the introducer sheath of pulmonary artery catheters in cardiac output measurement. Crit Care Med 1994;22:1132.

Califf RM, Fulkerson WJ, Jr, Vidaillet H, et al. The effectiveness of right-heart catheterization in the initial case of critically ill patients. JAMA 1996;18:889.

Clark SL, Cotton DB. Clinical opinion: clinical indications for pulmonary artery catheterization in severe pregnancy induced hypertension. Am J Obstet Gynecol 1988;158:453.

Clark SL, Cotton DB, Lee W, et al. Central hemodynamic assessment of normal term pregnancy. Am J Obstet Gynecol 1989;161:1439.

Clark SL, Horenstein JM, Phelan JP, et al. Experience with the pulmonary artery catheter in obstetrics and gynecology. Am J Obstet Gynecol 1985;152:374.

Clark SL, Southwick J, Pivarnik JM, et al. A comparison of cardiac index in normal term pregnancy using thoracic electrical bioimpedance and oxygen extraction (Fick) technique. Obstet Gynecol 1994;83:669.

Cockroft S, Withington PS. The measurement of right ventricular ejection fraction by thermodilution. A comparison of values obtained using differing injectate ports. Anaesthesia 1993;48:312.

Coles NA, Hibberd M, Russell M, et al. Potential impact of pulmonary artery catheter placement on short term management decisions in the medical intensive care unit. Am Heart J 1993;126:815.

Cotton DB, Gonik B, Dorman K, et al. Cardiovascular alterations in severe pregnancy induced hypertension: relationship of central venous pressure to pulmonary capillary wedge pressure. Am J Obstet Gynecol 1985; 151:762.

Easterling T, Watts D, Schmucker B, et al. Measurement of cardiac output during pregnancy: validation of Doppler technique and clinical observations in preeclamplsia. Obstet Gynecol 1987;69:845.

Ensing G, Seward J, Darragh R, et al. Feasibility of generating hemodynamic pressure curves from noninvasive Doppler echocardiographic signals. J Am Coll Cardiol 1994;23:434.

European Society of Intensive Care Medicine. Expert panel: the use of the pulmonary artery catheter. Intensive Care Med 1991;17:I–VIII.

Findling R, Lipper B. Femoral vein pulmonary artery catheterization in the intensive care unit. Chest 1994;105:874.

Iberti TJ, Daily EK, Leibowitz AB. Assessment of critical care nurses' knowledge of the pulmonary artery catheter. Crit Care Med 1994;22:1674.

Inomata S, Nishikawa T, Taguchi M. Continuous monitoring of mixed venous oxygen saturation for detecting alterations in cardiac output after discontinuation of cardiopulmonary bypass. Br J Anaesth 1994;72:11.

Jensen EW, Rosenberg D, Thomson JK, et al. Comparison of cardiac output techniques: Thermodilution, Doppler, $CO_2$ rebreathing and the direct Fick method. Acta Anaesthesiol Scand 1995;39:245.

Johnson MIC, Schuman L. Comparison of three methods of measurement of pulmonary artery catheter readings in critically ill patients. Am J Crit Care 1985;4:300.

Komadina KH, Schenk DA, LaVeau P, et al. Interobserver variability in the interpretation of pulmonary artery catheter pressure tracings. Chest 1991;100:1647.

Lanigan C, Cornwell E. Pulmonary artery catheter entrapment. Anaesthesia 1991;46:600.

Lee W, Leduc L, Cotton DB. Ultrasonographic guidance for central venous catheterization. Am J Obstet Gynecol 1989;161:1012.

Lefrant JY, Bruelle P, Ripart J, et al. Cardiac output measurement in critically ill patients: Comparison of continuous and conventional thermodilution techniques. Can J Anesth 1995;42:972.

Manager D, Connell GR, Lessin JL. Catheter induced pulmonary artery haemorrhage resulting from a pneumothorax. Can J Anaesth 1993;40:1069.

Mihaljevic T, von Segesser LK, Tonz M, et al. Continuous thermodilution measurement of cardiac output: in-vitro and in-vivo evaluation. Thorac Cardiovasc Surg 1994;42:32.

Mimoz O, Rauss A, Rekik N, et al. Pulmonary artery catheterization in critically ill patients: a prospective analysis of outcome changes associated with catheter-prompted changes in therapy. Crit Care Med 1994;22:573.

Moorthy SS, Tisinai KA, Speiser BS, et al. Cerebral air embolism during removal of a pulmonary artery catheter. Crit Care Med 1991;19:981.

Patel C, Labby V, Venus B, et al. Acute complications of pulmonary artery catheter insertion in critically ill patients. Crit Care Med 1986;14:195.

Pesola HR, Pesola GR: Room temperature thermodilution cardiac output. Central venous vs side port. Chest 1993;103:339.

Safcsak K, Nelson LD. Thermodilution right ventricular ejection fraction measurements: room temperature versus cold temperature injectate. Crit Care Med 1994;22:1136.

Santora T, Ganz W, Gold J, et al. New method for monitoring pulmonary artery catheter location. Crit Care Med 1991;19:422.

Schiller WR, Bay RC, McLachlan JG. Survival in major burn injuries is predicted by early response to Swan-Ganz-guided resuscitation. Am J Surg 1995;170:696.

Scott WL. Complications associated with central venous catheters. Chest 1988;91:1221.

Segal J, Gaudiani V, Nishimura T. Continuous determination of cardiac output using a flow directed Doppler pulmonary artery catheter. J Cardiothorac Vasc Anesth 1991;5:307.

Sherer DM, Abulafia O, DuBeshter B, et al. Ultrasonically guided subclavian vein catheterization in critical care obstetrics and gynecologic oncology. Am J Obstet Gynecol 1994;171:285.

Sheude K, Raab R, Lee P. Decreasing the risk of pulmonary artery rupture with a pressure relief balloon. J Cardiothorac Vasc Anesth 1994;8:30.

Soding PF, Klinck JR, Kong A. Infective endocarditis of the pulmonary valve following pulmonary artery catheterization. Intensive Care Med 1994;20:222.

Sola JE, Bender JS. Use of the pulmonary artery catheter to reduce operative complications. Surg Clin North Am 1993;73:253.

Sommers MS, Woods SL, Courtade MA. Issues in methods and measurement of thermodilution cardiac output. Nurs Res 1993;42:228.

Swan JHC, Ganz W, Forrester J, et al. Catheterization of the heart in man with use of a flow-directed balloon-tipped catheter. N Engl J Med 1970;283:447.

U.S. Food and Drug Administration. Precautions necessary with central venous catheters. FDA Drug Bulletin, July 1989;15.

Vaswani S, Garvin L, Matuschak GM. Postganglionic Horner's syndrome after insertion of a pulmonary artery catheter through the internal jugular vein. Crit Care Med 1991;19:1215.

Vender JS. Clinical utilization of pulmonary artery catheter monitoring. Int Anesthesiol Clin 1993;31:57.

Wadas TM. Pulmonary artery catheter removal. Crit Care Nurse 1994;14:63.

Yellin LB, Filler JJ, Barnette RE. Nominal hemoptysis heralds pseudoaneurysm induced by a pulmonary artery catheter. Anesthesiology 1991;74:370.

Weiss S, Calloway E, Cairo J, et al. Comparison of cardiac output measurements by thermodilution and thoracic electrical bioimpedance in critically ill vs. noncritically ill patients. Am J Emerg Med 1995;13:62.

# CHAPTER 6

# Arterial Access

Arterial cannulation may afford many advantages to the critically ill obstetrical patient: (1) assured access for repeating arterial blood sampling, (2) access for blood samples in general without need for venipuncture, and (3) ability to continuously monitor arterial BP. While discomfort with initial line insertion may exceed that of a single arterial puncture to obtain a blood gas, the discomfort is less than that in aggregate from multiple samplings over several days. Additionally, the integrity of the sample is assured, and one does not have to question whether abnormal values are a reflection of contamination with venous blood. A general management tenet, however, is that arterial catheters should be used for specific purposes and for as short a time as necessary.

## Sites

Arteries that are accessible to palpation can generally be cannulated: the radial, brachial, axillary, femoral, and dorsalis pedis arteries. An artery suitable for placing an indwelling catheter for continuous monitoring of intraarterial pressures should have the following characteristics:

1. The vessel should be large enough to measure pressure accurately without the catheter occluding the artery or producing thrombosis.

2. There should be adequate collateral circulation should vessel occlusion occur.
3. There should be easy site access for nursing care.
4. The site should be in an area not prone to contamination.

For safety purposes, the order of preference for arterial cannulation is

1. Radial
2. Dorsalis pedis
3. Femoral
4. Axillary
5. Brachial

## Contraindications to Arterial Cannulation

Due to the young age of the obstetric patient, atherosclerosis or stenosis of vessels and inadequate collateral flow such that distal ischemia would follow catheterization of the artery are unlikely. It is necessary, however, to assure that there is good pulsation of the vessel as well as adequate collateral flow. This is especially true with radial arterial cannulization. Adequate flow through the ulnar artery should be assured before catheter insertion into the radial artery. The importance of assessing the adequacy of collateral flow is demonstrated by occurrence of delayed ischemia of the hand, necessitating amputation after radial artery cannulation, despite a lack of signs of vascular compromise and the catheter's removal within 24 hours (Mangar, 1993). Other contraindications to arterial cannulation include infection or inflammation at the proposed site. Rare contraindications, such as existence of arterial-venous (AV) or aneurysmal malformations of the vessel or the presence of an arterial graft of the vessel under consideration, are unlikely to be encountered in the pregnant woman. Relative contraindications include coagulopathies, which, regardless of cause, merit greater concern as vessels become more proximal (i.e., axillary or femoral). However, coagulopathies are managed readily by pressure if peripheral access via the radial or dorsalis pedis vessels is attempted.

## Technique of Arterial Cannulation

### General Guidelines (All Sites)

Regardless of the site selected, the area should be prepared with Betadine (povidone-iodine) or a similar solution for a distance of several centimeters, both above and below the proposed puncture site. The site is next draped with sterile towels such that a sterile operating environment is retained. The operator should wear a mask, hat, and sterile gloves. The site is next anesthetized with 1% xylocaine using a 25-gauge needle.

Arteries can be cannulized by a variety of techniques. The earliest technique involved palpation and direct needle puncture, usually with advancement of a Teflon catheter over the needle and into the vessel. A second technique involves use of a guidewire. This technique, originally described by Seldinger (1953), was for replacement of the needle at percutaneous arteriography. Once the vessel has been punctured and pulsatile return of blood flow achieved, the needle is not advanced further, but rather a fine and flexible wire is inserted through the needle and into the lumen of the vessel. The sharp needle is then removed and a polyurethane-type catheter is threaded over the wire and into the vessel. Commercially produced catheters are available that incorporate an integral guidewire (a modified Seldinger technique). Beards and associates

(1994) compared all three insertion techniques in 69 critically ill patients. The direct puncture technique was associated with the highest failure rate, followed by the modified and classic Seldinger techniques, respectively. The direct puncture technique also took significantly longer, used more catheters, and required more punctures per successful insertion than did the modified or classic Seldinger technique. These authors also observed that polyurethane catheters were significantly less likely to block and require reinsertion than were the Teflon catheters. They strongly endorsed use of the classic Seldinger technique and polyurethane catheters.

Successful line placement can be confirmed by the appearance of pulsatile blood flow or, if any doubt exists, by blood gas analysis. The catheter is connected to a transducer with a three-way stopcock and high-pressure tubing connected to a pressure bag containing normal saline and heparin (1500 units/500 mL). We prefer to use a 6-cm segment of high-pressure tubing to connect the catheter itself to the three-way stopcock, because this produces less manipulation of the catheter itself during blood sampling. The high-pressure tubing is necessary to prevent damping of BP readings. The heparinized saline is administered through the pressurized bag at a rate of approximately 2 to 5 mL/hr to prevent the catheter from clotting off. It is critically important to purge all pressure lines and stopcocks prior to connecting the arterial line to prevent arterial air embolism. All set-ups should also have a purge or flush device that can be used to clear any blood that may back up into the pressure tubing as well as to clear the catheter itself and the stopcock after blood sampling.

Most arterial lines should be sutured into place to prevent accidental disconnection or withdrawal. The catheter itself is then covered with a sterile, waterproof occlusive dressing after application of an antibiotic ointment at the skin puncture site. The pressure tubing itself also should be taped to the patient some 10 to 12 cm above its connection to the catheter and three-way valve as yet another safeguard to prevent the line's accidental dislodging. When withdrawing blood samples through an arterial line, the deadspace in the system should be appreciated, and a sufficient quantity of blood to account for this should be withdrawn and discarded prior to actual specimen collection. It also is very important to purge the system after specimen collection, lest the line clot off.

## Radial Artery

The palmar arch is supplied by the radial and ulnar arteries; prior to cannulation of either, the adequacy of collateral circulation must be established. The patient's hand should be elevated and both arteries occluded simultaneously, following which the patient is instructed to make a fist repeatedly until the hand blanches. The ulnar artery is then released, following which the palm should regain its normal color within 6 seconds. Delay of color from 7 to 15 seconds indicates that ulnar artery filling is slow. Persistent blanching for up to 15 seconds or more indicates an incomplete or occluded ulnar arch. Failure to regain normal color promptly is presumptive evidence of inadequate collateral flow, and the radial artery should not be cannulated. In performing this test, care is taken not to hyperextend the wrist, which could falsely compromise ulnar flow.

The wrist is dorsiflexed slightly to optimize exposure of the artery. This may best be accomplished by use of an arm board and placement of a small gauze roll beneath the dorsal surface of the wrist, with tape placed across the patient's palm and upper forearm. When taping the upper forearm, care is taken not to constrict blood flow. Alternatively, an assistant may hold the patient's arm in place, but access to the puncture site is often obstructed in so doing.

Once positioned, the area is prepped and anesthetized as described previously. We prefer use of a 20- or 22-gauge angiocath. The needle is advanced at a 30-degree angle to the artery until a flash of blood appears in the hub (Fig 6-1). If using the direct puncture technique, the needle is now lowered and the catheter advanced while holding the needle stable. This can often be facilitated by rotating the catheter itself backward and forward, in a drilling action, as it is advanced. If the catheter fails to advance easily, it should not be forced, lest a traumatic pseudoaneurysm be produced. Often both walls of the vessel will have been punctured and the catheter will lie posterior to the vessel. Once the catheter has been advanced beyond the tip of the metal needle, the needle should never be advanced, because the catheter is unlikely to be straight, and accordingly, its back wall is prone to being punctured by the needle, making further advancement of the catheter impossible. Instead, completely remove the needle and then slowly withdraw the catheter until pulsatile flow is established, at which point one can gently try to advance the catheter or pass a 25-gauge vascular wire through the catheter, followed by advancement over the wire. If neither of these maneuvers meets with success, the catheter should be removed and discarded. The procedure is then repeated with a new needle and catheter.

As noted previously, the modified or classic Seldinger technique also can be employed. The needle is advanced until a flash of blood is observed in the hub of the catheter. The guidewire is then advanced through the needle until it is 2 to 3 cm into the artery. The catheter can then be advanced over both guidewire and needle, or the needle can be removed and the catheter advanced over just the guidewire. Once the catheter has been advanced, the guidewire and/or needle is removed, pulsatile flow is established, and the line is secured and connected, as previously discussed.

Rarely, cutdown and direct visualization will be required for radial artery catheterization. A 2-cm transverse incision is made 2 cm proximal to the wrist fold, and the vessel is located by blunt dissection with small hemostats. Skin hooks are helpful to hold the incision open. In general, the hemostats should be used to separate the tissues in a plane parallel to the vessels, because this will minimize vessel injury. The dissection also is guided by intermittent palpation to maintain orientation to the vessel. Once exposed, a 1.0- to 1.5-cm length of vessel should be cleaned and mobilized, following which 2-0 or 3-0 silk sutures are passed beneath it with a right-angle clamp. We prefer use of one suture proximal and one distal to the site of vessel puncture. The distal suture can be used to elevate the vessel for direct visual puncture. If not successful initially,

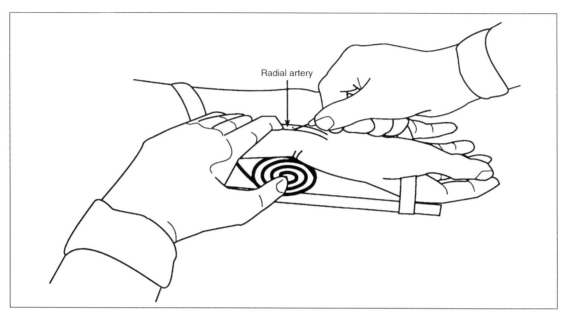

FIGURE   **6-1**

Radial arterial line insertion. The hand is dorsiflexed and secured on an arm board. The catheter is positioned by palpation of the artery. Initial needle insertion is at about 30 degrees to the skin.

traction on the proximal suture will stop the bleeding, allowing visualization of the vessel puncture site so that it can be catheterized without the necessity of another puncture. Once catheterized, both sutures are removed (not tied) and the skin closed. Pressure should be maintained on the cutdown site for 5 or 10 minutes to prevent hematoma formation.

## Brachial Artery

The brachial artery is the continuation of the axillary artery and gives rise to the radial and ulnar arteries. Collateral circulation is supplied by the ulnar collateral artery. This artery is best isolated just above the elbow crease medial to the biceps tendon. A 20-gauge, 2-inch catheter is inserted at a 30-degree angle to the skin until blood appears in the flash chamber. The vessel is then cannulated by either the direct or modified or classic Seldinger technique, as described previously. Use of an arm board is recommended to prevent flexion at the elbow and kinking of the catheter.

Use of the brachial artery entails greater risk than use of the radial artery: (1) Adequacy of collateral circulation is much more difficult to assure, (2) embolization could occlude either of the major arterial supplies to the hand, and (3) bleeding in the area of the median nerve may result in neuropathy and Volkmann's contracture. Bleeding may require fasciotomy (Hudson-Civetta, 1983). Cannulation of the brachial artery should not be attempted in patients with bleeding disorders.

## Axillary Artery

The axillary artery is the continuation of the subclavian artery. It enters the axilla from under the teres major and lies in the proximal groove between the biceps and triceps muscles medially in the arm. This artery is almost as large as the femoral artery and has significant collateral flow; axillary artery thrombosis does not lead to distal ischemia. Because the right axillary artery arises from the right brachiocephalic trunk in direct communication with the common carotid artery, air, clot, or particulate matter may embolize the brain during flushing. Thus, it may be safer to use the left axillary artery.

For cannulation, the patient can be positioned either with the hand beneath the head with the palm near the occiput or with the arm extended and externally rotated (Fig 6-2). The vessel is located by palpation, and an 18- or 20-gauge catheter, measuring at least 5 cm but preferably 16 cm, is inserted into the artery until pulsatile blood is observed in the flash chamber. The needle is inserted initially at about a 30-degree angle to the skin, and it is lowered once blood return is noted for direct advancement or guidewire insertion. The remainder of the procedure is as described previously. Location of the artery near the brachial plexus can result in nerve compression should a hematoma develop. Direct injury to the cords of the brachial plexus may occur during insertion attempts, because the axillary artery, vein, and three cords of the brachial

F I G U R E   **6-2**

Axillary arterial line insertion. The patient is positioned with the arm extended and externally rotated. The artery is palpated with one hand, and the needle is inserted at a 30-degree angle to the skin. The glide slope of the needle is projected to puncture the artery at or near the site of palpation by the opposite hand.

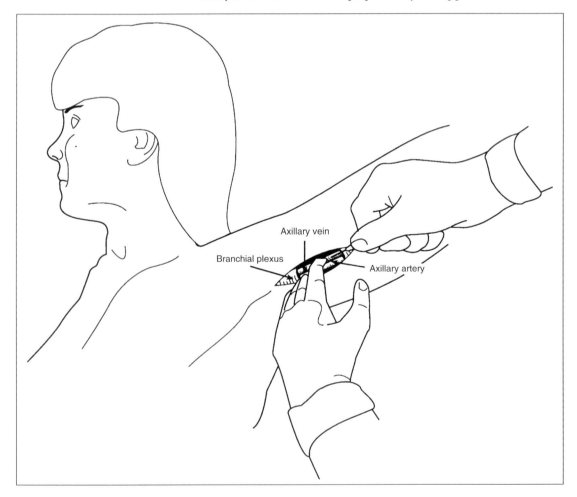

plexus form a neurovascular bundle within the axillary sheath. Similar to brachial cannulation, distal circulation should be checked regularly after axillary arterial line insertion.

## Dorsalis Pedis Artery

The dorsalis pedis artery is located on the dorsal aspect of the foot and is usually easily palpated, except in the 12% of people in whom it is congenitally absent. It is an extension of the anterior tibial artery. Collateral blood supply is usually good, and ischemia is uncommon following cannulation of this vessel. Collateral circulation, supplied by the lateral plantar artery, can be assessed by compression to occlusion of the dorsalis pedis artery, followed by pressure on the nail bed of the great toe until it blanches. On release of pressure on the nail bed, color should return within 2 to 3 seconds.

The patient's foot is held in a neutral position, and a 20- or 22-gauge needle is introduced into the artery at a shallow angle to the skin (Fig 6-3). Although any of the three techniques described previously may be used, guidewires are felt by many to be particularly useful for gaining

access to the dorsalis pedis. The remainder of the procedures is as described previously.

## Femoral Artery

The femoral artery is an extension of the external iliac artery. It lies just below the inguinal ligament midway along a line drawn from the superior iliac spine and symphysis pubis just lateral to the vein and medial to the nerve. The usual catheters employed range from 20 to 16 gauge, are 16 cm in length, and are attached to a 10-mL syringe. The needle is inserted about 2 cm below the inguinal ligament and at a 45-degree angle (Fig 6-4). Puncture often can be felt and is heralded by the ability to rapidly aspirate bright red blood. A gloved finger placed over the hub of the needle can usually feel the arterial pulsations. Once the vessel is punctured, the needle is lowered to between 15 and 30 degrees, and a J-tipped guidewire is inserted. The needle is removed, and direct pressure is applied to the insertion site to prevent bleeding or hematoma formation. The catheter is placed over the guidewire, but it is not advanced until the distal (external) tip of the guidewire itself has been secured. A scalpel nick

FIGURE  **6-3**

Dorsalis pedis arterial line insertion. The artery is palpated beneath two fingers of one hand. The skin is punctured about 1 to 2 cm distal to the site of palpation, and the needle is advanced at a 10-degree angle to puncture the vessel (beneath the fingers).

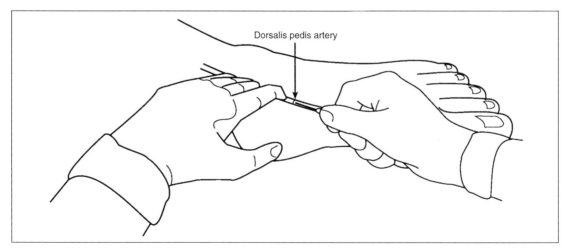

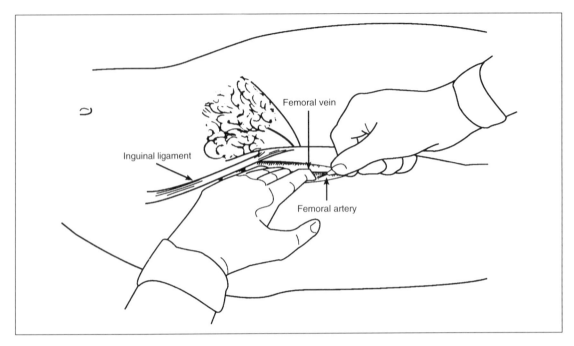

F I G U R E    **6-4**

Femoral arterial line insertion. The femoral artery is palpated distal to the inguinal ligament. The needle is inserted at a 45-degree angle to the skin. The hub of the needle is then dropped to between 15 and 30 degrees once the vessel is punctured. A J-tipped guidewire is then introduced, following which the catheter is slid over it and into the artery.

of the skin may be required for ease of passage of the catheter through the skin. The wire is then removed and the catheter connected and secured as detailed previously.

A complication peculiar to femoral vessel cannulation is puncture of the back wall of the vessel above the inguinal ligament, where blood may dissect into the retroperitoneal area; this is capable of masking a hemorrhage of up to several liters. Because of the large size of the femoral artery and vein, the likelihood of an AV fistula is higher than with smaller vessels, should both vessels be penetrated with a single insertion. Risk of AV fistula formation also relates to the much larger catheters used for femoral arterial cannulation. Similarly, the larger puncture site makes bleeding at the time of line removal more problematic. Pressure should be applied to the femoral site for 10 to 20 minutes at removal.

## Complications

As mentioned previously some complications are site-specific, while others are more general. Those that are more site-specific are covered in the technique section of this chapter (Table 6-1).

## Arterial Occlusion

Postcannulation radial arterial occlusion has been reported in up to 50% of patients in some series (Butt, 1987; Bedford, 1977). Ischemic and necrotic complications are much less common, occurring in less than 1% of patients with radial artery cannulas. Thrombosis appears to be related to the relative diameters of the catheter and vessel (Kaye, 1983), the material and whether the catheter is tapered (Beards, 1994), and duration

TABLE  **6-1**

Complications of arterial lines

Hematoma
Hemorrhage
Catheter
    Occlusion
    Dislocation
Infection
Embolism
    Thrombotic
    Air
Ischemic injury
Thrombosis
Pseudoaneurysm (traumatic)
AV fistulas

of insertion greater than 72 hours (Butt, 1987). The number of attempts before successful cannulation, low cardiac output, hypotension, use of vasopressors, peripheral vaso-occlusive processes, and Raynaud's disease all increase the risk of thrombosis. Fortunately, most thrombosed radial arteries recannalize within a few weeks (Hudson-Civetta, 1983). Generally, the smaller the catheter relative to the vessel, the lower the incidence of thrombosis.

## Embolism

Clots adherent to the catheter tip, or even the vessel lumen, can be dislodged by flushing of the arterial line or at the time of removal. To reduce this risk, some have proposed that intermittent flushing be limited to 1 to 2 seconds, despite any basis in data. Flush solutions are heparinized for the purpose of reducing the risk of thrombosis and subsequent embolization. Air embolism also can occur as a result of line flushing. Air emboli may present as seizures, hemiparesis, or focal neurologic findings. Treatment is supportive and involves either the administration of 100% oxygen or the institution of hyperbaric chamber dives.

## Skin Necrosis

Flow disturbances by the catheter in the small branches of any artery may produce ischemia and sloughing of the skin. Indeed, amputations of hands and feet have resulted from such complications. Blanching of the skin may occur with flushing of the catheter and indicate interference with skin circulation.

## Bleeding

Any disturbances of the coagulation mechanism may result in oozing or frank bleeding at the site of arterial puncture. When such abnormalities exist, or are likely to exist, use of peripheral sites (radial and dorsalis pedis) is much preferred to the more central sites (axillary, brachial, femoral). Local pressure and use of topical thrombin spray may be used to control bleeding, if peripheral. Ultimately, the goal is correction of the coagulopathy.

## Infection

Both local site infection and septicemia increase with the duration of catheterization (Band, 1979). The rate of bacteremia with cutdowns is almost 10 times that with percutaneous cannulation. To reduce risk of infection, the catheter site should be rotated every 4 days, and more often if there are local signs of infection (Spaccavento, 1982). Transducer, tubing, and infusion solutions should be changed every 48 hours.

**REFERENCES**

Band JD, Maki DG. Infections caused by arterial catheters used for hemodynamic monitoring. Am J Med 1979;67:735–741.

Beards SC, Doedens L, Jackson A, Lipman J. A comparison of arterial lines and insertion techniques in critically ill patients. Anaesthesia 1994;49: 968–973.

Bedford RF. Radial arterial function following percutaneous cannulation with 18 and 20 gauge catheters. Anesthesiology 1977;47:37–39.

Butt W, Shann F, McDonnel G. Effect of heparin concentration and infusion rate of patency of arterial catheters. Crit Care Med 1987;15:230–232.

Hudson-Civetta J, Caruthers-Banner TE. Intra-vascular catheters: current guidelines for care and maintenance. Heart Lung 1983;12:466–476.

Kaye A. Invasive monitoring techniques: arterial cannulation, bedside pulmonary artery catheterization and arterial puncture. Heart Lung 1983;12:395–427.

Mangar D, Laborde RS, Vu DN. Delayed ischaemia of the hand necessitating amputation after radial artery cannulation. Can J Anaesth 1993; 40:247–250.

Seldinger SI. Catheter replacement of the needle in percutaneous arteriography. Acta Radiol Diagn 1953;39:368–376.

Spaccavento LJ, Hawley HG. Infections associated with intra-arterial lines. Heart Lung 1982;11: 118–122.

# CHAPTER 7

# Venous Access: Techniques for Difficult or Chronic Cases

*W*hile the need for prolonged intravenous (IV) access is rare in uncomplicated obstetrical practice, coexisting disease processes may require prolonged IV access in order to deliver total parenteral nutrition (TPN). The use of TPN in pregnancy is well described for such conditions as hyperemesis gravidarum, inflammatory bowel disease, cystic fibrosis, pancreatitis, and gastroparesis (Wolk, 1990; Hatjis, 1985; Levine, 1988; Lee, 1986; Lavin, 1990; Greenspoon, 1993, 1994; Korelitz, 1992; Abell, 1992; Gineston, 1984; Hew, 1980; Hanan, 1993; MacBurney, 1986; Watson, 1990; Kirby, 1988; Gray, 1989; Wiedner, 1993). Less commonly, prolonged IV access may be necessary for gravidas suffering from diseases requiring prolonged administration of parenteral medication, such as heparin, antibiotics, cytotoxic chemotherapy, or magnesium sulfate for preterm labor. Acute or chronic renal failure requiring hemodialysis also may necessitate prolonged IV access. Finally, obtaining IV access may be challenging in gravidas with a history of prolonged parenteral chemotherapy or IV drug abuse, or with severe hypovolemia in which suitable peripheral veins cannot be accessed easily. Table 7-1 lists indications for prolonged venous access in obstetric patients.

---

## Catheter Types and Placement Sites

Currently available IV catheters are of three types: short-term transcutaneous catheters, long-term transcutaneous catheters, and implanted subcutaneous catheters. Catheters are named *peripheral* or *central* based on the vein of insertion and the location of the catheter tip. Veins distal (based on the direction of venous blood flow) to and including the axillary and common femoral veins are considered central, while those further "upstream" are considered peripheral. Central vein cannulation is required to accommodate the large-bore catheters necessary for high-volume administration rates. When administering highly osmolar, sclerotic, or thrombotic IV fluids, most agree the catheter tip should be placed near the heart in the superior or inferior vena cava, although optimal placement has not been established in prospective human studies (McGee, 1993). When centrally placed, catheters have been most commonly placed into the superior vena cava via larger central veins in the thoracic inlet and neck(subclavian and jugular veins) and are available in single-, double-, and triple-lumen configurations. While the peripherally inserted central venous catheter (PICC) was first introduced in 1975 (Hoshal, 1975), the popularity of peripherally placed IV catheters of all types has increased in the past decade. Peripheral cannulation can generally be performed outside the operating room, and it eliminates some of the iatrogenic risks of central venous puncture (pneumothorax, hemothorax, thoracic duct laceration, etc.). Skilled nursing personnel are trained in peripheral IV access techniques in many institutions. All of these characteristics of peripherally placed

## Indications for prolonged venous access

### Conditions Requiring Parenteral Nutrition
Hyperemesis gravidarum
Inflammatory bowel disease
Gastroparesis
Pancreatitis
Cystic fibrosis
Short bowel syndrome

### Requirement for Prolonged Parenteral Drug Therapy
Heparin (heart valves, deep vein thrombosis)
Antibiotics (bacterial endocarditis, osteomyelitis)
Chemotherapeutic agents for malignancy
Magnesium sulfate

### Lack of Peripheral Access
Previous intravenous drug abuse
Previous prolonged chemotherapy

### Hemodialysis

catheters may make them less costly. Peripheral placement also is advantageous for patients suffering from a coagulopathy.

Short-term transcutaneous catheters are constructed of polyethylene, polyurethane, polycarbonate, vinyl chloride, or silicone and are available in multiple lengths, diameters, and lumen numbers. Generally, they are used for periods of less than 2 weeks. These catheters are suitable for most obstetric patients in the "difficult access" group (history of IV drug abuse, IV chemotherapy, hypovolemia) and for others with rapidly resolvable conditions. Because of the intended short duration of use, sites on the lower extremities, such as pedal, saphenous, and femoral veins, might be selected. Decreased patient mobility and the high risk of catheter dislodgement are among the generally accepted disadvantages of lower extremity access locations.

Long-term transcutaneous catheters are usually constructed of silicone and are passed through a subcutaneous tunnel between the points of venous insertion and exit from the skin. Frequently, these catheters incorporate a Dacron cuff, which is positioned during placement within the subcutaneous tunnel, just proximal to the skin exit site. Catheter tunneling and the Dacron cuff promote tissue ingrowth and fixation and limit the spread of skin exit-site colonization or infection. Long-term catheters may incorporate a Groshong valve tip (Pasquale, 1992; Delmore, 1989; Davidson, 1988). Such catheters are blind-ended but incorporate a side slit near the catheter tip. Positive pressure exerted through the catheter blows the slit walls open outwardly for fluid or medication administration, while negative pressure draws the slit walls inward for blood sampling. At rest, the catheter is closed, theoretically obviating the need for heparinization between catheter use periods.

Long-term transcutaneous catheters are generally indicated when IV access is required for 4 or more weeks, and when catheter use events will be very frequent and/or prolonged (Ray, 1996). Veins commonly utilized for insertion of these catheters include the subclavian, external and internal jugular, cephalic (in the deltopectoral groove), and facial, with the catheter tunneled to exit on the flat portion of the upper thorax. When the femoral or greater saphenous veins near the groin are used, the catheter is tunneled onto the lower chest or abdominal wall or onto the thigh. Peripherally placed central IV lines for long-term use are also inserted via the basilic, cephalic, and antecubital veins near the antecubital fossa.

The "implantables," catheters attached to reservoirs placed into subcutaneous pockets, are indicated for very long-term use (months to years), typically in patients requiring intermittent boluses or short infusions of parenteral medications. During catheter use, access to the reservoir is gained by transcutaneous placement of a special Huber-point needle (Fig 7-1). Huber-point needles have a noncoring tip that is less damaging to the silicone covers of reservoir chambers. Using implantables, patients have maximal mobility, freedom from worry about catheter dislodgement, and no external appliances in between catheter use events. Implantable reservoir pumps are also available (Blackshear, 1972). One such pump, the Infusaid pump (Norwood, MA) utilizes a metal shell surrounding two chambers separated by a diaphragm. One chamber houses the medication to be delivered, and the other, a volatile fluorocarbon, which exerts pressure on the diaphragm between the two chambers, forcing the medication from the reservoir.

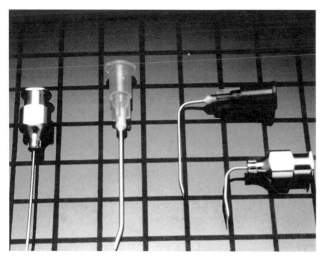

F I G U R E  **7-1**

Huber (noncoring) needle. Notice that the needle shaft is angled so the bevel remains parallel to the long axis of the needle, eliminating coring out of the silicone tops of reservoir chambers of implantable ports.

Implantable catheters are available in single- or double-lumen configurations for central use. The veins utilized for catheter insertion are generally the same as for the long-term transcutaneous catheters, but the reservoir should be placed in a secure, flat, nonmobile area, preferably overlying a rib, to facilitate reservoir puncture. Abdominal wall placement is thus less desirable. Reservoir systems for peripherally placed catheters have been developed, with the subcutaneous tunnel for the reservoir made overlying the muscles of the radial aspect of the proximal anterior forearm (Fig 7-2) (Starkhammer, 1990; Winters, 1990; Andrews, 1990; Pearl, 1991; McKee, 1991; Morris, 1991; Finney, 1992; Salem, 1993; Schuman, 1995).

## Catheter and Site Selection

The first considerations are the treatment requirements of the patient. How will the catheter be used—for TPN, medications, blood sampling, dialysis, or combinations of these? How frequently will the catheter be used? How long is the expected duration of treatment—weeks, months, years, lifelong? Is there a requirement for rapid

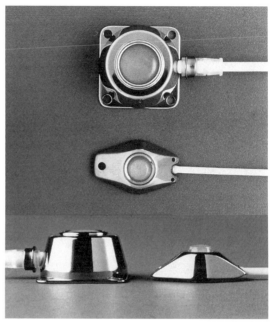

F I G U R E  **7-2**

Standard and peripherally placed implantable ports, as viewed from above and the side. (The larger standard port is superior-most in the view from above and is to the left in the side view.)

fluid volume administration? Is the planned infusate highly osmolar, sclerotic, or thrombogenic, favoring catheter tip placement in the superior or inferior vena cava? These concerns will usually identify the catheter type to be used and whether it should be placed peripherally or centrally or be implanted.

The second concerns are addressed in the patient physical assessment. Medical history points that should be considered include previous trauma, surgery, or radiation therapy involving potential catheterization sites; previous history and the site of catheterizations (or attempts), especially noting complications such as thrombosis and infection; history of coagulopathy or active infection; and any allergies, especially to antiseptic solutions, tape, and catheter materials. During the physical examination, the patient's general body habitus is assessed, as well as any deformities or immobility that could possibly affect catheter placement. Specific potential catheterization sites are inspected for scars, loss of skin integrity, and local infection, as well as for evidence of edema, developed collateral veins, or chronic skin changes typical of the postphlebitic syndrome, which may indicate previous venous thrombosis. Arteries nearby catheterization sites are assessed in the event of inadvertent injury. Finally, the patient's ability to tolerate the Trendelenburg position, as well as her ability to tolerate potential complications, such as pneumothorax, are assessed. The physical assessment, then, should allow selection and rank ordering of potential catheterization sites, in the event catheterization at the primary site is unsuccessful.

The final factor is the training, ability, and experience of the individual placing the catheter. With other factors being equal, the operator should choose the catheter, site, and placement technique with which he or she is most experienced and comfortable.

## Catheterization Techniques

Veins are cannulated either percutaneously or by direct surgical cutdown. Percutaneous catheter insertion has the advantages of decreased tissue trauma, lower infection risk, potential reusability of insertion sites, and simpler, more rapid performance (Nohr, 1994). Catheters may be percutaneously placed into the superior vena cava via the subclavian, internal or external jugular, median basilic, cephalic, and antecubital veins, and into the inferior vena cava via the femoral vein. Direct surgical cutdown techniques virtually eliminate the risks of pneumothorax or inadvertent puncture of other structures associated with the percutaneous technique. Dissected tissues and the vein to be cannulated are visualized directly, decreasing the bleeding risk in coagulopathic patients (Davis, 1984). Additionally, almost any suitable vein can be cannulated by surgical cutdown. In addition to the veins listed, the lateral thoracic, internal mammary, axillary, intercostal, azygous, inferior epigastric, iliac, greater saphenous, and gonadal veins all can be used to access either the superior or inferior vena cava by surgical cutdown technique.

In transcutaneous catheter placement by direct central venous puncture, the patient is first positioned properly. The patient should be in the Trendelenburg position, perhaps rolled slightly to the left in later stages of pregnancy when the inferior vena cava is susceptible to compression by the uterus. The legs should be raised if the patient is intolerant of the Trendelenburg position. For PICC cannulations, a tourniquet or BP cuff is placed proximally on the arm, and the arm is abducted 90 degrees from the trunk. The skin is widely prepared with a suitable disinfectant solution and is sterilely draped. The chosen vein is punctured with a needle attached to a syringe, with free blood return indicating entry into the vein. Pulsatile blood flow from the needle indicates arterial puncture, and the needle should be immediately removed and direct pressure applied to the site.

After correct venous puncture, the syringe is removed carefully, while the operator covers the needle hub to prevent excessive bleeding and entry of air (for central venous punctures). In the Seldinger technique (used for most direct central venous punctures), a guidewire is placed through the needle, and the needle is withdrawn. If not accomplished previously, local anesthetic is infused into the region prior to enlarging the puncture site slightly with a scalpel to accommodate the catheter or dilators. Local anesthetic also is infiltrated into the sites of incisions or dissection for subcutaneous pockets for Dacron cuffs or reservoirs. A stiff dilator is then generally threaded over the wire and passed one or more times to dilate the tract to the vein. The dilator is then removed and is placed through the slightly larger catheter. The dilator-catheter assembly is then threaded over the wire into correct position, and the wire and dilator are removed. Correct placement is supported by confirming free aspiration of blood from the catheter and free flow (by gravity alone) of an appropriate crystalloid solution into the catheter.

Long-term transcutaneous catheters are generally placed using a peel-away sheath modification of Seldinger's technique. The initial steps are identical. After dilation of the tract, the dilator is removed and placed through a slightly larger peel-away sheath. The dilator-sheath assembly is then advanced over the wire into the chosen vein, and the wire and dilator are removed. A silastic catheter is then threaded through the peel-away sheath into the proper position. After correct positioning, the handles on the peel-away sheath are rotated perpendicularly to its long axis until the sheath cracks along its sides. Pulling the sheath handles apart, the sheath is then simultaneously peeled in half along its long axis and removed, while carefully holding the catheter in place.

The catheter-through-the-needle technique is also utilized, primarily for short-term transcutaneous catheterizations of central veins, and for PICC placement. The initial steps are again identical to those described previously. A relatively larger needle is used for the venipuncture. Following venipuncture, a catheter of appropriate size is fed directly through the needle into proper position. Extreme caution must be taken to never pull the catheter back out through the needle, or the catheter may be sheared and catheter embolus occurs. Following positioning, a plastic sheath is snapped into position around both the needle and the catheter, and both are secured in place. Alternatively, PICC systems allow the needle to be peeled away.

The jugular, subclavian, and femoral veins are utilized for direct central venous access, and two excellent references are available for descriptions of anatomic landmarks and specific technique (Nohr, 1994; Agee, 1992). When utilized, the external jugular vein is usually visible coursing from the parotid area near the angle of the mandible to the mid-clavicular region (Fig 7-3).

The internal jugular vein is usually approached between the sternal and clavicular heads of insertion of the sternocleidomastoid muscle, puncturing the skin at a 30- to 45-degree angle and aiming toward the ipsilateral nipple (middle approach) (Fig 7-4). Alternatively, the vein may be approached from a more cephalad point, posterior to the sternocleidomastoid muscle, where it is crossed by the external jugular vein, while aiming for the sternal notch (posterior approach) (Fig 7-5).

The subclavian vein is usually cannulated via an infraclavicular approach, beneath the middle third of the clavicle. The skin puncture site is approximately 1 cm beneath the clavicle but should be further from the clavicle to lessen the risk of pneumothorax in patients with a thick chest wall. This increased distance from the clavicle allows the needle to scythe closely along the posterior surface of the clavicle. The needle is aimed toward the sternal notch. A supraclavicular approach is also described (Conroy, 1990).

The femoral vein lies just medial to the femoral artery and is deep to the inguinal ligament running between the pubic tubercle and anterior superior iliac spine. The skin is punctured 2 to 3 cm caudal to the inguinal ligament to ensure the vein is cannulated in the thigh (Fig 7-6).

For central venous access via a surgical cutdown, the cephalic vein is most often utilized.

FIGURE  **7-3**

External jugular vein anatomy.

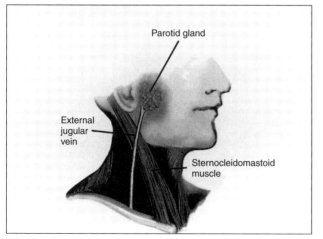

FIGURE  **7-4**

Middle approach to internal jugular vein catheterization.

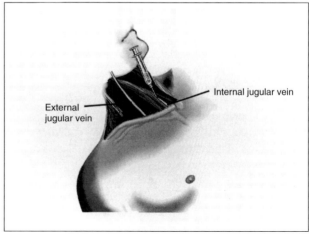

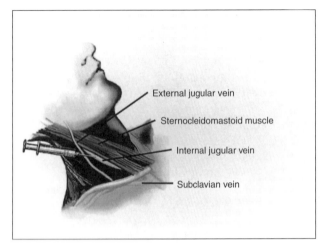

FIGURE 7-5

Posterior approach to internal jugular vein catheterization.

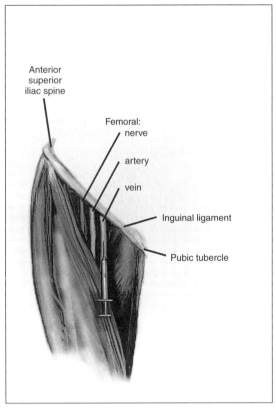

FIGURE 7-6

Infrainguinal femoral vein catheterization.

The cephalic vein is found deep to the clavipectoral fascia, in the deltopectoral groove (Fig 7-7). The deltopectoral groove runs vertically, just medial to the coracoid process of the scapula.

Long-term transcutaneous, surgical cutdown, and implanted catheters are generally inserted following prophylactic antibiotic administration in an operating theater or outpatient surgical suite, maximizing sterility. Several authors have described utilizing real-time ultrasonography to facilitate venous location and puncture and to lessen the incidence of puncture-related complications (Denys, 1991; Sherer, 1993). Fluoroscopic guidance is used frequently to speed and simplify correct catheter positioning. Right atrial electrocardiography is also described for facilitating proper catheter tip placement (McGee, 1993). Peripherally inserted central venous catheters are most often placed at the patient's bedside or in a clinic setting. Some PICC systems utilize an electronic catheter tip finder wand to facilitate catheter placement (Fig 7-8) (McKee, 1991; Morris, 1991). Postprocedure chest radiographs should be performed after all central venous catheterizations to confirm correct catheter positioning and to assess for complications (Nohr, 1994; Agee, 1992; Baranowski, 1993).

FIGURE 7-7

Cephalic vein course via cutdown in the deltopectoral groove.

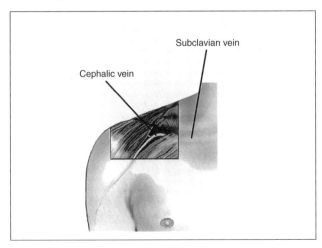

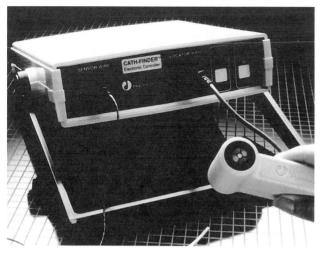

F I G U R E   **7-8**

Electronic catheter tip finder system, including finder wand, an alternative to fluoroscopy to locate the catheter tip during catheter insertion.

## Catheter Care

Although essentially all authors profess the value of catheter teams to insert and care for long-term and central venous catheters, there is little universal agreement on most other aspects of catheter use and care, including recommended length of use, catheter site care procedures, dressing type, catheter flushing protocols, treating the occluded catheter, catheter management in the patient with fever or suspected infection, or even how to define catheter-related infection. The confusion exists largely because of the paucity of prospective, randomized clinical trials and because of the differing populations studied in the available published studies. One of the best overall discussions is the very well referenced publication of Baranowski (1993). In the absence of a clear consensus on these aspects of catheter care, it is recommended that hospitals and practitioners establish practice guidelines and/or protocols that can be subsequently studied and modified within a quality improvement program.

## Complications

Complications associated with IV catheters are of two general types: those associated with venipuncture and catheter insertion (immediate complications) and those associated with catheter use (delayed complications) (Table 7-2). The risk of immediate complications is highest with direct central vein catheterization and is minimized with external jugular vein or PICC utilization and with surgical cutdown techniques. General catheter-use guidelines published by the Food and Drug Administration are directed at reducing catheter-related complications (FDA Drug Bulletin, 1989).

## Failed Catheterization

Ninety-five percent of direct central venous and surgical cutdown catheterizations are accomplished successfully, while external jugular venous catheterization is successful only 70% of the time

T A B L E   **7-2**

Complications of central venous catheters

| Immediate Complications | Delayed Complications |
| --- | --- |
| Insertion failure | Venous thrombosis |
| Malposition | Pulmonary embolism |
| Air embolism | Superior vena caval |
| Catheter embolism | syndrome |
| Cardiac arrhythmia | Venous stenosis |
| Pneumothorax | Arteriovenous fistula |
| Hemothorax | Arterial pseudo- |
| Hydrothorax/ | aneurysm |
| chylothorax | Catheter thrombosis |
| Tracheal injury | Catheter dislodgement/ |
| Esophageal injury | breakage |
| Femoral nerve injury | Catheter-associated |
| Brachial plexus injury | bacteremia |
| Phrenic nerve injury | Catheter tunnel |
| Vagus nerve injury | infection |
| Recurrent laryngeal | Endocarditis |
| nerve injury | Cardiac perforation |
| Stellate ganglion injury | Cardiac tamponade |
| | Thrombophlebitis |
| | Suppurative |
| | thrombophlebitis |
| | Clavicular osteomyelitis |

(Agee, 1992). Most PICC studies do not report failed catheterizations, but one reported a 15.4% incidence (Merrell, 1994).

## Catheter Malposition

Although optimal catheter tip location has not been established by any prospective human study, most believe the superior vena cava, proximal to the right atrium, to be the ideal location (McGee, 1993). With catheter tips located in smaller, more proximal veins, the complications of venous thrombosis and stenosis may be more likely, while catheter tips positioned in the heart may lead to cardiac arrhythmias, perforation, tamponade, valvular injury, or endocarditis. Catheter tip malposition is most frequently seen following PICC insertion from the antecubital approach, ranging from 21% to 55% nationally. Most of these malpositioned catheters reposition spontaneously, or they may be repositioned successfully by forceful saline injection through the catheter or with radiologic guidance (Lum, 1989; Goodwin, 1993; James, 1993). The tips of PICCs may move as much as 10 cm with arm and neck positioning (McGee, 1993). Fluoroscopic guidance during insertion facilitates correct placement of all types of central venous catheters, as does right atrial electrocardiography (McGee, 1993), ultrasonography (Sherer, 1993), and electronic catheter tracking systems (McKee, 1991; Morris, 1991). Postinsertion chest radiographs are recommended universally (Nohr, 1994; Agee, 1992; Baranowski, 1993; James, 1993; LaFortune, 1993).

## Catheter Dislodgement

Although little discussed, several PICC series report the incidence of accidental catheter dislodgement at between 0.8% and 10.4% (Hoshal, 1975; Merrell, 1994; Goodwin, 1993; James, 1993; Lam, 1994; Loughran, 1992). The method of catheter fixation utilized in the series with the highest accidental dislodgement rate was not specified (Lam, 1994), but the high overall incidence of this complication is a topic for concern and future research.

## Pneumothorax

The risk of pneumothorax is 1% to 6% in direct subclavian vein catheterization, is less following direct catheterization of other central veins, and is essentially eliminated with PICC and surgical cutdown techniques (Nohr, 1994; Collin, 1994). Collin and Clarke (1994) reviewed the occurrence of delayed or late pneumothorax following central venous catheterization and recommended that postinsertion chest radiographs be expiratory and in the upright position. Repeat or delayed chest radiographs are indicated following catheterizations requiring multiple insertion attempts, for suspicion of pneumothorax despite an initially normal postinsertion radiograph, for persistent (pleuritic or back) pain or respiratory symptoms following catheterization, in the preoperative assessment in any patient having had a central venous catheter inserted, and for patients requiring intraoperative catheterizations.

## Hemothorax and Other Bleeding Complications

Hemothorax, an infrequent complication primarily of direct subclavian vein catheterization, occurs following puncture or laceration of an intrathoracic vein or artery and the parietal pleura. Because intrathoracic vascular structures are inaccessible for direct compression, subclavian and, to a lesser degree, internal jugular direct venous catheterization is contraindicated in patients with a coagulopathy.

Extrapleural arterial puncture results in an extrapleural hematoma that may be visible on a chest radiograph. Erosion through the heart by a malpositioned catheter tip may result in life-threatening pericardial tamponade from either infusate or blood. Arterial puncture during femoral venous catheterization may cause retroperitoneal hemorrhage.

## Catheter Thrombosis and Occlusion

Catheter occlusion usually results from the formation of a fibrin plug at the catheter tip (Nohr, 1994). This is part of a fibrin sleeve that forms around essentially all IV catheters present for more than a week (Lowell, 1991). Flushing protocols, with and without heparin, have been devised to reduce catheter thrombosis (Baranowski, 1993; Fry, 1992), and fibrinolytic agent administration through the catheter is frequently successful to reopen thrombosed catheters (Tschirhart, 1988; Lawson, 1991; Wachs, 1990; Holcombe, 1992; Lawson, 1982; Bjeletich, 1987; Haire, 1990; Atkinson, 1990). Precipitate occlusions resulting from administering multiple incompatible medications via a catheter may be dissolved with 0.1 N hydrochloric acid (Shulman, 1988; Duffy, 1989; Breaux, 1987), and lipid aggregation may be cleared with 70% ethyl alcohol (Pennington, 1987).

The longer length and frequently the smaller diameter of PICCs may place these catheters at higher risk for thrombosis or occlusion. The reported incidence of PICC occlusion is between 1.0% and 8.2% (Merrell, 1994; Goodwin, 1993; James, 1993; Loughran, 1992). Incorporation of a Groshong valve reduces catheter thrombosis or occlusion and the need for heparin flushes (Pasquale, 1992; Baranowski, 1993; Fry, 1992).

## Thrombophlebitis

Mechanical phlebitis within the first week after catheterization is the most common complication seen with PICCs (Baranowski, 1993), occurring in 4.7% to 11.4% of patients (Merrell, 1994; Goodwin, 1993; James, 1993; Loughran, 1992). Most mechanical phlebitis will resolve with heat and elevation and does not necessitate catheter removal.

## Venous Thrombosis and Stenosis

Thrombosis of the great veins utilized in central venous catheterization is frequently asymptomatic and therefore underrecognized and -reported (Nohr, 1994; Baranowski, 1993). In subclavian venous catheterization, the complication is clinically diagnosed with a frequency of less than 5% but is diagnosed in 20% to 40% of patients by contrast venography (Nohr, 1994). Venous stenosis has been likewise detected in more than 20% of patients undergoing prolonged venous catheterization (Wanscher, 1988). Although infrequent, pulmonary embolism from catheter-related venous thrombosis can occur (Leiby, 1989). Particularly for the longer-length PICCs, keeping catheters scrupulously clean during insertion, using powderless or rinsed gloves, is advocated to reduce thrombogenicity (Hoshal, 1975). Treatment of catheter-related deep vein thrombosis involves catheter removal, anticoagulant administration, and possibly fibrinolytic administration (Nohr, 1994; Baranowski, 1993; Haire, 1990; Clarke, 1990; Steed, 1986; Faschini, 1987; Barclay, 1991). Because it is naturally occurring in humans, has a very short plasma half-life of 5 minutes, and does not cross the placenta, tissue plasminogen activator may be well-suited for fibrinolytic use during pregnancy (Barclay, 1991).

## Catheter-Related Infection

Catheter-related infections (CRIs) include a number of entities: exit-site and tunnel infections, catheter-related bacteremia, catheter-related sepsis, suppurative thrombophlebitis, endocarditis, and clavicular osteomyelitis. Coagulase-negative staphylococci, *Staphylococcus aureus*, and *Candida* species arising from the skin and colonizing the catheter and catheter tunnel are the most common etiologic agents of CRIs (Baranowski, 1993; Kruse, 1993; Egebo, 1996). These infections occur with an estimated overall incidence of approximately 10% to 40% (Nohr, 1994; Bozzetti, 1985; Maki, 1973) and include more than 80% of the intravascular device-related bacteremias in hospitals (Baranowski, 1993; Nystrom, 1983). The marginal cost of treating a case of catheter-related sepsis has been estimated at more than $6000 (Maki, 1988).

Despite the obvious importance of CRIs when considering their frequency, resultant patient morbidity, and cost, there is little universal agreement over the relative importance of the potential predisposing factors for CRI. There also are few areas of agreement regarding catheter use guidelines as related to CRI. This confusion arises from the general dearth of prospective randomized controlled studies pertaining to CRI. Additionally, comparison of existing studies is hampered by important study differences, such as study populations, type and indication for the catheter used, definitions of CRIs employed, and methods of catheter care and management. Thus, many basic questions remain unanswered with regard to catheter use and CRIs, such as which catheter type and site to use; whether to use single-, double-, or triple-lumen catheters; what catheter care regimen is ideal; whether to change catheters (and sites) at predetermined intervals; and what is appropriate catheter management during suspected infection or CRI.

There are, however, a few areas of general agreement. First, hospital-based catheter care or management teams reduce the incidence of catheter-related complications (Baranowski, 1993; Kruse, 1993; Maki, 1973; Goldman, 1973; Nehme, 1980; Moyer, 1983; Faubion, 1986; Puntis, 1990; Ena, 1992; Nelson, 1986). Second, maximal sterile technique and barrier precautions and educational programs detailing these procedures reduce CRIs (Nehme, 1980; Faubion, 1986; Puntis, 1990; Raad, 1994; Maki, 1994; Parras, 1994; Ryan, 1974; Snydman, 1982). Data from clinical and basic science studies strongly suggest the superiority of chlorhexadine over other available skin disinfectants (Maki, 1991a; Sheikh, 1986; Lowbury, 1974). Given these data, the less than universal use of chlorhexadine (compared with other disinfectants, such as povidone-iodine) most likely stems from the lack of practical commercially prepared single-use packaging of this disinfectant (Baranowski, 1993).

Catheter-related infection is usually suspected by recognizing local signs of infection (erythema, tenderness, purulent drainage) at the catheter exit site or systemic signs of infection (fever, rigors, fluid sequestration, rising WBC count), particularly in patients lacking another likely source of infection. The diagnosis of local exit-site and tunnel infections is most often made clinically, with cultures necessary only to define antibiotic treatment, if needed. Exit-site infections may be treated successfully with local care and antibiotics in many instances; tunnel infections, however, generally also require catheter removal (Nohr, 1994; Baranowski, 1993; Clarke, 1990; Benezra, 1988). When suspected clinically, catheter-related bacteremia and sepsis are usually diag-

nosed by examining the results of catheter tip and blood cultures, as described by Nohr (1994). By this method, no infection is present when all cultures are "no growth," and no treatment is required. Infection unrelated to the catheter is present if peripheral blood cultures have growth, but catheter tip cultures are without growth. Treatment for the non-CRI is indicated. Catheter colonization or infection exists if catheter tip and/or aspirated blood cultures have growth, but peripheral blood cultures yield "no growth." Some authors would change nontunneled catheters over a wire in this instance, or administer specific antibiotics through tunneled catheters. Nohr and others recommend catheter removal should the involved organism be fungi, *S. aureus*, or other virulent bacteria (Benezra, 1988; Rotstein, 1995; Dugdale, 1990; Pizzo, 1993). Finally, catheter-related bacteremia or sepsis exits if peripherally drawn blood cultures and catheter tip and/or aspirated blood cultures yield the same organisms. In this instance, 10 or more days of appropriate antibiotic therapy and catheter removal are required. Catheter removal is also generally recommended in catheterized patients whose presumed catheter-unrelated infections fail to rapidly improve with appropriate treatment.

Other methods are employed, particularly during research, to diagnose CRIs. Most commonly cited is the quantitative culture technique for catheter tip culture described by Maki (Snydman, 1982a; Maki, 1977; Curtas, 1991). Catheter colonization or infection is indicated by growth of 15 or more colony-forming units. This technique has the disadvantage of requiring catheter change or removal. Others have used a Gram staining technique of either the catheter tip or skin at the catheter exit site (Cooper, 1985; Collignon, 1987; McGeer, 1987). In a small study population, McGeer and Righter (1987) showed complete correlation between catheter site and quantitative catheter cultures. This method has the advantage of not requiring catheter change or removal. Others have quantitatively cultured blood aspirated through catheters to diagnose CRI, another diagnostic technique not requiring catheter manipulation (Moyer, 1983; Capdevila, 1992; Wing, 1979). Skin and catheter hub culture results are used by some authors to predict CRI

(Guidet, 1994; Snydman, 1982a); Bjornson, 1982; Linares, 1985; Cheesbrough, 1986; Fan, 1988; De Cicco, 1989; Cercenado, 1990; Moro, 1994). Rush-forth et al (1993) evaluated three relatively rapid tests (acridine orange leukocyte cytospin [AOLC], nitroblue tetrazolium, and C-reactive protein) against quantitative blood culture data in a population of neonates and children, and found the AOLC test 87% sensitive and 94% specific for catheter-related bacteremia, supporting results from a previous study in neonates (Kite, 1988). Given the absence of a clear consensus on the best method of diagnosing CRIs, developing and evaluating hospital-specific guidelines, giving consideration to the user population and catheter use patterns, seems appropriate.

Technologic advancements may further reduce the incidence of CRIs. Although study results have not been uniformly favorable, attachable silver-impregnated cuffs implanted under the skin at the catheter exit site may have efficacy (Nystrom, 1983; Kite, 1988; Dahlberg, 1995; Flowers, 1989; Rafkin, 1990). Antiseptic-coated catheters are available, and studies have documented their reduction of catheter-related bacteremias (Maki, 1991b; Bach, 1992; Mimoz, 1996). Treating catheters with substances such as triiododecyl-methylammonium chloride and poly-N-vinylpyr-rolidine allows binding with antibiotics (Jansen, 1992) and may reduce CRIs (Trooskin, 1985; Kamal, 1991; Thornton, 1996).

Others have investigated the efficacy of thrombolytic therapy in treating catheter colonization or infection (Fishbein, 1990), a therapy that also may be necessary to medically treat septic thrombophlebitis (Clarke, 1990). Still others have begun investigating the prophylactic use of antibiotics to reduce the incidence of CRIs (Spafford, 1994; Schwartz, 1990; Hartman, 1989; Lim, 1991). Bullard (1996) and Civetta (1996) have reviewed techniques for prevention, diagnosis, and treatment of catheter-related infections.

## Conclusion

Prolonged IV access is occasionally vital to the successful outcome of a pregnancy, particularly for the provision of TPN. A variety of IV devices are available, with more assuredly just over the horizon. The proper and safe use of these devices requires understanding of their indications, skill in their insertion, and competence in recognizing and treating their associated complications. Given evolving trends in the practice of medicine, it seems likely that more research will focus on the cost-effectiveness of IV catheters and practices and their adaptability for home use (Mannel, 1994; Kravitz, 1993; Stokes, 1988; Boutin, 1992). Increasingly, health-care providers will require familiarity with these aspects of IV access.

**REFERENCES**

Abell TL, Riely CA. Hyperemesis gravidarum. Clin Gastroenterol 1992;21:835.

Agee KR, Balk RA. Central venous catheterization in the critically ill patient. Crit Care Clin 1992; 8:677.

Andrews JC, Walker-Andrews S, Ensminger WD. Long-term central venous access with a peripherally placed subcutaneous infusion port: initial results. Radiology 1990;176:45.

Atkinson JB, Bagnall HA, Gomperts E. Investigational use of tissue plasminogen activator (t-PA) for occluded central venous catheters. JPEN 1990;14:310.

Bach A, Bohrer H, Motsch J, et al. Prevention of catheter-related infections by antiseptic coating. Anesthesiology 1992;77:A259. Abstract.

Baranowski L. Central venous access devices: current technologies, uses, and management strategies. J Intravenous Nurs 1993;16:167.

Barclay GR, Allen K, Pennington CR. Tissue plasminogen activator in the treatment of superior vena caval thrombosis associated with parenteral nutrition. Postgrad Med J 1991;66:398.

Benezra D, Kiehn TE, Gold JWM, et al. Prospective study of infections in indwelling central venous catheters using quantitative blood cultures. Am J Med 1988;85:495.

Bjeletich J. Declotting central venous catheters with urokinase in the home by nurse clinicians. NITA 1987;Nov/Dec:428.

Bjornson HS, Colley R, Bower RH, et al. Association between microorganism growth at the catheter insertion site and the colonization of the catheter in patients receiving total parenteral nutrition. Surgery 1982;92:1385.

Blackshear PJ, Dorman FD, Blackshear PL Jr, et al. The design and initial testing of an implantable infusion pump. Surg Gynecol Obstet 1972; 134:51.

Boutin J, Hagan E. Patients' preference regarding portable pumps. J Intravenous Nurs 1992;15: 230.

Bozzetti F. Central venous catheter sepsis. Surg Gynecol Obstet 1985;161:293.

Breaux CW, Duke D, Georgeson KE, et al. Calcium phosphate crystal occlusion of central venous catheters used for total parenteral nutrition in infants and children: prevention and treatment. J Pediatr Surg 1987;22:829.

Bullard KM, Dunn DL. Diagnosis and treatment of bacteremia and intravascular catheter infections. Am J Surg 1996;172:13(s).

Capdevila JA, Planes AM, Palomar M, et al. Value of differential quantitative blood cultures in the diagnosis of catheter-related sepsis. Eur J Microbiol Infect Dis 1992;11:403.

Cercenado E, Ena J, Rodriguez-Creixems M, et al. A conservative procedure for the diagnosis of catheter-related infections. Arch Intern Med 1990;150:1417.

Cheesbrough JS, Finch RG, Burden RP. A prospective study of the mechanisms of infections associated with hemodialysis catheters. J Infect Dis 1986;154:579.

Civetta JM, Hudson-Civetta J, Bull S. Decreasing catheter-related infections and hospital costs by continuous quality improvement. Crit Care Med 1996;24:1660.

Clarke DE, Raffin TA. Infectious complications of in-dwelling long-term central venous catheters. Chest 1990;97:966.

Collignon P, Chan R, Munro R. Rapid diagnosis of intravascular catheter-related sepsis. Arch Intern Med 1987;147:1609.

Collin GR, Clarke LE. Delayed pneumothorax: a complication of central venous catheterization. Surg Rounds 1994;17:589.

Conroy JM, Rajagopalan PR, Baker JD III, et al. A modification of the supraclavicular approach to the central circulation. South Med J 1990;83: 1178.

Cooper GL, Hopkins CC. Rapid diagnosis of intravascular catheter-associated infection by direct gram staining of catheter segments. N Engl J Med 1985;312:1142.

Curtas S, Tramposch K. Culture methods to evaluate central venous catheter sepsis. Nutr Clin Pract 1991;6:43.

Dahlberg PJ, Apper WA, Singer JR, et al. Subclavian hemodialysis catheter infections: a prospective, randomized trial of an attachable silver-impregnated cuff for prevention of catheter-related infections. Infect Control Hosp Epidemiol 1995;16:506.

Davidson H, Bowersox J, Lee R. Experience with Groshong versus Hickman central venous catheters. Proc Am Soc Clin Oncol 1988;7:289.

Davis SJ, Thompson JS, Edney JA. Insertion of Hickman catheters: a comparison of cutdown and percutaneous techniques. Am Surg 1984;50:673.

De Cicco M, Chiaradia V, Veronesi A, et al. Source and route of microbial colonization of parenteral nutrition catheters. Lancet 1989;2:1258.

Delmore JE, Horbelt DV, Jack BL, et al. Experience with the Groshong long-term central venous catheter. Gynecol Oncol 1989;34:216.

Denys BG, Uretsky BF, Reddy PS, et al. An ultrasound method for safe and rapid central venous access. N Engl J Med 1991;324:566. Letter.

Duffy LF, Kerzner B, Gebus V, et al. Treatment of central venous catheter occlusions with hydrochloric acid. J Pediatr 1989;114:1002.

Dugdale DC, Ramsey PG. *Staphylococcus aureus* bacteremia in patients with Hickman catheters. Am J Med 1990;89:137.

Egebo K, Toft P, Jakobsen CJ. Contamination of central venous catheters: The skin insertion wand is a major source of contamination. J Hosp Infect 1996;32:99.

Ena J, Cercenado E, Martinez D, et al. Cross-sectional epidemiology of phlebitis and catheter-related infections. Infect Control Hosp Epidemiol 1992;13:15.

Fan ST, Teoh-Chan CH, Lau KF, et al. Predictive value of surveillance skin and hub cultures in central venous catheter sepsis. J Hosp Infect 1988;12:191.

Faschini G, Jadeja J, Lawson M, et al. Local infusion of urokinase for the lysis of thrombosis associated with permanent central venous catheters in cancer patients. J Clin Oncol 1987;5:672.

Faubion WC, Wesley JR, Khalidi N, et al. Total parenteral nutrition catheter sepsis: impact of the team approach. JPEN 1986;10:642.

FDA Drug Bulletin. 1989;19:15.

Finney R, Albrink M, Hart M, et al. A cost-effective peripheral venous port system placed at the bedside. J Surg Res 1992;53:17.

Fishbein HD, Friedman HS, Bennett BB, et al. Catheter-related sepsis refractory to antibiotic treated successfully with adjunctive urokinase infusion. Pediatr Infect Dis 1990;9:676.

Flowers RH, Schwenzer KJ, Kopel RF, et al. Efficacy of an attachable subcutaneous cuff for the prevention of intravascular catheter-related infection. A randomized, controlled trial. JAMA 1989;261:878.

Fry B. Intermittent heparin flushing protocols. A standardization issue. J Intravenous Nurs 1992; 15:160.

Gineston JL, Capron JP, Delcenserie R, et al. Prolonged total parenteral nutrition in a pregnant woman with acute pancreatitis. J Clin Gastroenterol 1984;6:249.

Goldman DA, Maki DG. Infection control in total parenteral nutrition. JAMA 1973;223:1341.

Goodwin ML, Carlson I. The peripherally inserted central catheter. J Intravenous Nurs 1993; 16:92.

Gray DS, Cabaniss ML. Home total parenteral nutrition in a pregnant diabetic after jejunoileal bypass for obesity. JPEN 1989;13:214.

Greenspoon JS, Rosen DJD, Ault M. Use of the peripherally inserted central catheter for paren-teral nutrition during pregnancy. Obstet Gynecol 1993;81:831.

Greenspoon JS, Safarik RH, Hayashi JT, et al. Parenteral nutrition during pregnancy: lack of association with idiopathic preterm labor or preeclampsia. J Reprod Med 1994;39:87.

Guidet B, Nicola I, Barakett V, et al. Skin versus hub cultures to predict colonization and infection of central venous catheter in intensive care patients. Infection 1994;22:43.

Haire WD, Lieberman RP, Lund GB, et al. Obstructed central venous catheters. Restoring function with a 12-hour infusion of low-dose urokinase. Cancer 1990;66:2279.

Hanan, IM. Inflammatory bowel disease in the pregnant woman. Compr Ther 1993;19:91.

Hartman LC, Urba WJ, Steis RG, et al. Use of prophylactic antibiotics for prevention of intravascular catheter-related infections in interleukin-2-treated patients (letter). JNCI 1989;81:1190.

Hatjis CG, Meis PJ. Total parenteral nutrition in pregnancy. Obstet Gynecol 1985;66:585.

Hew LR, Deitel ML. Total parenteral nutrition in gynecology and obstetrics. Obstet Gynecol 1980;55:464.

Holcombe BJ, Forloines-Lynn S, Garmhausen LW. Restoring patency of long-term central venous access devices. J Intravenous Nurs 1992;15:36.

Hoshal VL Jr. Total intravenous nutrition with peripherally inserted silicone elastomer central venous catheters. Arch Surg 1975;110:644.

James L, Bledsoe L, Hadaway LC. A retrospective look at tip location and complications of peripherally inserted central catheter lines. J Intravenous Nurs 1993;16:104.

Jansen B, Jansen S, Peters G, et al. In-vitro efficacy of a central venous catheter ("hydrocath") loaded with teicoplanin to prevent bacterial colonization. J Hosp Infect 1992;22:93.

Kamal GD, Pfaller MA, Rempe LE, et al. Reduced intravascular infection by antibiotic bonding. JAMA 1991;265:2364.

Kirby DF, Fiorenza V, Craig RM. Intravenous nutritional support during pregnancy. JPEN 1988; 12:72.

Kite P, Millar MR, Gorham P, et al. Comparison of five tests used in diagnosis of neonatal bacteraemia. Arch Dis Child 1988;63:639.

Korelitz BI. Inflammatory bowel disease in pregnancy. Clin Gastroenterol 1992;21:827.

Kravitz GR. Advances in IV delivery. Outpatient parenteral antibiotic therapy. Hosp Pract 1993; 28(suppl):21.

Kruse JA, Shah NJ. Detection and prevention of central venous catheter-related infections. Nutr Clin Pract 1993;8:163.

LaFortune S. The use of confirming x-rays to verify tip position for peripherally inserted catheters. J Intravenous Nurs 1993;16:246.

Lam S, Scannell R, Roessler D, et al. Peripherally inserted central catheters in an acute-care hospital. Arch Intern Med 1994;154:1833.

Lavin PL. Nutrition support in obstetric patients. Nutr Clin Pract 1990;5:138.

Lawson M. Partial occlusion of indwelling central venous catheters. J Intravenous Nurs 1991; 14:157.

Lawson M, Bottino JC, Hurtubise MR, et al. The use of urokinase to restore the patency of occluded central venous catheters. Am J Intravenous Ther Clin Nutr 1982;9:29–30, 32–34.

Lee RV, Rodgers BD, Young C. Total parenteral nutrition during pregnancy. Obstet Gynecol 1986;68:563.

Leiby JM, Purcell H, DeMaria JJ, et al. Pulmonary embolism as a result of Hickman catheter-related thrombosis. Am J Med 1989;86:228.

Levine MG, Esser D. Total parenteral nutrition for treatment of severe hyperemesis gravidarum: maternal nutritional effects and fetal outcome. Obstet Gynecol 1988;72:102.

Lim SH, Smith MP, Salooja N, et al. A prospective randomized study of prophylactic teicoplanin to prevent early Hickman catheter-related sepsis in patients receiving intensive chemotherapy for haematological malignancies. J Antimicrob Chemother 1991;28:109.

Linares J, Sitges-Serra A, Garau J, et al. Pathogenesis of catheter sepsis: a prospective study with quantitative and semiquantitative culture of catheter hub and segments. J Clin Microbiol 1985;21:357.

Loughran SC, Edwards S, McClure S. Peripherally inserted central catheters. Guidewire versus nonguidewire use: a comparative study. J Intravenous Nurs 1992;15:152.

Lowbury EJL, Lilly HA. The effect of blood on disinfection of surgeon hands. Br J Surg 1974;61:19.

Lowell JA, Bothe A Jr. Venous access: preoperative, operative, and postoperative dilemmas. Surg Clin North Am 1991;71:1231.

Lum P, Soski M. Management of malpositioned central venous catheters. J Intravenous Nurs 1989;12:356.

MacBurney M, Wilmore DW. Parenteral nutrition in pregnancy. In: Rombeau JL, Caldwell MD, eds. Parenteral nutrition. 2nd ed. Philadelphia: WB Saunders, 1986:615.

Maki DG. Yes, Virginia, aseptic technique is very important: maximal barrier precautions during insertion reduce the risk of central venous catheter-related bacteremia. Infect Control Hosp Epidemiol 1994;15:227.

Maki DG, Cobb L, Garman JK, et al. An attachable silver-impregnated cuff for prevention of infection with central venous catheters: a prospective randomized multicenter trial. Am J Med 1988;85:307.

Maki DG, Goldman DA, Rhame FS. Infection control in intravenous therapy. Ann Intern Med 1973;79:867.

Maki DG, Ringer M, Alavarado CJ. Prospective randomized trial of povidone-iodine, alcohol, and chlorhexidine for prevention of infection associated with central venous and arterial catheters. Lancet 1991a;338:339.

Maki DG, Wheeler SJ, Stolz SM, et al. Study of a novel antiseptic-coated central venous catheter. Crit Care Med 1991b;19(suppl):S99. Abstract.

Maki DG, Weise CE, Saratin HW. A semi-quantitative culture method for identifying intravenous catheter related infection. N Engl J Med 1977; 298:1305.

Mannel RS, Manetta A, Hickman RL Jr, et al. Cost analysis of Hickman catheter insertion at bedside in gynecologic oncology patients. J Am Coll Surg 1994;179:558.

McGee WT, Ackerman BL, Rouben LR, et al. Accurate placement of central venous catheters: a prospective, randomized, multicenter trial. Crit Care Med 1993;21:1118.

McGeer A, Righter J. Improving our ability to diagnose infections associated with central venous catheters: value of Gram's staining and culture of entry site swabs. Can Med Assoc J 1987; 137:1009.

McKee J. Future dimension in vascular access. Peripheral implantable ports. J Intravenous Nurs 1991;14:387.

Merrell SW, Peatross BG, Grossman MD, et al. Peripherally inserted central venous catheters. Low-risk alternatives for ongoing venous access. West J Med 1994;160:25.

Mimoz O, Pleroni L, Lawrence C, et al. Prospective randomized trial of two antiseptic solutions for prevention of central venous catheterization of arterial colonization and infection. Crit Care Med 1996;24:1818.

Moro ML, Vigano EF, Lepri AC, et al. Risk factors for central venous catheter-related infections in surgical and intensive care units. Infect Control Hosp Epidemiol 1994;15:253.

Morris P, Buller R, Kendall S, et al. A peripherally implanted permanent central venous access device. Obstet Gynecol 1991;78:1138.

Moyer MA, Edwards LD, Farley L. Comparative culture methods on 101 intravenous catheters. Routine, semi-quantitative, and blood cultures. Arch Intern Med 1983;143:66.

Nehme AE. Nutritional support of the hospitalized patient. The team concept. JAMA 1980;243:1906.

Nelson DB, Kien CL, Mohr B, et al. Dressing changes by specialized personnel reduce infection rates in patients receiving central venous parenteral nutrition. JPEN 1986;10:220.

Nohr C. Care of the surgical patient. Perioperative management and techniques. 2. Elective care. Vol. 2. Surgical techniques, Supplement 3. Vascular access. Scientific American, Inc. Winter, 1994.

Nystrom B, Larsen SO, Dankert J, et al. Bacteremia in surgical patients with intravenous devices: a European multicenter incidence study. J Hosp Infect 1983;4:338.

Parras F, Ena J, Bouza E, et al. Impact of an educational program for the prevention of colonization of intravascular catheters. Infect Control Hosp Epidemiol 1994;15:239.

Pasquale MD, Campbell JM, Magnant CM. Groshong versus Hickman catheters. Surg Gynecol Obstet 1992;174:408.

Pearl JM, Goldstein L, Ciresi KF. Improved methods in long term venous access using the P.A.S. port. Surg Gynecol Obstet 1991;173:313.

Pennington CR, Pithie AD. Ethanol lock in the management of catheter occlusion. JPEN 1987; 11:507.

Pizzo PA. Management of fever in patients with cancer and treatment-induced neutropenia. N Engl J Med 1993;328:1323.

Puntis JWL, Holden CE, Finkel Y, et al. Staff training: a key factor in reducing intravascular catheter sepsis. Arch Dis Child 1990;65:335.

Raad II, Hohn DC, Gilbreath BJ, et al. Prevention of central venous catheter-related infections by using maximal sterile barrier precautions during insertion. Infect Control Hosp Epidemiol 1994;15:231.

Rafkin HS, Hoyt JW, Crippen DW. Prevention of certified venous catheter-related infection with a silver-impregnated cuff. Chest 1990;98:117S. Abstract.

Ray S, Stacey R, Imrie M, Filshie J. A review of 560 Hickman catheter insertions. Anesthesia 1996; 51:981.

Rotstein C, Brock L, Roberts RS. The incidence of first Hickman catheter-related infection and predictors of catheter removal in cancer patients. Infect Control Hosp Epidemiol 1995;16:451.

Rushforth JA, Hoy CM, Puntis JWL. Rapid diagnosis of central venous catheter sepsis. Lancet 1993;342:402.

Ryan JA, Abel RM, Abbott WM, et al. Catheter complications in total parenteral nutrition. A prospective study in 200 consecutive patients. N Engl J Med 1974;290:757.

Salem R, Ward B, Ravikumar T. A new peripherally implanted subcutaneous permanent central venous access device for patients requiring chemotherapy. J Clin Oncol 1993;11:2181.

Schuman E, Ragsdale J. Peripheral ports are a new option for central venous access. J Am Coll Surg 1995;180:456.

Schwartz C, Henrickson KJ, Roghmann K, et al. Prevention of bacteremia attributed to luminal colonization of tunneled central venous catheters with vancomycin-susceptible organisms. J Clin Oncol 1990;8:1591.

Sheikh W. Comparative antibacterial efficacy of Hibiclens and Betadine in the presence of pus derived from human wounds. Curr Ther Res 1986;40:1096.

Sherer DM, Abulafia O, DuBesher B, et al. Ultrasonographically guided subclavian vein catheterization in critical care obstetrics and gynecologic oncology. Am J Obstet Gynecol 1993;169:1246.

Shulman RJ, Reed T, Pitre D, et al. Use of hydrochloric acid to clear obstructed central venous catheters. JPEN 1988;12:509.

Snydman DR, Gorbea HF, Pober BR, et al. Predictive value of surveillance skin cultures in total-parenteral-nutrition-related infections. Lancet 1982a;2:1385.

Snydman DR, Murray SA, Kornfield SJ, et al. Total parenteral nutrition-related infections. Prospective epidemiologic study using semi-quantitative methods. Am J Med 1982b;73:695.

Spafford PS, Sinkin RA, Cox C, et al. Prevention of central venous catheter-related coagulase-negative staphylococcal sepsis in neonates. J Pediatr 1994;125:259.

Starkhammer H, Bengtsson M, Gain T, et al. A new injection portal for brachially inserted central venous catheter. A multicenter study. Med Oncol Pharmacol 1990;4:281.

Steed DL, Teodori MF, Peitzman AB, et al. Streptokinase in the treatment of subclavian vein thrombosis. J Vasc Surg 1986;4:28.

Stokes MA, Irving MH. How do patients with Crohn's disease fare on home parenteral nutrition? Dis Colon Rectum 1988;31:454.

Thornton J, Todd NJ, Webster NR. Central venous line sepsis in the intensive care unit: A study comparing antibiotic-coated with plain catheters. Anaesthesia 1996;51:1018.

Trooskin SZ, Donetz AP, Harvey RA, et al. Prevention of catheter sepsis by antibiotic bonding. Surgery 1985;97:547.

Tschirhart JM, Rao MK. Mechanism and management of persistent withdrawal occlusion. Am Surg 1988;54:326.

Wachs T. Urokinase administration in pediatric patients with occluded central venous catheters. J Intravenous Nurs 1990;13:100.

Wanscher M, Frifelt JJ, Smith-Sivertsen C, et al. Thrombosis caused by polyurethane double-lumen subclavian vena cava catheter and hemodialysis. Crit Care Med 1988;16:624.

Watson LA, Bommarito AA, Marshall JF. Total peripheral parenteral nutrition in pregnancy. JPEN 1990;14:485.

Wiedner LC, Fish J, Talabiska DG, et al. Total parenteral nutrition in pregnant patient with hyperemesis gravidarum. Nutrition 1993;9:446.

Wing EJ, Norden CW, Shadduck RK, et al. Use of quantitative bacteriologic techniques to diagnose catheter-related sepsis. Arch Intern Med 1979;139:482.

Winters V, Peters B, Coila S, et al. A trial with a new peripheral implanted vascular access device. Oncol Nurs Forum 1990;17:891.

Wolk RA, Rayburn WF. Parenteral nutrition in obstetric patients. Nutr Clin Pract 1990;5:139.

# Ventilator Therapy and Airway Management

*T*raditionally, obstetricians have been reliant on other medical specialties during mechanical ventilation of pregnant patients. This chapter focuses on the interrelation of pregnancy and mechanical ventilation. Our aim is to provide a framework of understanding for the clinician not usually exposed to mechanical ventilators.

## Basic Concepts

### Pulmonary Physiology

As detailed in previous chapters of this book, pregnancy results in several alterations in respiratory homeostasis germane to mechanical ventilation. Pregnancy induces a compensated respiratory alkalosis. The respiratory alkalosis of pregnancy is due to a progesterone-mediated increase in minute volume. While respiratory rate increases somewhat, the predominant factor producing the increase in minute volume is an increase in tidal volume (Lucius, 1970). Alveolar volume (or ventilation), that portion of tidal volume (ventilation) that is actually used for gas exchange, is increased as well (Myers, 1992). Dead space ventilation, the antithesis of alveolar ventilation, is that portion of tidal ventilation that does not participate in gas exchange. Normally, "dead space" as such, is mostly a consequence of the nonfunctional lung volume of the conducting air-

ways. This "anatomic dead space" is modestly increased during pregnancy because of large airway bronchodilation (Hyman, 1978). Physiologic dead space is a result of the ventilation of poorly perfused alveolar segments. As we will see in subsequent sections of this chapter, physiologic dead space is altered by both the normal physiology of pregnancy and the various pathophysiologic states encountered during pregnancy. Generally speaking, mechanical ventilation of patients with pulmonary disease often occurs in the face of increased physiologic dead space. The relation of dead space to tidal volume ($V_D/V_T$) thereby determines the relative amount of a given tidal volume that is actually used in gas exchange.

Another important concept germane to mechanical ventilation involves functional volume (FRV), which is defined as the sum of expiratory reserve volume and residual volume. Functional volume decreases during pregnancy (Alaily, 1978). The operational result of decreased FRV is to bring the lung volumes used for normal tidal breathing at or near the volume in which an increasing number of alveolar units collapse (Russell, 1981). When perfused alveolar units are deprived of gas exchange, the resulting intrapulmonary shunt increases. Shunted blood, deprived of the opportunity for gas exchange, results in a defect not correctable per se by increasing inhaled oxygen. Positive end-expiratory pressure (PEEP) works by increasing FRV through recruitment of alveoli (Gattinoni, 1993). Conversely, in addition to pregnancy

**143**

itself, postural change and pulmonary disease may contribute to an increase in intrapulmonary shunt through a decrease in FRV.

Another important concept in pulmonary physiology is lung compliance. Compliance is determined as a relative change in volume per given change in pressure (West, 1995). Therefore, compliance is a quantitative measurement of distensibility. Just as myocardial compliance may change at different relative ventricular volumes, pulmonary compliance is not uniform over all attainable lung volumes. Emphysema can increase lung compliance. Conversely, acute (adult) respiratory distress syndrome (ARDS) reduces lung compliance. Furthermore, the relative difference in compliance at different lung volumes may be exaggerated by pulmonary diseases. Finally, different alveolar units may exhibit different compliance at different volumes. Compliance is usually not uniform throughout the diseased lung. In that gases flow from higher to lower pressure, dishomogeneity in compliance can result in altered gas exchange, over or under distention of alveolar units and/or segmental barotrauma (Gattinoni, 1993).

All of the aforementioned effects result in alterations of ventilation, perfusion, and pressure. Pulmonary pathophysiology accentuates the interrelationship between compliance, shunt, dead space, and ventilation. As stated previously, gas exchange is critically affected by blood-flow to the alveolar units participating (or not participating) in ventilation. The lung is operationally made up of a large number of units with varying degrees of ventilation and/or perfusion. West describes different regions of ventilation perfusion matching as characterized by Figure 8-1 (West, 1995). Postural change, perfusion alterations (alterations in cardiac output or BP), pulmonary pathophysiology, and pregnancy itself all alter the relative number of lung segments in any given "West Zone." What is often less recognized is that the relative pressure/volume relationship (compliance) of alveolar units at any given lung volume may also affect ventilation/perfusion. Once again, the application of PEEP or the selection of a different relative change in lung volume during mechanical ventilation may favorably or adversely influence the overall ventilation/perfusion relationship.

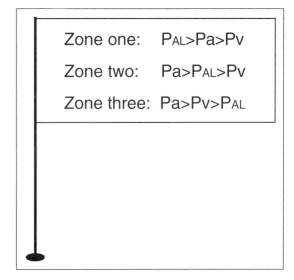

F I G U R E **8-1**
**West zones of lung perfusion.** Pa, pulmonary artery pressure; Pv, pulmonary venous pressure; $P_{AL}$, alveolar pressure. (Adapted from West JB. Respiratory physiology—the essentials. 5th ed. Baltimore: Williams and Wilkins, 1995:41.)

## Ideal Alveolar Gas Equation

The amount of gas that can be transferred across the alveolus to the pulmonary capillary is dependent on the quantity of that gas in the alveolus. The amount of oxygen present in an alveolar unit ($P_{A}O_2$) is determined by the alveolar gas equation (Aldrich, 1994):

$$P_{A}O_2 = F_IO_2(P_{Atm} - P_{H_2O}) - P_{A}CO_2/R$$

The partial pressure of oxygen in an alveolus is determined by the product fraction of inspired oxygen ($F_IO_2$) and the atmospheric pressure ($P_{Atm}$), with subtraction of the component of atmospheric pressure occupied by water vapor ($P_{H_2O}$). Equally important is the contribution carbon dioxide ($CO_2$) makes to the ultimate availability of oxygen in a given alveolar unit. Carbon dioxide is freely diffusible in and out of the alveolus and the bloodstream. Therefore, carbon dioxide in the alveolus is determined by the relative amount dissolved in pulmonary blood. The relative amount of production and elimination of carbon dioxide affects dissolved arterial carbon dioxide, thereby affecting alveolar carbon dioxide. The respiratory quotient describes the ratio between carbon dioxide production and carbon dioxide elimination. In normally resting and non-starving pregnant and nonpregnant women, a respiratory quotient of 0.8 is typically measured (Bryan Brown, 1995). Therefore, alveolar carbon dioxide ($PA_{CO_2}$) is determined by arterial carbon dioxide ($Pa_{CO_2}$) divided by the respiratory quotient (0.8).

As the alveolar gas equation shows, $PA_{O_2}$ is dependent on both the amount of oxygen available in whatever gas mixture is inhaled and the $PA_{CO_2}$ (or $Pa_{CO_2}$). Alveolar hyperventilation will cause an increase in $PA_{O_2}$, while hypoventilation will result in a lower $PA_{O_2}$ (and $Pa_{O_2}$). The relationship between ventilation and alveolar oxygenation explains the small increase in $Pa_{O_2}$ seen early in pregnancy. Minute ventilation increases early in pregnancy, resulting in a lower $Pa_{CO_2}$ and a higher $Pa_{O_2}$. The interrelationship between ventilation and oxygenation is usually not important in normal, healthy individuals. In patients with increased dead space ventilation and impaired oxygen exchange, however, an understanding of this interaction is crucial.

## Initiation of Mechanical Ventilation

Several indications dictate the requirement for mechanical ventilation. Not all patients receiving mechanical ventilation require it for hypoxemia or pulmonary hypoventilation. It is crucial to understand the indications for initiating mechanical ventilation, because the indications may dictate the modality, the type of ventilator used, the type of airway used, and the adjunctive measures necessary to maintain appropriate mechanical ventilatory support.

## Hypoxia and Hypoventilation

Indications for mechanical ventilation can be grouped into several broad categories (Slutsky, 1993) (Table 8-1). The two most intuitive circumstances necessitating mechanical ventilation are

T A B L E   **8-1**

Indications for mechanical ventilation

Pulmonary hypoventilation
  Apnea
  Acute ventilatory failure
  Impending acute ventilatory failure
Hypoxia
Airway control
Increased work of breathing
Nonphysiologic ventilatory management

hypoxic respiratory failure and pulmonary hypoventilation. Hypoxia ($Pa_{O_2}$ <60 mm Hg on 50% or greater $FI_{O_2}$) and hypoventilation ($Pa_{CO_2}$ >60 mm Hg) must be taken in clinical context and not as absolutes. Hypoxia, as described, in the face of limited hope for improvement or with significant risk of deterioration, may dictate initiation of mechanical ventilation. Conversely, as outlined in the section on weaning, a $Pa_{O_2}$ of more than 60 mm Hg on 50% or less $FI_{O_2}$ may be a positive indicator for extubation! Hypoventilation also is interpreted in the clinical context of the situation. The underlying blood gas changes of pregnancy affect the clinical recognition of hypoventilation. An example would be in the blood-gas interpretation of the patient with chronic obstructive lung disease. Such a patient may usually function with a relatively high $Pa_{CO_2}$. Therefore, the relative change in $Pa_{CO_2}$ rather than the absolute value would be used as the requirement for mechanical ventilation. Asthmatic respiratory failure during pregnancy is an obstetric example of this phenomenon. Arterial blood gas values indicative of respiratory failure during acute exacerbations of asthma during pregnancy are significantly different from those values predictive of respiratory failure in the nonpregnant individual (Barth, 1991). In pregnancy, given the preexisting compensated respiratory alkalosis, a $Pa_{CO_2}$ within or just above the normal range in an asthmatic could be indicative of impending ventilatory respiratory failure. In summary, it is most important to interpret hypoxemia and hypoventilation in relative as well as in absolute terms.

## Airway Control

Airway control is an often used, but seldom thought of, indication for mechanical ventilation. Airway control is used daily as the reason for intubation during initiation of general anesthesia and in patients with altered levels of consciousness. It is important to recognize that intubation and ventilation for the sole purpose of airway control is a situation in which ventilatory support is begun on a patient with normal (or relatively normal) pulmonary function. (Airway management is discussed briefly later in this chapter.) Review of other references concerning this extensive topic is suggested.

## Work of Breathing

Many pulmonary diseases result in decreased pulmonary compliance and increased airway resistance. The end result of decreased compliance or increased airway resistance is an increase in the work or effort necessary to effect adequate gas exchange. If the amount of effort exceeds either the capacity or the endurance of the respiratory muscles, respiratory failure can result. Respiratory failure due to an increased work of breathing is manifested by ventilatory respiratory failure and ultimately hypoxemia. Unfortunately, hypoxemia and hypercarbia may be relatively late indicators of respiratory collapse (Corre, 1985; Rodriguez-Roisin, 1989). It is always preferable to electively rather than emergently intubate and mechanically ventilate a patient. Therefore, recognition of increased work of breathing prior to development of hypercarbia (hypoventilation) or hypoxemia is important. Tachypnea (respiratory rate > 30–35 times per minute), use of accessory muscles of respiration, anxiousness, shallow breathing, and auscultation of turbulent airway flow (ronchi or wheezes) all are potential indicators of increased work of breathing. Shallow, rapid tidal breathing, even if tolerated from a mechanical standpoint, may not be tolerated because of secondary atelectasis. Secondary atelectasis significantly furthers respiratory compromise via FRV-mediated changes. Pulmonary pathophysiology that causes diminished compliance also alters FRV. In composite, low compliance and diminished FRV result in shallow and rapid tidal breathing that may well be conducted within the range of lung volumes that produce airway collapse (critical closing volumes). With progressive airway collapse, pulmonary segments are perfused but not ventilated and result in intrapulmonary shunt. Besides increasing pulmonary shunt, secondary atelectasis may lead to further decreases in both compliance and FRV, thereby perpetuating further atelectasis. A self-perpetuating process of increasing shunt, increasing work of breathing, and increased atelectasis ensues (West, 1995; Hirsch, 1991). The relationships between lung volume, compliance, and atelectasis are illustrated in Figures 8-2 and 8-3.

## Nonpulmonary Indications

All mechanical ventilation is therapeutic in that its use addresses the goals of gas exchange, oxygenation, airway protection, and relief of work of breathing. However, an additional indication for subjecting a patient to the rigors of mechanical ventilation may be to affect a specific physiologic endpoint in treatment of a nonpulmonary process. An example of such an indication would be controlled hyperventilation for the purpose of temporarily reducing intracranial hypertension (Crockard, 1973; Muizelaari, 1991). Other indications include the augmentation of oxygen delivery for sepsis or trauma treatment (Shoemaker, 1985, 1992), independent lung ventilation in the management of bronchopulmonary fistula (Benjaminsson, 1981), decreased myocardial oxygen consumption in unstable angina (Aubier, 1981),

F I G U R E  **8-2**

**Diminished compliance reducing tidal breathing. Diminished compliance may self-perpetuate as a result of atelectasis.**

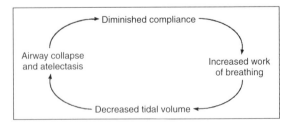

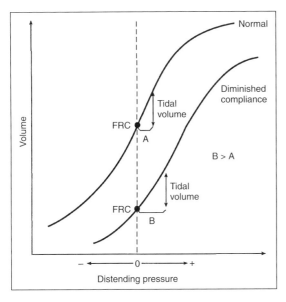

FIGURE   **8-3**

**Altered pressure volume relationships in poorly compliant lungs. Altered compliance may affect relative and absolute pulmonary distensibility.** FRC, functional residual volume (capacity) (dotted line denotes FRC location); A, pressure change for tidal breathing (normal); B, pressure change for tidal breathing (abnormal).

and stabilization of the chest wall (as in massive flail chest) (Slutsky, 1993).

Intubation and mechanical ventilation is a serious process that should be undertaken with clear indications, goals, and outcomes in mind. Initiation of mechanical ventilation is best begun *electively* rather than *emergently*. Prompt recognition of the need for mechanical ventilation will clearly reduce the morbidity associated with the induction of ventilation. Table 8-2 lists *minimum* equipment necessary for intubation and mechanical ventilation. Suction, airway control, oxygenation, bag-mask and machine methods of gas exchange, nasogastric emptying, and medications for sedation and, potentially, paralysis are recommended. Pulse oximetry monitoring is recommended for moment-to-moment appraisal of oxyhemoglobin saturation. End-tidal $CO_2$ measurement, postintubation auscultation of breath sounds, and chest x-ray confirmation of endotracheal tube position (normally 4–7 cm above the

| TABLE   **8-2** |
| --- |
| **Equipment list for intubation and mechanical ventilation** |
| Oropharyngeal suction equipment |
| Working (and tested) endotrachael tube(s) |
| Stylet |
| Working (and tested) laryngoscope with blades |
| Correctly sized mask |
| Alternate oxygen source |
| Manual inflation bag |
| Sedation and paralysis medications |
| Qualified personnel |
| Anticipated plan of action if primary method of intubation fails |
| Pulse oximetry |
| Mechanism for ensuring correct endotracheal tube placement |
| Cardiac (ECG) and BP monitoring |

carina) help assure endotracheal intubation (Brunel, 1989). Evacuation of gastric contents before or after intubation also may be required.

## Basic Modes of Mechanical Ventilation

Three basic modes of mechanical ventilation are available: assist-control ventilation, intermittent mandatory volume ventilation, and pressure-support ventilation. In rare circumstances, other modes of ventilation are often required or modalities are combined. Nonetheless, these basic modes of ventilation are the underlying foundations of advanced methods of ventilation. An understanding of and familiarity with basic mechanical ventilation are, therefore, important prerequisites to a thorough understanding of advanced mechanical ventilation.

## Assist/Controlled Mechanical Ventilation

Controlled mechanical ventilation (CMV) is a technique of ventilation in which a given volume (or pressure) is delivered at a given rate, thereby resulting in a given minute ventilation. When combined with the feature of patient-initiated triggering of the ventilator, the mode becomes one of assist/control mechanical ventilation (ACMV). Volume-set ACMV, with a given tidal volume delivered at a given rate and curve, has been a well-studied technique of ventilation. Using ACMV, an underlying minimum minute ventilation is set by the operator. This "backup rate" ensures a minimum number of breaths at the set tidal volume regardless of whether the patient triggers the ventilator. Figure 8-4 illustrates ACMV ventilation. An important concept with ACMV is that patient initiation of ventilatory effort above and beyond the number of backup breaths desired will result in a minute ventilation (number of breaths) above that amount set on the ventilator. In ACMV, the ventilator guarantees the set tidal volume with every breath initiation by the patient. In many patients undergoing mechanical ventilation, ACMV will allow ventilation to a level set by the patient. This mode is, therefore, potentially advantageous for use in the nonparalyzed patient with intact central ventilatory control who is without the requirement for nonphysiologic minute ventilation. Alternatively, ACMV may not be the ideal choice in spontaneously hyperventilating subjects (Mador, 1994).

Although work of breathing is not as low as it was formerly thought to be (Marini, 1985), ACMV is one of the least strenuous of the patient-influenced modalities. The work of breathing associated with ACMV is principally determined by the sensitivity and nature of the demand valve used by the ventilator itself and the airway resistance of the ventilatory circuit and endotracheal tube. Work of breathing also may be influenced by inspiratory flow. Inadequate inspiratory flow may result in an increased work of breathing.

The lack of regulation and modulation of work of breathing can potentially cause increased complexity during the weaning of long-term mechanical ventilator recipients. Because ACMV is a modality that cannot be adjusted to provide the gradual alteration (increase) in work of breathing, another modality, or progressive "T-bar trials," is generally used (Tobin, 1990; Tomlinson, 1989). Other potential drawbacks to ACMV include the potential increase in air trapping that may occur in chronic obstructive pulmonary disease (COPD) subjects receiving the modality, lack of synchrony that may be evident in anxious or uncooperative patients, and the lessened ability to manipulate peak airway pressure during volume-regulated ACMV. Pressure-regulated ACMV will be discussed in the section on pressure-controlled ventilation.

F I G U R E **8-4**

**Modes of ventilation**: 1, patient initiation of breath; 2, inspiration; 3, expiration; A, B, patient-triggered breaths; C, machine-triggered breaths. **Synchronized intermittent mandatory ventilation**: 1, machine breath inspiration; 2, machine breath expiration; 3, spontaneous inspiration; 4, spontaneous expiration; A, patient breath; B, patient breath; C, synchronized machine breath.

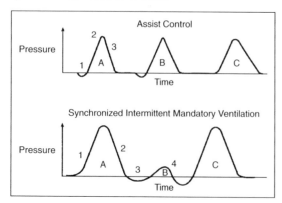

## Synchronized Intermittent Mandatory Ventilation

Synchronized intermittent mandatory ventilation (SIMV) is a widely used basic method of mechanical ventilation. In SIMV (see Fig 8-4), a tidal volume and respiratory rate are set as in ACVM. Unlike ACMV, any patient-initiated breath above the set rate will result in whatever tidal volume the patient herself can generate. Subsequently, any patient-supplied portion of total minute ventilation will depend on spontaneous respiratory drive, respiratory muscle strength, airway (and ventilator circuit) resistance, and pulmonary compliance. Synchronized intermittent mandatory ventilation is synchronized in that spontaneous inspiratory efforts are integrated within set machine breaths, a key difference between SIMV and the now rarely found nonsynchronous IMV modality (Luce, 1981; Slutsky, 1993).

Tidal volume–based SIMV enjoys a convenient advantage over ACMV ventilation during attempts at ventilator weaning. The component of patient-supplied ventilatory effort can easily and gradually be increased during short or prolonged attempts at weaning. As stated in the section on weaning, it is important to note that neither modality has proven conclusively better at successful weaning. The main disadvantage of volume-targeted SIMV relates to work of breathing (Marini, 1988). Excessive work of breathing can pose disadvantages in the ventilation of the seriously ill patient. With SIMV ventilation, each patient-generated breath is at a cost of work done, which may be useful (as in weaning) or deleterious. Therefore, patients with significant metabolic derangement, or increased intrinsic work requirements (e.g., decreased pulmonary compliance, obesity), or with the inability to "cooperate" with the ventilator may require either sedation and paralysis, an alternative mode of ventilation, or the use of adjuncts such as pressure support (Beydon, 1991; Lemaire, 1988).

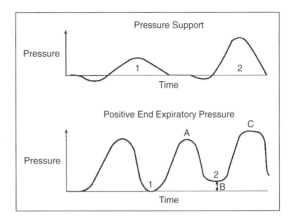

F I G U R E  **8-5**

**Pressure support, positive end expiratory pressure:** 1, SIMV breath (pressure support off); 2, SIMV breath (pressure support on). **Positive end expiratory pressure:** 1, PEEP off; 2, PEEP on; pressure at C, pressure A + pressure B (refer to text).

## Pressure Support Ventilation

Pressure support ventilation (PSV), when used alone, is not time cycled or volume targeted (as are volume-set ACMV and volume-set SIMV). Instead, PSV is flow cycled (triggered) and pressure targeted (McIntyre, 1986). Unless used in combination with another modality, each and every breath generated during PSV is initiated by the patient herself. Respiratory rate is a function of inspiratory effort. Minute ventilation is determined by endogenous respiratory rate and derived tidal volume. Derived tidal volume is dependent on pulmonary compliance, pressure support level, and respiratory muscle effort. Pressure support use on a spontaneously ventilating patient is illustrated in Figure 8-5.

Pressure support ventilation can be added to other ventilatory modalities. When added to volume-set, time-cycled ventilators, machine breaths will be of tidal volumes chosen by the operator, providing that the level of pressure support is *less* than the peak pressure required to generate the tidal volume set on the ventilator

(Brochard, 1987). Spontaneous tidal volumes will be based on the factors described at the end of the previous paragraph. At any point that the set peak pressures are exceeded, the baroventilator cycle is terminated, reducing base trauma.

Because PSV is flow-based, a significant indication for its use is to improve patient comfort. Small amounts (5–10 cm $H_2O$) will help overcome the resistance of the endotracheal tube and ventilator circuit (Brochard, 1991). Pressure support ventilation provides another way to wean a patient from the ventilator. Relatively large amounts of PSV are used initially, and over time the PSV level is gradually reduced to increase patient-supplied work of breathing (Kacmarek, 1988).

The major disadvantage of PSV is that unless otherwise accounted for, minute volume is not controlled. Tidal volume will change in parallel with pulmonary compliance. Finally, patients with disorders of increased airway resistance may not tolerate the flow parameters of PSV.

## Positive End-Expiratory Pressure

Positive end-expiratory pressure is not an independent method of mechanical ventilation. However, because of its widespread use, or misuse, with most modalities of mechanical ventilation, PEEP will be discussed in this section.

Positive end-expiratory pressure (see Fig 8-5) is an outgrowth of face mask continuous positive airway pressure breathing (CPAP) (Ashbaugh, 1969; Ferguson, 1993). Both PEEP and CPAP instill a continuous airway pressure above baseline. In the patient receiving CPAP, airway pressure is increased a predetermined amount throughout spontaneous respiration. In PEEP, end-expiratory pressure is elevated by some degree during machine and spontaneous respirations. Through elevation of end-expiratory pressure, the lung volume found at end-expiration is altered (elevated) over what the volume would normally be. In alteration of the "resting" (sic) lung volume, PEEP may afford a relative change in the pressure-volume relationship of the pulmonary alveolar units. Lung volume may be elevated above critical closing volume, allowing for a decrease in the amount of pressure necessary to change lung volume (compliance is increased), and otherwise non-ventilated alveoli may thereby be recruited. The use of PEEP may improve gas exchange and oxygenation through this basic mechanism (Gattinoni, 1988; Dall'ava-Santucci, 1990).

"Physiologic PEEP" is the theoretical amount of residual end-expiratory pressure produced during normal exhalation as a by-product of glottic closure. It is unclear whether physiologic PEEP truly exists or what its importance is. Nonetheless, in attempts to reduce atelectasis, many clinicians will place patients using mechanical ventilators on 3 to 5 cm $H_2O$ of baseline PEEP. Higher levels of PEEP have been used to promote airway recruitment in patients with significant pulmonary disease. Through the appropriate use of PEEP and airway recruitment, intrapulmonary shunt is often reduced, effecting an improvement in oxygenation (Suter, 1975).

Several important tenants need to be recognized during the application of PEEP. First and foremost is that extrinsic PEEP in effect adds to the baseline and peak airway and intrapleural pressures generated during volume-based ventilation. Barotrauma is, therefore, a by-product of high levels of PEEP. Furthermore, because flow of any liquid or gas is dependent on the pressure gradient across the flow unit, elevation of trans-

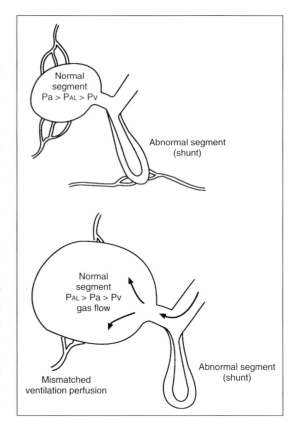

FIGURE **8-6**

Overdistention from PEEP. Gas flows preferentially to high-compliance alveolar units, thereby adversely altering pulmonary ventilation to perfusion relationships. Pa, pulmonary arterial pressure; PA, alveolar pressure; PV, pulmonary venous pressure.

mural intrapleural pressure alters great vessel blood flow and ventricular preload and afterload. Pronounced elevations in PEEP usually decrease cardiac output. Because, by convention, pulmonary capillary wedge pressure is measured at end-expiration, addition of PEEP may alter pulmonary artery and/or other intracardiac pressures. The degree and amount of PEEP-induced alteration is determined by the amount of PEEP and the relative compliance of the pulmonary and vascular tissues.

Because oxygen delivery is dependent on both the content of oxygen carried in a given unit of blood and the rate of flow or delivery (cardiac output) of the blood through the interchange areas of the body, PEEP may improve Pao$_2$ (and arterial oxygen content) while actually diminishing oxygen delivery by decreasing cardiac output. Similarly, PEEP may have a variable influence on gas exchange through non-uniform over- or underdistention of alveolar segments (Fig 8-6), either of which may increase shunt. Because lung injury is rarely uniform, given alveolar units may exhibit normal compliance, diminished compliance, or total absence of ventilation (Maunder, 1986). Under PEEP therapy, relatively normal alveolar units may preferentially become overdistended and produce lung injury and/or alteration of ventilation-perfusion ratios. Concomitantly, poorly distensible lung units may remain undistended (Benito, 1990). The effects of PEEP on oxygen delivery are, therefore, variable and complex.

Positive end-expiratory pressure has been studied extensively in both animal and human pulmonary pathophysiology. The basic premise on which the use of PEEP in ARDS was based is the philosophy of limiting lung damage due to hyperoxia. Unfortunately, animal data and human pathophysiologic correlation infer that the mechanisms of hyperoxia and barotrauma may be interrelated (Resister, 1987). Nonetheless, PEEP remains a basic tool in the mechanical ventilation of the hypoxic patient (Marini, 1992a).

## Advanced Modes of Mechanical Ventilation

Despite advances in intensive care, the basic mortality rate from ARDS remains at approximately 50% (Trottier, 1995). Because of improvements in the initial resuscitation and clinical support of patients with ARDS, end-stage and irreversible pulmonary injury predominate as causes of its morbidity and mortality. Several advanced modes of mechanical ventilation have been developed to attempt to reduce both mortality and residual lung disease. Nonpulmonary adjuncts to mechanical ventilation (e.g., intravenous oxygenation, extracorporeal membrane oxygenation, and partial liquid ventilation) also have been utilized. A brief description of several of the more commonly available advanced modes of ventilation will be discussed.

## Pressure-Regulated Ventilation

Pressure-regulated ventilation (PRV) encompasses an endpoint pressure rather than volume in the accomplishment of positive pressure ventilation. Pressure-regulated ventilation use was widespread in the early days of mechanical ventilation. The modality still enjoys widespread use in neonatology. With the emergence of philosophies aimed at limiting barotrauma, PRV is now more frequently used in adult patients (Hickling, 1990). It is available with ACMV and SIMV regulation, the difference being that with use of PRV-ACMV or SIMV-ACMV, ventilator tidal breathing is pressure rather than volume based.

In PRV, tidal volume is related directly to inspiratory time, gas flow over inspiratory time, and lung compliance. Consequently, if inspiratory time, ventilator flow rate, airway resistance, or pulmonary compliance is changed, tidal volume and, therefore, minute ventilation are altered. Improvement or worsening of underlying pulmonary pathophysiology can have pronounced effects on minute ventilation. The chief advantage of PRV is limitation of peak airway pressure. By sequential adjustment of flow rate and inspiratory time, peak airway pressure can usually be maintained at less than 35 to 40 cm H$_2$O, which is thought to be the upper limit of pressure that will not produce irreversible barotrauma (Tobin, 1994). Pressure-regulated ventilation also can be used to increase intrinsic PEEP.

## Intrinsic Peep

Conventionally applied PEEP is added to the distending pressure necessary to generate a given tidal volume. The method is, therefore, referred to as extrinsic PEEP. Intrinsic PEEP (also known euphemistically by the manner in which it is produced as "air-trapping PEEP" or "auto-PEEP") produces end-expiratory pressure through initiation of a new inspiration before all of a previous tidal volume is exhaled (Fig 8-7) (Lain, 1989).

During normal spontaneous respiration, inspiration is accomplished more rapidly than expiration. During normal spontaneous respiration

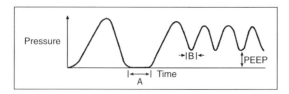

F I G U R E  **8-7**

**Intrisinc PEEP.** A, normal inspiratory time; B, short-ened inspiratory time (refer to text).

and conventional mechanical ventilation, the ra-tio of inspiration to expiration (I:E ratio) is nor-mally 1:1.2 to 1.5. "Reversal" of the I:E ratio oc-curs when the ratio is 1:1 or less. I:E reversal (inverse ratio ventilation [IRV]) may be a conse-quence of reactive airway disease (asthma) or any other condition that alters expiratory flow. Inverse ratio ventilation is poorly tolerated by the awake and unsedated patient. During institution of intrinsic PEEP, respiratory rate is often in-creased and tidal volumes are generally low in an effort to reduce barotrauma. In the process of air trapping, I:E reversal is often produced with ra-tios of up to 1:0.3 not uncommon. Consequently, sedation and paralysis are often necessary.

Although difficult to quantify and in certain circumstances advantageous, intrinsic PEEP may be an unfortunate by-product of conventional me-chanical ventilation. The chief theoretical advan-tage of intrinsic PEEP is when combined with PRV. Pressure-regulated ventilation–inverse ratio ventilation (PRV-IRV) may allow adequate venti-lation without excessively increasing peak airway pressure, although mean airway pressure is in-creased (Lain, 1989; Parker, 1993; Marini, 1992b). In nonpregnant patients with ARDS, PRV-IRV has produced mixed results (Perel, 1987). We use this mode in patients with noncompliant lungs and recalcitrant hypoxemia. While it is difficult to determine if survival is favorably influenced, complications of barotrauma, to include pneu-mothorax and subcutaneous emphysema, are less frequent.

## High-Frequency Ventilation

*High-frequency ventilation* (HFV) is defined as ventilation occurring at frequencies greater than 60 breaths per minute and is subdivided into three distinct types. High-frequency positive-pressure ventilation (HFPPV) is otherwise conventionally applied mechanical ventilation at rates of 60 to 100 breaths per minute. Tidal volumes of 3 to 5 mL/kg of body weight are typically used, and HFPPV can be instituted with some types of con-ventional ventilators, although low-compliance ventilator circuit equipment must be used. High-frequency jet ventilation (HFJV) and high-frequency oscillation (HFO) are accomplished at respiratory rates of 100 to 150 and 150 to 2400 breaths per minute, respectively. They require special endotracheal tubes and ventilators with the special ability to provide high rate flow (Froese, 1987).

These latter types of ventilation are accom-plished with very low tidal volumes (2–5 mL/kg with HFJV and <3 mL/kg with HFO). While con-ventional mechanical ventilation and HFPPV pre-dominantly employ bulk (convective) flow in gas movement, HFJV and HFO employ varying de-grees of convective flow, direct alveolar ventila-tion, Pendelluft asymmetric velocity profile flow, Taylor dispersion, cardiogenic oscillations, and molecular diffusion. Suffice it to say that gas ex-change characteristics of HFJV and HFO are com-plex (Chang, 1984; Standiford, 1989). In contrast, HFPPV is reasonably intuitive and straightforward.

High-frequency ventilation has been used with some degree of success in neonates (de-Lemos, 1992); success not generally achieved in adults. In adults, HFJV and HFO are reserved for refractory, severe hypoxemia and ventilatory res-piratory failure. High-frequency ventilation is es-pecially useful in the ventilation of patients with bronchopleural fistulas (Bishop, 1987). Only on a case-by-case exception is HFV the modality of choice for ventilating adults.

## Airway Pressure Release Ventilation

Airway pressure release ventilation (APRV) pro-duces exhalation through release of CPAP. Inspi-ration is through reinstitution of the selected level of CPAP. Because the peak airway pressure reached is never greater than the level of CPAP selected, APRV theoretically reduces barotrauma while simultaneously maintaining lung volume within the optimal range for gas exchange and ventilation. For a given degree of increase in mean airway pressure, APRV offers no advantage in hemodynamic stability. However, because lower mean and peak airway pressures may be possible, for a given degree of ventilation, APRV may hold hemodynamic advantages over conventional ventilation. It may be applied by mask and allow extubation of patients who are otherwise unable to be extubated. A modification of APRV, in which PSV is added to CPAP/APRV, is referred to as intermittent mandatory pressure release ventilation. Airway pressure release ventilation holds great promise as the technique is further developed (Davis, 1993).

## Partial Liquid Ventilation

Liquid ventilation was developed as an outgrowth of advancements in underwater breathing equipment and semisynthetic blood products and employs the oxygen carrying capacity of perfluorochemicals (PFCs). Liquid ventilation involves the infusion of PFCs into the patient's airway in conjunction with low-pressure conventional ventilation. Perfluorochemical is instilled up to an amount estimated to comprise the patient's FRV. Total or complete liquid ventilation is much less frequently used and developed. Perfluorochemical promotes gas exchange directly, recruits otherwise atelectatic airways, and may serve as an antiinflammatory lavage for the injured lung. Clinical trials are under way using partial liquid ventilation in adults (Hirsch, 1991; Hirsch, 1995; Hirsch, 1996).

## Extracorporeal Membrane Oxygenation

Extracorporeal membrane oxygenation (ECMO) was first used successfully in the treatment of ARDS in 1972 (Hill, 1972). It evolved as a refinement of intraoperative cardiopulmonary bypass. Because ECMO involves perfusion as well as gas exchange, the term *extracorporeal life support* is probably a more apt description for the technique. This technique is administered in two broad categories. Venoarterial bypass provides

both cardiac output and oxygenation through removal of venous blood, which is oxygenated and returned as arterial blood. Venovenous bypass provides respiratory support only (i.e., exchange of $CO_2$ but not $O_2$). To provide access, large-bore catheters are placed into the appropriate venous or arterial access sites. The internal jugular vein is the preferred venous site, while the common carotid artery is the preferred arterial site. In venovenous bypass, oxygenated blood is usually returned to the internal jugular, femoral, or iliac vein. In either method, full anticoagulation is required. The bypass circuit also can be used for ultrafiltration or hemodiafiltration (Presenti, 1988).

The largest group to receive ECMO has been neonates with respiratory distress. Survival rates up to 90 + % have been reported by some investigators (ECMO Quarterly Report, 1994). The efficacy of ECMO in treatment of acute respiratory disease in adults is less clear. The National Institutes of Health sponsored a multicenter investigation of ECMO in the treatment of adult ARDS (Anderson, 1995). Compared with conventional mechanical ventilation methods in use at the time, ECMO offered no advantage. Some, however, still feel that advances in both ECMO itself and in the mechanical ventilation techniques used in patients who would require ECMO hold promise. The extracorporeal life support organization reports adult ARDS survival rates between 50% and 65% (Anderson, 1992). Extracorporeal membrane oxygenation is an option for patients with potentially reversible pulmonary disease and who require significant ventilatory support based on specific parameters (compliance $< 0.5$ mL cm $H_2O^{-1}$ kg$^{-1}$, transpulmonary shunt $> 30\%$ on $FIo_2 \geq 0.6$), and who have required mechanical ventilation less than a total of 10 days (Anderson, 1995). Advanced age, prolonged prior mechanical ventilation, absolute contraindication to anticoagulation, necrotizing pneumonia, or predicted poor quality of life are contraindications to the use of ECMO (Bartlett, 1990).

We have used ECMO in one postpartum patient with ARDS complicating sickle SC pulmonary sequestration disease. After some 3 months of conventional mechanical ventilation and ECMO, she eventually regained full recovery. Her case underscores an important point in the often inevitably anecdotal treatment of the pregnant and immediately postpartum patient. Because women of childbearing age are usually younger and tend to be without the multisystem disease typical of many adult ARDS study subjects, attempts at advanced measures may sometimes be indicated in the pregnant/postpartum patient not otherwise or not usually considered as a candidate for such interventions. Hopefully, newer well-designed controlled trials will replace older data on ECMO in adults.

## Other Advanced Methods of Mechanical Ventilation

Many other techniques of mechanical ventilation have been attempted to include intravenous oxygenation (Conrad, 1993), permissive hypercapnia (Hickling, 1990), inhaled nitric oxide (Rossaint, 1993), and computer-modulated mechanical ventilation. Each at this point remains experimental.

## Care of the Patient Receiving Mechanical Ventilation

During initiation and maintenance of mechanical ventilation, particular attention must be paid to aspects necessary to the support of the patient. While an extensive review of all of the secondary aspects of support during mechanical ventilation is beyond the scope of this text, we will review pertinent aspects critical to successful mechanical ventilation.

### Airway

Indications for intubation and mechanical ventilation are listed in Table 8-3, and do not vary significantly with pregnancy. In addition to the criteria in Table 8-3, one should include apnea, upper airway obstruction, inability to protect the airway, respiratory muscle fatigue, mental status deterioration, and hemodynamic instability.

Intubation of the pregnant patient should be accomplished by skilled personnel. Intubation of pregnant patients differs only slightly from that of nonpregnant patients. Pregnancy, particularly at term, has been associated with slow gastric emptying and increased residual gastric volume (Sutherland, 1986). This implies a slightly increased risk of aspiration of gastric contents during intubation of the gravid patient. The use of Bicitra preoperatively neutralizes gastric contents (Gibbs, 1984). This should be administered prior to intubation if possible. In addition, intubation should proceed using techniques that preserve airway reflexes (e.g., awake intubation). Alternatively use "rapid-sequence" induction of anesthesia and Sellick's maneuver (cricoid pressure) to prevent passive reflux of gastric contents into the pharynx (Sellick, 1961). Another difference is that hyperemia associated with pregnancy can narrow the upper airways sufficiently that patients are at increased risk for upper airway trauma during intubation (Cheek, 1987). Relatively small endotracheal tubes may be required (6–7 mm). Nasal tracheal intubation should probably be avoided as well.

Decreased functional residual capacity in pregnancy may lower oxygen reserve such that, at the time of intubation, a short period of apnea may be associated with a preciptious decrease in the $P_{O_2}$ (Cheek, 1987). Therefore, 100% oxygen should be administered either by mask or by Ambu bag when the patient requires intubation. Overenthusiastic hyperventilation should be avoided because the associated respiratory alkalosis may actually decrease uterine blood flow. If intubation is not successful after 30 seconds, one should stop and resume ventilation with bag and mask and then repeat the attempt in order to avoid prolonged hypoxemia. Complications of endotracheal intubation are listed in Table 8-4.

Once intubation is performed, tube placement may be confirmed by end-tidal carbon dioxide measurement, direct auscultation, and chest x-ray (Heffner, 1990). Both early and late complications of endotracheal intubation may occur. Early complications include malposition of the endotracheal tube, aspiration, inability to intubate, hypertensive sequelae, dental or nasopharyngeal trauma, and bleeding. Late complications include dysphonia, infection (sinusitis with nasotracheal intubation), bleeding, fistula, and tracheal stenosis (Colice, 1989; Tonkin, 1989). The

T A B L E   **8-3**

Definition of acute respiratory failure: indications
for mechanical ventilation

| Parameter | Normal Range | Indication for Ventilatory Assistance |
|---|---|---|
| *Mechanics* | | |
| Respiratory rate (breaths/min) | 12–20 | >35 |
| Vital capacity (mL/kg body weight)[a] | 65–75 | <15 |
| Inspiratory force (cm $H_2O$) | −75–100 | <−25 |
| Compliance (mL/cm $H_2O$) | 100 | <25 |
| $FEV_1$ (mL/kg body weight)[a] | 50–60 | <10 |
| *Oxygenation* | | |
| $Pao_2$[b] (mm Hg) | 80–95 | <70 |
| (kPa) | 10.7–12.7 | <9.3 |
| $P(A\text{-}a)o_2$[c] (mm Hg) | 25–50 | >450 |
| (kPa) | 3.3–6.7 | >60 |
| Qs/Qt (%) | 5 | >20 |
| *Ventilation* | | |
| $Paco_2$ (mm Hg) | 35–45 | 55[d] |
| (kPa) | 4.7–6.0 | 7.3 |
| $V_D/V_T$ | 0.2–0.3 | 0.60 |

[a]Use ideal body weight.

[b]Room air.

[c]$FIo_2 = 1.0$.

[d]Exception is chronic lung disease.

$FEV_1$, forced expiratory volume in 1 min; $P(A\text{-}a)o_2$, alveolar-arterial oxygen
   tension gradient; Qs/Qt, shunt function; $V_D/V_T$, dead space to tidal volume ratio.

use of low-pressure, high-compliance endotracheal cuffs, inflated to less than 20 mm Hg, will reduce the incidence of proximal tracheal injury (Abbey, 1977; Joh, 1987). Opinion is divided as to how long an endotracheal tube can remain in situ. Clearly, the longer cuffed endotracheal intubation is used, the greater the risk of morbidity. Meticulous care and attention to tube position and cuff pressure is important in preventing late complications (Lee, 1992). It is our practice to reserve surgical airway placement (tracheostomy) for patients deemed to require mechanical ventilation longer than 21 days. Still, reports of longer periods of endotracheal cuff intubation without morbidity suggest some ability to individualize in any given case.

Tracheostomy as a controlled-elective procedure is generally reserved for long-term ventilation. Patient comfort concerns in the awake, alert, intubated subject clearly favor tracheostomy over endotracheal intubation. The most frequent complication of tracheostomy is infection (75%). Much less frequent complications include tracheostenosis (1%–2%) and life-threatening hemorrhage (1%) (Gungwardana, 1992; Rodriguez, 1990).

Immediately available expertise in airway control is necessary to safely conduct mechanical ventilation. Skill at suctioning, airway positioning, breath sound auscultation, and reintubation are prerequisites for care of the mechanically ventilated patient. The ability and equipment necessary to immediately bag and mask ventilate is another prerequisite to the conduct of mechanical ventilation.

The recommended initial ventilator settings are as follows: $F_Io_2$: 0.9 to 1.0 and a rate of 12 to 20 breaths per minute. Traditionally, a tidal volume ($V_T$) of 10 to 15 mL/kg was recommended.

TABLE 8-4

Complications of endotracheal intubation

*During Intubation: Immediate*
Failed intubation
Main stem bronchial or esophageal intubation
Laryngospasm
Trauma to naso/oropharynx or larynx
Perforation of trachea or esophagus
Cervical spine fracture
Aspiration
Bacteremia
Hypoxemia/hypercarbia
Arrhythmias
Hypertension
Increased intracranial/intraocular pressure

*During Intubation: Later*
Accidental extubation
Endobronchial intubation
Tube obstruction or kinking
Aspiration, sinusitis
Tracheoesophageal fistula
Vocal cord ulcers, granulomata

*On Extubation*
Laryngospasm, laryngeal edema
Aspiration
Hoarseness, sore throat
Noncardiogenic pulmonary edema
Laryngeal incompetence
Swallowing disorders
Soreness, dislocation of jaw

*Delayed*
Laryngeal stenosis
Tracheomalacia/tracheal stenosis

Source: Modified from Stehling LC: Management of the airway. In: Barash PG, Cullen BF, Stoelting RK, eds. Clinical anesthesia. Philadelphia: JB Lippincott, 1992:685–708.

It has now been recognized that those volumes result in abnormally high airway pressures and volutrauma. Therefore, $V_T$ should be instituted at 5 to 8 mL/kg to prevent excessive alveolar distention (Bidani, 1994).

## Monitoring

Close monitoring of the patient receiving mechanical ventilation is required. Skilled, trained critical care nursing and respiratory therapy support are cornerstones of the successful practice of mechanical ventilation. Monitoring of the mechanically ventilated patient should include continuous digital pulse oximetry to assess oxyhemoglobin saturation. Oximetry will provide real-time assessment of relative arterial oxygen content but must be interpreted in clinical context. Periodic arterial blood gas determination also is necessary, especially during significant ventilator changes. Blood pressure monitoring is recommended by continuous arterial pressure transducer or by frequent noninvasive means. We employ continuous electronic fetal heart rate monitoring in patients at greater than 24 weeks' gestation during acute or unstable circumstances. If not indicated for obstetric reasons and with a stable patient, we do not necessarily perform continuous fetal monitoring during mechanical ventilation.

## Sedation/Paralysis

Because of the discomfort inherent in receiving mechanical ventilation and intensive care, appropriate use of anxiolytics, analgesics, and sedatives is important to the welfare of the critically ill patient. Furthermore, pain relief may be necessary to render mechanical ventilation effectively. Conversely, inappropriate use of sedatives, anxiolytics, and/or analgesics may delay extubation, produce hemodynamic instability, or contribute to mental status abnormalities. Specific fetal side effects of these drugs have been referenced comprehensively (Briggs, 1994; Rayburn, 1992).

Narcotics are useful for pain relief, sedation, and anxiolysis (Balestrieri, 1995). Morphine sulfate is used frequently as a primary agent of pain relief. In usually administered amounts, morphine sulfate has relatively few adverse cardiovascular effects (Lowenstein, 1969). Intravenous administration is preferred over other parenteral routes, either intermittently or by continuous administration. Side effects relating to histamine release or cardiovascular interactions are uncommon. Potent synthetic narcotics such as fentanyl, alfentanil, and sufentanil are useful for continuous infusions as well. Ileus and tolerance are long term side effects of narcotic administration.

Short- and intermediate-action benzodiazepines, such as midazolam, lorazepam, and diazepam, are useful anxiolytic/hypnotics in long-term mechanical ventilation. While not singularly effective at providing pain relief, the hypnotic effects of the agents are additive with the effects of narcotics. Midazolam is useful for acute events because of its relatively short half-life. Midazolam can produce delayed hypotension. Lorazepam carries the advantage of glucuronidase metabolism, which is well preserved and remains effective even in patients who have moderate degrees of liver disease. Diazepam has a rapid onset and a long half-life. For sporadic use, diazepam is an effective and inexpensive choice. For continued use, intermittent bolus or continuous infusions of midazolam or lorazepam is preferred (Balestrieri, 1995).

Because of haloperidol's relatively large margin of safety and minimal hemodynamic and sedating side effects, it is the antipsychotic of choice in chronically mechanically ventilated patients. Agents such as haloperidol are useful for treatment of delirium and psychosis that is often a consequence of prolonged intensive care (Ayd, 1978).

For the long-term sedation often necessary for advanced modes of mechanical ventilation, propofol is in many ways an ideal agent. Given by continuous intravenous infusion, propofol has a very short single-dose half-life of 2 to 3 minutes. Rapid induction and emergence from anesthesia is possible with propofol. Because hypotension invariably occurs when sufficient doses are used to provide surgical anesthesia, propofol is not recommended for use in induction of anesthesia for delivery. In continuously infused doses necessary for mechanical ventilation, however, hypotension is less problematic. Propofol clearance is not appreciably altered in renal or hepatic disease states (Sebel, 1989).

Skeletal muscle paralysis is necessary under two broad circumstances. The first circumstance is when temporary paralysis is required for intubation. The second situation is when paralysis is a necessary addition to sedation for advanced mechanical ventilation when skeletal muscle paralysis for tolerance of mechanical ventilation is required. Intermittent or continuous doses of nondepolarizing muscle relaxants are generally employed. A nondepolarizing block is produced when the postjunctional membrane receptors are reversibly bound with the drug. The duration of the block depends on the rate at which the relaxant is redistributed. The relaxant effects of nondepolarizing drugs are reversed by anticholinergic-blocking drugs such as neostigmine (Cullen, 1995).

Of the several nondepolarizing agents available, pancuronium, vecuronium, and atracurium are most used. Pancuronium is effective for 60 to 90 minutes after an intubating dose is given. Anticholinergic effects of the drug may result in tachycardia and rarely hypotension (Cullen, 1995; Duvaldstein, 1978). Vecuronium produces a clinical effect for 30 to 60 minutes after an intubating dose. Hemodynamic effects are usually absent after typically used doses. Both vecuronium and pancuronium may have prolonged action in the presence of hepatic failure (Miller, 1984). Atracurium has a relatively short duration of action and is degraded non-enzymatically. It is, therefore, useful in patients with hepatic or renal failure. Any of the agents can be given by intermittent bolus or continuous infusion. Monitoring of the level of paralysis with nerve stimulator equipment ("twitch monitoring") is recommended during prolonged administration of paralytics. Because muscle relaxants paralyze without affording the patient any analgesia or sedation, appropriate monitoring for the adequacy of sedation is required any time a patient is pharmacologically paralyzed. Nonetheless, because of the potential for paralysis while awake, muscle relaxants must be used only when clearly necessary (Cullen, 1995; Ward, 1988).

Table 8-5 lists agents commonly used for sedation, pain relief, and paralysis of the mechanically ventilated patient. Pain relief and sedation are very important parts of the total care given to the ventilator "recipient." In many cases, otherwise difficult to ventilate patients have dramatically benefited from simple pain relief. Therefore, familiarity with the doses' interactions, side effects, and indications for analgesics, anxiolytics, nondepolarizing muscle relaxants, and antipsychotics is an important part of mechanical ventilation.

T A B L E   **8-5**

Sedation and paralysis in mechanical ventilation

*Narcotics*
Morphine
Fentanyl

*Anxiolytics*
Midazolam
Diazepam

*Anesthetics*
Propofol

*Nondepolarizing Muscle Relaxants*
Vercuronium
Pancuronium
Atracurium

Thorough familiarity with any pharmacologic agent is necessary prior to its use.

## Weaning from Mechanical Ventilation

Discontinuation of mechanical ventilation should be a goal considered concomitant with its initiation. While most patients with severe pulmonary pathophysiology require mechanical ventilation for several days, the philosophy of continually assessing the need for mechanical ventilation is prudent.

Discontinuation or weaning from mechanical ventilation may encompass several situations. The first circumstance entails the completion of or recovery from a specific event necessitating mechanical ventilation. An example of such an immediately reversible process would be extubation after general anesthesia from an uncomplicated surgical procedure. The second set of events in which weaning occurs is after 1 to 5 days of mechanical ventilation for an acute illness that is rapidly reversible. Situations in which 1 to 5 days of mechanical ventilation would be required include many pregnancy-related disorders (e.g., recovery from tocolytic or pre-eclampsia-induced pulmonary edema). The third and most difficult broad category of mechanical ventilation weaning follows recovery from a prolonged illness (many days or weeks), such as ARDS. While each situation entails different concerns and predictors of success, several

generalizations can be used to predict the success of sustained extubation. Obviously, the clinical circumstances surrounding each particular patient are as, if not more, important, in predicting successful extubation.

Prediction of success of weaning extubation involves assessment of oxygenation, gas exchange, respiratory muscle strength and endurance, and metabolic factors that may influence outcome (Weinberger, 1995). In prediction of oxygenation and gas exchange, $Pao_2$ greater than or equal to 60 mm Hg on an $FIo_2$ of 35% or less is positively predictive of success. More specific indicators include $Pao_2/FIo_2$ ratios of more than 200 (90% positive predictive value with 10% negative predictive value) (Krieger, 1988). Alveolar-arterial $Po_2$ gradients of less than 350 mm Hg and the arterial-alveolar tension ratio of 0.35 or greater have also been used successfully (Yang, 1991).

In many patients who have received longer-term mechanical ventilation, respiratory muscle strength and endurance are the most important predictors of extubation success. The reason for the importance of muscle strength and endurance lies in both the fact that most pulmonary disease causes a reduction in compliance (a greater amount of work is required for a given degree of ventilation) and the inevitability of respiratory muscle atrophy or weakening as a consequence of longer-duration mechanical ventilation. A demonstrated vital capacity of at least 10 to 15 mL/kg, a resting minute ventilation of less than 10 liters/min, and the ability to voluntarily double one's resting minute ventilation (maximum minute ventilation) are all indicators of reserve and strength (Feeley, 1975). A maximum negative inspiratory pressure of at least −30 cm $H_2O$ also is an indicator of respiratory muscle strength (Sahn, 1973). Table 8-6 outlines various weaning parameters. Unfortunately, all of these methods will exhibit poor positive and negative prediction value of success at extubation if taken at face value alone (Tahuanainen, 1983). Clinical judgment and assessment remain of signal importance!

More difficult to quantify is how any given ventilated patient will respond to trials of increased work of breathing. Rapid shallow ventilation, "tiring" while on minimal ventilator support, and

T A B L E   **8-6**

Variables used to predict weaning success

*Gas Exchange*

$Pao_2$ of $\geq 60$ mm Hg with $FIo_2$ of $\leq 0.35$

Alveolar-arterial $Po_2$ gradient of $< 350$ mm Hg

$Pao_2/FIo_2$ ratio of $> 200$

*Ventilatory Pump*

Vital capacity of $>10$–$15$ mL/kg body weight

Maximum negative inspiratory pressure

  $> -30$ cm $H_2O$

Minute ventilation $< 10$ liters/min

Maximum voluntary ventilation more than twice resting minute ventilation

Reproduced by permission from Tobin MJ, Yang K. Weaning from mechanical ventilation. Crit Care Clin 1990;6:733.

iatrogenic tiring (by prolonged high work of breathing through a highly resistant ventilator circuit) all can hinder attempts at successful extubation. Prolonged insomnia, fever (which increases spontaneous minute ventilation requirement), patient position (especially important in the supine obstetric patient), overuse of sedatives, residual CNS disease, and patient anxiety all may contribute to unsuccessful extubation (Lee, 1994; Weinberger, 1995).

An extremely important issue in ventilator weaning after intermediate or long-term mechanical ventilation is nutritional support. Parenteral, or preferably enteral, feeding provides caloric support to the muscles of respiration. An added advantage of enteral nutrition is a potential decrease in gastrointestinal bacterial translocation (Moore, 1992). Early and appropriate feeding may serve to attenuate the respiratory muscle atrophy that so often occurs in highly catabolic diseases such as ARDS. Nutritional requirements must be determined and met. Severe illness alters metabolic needs significantly. While the caloric requirements of normal pregnancy are well described, the changes that catabolic pathophysiology imposes on the nutritional requirements during pregnancy are not well studied. Both overfeeding and underfeeding may be detrimental. Overfeeding may adversely affect successful weaning by providing excessive carbohydrate substrate. During high-carbohydrate feeding, carbon dioxide pro-

duction is increased, and the excessive production of carbon dioxide may impede successful weaning. To accurately measure nutritional needs, indirect calorimetry and component requirements of the pregnant ventilator patient may be used (Durnin, 1987).

Several different methods of weaning have been proposed and used in the past 25 years (Tobin, 1994). Each is based on progressive reduction in the contribution of the ventilator and a progressive increase in the patient's contribution to ventilation (Weinberger, 1995). Successful weaning is more difficult in the patient ventilated for prolonged periods and for those with more intrinsic pulmonary disease. Intermittent T-bar trials, in which the patient is taken off mechanical ventilation for gradually increasing periods of time, was the traditional method of ventilator weaning. Because it is less labor-intensive, SIMV weaning to 4 or fewer breaths per minute is more commonly used. Pressure support ventilation, with a gradual decrease in supported pressure, also is used. Pressure support ventilation is sometimes combined with SIMV weaning to overcome the work of breathing inherent in ventilator circuits. Single daily trials of spontaneous breathing also have been tried (Esteban, 1995). No method has proven to be clearly superior over any other (Weinberger, 1995). We prefer to convert our patients to SIMV with 5 to 10 cm $H_2O$ of PSV. The SIMV rate is gradually reduced to a minimal amount. Blood gases are checked 30 to 45 minutes after each ventilator change, and the patient is weaned to an SIMV of 0 with 5 to 10 cm $H_2O$ of PEEP. This, in effect, provides CPAP with a small amount of pressure support. When the patient tolerates this level of work, we extubate her. A general schemata for SIMV weaning is shown in Figure 8-8.

Other factors necessary for effective extubation include an empty stomach (nasogastric suctioning and no gastric feeds prior to extubation), normal electrolytes (hypokalemia and hypomagnesemia may prevent extubation), airway suctioning immediately before extubation, and aggressive respiratory toilet after extubation. Always be prepared to reintubate immediately, if necessary! Place the extubated patient on 40% to 50% humidified mask oxygen, and evaluate ventilation

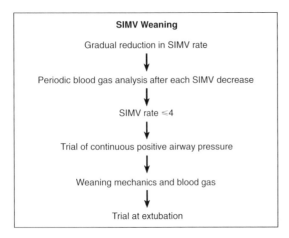

**SIMV Weaning**

Gradual reduction in SIMV rate

↓

Periodic blood gas analysis after each SIMV decrease

↓

SIMV rate ≤4

↓

Trial of continuous positive airway pressure

↓

Weaning mechanics and blood gas

↓

Trial at extubation

F I G U R E  **8-8**

Weaning strategies. Pressure support of 5 to 10 cm $H_2O$ causes reduction in airway circuit work of breathing. Standard SIMV weaning is illustrated.

and oxygenation with blood gas analysis frequently after extubation. It is not a failure to be required to reintubate a patient thought to be ready for extubation. It is a failure to not be prepared to or not recognize the need to reintubate a recently extubated patient.

## Complications of Mechanical Ventilation

Complications related to the use of mechanical ventilation include adverse hemodynamic effects, abnormal acid/base/gas exchange events, barotrauma, ventilator malfunction, and infection.

### Hemodynamic Effects

Because most mechanical ventilation is positive-pressure ventilation, profound alterations of the transmural pressures evident in the heart and great vessels may be seen. With the use of high ventilatory pressures and PEEP often necessary in the profoundly ill patient, a decrease in right and left ventricular preload coupled with an increase in pulmonary and systemic afterload may occur (Conway, 1975). The effects are variable because of non-uniformity in intrapulmonary compliance at different lung volumes. The con-

sequence of the inherent nonlinearity of compliance is a volume-dependent variation in transmural pressure transfer. In effect, ventilation at different lung volumes may have varying effects on ventricular preload and afterload (Brechar, 1955; Lloyd, 1982). Furthermore, measurement of left and right ventricular filling pressures may be spuriously altered by elevated pulmonary pressures (Pinsky, 1991). Increases in filling pressures by volume administration, pressors, inotropes, and/or reduction of PEEP may be necessary (Wallis, 1983). Measurement of oxygen delivery is a more reliable indicator of endpoint goals of mechanical ventilation than is assessment of $PaO_2$, $SaO_2$, or shunt!

### Acid/Base/Gas Exchange Alteration

Acid-base abnormalities while a patient is undergoing mechanical ventilation are common and have multiple possible causes. Simple misadjustment of the ventilator can lead to respiratory acidosis or alkalosis and can be determined relatively quickly. Hypoxemia can result from inadvertent extubation or endotracheal tube obstruction. A therapeutic maneuver that will bypass the mechanical ventilator and assist in diagnosing the location and patency of the endotracheal tube is to manually bag the patient through the endotracheal tube. Breath sounds can be auscultated and localized. Other causes of hypoxemia can present more insidiously. From a respiratory care standpoint, endotracheal suctioning and evaluation/treatment for bronchospasm should be considered early in the evaluation of hypoxemia. If hemodynamically tolerated, sedation will often remove asynchronicity in ventilation caused by an agitated patient (Strieter, 1988).

All of the previously described maneuvers should be undertaken immediately on a rapidly worsening hypoxemic patient. Chest x-ray and ECG evaluation should not delay initial therapies. If hypoxemia is worsening, pneumothorax and hemothorax need to be considered. Both may present with unilateral breath sounds, hypotension, mediastinal shift, and predisposing circumstances (barotrauma, recent thoracic venous catheter placement, or difficult to manipulate pulmonary artery catheter). Needle thoracostomy, or preferably drainage tube thoracostomy, should be performed in the face of clinical suspicion of pneumothorax. The necessary equipment to place a thoracostomy tube should be on the unit. Pulmonary hemorrhage is also a consideration (and is much more difficult to treat); differential lung ventilation or emergency thoracotomy is often necessary (Slutsky, 1993; Haake, 1987).

Pulmonary embolism, for which critically ill and bedridden patients are at risk, can produce hypoxemia and altered gas exchange. In suspected severe cases of pulmonary embolism, anticoagulation is often carried out, even prior to confirmation of the diagnosis, because it may reduce further deterioration in a patient already requiring mechanical ventilation. Open thoracotomy, embolectomy, and intravenous thrombolytics are reserved for unstable or unresponsive cases (Hyers, 1992).

Many other factors may alter oxygenation and ventilation. Altered production or delivery of carbon dioxide or oxygen can change blood gas homeostasis. Metabolic circumstances such as overfeeding, starvation, and fever may affect blood gases. Either worsening or improvement of the pathophysiology that initiated the pulmonary insult may produce segmental heterogenicity in gas exchange. Mere alteration of intrapulmonary blood flow, as might occur with alteration of patient position, may produce profound acid-base or oxygenation changes. Careful clinical assessment and consideration of all recent interventions will often provide important clues as to why a particular blood gas derangement occurred (Slutsky, 1993).

## Barotrauma

Barotrauma is often an unavoidable consequence of positive-pressure ventilation. Morbidity and mortality from barotrauma can be divided into two broad categories. Catastrophic effects from air extravasation (pneumothorax, pneumomediastinum, subcutaneous emphysema) are intuitively recognized as consequences of mechanical ventilation (Haake, 1987). What may not be as apparent is the heterogeneity of pulmonary injury that may exist in any given adjacent alveolar units. Overdistention of relatively normal alveolar units may cause large transmissions of pressure hemodynamically and extrathoracically. Both catastrophic and insidious effects may result from this overdistention. Insidious effects include injury of what were relatively uninjured alveolar units and alteration of ventilation/perfusion due to increased transmural pressure (Marini, 1992b). Pneumothorax, on the other hand, is usually quite apparent.

Barotrauma has always been recognized as a factor in acute lung injury. Recently, new emphasis on barotrauma reduction has emerged as a major concern in the treatment of ARDS. Unification in the classification and description of ARDS has allowed for uniformity in the performance of clinical trials (Murray, 1988). Subsequently, new insight into ventilatory management of ARDS patients has slowly emerged. Traditionally (as implied elsewhere in this chapter), ventilatory support in patients with low-compliance respiratory failure was based on experience gained through mechanical ventilation of postoperative patients. Tidal volumes of 10 to 15 mL/kg were used to prospectively prevent the development of progressive atelectasis. Treatment goals were primarily normalization of $Paco_2$ and $Pao_2$ (at the expense of airway distention pressure) (Pierson, 1995).

Animal data from high tidal volume mechanical ventilation show pathophysiologic changes similar to human ARDS (Kolobow, 1987; Webb, 1974). More importantly, it was shown that distending volume, not airway pressure, was particularly central to the progression of ARDS pathophysiology (Dreyfuss, 1988). In humans, because of the lack of uniformity of alveolar injury, hyperinflation of pulmonary segments occurs in patients with ARDS. It has been postulated that in such patients, mechanical ventilation at 10 to 15 mL/kg tidal volumes may result in some alveolar units receiving as many as 40 to 50 mL/kg tidal volumes (Pierson, 1995). Furthermore, alveolar recruitment is nonlinear, and the pressure volume relationship in the injured lung is critically non-uniform (Fig 8-9) (Maunder, 1986; Gattinoni, 1987).

To combat overdistention, several strategies have been developed. As mentioned elsewhere

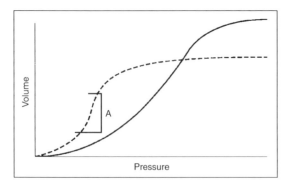

F I G U R E **8-9**

Pressure volume relationship in ARDS. A goal in the mechanical ventilation of poorly compliant lungs is to maintain lung volume within the optimum range of pressure-to-volume relationships. Broken line, ARDS; unbroken line, normal lung; A, target tidal lung volume (in mechanical ventilation).

in this chapter, pressure-controlled ventilation, permissive hypercapnia, conscious application of PEEP, and use *or* avoidance of auto PEEP (depending on the circumstances and ventilatory mode) have all been employed in an effort to control barotrauma (Pierson, 1995; Marini, 1994). These techniques are listed in Table 8-7.

The application of these techniques to pregnant and postpartum patients is presently anecdotal. Avoidance of barotrauma and hyperoxia, however, are central to the mechanical ventilation of any patient with low-compliance pulmonary injury.

It is nearly impossible to eliminate all barotrauma. A conscious policy of lower tidal volumes (6–10 mL/kg), minimal levels of PEEP, limitation of peak airway pressure to 35 to 40 cm $H_2O$, and decreased peak airway pressure at the expense of higher mean airway pressure and decreased ventilation (permissive hypercapnea) will sometimes limit barotrauma (Fu, 1990; Parker, 1993). $FIO_2$ should be reduced to less than 0.5 (50%) as soon as practicable. If possible, in patients with progressive lung injury, lower $FIO_2$s may be desirable, providing adequate oxyhemoglobin saturation is produced. It should be emphasized that *both* hyperoxia and barotrauma contribute to propagation of pulmonary injury. It also should be emphasized that arterial oxygen con-

tent does not appreciably increase above a $Pao_2$ of 60 to 70 mm Hg. Therefore, with barotrauma and hyperoxia, "too much of a good thing" may be just as deleterious as too little!

## Oxygen Toxicity

A variety of gross and histopathologic lesions have been described in human and experimental animal lung tissues that have been exposed to increased concentrations of oxygen in the airways (Bezzant and Mortensen, 1994). Free oxygen radicals generated by high concentrations of oxygen in and along the airways and alveoli attach intracellular enzyme systems, damage DNA, destroy lipid membranes, and increase microvascular permeability. The duration of exposure of lungs to increased oxygen concentrations is related directly to the incidence and severity of resultant lung injury. No definitive data are available to establish the upper limits of concentration of oxygen in inspired air that can be considered safe (Bezzant and Mortensen, 1994). General consensus, however, seems to be that oxygen concentrations greater than 50% in inspired air are undesirable and should be avoided if clinical circumstances permit. Therefore, one should institute measures to ensure that the lowest possible concentration of oxygen is used during ventilatory support.

When oxygenation is inadequate, sedation, paralysis, and position change are possible therapeutic measures. Other factors in oxygen delivery (i.e., cardiac output and hemoglobin) also should be considered. In some clinical situations, when significant concerns over both elevated plateau pressure and high $FIO_2$ exists, consideration for accepting an $Sao_2$ slightly less than 90% is reasonable (Slutsky, 1994).

## Oxygen Delivery Systems

A wide range of oxygen delivery systems exists, from standard nasal cannula, which delivers low and unpredictable concentrations of oxygen, to intubation, which can reliably deliver an $FIO_2$ of up to 100%. Each has benefits and limitations of which the clinician should be aware (Table 8-8).

T A B L E   **8-7**

The new "lung-protective" ventilation strategy
for managing ARDS

| Aspect of Management | Previous Practice | New Strategy |
|---|---|---|
| *Tidal Volume* | 10–15 mL/kg | 5–8 mL/kg |
| *PEEP* | | |
| Minimum set PEEP level | No minimum PEEP level | Above lower inflection point (in most patients about 8 cm $H_2O$) |
| Maximum set PEEP level | Whatever it took to achieve target $Po_2$ (often >20 cm $H_2O$) | Below upper inflection point (in most patients $\leq$15 cm $H_2O$) |
| *Rate* | Whatever it took to keep $Pco_2$ normal | 15–25 breaths/min (back off if auto-PEEP develops) |
| *Inspiratory Time* | No consensus; commonly 0.33 | Usually 0.33; increase cautiously if needed to improve oxygenation; back off if auto-PEEP develops |
| *Airway Pressures* | | |
| Relevant airway pressure goal | Peak inspiratory pressure (PIP) | End-inspiratory plateau pressure |
| | Avoid PIP >50 cm $H_2O$ | Keep $P_{plat}$ 35 cm $H_2O$ or less |
| *Oxygenation* | | |
| Relevant measure | Arterial $Po_2$ | Arterial $O_2$ saturation; arterial $O_2$ content |
| Target value | Normal $Po_2$ (e.g., >80 mm Hg) | $Sao_2$ 90 $\pm$ 5%; consider RBC transfusion if maintaining $Sao_2$ requires high $FIo_2$ and hct <30 |
| *Arterial $Pco_2$* | Normal (40 $\pm$ 5 mm Hg) | Accept hypercapnia (e.g., $Pco_2$ 50–70 mm Hg or higher) if above measures do not result in normal value* |
| *Arterial pH* | Normal (7.4 $\pm$ 0.05 units) | Accept acidemia (e.g., pH 7.20–7.30) if above measures do not result in normal value* |

*Exceptions: Acute intracranial pathology and potentially life-threatening arrhythmias.

## Infection

Pulmonary colonization and infection rates approach 100% after prolonged ventilation. Ventilator-induced atelectasis and early infiltrates are often difficult to discern radiographically. Unexplained febrile morbidity is commonly seen in ventilated patients. Colonization of the upper airway of intubated or tracheostomized patients may or may not correlate with pulmonary microbiology. Sinusitis may be a source in patients with nasotracheal tubes in place for long periods. Very few currently available strategies have significantly reduced the infection rate in mechanically venti-

lated patients. Promise is held in the strategy of reduction of bacterial microaspiration through selective oral decontamination and aggressive enteral feeding. Until further progress is made, however, meticulous respiratory care, aggressive pulmonary toilet, and bronchoscopic diagnosis of respiratory infection are the mainstays in control of hospital-acquired "ventilator" pneumonia (Craven, 1989; Sumner, 1989; Pingleton, 1988).

## Nutritional Complications

Nutritional complications in acute respiratory failure patients include the adverse effects of

TABLE **8-8**

Oxygen delivery systems

| Type | FIo$_2$ Capability | Comments |
|------|-------------------|----------|
| *Nasal Cannula* | | |
| Standard | True FIo$_2$ uncertain and highly dependent on inspiratory flow rate | Flow rates should be limited to <5 liters/min |
| Reservoir type | True FIo$_2$ uncertain and highly dependent on inspiratory flow rate | Severalfold less flow required than with standard cannula |
| Transtracheal cannula | FIo$_2$ less dependent on inspiratory flow rate | Usual flow rates of 0.25–3.0 liters/min |
| Ventimask | Available at 24%, 28%, 31%, 35%, 40%, and 50% | Less comfortable, but provides a relatively controlled FIo$_2$. Poorly humidified gas at maximum FIo$_2$. |
| *High-Humidity Mask* | Variable from 28% to nearly 100% | Levels >60% may require additional oxygen bleed-in. Flow rates should be 2–3 times minute ventilation. Excellent humidification. |
| *Reservoir Mask* | | |
| Nonrebreathing | Not specified, but about 90% if well fitted | Reservoir fills during expiration and provides an additional source of gas during inspiration to decrease entrainment of room air. |
| Partial rebreathing | Not specified, but about 60%–80% | |
| *Face Tent* | Variable; same as high-humidity mask | Mixing with room air makes actual O$_2$ concentration inspired unpredictable. |
| *T Tube* | Variable; same as high-humidity mask | For spontaneous breathing through endotracheal or tracheostomy tube. Flow rates should be 2–3 times minute ventilation. |

malnutrition on the thoracic-pulmonary system as well as complications associated with administration of nutritional support (Pingleton, 1988). Nutritionally associated complications can occur with enteral and total parenteral nutrition (Ang, 1986). Poor nutritional status does not appear to predispose to the need for mechanical ventilation. Malnourished patients who require mechanical ventilation, however, have a significantly higher mortality than well-nourished patients who require mechanical ventilation. Poor nutritional status can adversely effect thoracic-pulmonary function impairment of respiratory muscle function, ventilatory drive, and pulmonary defense mechanisms (Rochester, 1984).

The diaphragm is the critical respiratory muscle; malnutrition reduces diaphragmatic muscle mass (Pingleton, 1988). Underweight patients with reduction of diaphragmatic mass may have contractile force reductions out of proportion to the reduction of muscle mass (Pingleton, 1988). Hypophosphatemia or decreased inorganic phosphate precursors also may be responsible for respiratory muscle weakness. Nutritional repletion can improve altered respiratory muscle strength in some patients. Increases in maximal inspiratory pressure and body cell mass were noted in critically ill patients given parenteral nutrition for 2 to 4 weeks (Kelly, 1984). Malnutrition reduces ventilatory drive and influences the immune system. Systemic effects of malnutrition are most profound in cell-mediated immunity, because malnourished patients have suppressed delayed cutaneous hypersensitivity and impaired T-lymphocyte transformation in response to mitogens (Martin, 1987). Nutritional support can be instituted either by the enteral route or with total parenteral nutrition. Nutritionally associated hypercapnia can occur in patients receiving enteral feeding or total parenteral nutrition. This develops when excess carbohydrate calories are given (Pingleton, 1988). Carbon dioxide production is increased because calories in excess of energy needs result in lipogenesis and a markedly increased respiratory quotient (Pingleton, 1988). The respiratory quotient is defined as the ratio of carbon dioxide production to oxygen consumption during substrate utilization. Hypercapnia from increased carbon dioxide production is avoided in normal persons by a compensatory increase in ventilation. Patients with compromised ventilatory status may not be able to increase ventilation appropriately, and hypercapnia may result (Pingleton, 1988). The practical significance of this potential complication is not entirely known.

## Mechanical Ventilation of Obstetric Patients

Limited published data exist on the specific conduct of mechanical ventilation of the pregnant patient. Two outcome studies were conducted on critical illness in pregnancy and ARDS in pregnancy, respectively. Mabie et al (1992) reviewed 16 patients treated between 1986 and 1992. Each patient met defining features of ARDS. Maternal mortality was 44%, and perinatal mortality was 20%. Specifics regarding the type of mechanical ventilation were not included. Collop and Sahn reviewed a heterogeneous group of patients admitted to a medical intensive care unit; 60% of the patients in their series required mechanical ventilation. Maternal mortality was 20%. The authors felt that despite being younger than the usual medical intensive care patients, critically ill pregnant patients appeared to have as great a risk of dying as their older nonpregnant counterparts. Specifics regarding the nature of the mechanical ventilation were, again, not supplied (Collop, 1993).

At our institution, we utilize an integral perinatal special care unit and conduct mechanical ventilation of pregnant and postpartum patients using conventional mechanical ventilation for postoperative patients and advanced mechanical

ventilation for patients with ARDS. Preliminary results regarding weaning and intrapulmonary shunt have been presented (Van Hook, 1995). Despite the relative frequency with which we mechanically ventilate pregnant patients, the heterogeneity of their diseases coupled with the relatively small numbers of patients makes nonanecdotal analysis difficult.

The nosocomial pathogens that infect our patients by and large appear to be normal community pathogens instead of resistant organisms. The general makeup of our unit, consisting of a large majority of relatively healthy patients undergoing childbirth, probably lessens the chance for cross-infection with hospital-acquired organisms.

Table 8-9 details suggested initial settings in conventional mechanical ventilation. In cases in which decreased compliance may preclude safe high tidal volume ventilation, we generally recommend a schema similar to that in Table 8-7. Important in the mechanical ventilation of pregnant patients is the recognition of the potential for recovery when coupled with early and aggressive use of advanced means of support. In nonobstetric units, the obstetrician must function as

T A B L E   **8-9**

''Typical'' initial ventilator settings

*8A: Normal Compliance—SIMV*

| | |
|---|---|
| Tidal volume | 10–15 mL/kg |
| Respiratory rate | 10/min |
| PEEP | 5 cm $H_2O$ |
| Flow rate | 60 liters/min |
| Pressure support | 10 cm $H_2O$ |
| *Fraction Inspired Oxygen* | 100% |

*8B: Decreased Compliance*

| | |
|---|---|
| Fraction inspired oxygen | 100% |

Goal-directed ventilation settings
   Peak plateau inspiratory pressure less than
     35–40 cm $H_2O$
   $Pao_2$ >60 mm Hg
   $Paco_2$ <45 mm Hg*
   Tidal volume 5–8 mL Hg

Note: Different ventilators and different circumstances could markedly alter what would be appropriate for any single patient. These settings are for illustrative purposes only.

*If possible.

an ombudsman for his or her patient. Many consultants are just as unfamiliar with the unique circumstances of pregnancy as the obstetrician may be with intensive care. Adequate communication, early consultation, and early referral are key in optimization of outcome.

## Conclusion

Even under "normal" circumstances, mechanical ventilation is a challenging and labor-intensive undertaking. Mechanical ventilation of the pregnant or recently pregnant individual carries special considerations that are seldom encountered by either the intensivist or the obstetric provider. We do not endorse unsupervised mechanical ventilation of the pregnant patient by either specialty. Instead, we recommend an interactive multidisciplinary approach to the mechanical ventilation of the critically ill pregnant patient. Only through the combined efforts of a properly functioning interrelationship between the two disciplines can the successful care of the pregnant patient be achieved. We recommend early transfer to tertiary care institutions familiar with critical care obstetrics for most cases in which mechanical ventilation is required during pregnancy.

**REFERENCES**

Abbey NC, Green DE, Cicale MJ. Massive tracheal necrosis. Complicating endotracheal intubation. Chest 1977;72:776.

Abu SD, Daly JM. Potential complications and monitoring of patients receiving total parenteral nutrition. In: Rowbeau JL, Caldwell MD, eds. Parenteral nutrition. Philadelphia: Saunders, 1986.

Alaily AB, Carrol KB. Pulmonary ventilation in pregnancy. Br J Obstet Gynecol 1987;85:518.

Aldrich TK, Prezant DJ. Indications for mechanical ventilation. In: Tobin MJ, ed. Principles and practice of mechanical ventilation. New York: McGraw-Hill, 1994:168.

Anderson HL III, Bartlett RH. Extracorporeal and intravascular gas exchange devices. In: Ayres SM, Gsenvik A, Holbrook PR, Shoemaker WC, eds. Textbook of critical care, 3rd ed. Philadelphia: WB Saunders, 1995:943–951.

Anderson HL III, Decius RE, Sinard JM, et al. Early experience with adult extracorporeal membrane oxygenation in the modern era. Ann Thorac Surg 1992;53:553.

Ashbaugh DG, Petty TL, Biselow DG, et al. Continuous positive pressure breathing (CPPB) in adult respiratory distress syndrome. J Thorac Cardiovasc Surg 1969;57:31.

Aubier M, Trippenbech T, Roussos C. Respiratory muscle fatigue during cardiogenic shock. J Appl Physiol 1981;51:499.

Ayd FJ Jr. Intravenous haloperidol therapy. Int Drug Ther Newslett 1978;13:20.

Barth WH, Hankins GDV. Severe acute asthma in pregnancy. In: Clark SL, Cotton DB, Hankins GDV, Phelan JP, eds. Critical care obstetrics. 2nd ed. Oxford: Blackwell Scientific, 1991:377.

Balestrieri F, Fisher S. Analgesics. In: Chernow B, ed. The pharmacologic approach to the critically ill patient. Baltimore: Williams and Wilkins, 1995:640–650.

Bartlett RH. Extracorporeal life support for cardiopulmonary failure. Curr Probl Surg 1990;27:621.

Benito S, Lemaire F. Pulmonary pressure volume relationship in acute respiratory distress syndrome in adults: role of positive and expiratory pressure. J Crit Care 1990;5:27.

Benjaminsson E, Klain M. Intraoperative dual-mode independent lung ventilation of a patient with bronchopleural fistula. Anesth Analg 1981; 60:118.

Beydon L, Cinotti L, Rekik N, et al. Changes in the distribution of ventilation and perfusion associated with separation from mechanical ventilation in patients with obstructive pulmonary disease. Anesthesiology 1991;75:730.

Bezzant TB, Mortensen JD. Risks and hazards of mechanical ventilation: A collective review of published literature. DM 1994;40:581.

Bidani A, Tzouanakis AE, Cardenas VJ, et al. Permissive hypercapnia in acute respiratory failure. JAMA 1994;272:957.

Bishop MJ, Benson MS, Satyo P, et al. Comparison of high frequency ventilation with conventional ventilation for bronchopleural fistula. Anesth Analg 1990;70:375.

Brecher GA, Hobay CA. Pulmonary blood flow and venous return during spontaneous respiration. Cir Res 1955;3:210.

Briggs GG, Freeman RK, Yaffe SJ. Drugs in pregnancy and lactation. 4th ed. Baltimore: Williams and Wilkins, 1994.

Brochard L, Pluskwa F, Lemaire F. Improved efficacy of spontaneous breathing with inspiratory pressure support. Am Rev Respir Dis 1987; 136:411.

Brochard L, Rua F, Lorino H, et al. Inspiratory pressure support compensates for additional work of breathing caused by the endotracheal tube. Anesthesiology 1991;75:739.

Brunel SW, Coleman DL, Schwartz DE. Assessment of routine chest roentgenograms and the physical examination to confirm endotracheal tube position. Chest 1989;96:1043.

Bryan CL, Jenkins SG. Oxygen toxicity. Clin Chest Med 1988;9:141.

Bryan-Brown CW, Gutierrez G. Pulmonary gas exchange, transport and delivery. In: Ayres SM, Grenvit A, Holbrook PR, Shoemaker WC, eds. Textbook of critical care. 3rd ed. Philadelphia: WB Saunders, 1995:777.

Chang HK. Mechanisms of gas transport during ventilation by high-frequency oscillation. J Appl Physiol 1984;56:553.

Cheek TG, Gutsche BB. Maternal physiologic alterations during pregnancy. In: Anesthesia for Obstetrics. Baltimore: Williams and Wilkins, 1987.

Colice GL, Stokes TA, Dain B. Laryngeal complications of prolonged intubation. Chest 1989; 96:877.

Collop NA, Sahn SA. Critical illness in pregnancy: an analysis of 20 patients admitted to a medical intensive care unit. Chest 1993;103:1548.

Conrad SA, Eggerstedt JM, Morris JF, et al. Prolonged intracorporeal support of gas exchange with an intravenous oxygenator. Chest 1993;103:158.

Conway CM. Hemodynamic effects of pulmonary ventilation. Br J Anaesth 1975;47:761.

Corre KA, Rothstein RJ. Assessing severity of adult asthma and the need for hospitalization. Ann Emerg Med 1985;14:45.

Craven DE, Steger KA. Pathogenesis and prevention of nosocomial pneumonia in the mechanically ventilated patient. Respir Care 1989;34:85.

Crockard HA, Coppel DL, Morrow WFK. Evaluation of hyperventilation in treatment of head injuries. Br Med J 1973;4:634.

Cullen DJ, Bigatello LM, DeMonaco HJ. Anesthetic pharmacology and critical care. In: Charnow B, ed. The pharmacologic approach to the critically ill patient. 3rd ed. Baltimore: Williams and Wilkins, 1995:291–308.

Dall'ava-Santucci J, Armaganidis A, Brunet F, et al. Mechanical effects of PEEP in patients with adult respiratory distress syndrome. J Appl Physiol 1990;68:843.

Davis K, Johnson DJ, Branson RD, et al. Airway pressure release ventilation. Arch Surg 1993; 128:1348.

DeLemos R, Yoder B, McCurnin D, et al. The use of high frequency oscillatory ventilation (HFOV) and extracorporal membrane oxygenation (ECMO) in the management of the term/near term infant with respiratory failure. Early Hum Dev 1992;29:299.

Dreyfuss D, Soler P, Basset G, et al. High inflation pressure pulmonary edema. Am Rev Respir Dis 1988;137:1159.

Durnin JV. Energy requirements of pregnancy—an integration of the longitudinal data from the five-country study. 1987;B568:1131.

Duvaldstein P, Agoston S, Henzel D, et al. Pancuronium pharmacokinetics in patients with liver cirrhosis. Br J Anaesth 1978;50:1131.

ECMO Quarterly Report. Ann Arbor, MI: ECMO Registry of the Extracorporeal Life Support Organization (ELSO) May, 1994.

Esteban A, Frutos F, Tobin MJ, et al. A comparison of four methods of weaning patients from mechanical ventilation. N Engl J Med 1995;332:345.

Feeley TW, Hedley-White J. Weaning from controlled ventilation and supplemental oxygen. N Engl J Med 1975;292:903.

Ferguson GT, Benoist J. Nasal continuous positive airway pressure in the treatment of tracheobronchomalacia. Am Rev Respir Dis 1993; 137:457.

Froese AB, Bryan AC. High frequency ventilation. Am Rev Respir Dis 1987;135:1363.

Fu Z, Costello ML, Tskimoto K, et al. Tidal ventilation at low airway pressures can cause pulmonary barotrauma. Am Rev Respir Dis 1990; 142:321. Abstract.

Gattinoni L, Pesenti A, Avalli L, et al. Pressure volume curve of total respiratory system in acute respiratory failure. Am Rev Respir Dis 1987; 136:730.

Gattinoni L, Pesenti A, Bombino M, et al. Relationships between lung computed tomographic density, gas exchange, and PEEP in acute respiratory failure. Anesthesiology 1988;69:824.

Gattinoni L, D'Andrea L, Pelosi P, et al. Regional effects and mechanism of end-expiratory pressure in early adult respiratory positive distress syndrome. JAMA 1993;269:2122.

Gibbs CP, Banner TC. Effectiveness of Bicitra/Pr as a preoperative antacid. Anesthesiology 1984; 61:97.

Gungwardana RH. Experience with tracheostomy in medical intensive care patients. Postgrad Med J 1992;68:338.

Haake R, Schlichtig R, Ulstad DR, et al. Barotrauma pathophysiology, risk factors, and prevention. Chest 1987;91:608.

Heffner JE. Airway management in the critically ill patient. Crit Care Clin 1990;6:533.

Hickling KG, Henderson SJ, Jackson R. Low mortality associated with low volume, pressure limited ventilation with permissing hyperpnea in severe adult respiratory distress syndrome. Intensive Care Med 1990;16:372.

Hill JD, O'Brian TG, Murray JJ, et al. Extracorporeal oxygenation for acute post-traumatic respiratory failure (shock-lung syndrome): use of the Bramson membrane lung. N Engl J Med 1972;286:629.

Hirsch C, Kacmarek RM, Stanek K. Work of breathing CPAP and PSV imposed by the new generation mechanical ventilators: a long model study. Respir Care 1991;36:815.

Hirschl RB, Pranikoff T, Wise C, et al. Initial experience with partial liquid ventilation in adult patients with the acute respiratory distress syndrome. JAMA 1996;275:383.

Hirschl RB, Parent AB, Tooley R, et al. Liquid ventilation improves pulmonary function, gas exchange, and lung injury in a model of respiratory failure. Ann Surg 1995;221:79.

Hyers TN, Holl RD, Wes JG. Antithrombotic therapy for venous thromboembolic disease. Chest 1992;102:3915.

Hyman AL, Spannhake EW, Kapowitz PF. Prostaglandins and the lung: state of the art. Am Rev Respir Dis 1978;117:111.

Joh S, Matsuusa H, Kotani Y, et al. Change in tracheal blood flow during endotracheal intubation. Acta Anesthesiol Scand 1987;31:300.

Kacmarek RM. The role of pressure support in reducing the work of breathing. Respir Care 1988;33:99.

Kelly SM, Rosa A, Field S, et al. Inspiratory muscle strength and body composition in patients receiving total parenteral nutrition therapy. Am Rev Respir Dis 1984;130:33.

Knott-Craig CT, Oostuizen JE, Rossouw G, et al. Management and prognosis of massive hemoptysis. J Thorac Cardiovasc Surg 1993;105:394.

Kolobow T, Moretti MP, Fumagalli R, et al. Severe impairment in lung function induced by high peak airway pressure during mechanical ventilation—an experimental study. Am Rev Respir Dis 1987;135:312.

Kreiger BP, Ershowsky P. Noninvasive detection of respiratory failure in the intensive care unit. Chest 1988;94:254.

Lain DC, DiBenedetto R, Nguyen AV, et al. Pressure control inverse ratio ventilation as a method to reduce postinspiratory pressure and provide adequate ventilation and oxygenation. Chest 1989;95:1081.

Lee KH, Hui KP, Chan TB, et al. Rapid shallow breathing (frequency-tidal volume ratio) did not predict extubation outcome. Chest 1994;105:504.

Lee TS. Routine monitoring of intracuff pressure. Chest 1992;102:1309.

Lemaire F, Teboul J, Cinotti L, et al. Acute left ventricular dysfunction during unsuccessful weaning from mechanical ventilation. Anesthesiology 1988;69:171.

Lloyd TC Jr. Mechanical cardiopulmonary interdependence. J Appl Physiol 1982;52:333.

Lowenstein E, Hallowell P, Levine FH, et al. Cardiovascular response to large doses of intravenous morphine in man. N Engl J Med 1969;281:1389.

Luce JM, Pierson DJ, Hodson LD. Intermittent mandatory ventilation. Chest 1981;79:678.

Lucius H, Gahlenbeck H, Klein HO, et al. Respiratory functions, buffer systems, and electrolyte concentrations of blood during human pregnancy. Respir Physiol 1970;9:3111.

Mabie WC, Barton JR, Sibai BM. Adult respiratory distress syndrome in pregnancy. Am J Obstet Gynecol 1992;167:950.

Mador MJ. Assist-control ventilation. In: Tobin MJ, ed. Principles and practice of mechanical ventilation. New York: McGraw-Hill, 1994:207–220.

Marini JJ. New approaches to the ventilatory management of the adult respiratory distress syndrome. J Crit Care 1992a;87:256.

Marini JJ, Kelson SE. Retargeting ventilatory objectives in adult respiratory distress syndrome. New treatment prospects—persistent questions. Am Rev Respir Dis 1992b;146:2.

Marini JJ. Pressure targeted, lung protective ventilatory support in acute lung injury. Chest 1994;105(suppl):1095.

Marini JJ, Capps JS, Colver BH. The inspiratory work of breathing during assisted mechanical ventilation. Chest 1985;87:612.

Marini JJ, Smith TC, Lamb VJ. External work output and force generation during synchronized intermittent mechanical ventilation: effect of machine assistance on breathing effort. Am Rev Respir Dis 1988;138:1169.

Martin TR. Relationship between malnutritional lung infections. Clin Chest Med 1987;3:359.

Mathru M, Rao TL, El-Etr AA, et al. Hemodynamic response to changes in ventilatory patterns in patients with normal and poor left ventricular reserve. Crit Care Med 1982;10:423.

Maunder RJ, Shuman WP, McHugh JW, et al. Preservation of normal lung regions in the adult respiratory distress syndrome—analysis by computed tomography. JAMA 1986;255:2463.

McIntyre NR. Respiratory function during pressure support ventilation. Chest 1986;89:677.

Miller RD, Rupp SM, Fisher DM. Clinical pharmacology of vecuronium and atracurium. Anesthesiology 1984;61:444.

Moore FA, Feliciano DV, Andrassy RJ, et al. Early enteral feeding, compared with parenteral, reduces postoperative septic complications. Ann Surg 1992;216:172.

Muizelaari JP, Mamaron A, Ward JD, Choi SC, et al. Adverse effects of prolonged hyperventilation in patients with severe head injury: a randomized clinical trial. J Neurosurg 1991;75:731.

Murray JF, Matthay MA, Luce JM, et al. An expanded definition of the adult respiratory distress syndrome. Am Rev Respir Dis 1988;138:720.

Myers SA, Gleicher N. Physiologic changes in normal pregnancy. In: Gleicher N, Gall SA, Sibai BM, et al, eds. Principles and practice of medical therapy in pregnancy. 2nd ed. Norwalk, CT: Appleton and Lang, 1992:35–51.

Parker JC, Hernandez CA, Peevy KJ. Mechanisms of ventilator-induced lung injury. Crit Care Med 1993;21:131.

Perel A. Newer ventilator modes—temptations and pitfalls. Crit Care Med 1987;15:707.

Pierson DJ. Ventilator management of ARDS: emerging concepts. Crit Care Alert 1995;3:68.

Pingleton SK. Complications of acute respiratory failure. Chest 1988;84:A343.

Pinsky MR, Vincent JL, Pesmer JM. Estimating left ventricular filling pressure during positive end expiratory pressure in humans. Am Rev Respir Dis 1991;143:25.

Presenti A. Target blood gases doing ARDS ventilatory management. Intensive Care Med 1990; 16:349. Editorial.

Presenti A, Gattinoni L, Kolobow T, et al. Extracorporeal circulation in adult respiratory failure. ASAIO Trans 1988;34:43.

Rayburn WF, Zuspan FP, eds. Drug therapy in obstetrics and gynecology. 3rd ed. St Louis: Mosby Year Book, 1992.

Resister SD, Downs JB, Stock MC, et al. Is 50% oxygen harmful? Crit Care Med 1987;15:598.

Rochester DF, Esau SA. Malnutrition and respiratory system. Chest 1984;85:411.

Rodriguez JL, Steinberg SM, Luchetti FA, et al. Early tracheostomy for primary airway management in the surgical critical care setting. Surgery 1990;108:655.

Rodriguez-Roisin R, Ballester E, Roca J, et al. Mechanisms of hypoxemia in patients with status asthmaticus requiring mechanical ventilation. Am Rev Respir Dis 1989;139:732.

Rossaint R, Falke KJ, Lopez F, et al. Inhaled nitric oxide for the adult respiratory distress syndrome. N Engl J Med 1993;328:399.

Russell IF, Chambers WA. Closing volume in normal pregnancy. Br J Anaesth 1981;53:1043.

Sahn SA, Lakshminarayan S. Bedside criteria for discontinuation of mechanical ventilation. Chest 1973;63:1002.

Sebel PS, Lowdon JD. Propofol: a new intravenous anesthetic. Anesthesiology 1989;71:260.

Sellick BA. Cricoid pressure to control regurgitation of stomach contents during induction of anesthesia. Lancet 1961;2:404.

Shoemaker WC, Appel PL. Pathophysiology of adult respiratory distress syndrome following sepsis and surgical operations. Crit Care Med 1985; 13:166.

Shoemaker WC, Appel PL, Kram HB. Role of oxygen debt in the development of organ failure, sepsis and death. Chest 1992;102:208.

Slutsky AS, Brochard L, Dellinger RP, et al. ACCP consensus conference—mechanical ventilation. Chest 1993;104:1833.

Slutsky AS. Consensus conference on mechanical ventilation. Int Case Med 1994;20:64.

Standiford T, Morganroth ML. High-frequency ventilation. Chest 1989;96:1380.

Strieter RM, Lynch JP III. Complications in the ventilated patient. Clin Chest Med 1988;9:127.

Sumner WR, Nelson S. Nosocomial pneumonia characteristics of the patient-pathogen interaction. Respir Care 1989;34:116.

Suter PM, Fairley HB, Isenberg MD. Optimum end expiratory pressure in patients with acute pulmonary failure. N Engl J Med 1975;292:284.

Sutherland AD, Stock JG, Davies JM. Effects of preoperative fasting on morbidity and gastric contents in patients undergoing day-stay surgery. Br J Anaesth 1986;58:876.

Tahuanainen J, Salenpera M, Nikki P. Extubation criteria after weaning from intermittent mandatory ventilation and continuous positive airway pressure. Crit Care Med 1983;11:702.

Tobin MJ. Current concepts—mechanical ventilation. N Engl J Med 1994;330:1056.

Tobin MJ, Lodato RF. PEEP, auto PEEP and waterfalls. Chest 1989;96:449.

Tobin MJ, Yang K. Weaning from mechanical ventilation. Crit Care Clin 1990;6:725.

Tomlinson JR, Miller KS, Lorch DG, et al. A prospective comparison of IMV in T-piece weaning from mechanical ventilation. Chest 1989;96:348.

Tonkin JP, Harrison GA. The effect on the larynx of prolonged intubation. Chest 1989;96:877.

Trottier SJ, Taylor RW. Adult respiratory distress syndrome. In: Ayres SM, Grenvik A, Holbrook PR, Shoemaker WC, eds. Textbook of critical care. 3rd ed. Philadelphia: WB Saunders, 1995:819.

Van Hook JW, Harvey CJ, Uckan E. Mechanical ventilation in pregnancy and postpartum minute ventilation and weaning. Am J Obstet Gynecol 1995;172:326 (part 2). Abstract.

Wallis TW, Robotham JL, Compeon R, et al. Mechanical heart lung interaction with positive end expiratory pressure. J Appl Physiol 1983;54:1039.

Ward ME, Corbeil C, Gibbons W, et al. Optimization of respiratory muscle relaxation during mechanical ventilation. Anesthesiology 1988;69:29.

Webb HM, Tierney DF. Experimental pulmonary edema due to intermittent positive pressure ventilation with high inflation pressures. Protection by positive end-expiratory pressure. Am Rev Respir Dis 1974;110:556.

Weinberger SE, Weiss JW. Weaning from ventilatory support. N Engl J Med 1995;332:388.

West JB. Mechanics of breathing. In: Respiratory physiology—the essentials. 5th ed. Baltimore: Williams and Wilkins, 1995, chapter 7.

Yang K, Tobin MJ. A prospective study of indexes predicting outcome of trials of weaning from mechanical ventilation. N Engl J Med 1991; 32:1445.

# CHAPTER  9

# Dialysis

The need for dialytic support in pregnancy, while uncommon, is by no means a rarity. There are many case reports throughout the literature of dialysis during pregnancy. Dialysis may be required in the setting of acute renal failure (ARF), end-stage renal disease (ESRD), or deterioration of chronic renal failure (CRF) in pregnancy. Additionally, prophylactic dialysis has been instituted in the setting of CRF in the hopes of improving maternal and fetal outcomes. Both peritoneal and hemodialysis have been used successfully in pregnancy, although controlled prospective trials to determine the optimal therapy have not been done.

## Overview of Dialysis

*Dialysis* refers to renal replacement therapy designed to correct electrolyte abnormalities and remove excess fluids and toxic products of protein metabolism. In the setting of CRF, dialysis is usually initiated when the glomerular filtration rate (GFR), as determined by the 24-hour urine creatinine clearance, reaches 5 to 10 mL/min. At this level of renal function, biochemical abnormalities such as hyperkalemia and metabolic acidosis are likely to develop, as are fluid overload

and uremic complications (Table 9-1). In patients with diabetes who often have other end-organ damage, including autonomic neuropathy and vascular disease, dialytic support may be required even earlier, when GFR reaches 15 mL/min.

The physiology of dialysis is based on diffusive and convective transport. *Diffusion* refers to the random movement of a solute down its concentration gradient. It is by this means that the majority of urea and solute clearance is achieved. Convection is that solute movement that occurs by means of solvent drag as water is removed, either by hydrostatic or osmotic force. A lesser degree of clearance is obtained during fluid removal by ultrafiltration.

## Modes of Dialysis

Options for dialysis include hemodialysis and peritoneal dialysis, with the latter consisting of continuous ambulatory peritoneal dialysis (CAPD), continuous cycling peritoneal dialysis (CCPD), and nocturnal intermittent peritoneal dialysis (NIPD).

### Hemodialysis

Hemodialysis requires a vascular access for extracorporeal therapy. This is usually a surgically created artificial arteriovenous (AV) shunt or a native AV fistula, although dual lumen central venous catheters can be used temporarily (Fig 9-1).

The opinions or assertions contained herein are the private views of the author and are not to be construed as official or as reflecting the views of the Department of the Army or the Department of Defense.

T A B L E   **9-1**

Indications for initiation of dialysis

Hyperkalemia
Metabolic acidosis
Volume overload
Uremic pericarditis
Uremic encephalopathy
GFR 5–10 mL/min

Products of protein metabolism, such as urea nitrogen, potassium, and phosphate, are removed by both diffusion and convection across a semipermeable dialyzer membrane, while ions such as bicarbonate and calcium diffuse into the blood. Fluid removal is accomplished by applying hydrostatic pressure across the dialyzer membrane. The dialysis prescription for nonpregnant patients generally consists of 3 to 4 hours of hemodialysis thrice weekly, depending on urea generation rate and dialyzer solute clearance. Heparinization is generally employed throughout the dialysis treatment.

## Peritoneal Dialysis

The various forms of peritoneal dialysis have in common the removal of these same metabolites and excess fluid, albeit by diffusion and convective flow across the peritoneal membrane. Surgical placement of a peritoneal catheter allows repeated access to the peritoneal cavity (Fig 9-2). Removal of fluid by osmotic force is achieved by instilling a hypertonic dialysate such as dextrose solution into the peritoneal cavity. Urea and other ions present in high concentrations diffuse from the peritoneal vasculature into the dialysate, while calcium and a bicarbonate source such as lactate

move in the opposite direction. Depending on the mode of peritoneal dialysis selected, dialysate is instilled and drained either manually or automatically at repeated intervals throughout the day. Continuous ambulatory peritoneal dialysis consists of approximately four manual exchanges per day: the peritoneum is filled with several liters of dialysate with each exchange, and the fluid is drained 4 to 6 hours later. Both CCPD and NIPD utilize an automated cycler to repeatedly fill and drain the peritoneum at shorter intervals throughout the night. Continuous cycling peritoneal dialysis differs in that it also includes a daytime dwell for added clearance.

## Dialysis and Pregnancy

### Hemodialysis Versus Peritoneal Dialysis

Both hemodialysis and peritoneal dialysis have been used successfully in pregnancy. Although the reports consist of small numbers, women receiving peritoneal dialysis appear to have a higher success rate in terms of fetal survival than those treated with hemodialysis: 67% versus 20% (Gadallah, 1992), 83% versus 42% (Hou, 1994b), and 63% versus 20% historical controls (Redrow, 1988). There are many theoretical reasons to utilize peritoneal dialysis in pregnancy, most notably of which is the steady-state removal of uremic toxins (Table 9-2). This, coupled with easier fluid removal, should minimize episodes of hypotension and perhaps placental insufficiency. Additional advantages of peritoneal dialysis often include less severe anemia, as well as better BP control and more liberal dietary restrictions due

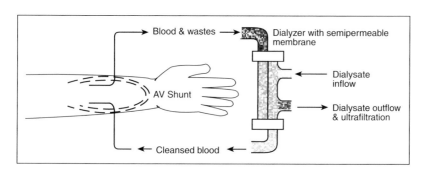

F I G U R E   **9-1**

Hemodialysis.

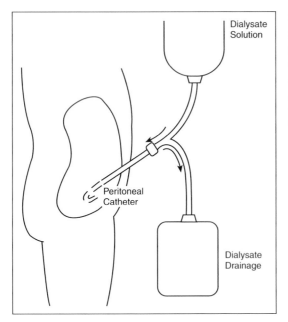

FIGURE **9-2**
Peritoneal dialysis.

to the continuous nature of the therapy. Furthermore, peritoneal dialysis obviates the need for systemic anticoagulation. In diabetic patients, the use of intraperitoneal insulin can facilitate strict glycemic control. There have also been several case reports of successful intraperitoneal magnesium administration for the treatment of preeclampsia, maintaining a steady-state magnesium serum level of approximately 5 mEq/liter, although generally, alternative therapy is recom-

mended in renal failure to avoid magnesium toxicity (Redrow, 1988; Elliott, 1991). Despite these apparent advantages of peritoneal dialysis, several complications are unique to it. These include catheter-related complications such as laceration of the uterine vessels (Hou, 1993b) and peritonitis. Hou reported on precipitation of preterm labor and delivery in two of three patients with peritonitis. Peritoneal dialysis catheters have been placed as late as 29 weeks' gestation. In some patients, however, repeated difficulties with catheter obstruction and failure to drain necessitated placement of multiple catheters or a change to hemodialysis. It is difficult to determine whether either method of dialysis actually precipitates preterm labor, because it has been described in patients utilizing both hemodialysis and peritoneal dialysis, and in those with CRF alone.

## Intensive Dialysis

Generally, modification of the dialysis prescription in pregnancy has been required in patients treated with both hemodialysis and peritoneal dialysis. Although there are no firm guidelines, it is the belief of most nephrologists that more intensive dialytic support is required during pregnancy to minimize fetal exposure to uremic toxins and improve outcome. This is based in part on the fact that pregnancy outcome appears to be better in those women with significant residual renal function and those women

TABLE **9-2**
Mode of dialysis: Advantages in pregnancy

| Hemodialysis | Peritoneal Dialysis |
|---|---|
| Less work intensive for patient | Stable biochemical environment |
| No risk of peritoneal catheter–related complications | Continuous fluid removal avoids hypotension |
| | Allows liberal fluid intake |
| Adequate clearances late in gestation readily obtained | Permits continuous insulin administration in diabetes mellitus |
| No interruption in therapy needed after cesarean section | No anticoagulation necessary |
| | Permits administration of intraperitoneal $MgSO_4$ in preeclampsia |
| | Hypertension easier to control |
| | Less severe anemia |

who require dialysis due to a deterioration of renal function during pregnancy than in those on dialysis prior to conception (Hou, 1994b). Furthermore, pregnancy appears to be most common during the first year of dialysis, presumably related to the greater residual renal function often present at the initiation of renal replacement therapy. However, there are reports of successful pregnancies in severely uremic patients, as well as failures in women who have been treated with intensive dialysis. Studies to assess optimal dialysis strategy in pregnancy have not been performed.

Intensive dialysis corresponds to initiation of dialysis at levels of BUN and serum creatinine between 60 and 70 mg/dL and 6 and 7 mg/dL, respectively, maintaining levels less than 50 mg/dL and 5 mg/dL, respectively (Hou, 1994b). To maintain such low levels of azotemia in pregnancy, dialysis patients may require a significant increase in total treatment time. This is especially true in the third trimester when fetal urea production increases and may account for as much as 540 mg per day (Hou, 1990b), or a 10% increase. For women on hemodialysis, daily treatments of 5 or more hours may be necessary to obtain adequate clearances late in gestation. As with hemodialysis, a patient's treatment requirements may increase markedly in peritoneal dialysis as well, especially because women in the latter half of gestation may be unable to tolerate the standard dwell volumes due to abdominal fullness. A switch to CCPD with an increased frequency of small volume exchanges and supplemental manual exchanges is often required late in gestation to obtain adequate clearance. A combination of hemodialysis and peritoneal dialysis may even be indicated. No guidelines exist with regard to evaluating the adequacy of dialysis, although a minimum combined renal and dialytic clearance of 15 mL/min is recommended. In one patient studied there was no apparent change in peritoneal physiology or peritoneal blood flow as assessed by the standard peritoneal equilibration test of glucose and creatinine (Lew, 1992). Similarly, Redrow and colleagues reported excellent ultrafiltration in all patients throughout pregnancy, and less than a one third decrease in peritoneal solute clearance in three patients studied (Redrow, 1988).

An additional benefit of intensive dialysis is that a low level of azotemia should minimize the risk of polyhydramnios, although it is not known if this will lead to improved outcome or a decreased incidence of preterm labor. Polyhydramnios has been ascribed to the urea diuresis that normally occurs in utero due to high fetal levels of urea nitrogen, as well as to fluid shifts that accompany intermittent hemodialysis (Nageotte, 1988; Hou, 1994a). An increased frequency of hemodialysis in particular limits the large interdialytic weight gains often seen in hemodialysis patients, thus avoiding hypotension and enabling better BP control by minimizing that component of hypertension that is volume-mediated.

## Modification of the Dialysis Prescription

With respect to hemodialysis, certain parameters of the dialysis prescription may warrant adjustment. Specifically, a lower sodium dialysate of 134 mEq/liter is recommended due to the mild physiologic hyponatremia of pregnancy. Similarly, a bicarbonate concentration as low as 25 mEq/liter may be necessary to avoid alkalemia, due to the repeated exposure to a bicarbonate dialysate and the concomitant respiratory alkalosis seen in pregnancy. Acetate dialysis is not generally recommended because it has been associated with an increased frequency of hypotension, although there are no data in pregnancy. There are no data on the use of the newer more permeable membranes, nor on high-flux dialysis, although the latter is probably best avoided due to a greater propensity for hypotension. A standard calcium dialysate can be used with both hemodialysis and peritoneal dialysis, thus ensuring a net positive calcium balance sufficient to meet fetal requirements. Due to placental production of calcitriol, however, there is augmented gastrointestinal absorption of calcium from calcium-containing antacids; thus, serum calcium levels must be monitored to avoid hypercalcemia (Grossman, 1994). With both methods of dialysis, one must also monitor closely for hypokalemia, which may develop with frequent dialysis.

## Dialysis and Uteroplacental Perfusion

Doppler flow velocity measurements have been performed during and after hemodialysis in an attempt to assess the effect of hemodialysis on uteroplacental blood flow. Results have been conflicting, with studies reporting unchanged, worsened, and improved perfusion during dialysis as assessed by the systolic-diastolic ratio or resistance index (Weiner, 1991; Jakobi, 1993; Krakow, 1993). In those patients studied, however, there was no evidence of uterine irritability or fetal distress as measured by external fetal monitoring during hemodialysis.

## Mode of Delivery

There are no data to support any particular mode of delivery in pregnant dialysis patients. Rates of cesarean section range from 24% to nearly 50% (Registration Committee of the EDTA, 1980; Yasin, 1988; Hou, 1993a). In peritoneal dialysis patients requiring cesarean section, both standard and extraperitoneal approaches have been utilized (Redrow, 1988; Hou, 1990b). In either case, it may be necessary to interrupt peritoneal dialysis for several days to allow healing of the abdominal wall and prevent dialysate leak or hernia formation. Peritoneal dialysis can be reinitiated using smaller dwell volumes initially, with a progressive increase in volume as tolerated. If necessary, temporary hemodialysis can be performed in the interim. Cesarean delivery should be performed for standard obstetric indications of maternal or fetal distress.

## Incidence of Pregnancy in End-Stage Renal Disease

The exact incidence of pregnancy in ESRD is unknown, although Hou reported an incidence of 1.5% over a 2-year period (Hou, 1994a). This estimate was based on a survey of 206 dialysis units, representing 10% of all U.S. dialysis units. This survey documented sixty pregnancies in 1281 women between the ages of 18 and 44, with 20 pregnancies occurring during the survey period of 1990 to 1991. Prior to this, the European Dial-

ysis and Transplant Association (EDTA) had reported on 115 pregnancies in approximately 8500 women on dialysis between the ages of 15 and 44 through 1978 (Registration Committee of the EDTA, 1980). Similarly, Gadallah et al reported an incidence of 3.6% in hemodialysis patients (Gadallah, 1992), and a retrospective survey of pregnancy in hemodialysis patients in Saudi Arabia between 1985 and 1990 revealed an incidence of less than 1% (Souqiyyeh, 1992). These statistics, however, are likely to underestimate the true incidence of conception in ESRD because many pregnancies in dialysis patients end in early miscarriage and therefore remain undetected, and many groups fail to report unsuccessful outcomes.

Women with CRF or ESRD are often uninformed of the potential for conception and the need for birth control. Similarly, many physicians remain unaware of this possibility as well. Amenorrhea or irregular menses are often seen in CRF along with a markedly decreased fertility, in part related to hyperprolactinemia. However, pregnancy is possible. Symptoms of early pregnancy may be confused with uremic symptoms, thus delaying the diagnosis (Table 9-3). Furthermore, laboratory tests including serum pregnancy tests may be difficult to interpret in this population due to impaired excretion of human chorionic gonadotropin in renal failure (Schwarz, 1985). Thus, confirmation of pregnancy and assessment of gestational age depend on ultrasound. The mean gestational age at diagnosis of pregnancy is 16.5 weeks in women with ESRD (Hou, 1993a). There is no information regarding fertility differences among women utilizing peritoneal versus hemodialysis for ESRD.

## Maternal Complications

In the past, women with severe renal disease were often advised to terminate pregnancies due to the belief that pregnancy carried a high risk of maternal complications, as well as a low success rate. These potential complications include an accelerated decline in renal function, accelerated hypertension, an increased risk of superimposed preeclampsia, worsened anemia often requiring transfusion, hemodialysis access thrombosis, and

T A B L E  **9-3**

Signs and symptoms of uremia

| Organ Involvement | Subjective Complaints | Objective Findings |
|---|---|---|
| Neurologic | Cognitive difficulties<br>Sleep-wake reversal<br>Dysesthias | Hyperreflexia, asterixis<br>Seizures<br>Encephalopathy<br>Peripheral neuropathy |
| Hematopoietic | Easy bruising and bleeding<br>Fatigue | Anemia<br>Prolonged bleeding time |
| Gastrointestinal | Dysgeusia, metallic taste<br>Constipation<br>Nausea | Angiodysplasia |
| Musculoskeletal | Weakness<br>Bone pain | Carpal tunnel syndrome<br>Bone fractures<br>Myopathy |
| Cardiovascular | Dyspnea<br>Chest pain | Hypertension<br>Pulmonary edema<br>Pericarditis |
| Dermatologic | Pruritus | Cutaneous calcifications |
| Endocrine | Decreased libido<br>Impotence | Decreased fertility<br>Dysmenorrhea or amenorrhea |

an increased incidence of abruptio placentae (Table 9-4). The latter cannot be ascribed solely to the use of heparin during hemodialysis because it has been seen with greater than normal frequency in patients on peritoneal dialysis as well.

Pregnancy has been associated with a permanent decline in renal function in a relatively small percentage of patients with mild renal failure, defined as serum creatinine less than 1.5 mg/dL. This risk may be increased significantly in those women with moderate or severe renal failure, especially in the setting of uncontrolled hypertension. It is always important to rule out readily reversible causes of declining renal function, such as volume depletion, infection, and obstruction. One report of 37 pregnant women with moderate or severe renal failure, defined as a serum creatinine greater than 1.4 mg/dL, noted a deterioration in renal function, defined as greater than a 50% rise in creatinine, in 16% (Cunningham, 1990). Five of these six women also suffered from poorly controlled chronic hypertension. A clinical diagnosis of superimposed preeclampsia was established in nearly 60% overall. Similarly, a more recent review encompassing more than 80 pregnant women with renal failure demonstrated accelerated hypertension in nearly 50% and an accelerated decline in renal function in more than one third (Imbasciati, 1991). However, there have been no maternal deaths reported in women requiring dialysis during pregnancy (Hou, 1994b).

T A B L E  **9-4**

**Renal failure and pregnancy:
Maternal complications**

Accelerated decline in renal function
Accelerated hypertension
Superimposed preeclampsia
Preterm labor
Worsened anemia
Hemodialysis access thrombosis
Abruptio placentae
Spontaneous abortion and second-trimester fetal
   loss

## Fetal Complications

The likelihood of fetal survival beyond the neonatal period is better than previously believed (Table 9-5). Surveys conducted by the EDTA (Registration Committee of the EDTA, 1980), the American Nephrology Nursing Association (Hou, 1994b), as well as a group in Saudi Arabia (Souqiyyeh, 1992) reported a fetal viability of 20% to 30% in those pregnancies that were not electively terminated. The EDTA survey revealed that greater than 50% of pregnancies resulted in spontaneous abortion (Registration Committee of the EDTA, 1980). Hou, in a more recent U.S. survey, noted a comparable incidence of 54% fetal loss, including spontaneous abortion, stillbirth, and neonatal death (Hou, 1994a). Furthermore, virtually all infants delivered were premature, and approximately 20% were growth-retarded. When stratified according to date, however, survival was greater than 50% in those pregnancies occurring since 1990. The increased frequency of CAPD in recent years did not account for this difference, because survival was improved in hemodialysis patients as well. As noted previously, polyhydramnios attributed to the fetal urea diuresis is seen with greater frequency in renal failure and may contribute to the high incidence of prematurity. Additionally, a urea-induced diuresis following delivery may result in volume depletion in the neonatal period. There does not appear to be an increased incidence in congenital anomalies (Registration Committee of the EDTA, 1980; Hou, 1994b). Unfortunately, there is little long-term follow-up on infants exposed to azotemia in utero with regards to physical and intellectual development.

## Anemia

Anemia develops during pregnancy largely due to an increase in plasma volume without a corresponding increase in red-cell mass. In renal failure, the picture is complicated by a relative deficiency in erythropoietin production by the diseased kidneys, as well as shortened red-cell survival, bone marrow suppression by uremic tox-

TABLE  **9-5**

**Renal failure and pregnancy: Fetal complications**

Spontaneous abortion and fetal loss (50%)
Preterm delivery (>90%)
Intrauterine growth retardation (20%)
Polyhydramnios

ins, and possible superimposed nutritional deficiencies. The severe anemia that was typical of ESRD in the past is now treated successfully in most cases with recombinant human erythropoietin (rHuEpo). Furthermore, correction of the anemia of ESRD may result in return of regular menses due to resolution of hyperprolactinemia (Hou, 1993a).

Recombinant human erythropoietin has been studied in pregnant animals at doses used clinically without apparent complications. Hou reported on eleven patients with CRF treated with Epogen in whom no congenital anomalies were seen and no rHuEpo could be detected in the cord blood (Hou, 1994b). All of the women required an increase in their dose of rHuEpo, as compared with prepregnancy, and three still required blood transfusions during pregnancy. Only one woman experienced severe hypertension complicating therapy, although several required additional antihypertensive medication. Additional reports have yielded similar results (Barth, 1994; Scott, 1995). It is accepted by most obstetricians that a hemoglobin less than 6 g/dL is associated with increased perinatal mortality and maternal morbidity secondary to high-output failure. Given this fact, as well as the increased risk of bleeding complications in uremia due to platelet dysfunction, and the overwhelming likelihood of preterm delivery, the recommendation for women with renal disease is an empirical 50% increase in rHuEpo dose once the pregnancy is detected, with a goal of maintaining the hemoglobin at more than 10 g/dL (Hou, 1994b). Most patients require oral iron supplementation or intermittent intravenous iron as well, because iron deficiency eventually develops in most patients successfully treated with rHuEpo.

## Dietary Guidelines

Dietary restrictions in renal failure generally consist of modest protein restriction, as well as to restrictions of potassium, phosphate, and sodium intake. Fluids are restricted to 1 liter daily, with more liberal intake permitted in those with substantial residual urine output. In pregnancy, however, protein intake is liberalized to allow for normal fetal development. The recommended protein intake is 1 g/kg/day in hemodialysis and 1.5 g/kg/day in peritoneal dialysis, with an additional 20 g/day allowed for pregnancy (Hou, 1994b). Increasing delivery of dialysis is recommended for worsening azotemia rather than strict protein restriction. Supplementation of water-soluble vitamins, which are removed during dialysis, is recommended, as well as supplementation with folate, zinc, and iron. Standard prenatal vitamins, which may contain excess vitamin A, are best avoided.

## Pregnancy and Acute Renal Failure

Most of the literature pertaining to dialysis in pregnancy concerns those women with CRF or ESRD. There are, however, a number of case reports of dialysis for ARF in pregnancy. Hemodialysis has been the primary form of dialysis utilized, both for ARF and acute ingestion of toxic substances (Trebbin, 1988; Kleinman, 1991; Devlin, 1994). Because the incidence of ARF itself has fallen to less than 1% of pregnancies in developed countries, the need for acute dialysis is rare (Krane, 1988).

## Summary

Although pregnancy remains uncommon in women with severe CRF or ESRD, it is possible. With intensive management on the part of the obstetrician as well as the nephrologist, the likelihood of a favorable outcome can be maximized. This may entail early initiation of dialysis in women with CRF or intensified dialytic therapy in those already requiring renal replacement therapy. It is not clear whether peritoneal dialysis offers a true advantage over hemodialysis in terms of better fetal outcome, although the preliminary data are encouraging. While most nephrologists do not advocate a change to peritoneal dialysis in those patients already receiving hemodialysis, there is a tendency to recommend peritoneal dialysis as first-line therapy in those patients who develop a need for chronic dialysis during pregnancy.

**REFERENCES**

Asrat T, Nageotte MP. Renal failure in pregnancy. Semin Perinatol 1990;14:59–67.

Barth W, Lacroix L, Goldberg M, Greene M. Recombinant human erythropoietin (rHEpo) for severe anemia in pregnancies complicated by renal disease. Am J Obstet Gynecol 1994;170:329A.

Cunningham FG, Cox SM, Harstad TW, et al. Chronic renal disease and pregnancy outcome. Am J Obstet Gynecol 1990;163:453–459.

Davison JM. Dialysis, transplantation, and pregnancy. Am J Kidney Dis 1991;17:127–132.

Devlin K. Pregnancy complicated by acute renal failure requiring hemodialysis. Anna Journal 1994;27:444–445.

Elliot JP, O'Keeffe DF, Schon DA, Cherem LB. Dialysis in pregnancy: a critical review. Obstet Gynecol Surv 1991;46:319–324.

Ferris TF. Pregnancy complicated by hypertension and renal disease. Adv Intern Med 1990;35:269–288.

Gadallah MF, Ahmad B, Karubian F, Campese VM. Pregnancy in patients on chronic ambulatory peritoneal dialysis. Am J Kidney Dis 1992;20:407–410.

Grossman S, Hou S. Obstetrics and gynecology. In: Daugirdas JT, Ing TS, eds. Handbook of dialysis. New York: Little, Brown, 1994:649–661.

Hou SH. Peritoneal dialysis and haemodialysis in pregnancy. Bailliere's Clin Obstet Gynaecol 1987;1:1009–1025.

Hou SH. Pregnancy in continuous ambulatory peritoneal dialysis (CAPD) patients. Perit Dial Int 1990a;10:201–204.

Hou SH, Grossman SD. Pregnancy in chronic dialysis patients. Semin Dial 1990b;3:224–229.

Hou SH, Orlowski J, Pahl M, et al. Pregnancy in women with end-stage renal disease: treatment of anemia and premature labor. Am J Kidney Dis 1993a;21:16–22.

Hou SH. Pregnancy and birth control in CAPD patients. Adv Perit Dial 1993b;9:173–176.

Hou SH. Pregnancy in women on haemodialysis and peritoneal dialysis. Bailliere's Clin Obstet Gynaecol 1994a;8:481–500.

Hou SH. Frequency and outcome of pregnancy in women on dialysis. Am J Kidney Dis 1994b; 23:60–63.

Imbasciati E, Ponticelli C. Pregnancy and renal disease: predictors for fetal and maternal outcome. Am J Nephrol 1991;11:353–362.

Jakobi P, Weiner Z, Geri R, Zaidise I. Umbilical and arcuate uterine artery flow velocity measurements during acute hemodialysis. Gynecol Obstet Invest 1993;37:247–248.

Kleinman GE, Rodriquez H, Good MC, Caudle MR. Hypercalcemic crisis in pregnancy associated with excessive ingestion of calcium carbonate antacid (milk-alkali syndrome): successful treatment with hemodialysis. Obstet Gynecol 1991; 78:496–499.

Krakow D, Castro LC, Schwieger J. Effect of hemodialysis on uterine and umbilical artery Doppler flow velocity waveforms. Am J Obstet Gynecol 1993;170:1386–1388.

Krane NK. Acute renal failure in pregnancy. Arch Intern Med 1988;148:2347–2357.

Lew SQ, Watson JA. Urea and creatinine generation and removal in a pregnant patient receiving peritoneal dialysis. Adv Perit Dial 1992;8:131–135.

McGregor E, Stewart G, Junor BJR, Rodger RSC. Successful use of recombinant human erythropoietin in pregnancy. Nephrol Dial Transplant 1991;6:292–293.

Nageotte MP, Grundy HO. Pregnancy outcome in women requiring chronic hemodialysis. Obstet Gynecol 1988;72:456–459.

Narva AS. Peritoneal dialysis in a pregnant woman with chronic renal failure. Semin Dial 1990; 3:249–251.

Packham DK. Aspects of renal disease and pregnancy. Kidney Int 1993;44:S64–S67.

Redrow M, Lazaro C, Elliot J, et al. Dialysis in the management of pregnant patients with renal insufficiency. Medicine 1988;67:199–208.

Registration Committee of the European Dialysis and Transplant Association. Successful pregnancies in women treated by dialysis and kidney transplantation. Br J Obstet Gynaecol 1980; 87:839–845.

Schwarz A, Post KG, Keller F, Molzahn M. Value of human chorionic gonadotropin measurements in blood as a pregnancy test in women on maintenance hemodialysis. Nephron 1985;39:341–343.

Scott LL, Ramin SM, Richey M, et al. Erythropoietin use in pregnancy: two cases and a review of the literature. Am J Perinatol 1995;12:22–24.

Souqiyyeh MZ, Huraib SO, Saleh AG, Aswad S. Pregnancy in chronic hemodialysis patients in the Kingdom of Saudi Arabia. Am J Kidney Dis 1992;19:235–238.

Trebbin WM. Hemodialysis and pregnancy. JAMA 1979;241:1811–1812.

Weiner Z, Thaler I, Ronen N, Brandes JM. Changes in flow velocity waveforms in umbilical and uterine artery following haemodialysis. Br J Obstet Gynaecol 1991;98:1172–1173.

Yasin SY, Bey Doun SN. Hemodialysis in pregnancy. Obstet Gynecol Surv 1988;43:655–668.

# CHAPTER 10

# Hyperalimentation

*P*regnancy constitutes one of the most profound physiologic stresses that a woman will experience. The length of pregnancy as well as the unique nature of the fetomaternal unit requires that significant adaptation be made by the mother to assure optimal fetal and maternal outcomes (Table 10-1). Most women make these adaptations with minimal need for supplementation other than with a few minerals and vitamins. Occasionally, the mother may be unable to meet this challenge, thereby necessitating medical intervention. The period of deficient food intake is usually brief and readily ameliorated by dietary adjustment and/or pharmacotherapy. When these measures fail, or in a prolonged critical illness, nutritional support must be provided by the enteral or parenteral route.

In 1972, Lakoff and Feldman published the first report of parenteral feeding during pregnancy in a woman with anorexia nervosa (Lee, 1986). Since then, there have been several case reports of successful use of enteral, total parenteral, and total peripheral parenteral nutrition in pregnancy for various indications.

## Normal Nutrition in Pregnancy

Our understanding of the crucial relationship between maternal nutritional status and perinatal outcome has improved substantially in the last three decades. Maternal prepregnancy weight and weight gain during pregnancy are important determinants of fetal growth and perinatal mortality. Low prepregnancy weight and poor weight gain during pregnancy are associated with a lower average birth weight, higher incidence of low birth weight ($< 2500$ g) and higher perinatal morbidity (Taffel, 1986; Institute of Medicine, 1990; Abrams, 1991; Abrams, 1989).

In the normal singleton pregnancy, the average total extra energy necessary to meet the metabolic demands of the fetus, placenta, and uterus is about 80,000 kcal or about 300 kcal/day in addition to maternal basal needs (National Research Council, 1989). In the pregnant adolescent, slightly more calories are required (National Research Council, 1989). This should result in a total weight gain of about 11 to 14 kg. This increased demand for calories is not distributed uniformly throughout pregnancy (Fig 10-1). In the first half of pregnancy—the anabolic phase—under the predominant influence of progesterone and aldosterone, there is maternal accumulation and storage of fat, protein, minerals, and fluid, which accounts for most of the weight gain (Dunnihoo, 1990). Thereafter, under the influence of human placental lactogen, cortisol, estrogen, and deoxycorticosterone—the catabolic phase—depletion of maternal glycogen, fat, and protein stores occurs to provide glucose, free fatty acids, and free amino acids for fetal accumulation of fat and protein and placental growth (Dunnihoo, 1990). Fetal fat depots are important storage sites for high-calorie density tissue, fat-soluble vitamins, and essential fatty acids, which are necessary for brain growth

T A B L E    **10-1**

### Changes in pregnancy that relate to nutrition

Weight gain (11–14 kg)
Fetal and placental growth
Increased fat stores
Increased total body water (6–9 liters)
Increased extracellular volume
    Vascular space increased 40%–55%
    RBC mass increased 25%
    Dilutional anemia and normal MCV (normal
        hemoglobin >10 g/dL, hct >30%)
    Dilutional hypoalbuminemia
Increased clotting factor production
Retention of sodium (1000 mEq) and potassium
    (350 mEq)
Increased cardiac output (50%), heart rate (20%),
    stroke volume (25%–40%) with reduced sys-
    temic vascular resistance (20%)
Increased renal blood flow (50%) and glomerular
    filtration rate (50%) with increased clearance
    of glucose urea and protein
    Creatinine clearance increased (100–180 mL/
        min)
Increased serum lipids
Increased total iron-binding capacity (40%)
    Increased serum iron (30%)
Hypomotility of gastrointestinal tract
    Delayed gastric emptying
    Gastroesophageal reflux
    Constipation

MCV, mean corpuscular volume; hct, hematocrit.

and metabolism in the perinatal period. Amino acids are fundamental building blocks for organ development and enzyme synthesis. Aberration of this process may result in abnormal fetal growth.

Any discussion on fetomaternal nutrition is incomplete without special emphasis on the critical role played by the placenta in the successful outcome of pregnancy. The earlier perception of the placenta as a biologic pipeline passively directing nutrients from the mother to fetus has been replaced by a keen awareness of its important endocrine, metabolic, and nutritional roles. Placental human chorionic gonadotropin is crucial in the maintenance of the corpus luteum of early pregnancy. Progesterone, produced from the corpus luteum, exerts a glucose-sparing effect in the placenta, and thus makes more glucose available to the developing embryo.

Human placental lactogen stimulates lipolysis, which results in free fatty acid release into the maternal circulation. By serving as a caloric source, free fatty acids spare amino acids and glucose to be passed transplacentally to the actively growing fetus. Placental estrogen stimulates protein synthesis for uterine growth. Together with progesterone, estrogen is responsible for the systematic vasodilatation necessary to maintain uteroplacental blood flow.

The placenta has well-developed mechanisms to control passage of substrate to the fetus (Table

F I G U R E    **10-1**

**Pattern and components of maternal weight gain during pregnancy.** (Adapted from Pitkin RM. Obstetrics and gynecology. In: Anderson CE, Coursin DB, Schneider HA, eds. Nutritional support of medical practice. Hagerstown, MD: Harper & Row, 1977.)

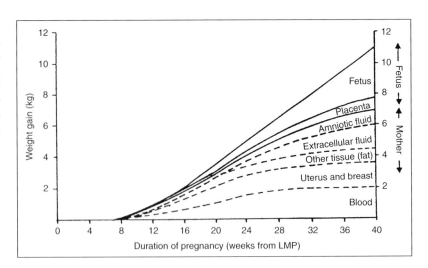

10-2). The effectiveness of passage of any substance across the syncytiotrophoblast depends on

- Maternal-fetal concentration gradient
- Physical properties of the substrate
- Placental surface area
- Uteroplacental blood flow
- Nature of transport mechanism (passive vs active transport)
- Specific binding or carrier proteins in maternal or fetal circulation
- Placental metabolism of the substance

## Malnutrition in Pregnancy

Our knowledge of the effects of nutritional deprivation in pregnancy are based primarily on animal studies and unfortunate human circumstance. Although several well-designed experiments studying the effects of starvation in pregnant rats are available, the suitability of using the rodent model for studying the primate pregnancy has been questioned (Payne, 1968). One would

T A B L E   **10-2**

**Substances that cross the placenta and currently accepted mechanisms of transport**

| Transport Mechanism | Substances Transported |
| --- | --- |
| Passive diffusion | Oxygen |
| | Carbon dioxide |
| | Fatty acids |
| | Steroids |
| | Nucleosides |
| | Electrolytes |
| | Fat-soluble vitamins |
| Facilitated diffusion | Sugars |
| Active transport | Amino acids |
| | Some cations |
| | Water-soluble vitamins |
| Solvent drag | Electrolytes |
| Pinocytosis, breaks in membrane | Proteins |

Reproduced by permission from Martin R, Blackburn G. Hyperalimentation in pregnancy. In: Berkowitz R, ed. Critical care of the obstetric patient. Churchill Livingstone, New York, 1983.

expect, intuitively, that the consequences of nutritional deprivation to the mother or fetus in a multifetal gestation of short duration (the typical rodent gestation) should differ from one of a singleton gestation of long duration (the typical human pregnancy). Pond et al (1969) following their experiments in swine, concluded the following: All gravidas fed protein-deficient diets lost weight. The earlier the protein deficiency began, the more severe the adverse effects. Protein deficiency during periods of fetal growth may affect DNA/RNA synthesis in vital organs (brain, liver) or enzyme systems. Maternal prepregnant labile protein reserve may mitigate the effect of protein deprivation in pregnancy. Riopelle et al (1975) made the following observations of the rhesus monkey: Although protein deficiency tends to increase fetal morbidity and mortality, the precise effect is dependent on several interacting factors. The improvement in metabolic efficiency in response to starvation is greater in the pregnant than the nonpregnant monkey. Antonov (Antonov, 1947) reported that birth weight was reduced by 400 to 600 g when pregestational nutrition was poor during the war in Leningrad. Reporting on undernourished women during a famine in Holland, Smith and Stein and Susser (Smith, 1947; Stein, 1975) observed that birth weight declined 10% and placental weight 15% when poor nutrition occurred in the third trimester with caloric intake less than 1500 g/day.

Generalized caloric intake reduction, as well as specific deficiencies like protein, zinc, folate and oxygen, have been implicated in the etiology of fetal growth restriction (Goldenburg et al, 1992; Neggars, 1991). Winick's hypothesis is particularly helpful in understanding the effect of maternal malnutrition on fetal growth (Winick, 1971). There are three phases of fetal growth: cellular hyperplasia, followed by both hyperplasia and hypertrophy, and then predominantly hypertrophy. Fetal malnutrition early in pregnancy is likely to cause a decrease in cell size and number, resulting in symmetric growth failure, while a later insult affects only cell size and not number, resulting in an asymmetric growth failure. This difference is of prognostic importance because postnatal catch-up growth is more likely with asymmetric rather than symmetric intrauterine growth retardation. Even when low total fetal body weight suggests growth retardation, the severity varies with organ systems, the adrenal and heart being more severely affected than the brain or skeleton (Lafever, 1979).

## Nutritional Assessment During Pregnancy

Several protocols have been proposed to evaluate the malnourished gravida. Some of these are based on parameters including maternal morphometry, serum biochemistry, and provoked immune responses (Wolk, 1990; Martin, 1983). In practice, however, such techniques have limited utility due to the following factors:

1. Normal values obtained in nonpregnant patients cannot be extrapolated readily to the hemodiluted pregnant patient.
2. Immune function is known to be impaired in normal pregnancy.
3. Nutritional supplementation is generally initiated in pregnant patients whose food intake is inadequate before these observations can be made.
4. Although nitrogen balance and creatinine clearance may be effective methods to assess protein status in the nonpregnant patient, both are altered markedly by the change in glomerular filtration rate that occurs in normal pregnancy.

## Routes for Nutritional Support

The decision on the route for nutritional support is best made by a multidisciplinary team composed of the obstetrician, intensivist, clinical nutritionist, and the patient herself, if possible. The enteral route should be the first consideration unless it is impractical, ineffective, or intolerable. It is not only associated with fewer complications than TPN but also is more physiologic, maintains bowel function, causes fewer maternal metabolic derangements, and is less expensive to deliver and monitor. The delayed gastric emptying typical of pregnancy should be considered when adjusting feeding solution delivery rates, to prevent regurgitation and aspiration.

Total peripheral parenteral nutrition (TPPN) has been proposed as an alternative to conventional total (central)-parenteral nutrition (TPN) in pregnant patients needing nutritional support. Watson et al (1990) reported favorably on the tolerance and efficacy of hypercaloric, hyperosmotic 3-in-1 peripheral parenteral nutrition in pregnant patients. The precise indications and potential side effects still remain to be clearly defined (Watson, 1990).

The majority of pregnant patients requiring nutritional support will receive TPN. Some of the more common indications for its use in pregnant patients are shown in Table 10-3. Total parenteral nutrition is generally well tolerated by the gravida and convenient for the medical staff, delivers a precise mixture of nutrients directly to the bloodstream, and allows a mixture of necessary medications (e.g., insulin, heparin). The disadvantages

TABLE **10-3**

**Possible criteria for consideration of pregnant patients for total parenteral nutrition**

I. Inaccessible or inadequate gastrointestinal nutritional route for any reason
II. Maternal malnutrition
  A. Weight loss greater than 1 kg/wk for 4 wk consecutively
  B. Total weight loss of 6 kg or failure to gain weight
  C. Underlying chronic disease which increases basal nutritional requirements, including preconception malnutrition
  D. Biochemical markers of malnutrition
    1. Severe hypoalbuminemia less than 2.0 g/dL
    2. Persistent ketosis
    3. Hypocholesterolemia
    4. Lymphocytopenia
    5. Macrocytic anemia: diminished folic acid
    6. Microcytic anemia and decreased serum Fe
    7. Negative nitrogen balance
  E. Anthropometric markers of malnutrition
    1. Weight and height
    2. Growth rate
      a) Poor weight gain
      b) Delayed growth of adolescent
    3. Skin fold thickness
    4. Head, chest, waist, and arm circumference
  F. Intrauterine growth retardation of fetus

Reprinted with permission from The American College of Obstetricians and Gynecologists (Obstetrics and Gynecology, 1982, vol. 59, pp. 660–664).

include the necessity for central venous cannulation, possibility of maternal metabolic derangements, and expense of delivery and monitoring.

## Calculation of Nutritional Requirements

The first step in assessing nutritional needs requires the estimation of total caloric needs. Maintenance needs, described as resting energy expenditure (REE), can be calculated using Wilmore's normogram (Willmore, 1980) or the Harris-Benedict equation for women (Harris, 1919).

$$REE(kcal) = 655 + 9.563(W) + 1.85(H) - 4.676(A)$$

where
W = weight in kilograms
H = height in centimeters
 A = age in years

During pregnancy this value translates to the following approximate patient-specific calorie requirement:

Maintenance therapy: REE(kcal) × 1.2

Anabolic therapy

Parenteral: REE(kcal) × 1.75

Enteral: REE(kcal) × 1.50

Ideally, estimation of caloric requirements should be individualized according to the patient's current metabolic rate. Commercially available metabolic carts, which base estimation of caloric requirement on oxygen consumption and carbon dioxide production, have recently become available for clinical use. These are generally quite accurate except at very high $FIO_2$ values (60%). Although the recommended dietary allowance is an additional 300 kcal/day in the second and third trimesters, a previously malnourished woman may require even more supplementation.

Though less precise than described in the equation, a useful rule is that at least 36 kcal/kg/day should provide enough calories to maintain a positive nitrogen balance (Oldham, 1957). Adequacy of supplementation is best assessed by plotting maternal weight gain against standard charts and serial sonographic estimation of fetal growth. The American Academy of Pediatrics and the American College of Obstetrics and Gynecology recommend a weight gain of 1 to 2 kg for the first trimester, with 0.4 kg/wk and 0.35 kg/wk in the second and third trimesters, respectively (Little, 1988). Fetal growth can be evaluated against appropriate normograms. A sample calculation of TPN requirements for a 60-kg pregnant patient is described in Table 10-4.

## Amino Acids

Nitrogen and energy intake are the dominant factors influencing positive nitrogen balance, provided intake of other nutrients is adequate. Protein catabolism tends to rise with an increase in metabolic rate. Protein need is dependent on previous nutritional status, provision of nonprotein energy, and the rate of desired replacement. More protein is required in pregnancy because of the expansion of blood volume and growth of the uterus, fetus, and placenta. The minimum daily protein requirement in pregnancy is approximately 1 g/kg. This should be provided throughout the pregnancy to meet maternal and fetal needs adequately. Adequacy of protein provision is best assessed by measuring serum protein levels and urea nitrogen excretion. Most commercially

T A B L E    **10-4**

**Sample calculation of total parenteral nutrition requirements for 60-kg patient**

Total protein requirements = 1.5 g/kg = 1.5 × 60
= 90 g/day

Total caloric requirements = 36 kcal/kg = 36 × 60
= 2160 kcal/day

If calories are provided in a ratio of 70%:30%, dextrose:lipid,

Daily dextrose requirement = (2160 × 0.7) (3.4 kcal/g)
= 445 g

Daily lipid requirement = (2160 × 0.3) (9 kcal/g)
= 72 g

Infusion is usually begun at about 50% of total estimated needs and increased gradually to target values at a rate that ensures minimal maternal metabolic derangement.

available amino acid products have been used successfully to maintain normal fetal growth. It is important to emphasize that in certain situations (e.g., renal failure), protein and caloric requirements are increased significantly, and frequent dialysis may increase these needs even further. Survival rates in these situations correlate significantly with adequate caloric intake. Rates of up to 2 g/kg may be necessary to maintain normal nitrogen balance.

## Carbohydrates

Dextrose is the energy source most commonly used because it is easily metabolized, promotes nitrogen retention, is readily miscible with other additives, is available in many strengths, and is relatively inexpensive. The disadvantages include increased oxygen consumption, increased carbon dioxide production, and prolonged hyperglycemia. Dextrose concentrations greater than 10% (600 mosm) should not be administered peripherally, to avoid osmolarity-induced phlebitis and venospasm. The low caloric potency of dextrose (3.4 kcal/kg) precludes its use as the sole source of energy. It is necessary, therefore, to access the central venous circulation for infusion of hyperosmolar solutions and utilize alternative energy substrates. Although infusion rates of 4 to 6 mg/kg/min reduce the severity of the aforementioned problems, it may be necessary to administer insulin to maintain serum glucose between 60 and 120 mg/dL. There is no evidence that parenteral hypertonic dextrose given over prolonged periods has adverse fetal effects, provided euglycemia is maintained.

## Fat Emulsions

Lipids are an important component of TPN in the pregnant patient for the following reasons:

1. They are an excellent energy source (approximately 9 kcal/g)
2. Essential fatty acids are utilized for fetal fat depot formation, brain development and myelination, and lung surfactant synthesis.
3. Fatty-acid metabolism requires less oxygen and produces less carbon dioxide than glucose metabolism.

Most commercially available solutions are a suspension of chylomicrons of arachidonic acid precursors and essential fatty acids in a base of safflower or soybean oil. Emulsions are available in concentrations of 10% and 20%. Infusion is usually limited to 12 hours a day, both because chylomicrons may remain in the maternal circulation for up to 8 to 10 hours after administration and due to concern about possible bacterial contamination of solution when infusion is prolonged. Placental transport of fatty acids is primarily by passive diffusion. It is necessary, therefore, to maintain a high maternal fetal concentration gradient to ensure adequate transfer. Overt signs of essential fatty-acid deficiency may not appear until 4 weeks or more of nutritional depletion (Parenteral and Enteral Nutrition Team, 1988). Maternal serum hypertriglyceridemia and ketosis are important complications of lipid use that should be sought and corrected. Initial concerns about preterm labor and placental infarction from fat embolism (Heller, 1988) have failed to materialize with the concentrations of lipid commonly used for TPN (i.e., 30%–40% of total caloric requirements) (Elthick, 1978).

## Fluids and Electrolytes

The increased requirement for fluid in pregnancy is significant. Over the course of a term singleton pregnancy, total body water increases by about 8 to 9 liters. This requirement is for expansion of extracellular volume (including intravascular volume), fetal needs, and amniotic fluid formation. Inadequate plasma volume expansion adversely affects fetal well-being (Rosso, 1992; Daniel, 1989). An additional 30 mL/day over standard maintenance fluids is considered sufficient to meet these needs (National Research Council, 1989).

Care should be taken to match any additional losses (e.g., gastrointestinal fluid from hyperemesis) with the appropriate solutions. Fluid replacement should be separate from hyperalimentation solution to prevent complications due to changes in rate and contents of TPN delivered. Suggested electrolyte and vitamin requirements for obstetric patients are displayed in Tables 10-5 and 10-6. These are based on estimates of oral

T A B L E   **10-5**

Electrolyte requirements in the obstetric patient on total parenteral nutrition

| Electrolyte | Daily Range |
|---|---|
| Calcium | 10–15 mEq |
| Magnesium | 8–24 mEq |
| Potassium | 90–240 mEq |
| Sodium | 60–150 mEq |
| Acetate | 80–120 mEq |
| Chloride | 60–150 mEq |
| Phosphorus | 0–50 mmol |

Modified from Parenteral and Enteral Nutrition Manual, 5th edition; and Rayburn et al. Parenteral nutrition in obstetrics and gynecology. Obstetrics and Gynecology Survey. 1986;41:200–214.

T A B L E   **10-6**

Vitamins, trace elements, and drug additives for obstetric patients

**Daily Recommendation**

| *Standard Multivitamins Package (Per Day)* | | *Typical Trace Element Package* | |
|---|---|---|---|
| Ascorbic acid | 100.0 mg | Zinc | 4.0 mg (plus an additional 2 mg required for pregnancy) |
| Vitamin A | 1000.0 µg | | |
| Vitamin D | 5.0 µg | | |
| Thiamine HCl | 3.0 mg | Copper | 1.0 mg |
| Riboflavin | 3.6 mg | Manganese | 0.8 mg |
| Pyridoxine HCl | 4.0 mg | Chromium | 0.010 mg |
| Niacinamide | 40.0 mg | *Other Trace Elements* | |
| Pantothenic acid | 15.0 mg | Selenium | 55 µg |
| Vitamin E | 10 mg | Iodine | 2–3 µg/kg (long-term) |
| Biotin | 60 µg | Iron | 25 mg (weekly) |
| Folic acid | 400 µg | *Drugs* | |
| Cyanocobalamin (Vitamin $B_{12}$) | 5.0 µg | Heparin | 1000 units/liter |
| *Phytonadione (Vitamin $K_1$)* | 5–10 mg (per week) | Insulin, regular (if necessary) | 0.5 units/10 g infused glucose (initially) |

Adapted from Parenteral and Enteral Nutrition Manual, 5th edition; and Rayburn et al. Parenteral nutrition in obstetrics and gynecology. Obstetrics and Gynecology Survey. 1986;41:200–214.

T A B L E   **10-7**

Monitoring during total parenteral nutrition

| | |
|---|---|
| Daily weights | Liver function assessment, calcium, $PO_4$, magnesium, albumin (2–3 times/wk) |
| Strict I/O | |
| Urine sugar and ketones | Weekly nitrogen balance |
| Serum glucose monitoring (every 6–12 hr) | Fetal growth assessment (every 2–4 wk) |
| Daily electrolytes | |

I/O, input/output.

recommended dietary allowances actually absorbed. Commercially available intravenous vitamin preparations have proven to be adequate for normal fetal growth.

## Monitoring and Complications

A suggested protocol for monitoring the pregnant patient receiving TPN is outlined in Table 10-7. Commonly encountered complications of therapy are detailed in Table 10-8.

T A B L E **10-8**

## Complications of total parenteral nutrition in the obstetric patient

*Catheter-Related*
Pneumothorax
Arterial laceration
Mediastinal hematoma
Malposition
Brachial plexus/phrenic nerve palsy
Catheter sepsis
Subclavian vein thrombosis
Hydro/chylothorax

*Metabolic*
Deficiencies of vitamins, minerals, electrolytes,
    trace metals, or essential fatty acids
Hyperglycemia
Hepatic dysfunction and fatty infiltration
Carbon dioxide retention
Over/underhydration

*Other*
Bowel atrophy
Cholecystitis
Heparin-related complications (e.g., hemorrhage,
    thrombocytopenia, or osteopenia)

*Neonatal*
Maternal diabetes syndrome (e.g., macrosomia,
    postnatal hypoglycemia)
Growth retardation

**REFERENCES**

Abrams B, Newman V, Key T, Parker J. Maternal weight gain and preterm delivery. Obstet Gynecol 1989;74:577–583.

Abrams B, Newmann V. Small-for-gestational age birth: maternal predictors and comparison with risk factors of spontaneous preterm delivery in same cohort. Am J Obstet Gynecol 1991; 164:785.

Antonov AN. Children born during siege of Leningrad in 1942. J Pediatr 1947;30:250–259.

Benny P, Legge M, Aickin D. The biochemical effects of maternal hyperalimentation during pregnancy. NZ Med J 1978;88:283–285.

Breen K, McDonald I, Panelli D, Ihle B. Planned pregnancy in a patient who was receiving home PN. Med J Aust 1987;146:215–217.

Buchman AL. Total peripheral parenteral nutrition in pregnancy. JPEN 1990;16:189. Letter.

Cole B, Seltzer M, Kassabian J, Abboud S. PN in a pregnant cystic fibrosis patient. JPEN 1987; 11:205–207.

Cox K, Byrne W, Amenet M. Home total parenteral nutrition during pregnancy: a case report. JPEN 1981;5:246–249.

Daniel SS, James LS, Stark RI, et al. Prevention of the normal expansion of maternal plasma volume: a model for chronic fetal hypoxemia. J Dev Physiol 1989;11:225–228.

Di Constanzo J, Martin J, Cano N, et al: Total parenteral nutrition with fat emulsions during pregnancy—nutritional requirements: a case report. JPEN 1982;6:534–538.

Dunnihoo D. Fundamentals of gynecology and obstetrics. Philadelphia: JB Lippincott, 1990:164–176.

Elphick MC, Filshie GM, Hull D. The passage of fat emulsion across the human placenta. Br J Obstet Gynaecol 1978;85:610–618.

Gineston J, Carpon J, Delcenserie R, et al. Prolonged total parenteral nutrition in a pregnant woman with acute pancreatitis. J Clin Gastroenterol 1984;6:249–252.

Goldenberg RL, Tamura T, Cliver SP, et al. Serum folate and fetal growth retardation: a matter of compliance? Obstet Gynecol 1992;79:719–722.

Gray D, Cabaniss M. Home total parenteral nutrition in a pregnant diabetic after jejunoileal bypass for obesity. JPEN 1989;13:214–217.

Harris J, Benedict F. Biometric studies of basal metabolism in man. Washington, DC: Carnegie Institute of Washington, 1919, publication no. 279.

Heller L. Clinical and experimental studies in complete parenteral nutrition. Scand J Gastroenterol 1968;4(suppl):4–7.

Herbert W, Seeds K, Bowes W, Sweeney C. Fetal growth response to total parenteral nutrition in pregnancy: a case report. J Reprod Med 1986;31:263–266.

Hew L, Dietal M. Total parenteral nutrition in gynecology and obstetrics. Obstet Gynecol 1980; 55:464–468.

Institute of Medicine, Committee on Nutritional Status During Pregnancy and Lactation. National Academy of Sciences. Nutrition during pregnancy. Washington, DC: National Academy Press, 1990.

Jacobson L, Clapp D. TPN in pregnancy complicated by Crohn's disease. JPEN 1987;11:93–96.

Karamatsu J, Boyd A, Cooke J, et al. Intravenous nutrition during twin pregnancy. JPEN 1987; 11:499–501.

Klein F, Lin C, Lowensohn R. Total parenteral nutrition during pregnancy. American Dietary Association 66th Annual Meeting, September 12–15, 1983;147.

Lafever HN, Jones CT, Rolph TP. Some of the consequences of intrauterine growth retardation. In: Visser HKA, ed. Nutrition and metabolism of the fetus and infant. The Hague: Martinus Nijhoff, 1979:43.

Lakoff KM, Feldman JD. Anorexia nervosa associated with pregnancy. Obstet Gynecol 1972; 39:699.

Lavin J, Gimmon Z, Miodovnik M, et al. Total parenteral nutrition in a pregnant insulin requiring diabetic. Obstet Gynecol 1982;59:660–664.

Lee R, Rodger B, Young C, et al. Total parenteral nutrition in pregnancy. Obstet Gynecol 1986; 68:563–571.

LeGrix A, Colin R, Galmiche J, et al. Acute outbreak of haemorrhagia rectocolitis in a pregnant woman treated with prolonged total parenteral nutrition. I. Nouv Presse Med 1978;7:30–44. Letter.

Lipkin E, Benedetti T, Chait A. Successful pregnancy outcome using total parenteral nutrition from the first trimester of pregnancy. JPEN 1986; 10:665–669.

Little G, Frigolette F, eds. Guidelines for perinatal care. 2nd ed. Washington, DC: American College of Obstetrics and Gynecologists, 1988.

Loiudice T, Chandrakaar C. Pregnancy and jejunoileal bypass: treatment of complications with total parenteral nutrition. South Med J 1980;73:256–261.

Luke B. Maternal nutrition. In: Medicine of the fetus and mother. Reece A, et al, eds. Philadelphia: Lippincott, 1992:869.

Main A, Shenkin A, Black W, et al. Intravenous feeding to sustain pregnancy in patient with Crohn's disease. Br Med J 1981;283:1221–1222.

Martin R. Hyperalimentation during pregnancy. Clin Consult Nutr 1982;25:9–12.

Martin R, Blackburn G. Hyperalimentation in pregnancy. In: Berkowitz R, ed. Critical care of the obstetric patient. Churchill Livingstone, 1983;133–163.

National Research Council. Subcommittee on the Tenth Edition of the RDA's Food and Nutrition Board. Commission on Life Sciences. Washington, D.C.: National Academy Press, 1989.

Neggars YH, Cutter GR, Alvarez JO, et al. The relationship between maternal serum zinc levels during pregnancy and birthweight. Early Hum Dev 1991;25:75–85.

Nugent F, Rajala M, O'Shea, et al. TPN in pregnancy: conception to delivery. JPEN 1987;11:424–427.

Nuutinen L, Alahuhta S, Heikkinen J. Nutrition during ten-week life support with successful fetal outcome in a case with fatal maternal brain damage. JPEN 1989;13:432–435.

Oldham H, Shaft B. Effect of caloric intake on nitrogen utilization during pregnancy. J Am Diet Assoc 1957;27:847.

Parenteral and Enteral Nutrition Team. Parenteral and enteral nutrition manual. 5th ed. Ann Arbor, MI: University of Michigan Hospitals, 1988.

Payne PR, Wheeler EF. Comparative nutrition in pregnancy and lactation. Proc Nutr Soc 1968; 27:129–138.

Pitkin RM. Obstetrics and gynecology. In: Schneider HA, Anderson CE, Coursin DB, eds. Nutritional support of medical practice, 2nd ed. Hagerstown, MD: Harper & Row, 1983:491–506.

Pond WG, Strachan DN, Sinha YN, et al. Effect of protein deprivation of the swine during all or part of gestation on birth weight, postnatal growth rate, and nucleic acid content of brain and muscle of progeny. J Nutr 1969;99:61.

Riopelle AJ, Hill CW, Li SC. Protein deprivation in primates versus fetal mortality and neonatal status of infant monkeys born of deprived mothers. Am J Clin Nutr 1975;28:989–993.

Rivera-Alsina M, Saldana L, Steipger C. Fetal growth sustained by parenteral nutrition in pregnancy. Obstet Gynecol 1984;64:138–141.

Rosso P, Danose E, Braun S, et al. Hemodynamic changes in underweight pregnant women. Obstet Gynecol 1992;79:908–912.

Schoenbeck J, Segerbrand E. Candida albicans septicaemia during first half of pregnancy, successfully treated with 5 fluorocytosine. Br Med J 1973;4:337–338.

Smith C, Refleth P, Phelan J, et al. Long-term hyperalimentation in the pregnant woman with insulin-dependent diabetes: a report of two cases. Am J Obstet Gynecol 1981;141:180–183.

Smith CA. Effects of maternal undernutrition upon newborn infants in Holland: 1944–1945. J Pediatr 1947;30:229–243.

Stein Z, Susser M. The Dutch famine 1944–1945, and the productive process. I. Effects on six indices at birth. Pediatr Res 1975;9:70.

Stellato T, Danziger L, Burkons D. Fetal salvage with maternal TPN: the pregnant mother as her own control. JPEN 1988;12:412–413.

Stowell J, Bottsford J, Rubel H. Pancreatitis with pseudocyst and cholelithiasis in third trimester of pregnancy: management with total parenteral nutrition. South Med J 1984;77:502–504.

Taffell SM, National Center of Health Statistics. Maternal weight gain and the outcome of pregnancy: United States; 1980. Vital and Health Statistic Series 21-No. 44. DHHS (PHS) 86, Public Health Service, Washington, DC: U.S. Government Printing Office, 1986.

Tresadern J, Falconar G, Turnberg L, et al. Maintenance of pregnancy in a home parenteral nutrition patient. JPEN 1984;8:199–202.

Voight H, Sailer D, Kolb S, Frobenius W. Conception and pregnancy without complications in parenteral home nutrition 7. Geburtsch Perinatol 1989;193:198–202. Abstract.

Watson LA, Bermarilo AA, Marshall JF. Total peripheral parenteral nutrition in pregnancy. JPEN 1990;14:485–489.

Webb G. The use of hyperalimentation and chemotherapy in pregnancy: a case report. Am J Obstet Gynecol 1980;137:263–265.

Weinberg R, Sitrin M, Adkins G, et al. Treatment of hyperlipidemic pancreatitis in pregnancy with total parenteral nutrition. Gastroenterology 1982;83:1300–1305.

Wilmore D. The metabolic management of the critically ill. New York: Plenum, 1980.

Winick M. Cellular changes during placental and fetal growth. Am J Obstet Gynecol 1971;109:166–176.

Wolk RA, Rayburn WF. Parenteral nutrition in obstetric patients. Nutr Clin Pract 1990;5:139–152.

Young K. Acute pancreatitis in pregnancy: two case reports. Obstet Gynecol 1982;60:653–657.

# CHAPTER 11

# Blood Component Replacement Therapy

*T*his chapter is intended as a brief summary of blood products and their indications in acute obstetric care. Potential complications of and alternatives to allogeneic transfusion also will be discussed. Frequent reference will be made to the standards of the American Association of Blood Banks (Standards Committee, 1994). Blood products (e.g., liquid plasma, plasma derivatives, granulocytes) and procedures (e.g., autotransfusion), which are infrequently used in obstetric critical care, will not be covered. The interested reader is referred to standard blood banking texts for information about these products and procedures.

## Blood Collection and Storage

### Donors

The American Association of Blood Banks (AABB) frequently updates the standards required of all blood banks regarding donor selection and blood collection (Standards Committee, 1994). In addition to requirements protecting the potential recipient (Table 11-1), selection criteria are also designed to protect the potential donor. Potential donors must be in good health. Those having heart, liver, or lung disease, as well as those having a history of cancer or bleeding tendency, are usually excluded. Age, weight, pulse, and BP requirements also are stipulated. A minimum donor hemoglobin of 12.5 g/dL or hematocrit of 38% is required. Only with physician approval may an obstetric patient donate blood prior to 6 weeks following pregnancy, and then only for purposes of autologous collection or transfusion to the infant.

It is noteworthy that while a number of decisions regarding blood donation and collection have been scientifically based (e.g., self-deferral of at-risk donors, routine HIV testing), others have been in response to political, legal, and social pressures (e.g., directed donor options) (Hanson, 1994; Schmidt, 1994).

## Collection

Although separation of components at the time of blood donation has been explored (Valbonesi, 1994), contemporary blood banking practice requires the separation of blood into its components following removal of the unit of whole blood from the donor. Whole blood is initially collected in a bag containing a storage solution. Within 6 hours of collection, the blood is separated by centrifuging into RBCs and platelet-rich plasma. The latter, which contains about 70% of the platelets in the original unit of whole blood, is then again centrifuged at a higher speed in order to create a "pellet" of platelets. These platelets are resuspended in 50 mL of the plasma. The remaining supernatant plasma is frozen at or below $-18°C$. This fresh frozen plasma (FFP) may be

T A B L E  **11-1**

Some AABB exclusion criteria based on routine testing of all prospective blood donors

*Indefinite Exclusion as a Donor*

History of viral hepatitis after age 11 and/or a positive test for hepatitis B surface antigen or antibodies to hepatitis B core

Past or present clinical or laboratory evidence of infection with hepatitis C virus, human T-cell lymphotropic virus type I/II, or HIV

Persons whose responses to questions indicate high risk for HIV infection

History of babesiosis or Chagas' disease

Stigmata of parenteral drug use

Alcohol intoxication or stigmata of alcohol habituation

*Deferral as a Donor for 12 Months*

Following receipt of hepatitis B immune globulin

Following receipt of blood

Following application of a tattoo

Following nonsterile skin penetration with instruments contaminated with blood or body fluids

Following sexual contact with viral hepatitis or HIV

Following syphilis or gonorrhea

*Other Deferrals*

Three years following the most recent symptom of malaria, and/or 3 years after departure from an endemic area

Four weeks following vaccination for rubella

Two weeks following vaccination for rubeola, mumps, polio (oral), or yellow fever

Source: Data from Standards Committee, American Association of Blood Banks. Standards for blood banks and transfusion services. 16th ed. Bethesda, MD: American Association of Blood Banks, 1994.

thawed to 4°C. The cryoprecipitate that forms at this temperature is then separated and refrozen to −18°C or below. The steps involved in the separation of components are illustrated in Figure 11-1.

Blood components also may be obtained by apheresis. Apheresis is the procedure in which whole blood is withdrawn from the donor, a portion retained, and the remainder retransfused to the donor. Both cellular (red cells, granulocytes, and platelets) and plasma components may be removed by either manual or mechanical apheresis (Standards Committee, 1994; Hogman, 1987).

## Storage

Platelets may be stored under constant agitation at 20°C to 24°C for up to 5 days. Fresh frozen plasma and cryoprecipitate may remain frozen for up to 12 months following collection (Standards Committee, 1994). The shelf life of red-cell products depends on the selection of storage solution.

Storage solutions contain an anticoagulant (e.g., citrate) and nutritive substrates (e.g., dextrose, adenine) to maintain red cell viability. By chelating calcium, citrate inhibits the coagulation cascade. Dextrose provides a substrate for anaerobic glycolysis, which in turn promotes RBC production of adenosine triphosphate (ATP). The ATP prevents deformation of the red cell and preserves membrane function. Storage solutions containing citrate and dextrose (anticoagulant citrate dextrose, or ACD, and citrate phosphate dextrose, or CPD) are slightly acidic. The acidity helps to maintain cell nucleotides, which in turn maintain red cell viability (Hogman, 1987). Red

F I G U R E  **11-1**

**Preparation of blood components.** WB, whole blood; CPDA-1, citrate phosphate dextrose adenine; pRBCs, packed red blood cells; HCT, hematocrit. (Reproduced by permission from Fakhry SM, Sheldon GF. Blood administration, risks, and substitutes. Adv Surg 1995;28:71–92.)

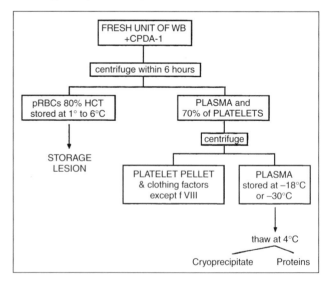

cells stored in ACD or CPD expire 21 days following collection. The addition of adenine to the storage solution (as in CPDA-1) allows the resynthesis of ATP and prolongs the shelf life of the unit to 35 days. The addition of mannitol to the storage solution (e.g., in SAGM) stabilizes the red-cell membrane and prolongs the shelf life of the unit to 42 days (Standards Committee, 1994).

Stored blood undergoes certain metabolic changes over time. The increase in potassium concentration must be considered in transfusing patients who are already hyperkalemic or who have compromised renal function. The progressive decline in pH, which can occur over time, may contribute to red-cell deformation, which may in turn lead to difficulties in the passage of transfused red blood cells through the recipient's microcirculation. 2,3-Diphosphoglycerate (2,3-DPG), an enzyme found in red cells, decreases their affinity for oxygen. As 2,3-DPG levels decline with storage, the ability of transfused cells to deliver oxygen to the recipient's tissues also declines. However, this enzyme is usually regenerated fairly rapidly following transfusion. Finally, because of the increase in ammonia concentration in stored blood, it is advisable to transfuse blood that is less than a week old to those patients having severely compromised hepatic function (Pisciotto, 1993).

## Blood Components and Their Indications and Administration

### Products Containing Red Cells

#### Whole Blood

A unit of whole blood contains approximately 450 mL of blood and 63 mL of a storage solution. Maintenance at 1°C to 6°C prolongs the shelf life of stored red cells by decreasing the rate of glycolysis. Typically, the hematocrit of a unit varies from 36% to 44%. A unit transfused to an adult will raise the recipient's hematocrit by 3% to 4% or the hemoglobin concentration by 1 g/dL. Whole blood contains red cells but is relatively deficient in functioning platelets and granulocytes. While stable clotting factors are maintained during stor-

age of whole blood, labile clotting factors V and VIII decrease over time (Pisciotto, 1993). Whole blood has the advantage of providing oxygen carriage as well as volume expansion from a single donor. However, because volume expansion may be achieved with crystalloid or colloid and because storage of whole blood precludes its use for component preparation, its use is currently quite limited (Fakhry, 1995). It may occasionally be indicated for the patient who has lost 25% of her blood volume and continues to actively bleed (Pisciotto, 1993). Whole blood is contraindicated in patients who are normovolemic and require only an increase in RBC mass.

### Red Blood Cells

Red blood cells are prepared from whole blood by gravitational or centrifugal separation from the plasma. Each unit has a volume of 250 to 300 mL. Like whole blood, this product is stored at 1°C to 6°C. The hematocrit of the unit varies with the storage solution. Red blood cells stored in CPDA-1 have hematocrits of 70% to 80%, while those stored in additive solutions (e.g., SAGM) have hematocrits of 52% to 60% (Pisciotto, 1993). A unit of RBCs provides the same oxygen-carrying capacity as a unit of whole blood. Because of the reduction in plasma, however, RBCs carry with them a reduced risk of circulatory overload, allergic reactions, and metabolic complications (Miller, 1995).

### Leukocyte-Reduced Red Blood Cells

The transfusion of "passenger" donor leukocytes during an RBC transfusion has been associated with a number of potential deleterious effects. These include graft-versus-host disease (GVHD) and transmission of bacteria and viruses. While these complications are encountered infrequently in transfusing an obstetric patient, a febrile nonhemolytic transfusion reaction resulting from an alloimmune response to transfused donor leukocyte antigens may be seen more often (Miller, 1995). An isolated febrile nonhemolytic reaction is unlikely to recur. Thus, leukocyte-reduced RBC products are useful primarily for patients who have experienced recurrent reactions.

Among those likely to develop alloimmunization to leukocyte antigens are those patients who have received multiple transfusions and women who have had several pregnancies (Pisciotto, 1993).

Leukocyte reduction has been accomplished through the development of blood filters made of small-diameter, high-density synthetic fibers. In addition to a reduction in pore size, the material used in filters designed for red-cell components binds leukocytes and platelets preferentially and allows passage of red cells. This combination of barrier retention and leukocyte adsorption allows reduction of donor leukocytes to less than 5 × 108, the concentration necessary to reduce the incidence of febrile nonhemolytic transfusion reactions (Klein, 1992). Prestorage leukocyte reduction has the added advantage of prevention of transfusion of undesirable leukocyte breakdown products, which may not be removed during filtration of stored blood. These products include histamines, membrane fragments, cytokines, and proteases (Klein, 1992).

### Washed Red Blood Cells

Machine-washing RBCs in sterile saline will remove platelets, cellular debris, and 98% of plasma and will reduce the concentration of leukocytes (Pisciotto, 1993). The product remaining after washing has a volume of approximately 180 mL. Washed RBCs have a number of disadvantages. Because the washing takes place in an "open" system, once prepared, the unit has a shelf life of only 24 hours. At least 80% of the original RBCs must be retained after washing.

Because the preparation is expensive and wasteful, there are currently few indications for this product. The development of efficient leukocyte-reduction filters has obviated the need for washed RBCs to prevent febrile nonhemolytic transfusion reactions. Patients who have antibodies to immunoglobulin-A (IgA) may benefit from transfusion with washed RBCs, although deglycerolized RBCs have more plasma removed (American Red Cross, 1994). The only remaining indication for washed RBCs is the rare patient who has recurrent or severe transfusion reactions.

### Frozen and Deglycerolized Red Blood Cells

To prepare this product, varying amounts of glycerol, a cryoprotective agent, is added to a unit of RBCs that is less than 6 days old. The unit may then be frozen at $-65°C$ to $-200°C$ (depending on the concentration of glycerol) and stored for up to 10 years. When needed, the unit is first thawed and then washed with a series of saline-glucose solutions to remove the glycerol. After reconstitution in saline, the unit may be stored at 1°C to 6°C. The unit must be used within 24 hours of deglycerolizing, because washing takes place in an "open" system. An additional risk of intravascular hemolysis exists if the glycerol has been incompletely removed in the process of washing.

As previously mentioned, thawed, deglycerolized RBCs may be used for the rare patient who has antibodies to IgA. They also may be useful for transfusion to patients who have uncommon red-cell phenotypes (Pisciotto, 1993; American Red Cross, 1994).

## The Transfusion Trigger

Deciding at which point the patient who is undergoing an obstetric hemorrhage requires an RBC transfusion is an exceedingly difficult task. Acute blood loss initiates a number of interrelated physiologic changes. These changes occur rapidly and in close temporal sequence in the body's attempt to preserve adequacy of tissue oxygenation. They may be considered as two primary adaptations: increased oxygen release to tissues and increased cardiac output.

As hemoglobin concentration falls below 9 g/dL, the oxygen-hemoglobin dissociation curve shifts to the right, allowing RBCs to give up oxygen to tissues at lower levels of oxygen tension. This rightward shift is caused by two mechanisms. Acutely, the Bohr effect (the increased release of oxygen from hemoglobin due to high concentrations of carbon dioxide and hydrogen ion) is activated. It is speculated that intracellular erythrocyte acidosis may initiate the Bohr effect (Welch, 1992). Over 12 to 36 hours of declining hemoglobin levels, an increase in 2,3-DPG concentrations in erythrocytes allows these cells to more readily give up oxygen to the tissues. Tissue oxygen extraction is contingent on tissue oxygen delivery ($Do_2$) and tissue oxygen consumption ($Vo_2$). For the 70-kg individual at rest, the normal $Do_2$ is 1000 mL/min and the normal $Vo_2$ is 250 mL/min. The overall oxygen extraction ratio (ER) is, therefore, 25%. However, individual organs extract oxygen at different rates. For example, the ER for the heart is 55% and for the kidney is 10% (Stehling, 1994a). As $Do_2$ decreases due to a fall in hemoglobin, the ER increases to maintain tissue oxygen consumption (Spence, 1993).

The cardiovascular changes that accompany acute blood loss function to maintain oxygen supply to essential organs. The body's first responses to sudden loss of blood include adrenergically mediated constriction of venules and small veins. This mobilization of blood from these capacitance vessels increases venous return to the heart (increased preload). The increase in preload is accompanied initially by systemic hypotension. The resultant decreased capillary hydrostatic pressure promotes movement of fluid from the interstitial space into the intravascular space. Not only may this fluid mobilization restore up to 50% of the intravascular volume, but it also serves to decrease viscosity of circulating blood. The combination of systemic vasodilatation and decreased blood viscosity has the net effect of decreasing the work the heart must perform to maintain adequacy of circulation (decreased afterload). The combination of increased preload with diminished afterload serves to increase the volume of blood pumped with every contraction of the heart (stroke volume). Although an increase in heart rate also increases circulation of RBCs, the major contribution to increased cardiac output in this acute phase of blood loss is the increase in stroke volume (Table 11-2) (Welch, 1992; Stehling, 1994b). As blood loss continues, selective arterial constriction is found in the circulatory beds of the skin, skeletal muscle, kidney, and splanchnic organs. The resultant anaerobic metabolism in these organs causes the release of fixed acids, lowering systemic pH. Systemic acidemia stimulates hyperventilation as the body attempts to compensate through the respiratory system for a metabolic acidosis. The accompanying increase in negative intrathoracic pressure serves to fur-

T A B L E   **11-2**

Hemoglobin and oxygen interactions

Cardiac output (CO) = stroke volume (SV)
$\qquad \times$ heart rate (HR)

Oxygen content ($Cao_2$) = $(1.39 \times So_2 \times Hgb$
$\qquad + 0.003 \times Po_2)$
$\qquad \times 10$ mL $O_2$/liter

where
$So_2$ = oxygen saturation and
Hgb = hemoglobin concentration in g/dL

Oxygen delivery ($Do_2$) = CO $\times Cao_2$ mL $O_2$/min

Oxygen consumption ($Vo_2$) = CO $\times$ ($Cao_2$
$\qquad - Cvo_2$) mL $O_2$/min

where
$Cao_2$ = arterial oxygen content and
$Cvo_2$ = mixed venous oxygen content

Oxygen extraction ratio ($O_2$ER) = $Vo_2/Do_2$

Hgb, hemoglobin.

Reproduced by permission from Spence R, Cernaianu A, Carson J, DelRossi A. Transfusion and surgery. Curr Probl Surg 1993;30:1101–1180.

ther increase venous return to the heart. In addition, this selective systemic vasoconstriction is accompanied by redistribution of blood flow to the brain and the coronary vessels (Welch, 1992; Stehling, 1994).

From this brief discussion it should be evident that a number of interrelated physiologic changes take place rapidly in response to acute blood loss (see Table 11-2). Some of these parameters are readily ascertainable (e.g., hemoglobin concentration), while others require sophisticated calculations (e.g., oxygen ER). It is not clear which of these parameters is more predictive of survival or of quality of survival.

Likely because of ease of ascertainment, much attention has been focused on the hemoglobin concentration as a transfusion trigger. Experiments in healthy animals undergoing normovolemic hemodilution have found the absence of depressed ventricular function, lactate production, and death in those maintaining hemoglobins above 5 g/dL (Carson, 1993). A study of 125 patients undergoing elective and emergency surgical procedures who refused blood found no deaths among those who had a preoperative hemoglobin concentration above 8 g/dL and who lost fewer than 500 mL intraoperatively. A multivariate analysis of these data, controlling for factors potentially influencing outcome (e.g., systemic disease, type of procedure) confirmed both preoperative hemoglobin and intraoperative blood loss as variables that are independently associated with postoperative mortality (Carson, 1988). Another review of 134 medical and surgical patients who declined transfusion found that there were no deaths among noncardiac patients who maintained hemoglobin concentrations above 5 g/dL. Of the eight obstetrics-gynecology patients in the latter series, the seven survivors had minimum hemoglobins ranging from 1.4 to 7.8 g/dL (Viele, 1994). Women who had an intraoperative hemorrhage at cesarean delivery of over 1500 mL and/or a fall in hematocrit of more than 10 points and/or a postoperative hematocrit below 24% had no difference in hospital stay, infection, and wound complications, regardless of whether they received an RBC transfusion (Naef, 1995).

Pregnant women normally undergo changes that may impact on the physiologic parameters used as transfusion triggers. Heart rate, stroke volume, and, thus, cardiac output increase progressively with advancing pregnancy. The concentration of most coagulation factors also increases progressively. The disproportionate expansion of plasma volume relative to red-cell mass accounts for the "physiologic anemia of pregnancy" (Mattison, 1993; Alving, 1993). It should be evident, therefore, that the physiologic changes unique to pregnancy may render inapplicable recommendations regarding RBC transfusion derived from nonpregnant patients. The superimposition of cardiovascular or hematologic disease on pregnancy may make this decision all the more difficult.

As a practical point, acute obstetric hemorrhage offers little time for quantification of and reflection on the numerous accompanying physiologic changes. Although not designed specifically for pregnancy, the guidelines proposed by the American College of Physicians offer a reasonable approach to RBC transfusion decision making (American College of Physicians, 1992). In the absence of patient risks (e.g., cardiac disease, previous thrombotic stroke, history of transient ischemic attacks), acute blood loss should first be managed by restoration of intracellular volume. While crystalloids are less expensive for

this purpose than are colloids, a smaller volume of the latter is sometimes used to achieve a given endpoint in intravascular volume expansion (Donaldson, 1992). Patients should not be transfused if volume expansion alone restores or maintains normal vital signs. If despite reestablishment of normovolemia, such signs and symptoms as syncope, dyspnea, postural hypotension, tachycardia, or angina persist, transfusion is indicated. The volume of RBCs transfused should be only that amount sufficient to correct these signs and symptoms. Single-unit transfusions are acceptable under these guidelines (American College of Physicians, 1992). Flexibility and intuitive judgment should be exercised in the application of these guidelines. For example, RBCs might be transfused prior to deterioration of vital signs in those patients whose massive blood loss continues unabated and in those with myocardial disease (Hasley, 1994).

## Blood Ordering Practices

Once the decision has been made to make blood available for the patient, the physician must decide whether to request a type and screen or type and crossmatch (Fig 11-2). In a *type and screen*, the potential recipient's ABO and Rh type are first determined. Her serum is then mixed with reagent red cells, which must contain antigens with which most clinically significant antibodies will react. Following incubation at 37°C, excess antibody is removed by washing the cells with saline. The red cells are then mixed with antihuman globulin and centrifuged. The presence of agglutination indicates that the potential recipient has antibodies in her serum to at least one of the antigens on the reagent red cells. This (these) antibody(ies) is/are then identified. A *major crossmatch*, consisting of mixing the recipient's serum with donor RBCs, is required prior to all but emergency transfusions (Standards Committee, 1994). In previous years, the only acceptable means of crossmatching required an antiglobulin phase, in which the donor cells–recipient serum mixture is mixed with antihuman globulin and then centrifuged (see Fig 11-2). However, an *abbreviated crossmatch*, consisting of a type and screen followed by an immediate spin (centrifuging a mixture of donor cells and recipient serum and

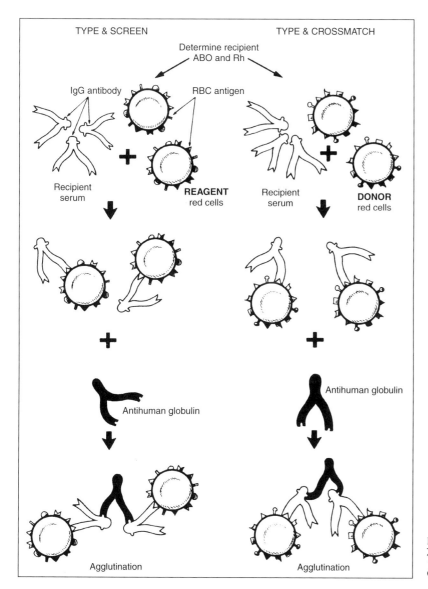

TYPE & SCREEN                    TYPE & CROSSMATCH

Determine recipient
ABO and Rh

IgG antibody          RBC antigen

Recipient                    REAGENT
serum                        red cells

Recipient                    DONOR
serum                        red cells

Antihuman globulin

Antihuman globulin

Agglutination                 Agglutination

F I G U R E   **11-2**
Type and screen versus type and
crossmatch.

then inspecting for hemolysis or agglutination), has been shown to be 99.9% effective in preventing incompatible transfusions (Raichle, 1994). Therefore, it is an acceptable alternative to an antiglobulin crossmatch when no clinically significant antibodies are detected with screening and there are no previous records of such antibodies (Standards Committee, 1994). Another option is a *computer crossmatch*, in which recent ABO serologic results on file for both the donor and the potential recipient are used to determine compatibility (Raichle, 1994). This method is acceptable, provided there

have been two determinations of the recipient's ABO group (Standards Committee, 1994).

Blood banks are required to have ABO- and Rh-compatible donor blood available for patients who are typed and screened. If a transfusion becomes necessary, donor cells may be given following only an immediate spin of donor cells and recipient serum if no antibodies were found on screening (Raichle, 1994). The potential recipient whose screen demonstrates the presence of antibodies must have a major crossmatch prior to transfusion (Standards Committee, 1994).

From Figure 11-2, it should be evident that the possibility of an antibody-mediated reaction following transfusion of ABO- and Rh-compatible blood that has been typed and screened but not crossmatched exists only for those recipients who have antibodies to RBC antigens that are present on the actual donor RBCs but not on the reagent RBCs. The likelihood of such an occurrence is remote (Boral, 1979). It is, therefore, an acceptable practice to transfuse screened, uncrossmatched blood in an emergency (Pisciotto, 1993).

Though the need for transfusion arises infrequently, obstetric hemorrhage is most often unpredictable and is often massive (Sherman, 1993). Historically, the decisions about whether to type and crossmatch, type and screen, and, ultimately, whether to transfuse have been largely based on local custom, personal experience, and peer pressure (Salem-Schatz, 1990). A survey of 89 obstetrics units in the United Kingdom found a wide variation in typing and screening versus typing and crossmatching for identical obstetric indications. These practices were not influenced by whether the facility was a teaching hospital, had 24-hour blood bank technicians, or was at a location remote from the nearest blood bank (Clark, 1993). Likely because of increased awareness of the potential risks of transfusion since the AIDS epidemic, the rate of transfusion for certain procedures has abated in recent years (Camann, 1991). Both formal and informal provider education has probably played a role in instituting these changes. Requiring the ordering physician to fill out a checklist that notes the indication for the transfused blood product has been shown to be a useful tool (Morrison, 1993).

The maximum surgical blood order schedule (MSBOS) has been found to be an effective tool to improve the utilization of blood resources for elective procedures (e.g., elective repeat cesarean delivery, postpartum tubal sterilization) (Pisciotto, 1993; Galea, 1994). An MSBOS is institution-specific. The schedule is developed by comparing the ratio of units crossmatched to units transfused (the C/T ratio) for specific surgical procedures. Those procedures having a C/T ratio of greater than 2.0 are considered to have had an excessive number of units typed and crossmatched (Stehling, 1994b). Surgical procedures requiring less than 0.5 units of blood per operation (Pisciotto, 1993) and those whose C/T ratio exceeds 2.0 should be considered for typing and screening instead of typing and crossmatching.

## Blood Products Not Containing Red Blood Cells

### Fresh Frozen Plasma

The preparation and storage of FFP was detailed in the Collection section. A unit of FFP has a volume of approximately 200 to 250 mL. Fresh frozen plasma contains all coagulation factors, including labile factors V and VIII. It must be thawed to 30°C to 37°C prior to transfusion. It must be transfused within 24 hours of thawing if it is to serve as a source of labile clotting factors. After thawing, it may be stored at 1°C to 6°C. Compatibility testing is not required, but ABO-compatible FFP should be used to minimize the risk that antibodies in the transfused plasma will hemolyze recipient RBCs (Pisciotto, 1993; American Red Cross, 1994).

The indications for FFP in obstetric critical care are limited. It is useful for the patient with coagulation factor deficiencies secondary to liver disease. In instances of disseminated intravascular coagulation (DIC) and massive transfusion, the risks of FFP must be weighed against the possibility of limiting blood loss without the use of FFP, respectively, by the removal of the source of the DIC or the medical and surgical arrest of bleeding. The suggestion has been made that, prior to transfusing FFP in a bleeding patient, documentation of its need should be supplied by a prothrombin time (PT) greater than 1.5 times normal (usually > 18 sec) and an activated partial thromboplastin time (aPTT) greater than 1.5 times the mean normal value (usually > 55 sec) (Stehling, 1994b; College of American Pathologists, 1994). Fresh frozen plasma should be given when such test results are not available in the face of continued microvascular (small vessel) bleeding (Stehling, 1994b). The usual starting dose of FFP is 2 units. However, if platelets also are being administered, the volume of plasma in which they are being administered may justify a reduction in the FFP dose. Serial PT and/or aPTT assessments may be useful in determining the need for further FFP transfusions.

## Cryoprecipitate

Cryoprecipitate, or cryoprecipitated antihemophilic factor (Pisciotto, 1993), is prepared from FFP (see Collection section). A unit of cryoprecipitate has a volume of 10 to 15 mL. It contains fibrinogen, factor VIII:C (procoagulant), factor VIII:vWF (von Willebrand factor), and factor XIII. Cryoprecipitate must be thawed to 30°C to 37°C prior to transfusion.

The use of cryoprecipitate in obstetrics is severely limited. Hemophilia A, an X-linked recessive disorder, is extremely unusual in pregnancy, as is factor XIII deficiency. The current management for all forms of von Willebrand's disease except type IIB is the administration of desmopressin (DDAVP). The latter avoids the infectious risks of cryoprecipitate. Another potential use of cryoprecipitate requires its mixture with bovine thrombin to form the surgical adhesive, fibrin glue. As with FFP, it is desirable that transfused cryoprecipitate should be ABO-compatible with the recipient (Pisciotto, 1993; American Red Cross, 1994; College of American Pathologists, 1994).

## Platelets

The collection and preparation of a unit of *platelets* was described under the heading of Collection. Once collected, a unit of platelets should contain no fewer than $5.5 \times 10^{10}$ platelets suspended in a sufficient amount of plasma to maintain a pH of greater than 6.0 (usually 40–70 mL). The unit is stored at 2°C to 24°C with constant gentle agitation. The shelf life of a unit is approximately 5 days (Standards Committee, 1994; Pisciotto, 1993; American Red Cross, 1994).

As with other transfused coagulation factors, the need for platelet transfusion in obstetrics is uncommon. Thrombocytopenia secondary to bone marrow hypoplasia due to tumor invasion, chemotherapy, or primary aplasia is, fortunately, rarely encountered. The same cautions expressed about the use of FFP for DIC and massive bleeding apply to the use of platelets for these indications. It must be remembered that bleeding will generally not result from thrombocytopenia unless the platelet count falls below 5000 to 10,000/$\mu$L in a surgical patient or below 50,000/$\mu$L in a woman with an intact circulation. Because of rapid antibody-mediated platelet destruction in autoimmune thrombocytopenic purpura, the transfusion of platelets in this disease should be limited to patients with life-threatening hemorrhage (Stehling, 1994a,b; College of American Pathologists, 1994; British Committee for Standards in Haematology, 1992).

A single unit of platelets will increase the platelet count for a 70-kg adult by approximately $5 \times 10^9$/liter. The usual dose for a thrombocytopenic bleeding adult is 6 to 10 units of platelets.

Because of the risks of exposure to multiple donors, platelets obtained by cytapheresis from a single donor (platelets, pheresis) are an alternative to conventionally obtained platelets. A single unit of platelets, pheresis contains at least $3 \times 10^{11}$ platelets (i.e., the same number of platelets as is found in 5.5 conventional units). The plasma volume of this product varies from 200 to 500 mL. Platelets, pheresis are also useful for those patients who are refractory to platelet transfusion on the basis of anti-human leukocyte antigen (HLA) antibodies; HLA-compatible donors should be obtained for these recipients (Pisciotto, 1993; British Committee for Standards in Haematology, 1992).

Because in the separation of platelets from whole blood some RBCs or RBC fragments may remain with the platelets, Rh-negative patients should ideally be transfused with platelets from only Rh-negative donors. If an Rh-negative woman must receive platelets from an Rh-positive donor, consideration should be given to the use of Rh-immune globulin (Pisciotto, 1993).

## Massive Transfusion

Massive transfusion may be defined as either the acute replacement of 1.5 times the patient's blood volume or as the replacement of one or more blood volumes within 24 hours (Pisciotto, 1993; Donaldson, 1992). In a 70-kg adult, one blood volume is estimated as 75 mL/kg, or approximately 5000 mL. Transfusion with whole blood may be considered in the face of acute massive hemorrhage. Given current blood banking practices, however, it is unlikely that an adequate supply of this product will be readily available. It is more likely that initial resuscitation will require the administration of RBCs, with volume expansion being provided by either crystalloids (e.g., saline or lactated Ringer's solution) or colloids (e.g., albumen, dextrans, hydroxyethyl starch). While the debate surrounding the respective merits of emergency administration of these fluids continues, a few facts appear to have been clearly established. By volume, about 50% to 75% less colloid than crystalloid is required to achieve fluid resuscitation. The administration of a large volume of room-temperature crystalloid may increase thermal stress. On the other hand, colloids are more often associated with allergic reactions than are crystalloids. Furthermore, although both solutions contribute to a dilution of clotting factors, hydroxyethyl starch and dextrans both accelerate the reduction in factor VIII concentrations. They are also incorporated into polymerizing fibrin fibers, resulting in large clots that stimulate enhanced fibrinolysis (Donaldson, 1992).

There are no controlled studies supporting the formulaic transfusion of coagulation factors following the transfusion of a certain number of units of red-cell products. It is unusual for a coagulation disorder to develop in the face of massive hemorrhage exclusively on the basis of dilution of clotting factors. Stress, tissue injury, bacteremia, and shock may individually or collectively contribute to a depletion of coagulation factors. Physiologic changes that accompany blood loss, such as metabolic acidosis, hypothermia, hypocalcemia, and hypokalemia, may also inhibit coagulation, and will improve when corrected. Thus the decision to transfuse FFP, cryoprecipitate, or platelets should depend primarily on the finding of microvascular bleeding, supported, as time allows, by laboratory tests (e.g., aPTT, PT, and platelet counts) (Pisciotto, 1993; Donaldson, 1992).

# Administration of Blood

## Issue of Blood and Components

Because most fatal transfusion reactions result from clerical errors in the identification of specimens, components, and recipients, the Food and Drug Administration has specified labeling requirements intended to minimize these errors (Code of Federal Regulations, 1986). A transfusion record must be completed for each unit of donor blood or component. This record must bear the intended recipient's name, identification number, ABO group, and Rh type; and the donor unit number, donor ABO group and Rh type, and results of crossmatch tests. A sample of each donor RBC product and of each recipient's blood must be stored at 1°C to 6°C for at least 7 days following transfusion. If blood that has been issued by the blood bank has not been opened, it may be reissued, provided that it has not been warmed above 10°C or cooled below 1°C (Standards Committee, 1994).

## Duration of Transfusion

Because of the risk of bacterial contamination of blood kept at room temperature, each unit of a blood product should be transfused over fewer than 4 hours. If the clinical situation requires infusion of the unit over a period of greater than 4 hours, that unit should be divided into aliquots and each infused over no more than 4 hours. It is also advisable to change blood filters every 4 hours (Pisciotto, 1993).

## Warming of Blood

Cold blood infused to adults at rates exceeding 100 mL/min has been associated with cardiac arrest. Therefore, the rapid infusion of large volumes (>50 mL/kg/hr) should be accomplished with warmed blood. Both the water-bath and electric heating plate types of warmers should be equipped with a visible thermometer and, ideally, an audible alarm. Blood must not be warmed above 42°C, because overheating may result in hemolysis (Standards Committee, 1994).

## *Intravenous Solutions*

Only normal saline (0.9% USP) may be infused along with blood products. Solutions containing glucose may be hypotonic and cause hemolysis. The calcium in lactated Ringer's solution may coagulate citrated blood. For a variety of reasons, medications should never be added to a unit of blood. Because of their high pH, some drugs cause hemolysis. If a reaction occurs, it will be impossible to determine if its source is the drug or the transfused component. If transfusion of a unit is interrupted, it will not be possible to determine exactly what portion of the intended dose of medication the recipient received (Pisciotto, 1993).

## *Filters*

All blood products must be given through a filter. Standard blood filters, which have a pore size of about 170 μm, remove most macroaggregates (e.g., clots and debris). Microaggregates, which form in blood that has been stored for over 5 days, may lodge in the pulmonary circulation. However, the clinical significance of this finding is unclear. Because of this and because of the risk of microaggregate filters (pore size, 20–40 μm) becoming clogged and therefore inhibiting rapid transfusion, some feel that their selective use should be determined by the hospital's transfusion committee (Pisciotto, 1993). Others (Klein, 1992) feel that microfilters should be used routinely for patients who are thrombocytopenic and for those receiving massive transfusions.

## Complications of Blood Transfusions

### Infectious Disease Transmission

#### *Viral Infections: Donor Deferral*

Most blood-borne viral infections have potentially serious consequences for recipients should they become infected. Evidence of, or the possibility of, infection with the viruses discussed in this section is grounds for indefinite deferral as a blood

donor (Standards Committee, 1994). The risk of transfusion-related viral infections has recently been reviewed by Schreiber and colleagues (1996). Unfortunately, 1% to 2% of blood donors have unreported risk factors at the time of blood donation (Williams, 1997).

**Human Immunodeficiency Virus**   Likely more than any other development, the recognition by the medical community of the potential for transfusion-associated transmission of HIV and subsequent patient and consumer activism have contributed to a cautious reexamination of blood collection, storage, and transfusion policies (Crosby, 1992). In 1985, when tests for antibody to HIV were licensed, the U.S. Public Health Service recommended that all donated blood or plasma be tested for HIV antibody. In the United States, the incidence of transfusion-acquired HIV infection decreased from 714 cases in 1984 to 288 in 1985 to fewer than 20 per year from 1986 to 1991 (Selik, 1993). A 1993 report from Australia found no new cases of transfusion-associated HIV transmission since 1985 (Wylie, 1993).

Because the tests used to screen for HIV are assays for antibody, it is theoretically possible to donate infected blood during the "window" period between infection and antibody development. While screening for viral antigen, therefore, seems logical, at least two studies failed to identify p24 antigen in the absence of HIV antibody (Alter, 1990; Roberts, 1991). One case, however, has been reported in which blood that screened antibody-negative by four of five ELISA tests was found to contain HIV p24 antigen and genomeric RNA material (Roberts, 1994). In 1996, p24 antigen testing of donor blood became a requirement.

A recent estimate of blood-borne HIV transmission is one case per 450,000 to 660,000 donations of screened blood (Lackritz, 1995). Although the risk of transmission-associated HIV infection is low, it must be remembered that because of the division of whole blood into components (see Fig 11-1), one infected donor may potentially infect several recipients. A further reduction in the transmission of this lethal virus awaits the development of more sensitive screening tests and, perhaps, further scrutiny of existing transfusion policies.

**Hepatitis** Jaundice following within 1 to 4 months of a blood transfusion was first recognized in 1943 (Crosby, 1992). Subsequently, the causal relationship between antecedent transfusion and subsequent hepatitis was clearly recognized. Although HIV infection has attracted the fear and concern of both the medical community and the lay public, non-A, non-B hepatitis is much more likely to be a cause of death following transfusion than is HIV infection (Spence, 1993).

A number of variables affect calculations of the incidence and prevalence of posttransfusion hepatitis (PTH). Most PTH is anicteric. Therefore, studies relying on clinical diagnosis might underestimate the prevalence of the virus among transfusion recipients. Depending on the causal virus, the responsible blood product, and the test sensitivity, the timing of testing relative to the transfusion and frequency of repeat testing will likely alter the ability to detect the disease. Finally, products derived from large donor pools (e.g., factor concentrates) or those from multiple donors given at one time (e.g., platelets) will have a higher risk of disease transmission than will those from single donors (Crosby, 1992).

The clinical courses of hepatitis B and C infections differ substantially. Approximately 85% of patients with hepatitis B resolve spontaneously. The remaining 9% progress to chronic persistent hepatitis, 3% to chronic active hepatitis, 1% to cirrhosis, 1% to fulminant hepatitis, and 1% to hepatocellular carcinoma. In contrast, only 48% of hepatitis C infections resolve spontaneously. The remaining 28% progress to chronic persistent hepatitis, 13% to chronic active hepatitis, 10% to cirrhosis, and 1% to fulminant hepatitis. The relationship between hepatitis C and hepatocellular carcinoma is unclear (Carson, 1993; Takano, 1994; Walker, 1987; Alter, 1994a,b; Heymann, 1993).

The development of serologic tests for hepatitis B and C has had a marked impact on the incidence of PTH. A test for hepatitis B surface antigen became available in the 1970s. However, the removal of hepatitis B carriers from the donor pool decreased the incidence of PTH by only 10%. It rapidly became evident that the majority of PTH was due to a virus that was not detectable by serologic tests for either hepatitis A or B. In the 1980s, data emerged that suggested the presence of hepatitis B core antibody (HBcAb) and/or elevated alanine aminotransferase (ALT) was associated with an increased risk of non-A, non-B hepatitis (Seef, 1988; Koziol, 1986). The use of these surrogate markers to eliminate infected donors decreased, but did not eliminate PTH (Morris, 1994). The development of tests for the detection of antibody to hepatitis C in the 1990s was a major advance. Retrospective analysis has demonstrated that virtually all transfusion-associated non-A, non-B hepatitis is due to hepatitis C (Ismay, 1995). Screening all potential blood donors for antibody to hepatitis C has resulted in a reduction in the incidence of PTH to 0% to 2% per transfusion (Gonzalez, 1995; Huang, 1994; Wang, 1994).

The availability of sensitive second-generation tests for hepatitis C antibody draws into question the continued use of surrogate markers as a screening tool to eliminate potential blood donors. At issue is the ability of these tests to narrow the window of detectability in persons with recent-onset hepatitis C infection and to detect other causes of clinically significant PTH. Available data suggest that neither purpose is served, but that continued screening for elevated ALT and HBcAb results in the needless elimination of potential donors (Alter, 1994a,b; Blajchman, 1995).

Other types of hepatitis are infrequently transmitted by blood transfusion. Transmission of hepatitis A virus by pooled plasma derivatives has been reported in hemophiliacs (Mosley, 1994). Hepatitis D is transmitted by the delta agent, an RNA virus that is dependent on hepatitis B for its replication. Delta hepatitis infection may be concurrent with hepatitis B infection (coinfection) or may be found in a hepatitis B carrier (superinfection). Prevention of delta hepatitis transmission is accomplished by prevention of transmission of hepatitis B (Wylie, 1993).

**Human T-lymphotropic Virus Types I and II** Both human T-lymphotropic virus types I and II (HTLV-I and HTLV-II) are retroviruses related to HIV. One characteristic that differentiates HIV and the HTLVs is that the former results in cell lysis, while the latter results in cell proliferation (Crosby, 1992). Unlike HIV, which is found in all blood components, HTLV infections are transmitted exclusively by cellular blood components. Thus, recipients of acellular components (e.g., plasma) are not at risk of HTLV infections. In addition, blood stored for over 10 days will not transmit this infection, probably because of the loss of the virus' ability to proliferate in lymphocytes that have undergone prolonged storage (Donegan, 1994).

Available testing for the HTLVs is complicated by the lack of simple, inexpensive tests to distinguish type I from type II (Wylie, 1993). This distinction has some clinical importance: HTLV-I may cause T-cell leukemia, tropical spastic paraphe-resis, and HTLV-I-associated myelopathy. The potential for infected blood products to cause clinical disease is, however, unknown (Crosby, 1992). HTLV-II has been found in patients with T-cell hairy-cell leukemia (Wylie, 1993). Although the risk of HTLV-I infection is largely related to geography, with the disease being endemic to Japan, parts of Papua, New Guinea; Africa; and the Caribbean, the distribution of HTLV-II infection is associated more with injected drug use than with geography (Dodd, 1995).

**Jakob-Creutzfeldt Disease** First described in 1920, this diffuse degenerative disorder of the cerebellar and cerebral cortex is characterized by progressive dementia, spasticity or rigidity, and ataxia. Transmission of the virus causing this disease to recipients of human pituitary hormone extracts has been reported. Although no transmission of Jakob-Creutzfeldt disease by a blood transfusion has ever been reported, individuals who have received human pituitary growth hormone may not donate blood (Standards Committee, 1994; Wylie, 1993).

---

### Other Viral Infections

Other viruses may be transmitted by blood components but are not grounds for deferral as a blood donor. A few of those that have relevance to perinatal medicine will be discussed.

**Cytomegalovirus** Cytomegalovirus (CMV) is a ubiquitous DNA virus that, depending on geographic location, has a prevalence of from 40% to 100% (Wylie, 1993). Its distribution is also a function of demographics, being found more often

among densely populated, lower socioeconomic groups (Bowden, 1995). Following primary infection, the virus remains latent (presumably in leukocytes) for life and may cause recurrent infection when reactivated. Most infections caused by CMV are either minor or totally asymptomatic. Those individuals whose immune response is impaired, however, may suffer significant morbidity and mortality from CMV-induced pneumonia, hepatitis, gastroenteritis, retinitis, and disseminated disease (Sayers, 1994; Tegtmeier, 1994). The latter includes recipients of solid organ or bone marrow transplants, patients receiving immunosuppressive chemotherapy, splenectomized patients, and those suffering from AIDS. Maternal acquisition of CMV infection during pregnancy may result in a severely infected neonate. Cytomegalovirus remains the major congenital infection that causes mental retardation and deafness (Wylie, 1993).

It is clear that leukocytes are the vehicle for transmission of CMV infections in blood transfusion. Thus, acellular products, such as plasma and cryoprecipitate, will not transmit CMV. Measures for prevention of transmission of CMV should be activated for all blood recipients, including seronegative pregnant women, who are at risk for serious CMV infection. These measures include the transfusion of cellular blood products from CMV-negative donors. When a CMV-negative donor cannot be located, alternatives include transfusion of frozen and deglycerolized red cells or leukocyte-reduced RBCs. To effectively decrease the risk of CMV transmission, the latter must have a leukocyte count no greater than $5 \times 10^6$ (Standards Committee, 1994; Pisciotto, 1993; Bowden, 1995; Sayers, 1994).

**Parvovirus B19** Human parvovirus B19 is a nonenveloped, single-stranded DNA virus. Antibodies to B19 are found in 50% of adults. The virus is usually transmitted via respiratory secretions. Transmission of the virus by transfused blood products, however, has been documented (Sayers, 1994; Tegtmeier, 1994; Luban, 1994). Because the virus does not have a lipid envelope and is heat-stable, it is resistant to methods currently used to inactivate viruses, such as solvent/detergent and heat treatment. Thus, clotting factor concentrates that have undergone such treatment (e.g., factors VIII and IX) have transmitted the virus (Tegtmeier, 1994; Luban, 1994).

The disease caused by parvovirus B19 is usually benign. The virus, however, does have an affinity for late erythroid progenitor cells. While the hemolytic anemia caused by parvovirus B19 is usually transient, concern has been expressed about transmission of the virus to three subsets of patients. Those who have a chronic hemolytic anemia run the risk of aplastic crises when infected with the virus. A chronic form of parvovirus B19 infection has been reported in patients who have both congenital (e.g., Nezeloff's syndrome) and acquired (e.g., leukemia, AIDS) immunocompromise (Sayers, 1994; Luban, 1994). Parvovirus B19 infection during pregnancy has been identified as a cause of transient fetal aplastic crisis, which may result in fetal hydrops and death (Porter, 1988). Currently, there are no blood-banking standards or guidelines with regard to avoidance of parvovirus B19 transmission.

## Protozoal Infections

**Malaria** Malaria is a disease characterized by high spiking fevers and severe shaking chills. It is caused by protozoa of the *Plasmodium* genus (falciparum, vivax, ovale, and malariae). Although these are obligate intracellular parasites, transmission has been reported from cryoprecipitate as well as RBCs and platelets (Wylie, 1993). Unlike malaria transmitted by infected mosquitoes, transfusion-transmitted parasites bypass the exoerythrocytic stage in the life cycle of the plasmodium and, therefore, do not cause relapses.

In malaria-endemic areas, most blood recipients will have antibodies to the *Plasmodium* species and, therefore, are unlikely to be infected by blood from an infected donor. Infection is most likely if a donor who has lived in or traveled to an endemic area gives blood for a recipient in a non-endemic area (Tegtmeier, 1994). In the United States, prospective donors who have had a diagnosis of malaria are deferred for 3 years after becoming asymptomatic. Immigrants, refugees, and citizens from endemic areas who have been asymptomatic for 3 years following departure from the endemic area are acceptable as blood donors. Travelers from countries where malaria is non-endemic who have been to areas where the disease is endemic may donate blood 1 year after return, provided that they have remained asymptomatic (Standards Committee, 1994).

**Chagas' Disease** Chagas' disease is caused by *Trypanosoma cruzi*, a protozoon that has a predilection for myocardial cells and smooth muscle cells in the colon and the esophagus. The acute form of the disease may be fatal. Survivors may progress to subacute and chronic forms. Although the disease is classically transmitted to humans from infected wild and domestic animals by insects, the risk of blood-borne disease transmission is 12% to 50% (Wylie, 1993). Chagas' disease is endemic to South and Central America and Mexico. Likely because of migration from these areas, transmission via blood transfusion has been reported in the United States and Canada (Tegtmeier, 1994). A history of Chagas' disease requires permanent deferral as a blood donor (Standards Committee, 1994).

**Babesiosis** Human babesiosis is caused by the intraerythrocytic protozoan *Babesia microti*. Because the illness caused by this protozoa in the immunocompetent host is so mild, it has likely been underreported (Shulman, 1994). *Babesia* infection is endemic to coastal lands and islands of the northeastern United States. The usual route of infection is tick-borne from wild and domestic animals to humans. However, blood-borne infection also has been reported (American Red Cross, 1994). Because of this, a history of babesiosis is grounds for permanent exclusion as a blood donor (Standards Committee, 1994).

## Spirochete Infections

**Syphilis** *Treponema pallidum*, the spirochete that causes syphilis, cannot survive for more than 72 to 96 hours at temperatures below 4°C. Because most blood products are stored for longer periods and at lower temperatures than those at which this organism can survive, transmission of syphilis by a blood transfusion is quite rare (Berkman, 1988). Potential blood donors who have a history of syphilis or a reactive test for syphilis in the absence of a negative confirmatory test are deferred for 1 year after completion of treatment (Standards Committee, 1994).

## Other Nonbacterial Infections

A variety of other viruses, protozoa, and spirochetes may be transmitted by transfusion of blood components. Not all of these are known to cause serious disease. A list of these organisms is found in Table 11-3.

## Bacterial Infections

A patient who experiences chills, high fever, and cardiovascular collapse during or immediately following a blood transfusion should be suspected of having received a product that is contaminated with bacteria (American Red Cross, 1994; Sazama, 1994; Blajchman, 1994). Investigation of the source of contamination requires immediate collection of blood samples from the recipient for culture, the blood container, and the filter. A Gram

T A B L E   **11-3**

Nonbacterial infectious organisms that may be transmitted by blood transfusions

| Viruses | Protozoa | Spirochetes |
|---|---|---|
| Colorado tick fever | *Toxoplasma gondii* | *Borrelia* species |
| Dengue virus | *Leishmania species* | |
| Ebola virus | | |
| Ebstein-Barr virus | Filarial infections | |
| Hepatitis E | | |
| Herpesvirus 6 | | |
| Lassa virus | | |
| Rift valley fever | | |

The potential for transfusion transmission and/or serious disease for many of these organisms is unknown.

Sources: Data from American Red Cross, Council of Community Blood Centers, American Association of Blood Banks. Circular of information for the use of human blood and blood components. Bethesda, MD: American Association of Blood Banks, 1994; Sayers MH. Transfusion-transmitted viral infections other than hepatitis and human immunodeficiency virus infection. Arch Pathol Lab Med 1994;118:346–365; Schulman IA. Parasitic infections and their impact on blood donor selection and testing. Arch Pathol Lab Med 1994;118:366–370; and Wylie BR. Transfusion transmitted infection: viral and exotic diseases. Anaesth Intensive Care 1993;21:24–30.

stain of the blood left in the container should be examined promptly. Therapeutic measures include stopping the transfusion, broad-spectrum antibiotics, vasopressors, and intravenous fluids (Standards Committee, 1994; Sazama, 1994).

Serious morbidity and mortality due to bacterial contamination of transfused blood products have been reported (Table 11-4) (Sazama, 1994; Blajchman, 1994; Haditsch, 1994). Measures proposed to limit bacterial contamination include improved donor screening, reduced storage time, and improved physical and chemical sterilization of blood products (Sazama, 1994; Blajchman, 1994). The limitation of bacterial contamination may be an unexpected benefit of solvent/detergent viral inactivation of FFP (Sazama, 1994; Thomas, 1994).

## Complications of Massive Transfusions

The inability of older equipment to transfuse large volumes of blood within a short period, coupled with the rapid adaptations of transfused blood products to their new hosts, relegated the identification of problems unique to massive transfusions to the realm of the theoretical. However, technologic advances now permitting the transfusion of up to four blood volumes per hour (Crosby, 1992) require knowledge of prevention, recognition, and treatment of complications unique to massive transfusions. In addition, the synergistic effect of simultaneously occurring complications (e.g., acidosis, hypocalcemia, hypothermia) must be borne in mind.

## Hypocalcemia and Citrate Toxicity

Each unit of RBCs contains approximately 3 g of citrate. Ordinarily, this citrate is rapidly metabolized in the liver to bicarbonate. However, compromised hepatic function due to liver disease, hypothermia, or low cardiac output, as well as transfusion rates in excess of 1 unit every 5 minutes may overwhelm the body's ability to metabolize citrate. The resultant hypocalcemia may become manifest clinically as hypotension, elevated diastolic and central venous pressures, and narrow pulse pressure. It is unusual for the inhibiting effect of citrate on coagulation pathways to result in clinical bleeding until calcium levels have

TABLE **11-4**

Reported bacterial contaminants of blood components resulting in fatalities.

| Gram-positive Bacteria | Gram-negative bacteria |
| --- | --- |
| Alpha-hemolytic streptococcus | *Enterobacter cloacae* |
| *Bacillus cereus* | *Klebsiella oxytoca* |
| *Bacillus subtilis* | *Klebsiella pneumoniae* |
| *Clostridium perfringens* | *Klebsiella* species |
| *Clostridium* species | *Proteus mirabilis* |
| *Propionibacterium acnes* | *Pseudomonas aeruginosa* |
| *Staphylococcus aureus* | *Pseudomonas* species |
| *Staphylococcus epidermidis* | *Salmonella choleraesuis* |
| *Staphylococcus warneri* | *Salmonella,* type B |
| *Streptococcus mitis* | *Serratia marcescens* |
| | *Yersinia enterocolitica* |

Source: Data from Sazama K. Bacteria in blood for transfusion. Arch Pathol Lab Med 1994;118:350–365.

fallen to a level sufficient to cause cardiac arrest. Electrocardiograph monitoring may be useful in the early detection of hypocalcemia. Hypotension following correction of hypovolemia provides a clinical clue to this complication. Calcium chloride may be cautiously given to patients exhibiting ECG changes and/or who demonstrate a measured decrease in ionic calcium (American Red Cross, 1994; Donaldson, 1992; Crosby, 1992).

### Hyperkalemia and Hypokalemia

After 2 weeks of storage, RBC-containing products have a high potassium concentration. Following transfusion, viable red cells restore their capacity to pump potassium from the extracellular space into the RBC. While hyperkalemia following massive transfusion of stored blood is unusual, *hypokalemia* resulting from metabolic alkalosis secondary to the production of bicarbonate from citrate is not. Lethal cardiac arrhythmias found coincident with transfusion-associated hyperkalemia have been reported (Donaldson, 1992; Crosby, 1992). The use of ECG monitoring during massive transfusions, therefore, seems prudent.

### Acid-Base Disturbances

Stored citrated blood accumulates an acid load both because of the anticoagulant citric acid and

the lactate generated by RBCs during storage. Theoretically, the transfusion of stored blood into a patient already undergoing a metabolic acidosis due to hypotension and tissue hypoxia may aggravate the acidosis. Following transfusion, however, the citrate is usually rapidly metabolized to bicarbonate, which may produce a metabolic alkalosis. In addition, the restoration of circulating volume and oxygen-carrying capacity usually results in a reduction of endogenous lactate production. The acid-base changes accompanying massive transfusion are, therefore, usually well tolerated.

### Hypothermia

The administration of 1 to 2 units of RBCs taken directly from storage at 1°C to 6°C is not likely to pose a risk to the recipient. However, a number of potentially serious metabolic effects may attend the rapid transfusion of a large volume of cold blood into a hypovolemic recipient. Energy expenditure in the amount of 300 kcal may be required to restore normothermia. A drop in core temperature has been associated causally with a decrease in cardiac output and an increase in metabolic acidosis. Transfusion-induced hypothermia in the operating room may be aggravated further by heat loss from skin or exposed body cavities. Patients who become hypothermic during massive transfusions have a higher mortality than those who maintain normothermia (Donaldson, 1992; Crosby, 1992). Normal body temperature in the face of massive transfusion may be maintained by using blood warmers. Additional measures include placing the patient on a warming mattress and by warming and humidifying all ventilatory gases used during surgery (Donaldson, 1992).

## Immune-Mediated Complications

### Transfusion Reactions

A transfusion reaction may be defined broadly as any untoward occurrence directly attributable to an infused blood product. Such reactions may be classified relative to both the time of transfusion (acute or delayed) and to the site of hemolysis (intravascular or extravascular). Transfusion reactions may be noted in up to 10% of all recipients (Pisciotto, 1993). While the overwhelming majority are not life-threatening, acute intravascular hemolytic reactions are the most common cause of transfusion-associated deaths (Donaldson, 1992).

**Acute Hemolytic Reactions**  Acute intravascular hemolytic reactions result from the transfusion of either incompatible cells or plasma. These, in turn, are most often due to individual and systematic errors, such as collection of the blood sample from the wrong person, incorrect identification of samples, incorrect data recording, release of the incorrect unit, and administration of blood to the wrong recipient (Linden, 1994; Taswell, 1994). Although computerization of records and computer-generated labels have helped reduce the incidence of these life-threatening reactions, minimizing human error remains a challenge to blood banks and clinical services (Crosby, 1992; Taswell, 1994).

The mechansims underlying acute hemolytic transfusion reactions are complex. Every type O recipient has "naturally occurring" antibodies to type A, B, or AB antigens in plasma and in the extravascular space. Thus, the transfusion of types A, B, or AB cells to a type O recipient initiates the immunologic processes at the core of a hemolytic reaction. By the same mechanism, but to a lesser extent, the transfusion of plasma products from a type O donor to a type A, B, or AB recipient may also result in an acute hemolytic transfusion reaction (Pisciotto, 1993; Crosby, 1992).

Because the majority of life-threatening transfusion reactions occur within minutes of initiating a transfusion, a patient receiving a blood product should be monitored carefully throughout the transfusion. In an acute hemolytic reaction, IgM antibodies complex with corresponding RBC antigens. These antigen-antibody complexes and/or complement-fixing IgG then activate complement. The binding of the C5-9 component of complement (the membrane attack complex) results in the formation of a pore in the RBC membrane. Hemoglobin leaks through this pore into the serum. The free hemoglobin is bound initially by circulating haptoglobin and albumen. As these proteins rapidly become saturated, however, hemoglobin is cleared by the kidney, and hemoglobinuria may be noted. Complement activation also results in the generation of complement fragments. Vasoactive fragment C3a causes hypotension and often rebound tachycardia. Fragment C5a activates granulocytes and causes migration and adhesion of neutrophils to the pulmonary capillary bed, thus interfering with the normal exchange of oxygen and carbon dioxide. The deposition of antibody-coated red-cell stroma in the kidney produces renal vasoconstriction, which in turn may lead to acute tubular necrosis and renal failure. Complement fragments are also responsible for thrombin generation and platelet activation, which may, in turn, precipitate disseminated intravascular coagulation. Cytokines, a group of non-antibody proteins that are activated by antigens, may also play a role in acute hemolytic transfusion reactions. In an experimental model of ABO-incompatible reactions, interleukins (IL-)1, 6, and 8 as well as tumor necrosis factor-$\alpha$ (TNF-$\alpha$) were generated by lymphocytes. These cytokines may by their action cause or aggravate hypotension. In addition, IL-6, IL-8, and TNF-$\alpha$ are pyrogens that are responsible for the fever sometimes found in these reactions (American Red Cross, 1994; Crosby, 1992; Snyder, 1994; Perkins, 1995).

The severity of an acute intravascular hemolytic transfusion reaction is dependent on both the rate of transfusion and the dose of transfused blood product. Prompt recognition is, therefore, imperative. The most common signs reported in fatal reactions are hemolysis, hemoglobinemia, hemoglobinuria, disseminated intravascular coagulation, hypotension, and oliguria with subsequent renal failure. An acute intravascular hemolytic transfusion reaction occurring during general anesthesia may present with more subtle findings; sudden urticaria, generalized bleeding, and hypotension disproportionate to blood loss may be the first clues (Crosby, 1992). Management of a reaction requires discontinuation of the transfused product, evaluation of its source, and support of the patient's vital functions (Table 11-5).

Most acute hemolytic transfusion reactions are intravascular. However, if the antibody does not fix complement, as is true of most IgG antibodies, or if it fixes only to C3, acute hemolysis may occur extravascularly (Piciotto, 1993).

Other nonimmunologically mediated causes must be borne in mind when evaluating the patient with acute hemolysis. These include hemolysis due to administration of hypotonic fluid, bacterial infection or contamination, and hemolysis of RBCs prior to transfusion by improper overheating or freezing (American Red Cross, 1994).

**Delayed Hemolytic Reactions** Delayed hemolytic transfusion reactions are due to the induction of an antibody response by transfused RBCs days or weeks following a transfusion. While a primary delayed transfusion reaction is usually manifested weeks following transfusion, an anamnestic response is frequently seen within days of the event. The latter should be suspected in patients who have had previous exposure to RBCs (e.g., women who have been pregnant previously and/or those who previously received blood products). Prevention of these reactions is likely not possible. Routinely performing a complete crossmatch for all donor units rather than an immediate spin crossmatch for potential recipients who on initial screening exhibited no antibodies has not been shown to decrease the risk of delayed hemolytic transfusion reactions (Pinkerton, 1992).

Because the antibodies involved in a delayed hemolytic transfusion reaction generally do not fix the C5-9 complement component, they are rarely of a magnitude that is life-threatening. If complement is fixed, the cascade usually stops at C3. C3 complement receptors in the liver remove

T A B L E   **11-5**

**Diagnostic evaluation and clinical management of a suspected acute intravascular hemolytic transfusion reaction**

*Immediate Management*

Stop transfusion.

Aggressive fluids (crystalloids or colloids) to maintain adequate circulatory volume.

Maintain adequate ventilation.

Maintain renal perfusion; osmotic diuretics as needed.

Consider platelet and plasma transfusion if DIC producing uncontrolled bleeding.

Consider plasma exchange to remove large volumes of free hemoglobin.

Collect specimens for blood bank work-up.

Consider blood cultures, especially if febrile.

*Blood Bank Work-up*

Examine label on blood containers and all other records to detect a possible error in identifying the patient or the blood.

Send new, properly labeled postreaction blood and urine samples from the patient to the blood bank.

Send the blood container and attached transfusion set and intravenous solutions to the blood bank.

Evaluate postreaction plasma for hemoglobinuria. The prereaction sample may be used for comparison.

Perform a direct antiglobulin (Coombs') test on the postreaction sample. If positive, a prereaction sample should be compared.

Repeat crossmatch.

Analyze urine for hemoglobinuria.

Sources: Data from Standards Committee, American Association of Blood Banks. Standards for blood banks and transfusion services. 16th ed. Bethesda, MD: American Association of Blood Banks, 1994; Pisciotto PT. Blood transfusion therapy. A physician's handbook. Bethesda, MD: American Association of Blood Banks, 1993; Crosby ET. Perioperative haemotherapy: II. Risks and complications of blood transfusion. Can J Anaesth 1992;39:822–837.

RBCs, while IgG-coated RBCs are removed in the spleen (Piciotto, 1993). Thus the majority of delayed hemolytic reactions occur extravascularly. Most delayed reactions are characterized merely by the appearance of an antibody, demonstrated by a positive direct antiglobulin test (American Red Cross, 1994; Crosby, 1992). Other manifestations may include a progressive fall in hemoglobin concentration, low-grade fever, and indirect hyperbilirubinemia. Free hemoglobinemia and hemoglobinuria are rare. Most delayed hemolytic transfusion reactions require no special treatment. The unusual patient who demonstrates findings consistent with a severe delayed hemolytic reaction should receive the same management as a patient with an acute intravascular hemolytic reaction (see Table 11-5).

**Febrile Nonhemolytic Reactions** Fever may be a manifestation of an acute or delayed hemolytic reaction. It may also accompany transfusion of a product contaminated by bacteria. However, the most common cause of fever that accompanies a transfusion is an antibody-mediated reaction to leukocyte antigens. This occurs in approximately 1% of all transfusions. It is characterized by a temperature elevation of 1°C or more, possibly associated with chills but rarely with hypotension (Pisciotto, 1993; American Red Cross, 1994). The diagnosis is one of exclusion. Antipyretics are the only treatment indicated. Given the seriousness of other differential diagnoses, however, it is sometimes appropriate to presumptively manage a transfused patient who develops a fever as one who has an acute intravascular hemolytic reaction (see Table 11-5).

Because febrile nonhemolytic reactions are mediated by antibodies to leukocytes, it was originally thought that transfusion with blood products that contain a reduced quantity of leukocytes (e.g., leukocyte-reduced or washed RBCs) would decrease the incidence of these reactions. While this did prove to be the case (Miller, 1995), the persistence of febrile reactions following transfusion with leukocyte-depleted products as well as following platelet transfusions suggested the possibility of other mechanisms causing the fever. It is now known that lymphocytes stored with either RBCs or platelets may generate cytokines that are pyrogens. Employing leukocyte-depleting filters at the time of transfusion will not prevent these pyrogens from entering the recipient's circulation. Leukodepletion at the time of donation, however, may eliminate or markedly decrease the concentration of donor lymphocytes (Snyder, 1994).

**Allergic Reactions** Allergic reactions are immune-mediated clinical responses to transfused plasma proteins. Clinically, they run the gamut from minor urticaria to systemic anaphylaxis including bronchospasm and cardiovascular collapse (Piciotto, 1993; American Red Cross, 1994; Isbister, 1993). Most allergic reactions are mild and will respond to oral or intramuscular antihistamines. Because the severity of an allergic reaction is usually not dose- or duration-dependent, a unit of blood that is producing a mild, localized reaction may be continued after medication is given and the reaction subsides. In this instance, the risk of disease transmission from a new unit outweighs the risk of continuing the previous allergy-producing unit (Pisciotto, 1993).

A unique and more serious allergic reaction may be seen in the rare recipient who is deficient in all classes of IgA antibodies and who has a high titer of anti-IgA IgG antibodies. Reportedly 1 in 400 to 1 in 2000 people have a selective IgA deficiency; approximately 20% to 60% of these will develop anti-IgA antibodies (Crosby, 1992; Isbister, 1993). When such an IgA-deficient patient receives a blood product from a non-IgA-deficient donor, a severe systemic reaction may ensue. An IgA-deficient recipient who manifests such a reaction is likely to have another severe reaction following subsequent transfusion with a blood product containing plasma that has IgA. Prevention of anaphylaxis in these recipients may be accomplished by transfusing with autologous products, products obtained from IgA-deficient donors, or those from which plasma has been removed (washed RBCs, frozen/deglycerolized RBCs) (Pisciotto, 1993; American Red Cross, 1994; Crosby, 1992; Isbister, 1993).

### Graft-Versus-Host Disease

Graft-versus-host disease occurs as a consequence of the transfusion of viable T-lymphocytes present in donor cellular components (e.g., RBCs, platelets). These T cells engraft, proliferate, and then react against host tissues. The disease is found most often in recipients who have compromised immune systems, such as bone marrow transplant recipients, those with congenital immune deficiency syndromes, and fetuses in utero. It has also been reported in immunocompetent HLA heterozygous patients who receive cells from HLA homozygous donors. The latter is seen more often in recipients who are first- or second-degree relatives of the donors (Pisciotto, 1993; American Red Cross, 1994; Benson, 1994).

Probably because bone marrow is donor derived, GVHD in bone marrow recipients is usually benign and characterized by a diffuse maculopapular rash affecting predominantly proximal areas (Appleton, 1994). Transfusion-associated GVHD, however, which usually appears 6 to 10 days following transfusion, usually has a more fulminant course. In addition to the rash, fever, diarrhea, and hepatitis ensue. Bone marrow hypocellularity and pancytopenia are both common and fatal (Pisciotto, 1993; American Red Cross, 1994; Appleton, 1994). Gamma irradiation of donor cells prevents the proliferation of donor lymphocytes in the recipient. It is a blood banking standard that only irradiated cellular blood components are given to recipients at risk for GVHD. The latter include fetuses receiving intrauterine transfusions and recipients of donor units from a blood relative (Standards Committee, 1994).

### Transfusion-Related Lung Injury

Transfusion-related lung injury (TRALI) is a rare but potentially fatal complication of blood transfusions. It is characterized by noncardiogenic pulmonary edema, usually occurring within 4 to 8 hours of a transfusion. Symptoms include dyspnea, cough, chills, and fever. Physical findings include tachycardia, tachypnea, wheezing, crepitations, and cyanosis. Bilateral interstitial infiltrates are seen on chest x-ray. Central monitoring reveals normal pulmonary capillary wedge pressure and cardiac output, but pulmonary artery pressure may become elevated (Pisciotto, 1993; Malouf, 1993).

While the pathophysiology underlying this complication seems immunologically based, the specific mechanisms are unclear. The passive transfer of anti-HLA or anti-WBC antibodies as well as recipient alloimmunization have been implicated (Pisciotto, 1993). Factors involved in pulmonary injury may include activated complement, cytokines, and metabolites of arachidonic acid (Malouf, 1993).

The clinical management of suspected TRALI involves stopping the transfusion and providing supportive care. Recurrence of TRALI with a subsequent transfusion is not likely.

### Cancer Recurrence

Reviews of human and animal data suggest an immunosuppressive effect, however transient, by allogeneic blood transfusion (Spence, 1993; Blumberg, 1994). Whether this immunosuppression contributes to a shortening of life due to tumor recurrence in recipients who have a preexisting cancer is not clear. Clarification of the issue is hampered by the likelihood that it is the patient with advanced disease who is more likely to receive a transfusion. Retrospective studies controlling for such variables as cancer type and extent have produced conflicting results (Blumberg, 1994; Molland, 1995). The use of leukocyte-poor or autologous blood products for cancer patients has not been demonstrated to limit tumor recurrence (Blumberg, 1994).

## Autologous Donation

Autologous blood donation is the process of collecting and storing blood when the donor and the recipient are the same individual. Of the three methods of autologous collection (predonation, intraoperative salvage, and normovolemic hemodilution), only autologous predonation has a limited potential for application in obstetrics. It is useful for those patients who have rare blood types or for those who have antibodies that make it difficult to find compatible blood. Autologous blood has certain advantages for the donor-recipient. The risks of infectious disease transmission; alloimmunization to RBC, leukocyte, and platelet antigens; and hemolytic, allergic, febrile, and graft-versus-host reactions should be minimized (Pisciotti, 1993). However, autologous blood donation and reinfusion are not devoid of risks.

During donation of 450 mL of whole blood, BP decreases slightly but recovers within 10 minutes of donation (Walpoth, 1993). A severe hypotensive reaction occurs in about one of every 500 donations (AuBuchon, 1994). Because of this risk, some feel that patients with serious cardiac diseases (e.g., unstable angina, severe aortic stenosis, valvular heart disease, history of congestive heart failure) should not be considered for autologous predonation (Spence, 1993; Ereth, 1994). One study, however, found no statistically significant differences in hemodynamics or reaction severity in comparing high-risk with low-risk autologous donors. Only first-time donation and the use of cardiac glycosides were associated with a reaction at the time of autologous donation (Hillyer, 1994). Concern has been expressed that the few pregnant autologous donors who have hypotensive reaction might put their fetuses at risk. Transient fetal bradycardias and painless uterine contractions have been reported during maternal blood donations. However, no detrimental outcomes for newborns of mothers who had reactions at the time of donation have been reported (Gibson, 1993).

Reinfusion of stored autologous blood carries with it certain risks. Clerical error is as much a possibility with autologous as with homologous units. A major concern is the possibility of accidental transfusion of HIV-positive blood into an HIV-negative recipient. The likelihood of this happening is the product of the independent risk of transfusion to the wrong recipient and the rate of HIV seroprevalence in autologous units. That likelihood has been estimated to be 1:120,000,000 to 1:250,000,000. To date, there have been no documented instances of HIV infection having been transmitted in this fashion (Yomtovian, 1995). Clerical error may also result in a hemolytic reaction. Acute intravascular hemolysis may also occur following inadequate deglycerolization of previously frozen blood. Hypotension accompanying reinfusion of autologous blood has been attributed to hypersensitivity to stabilizers of sterilizing agents used in plastic bags and tubing (Stehling, 1994b). Bacterial contamination of any stored blood product may occur.

Criteria for donation for autologous blood are less stringent than those for homologous donation. The hemoglobin concentration of the donor-recipient's blood must be at least 11 g/dL and/or the hematocrit at least 33%. Bacteremia or a significant bacterial infection that may be associated with bacteremia is a reason for tempo-

rary deferral for autologous donation. Only autologous blood that will be transfused outside the collecting facility must be tested for HIV and hepatitis. There are no age or weight requirements for donation (Standards Committee, 1994).

During pregnancy, the uncertainty of both the date of delivery and the timing of transfusion pose the problem of appropriate frequency, timing, and storage of autologous blood. Of those obstetrics patients requiring transfusion, the majority will require 2 or fewer units (Pepkowitz, 1993). One approach is to collect blood during the last month of pregnancy and to store it in the liquid state at 1°C to 6°C for 35 to 42 days, depending on the storage solution used (O'Dwyer, 1993). Another approach is to collect blood earlier in pregnancy and to hold it in frozen storage (Pepkowitz, 1993). A third approach is the "leapfrog" technique, wherein blood is collected at a time remote from term. A unit that is about to expire is transfused back to the autologous donor, and she then donates 2 fresh units within a week of having received her almost-expired unit (Kuromaki, 1994).

The necessity of frequent autologous donation within a short period has given rise to the problem of rapid restoration of circulating red-cell mass. A randomized controlled trial of patients who were scheduled for orthopedic surgery was conducted to evaluate the use of recombinant erythropoietin (EPO) in autologous donors. Subjects donated a maximum of 6 units over 3 weeks. The study group received 600 units/kg of EPO twice weekly, along with oral iron. Those receiving EPO had a significant increase in daily RBC production (56 mL/day in the EPO group vs. 44 mL/day in the placebo group) (Fig 11-3) (Goodnough, 1992). A number of details of EPO use in autologous donation remain to be resolved. The optimal dose, route, and frequency of administration are unclear (Mercuriali, 1994; Biesma, 1994a,b). These issues have economic implications, because the cost of EPO to produce the equivalent of one unit of blood has been estimated at $840 (Goodnough, 1994a). The need for oral iron supplementation to maximize the effect of EPO raises the issue of patient compliance; intravenous iron has been suggested as an alternative (Walpoth, 1993; Biesma, 1994).

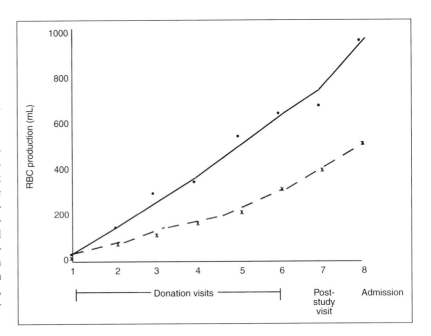

F I G U R E  **11-3**
Red blood cell production during autologous blood donation, in 23 placebo-treated (x) and 21 erythropoietin-treated (•) patients. Data points represent calculated RBC production (mL) at donation visits 1 through 6, the poststudy visit, and hospital admission. Red blood cell production is indicated by polynomial regression curve for each treatment group (n = 44 at each point). (Reprinted with permission from TRANSFUSION 1992;32:442, published by the American Association of Blood Banks.)

Potential side effects of EPO include exacerbation of hypertension and thrombotic events. The latter may be related to an EPO-augmented increase in hematocrit and blood viscosity (Goodnough, 1994a). Most importantly for the purposes of this discussion, EPO for use in autologous donors in pregnancy has not been investigated.

In an era of medical cost containment, priority has shifted from exclusive consideration of those procedures that serve the patients' best interests to determining those procedures whose costs and benefits compete successfully with others for limited resources (AuBuchon, 1994). Blanket substitution of autologous for allogeneic blood has not fared well under such scrutiny. Administrative costs for autologous blood are greater, and its collection is more labor-intensive than for allogeneic blood (AuBuchon, 1994; Etchason, 1995; Kruskall, 1994). Most blood donated for autologous use is discarded, because many of such units do not meet the more rigorous requirements for allogeneic donation, and the costs of "crossover" of autologous blood to the allogeneic pool are unreasonably high (Standards Committee, 1994; Etchason, 1995; Kruskall, 1994). Furthermore, the improved safety of the allogeneic blood supply limits the cost effectiveness of autologous programs (Etchason, 1995).

Certain considerations unique to obstetrics limit the efficiency of autologous programs for pregnant women. Except for the woman with a placenta previa, the need for blood transfusion may be anticipated in only a minority of patients (Sherman, 1993; Gibson, 1993; Pepkowitz, 1993). A multivariate analysis of 14,267 deliveries identified four factors, other than placenta previa, that were significantly and independently associated with peripartum RBC transfusion (preeclampsia, multiple gestation, elective cesarean delivery, and multiparity). Only 8% of those patients who had three or more risk factors received a transfusion. Even limiting autologous donation to those who have three or more risk factors, the calculated costs were $32,800 to prevent one case of posttransfusion hepatitis and $26,000,000 to prevent one case of HIV infection (Combs, 1992).

Some strategies have been proposed in an attempt to limit the costs of autologous transfusion practices. These include data-based interinstitutional practice comparisons (Renner, 1994), elimination of crossover of unused autologous units, storage of autologous whole blood rather than components, and the use of standardized indications for preoperative autologous blood collection and transfusion (Kruskall, 1994). Implementation of the latter suggestion may be problematic, because some state laws mandate offering autologous blood collection to all patients, regardless of how remote the likelihood of the need for transfusion (Goodnough, 1994b).

## Directed Donation

The donation of blood by friends or family for the exclusive use of a designated recipient is termed *directed donation.* Directed donors must meet all the requirements demanded of "altruistic" donors of allogeneic blood (Standards Committee, 1994). Some theoretical concerns have been raised about directed donation. Concern has been expressed about the risk of disease transmission from those whose donations have been coerced and who therefore might not be truthful in response to a predonation questionnaire (Pepkowitz, 1993; Klein, 1994). Another consideration is that the mere existence of a directed donor program might divert potential autologous donors (AuBuchon, 1994). However, the directed donation of blood by a sexual partner might potentially decrease the recipient's exposure to those infectious diseases that may be both sexually and hematogenously transmitted.

Repetitive donations of blood components from a single donor is a more recent development derived from directed donation. A waiver of the usual 6-week interval between donations has proven safe and effective in permitting dedicated single-donor collections (Herman, 1994). Both cellular and acellular products harvested from a single dedicated donor should decrease recipient exposure to blood-borne infections, antigens, and antibodies. However, use of a sexual partner of a reproductive-aged female recipient as a dedicated donor might enhance the possibility of the development of antibodies that may cause hemolytic disease of the newborn in subsequent progeny.

## Blood Substitutes

It must be acknowledged that blood, with all its cellular and liquid components, is too complex a solution to duplicate or replace. Thus, the term *blood substitutes* is essentially an oxymoron. For some time, efforts have been made to develop compounds that may transport oxygen, as do RBCs. The two broad classes of oxygen-carrying compounds that have been developed are those that contain hemoglobin, and the perfluorocarbons.

### *Hemoglobin-containing Compounds*

In the 1960s, investigation was begun on hemoglobin that had been removed from RBCs and then transfused. The infusion of free hemoglobin has been complicated by elevations in systemic and pulmonary vascular resistance. This effect is thought to be due to the binding of intravascular nitric oxide and free hemoglobin (Dracker, 1995). Renal dysfunction has also been noted in stroma-free hemoglobin recipients. The explanation for this finding is that hemoglobin, which exists as a tetramer consisting of two alpha and two beta chains within the RBC, dissociates into dimers when the RBC stroma is removed. These dimers are nephrotoxic. A variety of hemoglobin-containing compounds have been developed in an attempt to overcome this undesirable side effect. Intramolecular cross-linking of either the alpha or the beta chains has prevented dissociation of the hemoglobin tetramers. Intermolecular linkage has been used to produce hemoglobin polymers. The linkage of hemoglobin to albumen or to the other polymers has resulted in products that perform oxygen carriage and remain in the vascular space longer than simple stroma-free hemoglobin (Fratantoni, 1994). Other developments include attempts at encapsulating free hemoglobin into red-cell-like "neohemacytes," to which may be added 2,3-DPG, oxygen radical scavengers, dismutases, and the like (Dracker, 1995). To date, the utilization of these compounds has been hampered by undesired side effects and the difficulties and expense of their production.

### *Perfluorocarbons*

The perfluorocarbons are a class of hydrocarbons in which all the hydrogen ions are replaced by fluorine. Unlike hemoglobin, which binds oxygen, the perfluorocarbons carry oxygen in solution.

Thus, the degree of oxygen carriage by these compounds is contingent upon inspired oxygen tension. In contrast with hemoglobin in circulating RBCs, which is 95% saturated when exposed to room air, or 20% (Fratantoni, 1994). To raise oxygen carriage, the inspired oxygen tension must be increased. Perfluorocarbons have other limitations. Because they are immiscible in water, they must be emulsified prior to infusion. Capillary plugging may develop if the emulsified particle is too large. In addition, the ingestion of perfluorocarbons by macrophages and inhibition of neutrophil function may have undesirable consequences. Current efforts target the development of minimally toxic solutions that have improved oxygen solubility (Dracker, 1995; Fratantoni, 1994).

---

**REFERENCES**

Akingbola OA, Custer JR, Bunchman TE, Sedman AB. Management of severe anemia without transfusion in a pediatric Jehovah's Witness patient. Crit Care Med 1994;22:524–552.

Alter HJ, Epstein JS, Swenson SG. Prevalence of human immunodeficiency virus type 1 p24 antigen in US blood donors: an assessment of the efficacy of testing in donor screening. N Engl J Med 1990;323:1312–1317.

Alter HJ. Transfusion transmitted hepatitis C and non-A, non-B, non-C. Vox Sang 1994a;67(suppl 3):19–24.

Alter MJ. Review of serologic testing for hepatitis C virus infection and risk of posttransfusion hepatitis C. Arch Pathol Lab Med 1994b;118:342–345.

Alving BM. Management of congenital and acquired hemostatic disorders during pregnancy. In: Sachar RA, Brecher ME, eds. Obstetric transfusion practice. Bethesda, MD: American Association of Blood Banks, 1993:117–134.

American College of Physicians. Practice strategies for elective red blood cell transfusion. Ann Intern Med 1992;116:403–406.

American Red Cross, Council of Community Blood Centers, American Association of Blood Banks. Circular of information for the use of human blood and blood components. Bethesda, MD: American Association of Blood Banks, 1994.

Appleton AL, Sviland L, Pearson ADJ, et al. Diagnostic features of transfusion associated graft versus host disease. J Clin Pathol 1994;47:541–546.

Aubuchon JP. Minimizing donor exposure to hemotherapy. Arch Pathol Lab Med 1994;118:380.

Benson K, Marks AR, Marshall MJ, Goldstein JD. Fatal graft-versus-host disease associated with transfusions of HLA-matched, HLA-homozygous platelets from unrelated donors. Transfusion 1994;34:432–437.

Berkman SA. Infectious complications of blood transfusion. Blood Rev 1988;2:206–210.

Biesma DH, Kraaijenhagen RJ, Dalmulder J, et al. Recombinant human erythropoietin in autologous blood donors: a dose-finding study. Br J Haematol 1994a;86:30–35.

Biesma DH, Van de Wiel A, Beguin Y, et al. Erythropoietic activity and iron metabolism in autologous blood donors during recombinant human erythropoietin therapy. Eur J Clin Invest 1994b;24:426–432.

Blajchman MA, Ali AA, Richardson HL. Bacterial contamination of cellular blood components. Vox Sang 1994;67(suppl 3):25–33.

Blajchman MA, Bull SB, Feinman SV. Posttransfusion hepatitis: impact of non-A, non-B hepatitis surrogate tests. Lancet 1995;345:21–25.

Blumberg N, Heal JM. Effects of transfusion on immune function. Arch Pathol Lab Med 1994;118:371–379.

Boral LI, Hill SS, Apollon CJ, Folland A. The type and antibody screen, revisited. Am J Clin Pathol 1979;71:578–581.

Bowden RA. Transfusion-transmitted cytomegalovirus infection. Immunol Invest 1995;24:117–128.

British Committee for Standards in Haematology, Working Party of the Blood Transfusion Task Force. Guidelines for platelet transfusions. Transfus Med 1992;2:311–318.

Camann WR, Datta S. Red cell use during cesarean delivery. Transfusion 1991;31:12–15.

Carson JL, Spence RK, Poses RM, Bonavita G. Severity of anaemia and operative mortality and morbidity. Lancet 1988;1:727–729.

Carson JL, Willett SR. Is a hemoglobin of 10 g/dL required for surgery? Med Clin North Am 1993; 77:335–347.

Clark VA, Wardall GJ, McGrady EM. Blood ordering practices in obstetric units in the United Kingdom. Anaesthesia 1993;48:998–1007.

Code of Federal Regulations, Title 21 (vol 6, parts 600–799). Washington, DC: US Government Printing Office, 1986.

College of American Pathologists. Practice parameter for the use of fresh-frozen plasma, cryoprecipitate, and platelets. JAMA 1994;271:777–781.

Combs CA, Murphy EL, Laros RK. Cost-benefit analysis of autologous blood donation in obstetrics. Obstet Gynecol 1992;80:621–625.

Crosby ET. Perioperative haemotherapy: II. Risks and complications of blood transfusion. Can J Anaesth 1992;39:822–837.

Dodd RY. Viral contamination of blood components and approaches for reduction of infectivity. Immunol Invest 1995;24:25–48.

Donaldson MDJ, Seaman MJ, Park GR. Massive blood transfusion. Br J Anaesth 1992;69:621–630.

Donegan E, Lee H, Operskalski EA, et al. Transfusion transmission of retroviruses: human T-lymphotropic virus types I and II compared with human immunodeficiency virus type I. Transfusion 1994;34:478–483.

Dracker RA. The development and use of oxygen-carrying blood substitutes. Immunol Invest 1995;24:403–410.

Ereth MH, Oliver WC, Jr, Santrach PJ. Perioperative interventions to decrease transfusion of allogenic blood products. Mayo Clin Proc 1994;69:575.

Etchason J, Petz L, Keeler E, et al. The cost effectiveness of preoperative autologous blood donations. N Engl J Med 1995;332:719–724.

Fakhry SM, Sheldon GF. Blood administration, risks, and substitutes. Adv Surg 1995;28:71–92.

Fratantoni JC. Blood substitutes: problems and prospects. In: AuBuchon JP, Issitt LA, eds. Limiting donor exposure in hemotherapy. Bethesda, MD: American Association of Blood Banks, 1994:61–73.

Galea G, Urbaniak SJ. Blood transfusion practice in gynaecology and obstetrics. Vox Sang 1994; 67:323–325.

Gibson J. Autologous predeposit blood donation in pregnancy—a perspective. Aust NZ J Obstet Gynaecol 1993;33:276–279.

Gonzalez A, Esteban JI, Madoz P, et al. Efficacy of screening donors for antibodies to the hepatitis C virus to prevent transfusion-associated hepatitis: final report of a prospective trial. Hepatology 1995;22:439–445.

Goodnough LT, Price TH, Rudnick S, Soefiarso RW. Preoperative red cell production in patients undergoing aggressive autologous blood phlebotomy with and without erythropoietin therapy. Transfusion 1992;32:441–445.

Goodnough LT. Reducing the need to transfuse: applications of hematopoietic growth factors. In: AuBuchon JP, Issitt LA, eds. Limiting donor exposure in hemotherapy. Bethesda, MD: American Association of Blood Banks, 1994a:1–15.

Goodnough LT, Bodner MS, Martin JW. Blood transfusion and blood conservation: cost and utilization issues. Am J Med Qual 1994b;9:172–183.

Haditsch M, Binder L, Gabriel C, et al. *Yersinia enterocolitica* septicemia in autologous blood transfusion. Transfusion 1994;34:907.

Hanson, M. Blood donor screening. Factors influencing decision making. Arch Pathol Lab Med 1994;118:457–461.

Hasley PB, Lave JR, Kapoor WN. The necessary and the unnecessary transfusion: a critical review of reported appropriateness rates and criteria for red cell transfusions. Transfusion 1994;34:110–115.

Herman JH, Moolten DN, Peek CC. Collection and transfusion technologies to reduce donor exposure. In: AuBuchon JP, Issitt LA, eds. Limiting donor exposure in hemotherapy. Bethesda, MD: American Association of Blood Banks, 1994:75–95.

Heymann SJ, Brewer TF. The infectious risks of transfusions in the United States: a decision-analytic approach. Am J Infect Control 1993;21:174–182.

Hillyer CD, Hart KK, Lackey DA, et al. Comparable safety of blood collection in "high-risk" autologous donors versus non-high-risk autologous and directed donors in a hospital setting. Am J Clin Pathol 1994;102:275–277.

Hogman CF, Bagge L, Thoren L. The use of blood components in surgical transfusion therapy. World J Surg 1987;11:2–13.

Huang YY, Yang SS, Wu CH, et al. Impact of screening blood donors for hepatitis C antibody on posttransfusion hepatitis: a prospective study with a second-generation anti-hepatitis C virus assay. Transfusion 1994;34:661–665.

Isbister JP. Adverse reactions to plasma and plasma components. Anaesth Intensive Care 1993;21:31–38.

Ismay SL, Thomas S, Fellows A, et al. Post-transfusion hepatitis revisited. Med J Aust 1995;163:74–77.

Kitchens CS. Are transfusions overrated? Surgical outcome of Jehovah's Witnesses. Am J Med 1993;94:117–119.

Klein HG, Dzik WH, Strauss RG, Busch MP. Leukocyte-reduced blood component therapy. In: Hematology 1992. Anaheim California: American Society of Hematology, 1992:76–85.

Klein HG. Oxygen carriers and transfusion medicine. Artif Cells Blood Substit 1994;22:123–135.

Koziol DE, Holland PV, Alling DW, et al. Antibody to hepatitis B core antigen as a paradoxical marker for non-A, non-B hepatitis agents in donated blood. Ann Intern Med 1986;104:488–495.

Kruskall MS, Yomtovian R, Dzik WH, et al. On improving the cost-effectivenesss of autologous blood transfusion practices. Transfusion 1994;34:259–264.

Kuromaki K, Takeda S, Seki H, et al. Autologous blood transfusion for the patient with placenta previa complicated by placenta increta: a case report. Asia Oceania J Obstet Gynaecol 1994;20:155–159.

Lackritz EM, Satten GA, Aberle-Grasse J, et al. Estimated risk of transmission of the human immunodeficiency virus by screened blood in the United States. N Engl J Med 1995;333:1721–1725.

Linden JV, Kaplan HS. Transfusion errors: causes and effects. Transfus Med Rev 1994;8:169–183.

Luban NLC. Human parvoviruses: implications for transfusion medicine. Transfusion 1994;34:821–827.

Malouf M, Glanville AR. Blood transfusion related adult respiratory distress syndrome. Anaesth Intensive Care 1993;21:44–49.

Mattison DR. Anatomical, physiologic and biochemical adaptations to pregnancy. In: Sachar RA, Brecher ME, eds. Obstetric transfusion practice. Bethesda, MD: American Association of Blood Banks, 1993:1–19.

Mercuriali F, Inghilleri G, Biffi E, et al. Erythropoietin treatment to increase autologous blood donation in patients with low basal hematocrit undergoing elective orthopedic surgery. Clin Invest 1994;72:S16–S18.

Miller JP, Mintz PD. The use of leukocyte-reduced blood components. Hematol Oncol Clin North Am 1995;9:69–89.

Molland G, Dent OF, Chapuis PH, et al. Transfusion does not influence patient survivai after resection of colorectal cancer. Aust NZ J Surg 1995;65:592–595.

Morris JA, Wilcox TR, Reed GW, et al. Safety of blood supply. Surrogate testing and transmission of hepatitis C in patients after massive transfusion. Ann Surg 1994;219:317–326.

Morrison JC, Sumrall D, Chevalier SP, et al. The effect of provider education on blood utilization practices. Am J Obstet Gynecol 1993;169:1240–1245.

Mosley JW, Nowicki MJ, Kasper CK, et al. Hepatitis A virus transmission by blood products in the United States. Vox Sang 1994;67(suppl 1):24–28.

Naef RW, Washburne JF, Martin RW, et al. Hemorrhage associated with cesarean delivery: when is transfusion needed? J Perinatol 1995;15:32–35.

O'Dwyer G, Mylotte M, Sweeney M, Egan EL. Experience of autologous blood transfusion in an obstetrics and gynaecology department. Br J Obstet Gynaecol 1993;100:571–574.

Pepkowitz SH. Autologous blood donation and obstetric transfusion practice. In: Sacher RA, Brecher ME, eds. Obstetric transfusion practice. Bethesda, MD: American Association of Blood Banks, 1993:77–94.

Perkins H. Transfusion reactions: the changing priorities. Immunol Invest 1995;24:289–302.

Pinkerton PH, Coovadia AS, Goldstein J. Frequency of delayed hemolytic transfusion reactions following antibody screening and immediate-spin crossmatching. Transfusion 1992;32:814–817.

Pisciotto PT. Blood transfusion therapy. A physician's handbook. Bethesda, MD: American Association of Blood Banks, 1993.

Porter HJ, Khong TY, Evans MF, et al. Parvovirus as a cause of hydrops fetalis: detection by in situ DNA hybridisation. J Clin Pathol 1988;41:381–383.

Raichle LT, Paranto ME. Compatibility testing. In: Harmening DM, ed. Modern blood banking and transfusion practices. Philadelphia: FA Davis, 1994:256–287.

Renner SW. The use of Q-probes in modifying transfusion practice. Arch Pathol Lab Med 1994;118:438–441.

Roberts CR. Laboratory diagnosis of retroviral infections. Dermatol Clin 1991;9:453–464.

Roberts CR, Longfield JN, Platte RC, et al. Transfusion-associated human immunodeficiency virus type 1 from screened antibody-negative blood donors. Arch Pathol Lab Med 1994;118:1188–1192.

Salem-Schatz SR, Avorn J, Soumerai SB. Influence of clinical knowledge, organizational context, and practice style on transfusion decision making. JAMA 1990;264:471–475.

Sayers MH. Transfusion-transmitted viral infections other than hepatitis and human immunodeficiency virus infection. Arch Pathol Lab Med 1994;118:346–349.

Sazama K. Bacteria in blood for transfusion. Arch Pathol Lab Med 1994;118:350–365.

Schmidt PJ. Introducing new tests before transfusion. Who shall decide? Arch Pathol Lab Med 1994;118:454–456.

Schreiber GB, Busch MP, Kleinman SH, et al. The risk of transfusion-transmitted viral infections. N Engl J Med 1996;334:1685.

Seeff LB, Dienstag JL. Transfusion-associated non-A, non-B hepatitis: where do we go from here? Gastroenterology 1988;95:530–533.

Selik RM, Ward JW, Buehler JW. Trends in transfusion-associated acquired immune deficiency syndrome in the United States, 1982 through 1991. Transfusion 1993;33:890–893.

Sherman SJ, Greenspoon JS, Nelson JM, Paul RH. Obstetric hemorrhage and blood utilization. J Reprod Med 1993;38:929–934.

Shulman IA. Parasitic infections and their impact on blood donor selection and testing. Arch Pathol Lab Med 1994;118:366–370.

Snyder EL. Transfusion reactions: state-of-the-art 1994. Vox Sang 1994;67(suppl 3):143–146.

Spence R, Cernaianu A, Carson J, DelRossi A. Transfusion and surgery. Curr Probl Surg 1993;30:1101–1180.

Standards Committee, American Association of Blood Banks. Standards for blood banks and transfusion services. 16th ed. Bethesda, MD: American Association of Blood Banks, 1994.

Stehling L, Simon TL. The red blood cell transfusion trigger. Arch Pathol Lab Med 1994a;118:429–434.

Stehling L, Luban NLC, Anderson KC, et al. Guidelines for blood utilization review. Transfusion 1994b;34:438–448.

Takano S, Omata M, Ohto M, Satomura Y. Prospective assessment of incidence of fulminant hepatitis in post-transfusion hepatitis: a study of 504 cases. Dig Dis Sci 1994;39:28–32.

Taswell HF, Galbreath JL. Errors in transfusion medicine. Arch Pathol Lab Med 1994;118:405–410.

Tegtmeier GE. Infectious diseases transmitted by transfusion: a miscellanea. Vox Sang 1994;67(suppl 3):179–191.

Thomas DP. Viral contamination of blood products. Lancet 1994;343:1583–1584.

Valbonesi V, Frisoni R, Florio G, et al. Multicomponent collection (MCS): a new trend in transfusion medicine. Int J Artif Organs 1994;17:65–69.

Viele MK, Weiskopf RB. What can we learn about the need for transfusion from patients who refuse blood? The experience with Jehovah's Witnesses. Transfusion 1994;34:396–401.

Walker RH. Special report: transfusion risks. Am J Clin Pathol 1987;88:374–378.

Walpoth BH, Schwaller J, Hofstetter H, et al. Current problems with autologous blood supply. Infusionther Transfusionmed 1993;20:316–326.

Wang Y-J, Lee S-D, Hwang S-J, et al. Incidence of post-transfusion hepatitis before and after screening for hepatitis C virus antibody. Vox Sang 1994;67:187–190.

Welch HG, Meehan KR, Goodnough LT. Prudent strategies for elective red blood cell transfusion. Ann Intern Med 1992;116:393–402.

Williams AC, Thomson RA, Schreiber GB, et al. Estimate of infection disease risk factors in U.S. blood donors. JAMA 1997;277:967.

Wylie BR. Transfusion transmitted infection: viral and exotic diseases. Anaesth Intensive Care 1993;21:24–30.

Yomtovian R, Kelly C, Bracey AW, et al. Procurement and transfusion of human immunodeficiency virus-positive or untested autologous blood units: issues and concerns: a report prepared by the Autologous Transfusion Committee of the American Association of Blood Banks. Transfusion 1995;35:353–361.

# CHAPTER 12

# Cardiopulmonary Resuscitation

*N*early 10% of all maternal deaths result from cardiac arrest (Syverson, 1991). This suggests that obstetricians in large practices or maternal-fetal medicine specialists in tertiary referral centers are likely to encounter a "peripartum code" and should, therefore, have an understanding of the physiology and techniques of cardiopulmonary resuscitation (CPR), especially as applied to the pregnant woman and her fetus. Earlier this century, most maternal cardiac deaths stemmed from chronic illnesses. More recently, the leading causes include embolism, intrapartum cardiac arrest, complications of hypertensive disease, anesthetics, acute respiratory failure, sepsis, tocolysis, and hemorrhage.

Cardiopulmonary arrest is the abrupt cessation of spontaneous and effective ventilation and systemic perfusion. Cardiopulmonary resuscitation provides artificial ventilation and perfusion until advanced cardiac life support (ACLS) can be obtained and spontaneous cardiopulmonary function restored. Although closed chest circulatory support was reported in the 1800s, Kouwenho-

ven's landmark description of closed chest compressions in 1960 represents the birth of modern day cardiopulmonary resuscitation (Kouwenhoven, 1960). Emergency cardiac care (ECC) includes both basic life support (BLS) and ACLS. Cardiopulmonary resuscitation is an integral part of the life-saving process in both. National conferences co-sponsored by the American Heart Association and the National Academy of Sciences–National Research Council periodically review advances and research in ECC and publish texts in ACLS and BLS (American Heart Association, 1994a; American Heart Association, 1994b). The importance and acceptance of these conferences and their conclusions is emphasized by the fact that many medical centers require completion of AHA courses in BLS and ACLS as part of the physicians' credentials process.

Since the publication of the second edition of this text, a national conference on cardiopulmonary resuscitation has led to several important changes in the recommendations of the American Heart Association for the management of cardiopulmonary arrest (Satin, 1990). This chapter serves as an update while also reviewing maternal and fetal physiologies and their unique relationships, which require adjustment in both physical and pharmacologic aspects of ECC. Furthermore, we readdress the issue of perimortem cesarean and survival data for mother and infant.

## Physiology and Techniques of Cardiopulmonary Resuscitation

Passage of time drives all aspects of ECC and determines patient outcomes. Spontaneous ventilation and circulation must be restored quickly if the patient is to make a full neurologic recovery. Time is critical in cases of cardiac or pulmonary arrest. There is usually enough oxygen in the lungs and bloodstream to support life for up to 6 minutes (American Heart Association, 1994b). If breathing stops first, the heart often continues to pump blood for several minutes. When the heart stops, oxygen in the lungs and bloodstream cannot be circulated to vital organs. The patient whose heart and breathing have stopped for less than 4 minutes has an excellent chance for recovery if CPR is administered immediately and is followed by ACLS within 4 minutes (Eisenberg, 1979). By 4 to 6 minutes, brain damage may occur, and after 6 minutes, brain damage will almost always occur (American Heart Association, 1994a). The initial goals of CPR, therefore, are (1) delivery of oxygen to the lungs, (2) providing a means of circulating it to the vital organs (via closed-chest compressions), followed by (3) ACLS, with restoration of the heart as the mechanism of circulation. Practically speaking these goals are achieved by remembering the "A-B-C-Ds" of the primary and secondary survey (Table 12-1).

Delivery of oxygen is achieved by positioning the patient, opening the airway, and rescue breathing. In the absence of muscle tone, the tongue and epiglottis frequently obstruct the airway. The head-tilt with the chin-lift maneuver (Fig 12-1) or the jaw-thrust maneuver (Fig 12-2) may provide airway access. If foreign material appears in the mouth, it should be removed either manually or with active suction if available. If air does not enter the lungs with rescue breathing, reposition the head and repeat the attempt at rescue breathing. Persistent obstruction may require the Heimlich maneuver (subdiaphragmatic abdominal thrusts), chest thrusts, finger sweeps, and rescue breathing (Table 12-2). Importantly, the Heimlich maneuver cannot be used in the late stages of pregnancy or the obese choking victim. Airway obstruction may occur in a choking victim as well as a patient experiencing a cardiopulmonary arrest. The conscious woman with only partial airway obstruction should be allowed to attempt to clear the obstruction herself, and finger sweeps by the rescuer are avoided. Finally, failure of nonsurgical procedures to relieve the airway obstruction is an indication for emergency cricothyroidotomy or jet-needle insufflation, if appropriate equipment is available.

Abdominal thrusts are accomplished by wrapping your hands around the victim's waist, making a fist with one hand and placing the thumb-side of the fist against the victim's abdomen in the midline slightly above the navel and well below the top of the xiphoid process. The rescuer grasps the fist with the other hand and presses the fist into the victim's abdomen with quick, distinct, upward thrusts (Fig 12-3). The thrusts are continued until the object is expelled or the victim is unconscious. Abdominal thrusts may be prevented by the gravid uterus. The unconscious

T A B L E   **12-1**

The systematic survey approach to emergency cardiac care

|  |  | **Primary** | **Secondary** |
|---|---|---|---|
| A | **A**irway | Open | Intubate |
| B | **B**reathing | Positive-pressure ventilation | Assess bilateral chest rise and ventilation |
| C | **C**irculation | Chest compressions | Intravenous access, pharmacologic interventions |
| D |  | **D**efibrillate VF/pulseless VT | **D**ifferential diagnosis—treat reversible causes |

VF, ventricular fibrillation; VT, ventricular tachycardia.

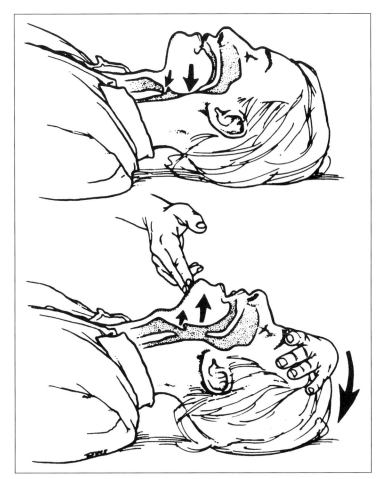

FIGURE **12-1**
Opening the airway. (Top) Airway obstruction produced by the tongue and epiglottis. (Bottom) Relief via head-tilt and chin-lift maneuvers. (Reproduced with permission. Textbook of Basic Life Support for Healthcare Providers, 1994. Copyright American Heart Association.)

FIGURE **12-2**
Jaw-thrust maneuver. Rescuer grasps the angles of the victim's lower jaw and lifts with both hands, one on each side, displacing the mandible forward while tilting the head backward. (Reproduced with permission. Basic Life Support for Healthcare Providers, 1994. Copyright American Heart Association.)

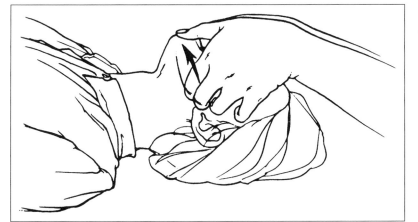

victim is placed supine (Fig 12-4), and the heel of one hand remains against the victim's abdomen, in the midline slightly above the navel but below the top of the xiphoid. The second hand lies directly on top of the first, and quick upward thrusts are administered.

The gravid uterus may necessitate the use of chest thrusts instead of abdominal thrusts. Chest

T A B L E    **12-2**

Management of a foreign-body obstruction

*Conscious Victim*

1. Perform the Heimlich maneuver (chest thrusts if in latter half of gestation).
2. Repeat until the obstruction is relieved or the victim is unconscious.

*Unconscious Victim*

1. Turn the victim on the back.
2. Open the mouth, position the head.
3. Perform a finger sweep, or use a Kelly clamp or Magill forceps if there is direct visualization of the foreign body.
4. Attempt ventilation, reposition the head, and repeat ventilation.
5. Repeat the sequence of Heimlich maneuver (chest thrusts), finger sweep, and attempt at ventilation until the obstruction is relieved.

thrusts in a conscious sitting or standing victim require placing the thumb side of the fist on the middle of the sternum, avoiding the xiphoid and the ribs. The rescuer then grabs her or his own fist with the other hand and performs chest thrusts until either the foreign object dislodges or the patient loses consciousness (Fig 12-5). The unconscious patient is placed supine. The rescuer's hand closest to the patient's head is placed two finger-breadths above the xiphoid. The long axis of the heel of the provider's hand rests in the long axis of the sternum (Fig 12-6). The other hand lies over the first, with fingers either extended or interlaced. The elbows are extended, and the chest is compressed 1.5 to 2 inches.

Rescue breathing may be facilitated by mouth-to-mouth, mouth-to-nose, mouth-to-mask, or bag valve-to-mask resuscitation, or ultimately by endotracheal intubation. Endotracheal intubation by direct laryngoscopy is the preferred method for maintaining airway patency for the gravid arrest victim. Alternative techniques for airway management include endotracheal intubation by lighted stylet, esophageal tracheal combitube, laryngeal mash airway, and transtracheal ventilation. The reader is referred to the extensive review by Reed (1995). Tracheal intubation offers

F I G U R E    **12-3**

**Heimlich maneuver administered to sitting or standing conscious victim.** (Reproduced with permission. Textbook of Basic Life Support for Healthcare Providers, 1994. Copyright American Heart Association.)

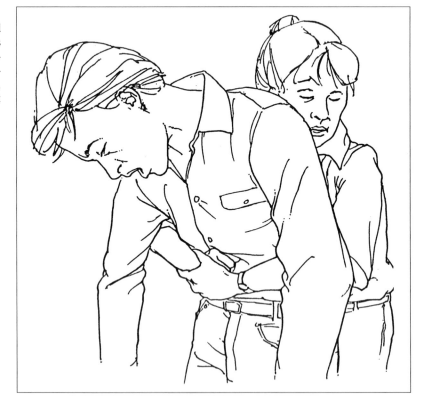

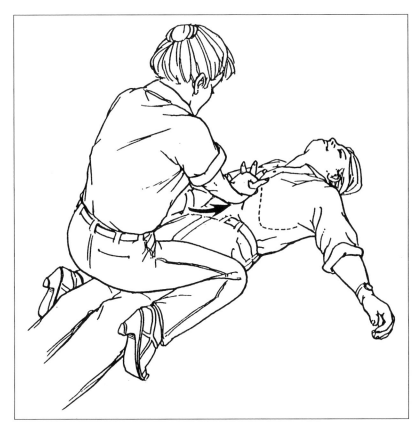

F I G U R E **12-4**
Heimlich maneuver administered to **supine unconscious victim.** (Reproduced with permission. Textbook of Basic Life Support for Healthcare Providers, 1994. Copyright American Heart Association.)

several advantages, including security and protection of the airway, as well as facilitation of oxygenation and ventilation, and it provides a route for administration of drugs during a cardiac arrest.

In the absence of a spontaneous heartbeat, external chest compressions provide a means of circulation. Kouwenhoven et al originally described this in 1960. They believed that the chest compressions caused a direct compression of the heart between the sternum and the spine, leading to a rise in ventricular pressure, a closure of the mitral and tricuspid valves, and a forcing of blood into the pulmonary artery and aorta. More recently, fluctuations in intrathoracic pressure and creation of an arteriovenous pressure gradient peripherally have been implicated as the mechanism of circulation with external chest compressions (Rudikoff, 1980). External chest compressions cause a rise in intrathoracic pressure, which is distributed to all intrathoracic structures. Competent venous valves prevent transmission of this

pressure to extrathoracic veins, whereas the arteries transmit the increased pressure to extrathoracic arteries, creating an arterial venous pressure gradient and forward blood flow (Fig 12-7). Werner et al (1981), using echocardiography, showed that the mitral and tricuspid valves remain open during CPR, supporting the concept of the heart as a passive conduit rather than a pump during CPR.

Basic life support guidelines call for a ratio of 2 ventilations to 15 compressions in one-person CPR and a 1:5 ratio in two-rescuer CPR, with a total of 80 to 100 compressions per minute in both circumstances. Advanced cardiac life support involves the addition of electrical and pharmacologic therapy, invasive monitoring, and therapeutic techniques to correct cardiac arrhythmias, metabolic imbalances, and other causes of cardiac arrest. Standard algorithms recommended by the American Heart Association are reviewed in Figures 12-8 through 12-14. Major changes in

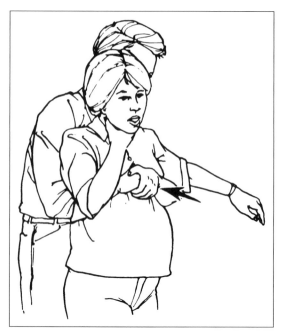

F I G U R E   **12-5**

**Chest thrusts administered to a standing conscious victim.** (Reproduced with permission. Textbook of Basic Life Support for Healthcare Providers, 1994. Copyright American Heart Association.)

ECC recommended by the national conference in 1992 are listed in Table 12-3.

## The Effect of Pregnancy on Cardiopulmonary Resuscitation

Pregnancy produces physiologic changes that have a dramatic effect on cardiopulmonary resuscitation (Table 12-4). Pregnancy represents a high-flow, low-resistance state with a high cardiac output (CO) and low systemic vascular resistance. Cardiac output increases to 150% of nonpregnant norms. The uterus, with minimum resistance, receives up to 30% of CO, as compared with 2% to 3% in the nongravid patient. The increase in CO satisfies the increase in oxygen demands of the growing fetus, the placenta, and the mother.

The enlarging uterus imposes changes on the respiratory system as well. Upward displacement of the diaphragm leads to a decrease in the functional residual capacity (FRC) of the lungs. Maternal minute ventilation increases, probably due to a central effect of progesterone (deSwiet, 1994). The decrease in FRC combines with the increase in oxygen demand to predispose the pregnant woman to a decrease in arterial and

F I G U R E   **12-6**

**The technique for chest thrusts for an unconscious supine victim of foreign body airway obstruction is identical to closed chest compressions for cardiac arrest.** (Reproduced with permission. Textbook of Basic Life Support for Healthcare Providers, 1994. Copyright American Heart Association.)

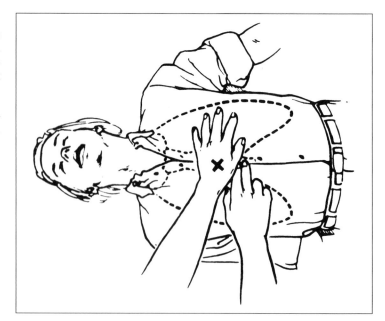

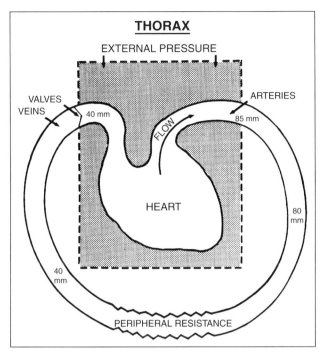

**THORAX**

EXTERNAL PRESSURE

VALVES
VEINS

40 mm

ARTERIES

85 mm

FLOW

HEART

80 mm

40 mm

PERIPHERAL RESISTANCE

F I G U R E   **12-7**

Hypothesized mechanism for circulation prompted by external chest compressions.

venous oxygen tension during periods of decreased ventilation. Furthermore, the increase in ventilation in pregnancy leads to a decline in arterial carbon dioxide tension. The maternal kidney compensates for this respiratory alkalosis by a fall in serum bicarbonate concentration. Maternal hypocapnia and respiratory alkalosis enhance renal excretion of carbon dioxide by the fetus. Hence, increases in maternal carbon dioxide may lead to fetal acidosis. The mother also compensates for hypoxia by decreasing uteroplacental blood flow. Therefore, during maternal cardiopulmonary arrest, the physiologic changes of pregnancy and tendency toward hypoxia in the presence of apnea make it more difficult to resuscitate the mother. Superimposed on an already compromised maternal circulation characterized by hypercarbia and hypoxia, normal physiologic compensatory mechanisms that decrease uteroplacental flow during the arrest lead to further fetal acidosis.

For the patient in the latter half of pregnancy, aortocaval compression by the gravid uterus

T A B L E   **12-3**

Recently recommended changes in basic life support and advanced cardiac life support*

*Basic Life Support*
The time taken during ventilation for filling the lungs is increased from 1.5 to 2 seconds.
The unresponsive victim with spontaneous respirations should be placed on her side.

*Advanced Cardiac Life Support*
Rapid defibrillation in cases of VF/pulseless VT should be used.
Although the initial dose of epinephrine for the pulseless victim remains unchanged, high-dose epinephrine (up to 0.1 mg/kg) should be considered if repetitive doses are necessary.
Sodium bicarbonate and calcium are not routinely recommended except in rare cases, such as hyperkalemia and calcium channel blocker overdose, respectively.
Adenosine is the drug of choice for PSVT.
Higher volumes of drugs should be used via the endotracheal tube.
Pulseless electrical activity replaces electromechanical dissociation as proper nomenclature.

*New, detailed protocols are outlined in subsequent tables.

VF, ventricular fibrillation; VT, ventricular tachycardia; PSVT, paroxysmal supraventricular tachycardia.

T A B L E   **12-4**

Maternal physiologic changes of pregnancy

| *Cardiovascular* | |
| --- | --- |
| CO | Increases |
| Blood volume | Increases |
| SVR | Decreases |
| COP | Decreases |
| *Respiratory* | |
| Minute ventilation | Increases |
| FRC | Decreases |
| *Gastrointestinal* | |
| Motility | Decreases |
| Lower esophageal sphincter tone | Decreases |

CO, cardiac output; SVR, systemic vascular resistance; COP, colloid oncotic pressure; FRC, functional residual capacity.

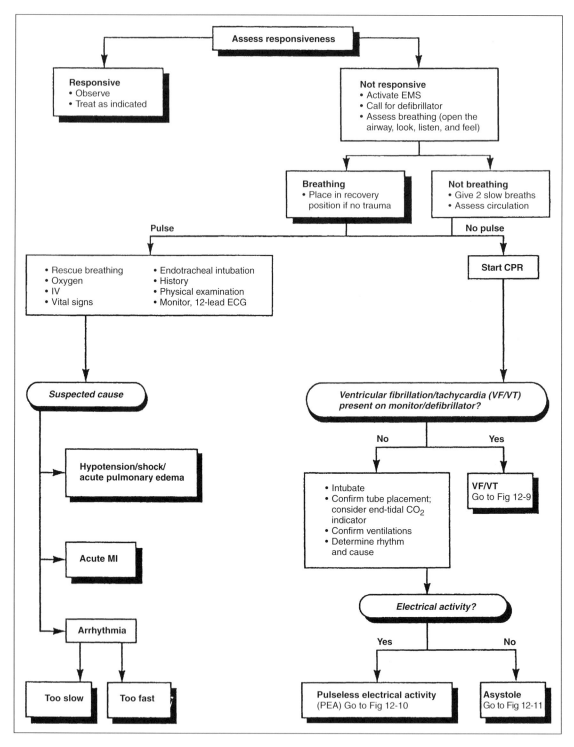

F I G U R E   **12-8**

Universal algorithm for adult emergency cardiac care.

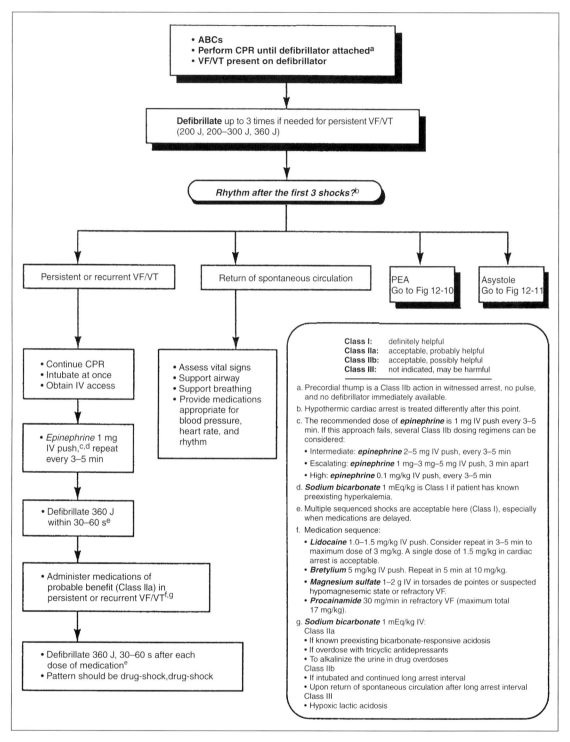

F I G U R E  **12-9**

Ventricular fibrillation/pulseless ventricular tachycardia (VF/VT) algorithm.

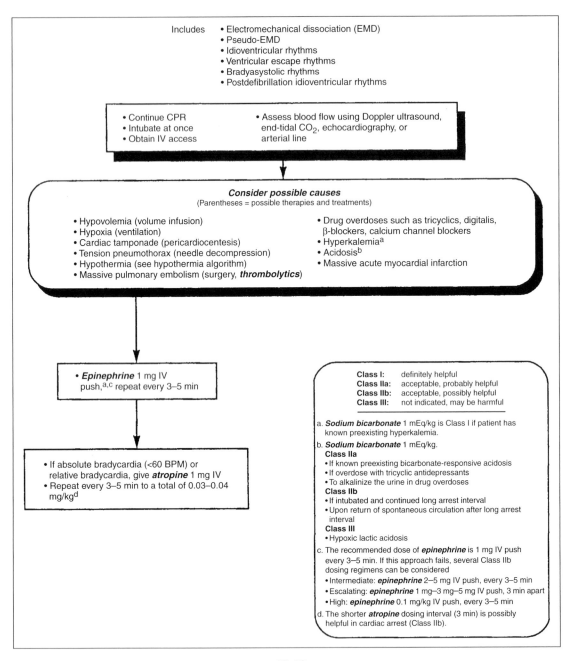

Includes
• Electromechanical dissociation (EMD)
• Pseudo-EMD
• Idioventricular rhythms
• Ventricular escape rhythms
• Bradyasystolic rhythms
• Postdefibrillation idioventricular rhythms

---

• Continue CPR
• Intubate at once
• Obtain IV access

• Assess blood flow using Doppler ultrasound, end-tidal $CO_2$, echocardiography, or arterial line

---

**Consider possible causes**
(Parentheses = possible therapies and treatments)

• Hypovolemia (volume infusion)
• Hypoxia (ventilation)
• Cardiac tamponade (pericardiocentesis)
• Tension pneumothorax (needle decompression)
• Hypothermia (see hypothermia algorithm)
• Massive pulmonary embolism (surgery, **thrombolytics**)

• Drug overdoses such as tricyclics, digitalis, β-blockers, calcium channel blockers
• Hyperkalemia[a]
• Acidosis[b]
• Massive acute myocardial infarction

---

• **Epinephrine** 1 mg IV push,[a,c] repeat every 3–5 min

---

| | |
|---|---|
| **Class I:** | definitely helpful |
| **Class IIa:** | acceptable, probably helpful |
| **Class IIb:** | acceptable, possibly helpful |
| **Class III:** | not indicated, may be harmful |

a. **Sodium bicarbonate** 1 mEq/kg is Class I if patient has known preexisting hyperkalemia.
b. **Sodium bicarbonate** 1 mEq/kg.
   **Class IIa**
   • If known preexisting bicarbonate-responsive acidosis
   • If overdose with tricyclic antidepressants
   • To alkalinize the urine in drug overdoses
   **Class IIb**
   • If intubated and continued long arrest interval
   • Upon return of spontaneous circulation after long arrest interval
   **Class III**
   • Hypoxic lactic acidosis
c. The recommended dose of **epinephrine** is 1 mg IV push every 3–5 min. If this approach fails, several Class IIb dosing regimens can be considered
   • Intermediate: **epinephrine** 2–5 mg IV push, every 3–5 min
   • Escalating: **epinephrine** 1 mg–3 mg–5 mg IV push, 3 min apart
   • High: **epinephrine** 0.1 mg/kg IV push, every 3–5 min
d. The shorter **atropine** dosing interval (3 min) is possibly helpful in cardiac arrest (Class IIb).

---

• If absolute bradycardia (<60 BPM) or relative bradycardia, give **atropine** 1 mg IV
• Repeat every 3–5 min to a total of 0.03–0.04 mg/kg[d]

F I G U R E    **12-10**

Pulseless electrical activity (PEA) algorithm (electromechanical dissociation [EMD]).

renders resuscitation more difficult than in her nonpregnant counterpart. It does so by decreasing venous return, causing supine hypotension, and decreasing the effectiveness of thoracic compressions. The pregnant uterus exerts pressure on the inferior vena cava, iliac vessels, and abdominal aorta. In the supine position, such uterine compression may lead to sequestration of up to 30%

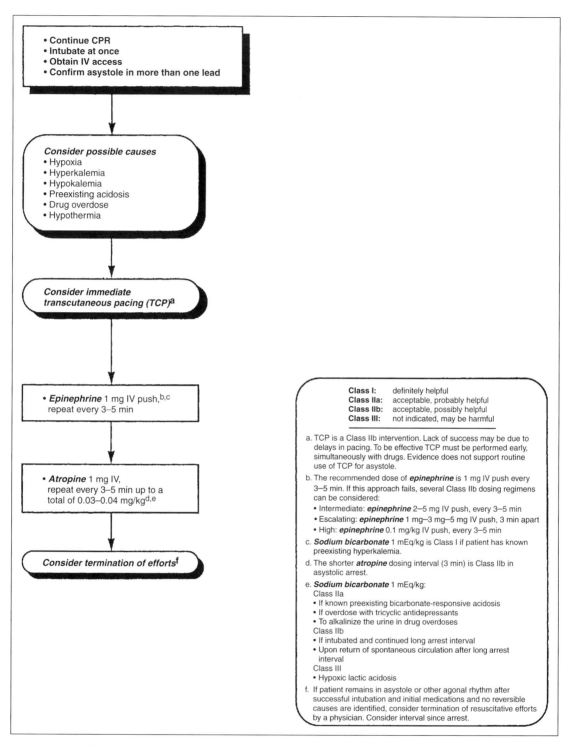

- Continue CPR
- Intubate at once
- Obtain IV access
- Confirm asystole in more than one lead

*Consider possible causes*
- Hypoxia
- Hyperkalemia
- Hypokalemia
- Preexisting acidosis
- Drug overdose
- Hypothermia

*Consider immediate transcutaneous pacing (TCP)[a]*

- *Epinephrine* 1 mg IV push,[b,c] repeat every 3–5 min

- *Atropine* 1 mg IV, repeat every 3–5 min up to a total of 0.03–0.04 mg/kg[d,e]

*Consider termination of efforts[f]*

| | |
|---|---|
| **Class I:** | definitely helpful |
| **Class IIa:** | acceptable, probably helpful |
| **Class IIb:** | acceptable, possibly helpful |
| **Class III:** | not indicated, may be harmful |

a. TCP is a Class IIb intervention. Lack of success may be due to delays in pacing. To be effective TCP must be performed early, simultaneously with drugs. Evidence does not support routine use of TCP for asystole.

b. The recommended dose of *epinephrine* is 1 mg IV push every 3–5 min. If this approach fails, several Class IIb dosing regimens can be considered:
   - Intermediate: *epinephrine* 2–5 mg IV push, every 3–5 min
   - Escalating: *epinephrine* 1 mg–3 mg–5 mg IV push, 3 min apart
   - High: *epinephrine* 0.1 mg/kg IV push, every 3–5 min

c. *Sodium bicarbonate* 1 mEq/kg is Class I if patient has known preexisting hyperkalemia.

d. The shorter *atropine* dosing interval (3 min) is Class IIb in asystolic arrest.

e. *Sodium bicarbonate* 1 mEq/kg:
   Class IIa
   - If known preexisting bicarbonate-responsive acidosis
   - If overdose with tricyclic antidepressants
   - To alkalinize the urine in drug overdoses
   Class IIb
   - If intubated and continued long arrest interval
   - Upon return of spontaneous circulation after long arrest interval
   Class III
   - Hypoxic lactic acidosis

f. If patient remains in asystole or other agonal rhythm after successful intubation and initial medications and no reversible causes are identified, consider termination of resuscitative efforts by a physician. Consider interval since arrest.

F I G U R E   **12-11**

Asystole treatment algorithm.

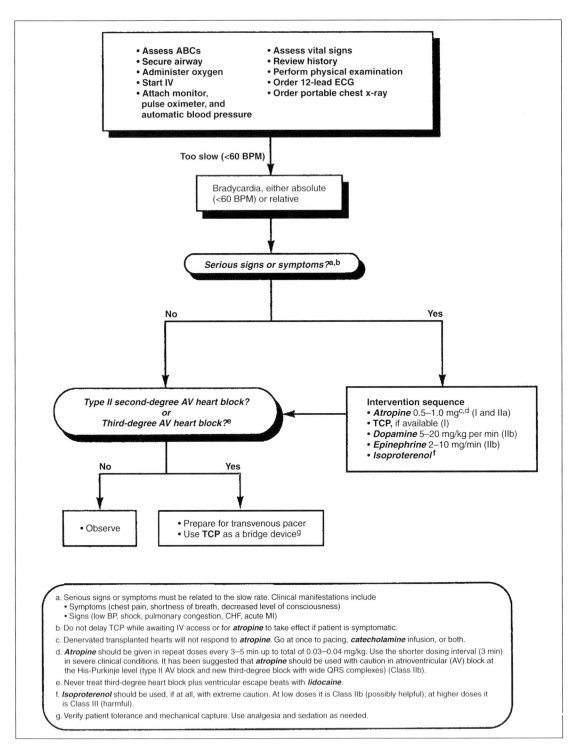

- **Assess ABCs**
- **Secure airway**
- **Administer oxygen**
- **Start IV**
- **Attach monitor, pulse oximeter, and automatic blood pressure**

- **Assess vital signs**
- **Review history**
- **Perform physical examination**
- **Order 12-lead ECG**
- **Order portable chest x-ray**

**Too slow (<60 BPM)**

Bradycardia, either absolute (<60 BPM) or relative

*Serious signs or symptoms?*[a,b]

No                                              Yes

*Type II second-degree AV heart block?*
*or*
*Third-degree AV heart block?*[e]

**Intervention sequence**
- *Atropine* 0.5–1.0 mg[c,d] (I and IIa)
- **TCP,** if available (I)
- *Dopamine* 5–20 mg/kg per min (IIb)
- *Epinephrine* 2–10 mg/min (IIb)
- *Isoproterenol*[f]

No                          Yes

- Observe

- Prepare for transvenous pacer
- Use **TCP** as a bridge device[g]

a. Serious signs or symptoms must be related to the slow rate. Clinical manifestations include
  - Symptoms (chest pain, shortness of breath, decreased level of consciousness)
  - Signs (low BP, shock, pulmonary congestion, CHF, acute MI)

b. Do not delay TCP while awaiting IV access or for *atropine* to take effect if patient is symptomatic.

c. Denervated transplanted hearts will not respond to *atropine*. Go at once to pacing, *catecholamine* infusion, or both.

d. *Atropine* should be given in repeat doses every 3–5 min up to total of 0.03–0.04 mg/kg. Use the shorter dosing interval (3 min) in severe clinical conditions. It has been suggested that *atropine* should be used with caution in atrioventricular (AV) block at the His-Purkinje level (type II AV block and new third-degree block with wide QRS complexes) (Class IIb).

e. Never treat third-degree heart block plus ventricular escape beats with *lidocaine*.

f. *Isoproterenol* should be used, if at all, with extreme caution. At low doses it is Class IIb (possibly helpful); at higher doses it is Class III (harmful).

g. Verify patient tolerance and mechanical capture. Use analgesia and sedation as needed.

F I G U R E    **12-12**

Bradycardia algorithm. The patient is not in cardiac arrest.

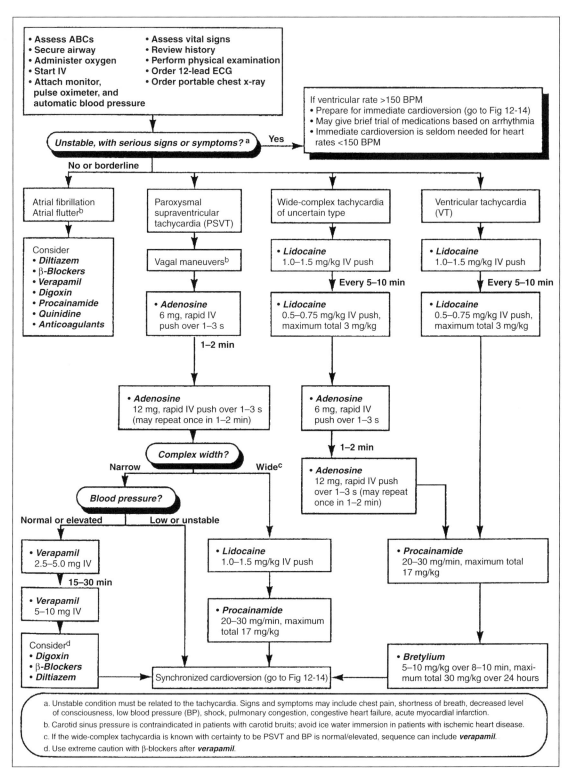

F I G U R E   **12-13**

Tachycardia algorithm.

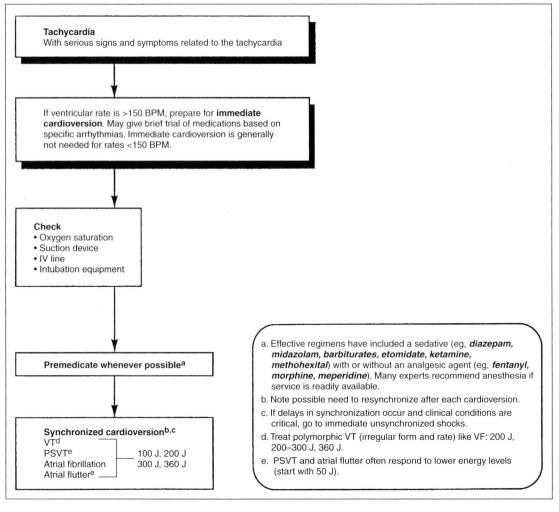

**Tachycardia**
With serious signs and symptoms related to the tachycardia

If ventricular rate is >150 BPM, prepare for **immediate cardioversion**. May give brief trial of medications based on specific arrhythmias. Immediate cardioversion is generally not needed for rates <150 BPM.

**Check**
• Oxygen saturation
• Suction device
• IV line
• Intubation equipment

**Premedicate whenever possible**[a]

**Synchronized cardioversion**[b,c]
VT[d]
PSVT[e]          100 J, 200 J
Atrial fibrillation   300 J, 360 J
Atrial flutter[e]

a. Effective regimens have included a sedative (eg, *diazepam, midazolam, barbiturates, etomidate, ketamine, methohexital*) with or without an analgesic agent (eg, *fentanyl, morphine, meperidine*). Many experts recommend anesthesia if service is readily available.
b. Note possible need to resynchronize after each cardioversion.
c. If delays in synchronization occur and clinical conditions are critical, go to immediate unsynchronized shocks.
d. Treat polymorphic VT (irregular form and rate) like VF: 200 J, 200–300 J, 360 J.
e. PSVT and atrial flutter often respond to lower energy levels (start with 50 J).

FIGURE  **12-14**

Electrical cardioversion algorithm. The patient is not in cardiac arrest.

of circulating blood volume (Lee, 1986). Furthermore, the enlarged uterus poses an obstruction to forward blood flow, particularly when arterial pressure and volume are decreased, as in a cardiac arrest.

Changes in the gravid woman's response to drugs and alterations in the maternal gastrointestinal system also hinder effective resuscitation. Vasopressors used in ACLS, especially alpha-adrenergic or combined alpha and beta agents are capable of producing uteroplacental vasocon-

striction, leading to decreased fetal oxygenation and carbon dioxide exchange. Decreases in gastrointestinal motility and relaxation of the lower esophageal sphincter lead to an increased risk of aspiration prior to or during endotracheal intubation. Thus, physiologic and anatomic changes of pregnancy involving the cardiac, respiratory, and gastrointestinal systems; the enlarging uterus; and the patient's response to pressors all adversely affect resuscitation of the pregnant patient.

## Modifications of Basic Life Support and Advanced Cardiac Life Support in Pregnancy

The anatomic and physiologic changes of pregnancy require several modifications in ECC (Table 12-5). Most important, to effect an increase in venous return and reduce supine hypotension, the uterus must be displaced to the left. Left lateral displacement can be achieved (1) by manual displacement of the uterus by a member of the resuscitation team, (2) by positioning the patient on an operating room table that can be tilted laterally, (3) by positioning a wedge under the right hip, (4) by using a Cardiff resuscitation wedge (Rees, 1988), or (5) by using a human wedge (Goodwin, 1992) (Figs 12-15 and 12-16). The human wedge kneels on the floor with the victim's back placed on the thighs of the human wedge. The wedge uses one arm to stabilize the victim's shoulder and the other arm to stabilize the pelvis. The human wedge maneuver has the

**TABLE 12-5**

Modifications in emergency cardiac care for the pregnant victim

Left uterine displacement
Aggressive airway management
Delivery within 5 minutes if fetus is viable
Aggressive restoration of circulatory volume if appropriate

advantage that it may be employed without equipment, utilizing an untrained person. Its obvious disadvantage is the wedge must be displaced when defibrillation is necessary.

While the maternal propensity for hypoxia and hypercapnia (which lead to decreases in uteroplacental perfusion) suggests that the pregnant patient may benefit from sodium bicarbonate in an arrest situation in order to keep maternal pH greater than 7.10, it must be kept in mind that sodium bicarbonate only very slowly crosses the placenta. Accordingly, with rapid correction

**FIGURE 12-15**

Cardiff resuscitation wedge, which tilts the patient such that the uterus is displaced to the patient's left side.

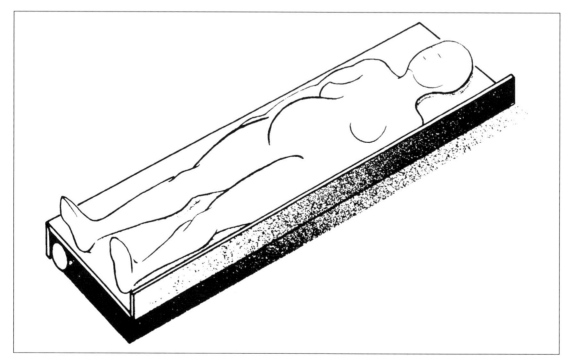

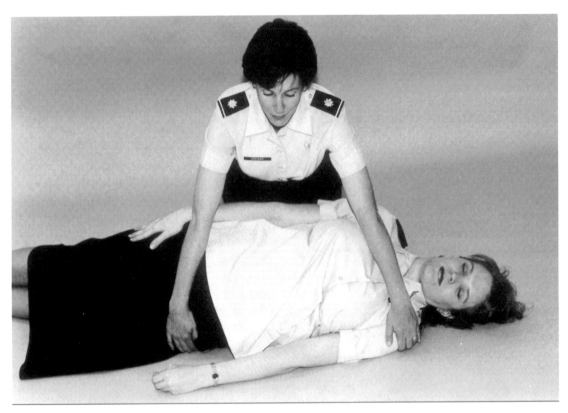

F I G U R E   **12-16**
Left uterine displacement achieved by a human wedge.

of maternal metabolic acidosis, her respiratory compensation will cease with normalization of her partial pressure of carbon dioxide ($pco_2$). If the maternal $pco_2$ increases from 20 mm Hg to 40 mm Hg as a result of bicarbonate administration, the fetal $pco_2$ will also increase. However, the fetus will not receive the benefit of the bicarbonate. If the fetal pH was 7.00 before maternal bicarbonate administration, the normalization of maternal pH will be achieved at the expense of increasing the fetal $pco_2$ by 20 mm Hg, with a resultant fall in fetal pH to approximately 6.84. Accordingly, the merits of such treatment must be questioned. Indeed, sodium bicarbonate is not indicated and is possibly harmful in patients with hypoxic lactic acidosis, such as occurs in nonintubated patients with prolonged cardiopulmonary arrest. Current understanding of the acid-base pathophysiology during cardiopulmonary arrest indicates that carbon dioxide generated in tissues is not well cleared by low blood flow (Adrogue, 1989). Adequate ventilation and restoration of perfusion are the mainstays of control of acid-base balance during cardiac arrest. Buffering the blood with bicarbonate does not benefit the patient (Adult Advanced Cardiac Life Support, 1992; Niemann, 1992).

Both the increased oxygen utilization in pregnancy and the increased risk of aspiration suggest that the airway should be managed aggressively, and prompt endotracheal intubation should be performed in all pregnant women during arrest situations. With an obstructed airway, abdominal thrusts must be avoided in the latter half of pregnancy and chest compressions substituted.

Clinical experience with the pharmacologic agents used in ACLS is limited in pregnancy. Importantly, the volume of distribution and drug metabolism may vary from nonpregnant norms.

If the victim does not respond to standard doses, higher doses should be considered to account for the expanded plasma volume of pregnancy. Although volume administration, which can lead to decreased cerebral and coronary blood flow, is generally not recommended during treatment of cardiac arrest, it should be strongly considered in cardiopulmonary arrest related to postpartum hemorrhage or circulatory collapse as seen with amniotic fluid embolism. In spite of theoretical concerns with some drugs used in ACLS, such as lidocaine inducing fetal acidosis and beta-blockers inducing fetal bradycardia, no adverse fetal effects have been shown (Briggs, 1990; Rubin, 1981). The agents used in ACLS are recommended in standard doses. However, if standard doses do not produce the predicted response, one should not hesitate to give higher doses to account for the expanded plasma volume of pregnancy.

## Complications of Cardiopulmonary Resuscitation During Pregnancy

Cardiopulmonary resuscitation during pregnancy may impose complications on both mother and fetus. Maternal injuries may include (1) fractures of ribs and sternum, (2) hemothorax and hemopericardium, (3) rupture of internal organs (especially the spleen and uterus), and (4) lacerations of organs (most notably the liver). Damaging effects to the fetus consist of CNS toxicity from medications, altered uterine activity, and reduced uteroplacental perfusion, with possible fetal hypoxemia and acidemia.

## Successful Resuscitation

In contrast to the image popularized in the media, CPR is rarely effective in restoring spontaneous circulation and permitting neurologically intact recovery to hospital discharge. Successful resuscitation is reported in 6% to 15% of patients suffering inhospital cardiac arrest (Karetzky, 1995; Diem, 1996). A recent report by Diem et al (1996) explored in detail this dichotomy between public perception and reality.

## Perimortem Cesarean Delivery

In ancient times, peripartum cesarean was performed postmortem, not to save the child but to remove it from the mother prior to burial. Numa Pompilus, the king of Rome (715–673 BCE) decreed that if a woman died while pregnant, the infant was to be immediately cut out of her abdomen (Ritter, 1961). This decree became part of the *Lex Regia* and subsequently part of the *Lex Caesare* (Emperor's law), hence, the origin of the "cesarean operation." By the first half of this century, the operation was performed in a desperate attempt to save the infant of a dying mother. By 1960, 120 successful postmortem cesareans were reported (Ritter, 1961). It was noted that fetal prognosis was better in cases of sudden maternal death than after chronic illnesses.

In the nineteenth edition of *Williams Obstetrics*, Cunningham and colleagues (1993) suggested that delivery within 5 minutes of cardiopulmonary arrest would not only benefit the infant but also may facilitate maternal resuscitation. This recommendation was based primarily on the report by Katz and colleagues (1986) who analyzed reports of successful results. They recognized that the gravid uterus may prevent proper CPR techniques from restoring adequate cardiac output. In the nonpregnant state, external chest compressions produce a cardiac output approximately 30% of normal. The gravid uterus in the supine position obstructs venous return and CO. Left lateral tilt causes the torso to roll, and part of the compression force is lost. Therefore, optimal chest compressions in pregnancy will yield less than 30% of normal cardiac output. Because without adequate cerebral perfusion irreversible brain damage from anoxia occurs within 4 to 6 minutes, they argue for cesarean within 4 to 5 minutes, especially when the woman is pulseless despite CPR. Pulselessness may persist until the uterus is evacuated (DePace, 1982; O'Connor, 1994). Delivery leads to a decrease in aortocaval obstruction, an increase in effectiveness of compressions, and in an increase in maternal CO.

Clearly, the timing of the operation is critical for infant survival, which appears proportional to the time between the mother's cardiac arrest and

TABLE 12-6

Perimortem cesarean delivery with the outcome of surviving infants from the time of maternal death until delivery

| Time Interval (min) | Surviving Infants | Intact Neurologic Status of Survivors |
|---|---|---|
| 0–5 | 45 | 98% |
| 6–15 | 18 | 83% |
| 16–25 | 9 | 33% |
| 26–35 | 4 | 25% |
| 36+ | 1 | 0% |

Source: Data from Katz VL, Dotters DJ, Droegemueller W. Perimortem cesarean delivery. Obstet Gynecol 1986;68:571 and Clark SL, Hawkins GDV, Dudley DA, et al. Amniotic fluid embolism: Analysis of the national registry. Am J Obstet Gynecol 1995;172:1939.

her delivery (Table 12-6). If delivery is accomplished within 5 minutes of maternal cardiac arrest, intact neurologic neonatal survival is the rule (Katz, 1986; Clark, 1995). Beyond 15 minutes, neonatal death or impaired survival is generally seen. Primate studies confirm brain damage in utero with as little as 6 minutes of complete asphyxia; severe cellular damage occurs by 8 minutes (Windle, 1968). Scattered reports describe infant survival at longer intervals following arrest, implying that cesarean delivery should be performed even several minutes postarrest if signs of fetal life are present (Selden, 1988; Kaiser, 1994).

Women with chronic illness are less likely to have a normal surviving infant by perimortem cesarean, as compared with those suffering an acute arrest. Because the latter is now relatively more common, a more compelling argument is made for a cesarean within minutes of an arrest. Thus, if a pregnant woman suffers a cardiopulmonary arrest beyond the stage of viability for a given institution, a perimortem cesarean delivery should be considered. The 4-minute limit to initiate delivery, as advocated by Katz et al (1986), the American College of Obstetricians and Gynecologists, and several texts, is derived from theoretical physiologic advantages for resuscitating the mother, as well as from extrapolation of data on infant survival. While such data suggest an ideal arrest-to-delivery interval, in actual practice these goals can be achieved only rarely. Further, it must be emphasized that no data exist to document actual maternal benefits of perimortem cesarean section; maternal death clearly remains, by far, the most likely outcome regardless of arrest-to-delivery interval.

## Conclusion

Since publication of the last edition of this text, two important changes have impacted clinical practice. The American Heart Association has made extensive revisions to ACLS algorithms (see Figs 12-8 through 12-14), and early as opposed to late perimortem cesarean has become more widely accepted. Late pregnancy requires certain modifications to ECC, including aggressive airway management and left lateral uterine displacement. Physiologic alterations of pregnancy suggest that larger doses of pharmacologic agents may be necessary and that once cardiopulmonary arrest is confirmed, initiation of delivery within 4 minutes appears to offer the best chance for both maternal and neonatal survival. It is important to recognize that these recommendations are based on few clinical data.

REFERENCES

Adrogue HJ, Rashad MN, Gorin AB, et al. Assessing acid-base status in circulatory failure: differences between arterial and central venous blood flow. N Engl J Med 1989;320:1312.

Adult Advanced Cardiac Life Support. JAMA 1992; 268:2199.

American Heart Association. Advanced cardiac life support. Dallas: American Heart Association, 1994a.

American Heart Association. Textbook of basic life support for healthcare providers. Dallas: American Heart Association, 1994b.

Briggs GG, Garite TJ. Effects on the fetus of drugs used in critical care. In: Clark SL, Cotton DB, Hankins GDV, Phelan J, eds. Critical care obstetrics. Oradell, NJ: Medical Economics, 1990:704.

Clark SL, Hankins GDV, Dudley DA, et al. Amniotic fluid embolism: Analysis of the national registry. Am J Obstet Gynecol 1995;172:1939.

Cunningham FG, MacDonald PC, Gant NF, et al. Williams obstetrics. 19th ed. Norwalk, CT: Appleton and Lange, 1993:1065.

DePace NL, Betesh JS, Kotler MN. "Postmortem" cesarean section with recovery of both mother and offspring. JAMA 1982;248:971.

deSwiet M. Pulmonary disorders. In: Creasy RK, Resnick R, eds. Maternal-fetal medicine principles and practice. Philadelphia: WB Saunders, 1994:891–904.

Diem SJ, Lantos JD, Tulsky JA. Cardiopulmonary resuscitation on television. Miracles and misinformation. N Engl J Med 1996;334:1578.

Eisenberg MS, Bergner L, Hallstrom A. Cardiac resuscitation in the community. JAMA 1979; 24:1905.

Goodwin APL, Pearce AJ. The human wedge. A manoeuvre to relieve aortocaval compression during resuscitation in late pregnancy. Anesthesia 1992;47:433.

Kaiser RT. Air embolism death of a pregnant woman secondary to orogenital sex. Academic Emerg Med 1994;1:555.

Karetzky M, Zubair M, Parikh J. Cardiopulmonary resuscitation in intensive care unit and nonintensive care unit patients: immediate and long term survival. Arch Intern Med 1995;155:1277.

Katz VL, Dotters DJ, Droegemueller W. Perimortem cesarean delivery. Obstet Gynecol 1986;68:571.

Kouwenhoven WB, Jude JR, Knickerbocker GG. Closed-chest cardiac message. JAMA 1960; 173:94.

Lee RV, Rogers BD, White LM, Harvey RC. Cardiopulmonary resuscitation of pregnant women. Am J Med 1986;81:311.

Niemann JT. Cardiopulmonary resuscitation. N Engl J Med 1992;327:1075.

O'Connor RL, Sevarino FB. Cardiopulmonary arrest in a pregnant patient: a report of a successful resuscitation. J Clin Anesth 1994;6:66.

Reed AP. Current concepts in airway management for cardiopulmonary resuscitation. Mayo Clin Proc 1995;70:1172.

Rees GAD, Willis BA. Resuscitation in late pregnancy. Anesthesia 1988;43:347.

Ritter JW. Postmortem cesarean section. JAMA 1961;175:715.

Rubin PC. Beta blockers in pregnancy. N Engl J Med 1981;305:1323.

Rudikoff MT, Maughan WL, Effon M, et al. Mechanisms of blood flow during cardiopulmonary resuscitation. Circulation 1980;61:345.

Satin AJ, Hankins GDV. Cardiopulmonary resuscitation in pregnancy. In: Clark SL, Cotton DB, Hankins GDV, Phelan J, eds. Critical care obstetrics. Oradell, NJ: Medical Economics, 1990:579.

Selden BS, Binke TJ. Complete maternal and fetal recovery after prolonged cardiac arrest. Ann Emerg Med 1988;17:346.

Syverson CJ, Chavkin W, Atrash HK, et al. Pregnancy related mortality in New York City, 1980 to 1984: causes of death and associated risk factors. Am J Obstet Gynecol 1991;164:603.

Werner JA, Greene HL, Janko CL, Cobb LA. Visualization of cardiac valve motion in man during external chest compressions using two-dimensional echocardiography: Implications regarding the mechanism of blood flow. Circulation 1981;63:1417.

Windle WF. Brain damage at birth. JAMA 1968; 206:1967.

# CHAPTER *13*

# Cardiopulmonary Bypass

*C*ardiopulmonary bypass (CPB) results in significant alterations in patient physiology. Virtually every organ system is affected by CPB. Some of the salient adverse effects include dramatic alterations in cardiovascular function (hypotension, nonpulsatile blood flow, cardioplegia, cardiac arrhythmias) and inflammatory and immune responses, which involve changes in coagulation as well as most cellular and protein components of blood. Especially in open heart procedures, systemic embolization of particulate material as well as air can also occur. In addition, the management of patients requiring CPB frequently includes the use of hypothermia, invasive monitoring and supportive techniques, and the use of a variety of cardiovascular pharmacologic agents. Not infrequently, complications involving one or more major organ systems are experienced.

The first reports of cardiac surgery during pregnancy were published in 1952 and involved 11 closed mitral commissurotomies performed during pregnancy (Brock, 1952; Cooley, 1952; Logan, 1952; Mason, 1952). In 1961, Harken and Taylor published a review of 394 published cases of cardiac surgery during pregnancy (Harken, 1961). In this series, a maternal mortality rate of 1.8% and a fetal mortality rate of 9% were reported. Maternal mortality was not different than that seen in nonpregnant patients during this period.

Most available reports of cardiac surgery during pregnancy involve valve repair or replacement.

Early collective experience in over 500 patients undergoing closed mitral valvotomy prior to 1965 was associated with maternal mortality of under 2% and fetal mortality under 10% (Ueland, 1965). In 1968, Knapp and Arden presented data on 27 additional pregnant patients undergoing this procedure. These investigators found no maternal mortality, but a 15% perinatal mortality rate. In 1983, Becker (1983) published results from a survey of 600 members of the Society of Thoracic Surgeons. One hundred one cases of closed mitral commissurotomy during pregnancy were described, most from centers outside the United States performed during the second trimester of pregnancy due to progressive congestive failure. No maternal deaths were reported, and the perinatal mortality rate was 3%. Bernal and Miralles (1986), in a review of the literature, reported maternal and fetal mortalities of less than 2% and 10%, respectively, in 394 patients undergoing closed commissurotomy. In 1987, Vosloo and Reichart (1987) described 41 patients undergoing closed mitral commissurotomy during pregnancy. As with most previous studies, no maternal mortality was seen; however, overall fetal wastage was 12%, and 17% for procedures performed in the third trimester. Today, with the availability of continuous electronic fetal heart rate monitoring during surgery and the possibility of simultaneous cesarean section should severe fetal compromise be detected, such losses would be rare.

Despite the potential advantages of closed commissurotomy (or, more recently, balloon valvuloplasty) during pregnancy, however, this approach is associated with a significant likelihood of patients requiring additional surgery at a later date; in the series of Vosloo and Reichart (1987), 22% of patients required an additional cardiac surgery during a follow-up period lasting from 5 to 17 years. Thus, a longer-lasting procedure would be desirable, if the generally good perinatal outcome seen with closed commissurotomy could be maintained.

Most surgeons in the United States advocate open valvuloplasty in pregnant patients (Chambers, 1994). In nonpregnant patients, open commissurotomy may be performed as safely as can closed procedures, with both better short- and long-term results (Roe, 1971). Such procedures, however, require cardiopulmonary bypass, a technique that introduces an entirely different set of fetal risks than do closed procedures.

The body of literature describing the experiences of pregnant patients undergoing cardiac operations with CPB is comprised of case reports and surveys with no one institution or team of individuals having a large experience (Chambers, 1994). No well-controlled studies have been reported assessing the impact or consequence of CPB and its various aspects on the pregnant patient, the fetoplacental unit, or fetal outcome. In addition, these reports date back to the late 1950s (Dubourg, 1959) and early 1960s. In comparison to approaches and techniques currently employed, the care that the pregnant cardiac patient has received has changed significantly over time. As a result of this, many conclusions regarding maternal care and fetal outcome must be regarded as tentative.

## Uteroplacental Perfusion and Bypass Physiology

Uteroplacental blood flow (UPBF) is the major determinant of oxygen and other essential nutrient transport to the fetus. A direct correlation between uterine blood flow (UBF) and fetal oxygenation has been demonstrated in both animal models and humans (Bilardo, 1990; Skillman,

1985). Uteroplacental blood flow is derived primarily from uterine arteries, with a smaller contribution of unknown significance coming from the ovarian arteries. The uterine arteries are branches of the internal iliac arteries. Uterine artery blood flow increases two- to threefold in pregnancy and can represent up to 12% of the cardiac output. Increases in UBF during pregnancy are due to both physical (increased diameter of the uterine artery) and physiologic (decreased responsiveness of the uterine artery to endogenous circulating vasoconstrictors) mechanisms. Selective uterine artery relaxation during pregnancy may be the result of vasodilators released from its endothelium, such as PGI2 or nitric oxide, or local hormonal actions, which diminish the activity of certain intracellular enzymes that mediate vasoconstriction.

UBF is related to perfusion pressure and vascular resistance according to the formula:

$$UBF = \frac{\text{Uterine arterial pressure} - \text{Uterine venous pressure}}{\text{Uterine vascular resistance}}$$

Under normal circumstances, the uterine arteries are maximally dilated, thus impairing potential blood flow autoregulation in response to diminished systemic BP. Although in the ovine model, placental blood flow and fetal perfusion changes do not always parallel alterations in uterine artery blood flow (UABF) (Landauer, 1986), in the human it is generally considered axiomatic that any significant fall in systemic pressure will result in a corresponding decrease in uterine and placental perfusion, with resultant fetal hypoxia. These considerations are of paramount concern when considering the potential pressure and flow alterations associated with cardiopulmonary bypass.

## Cardiopulmonary Bypass

### Anesthesia

Although some anesthetic agents may produce teratogenic effects, especially after prolonged administration in experimental models, modern anesthetics are considered to be safe for use in the pregnant surgical patient (Brodsky, 1980; Duncan, 1986; Mazze, 1989, 1991; Shnider, 1965;

Smith, 1963). However, there may be an increased risk of fetal loss with first-trimester exposure to general anesthesia, which can be accentuated by the trauma of surgery, especially with surgical procedures on or around the uterus (Brodsky, 1980; Duncan, 1986).

In the pregnant cardiac surgery patient, it is more likely that the immediate cardiovascular depressant actions of anesthetic agents constitute a greater risk to the fetus. For example, because of their sensitivity to the hemodynamic effects of many anesthetic agents resulting in a limited ability to tolerate usual doses of anesthetics, pregnant as well as cardiac surgical patients as a group are known to be at increased risk for awareness under anesthesia. This fact highlights the difficulty anesthesiologists encounter when trying to provide an adequate depth of anesthesia for pregnant cardiac patients without compromising hemodynamic function. Also, the myocardial depression and hypotension produced by anesthesia can interact with other factors (maternal anemia and respiratory alkalosis, exogenous catecholamines or vasoactive drugs, cardiac pathology) and alter uterine artery pressure or resistance and uteroplacental perfusion and exacerbate fetal hypoxia and acidosis. Anesthetic techniques and agents should be chosen after careful consideration of maternal cardiac pathology and cardiovascular status in an attempt to minimize adverse hemodynamic effects in the mother in order to maintain uteroplacental perfusion (Figs 13-1, 13-2, 13-3).

## Ventilation

Mechanical positive pressure ventilation is instituted routinely in patients undergoing cardiac surgery, and various degrees of hyperventilation are frequently produced, either intentionally or inadvertently. Blood gas disturbances can effect sympathetic activity and thus indirectly effect UBF. In addition, hyperventilation may decrease uteroplacental perfusion either through mechanical means by increasing intrathoracic pressure and decreasing cardiac output or through the induction of hypocapnia, which decreases UBF. Thus, hyperventilation should be carefully avoided in the pregnant surgical patient unless specifically indicated (see later discussion).

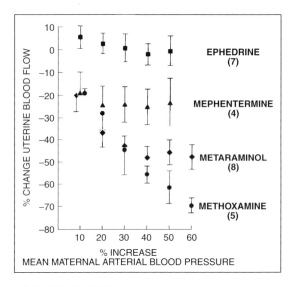

F I G U R E **13-1**

**Mean changes in uterine blood flow at equal elevations of mean arterial blood pressure following vasopressor administration.** (Reprinted with permission from Ralston DH, Snider SM, DeLorimer AA. Effects of equipotent ephedrine, metaraminol, mephentermine and methoxamine on uterine blood flow in the pregnant ewe. Anesthesiology 1974;40:354. Copyright © 1974, Williams & Wilkins Co.)

## Patient Positioning

Lateral uterine displacement during cardiac surgery is essential to avoid decreased cardiac output and thus the uteroplacental perfusion seen in the supine position (Clark, 1991). A lateral tilt of at least 30 to 40 degrees has been recommended during CPB (Becker, 1983; Nazarian, 1976). This is especially crucial because CPB often results in hypotension, even in the nonpregnant patient. A combination of a wedge and table tilt is generally adequate to achieve appropriate lateral uterine displacement.

## Cannulation

Cannulation of the inferior vena cava might partially obstruct blood flow in this vessel. While it is unlikely that such obstruction would lead to severe problems for mother or fetus, it could potentially impair uteroplacental perfusion due either to increases in uterine venous pressure or to

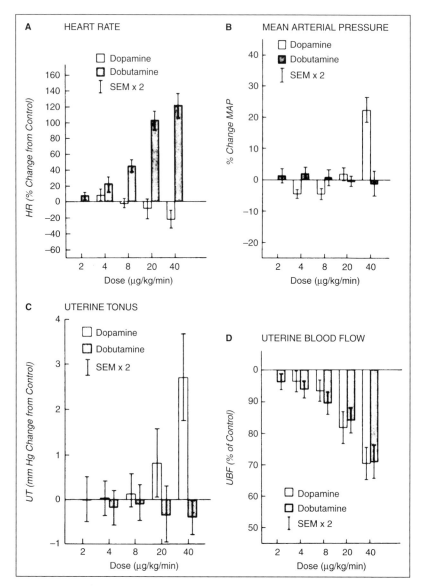

F I G U R E   **13-2**

Comparison of average changes in (A) HR, (B) MAP, (C) UT, and (D) UBF at various rates of dopamine and dobutamine infusion in pregnant ewes. HR, heart rate; MAP, mean arterial pressure; UT, uterine tonus; UBF, uterine blood flow. (Reproduced by permission from Fishburne JI, Meis PJ, Urban RB, et al. Vascular and uterine responses to dobutamine and dopamine in the gravid ewe. Am J Obstet Gynecol 1980;137:944.)

decreased blood return to the right heart and diminished cardiac output (Meffert, 1968).

## Cardiopulmonary Bypass Prime

Hemodilution is a mainstay of CPB. It decreases blood product utilization and its attendant costs and risks. Hemodilution also improves the rheology of blood by decreasing its viscosity, resulting in a lower arterial resistance and improved peripheral perfusion (Cooper, 1993). Other purported benefits of hemodilution during CPB include decreases in major organ complications, such as cerebral vascular accident, and renal and pulmonary dysfunction. In the pregnant cardiac surgical patient, however, the hemodilution produced by typical CPB prime solutions and volumes may compromise the oxygen-carrying capacity in these already relatively anemic patients. Whole blood or RBCs can be added to the prime of the CPB circuit so that the resultant hematocrit is no less than 21% to 26% (Becker,

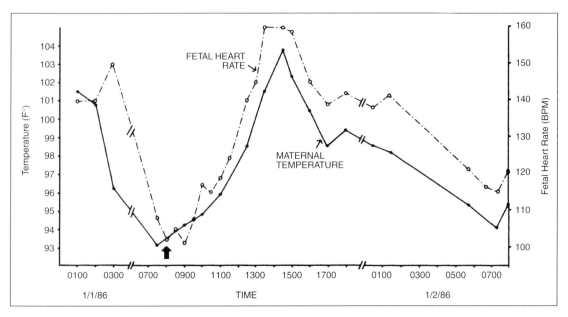

F I G U R E   **13-3**

Maternal temperature and fetal heart rate (FHR). The FHR plot directly parallels the maternal temperature. The arrow at 0800, 1/1/86, represents the nadir of maternal BP: 87/46 mm Hg (mean arterial pressure, 60). Within 20 minutes the BP was 94/57 mm Hg (mean arterial pressure, 69). The mean arterial pressure during the rest of the illustrated time ranged from 64 to 76. Previous and subsequent pressures during this pregnancy ranged from 90/50 to 110/65 mm Hg (mean arterial pressure, 63–80). BPM, beats per minute. (Reproduced by permission from Jadhon ME, Main EK. Fetal bradycardia associated with maternal hypothermia. Obstet Gynecol 1988;72:496.)

1983). Hemodilution and subsequent changes in hormone concentrations, such as a decrease in progesterone, may play a role in triggering uterine contractions (Korsten, 1989). Korsten et al (1989) suggested that the addition of progesterone to the prime may be helpful in avoiding preterm uterine activity, but this approach requires further investigation before incorporation into clinical practice.

## Oxygenator Type

Because bubble oxygenators may be associated with a greater incidence of embolic phenomena, membrane oxygenators are recommended for the conduct of CPB in the gravid patient.

## Hypothermia

Like hemodilution, hypothermia has long been considered an important component of CPB in order to decrease systemic oxygen consumption and minimize myocardial damage. In addition, some investigators have found an increased risk of neurologic injury to the patient if CPB is performed under normothermic conditions (McLean, 1996). In pregnant dogs, cooling to 28°C is associated with an increase in uterine tone (Assali, 1962). However, this did not result in any demonstrable effect on fetal survival, and pregnant ewes cooled to 29°C did not exhibit fetal distress as long as maternal acidosis and hypoxia were avoided (Matsuki, 1972). In humans, no adverse fetal effects have been demonstrated in pregnant patients undergoing cardiac and noncardiac surgery cooled as low as 25°C (Korsten, 1989; Boatman, 1958; Matsuki, 1972; Koh, 1975; Lamb, 1981; Levy, 1980; Mora, 1987). Although fetal heart rate has been reported to decrease in parallel with maternal temperature (see Fig 13-3), there is no evidence that hypothermic perfusion is deleterious to the fetus. However, rewarming is associated with increased frequency of uterine contractions (Becker, 1983). Thus, while normothermic or minimally hypothermic perfusion is probably ideal in the pregnant patient unless extended aortic clamp times are anticipated, actual risks of hypothermia are minimal, and its use should not be avoided if significant maternal benefits are likely to ensue due to the specifics of patient cardiovascular physiology or the preference or experience of the cardiovascular surgical team.

## Pulsatility

Nonpulsatile flow is most commonly employed during CPB. It can be argued that pulsatile flow would be superior, providing a more normal physiologic milieu and better tissue and organ perfusion than nonpulsatile blood flow. For example, differences in vascular resistance, oxygen delivery, and myocardial lactate production indicate the superiority of pulsatile CPB (Philbin, 1993; Trimakas, 1979). However, clinical outcome differences have not been demonstrated with pulsatile versus nonpulsatile CPB. In a pregnant patient receiving nonpulsatile CPB described by Farmakides et al (1987), Doppler velocimetry suggested the presence of pulsatile uterine artery flow, although these findings may have been affected by pump artifact (Strickland, 1991).

## Flow Rate

Because normal cardiac output in pregnant women is often greater than 6 liters/min (Clark, 1989), the usual (2.5 liters/m$^2$) flows employed during CPB may be too little. Changes in baseline fetal heart rate have been identified after initial flow rates as high as 80 mL/kg/min, even in the absence of maternal hypotension (Chambers, 1994). Increases in CPB flows to 3.0 to 4.0 liters/m$^2$

have been successfully (if only temporarily) employed during pregnancy, especially in response to fetal bradycardia (Becker, 1983; Lamb, 1981; Chambers, 1994). For example, Koh et al (1975) were the first to describe improvement in fetal bradycardia by increasing flow rate by 16%. Since that time, numerous other investigators have confirmed the value of increasing pump flow rate to improve fetal bradycardia (Korsten, 1989; Lamb, 1981; Trimakis, 1979; Werch, 1977; Veray, 1977; Bernal, 1986).

## Pressure

The ideal mean arterial pressure (MAP) during CPB in the pregnant patient has not been established and likely is highly variable. However, a consensus exists in the literature supporting the use of moderate to high arterial pressures during CPB. Mean arterial pressure should initially be maintained at a level of 70 mm Hg or greater. It is preferable to produce elevations in MAP with fluid volume administration and high flow rates as opposed to vasopressor administration, which would have an adverse effect on uteroplacental blood flow. It should be anticipated that on institution of CPB, transient but significant hypotension occurs and frequently produces fetal bradycardia (Koh, 1975; Lamb, 1981; Levy, 1980; Trimakas, 1979). This is generally correctable by appropriate manipulations of pump flow and pressure.

## Anticoagulation

Anticoagulation is essential during CPB. It is generally accomplished with heparin therapy and poses no risks to the fetus. Such anticoagulation is typically reversed with protamine sulfate following separation from CPB. There are no available data concerning the use of antifibrinolytics in the pregnant cardiac patient to improve hemostasis and decrease perioperative blood loss.

## Cardioplegia

The application of cardioplegia may need to be more frequent with the maintenance of high flows during CPB, especially if normothermia or only mild hypothermia is employed. Cardiac activity may return as frequently as every 10 minutes under these circumstances. Concomitant tocolytic therapy may potentially also increase the need for cardioplegia and is generally avoided unless absolutely essential.

## Acid-Base Status

Acid-base status may vary significantly during CPB. The most common approaches to the management of acid-base status during CPB are called pH STAT and alpha STAT. Briefly, alpha STAT management attempts to maintain normocarbia, as determined by blood gas analysis of a blood sample temperature of 37°C. pH STAT management usually involves the addition of carbon dioxide to the CPB oxygenator to maintain a calculated patient blood $pco_2$ of 40 mm Hg at any given patient temperature during hypothermic CPB. Although theoretical advantages and disadvantages have been suggested for both approaches, the superiority of one technique over another has not been demonstrated in studies performed to date.

The management of arterial carbon dioxide partial pressures has particular relevance for the pregnant patient undergoing CPB, because maternal hyperventilation can impair fetal oxygenation (Levinson, 1974; Motoyama, 1967). Levinson et al (1974) reported that in the unanesthetized pregnant ewe, mechanical hyperventilation with normocarbia maintained by the addition of carbon dioxide impaired UBF because of the intrathoracic effects of positive pressure on cardiac output. These authors found that respiratory alkalosis additionally impaired fetal oxygenation. On the other hand, after studying anesthetized ewes, Motoyama et al (1967) attributed impairment of fetal oxygenation solely to the respiratory alkalosis produced by hyperventilation and not the effects of positive pressure. Maternal metabolic alkalemia also impaired fetal oxygenation, while maternal hypercapnia with acidemia was associated with an increase in fetal oxygenation. These changes were due to a combination of alterations in oxygen transfer within the placenta and changes in umbilical blood flow. As summarized by Motoyama et al, reports in humans support the notion that the fetal effects of maternal hyperventilation can be deleterious. Based on available information, avoidance of significant disturbances in acid-base balance, especially respiratory alkalosis, is recommended.

## Cardiopulmonary Bypass Duration

The technical proficiency and speed of the cardiac surgical team have been well established as two of the primary determinants of outcome in cardiac surgery. With regards to the pregnant cardiac patient, fetal morbidity and mortality also appear to increase with CPB duration. Thus, it is essential that CPB time be minimized in the pregnant patient.

## Fetal Monitoring During Cardiopulmonary Bypass

In the previable fetus (< 24 wk), cesarean delivery would generally not be indicated, even if fetal compromise were detected during CPB. Even in the 24- to 26-week gestational age range, the potential risks of an additional major abdominal operation during the perioperative period in patients undergoing open heart surgery must be carefully weighed against the likelihood of intact neonatal survival. Because neonatal morbidity and mortality statistics are continually changing, consultation with a neonatologist is ideal to provide accurate information to the patient. However, even if non-intervention is elected, careful fetal monitoring is important, because alterations in pump flow and pressure may often enhance perinatal outcome in the face of bradycardia without the need to resort to operative delivery. Such monitoring is often most easily performed with continuous external electronic fetal heart rate monitoring, assuming fetal size and maternal habitus do not preclude such a technique. Otherwise, intermittent auscultation may allow the obstetric attendant to detect significant decreases in fetal heart rate and suggest the need for pump manipulation, if possible (Liu, 1985).

Other fetal heart rate features, such as diminished variability and a sinusoidal-like pattern, have also been described in association with CPB and may be amenable to pump manipulation, as described previously (Koh, 1975; Levy, 1980; Korsten, 1989; Burke, 1990). If technically feasible, uterine activity also should be monitored during CPB. If regular contractions appear, consideration may be given to tocolysis. Korsten et al (1989) reported uterine contractions that appeared shortly after the initiation of CPB and were decreased with the intravenous infusion of ritodrine hydrochloride. Terbutaline or magnesium sulfate may be appropriate alternative agents. However, given the lack of evidence of significant benefit of such tocolytic agents, even in bona-fide preterm labor, and the difficulty in distinguishing (in the short term) uterine irritability from preterm labor, great caution must be exercised in administering drugs with potent cardiovascular effects to a patient undergoing CPB. Such therapy is only appropriate given firm evidence of preterm labor in the fetus with gestational age below 32 to 34 weeks and with concurrence of the cardiovascular surgery team. During the postoperative period, careful fetal and uterine activity monitoring should be continued.

Actual fetal risks of CPB are difficult to establish, because evidence exists almost exclusively from compilations of case report data (Zitnik, 1969; Roussouw, 1993). Becker's survey of 68 CPB procedures performed during pregnancy by members of the Society of Thoracic Surgery suggested an overall fetal death rate of 16% (Becker, 1983) (Table 13-1). Westaby et al (1992) compiled a summary of reported cases of CPB during pregnancy between 1959 and 1990, with a cumulative fetal death rate of 17.4% (Table 13-2). Clearly, however, such figures have little meaning for counseling the pregnant patient today. These statistics may represent underreporting of bad outcomes, yet they are unjustifiably pessimistic, given the dramatic improvements in both cardiovascular and perinatal and neonatal care that exist today compared with those years in which many of these reported cases occurred. For the patient who has reached a stage of viability, where cesarean delivery may be considered, fetal death rate probably approaches zero, because ominous fetal heart rate patterns not promptly corrected by alterations in flow rate or pressure can be recognized and simultaneous cesarean performed (Martin, 1981). For patients with fetuses younger than 24 to 26 weeks, a 10% to 15% fetal mortality rate with heart surgery and CPB appears to be a

T A B L E    **13-1**

**Summary of cardiac procedures performed during pregnancy***

| Procedure | Total | Indication for Operation | Maternal Survivors | Fetal Survivors | Fetal Deaths |
|---|---|---|---|---|---|
| Closed mitral commissurotomy | 101 | CHF (96), emboli (3), hemoptysis (2) | 101 | 98 | 3 |
| Open mitral commissurotomy | 23 | CHF (23) | 23 | 22 | 1 |
| Mitral valve replacement | 19 | CHF (14), endocarditis (1), thrombosed prosthesis (4) | 18 | 15 | 4 |
| Aortic valve replacement | 10 | Aortic stenosis (7), endocarditis (3) | 10 | 6 | 4 |
| Pulmonary embolectomy | 3 | Shock (3) | 3 | 2 | 1 |
| Closure of atrial or ventricular septal defect | 8 | CHF (4), elective operation (4) | 8 | 7 | 1 |
| Coronary bypass | 3 | Unstable angina (3) | 3 | 3 | 0 |
| Myxoma removal | 2 | | 2 | 2 | 0 |

*Includes CPB and non-CPB procedures.

Source: Adapted from Becker RM. Intracardiac surgery in pregnant women. Ann Thorac Surg 1983;36:453–458.

T A B L E   **13-2**

Summary of reported cases of cardiac surgery performed with
cardiopulmonary bypass during pregnancy, 1959–1990

| Procedure | No. of Patients | Indication for Operation | Maternal Deaths | Fetal Deaths |
|---|---|---|---|---|
| Open mitral commissurotomy | 33 | CHF, 27* | 0 | 2 |
| Mitral valve replacement | 29 | CHF, 21; endocarditis, 1; thrombosed prosthesis, 7 | 1 | 6 |
| Aortic valve replacement | 15 | Aortic stenosis, 9; endocarditis, 6 | 0 | 5 |
| Pulmonary embolectomy | 4 | Shock, 4 | 0 | 1 |
| Closure of ASD or VSD | 22 | CHF, 8* | 1 | 6 |
| Coronary bypass | 4 | Unstable angina, 4 | 0 | 0 |
| Myxoma removal | 4 | — | | |
| Repair of thoracic aorta | 3 | Leaking/ruptured aneurysm, 3 | 0 | 0 |
| Tetralogy of Fallot | 1 | — | 0 | 0 |
| Total (%) | 115 | | 2 (1.7) | 20 (17.4) |

*Data in literature were incomplete.

CHF, congestive heart failure; ASD, atrial septal defect; VSD, ventricular septal defect.

Reproduced by permission from Westaby S, Parry AJ, Forfar JC. Reoperation for prosthetic valve endocarditis in the third trimester of pregnancy. Ann Thorac Surg 1992;53:263.

reasonable figure. For the term or near-term fetus, pre-CPB delivery would also be an appropriate option to avoid the potential need for concomitant cardiac and obstetric surgery.

## Postoperative Course

Patients undergoing CPB frequently suffer significant neurologic deficits and complications after heart surgery. These deficits can occur transiently in up to 50% of patients, with a much smaller (<5%) number experiencing permanent focal or cognitive problems (Borowicz, 1996; McLean, 1996). In pregnant patients, these problems are likely to be of greater concern for several reasons. Emergency procedures, and especially open heart operations, will increase neurologic complication rates. Systemic embolization and stroke will also be increased in pregnant patients if their condition includes rheumatic valvular disease with bacterial endocarditis and the presence of vegetations.

Once postoperative bleeding has resolved, and depending on the type of valvular prosthesis employed, mothers may require continued and consistent anticoagulation postoperatively. The complex issues surrounding the use of heparin versus coumadin derivatives in these patients is discussed in more detail in Chapters 15 and 17 of this volume.

Eventual delivery of the fetus may take place several months after cardiac operation. At the time of delivery, even if maternal outcome after surgery has been excellent, complete evaluation of the mother's cardiovascular status and advanced preparation for and treatment of problems (e.g., hemorrhage) should be made.

**R E F E R E N C E S**

Assali NS, Westin B. Effects of hypothermia on uterine circulation and on the fetus. Proc Soc Exp Biol Med 1962;109:485–488.

Becker RM. Intracardiac surgery in pregnant women. Ann Thorac Surg 1983;36:453–458.

Bernal JM, Miralles PJ. Cardiac surgery with cardiopulmonary bypass during pregnancy. Obstet Gynecol Surv 1986;41:1–6.

Bilardo CM, Nicolaides KH, Campbell S. Doppler measurements of fetal and uteroplacental circulations: relationship. Am J Obstet Gynecol 1990;162:115–120.

Boatman KK, Bradford VA. Excision of an internal carotid aneurysm during pregnancy employing hypothermia and a vascular shunt. Ann Surg 1958;148:271–275.

Borowicz LM, Goldsborough MA, Seines OA, McKhann GM. Neuropsychologic change after cardiac surgery: a critical review. J Cardiothorac Vasc Anesth 1996;10:105–112.

Brock RC. Valvulotomy in pregnancy. Proc R Soc Med 1952;45:538.

Brodsky JB, Cohen EN, Brown BW, et al. Surgery during pregnancy and fetal outcome. Am J Obstet Gynecol 1980;138:1165–1167.

Burke AE, Hurr D, Bolan JC, et al. Sinusoidal fetal heart rate pattern during cardiopulmonary bypass. Am J Obstet Gynecol 1990;163:17–18.

Chambers CE, Clark SL. Cardiac surgery during pregnancy. Clin Obstet Gynecol 1994;37:316–323.

Clark SL. Cardiac disease in pregnancy. Crit Care Clin 1991;7:777.

Clark SL, Cotton DB, Lee W, et al. Central hemodynamic assessment of normal term pregnancy. Am J Obstet Gynecol 1989;161:1439.

Cooley DA, Chapman DW. Mitral commissurotomy during pregnancy. JAMA 1952;150:1113.

Cooper JR Jr, Slogoff S. Hemodilution and priming solutions for cardiopulmonary bypass. In: Gravlee GP, Davis RE, Utley JR, eds. Cardiopulmonary bypass. Baltimore: Williams and Wilkins, 1993:124–137.

Dubourg G, Broustet P, Brigaud H, et al. Correction complete d'une Triade de Fallot, en circulation extra-corporelle, chez une femme enceinte. Arch Mal Coeur 1959;52:1389–1391.

Duncan PG, Pope WD, Cohen MM, Geer N. Fetal risk of anesthesia and surgery during pregnancy. Anesthesiology 1986;64:790–794.

Farmakides G, Schulman H, Mohtashemo M, et al. Uterine-umbilical velocimetry in open heart surgery. Am J Obstet Gynecol 1987;156:1221–1222.

Fishburne JI, Meis PJ, Urban RB, et al. Vascular and uterine responses to dobutamine and dopamine in the gravid ewe. Am J Obstet Gynecol 1980;137:944.

Harken DE, Taylor WJ. Cardiac surgery during pregnancy. Clin Obstet Gynecol 1961;4:697.

Jadhon ME, Main EK. Fetal bradycardia associated with maternal hypothermia. Obstet Gynecol 1988;72:496.

Koh KS, Friesen RM, Livingstone RA, Peddle LJ. Fetal monitoring during maternal cardiac surgery with cardiopulmonary bypass. Can Med Assoc J 1975;112:1102–1104.

Korsten HHM, Van Zundert AAJ, Moou PNM, et al. Emergency aortic valve replacement in the 24th-week of pregnancy. Acta Anaesthesiol Belg 1989;40:201–205.

Lamb MP, Ross K, Johnstone A, Manners JM. Fetal heart monitoring during open heart surgery. Br J Obstet Gynecol 1981;88:669–674.

Landauer M, Phernetton TM, Rankin JHG. Maternal ovine placental vascular responses to adenosine. Am J Obstet Gynecol 1986;154:1152–1155.

Levinson G, Shnider SM, deLorimier AA, Steffenson JL. Effects of maternal hyperventilation on uterine blood flow and fetal oxygenation and acid-based status. Anesthesiology 1974;40:340–347.

Levy DL, Warriner RAI, Burgess GE. Fetal response to cardiopulmonary bypass. Obstet Gynecol 1980;56:112–115.

Liu PL, Warren RM, Ostheimer GW, et al. Foetal monitoring in parturients undergoing surgery unrelated to pregnancy. Can Anaesth Soc J 1985;32:525–532.

Logan A, Turner RWD. Mitral valvulotomy during pregnancy. Lancet 1952;1:1286.

Martin MC, Pernoll ML, Boruszak AN, et al. Cesarean section while on cardiac bypass: report on a case. Obstet Gynecol 1981;57:41S–45S.

Mason J, Stable FE, Szekely PJ. Cardiac disease in pregnancy. J Obstet Gynecol Br Emp 1952; 59:569.

Matsuki A, Oyama T. Operation under hypothermia in a pregnant woman with an intracranial arteriovenous malformation. Can Anaesth Soc J 1972; 19:184–191.

Mazze RI, Kallen B. Reproductive outcome after anesthesia and operation during pregnancy: a registry study of 5405 cases. Am J Obstet Gynecol 1989;161:1178–1185.

Mazze RI, Kallen B. Appendectomy during pregnancy: a Swedish registry study of 778 cases. Obstet Gynecol 1991;77:835–840.

McLean RF, Wong BI. Normothermic versus hypothermic cardiopulmonary bypass: central nervous system outcomes. J Cardiothorac Vasc Anesth 1996;10:45–53.

Meffert WG, Stansel HC. Open heart surgery during pregnancy. Am J Obstet Gynecol 1968;102: 1116–1120.

Mora CT, Grunewald KE. Reoperative aortic and mitral prosthetic valve replacement in the third trimester of pregnancy. J Cardiothorac Anesth 1987;1:313–317.

Motoyama EK, Rivard G, Acheson F, Cook CD. The effect of changes in maternal pH and $Pco_2$ on the $Po_2$ of fetal lambs. Anesthesiology 1967; 28:891–903.

Nazarian M, McCullough GH, Fielder DL. Bacterial endocarditis in pregnancy. Thorac Cardiovasc Surg 1976;71:880–883.

Philbin DM. Pulsatile blood flow. In: Gravlee GP, Davis RF, Utley JR, eds. Cardiopulmonary bypass. Baltimore: Williams and Wilkins, 1993:323–337.

Ralston DH, Snider SM, DeLorimer AA. Effects of equipotent ephedrine, metaraminol, mephentermine and methoxamine on uterine blood flow in the pregnant ewe. Anesthesiology 1974;40:354.

Roe BB, Edmonds LH, Fishman NH, Hutchinson JC. Open mitral valvulotomy. Ann Thorac Surg 1971;12:483.

Rossouw GJ, Knott-Craig CJ, Barnard PM, et al. Intracardiac operation in seven pregnant women. Ann Thorac Surg 1993;55:1172–1174.

Shnider SM, Webster GM. Maternal and fetal hazards of surgery during prenancy. Am J Obstet Gynecol 1965;92:891–900.

Skillman CA, Plessinger MA., Woods JR, Clark KE. Effect of graded reductions in uteroplacental blood flow on the fetal lamb. Am J Physiol 1985;149:1098–1105.

Smith BE. Fetal prognosis after anesthesia during gestation. Anesth Analg 1963;42:521–526.

Strickland RA, Oliver WCJ, Chantigian RC, et al. Anesthesia, cardiopulmonary bypass, and the pregnant patient. Mayo Clin Proc 1991;66:411–429.

Trimakas AP, Maxwell KD, Berkay S, et al. Fetal monitoring during cardiopulmonary bypass for removal of a left atrial myxoma during pregnancy. John Hopkins Med J 1979;144:156–160.

Ueland K. Cardiac surgery and pregnancy. Am J Obstet Gynecol 1965;92:148.

Veray FX, Hernandez CJJ, Raffucci F, Pelegrina IA. Pregnancy after cardiac surgery. Conn Med 1970;34:496.

Vosloo S, Reichart B. The feasibility of closed mitral valvulotomy in pregnancy. J Thorac Cardiovasc Surg 1987;93:675.

Werch A, Lambert HM, Cooley D, Reed CC. Fetal monitoring and maternal open heart surgery. South J Med 1977;70:1024.

Westaby S, Parry AJ, Forfar JC. Reoperation for prosthetic valve endocarditis in the third trimester of pregnancy. Ann Thorac Surg 1992;53:263.

Zitnik RS, Brandenbug RO, Sheldon R, Wallace RB. Pregnancy and open-heart surgery. Circulation 1969;39(suppl I):I-257–I-262.

# PART III

# Disease Processes

# CHAPTER 14

# Complications of Preeclampsia

*P*regnancy-induced hypertension (PIH) is a complex disease process, the physiologic effects of which may range from simple hypertension to multiorgan failure. In the past, the term *preeclampsia* was reserved for those patients whose PIH was accompanied by renal tubular dysfunction and proteinuria, and the term *eclampsia*, for women with similar disease complicated by grand mal seizures. While deeply rooted in historic tradition, such distinctions may be confusing if taken to imply differing disease processes, rather than different clinical manifestations of the same condition (ACOG, 1996). In this chapter, the terms *pregnancy-induced hypertension* and *preeclampsia* are used interchangeably, with no implication of differing physiologies.

In the United States, preeclampsia occurs in 5% to 10% of pregnancies and is the second most common cause of maternal mortality in advanced gestations (Pritchard, 1985; Kaunitz, 1985; Grimes, 1994; Berg, 1996). Pathologic changes commonly affect the maternal cardiovascular, renal, hematologic, neurologic, and hepatic systems. Equally important are the adverse effects on the uteroplacental unit, resulting in fetal and neonatal complications (Lin, 1982; Sibai 1993a,b). The purpose of this chapter is to help guide the clinician in managing potentially severe complications of preeclampsia. Therapy for pregnant women with chronic hypertension is discussed elsewhere and will not be addressed in this chapter (Sibai, 1996).

## Etiology of Preeclampsia

Preeclampsia has been a recognized pathologic entity since the time of the ancient Greeks (Chesley, 1974, 1984). The inciting factor remains unknown, however, and an empty shield located on a portico at the Chicago Lying-In Hospital awaits inscription of the name of the person who discovers the etiology of the disease (Zuspan, 1978). A significant amount of investigation has been undertaken during the past 30 years to elucidate the cause and improve the treatment of this disease. In fact, 1935 documents were identified by computer search using the key word *preeclampsia* for the years 1966 through 1995. During the past 30 years of medical research, the number of published articles has literally grown in an exponential manner: 1966 to 1970 (n = 23), 1971 to 1975 (n = 26), 1976 to 1980 (n = 122), 1981 to 1985 (n = 284), 1986 to 1990 (n = 526), and 1991 to 1995 (n = 954).

Numerous risk factors are associated with the development of preeclampsia (Table 14-1), and several pathophysiologic mechanisms have been proposed as etiologic in the development of this disease process (Worley, 1984; Stone, 1994; Conde-Agudelo, 1994). An imbalance between the vasodilating, platelet-disaggregating prostaglandins ($PGI_2$ and PGE) and the vasoconstricting, platelet-aggregating prostaglandins (thromboxane $A_2$ and $PGF_2$) is thought to play an important role in the development of preeclampsia (Friedman,

T A B L E    **14-1**

Risk factors for the development of pregnancy-induced hypertension

| Risk Factor | Risk Ratio |
| --- | --- |
| Nulliparity | 3:1 |
| Age >40 yr | 3:1 |
| African-American race | 1.5:1.0 |
| Family history of PIH | 5:1 |
| Chronic hypertension | 10:1 |
| Chronic renal disease | 20:1 |
| Antiphospholipid syndrome | 10:1 |
| Diabetes mellitus | 2:1 |
| Twin gestation | 4:1 |
| Angiotensinogen gene T235 | |
|    Homozygous | 20:1 |
|    Heterozygous | 4:1 |

Source: Revised from American College of Obstetricians and Gynecologists. Hypertension in pregnancy. ACOG Technical Bulletin 219. Washington, DC: ACOG, 1996.

1988; Sorensen, 1993; Dadek, 1982; Downing, 1982; Lewis, 1981). In women at risk for PIH, low-dose aspirin therapy selectively suppresses maternal platelet thromboxane $B_2$ while sparing vascular prostacyclin; in one study, longer pregnancy duration and increased birth weight were observed, with maintenance of hemostatic competence in the fetus and newborn (Benigni, 1989). However, larger series involving prospective, randomized trials have shown that while the incidence of proteinuric hypertension may be decreased with low-dose aspirin, there is no improvement in maternal or perinatal outcome (CLASE, 1994; Dekker, 1993; Hauth, 1993; Imperiale, 1992). In a similar manner, a relative deficiency in calcium has been proposed as a contributing etiologic mechanism, while studies evaluating calcium supplementation for prevention of preeclampsia have shown mixed results (Belizaw, 1991; Sanches-Ramos, 1994).

Immunologic mechanisms also have been proposed as fundamental for the development of preeclampsia, because the disease is more common among primigravidas who have never been exposed to fetal antigens (Redman, 1981). There appears to be an inverse relationship between the duration of sexual cohabitation before conception and the incidence of PIH (Robillard,

1994). The role of circulating immune complexes in the pathophysiology of PIH is still unclear (Balasch, 1981; Rote, 1983; Massobrio, 1985).

One of the more striking clinical risk factors for the development of preeclampsia is the antiphospholipid syndrome. At the University of Utah, Branch and colleagues studied 43 women who presented with severe preeclampsia prior to 34 weeks of gestation and found 16% to have significant levels of antiphospholipid antibodies and none in normotensive controls of similar gestational age (Branch, 1989). They recommended that women with early-onset severe preeclampsia be screened for antiphospholipid antibodies and, if detected, be considered for prophylactic therapy in subsequent pregnancies. Branch and colleagues (1992) found a high incidence of preeclampsia (51%) and severe preeclampsia (27%) in 70 women with antiphospholipid syndrome whose pregnancies progressed beyond 15 weeks of gestation, despite various medical treatment protocols.

Increased vascular reactivity to vasoactive agents was demonstrated by Dieckman and Michael in 1937 (Dieckman, 1937). In 1961, Abdul-Karim and Assali found that normal pregnant women were less responsive to angiotensin II than nonpregnant women (Abdul-Karim, 1961). Gant published data in 1973 that demonstrated an early loss of refractoriness to angiotensin II in those patients who later were to develop PIH (Gant, 1973). Although clinical improvement may follow hospitalization and bed rest, vascular sensitivity to angiotensin II does not decrease until after delivery of the fetus (Whalley, 1983). Endothelial involvement and the role of tumor necrosis factor, β-carotene, and reduced antithrombia III, in preeclampsia have also been investigated, but remain incompletely understood (Friedman, 1994; Kupfermine, 1994; Mikhail, 1994; Rogers, 1988; Weiner, 1985; Weenink, 1984).

Easterling and Benedetti have proposed a hyperdynamic disease model of PIH, whereby a hyperdynamic increase in cardiac output produces renal hyperfusion and subsequent damage resulting in hypertension and proteinuria. Hyperperfusion, not limited to the renal vasculature, would result in endothelial damage with platelet aggregation and initiation of a positive feedback loop mediated by an altered thromboxane-prostacyclin ratio (Easterling, 1989).

An integrated model of the pathophysiology of PIH has been proposed by Romero and colleagues (Romero, 1988b). Abnormal placentation is thought to be the first step in the development of the disease, possibly related to immune mechanisms. Trophoblastic prostacyclin, which may be important with respect to trophoblast invasion and prevention of blood clotting in the intervillous space, becomes deficient. A relative decrease in the prostacyclin-thromboxane ratio allows platelet aggregation, thrombin activation, and fibrin deposition in systemic vascular beds. Thrombosis and vasospasm develop and lead to multiorgan involvement, including renal, hepatic, neurologic, hematologic, and uteroplacental dysfunction.

Subclinical blood coagulation changes (decreased endogenous heparin levels, decreased angiotensin III activity) occur within 15 days of development of preeclampsia and are particularly evident 1 to 7 days prior to the development of clinical signs of preeclampsia (Savelieva, 1995).

A molecular variant of the angiotensinogen gene (T235), found to be associated with essential hypertension, also has been associated with preeclampsia (Ward, 1993). These investigators propose that increased concentrations of plasma or tissue angiotensinogen could lead to increased baseline or reactive production of angiotensin II, chronically stimulating autoregulatory mechanisms, thus increasing vascular tone and producing vascular hypertrophy. These changes then may impede pregnancy-induced plasma volume expansion, which occurs in normal pregnancies, and result in general circulatory maladaptation.

All of the preceding theories still do not allow prediction of which gravidas will develop PIH, and an ideal screening test is currently not available (Conde-Agudelo, 1994; Massé, 1993). Furthermore, it is still not clear which process or processes separate mild disease from the development of critical illness and multiorgan dysfunction.

## Diagnosis of Preeclampsia

The diagnosis of PIH is often clinically confusing and erroneous (Sibai, 1988; Chesley, 1985; Fisher, 1981; Goodlin, 1976). Blood pressure criteria include a systolic blood pressure (SBP) of at least 140 mm Hg or a diastolic BP of at least 90 mm Hg. The relative rise from baseline values in systolic pressure of 30 mm Hg or diastolic pressure of 15 mm Hg appears to be of questionable value (Villar, 1989; Conde-Agudelo, 1993). Significant proteinuria is defined as at least 300 mg in a 24-hour period or at least 1 g per liter concentration in two random urine specimens collected 6 hours apart. Semiquantitative dipstick analysis of urinary protein is poorly predictive of the actual degree of proteinuria measured by 24-hour urinary collections; thus, classification of preeclampsia based on proteinuria should be confirmed with a 24-hour quantitative collection (Meyer, 1994). Edema must be generalized, or a weight gain of at least 5 pounds in 1 week confirmed. These changes must occur after 20 weeks of gestation, except when there exists extensive hydatidiform changes in the chorionic villi, such as seen with hydatidiform mole. In general, the serious end-organ involvement discussed in this chapter occurs in patients with both hypertension and proteinuria.

The signs and symptoms of severe preeclampsia are summarized in Table 14-2. The development of these severe manifestations of the disease necessitates careful evaluation and consideration of delivery (Pritchard, 1985).

TABLE **14-2**

**Diagnostic criteria for severe preeclampsia**

Blood pressure >160–180 mm Hg systolic or
  >110 mm Hg diastolic
Proteinuria >5 g per 24 hr
Oliguria defined as <500 mL per 24 hr
Cerebral or visual disturbances
Pulmonary edema
Epigastric or right upper quadrant pain
Impaired liver function of unclear etiology
Thrombocytopenia
Fetal intrauterine growth retardation or oligohydramnios
Elevated serum creatinine
Grand mal seizures (eclampsia)

Source: Revised from American College of Obstetricians and Gynecologists. Hypertension in pregnancy. ACOG Technical Bulletin 219. Washington, DC: ACOG, 1996.

Complications of severe pregnancy-induced hypertension

| | | |
|---|---|---|
| Cardiovascular | → | Severe hypertension, pulmonary edema |
| Renal | → | Oliguria, renal failure |
| Hematologic | → | Hemolysis, thrombocytopenia, disseminated intravascular coagulopathy |
| Neurologic | → | Eclampsia, cerebral edema, cerebral hemorrhage, amaurosis |
| Hepatic | → | Hepatocellular dysfunction, hepatic rupture |
| Uteroplacental | → | Abruption, intrauterine growth retardation, fetal distress, fetal death |

The remainder of this chapter focuses on the management of preeclampsia, as well as on the pathophysiology of specific complications (Table 14-3).

## General Management Principles for Preeclampsia

On making the diagnosis of PIH, several steps are initiated simultaneously to treat and further evaluate the mother and her fetus. A peripheral intravenous (IV) line is placed and meticulous fluid therapy initiated. Routine laboratory evaluation for PIH (Table 14-4) includes complete blood count with blood smear and platelet count, as well as serum creatinine and liver enzyme analyses (Weinstein, 1985; Romero, 1988a,b, 1989; Pritchard, 1976).

If delivery is not felt to be imminent, a 24-hour collection of urine should be started for volume, creatinine clearance, and total protein excretion. The patient should be placed in a lateral recumbent position and fetal assessment performed with a nonstress text, oxytocin challenge test, or biophysical profile, as indicated. Amniocentesis should be considered only in those cases in which fetal pulmonary maturity is in question and the disease process is not severe enough to mandate delivery.

When severe preeclampsia is diagnosed, immediate delivery, regardless of gestational age, is generally recommended (National, 1990). Under certain circumstances, however, conservative management may be appropriate in cases of extreme fetal immaturity (MacKenna, 1983). Thiagarajah et al managed 13 patients with manifestations of severe preeclampsia (Thiagarajah, 1984). Early delivery was effected for fetal maturity, fetal distress, or progressive thrombocytopenia. Betamethasone therapy was recommended in those cases with stable maternal-fetal status and fetal immaturity. Interestingly, these investigators also noted an improvement in platelet count and liver enzymes after corticosteroid therapy. Van Dam and colleagues developed a disseminated intravascular coagulopathy (DIC) scoring system to manage patients with HELLP syndrome, defined by *h*emolysis, *e*levated *l*iver enzymes, and *l*ow *p*latelets (Van Dam, 1989). They recommended that conservative therapy be reserved only for patients who present with proven fetal lung immaturity and no laboratory evidence of DIC. Expedient delivery was recommended in cases of suspected or diagnosed DIC to avoid additional maternal morbidity.

Sibai and colleagues retrospectively reviewed 60 cases of conservatively managed severe preeclampsia during the second trimester (18–27 weeks' gestation). They found a high maternal morbidity rate, with complications such as abruptio placentae, eclampsia, coagulopathy, renal failure, hypertensive encephalopathy, intracerebral hemorrhage, and ruptured hepatic hematoma. Additionally, an 87% perinatal mortality rate was

Laboratory evaluation for preeclampsia

Complete blood count
Platelet count
Liver function tests (SGOT, SGPT)
Renal function tests (creatinine, BUN)
Urinalysis and microscopy
24-hr urine collection for protein and creatinine
  clearance
Blood type and antibody screen

noted (Sibai, 1985b). In subsequent prospective studies, Sibai and colleagues reported improved perinatal outcomes with no increased rate of maternal complications in a select group of women with severe preeclampsia between 24 to 27 weeks of gestation and 28 to 32 weeks of gestation (Sibai, 1994) who were managed with intensive fetal and maternal monitoring under strict protocols in a tertiary care center. In another randomized controlled trial, expectant management in selected severe preeclamptics between 28 and 34 weeks of gestation was not associated with an increase in maternal complications, but did result in a significant prolongation of the pregnancy, reduction of neonates requiring ventilation, and a reduction in the number of neonatal complications (Odendaal, 1990).

In a stable maternal-fetal environment, in the absence of determining severe preeclampsia, steroid therapy may be considered if amniocentesis reveals fetal lung immaturity or the clinical situation is consistent with prematurity. The presence of PIH does not guarantee accelerated lung maturation, and a high incidence of neonatal respiratory complications has been associated with premature delivery for preeclampsia (Weinstein, 1982; Pritchard, 1984). Although delivery is generally indicated for severe PIH regardless of gestational age, we feel that conservative therapy is appropriate in select premature patients with proteinuria exceeding 5 g/24 hr, mild elevations of serum transaminase levels, or borderline decreases in platelet count and BP that is controllable.

## Fluid Therapy for Preeclampsia

Fluid management in severe PIH consists of crystalloid infusions of normal saline or lactated Ringer's solution, at a rate of 100 to 125 mL/hr. Additional fluid volumes, in the order of 1000 to 1500 mL, may be required prior to use of epidural anesthesia or vasodilator therapy to prevent maternal hypotension and fetal distress (Wasserstrum, 1986).

Epidural anesthesia appears to be safe and is the anesthetic method of choice in severe preeclampsia, if preceded by volume preloading to avoid maternal hypotension (Graham, 1980;

Jouppila, 1982; Newsome, 1986; Joyce, 1979; Gutsche, 1986). Likewise, severely hypertensive patients receiving vasodilator therapy may require careful volume preloading to prevent an excessive hypotensive response to vasodilators. Abrupt and profound drops in BP leading to fetal bradycardia and distress often occur in severe PIH when vasodilator therapy is not accompanied by volume expansion (Cotton, 1986b; Wasserstrum, 1989; Kirshon, 1988).

Intravenous fluids are known to cause a decrease in colloid oncotic pressure (COP) in laboring patients (Gonik, 1984). In addition, baseline COP is decreased in patients with PIH and may decrease further postpartum as a result of mobilization of interstitial fluids. This may be clinically relevant with respect to the development of pulmonary edema in patients who are receiving betamimetics or who have PIH (Cotton, 1984a). Therefore, close monitoring of fluid intake and output, hemodynamic parameters, and clinical signs must be undertaken to prevent an imbalance of hydrostatic and oncotic forces that potentiate the occurrence of pulmonary edema.

Kirshon and co-workers placed systemic and pulmonary artery catheters in 15 primigravid patients with severe PIH during labor (Kirshon, 1988b). A hemodynamic protocol requiring strict control of COP, pulmonary capillary wedge pressure (PCWP), and mean arterial pressure (MAP) throughout labor, delivery, and the postpartum period was followed. Low COP and PCWP were corrected with the administration of albumin. Mean arterial pressure was treated as needed with IV nitroglycerin, nitroprusside, or hydralazine. Furosemide was administered for elevated PCWP. These investigators found that the only benefit of such management was avoidance of sudden profound drops in SBP and fetal distress during antihypertensive therapy. The overall incidence of fetal distress in labor was not affected, however. Because of a significant requirement for pharmacologic diuresis to prevent pulmonary edema in the study group, these authors recommended that COP not be corrected with colloid unless markedly decreased (< 12 mm Hg) or a prolonged negative COP-PCWP gradient was identified. While the infusion of colloids has been shown to result in less of a decrease in COP when compared with crystalloids, there is no evidence of any clinical benefit of colloids over crystalloids for the pregnant patient (Jones, 1986). Thus, in the absence of a firm clinical indication for colloid infusion, carefully controlled crystalloid infusions appear to be the safest mode of fluid therapy in severe PIH.

## Seizure Prophylaxis for Preeclampsia

Magnesium sulfate ($MgSO_4 \cdot 7H_2O$ USP) has been used for the prevention of eclamptic seizures since the early twentieth century (Dorsett, 1926; Lazard, 1933; Eastman, 1945) and has long been the standard treatment of preeclampsia-eclampsia in the United States (Pritchard, 1955; Pritchard, 1975). The mechanism of action of magnesium sulfate remains controversial (Shelley, 1980). Some investigators feel that magnesium acts primarily via neuromuscular blockade, while others believe that magnesium acts centrally (Borges, 1978; Pritchard, 1979). Two separate investigations evaluating the effect of parenteral magnesium sulfate on penicillin-induced seizure foci in cats report conflicting data (Borges, 1978; Koontz, 1985). Koontz and Reid postulate that magnesium may be effective as an anticonvulsant only when the blood-brain barrier is disrupted (Koontz, 1985). Human data reveal that abnormal EEG findings are common in preeclampsia-eclampsia, and they are not altered by levels of magnesium considered to be therapeutic (Sibai, 1984b).

More recent studies, however, have demonstrated that $MgSO_4$ has a central anticonvulsant effect. Additionally, in a randomized placebo-controlled study, Belfort and co-workers evaluated the effect of magnesium sulfate on maternal retinal blood flow in preeclamptics by way of Doppler blood flow measurements of central retinal and posterior ciliary arteries (Belfort, 1992). Their findings suggested that magnesium sulfate vasodilates small vessels in the retina and proposed that this may reflect similar changes occurring in the cerebral circulation.

Magnesium sulfate regimens are illustrated in Table 14-5. Because a regimen of a 4-g IV loading dose followed by a 1- to 2-g/hr IV maintenance dose failed to prevent eclampsia in a significant number of preeclamptic women, Sibai and co-workers (1984a) modified this regimen to a 4-g IV loading dose followed by a 2- to 3-g/hr IV maintenance dose. Sibai compared Pritchard's regimen of a 4-g IV and a 10-g intramuscular (IM) loading dose, followed by a 5-g IM maintenance dose every 4 hours, with a 4-g IV loading dose, followed by a 1- or 2-g/hr continuous IV maintenance infusion. The IV loading dose with maintenance dose of one an hour did not produce adequate serum levels of magnesium (4–7 mEq/liter); thus, they recommended a 2- to 3-g/hr maintenance

T A B L E   **14-5**

Magnesium sulfate protocols

| | Loading Dose | Maintenance Dose |
|---|---|---|
| Pritchard, 1955, 1975 | | |
|     Preeclampsia | 10 g IM[a] | 5 g IM[a] q4hr |
|     Eclampsia | 4 g IV[b] and 10 g IM[a] | 5 g IM[a] q4hr |
| Zuspan, 1966 | | |
|     Severe preeclampsia | None | 1 g/hr IV |
|     Eclampsia | 4–6 g IV over 5–10 min | 1 g/hr IV |
| Sibai, 1984 | | |
|     Preeclampsia-eclampsia | 6 g IV[c] over 15 min | 2 g/hr |

[a]50% solution $MgSO_4$.

[b]20% solution $MgSO_4$.

[c]50% solution $MgSO_4$ diluted in $D_5W$.

IM, intramuscularly.

dose (Sibai, 1984a). We employ a regimen of a 4- to 6-g loading dose IV over 20 minutes, followed by a 2- to 3-g/hr continuous IV infusion. The maintenance infusion may be adjusted according to clinical parameters and serum magnesium levels. Pruett and co-workers found no significant effects on neonatal Apgar scores at these doses (Pruett, 1988).

There remains controversy regarding the best agent for eclampsia prophylaxis. In the United States, magnesium sulfate has been the agent of choice (Pritchard, 1984; Atkinson, 1991; National, 1990), whereas in the United Kingdom and in a few U.S. centers, conventional antiepileptic agents have been advocated (Donaldson, 1992; Hutton, 1992; Repke, 1992; Duley, 1994). In a randomized trial comparing magnesium sulfate with phenytoin for the prevention of eclampsia, Lucas and colleagues found a statistically significant difference ($p$ = 0.004) in the development of seizures between the magnesium sulfate group (0/1049) and the phenytoin group (10/1089), with no significant differences in eclampsia risk factors between the two study groups (Lucas, 1995).

The Eclampsia Trial Collaborative Group (Eclampsia, 1995) enrolled 1687 women with eclampsia in an international multicenter randomized trial comparing standard anticonvulsant regimens of magnesium sulfate, phenytoin, and diazepam. Women allocated magnesium sulfate had a 52% lower risk of recurrent convulsions than those allocated diazepam, and a 67% lower risk of recurrent convulsions than those allocated phenytoin. Women allocated magnesium sulfate were less likely to be ventilated, to develop pneumonia, and to be admitted to intensive care than those allocated phenytoin. Furthermore, the babies of mothers allocated magnesium sulfate were less likely to be intubated at delivery and less likely to be admitted to the newborn intensive care nursery when compared with babies of mothers treated with phenytoin. The Eclampsia Trial Collaborative Group concluded that magnesium sulfate is the drug of choice for routine anticonvulsant management of women with eclampsia, rather than diazepam or phenytoin, and recommended that other anticonvulsants be used only in the context of randomized trials.

Plasma magnesium levels maintained at 4 to 7 mEq/liter are felt to be therapeutic in preventing eclamptic seizures (Pritchard, 1985). Patellar reflexes usually are lost at 8 to 10 mEq/liter, and respiratory arrest may occur at 13 mEq/liter (Chesley, 1979; Pritchard, 1955). Urine output, patellar reflexes, and respiratory rates should be monitored closely during $MgSO_4$ administration. In those patients who have renal dysfunction, serum magnesium levels should be monitored as well. Calcium gluconate, oxygen therapy, and the ability to perform endotracheal intubation should be available in the event of magnesium toxicity (Chesley, 1979). Calcium will reverse the adverse effects of magnesium toxicity. Calcium gluconate is administered as a 1-g dose (10 mL of a 10% solution) IV over a period of 2 minutes (ACOG, 1996).

Bohman and Cotton (1990) reported a case of supralethal magnesemia (38.7 mg/dL) with patient survival and no adverse sequelae. They stated that the essential elements in the resuscitation and prevention of toxic magnesemia are (1) respiratory support as determined by clinical indicators; (2) use of continuous cardiac monitoring; (3) infusion of calcium salts to prevent hypocalcemia and the enhanced cardiotoxicity that is associated with concurrent hypocalcemia and hypermagnesemia; (4) use of loop or osmotic diuretics to excrete the magnesium ion more rapidly, as well as careful attention to fluid and electrolyte balances; (5) assurance that toxic magnesium is neither anesthetic nor amnestic to the patient; and (6) assurance that all magnesium infusions be administered in a buretrol-type system or by IM injection to prevent toxic magnesemia.

Magnesium sulfate is used to prevent or treat eclamptic seizures; it is not an antihypertensive agent (Pritchard, 1955). Administration of this agent produces a transient decrease in BP in hypertensive, but not normotensive, nonpregnant subjects (Mroczek, 1977). Young and Weinstein noted significant respiratory effects and a transient fall in maternal BP in patients who received a 10-g IM loading dose of magnesium sulfate followed by maintenance push doses of 2 g every 1 to 2 hours, but not in patients who received the 10-g loading dose followed by a 1-g/hr continuous infusion (Young, 1977). Cotton and co-workers observed a transient hypotensive effect related to bolus infusion, but not with continuous infusion in severe preeclampsia (Cotton, 1984b).

## Antihypertensive Therapy for Severe Preeclampsia

Markedly elevated systemic arterial BPs are one of the hallmarks of severe preeclampsia. Careful control of hypertension must be achieved to prevent complications such as maternal cerebral vascular accidents and placental abruption. Medical intervention is usually recommended when the diastolic BP exceeds 110 mm Hg (Lubbe, 1987; Naden, 1985; ACOG, 1996). The degree of systolic hypertension requiring therapy is less certain, but most would treat for a level exceeding the 160 to 180 mm Hg range, depending on the associated diastolic pressure. In the previously normotensive patient, cerebral autoregulation is lost and the risk of intracranial bleeding increases when the MAP exceeds 140 to 150 mm Hg (Fig 14-1) (Zimmerman, 1995). Although many different antihypertensive agents are available, we will

confine our discussion to those agents most commonly used for acute hypertensive crises in pregnancy (Table 14-6).

## Hydralazine Hydrochloride

Hydralazine hydrochloride (Apresoline) has long been the gold standard of antihypertensive therapy for use by obstetricians in the United States. Hydralazine reduces vascular resistance via direct relaxation of arteriolar smooth muscle, affecting precapillary resistance vessels more than postcapillary capacitance vessels (Koch-Weser, 1976). Assali et al noted the hypotensive effect to be marked and prolonged in preeclamptic patients, moderate in patients with essential hypertension, and slight in normotensive subjects (Assali, 1953). Using M-mode echocardiography, Kuzniar et al found an attenuated response to a 12.5-mg IV dose of hydralazine, in patients with preexisting hypertension, compared with those with severe preeclampsia (Kuzniar, 1985). Cotton and colleagues (1985) studied the cardiovascular alterations in six severe preeclamptics following the IV administration of a 10-mg bolus of hydralazine. They observed a significant increase in maternal heart rate and cardiac index (CI), with a decrease in MAP and systemic vascular resistance (SVR) index. There was a wide range of individual responses with respect to peak effects and duration of effects. Jouppila et al measured maternal-fetal effects with Doppler in severe preeclamptics receiving dihydralazine and demonstrated a fall in maternal BP with no change in intervillous blood flow and an increase in umbilical vein blood flow (Jouppila, 1985). Dihydralazine also has been shown to cross the placenta to the fetus (Liedholm, 1982). The administration of hydralazine may result in maternal hypotension and fetal distress (Spinnato, 1986). For this reason, we recommend an initial IV dose of 2.5 mg, followed by observation of hemodynamic effects. If appropriate change in BP is not achieved, 5- to 10-mg doses may be administered IV at 20-minute intervals to a total acute dose of 30 to 40 mg. Hypertension refractory to the preceding approach warrants the use of more potent antihypertensive agents (Cotton, 1986a; Clark, 1988).

FIGURE **14-1**

Cerebral blood flow remains constant over a wide range of pressures in normotensive individuals. This range is shifted to the right in individuals with chronic hypertension. (Modified from Zimmerman JL. Hypertensive crisis: emergencies and urgencies. In: Ayers SM, ed. Textbook of critical care. Philadelphia: WB Saunders, 1995.)

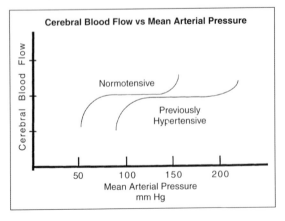

T A B L E    **14-6**

Pharmacologic agents for antihypertensive therapy in preeclampsia-eclampsia

| Agent (Generic) | Trade | Mechanism of Action | Dosage | Comment |
|---|---|---|---|---|
| Hydralazine hydrochloride | Apresoline | Arterial vasodilator | 5 mg IV, then 5–10 mg IV/20 min up to total dose of 40 mg; IV infusion 5–10 mg/hr, titrated | Must wait 20 min for response between IV doses; possible maternal hypotension |
| Labetalol | Normodyne Trandate | Selective alpha- and nonselective beta-antagonist | 20 mg IV, then 40–80 mg IV/10 min to 300 mg total dose; IV infusion 1–2 mg/min, titrated | Less reflex tachycardia and hypotension than with hydralazine |
| Nifedipine | Procardia Adalat | Calcium channel blocker | 10 mg by mouth, may repeat after 30 min | Oral route only; possible exaggerated effect if used with $MgSO_4$ |
| Nitroglycerin | Nitrostat IV Tridil Nitro-Bid IV | Relaxation of venous (and arterial) vascular smooth muscle | 5 μg/min infusion; double every 5 min | Requires arterial line for continuous BP monitoring; potential methemoglobinemia |
| Sodium nitroprusside | Nipride Nitropress | Vasodilator | 0.25 μg/kg/min infusion; increase 0.25 μg/kg/min/5 min | Requires arterial line for continuous BP monitoring; potential cyanide toxicity |
| Diazoxide | Hyperstat | Peripheral arteriolar vasodilator | 30–60 mg IV/ 5 min; IV infusion 10 mg/min, titrated | Possible rapid hypotension, hyperglycemia, decreased uterine contractility |
| Captopril Enalapril | Capoten Vasotec | Angiotensin-converting enzyme inhibitor | Oral route only | Contraindicated during pregnancy secondary to potential fetal side effects (anuria or renal failure) |
| Methyldopa | Aldomet | Dopa decarboxylase inhibitor | 1-g loading dose; then 250–500 mg IV/6 hr | Slow onset of action (4–6 hr) after IV injection; not ideal for hypertensive crises |

Source: Modified from Dildy GA, Cotton DB. Hemodynamic changes in pregnancy and pregnancy complicated by hypertension. Acute Care 1988; 89:14, 26.

## Diazoxide

Diazoxide (Hyperstat) is a benzothiadiazine derivative, which exerts its antihypertensive effect by reducing peripheral vascular resistance through direct relaxation of arterioles (Rubin, 1962). The commonly used 300-mg bolus injection to treat severe hypertension may induce significant hypotension with resultant morbidity. Minibolus diazoxide titration is clinically effective and relatively free of side effects in nonpregnant,

severely hypertensive adults; a suggested dose would be 30 to 60 mg IV in 5-minute intervals, titrating to desired clinical response. Thien and co-workers (1980) recommended that diazoxide for the treatment of severe preeclampsia/eclampsia be administered by the infusion method (15 mg/min; total amount, 5 mg/kg body weight) rather than by bolus injection (300 mg within 10 sec), because the infusion method results in a more gradual decline in BP and can be interrupted in cases of exaggerated drop in BP. No evidence of a benefit over hydralazine has been shown with diazoxide, and this agent should not be used in patients with PIH unless other agents (discussion follows) are not available.

## Calcium Channel Blockers

Calcium channel blockers such as nifedipine (Procardia, Adalat) lower BP primarily by relaxing arterial smooth muscle. An initial oral dose of 10 mg is administered, which may be repeated after 30 minutes, if necessary, for the acute management of severe hypertension; 10 to 20 mg may then be administered orally every 3 to 6 hours as needed (Naden, 1985). Principal side effects in severe preeclamptics include headache and cutaneous flushing. Care must be given when nifedipine is administered to patients receiving concomitant magnesium sulfate because of the possibility of an exaggerated hypotensive response (Waisman, 1988). Animal studies using nifedipine in pregnant sheep and rabbits have raised concerns regarding fetal acidosis and death. At Baylor College of Medicine, nifedipine was administered for the treatment of preterm labor in 10 laboring patients between 26 and 34 weeks' gestation. These patients received a 30-mg loading dose and then 20 mg 4 hours following the loading dose. A cordocentesis for cord pH was obtained 6 hours following the initial dose of nifedipine. The mean umbilical artery pH in three samples was $7.36 \pm 0.03$, and the mean umbilical venous pH was $7.39 \pm 0.02$ in seven samples (Adam, unpublished). Although the treatment of preterm labor does not exactly simulate the conditions of PIH, we feel that these data demonstrate that nifedipine by itself does not commonly cause fetal acidosis. If fetal acidosis does occur following nifedipine administration, it most likely represents the effects of excessive hypotension on the fetoplacental unit. In a randomized clinical trial, 49 women with severe preeclampsia and severe hypertension between 26 and 36 weeks of gestation were primarily treated with sublingual (then oral) nifedipine or IV (then oral) hydralazine (Fenakel, 1991). Effective control of BP (values consistently below 160/110 mm Hg) was achieved in 96% of the nifedipine group and 68% of the hydralazine group ($p < 0.05$), with acute fetal distress occurring more commonly in the hydralazine group. A beneficial effect may also be seen on urine output and MAP postpartum in women with severe preeclampsia who were treated with nifedipine.

Belfort and co-workers have evaluated the calcium channel blocker, nimodipine, which has specific vasodilatory effects on human cerebral vessels, in the management of preeclampsia (Belfort, 1994). Because of nimodipine's effectiveness in reducing high BP and its vasodilator effect on cerebral vessels, Belfort et al suggest that nimodipine may be particularly useful in treating preeclampsia and deserves further investigation as an antiseizure agent for the prevention of eclampsia.

## Labetalol

Labetalol (Normodyne, Trandate ) is a combined alpha- and beta-adrenoceptor antagonist that may be used to induce a controlled, rapid decrease in BP via decreased SVR in patients with severe hypertension (Lund-Johnson, 1983). Reports on the efficacy and safety of labetalol in the treatment of hypertension during pregnancy have been favorable (Riley, 1981; Lunell, 1981; Coevoet, 1980; Lamming, 1979; Michael, 1979; Mabie, 1987; Pickles, 1989). Mabie and co-workers compared bolus IV labetalol with IV hydralazine in the acute treatment of severe hypertension. They found that labetalol had a quicker onset of action and did not result in reflex tachycardia (Mabie, 1987). Labetalol also may exert a positive effect on early fetal lung maturation in patients with severe hypertension who are remote from term (Michael, 1979, 1982). An initial dose of 10 mg is given and is followed by progressively increasing doses (20, 40, 80 mg) every 10 minutes, to a total dose of 300 mg. Alternately, constant IV infusion may be started at 1 to 2 mg/min until therapeutic goals are achieved, then decreased to 0.5 mg/min or completely stopped (Naden, 1985). Lunell and co-workers studied the effects of labetalol on uteroplacental perfusion in hypertensive pregnant women and noted increased uteroplacental perfusion and decreased uterine vascular resistance (Lunell, 1984). Morgan and co-workers evaluated the effects of labetalol on uterine blood flow in the hypertensive gravid baboon and found that low doses (0.5 mg/kg) significantly reduced MAP without adversely affecting uterine blood flow (Morgan, 1993).

## Nitroglycerin

Nitroglycerin (Nitrostat IV, Nitro-Bid IV, Tridil) relaxes predominantly venous but also arterial, vascular smooth muscle. It has been shown to decrease preload at low doses and afterload at high doses (Herling, 1984). It is a rapidly acting potent antihypertensive agent with a very short hemodynamic half-life. Using invasive hemodynamic monitoring, Cotton and associates (1986a,b) noted that the ability to control BP precisely was dependent on volume status. Although larger doses of nitroglycerin were required following volume expansion, the ability to effect a smoother and more controlled drop in BP reduced prevasodilator hydration (Cotton, 1986b). Nitroglycerin is administered via an infusion pump at an initial rate of 5 µg/min and may be doubled every five minutes. Methemoglobinemia may result from high dose ($>7$ µg/kg/min) IV infusion. Patients with normal arterial oxygen saturation who appear cyanotic should be evaluated for toxicity, defined as a methemoglobin level greater than 3% (Herling, 1984).

## Sodium Nitroprusside

Sodium nitroprusside (Nipride, Nitropress) is another potent antihypertensive agent that may be used to control severe PIH. A dilute solution may be started at 0.25 µg/kg/min and titrated to the desired effect through an infusion pump by increasing the dose by 0.25 µg/kg/min every 5 minutes. The solution is light sensitive and should be covered in foil and changed every 24 hours (Pasch, 1983). Arterial blood gases should be monitored to watch for developing metabolic acidosis, which may be an early sign of cyanide toxicity. In nonpregnant subjects, sodium nitroprusside infusion rates in excess of 4 µg/kg/min led to RBC cyanide levels, which after 2 to 3 hours of administration extended into the toxic range of more than 40 nmol/mL; infusion rates of less than 2 µg/kg/min

for several hours remained nontoxic (Pasch, 1983). Treatment time should be limited because of the potential for fetal cyanide toxicity (Strauss, 1980). Correction of hypovolemia prior to initiation of nitroprusside infusion is essential to avoid abrupt and often profound drops in BP.

## Angiotensin-Converting Enzyme Inhibitors

Angiotensin-converting enzyme (ACE) inhibitors (Captopril, Enalapril) interrupt the renin-angiotensin-aldosterone system, resulting in a lowering of SBP (Oates, 1988). Experience in pregnant hypertensive patients is limited; however, the risk of inducing neonatal renal failure and other serious complications would contraindicate the use of ACE inhibitors during pregnancy (Hurault, 1987; Schubiger, 1988; Barr, 1991; Hanssens, 1991). Fetal abortion, possibly secondary to reduced uterine blood flow resulting from decreased prostaglandin $E_2$ ($PGE_2$) synthesis, has been reported in pregnant rabbits (Ferris, 1983). Additionally, the ACE inhibitors as a class do not appear to be useful in acute treatment of severe hypertension because of a 1- to 4-hour delay in achievement of peak serum levels after ingestion (Oates, 1988).

## Severe Hypertension

We recommend hydralazine for initial management of severe hypertension (BP $>180/110$ mm Hg). Hydralazine will be effective in restoring BP to a desired range (160–130/110–80 mm Hg) in the majority of cases. When maximum doses of hydralazine (40 mg) have not corrected severe hypertension, we then proceed to a calcium channel blocker or labetalol. In extremely rare cases, these agents are ineffective, and we resort to IV infusion of nitroglycerin or nitroprusside, which requires an intensive care setting.

## Analgesia-Anesthesia for Preeclampsia

The use of conduction anesthesia in PIH was, at one time, controversial. Concerns have been voiced by some authors that the sympathetic blockade and peripheral vasodilatation resulting from epidural anesthesia may lead to hypotension and fetal distress in patients who are already volume contracted (Pritchard, 1975, 1985; Lindheimer, 1985). However, induction of general endotracheal anesthesia is not without its own inherent risks. General anesthesia has been shown to result in significant rises in systemic arterial pressure in patients with severe PIH. An average increase in systolic arterial BP of 56 mm Hg during endotracheal intubation of 20 patients with hypertension was reported by Connell and co-workers (Connell, 1987).

Hodgkinson and associates evaluated 10 severe preeclamptic-eclamptic patients undergoing general anesthesia using the pulmonary artery catheter. They noted severe systemic and pulmonary hypertension during endotracheal intubation and extubation. Ten patients undergoing epidural anesthesia with 0.75% bupivacaine for cesarean section maintained stable systemic and pulmonary arterial pressures, with the exception of one patient who developed systemic hypotension that responded promptly to ephedrine (Hodgkinson, 1980).

Newsome et al demonstrated a drop in MAP and a slight but insignificant decrease in SVR without change in CI, peripheral vascular resistance (PVR), central venous pressure (CVP), or PCWP in 11 patients with severe PIH undergoing lumbar epidural anesthesia (Newsome, 1986). Jouppila et al measured intervillous blood flow in nine patients with severe preeclampsia during labor with lumbar epidural block and found a significant increase in uterine blood flow (Jouppila, 1982). Ramos-Santos (1991) studied the effects of epidural anesthesia on uterine and umbilical artery blood flow by way of Doppler velocimetry in mild preeclamptics, chronic hypertensives, and normal controls during active term labor. In the preeclamptic group, the uterine artery systolic/diastolic (S/D) ratios decreased to levels similar to those of the control group, suggesting a possible beneficial effect in reducing uterine artery vasospasm.

Deleterious hypotension may be avoided by lateral maternal tilt, thus preventing aortocaval occlusion, and preloading with crystalloid solu-

tion to compensate for peripheral vasodilatation (Jouppila, 1982). Contraindications to epidural anesthesia include patient refusal, fetal distress requiring immediate delivery, local infection, septicemia, severe spinal deformities, and coagulopathy (Gutsche, 1986). If preceded by volume loading, epidural anesthesia appears beneficial and safe in severe preeclampsia (Wasserstrum, 1986; Graham, 1980; Jouppila, 1982; Newsome, 1986; Joyce, 1979; Gutsche, 1986; Clark, 1988). Clark and Cotton state, "In skilled hands, a cautiously administered epidural anesthetic is, in our opinion, not only justified, but the method of choice for anesthesia in cesarean section or for control of the pain of labor in the patient with severe preeclampsia" (Clark, 1988). When general anesthesia is necessary, careful control of maternal BP, especially around the time of induction and awakening, is essential. Small doses of nitroglycerine or other similar agents are often useful in this regard.

## Hemodynamic Monitoring for Preeclampsia

The pulmonary artery catheter, introduced nearly 30 years ago, has been very useful in the management of critically ill patients (Swan, 1970). In cases of severe preeclampsia, most clinicians have obtained excellent results without invasive monitoring (Pritchard, 1984). However, invasive hemodynamic monitoring may be helpful in patients with severe preeclampsia complicated by profound oliguria, or pulmonary edema, or of uncertain etiology and/or hypertension unresponsive to conventional therapy (Clark, 1988). Protocols developed to study the central hemodynamic parameters of severe preeclampsia have revealed interesting data, which are sometimes confounded by differences in clinical patient management prior to and at the time of catheterization (Wasserstrum, 1986). Hemodynamic changes observed in normal pregnancies and pregnancies complicated by hypertension are summarized by Dildy and Cotton (1988, 1991). Central hemodynamic findings in severe preeclampsia are summarized by Clark and associates in Table 14-7 (Clark, 1988). A summary of hemodynamic

T A B L E    **14-7**

Hemodynamic findings in severe pregnancy-induced hypertension

1. CO is variable.
2. MAP is elevated. SVR is normal (early) or elevated (late).
3. CVP is usually low to normal and does not correlate with PCWP.
4. Pulmonary hypertension and pulmonary vascular resistance are not present, but low PAP may occur in the presence of hypovolemia.
5. PCWP may be low, normal, or high.
6. Oliguria may not reflect volume depletion.
7. Ventricular function is usually hyperdynamic, but it may be depressed in the presence of marked elevation in SVR.
8. COP is usually low.

PAP, pulmonary artery pressure.

Reproduced by permission from Clark SL, Cotton DB. Clinical indications for pulmonary artery catheterization in the patient with severe preeclampsia. Am J Obstet Gynecol 1988;158:453–458.

findings in nonpregnant, normal third-trimester pregnancy, and severe preeclamptics is provided in Table 14-8.

Current indications for the use of a pulmonary artery catheter in preeclampsia are listed in Table 14-9 (Clark, 1985, 1988; Cotton, 1988; Clark, 1985a). Routine use of a pulmonary artery catheter in uncomplicated severe preeclampsia is not recommended. In these cases, the potential morbidity of pulmonary artery catheterization does not appear to be justified. Known complications of invasive monitoring at the time of insertion include cardiac arrhythmias, pneumothorax, hemothorax, injury to vascular and neurologic structures, pulmonary infarction, and pulmonary hemorrhage. Later complications include balloon rupture, thromboembolism, catheter knotting, pulmonary valve rupture, and catheter migration into the pericardial and pleural spaces, with subsequent cardiac tamponade and hydrothorax (Kirshon, 1987; Cotton, 1980; Mitchell, 1979). It should be noted, however, that Clark and associates noted no significant complications from pulmonary artery catheterization in a series of 90 patients who underwent the procedure on an obstetrics-gynecology service (Clark, 1985a).

## Cardiopulmonary Complications of Preeclampsia

During normal pregnancy, plasma volume increases approximately 42% while RBC volume increases approximately 24% (Chesley, 1972). Earlier studies of cardiovascular changes in preeclampsia revealed increased vascular resistance, decreased circulatory volume, and decreased perfusion of various organ systems, most notably the renal and uteroplacental circulations, when compared with normal nonpregnant subjects (Zuspan, 1978; Hays, 1985). In pregnancies complicated by PIH, a reduction in plasma volume with hemoconcentration occurs in proportion to the severity of the disease (Chesley, 1972). More recent studies have demonstrated significant plasma volume depletion and reduction in circulating plasma protein, even prior to the clinical manifestations of preeclampsia (Bletka, 1970; Gallery, 1979; Hays, 1985).

Lees noted an increase in cardiac output (CO) in normotensive pregnant subjects during the first trimester, which remained elevated until a slight fall at the end of the third trimester. Heart rate remained static until a slight fall at the end of the third trimester. In subjects who developed hypertension during pregnancy, various degrees of increased CO and/or SVR were noted (Lees, 1979).

Although the precise cause of these changes remains unknown, further insight into the exact cardiovascular parameters associated with pregnancy-related disease states evolved around 1980, when obstetric and gynecologic indications for use of the pulmonary artery catheter were described, and measurements of CVP, pulmonary artery pressure (PAP), PCWP, CO, and mixed venous oxygen ($MVo_2$) became available (Cotton, 1980).

Rafferty and Berkowitz studied three preeclamptic patients with the pulmonary artery catheter and noted an increased left ventricular stroke work index (LVSWI) and normal pulmonary artery resistance. At delivery, the CI and PCWP increased in these patients, probably secondary to increased venous return. These investigators noted an increased PCWP postpartum, which also was felt to be secondary to increased circulatory

T A B L E 14-8

Hemodynamic profiles of nonpregnant women, normal women during the late third trimester, and severe preeclamptics

| | Normal Non-pregnant (n = 10)[a] (mean ± SD) | Normal Late Third Trimester (n = 10)[a] (mean ± SD) | Severe Pre-eclampsia (n = 45)[b] (mean ± SEM) | Severe Pre-eclampsia (n = 41)[c] (mean ± SEM) |
|---|---|---|---|---|
| Heart rate (beats/min) | 71 ± 10 | 83 ± 10 | 95 ± 2 | 94 ± 2 |
| Systolic BP (mm Hg) | — | — | 193 ± 3 | 175 ± 3 |
| Diastolic BP (mm Hg) | — | — | 110 ± 2 | 106 ± 2 |
| Mean arterial BP (mm Hg) | 86.4 ± 7.5 | 90.3 ± 5.8 | 138 ± 3 | 130 ± 2 |
| Pulse pressure (mm Hg) | — | — | 84 ± 2 | 70 ± 2 |
| Central venous pressure (mm Hg) | 3.7 ± 2.6 | 3.6 ± 2.5 | 4 ± 1 | 4.8 ± 0.4 |
| Pulmonary capillary wedge pressure (mm Hg) | 6.3 ± 2.1 | 7.5 ± 1.8 | 10 ± 1 | 8.3 ± 0.3 |
| Pulmonary artery pressure (mm Hg) | 11.9 ± 2.0[d] | 12.5 ± 2.0[d] | 17 ± 1 | 15 ± 0.5 |
| Cardiac output (liters/min) | 4.3 ± 0.9 | 6.2 ± 1.0 | 7.5 ± 0.2 | 8.4 ± 0.2 |
| Stroke volume (mL) | — | — | 79 ± 2 | 90 ± 2 |
| Systemic vascular resistance (dynes · sec · cm$^{-5}$) | 1530 ± 520 | 1210 ± 266 | 1496 ± 64 | 1226 ± 37 |
| Pulmonary vascular resistance (dynes · sec · cm$^{-5}$) | 119 ± 47 | 78 ± 22 | 70 ± 5 | 65 ± 3 |
| Serum colloid osmotic pressure (mm Hg) | 20.8 ± 1.0 | 18.0 ± 1.5 | 19.0 ± 0.5 | N/A |
| Body surface area (m$^2$) | — | — | — | — |
| Systemic vascular resistance index (dynes · sec · cm$^{-5}$ · m$^2$) | — | — | 2726 ± 120 | 2293 ± 65 |
| Pulmonary vascular resistance index (dynes · sec · cm$^{-5}$ · m$^2$) | — | — | 127 ± 9 | 121 ± 7 |
| Right ventricular stroke work index (g · m · M$^{-2}$) | — | — | 8 ± 1 | 10 ± 0.5 |
| Left ventricular stroke work index (gm · m · M$^{-2}$) | 41 ± 8 | 48 ± 6 | 81 ± 2 | 84 ± 2 |
| Cardiac index (liters · min$^{-1}$ · m$^2$) | — | — | 4.1 ± 0.1 | 4.4 ± 0.1 |
| Stroke volume index (mL · beat · m$^2$) | — | — | 44 ± 1 | 48 ± 1 |
| COP-PCWP (mm Hg) | 14.5 ± 2.5 | 10.5 ± 2.7 | — | — |

N/A, not available.

Sources:

[a]From Clark SL, Cotton DB, Lee W, et al. Central hemodynamic observations in normal third trimester pregnancy. Am J Obstet Gynecol 1989;161:1439–1442.

[b]From Cotton DB, Lee W, Huhta JC, Dorman KF. Hemodynamic profile of severe pregnancy-induced hypertension. Am J Obstet Gynecol 1988; 158:523–529.

[c]From Mabie WC, Ratts TE, Sibai BM. The central hemodynamics of severe preeclampsia. Am J Obstet Gynecol 1989;161:1443–1448.

[d]From Clark SL, et al. Unpublished data.

T A B L E   **14-9**

Indications for the use of pulmonary artery catheter in pregnancy-induced hypertension

Complications related to central volume status
Pulmonary edema of uncertain etiology
Pulmonary edema unresponsive to conventional therapy
Persistent oliguria despite aggressive volume expansion
Induction of conduction anesthesia in hemodynamically unstable patients
Medical complication that would otherwise require invasive monitoring

volume. These findings suggest that the pulmonary vasculature was not involved in the vasospastic process and that pulmonary hypertension was not present in severe preeclampsia (Rafferty, 1980).

Benedetti and associates studied 10 patients with severe preeclampsia in labor with the pulmonary artery catheter and noted an increased LVSWI, suggesting hyperdynamic ventricular function. The PAPs were normal. Central venous pressure was found to correlate poorly with PCWP (Benedetti, 1980a). The poor correlation of PCWP and CVP has been verified by subsequent investigations (Strauss, 1980; Cotton, 1985).

Subsequent hemodynamic studies have consistently demonstrated hyperdynamic left ventricular function in preeclamptic patients (Cotton, 1984b; Phelan, 1982; Henderson, 1984). Phelan and Yurth (1982) studied 10 severe preeclamptics and noted hyperdynamic cardiac function with elevated CO and variable elevation of SVR. Immediately postpartum, a transient fall in left ventricular function with a rise in CVP and PCWP was noted in six of 10 patients, possibly secondary to an autotransfusion effect. Hyperdynamic ventricular function returned 1 hour postpartum (Phelan, 1982). One criticism of this study as it related to CO is the fact that several of these patients received intrapartum hydralazine, which could account for the elevated CO.

Groenendijk et al noted a low CI, low PCWP, and high SVR in preeclamptics prior to volume expansion. Volume expansion resulted in an elevation of PCWP and CI to normal pregnant val-

ues, a drop in SVR, and no change in SBP. Vasodilatation using hydralazine then resulted in a further drop in SVR and SBP, with a rise in CI, and no change in PCWP (Groenendijk, 1984).

Eclamptics studied by Hankins and associates (1984) initially demonstrated hyperdynamic left ventricular function and elevated SVR, as well as low right and left ventricular filling pressures. Following labor management, consisting of fluid restriction, magnesium sulfate, and hydralazine, they observed a postpartum rise in PCWP in patients who did not have an early spontaneous diuresis. This rise in PCWP was thought to be secondary to mobilization of extravascular fluids before the diuresis phase. They concluded that the hemodynamic status was influenced by the severity and duration of the disease, other underlying disease states, and therapeutic interventions such as epidural anesthesia.

Cotton and associates summarized the hemodynamic profile in 45 patients with severe preeclampsia or eclampsia (Cotton, 1988). They observed a wide variety of hemodynamic measurements in these patients; however, the majority were found to have an elevated SBP, variably elevated SVR, hyperdynamic left ventricular function, normal to increased PCWP, and low CVP. They hypothesized that the elevated PCWP with decreased CVP was secondary to elevated left ventricular afterload, combined with a hypovolemic state. These findings are summarized by Clark and Cotton in Table 14-7 (Clark, 1988).

Clark and associates (see Table 14-8) documented for the first time central hemodynamic parameters in normotensive late third-trimester pregnant patients (Clark, 1989). They demonstrated that most reported patients with severe preeclampsia have SVR in the normal range for pregnancy, and that left ventricular function in normal pregnancy as assessed by LVSWI is not hyperdynamic. This supports the model of an initially hyperdynamic hypertension without vasospasm in preeclampsia. This may be followed by the development of elevated SVR associated with vasospasm and a secondary decline in CO and LVSWI. Such a phenomenon has been documented in untreated nonpregnant patients with essential hypertension (Lund-Johansen, 1983).

## Pulmonary Edema

Sibai and colleagues reported a 2.9% incidence of pulmonary edema in severe preeclampsia-eclampsia (Sibai, 1987). Seventy percent of these 37 cases developed postpartum. In 90% of the cases that developed antepartum, chronic hypertension was identified as an underlying factor. A higher incidence of pulmonary edema was noted in older patients, multigravidas, and patients with underlying chronic hypertension. The development of pulmonary edema was also associated with the administration of excess infusions, either colloids or crystalloids.

Reduction of COP, alteration of capillary membrane permeability, and elevated pulmonary vascular hydrostatic pressures all led to extravasation of fluids into the interstitial and alveolar spaces, resulting in pulmonary edema (Henderson, 1984). Cotton observed a negative COP-PCWP gradient in five preeclamptic patients who developed pulmonary edema (Cotton, 1985). Interestingly, Clark compared the hemodynamic alterations in severe preeclamptics and eclamptics and suggested that the occurrence of eclamptic seizures may have also been associated with decreased COP rather than with the intensity of peripheral vasospasm (Clark, 1985b).

The etiology of pulmonary edema in preeclamptic patients appears to be multifactorial, as illustrated by Benedetti's work involving 10 preeclamptic women with pulmonary edema (Benedetti, 1985). Eight of the 10 patients developed pulmonary edema in the postpartum period. Five patients had an abnormal COP-PCWP gradient, three demonstrated increased pulmonary capillary permeability, and two suffered left ventricular failure. Pulmonary edema secondary to capillary leak versus that due to increased hydrostatic pressure was distinguished by evaluating the ratio of edema fluid protein to plasma protein (Fein, 1979). The diagnosis of capillary leak was made in Benedetti's study when the ratio of protein in pulmonary edema fluid to serum protein was greater than 0.4 (Benedetti, 1985). Again, CVP was found not to correlate with PCWP. A decreased COP-PCWP gradient has long been correlated with the development of pulmonary edema in nonpregnant patients (Fein, 1979). Pregnancy is known to lower COP, and COP is lower in preeclamptic patients than in normal pregnant patients. Colloid osmotic pressure decreases further postpartum, secondary to supine positioning, bleeding at the time of delivery, and intrapartum infusion of crystalloid solutions (Weil, 1979). In 50% of Benedetti's preeclamptic patients, a lowered COP-PCWP gradient may have contributed to pulmonary edema (Benedetti, 1979).

From the foregoing discussion, it is clear that nonhydrostatic factors (pulmonary capillary leak and deceased COP) may cause or contribute to pulmonary edema in patients with preeclampsia. In other patients, highly elevated SVR may lead to decreased CO and LVSWI and secondary cardiogenic pulmonary edema. A similar hydrostatic pulmonary edema may have been seen with normal left ventricular function following iatrogenic fluid overload.

The diagnosis of pulmonary edema is made on clinical grounds. Symptoms of dyspnea and chest discomfort are usually elicited. Tachypnea, tachycardia, and pulmonary rates are noted on examination. Chest x-ray and arterial blood gases confirm the diagnosis. Other life-threatening conditions, such as thromboembolism, should be considered and ruled out as quickly as possible.

Initial management of pulmonary edema includes oxygen administration and fluid restriction. A pulse oximeter should be placed so that oxygen saturation may be monitored continuously. A pulmonary artery catheter may be considered for severe preeclamptic patients who develop pulmonary edema antepartum, in order to distinguish between fluid overload, left ventricular dysfunction, and nonhydrostatic pulmonary edema, each of which may require different approaches to therapy.

Furosemide (Lasix) administered in a 10- to 40-mg dose IV over 1 to 2 minutes represents the first line of conventional therapy for patients with pulmonary edema associated with fluid overload. If adequate diuresis does not commence within 1 hour, an 80-mg dose may be slowly administered to achieve diuresis. In severe cases of pulmonary edema, a diuresis of 2 to 3 liters needs to be achieved before oxygenation begins to improve. Again, the degree of diuresis appropriate for these hemodynamically complex patients may be clarified by complete hemodynamic evaluation, using parameters derived by a pulmonary artery catheter. An alternative approach in patients without evidence of fluid overload, but with congestive failure secondary to intense peripheral vasospasm (Strauss, 1980), involves the administration of IV nitroprusside. While hydrostatic derangements may be corrected quickly, rapid improvement in arterial oxygenation may not be seen (Herling, 1984; Cotton, 1986b). Continuous arterial BP monitoring is often helpful in this setting because of the potent activity of some arteriodilating agents.

When hypoxemia persists despite initial treatment, mechanical ventilation may be required for respiratory support, pending correction of the underlying problem. In all cases, close monitoring of the patient's respiratory status with frequent arterial blood gases should be performed. Fluid balance is maintained by careful monitoring of intake and output. An indwelling catheter with urometer should be placed to follow hourly urine output. Serum electrolytes should also be closely monitored, especially in patients receiving diuretics.

# Renal Complications of Preeclampsia

Renal plasma flow and glomerular filtration rate are diminished significantly in preeclamptic patients (Chesley, 1971). Renal biopsy of preeclamptic patients often demonstrates a distinctive glomerular capillary endothelial cell change, termed *glomerular endotheliosis*. Damage to the glomerular membrane results in renal dysfunction (Morris, 1964; Sheehan, 1980). Urinary sediment changes (granular, hyaline, red-cell, and tubular cell casts) are common in severe preeclampsia; they reflect renal parenchymal damage but do not correlate with or predict the clinical course of disease (Leduc, 1991; Gallery, 1993).

Acute renal failure in preeclamptic pregnancies is uncommon (Krane, 1988). In 245 cases of eclampsia reported by Pritchard et al, none required dialysis for renal failure (Pritchard, 1984). Among a group of 435 women with HELLP syndrome, however, 32 (7.4%) developed acute renal failure. Maternal and perinatal complications

were extremely high, although subsequent pregnancy outcome and long-term prognosis were usually favorable in the absence of preexisting chronic hypertension (Sibai, 1993a). Acute renal failure secondary to PIH is usually the result of acute tubular necrosis but may be secondary to bilateral cortical necrosis (Sibai, 1993a,b). Precipitating factors include abruption, coagulopathy, hemorrhage, and severe hypotension (Grunfeld, 1987). The urine sediment may show granular casts and renal tubular cells (Krane, 1988; Gallery, 1993). Renal cortical necrosis may be associated with preeclampsia and may present as anuria or oliguria. Renal failure presenting in association with preeclampsia may be secondary to other underlying medical disorders, especially in the older, multiparous patient (Fisher, 1981). Should acute renal failure occur, hemodialysis or peritoneal dialysis may be required, pending return of renal function (Krane, 1988).

# Oliguria

Severe renal dysfunction in preeclampsia is most commonly initially manifested as *oliguria*, defined as urinary output less than 25 to 30 mL/hr over 2 consecutive hours. This often parallels a rise in serum creatinine and BUN and a fall in creatinine clearance. Reversible hyperuricemia is a common feature of PIH and usually precedes the development of uremia and proteinuria (Redman, 1976). Significant alterations in albumin/creatinine ratio have also been described (Baker, 1994).

Clark and colleagues have described three different hemodynamic subsets of preeclamptic-eclamptic patients with persistent oliguria, based on invasive monitoring parameters (Clark, 1986b). The first group was found to have a low PCWP, hyperdynamic left ventricular function, and mild to moderately increased SVR. These patients responded to further volume replacement. This is the most common clinical scenario, and it is felt to be secondary to intravascular volume depletion.

The second group is characterized by normal or increased PCWP, normal CO, and normal SVR, accompanied by intense uroconcentration. The pathophysiologic basis of oliguria in this group is thought to be secondary to intrinsic renal arterial spasm out of proportion to the degree of generalized systemic vasospasm. Low-dose dopamine (1–5 μg/kg/min) has been shown to produce a significant rise in urine output in severe preeclamptic patients in this hemodynamic subgroup (Kirshon, 1988a). Alternatively, afterload reduction may also improve urine output in this setting.

The third group of oliguric patients has markedly elevated PCWP and SVR, with depressed ventricular function. These patients respond to volume restriction and aggressive afterload reduction. In many cases, a forced oliguria in this subgroup may often be accompanied by incipient pulmonary edema, with fluid accumulation in the pulmonary interstitial space. Such patients would certainly not benefit from further volume infusion, yet they may be clinically indistinguishable from patients in the first group, who do respond to additional fluid infusion. Central hemodynamic assessment will allow the clinician to distinguish the preceding subgroups and tailor therapy accordingly.

Lee and colleagues studied seven oliguria preeclamptic women, utilizing the pulmonary artery catheter, and also found that oliguria was not a good index of volume status. They determined that urinary diagnostic indices such as urine-plasma ratios of creatinine, urea nitrogen, and osmolality were clinically misleading if applied to fluid management. Five of seven patients were found to have urinary diagnostic indices consistent with prerenal dehydration, but PCWP consistent with euvolemia (Lee, 1987). Normal PCWPs in oliguria preeclamptics support the hypothesis that oliguria is often secondary to severe regional vasospasm (Pritchard, 1984; Lee, 1987).

Close monitoring of fluid intake and output is of paramount importance in all patients diagnosed with preeclampsia. If urine output falls below 25 to 30 mL/hr over 2 consecutive hours, oliguria is said to present, and a management plan should be instituted. Given the fact that plasma volume is diminished in preeclamptics, the cause of oliguria may be considered prerenal in most instances (Chesley, 1972; Gallery, 1979; Clark, 1986b). A fluid challenge of 500 to 1000 mL of normal saline or lactated Ringer's solution may be administered over 30 minutes. If urine output does not respond to an initial fluid challenge,

additional challenges should be withheld pending delivery, or the institution of pulmonary artery catheterization for a more precise definition of hemodynamic status (Clark, 1986b). If at anytime oxygen saturation drops during a volume challenge, pulmonary artery catheterization is indicated if further fluid is contemplated in an effort to resolve the oliguria (Clark, 1985a, 1986b, 1988; Cotton, 1988). Repetitive fluid challenges are to be avoided in the absence of close monitoring of oxygenation status. In the presence of oliguria, delivery is, of course, also indicated.

## HELLP Syndrome

HELLP syndrome is a variant of severe preeclampsia, affecting up to 12% of patients with preeclampsia-eclampsia (Table 14-10). In one study, the incidence of HELLP syndrome (442 cases) was 20% among women with severe preeclampsia (Sibai, 1993b). As mentioned earlier, HELLP syndrome is characterized by hemolysis, elevated liver enzymes, and low platelets (Weinstein, 1982). The acronym, HELLP syndrome, was coined by Weinstein in 1982, but the hematologic and hepatic abnormalities of three cases were described by Pritchard et al in 1954. Pritchard et al credited association of thrombocytopenia with severe preeclampsia to Stahnke in 1922, and hepatic changes to Sheehan in 1950. Despite the high maternal and perinatal mortality rates associated with the HELLP syndrome, considerable controversy exists as to the proper management of these patients, who constitute a heterogeneous group with a wide array of clinical and

T A B L E   **14-10**

**Differential diagnoses of HELLP syndrome**

Autoimmune thrombocytopenic purpura
Chronic renal disease
Pyelonephritis
Cholecystitis
Gastroenteritis
Hepatitis
Pancreatitis
Thrombotic thrombocytopenic purpura
Hemolytic-uremic syndrome
Acute fatty liver of pregnancy

laboratory manifestations. In addition, HELLP syndrome may be the imitator of a variety of non-obstetric medical entities (Killam, 1975; Goodlin, 1976) and serious medical-surgical pathology may be misdiagnosed as preeclampsia or HELLP syndrome (Goodlin, 1991).

Unlike most forms of preeclampsia, HELLP syndrome is not primarily a disease of primigravidas. For example, several studies have found that nearly half of HELLP syndrome patients were multigravidas, the incidence among multigravidas being almost twice that seen in primigravid patients (MacKenna, 1983; Sibai, 1986b; Weinstein 1985; Sibai, 1991).

Clinically, many HELLP syndrome patients do not meet the standard BP criteria for severe preeclampsia. In one series of 112 women with severe preeclampsia-eclampsia complicated by HELLP syndrome, admission diastolic BP was less than 110 mm Hg in 31% of cases and less than 90 mm Hg in 15% (Sibai, 1986c).

The multisystem nature of PIH is often manifested by hepatic dysfunction. Hepatic artery resistance is increased in patients with HELLP syndrome (Oosterhof, 1994). Liver dysfunction, as defined by an elevated SGOT, was identified in 21% of 355 patients with PIH, who were retrospectively reviewed by Romero et al (1988). Liver dysfunction has been associated with intrauterine growth retardation (IUGR), prematurity, increased cesarean section rates, and lower Apgar scores (Romero, 1988a). Using immunofluorescent staining, Arias and Mancilla-Jimenez found fibrin deposition in hepatic sinusoids of preeclamptic women, thought to be the result of ischemia secondary to vasospasm. Continued prolonged vasospasm may lead to hepatocellular necrosis (Shukla, 1978; Arias, 1976).

The clinical signs and symptoms of patients with HELLP syndrome are classically related to the impact of vasospasm on the maternal liver. Thus, the majority of patients present with signs or symptoms of liver compromise. These include malaise, nausea (with or without vomiting), and epigastric pain. In most series, hepatic or right-upper-quadrant tenderness to palpation is seen consistently in HELLP syndrome patients (Weinstein, 1982, 1985; MacKenna, 1983; Sibai, 1986c).

Laboratory studies often create the illusion of medical conditions unrelated to pregnancy or preeclampsia. Peripheral smears demonstrate burr cells and/or schistocytes with polychromasia, consistent with microangiopathic hemolytic anemia. Hemolysis can also be demonstrated by abnormal haptoglobin or bilirubin levels (Cunningham, 1978, 1985; Vardi, 1974; Gibson, 1982). Scanning electron microscopy demonstrates evidence of microangiopathic hemolysis in patients with HELLP syndrome (Cunningham, 1985). The microangiopathic hemolytic anemia is felt to occur secondary to passage of the red cells through thrombosed, damaged vessels (Romero, 1988a; Cunningham, 1978; Gibson, 1982; Entman, 1987; Burrows, 1987). Increased red-cell turnover has also been evidenced by increased levels of carboxyhemoglobin and serum iron (Entman, 1987). Although some degree of hemolysis is noted, anemia is uncommon.

*Thrombocytopenia* is defined as a platelet count of either less than 100,000 or less than $150,000/\mu L$. This process is not usually encountered in patients with essential hypertension (Pritchard, 1954). Thrombocytopenia in preeclampsia occurs secondary to increased peripheral platelet destruction, as manifested by increased bone marrow megakaryocytes, the presence of circulating megathrombocytes, evidence of reduced platelet life span, and platelet adherence to exposed vascular collagen (Gibson, 1982; Entman, 1987; Burrows, 1987; Hutt, 1994). Thrombocytopenia has been found in as many as 50% of preeclamptic patients studied prospectively for hemostatic and platelet function (Burrows, 1987). Evidence for platelet destruction, impaired platelet function, and elevated platelet-associated immunoglobulin G (IgG) were found in thrombocytopenic preeclamptics.

In a retrospective review of 353 patients with PIH, Romero and colleagues reported an 11.6% incidence of thrombocytopenia, defined as a platelet count less than $100,000/\mu L$. Patients with thrombocytopenia had an increased risk for cesarean section, blood transfusion, preterm delivery, IUGR, and low Apgar scores (Romero, 1989). Thrombocytopenia has also been reported to occur in the neonates of preeclamptic women (Weinstein, 1982, 1985; Klechner, 1977), although others have disputed these findings (Pritchard, 1987).

Clotting parameters, such as the prothrombin time (PT), partial thromboplastin time (PTT), fibrinogen, and bleeding time (BT), in the patient with HELLP syndrome are generally normal in the absence of abruptio placenta or fetal demise (Sibai, 1986). Platelet or fresh frozen plasma transfusion is necessary in only 8% to 10% of patients with HELLP syndrome (Pritchard, 1954; Sibai, 1986c).

Significant elevation of alkaline phosphatase is seen in normal pregnancy; elevation of SGOT and/or SGPT, however, indicate hepatic pathology. In HELLP syndrome, the SGOT and SGPT are rarely in excess of 1000 IU/liter; values in excess of this level suggest other hepatic disorders, such as hepatitis. HELLP syndrome progressing to liver rupture, however, may be associated with markedly elevated hepatic transaminases.

Laboratory abnormalities usually return to normal within a short time after delivery; it is not unusual, however, to see transient worsening of both thrombocytopenia and hepatic function in the first 24 to 48 hours postpartum (Neiger, 1991). An upward trend in platelet count and a downward trend in lactate dehydrogenase concentration should occur in patients without complications by the fourth postpartum day (Martin, 1991). Martin and colleagues (1991) evaluated postpartum recovery in 158 women with HELLP syndrome at the University of Mississippi Medical Center. A return to a normal platelet count (>100,000/μL) occurred in all women whose platelet nadir was below 50,000/μL by the eleventh postpartum day, and in all women whose platelet nadir was 50,000 to 100,000/μL by the sixth postpartum day.

HELLP syndrome can be a "great masquerader," and both clinical presentation and laboratory findings associated with this syndrome may suggest an array of clinical diagnoses (see Table 14-10). Because of the numerous misdiagnoses associated with this syndrome, and because a delay in diagnosis may be life threatening, a pregnant woman with thrombocytopenia, elevated serum transaminase levels, or epigastric pain should be considered to have HELLP syndrome until proven otherwise.

Complications associated with HELLP syndrome include placental abruption, acute renal failure and hepatic hematoma with rupture, and ascites. Placental abruption in HELLP syndrome patients occurs at a rate 20 times that seen in the general obstetric population; the reported incidence ranges from 7% to 20% (Pritchard, 1954; Sibai, 1986c; Cunningham, 1985; Messer, 1987). Abruption in the presence of HELLP syndrome is frequently associated with fetal death and/or consumptive coagulopathy.

A review of the literature discloses significantly elevated maternal and perinatal mortality rates associated with HELLP syndrome (Tables 14-11, 14-12). As with other severe preeclampsia variants, delivery is ultimately the treatment of choice. The timing of delivery, however,

T A B L E **14-11**

Maternal outcomes in HELLP syndrome

| Series | Location | Years | Cases (n) | Incidence (%) | Maternal Mortality | C/S Rate | |
|---|---|---|---|---|---|---|---|
| MacKenna, 1983 | Greenville, NC | 1978–1982 | 27 | 12[a] | 0/27 (0%) | — | |
| Weinstein, 1985 | Tucson, AZ | 1980–1984 | 57 | 0.67[b] | 2/57 (3.5%) | 33/57 | (58%) |
| Sibai, 1986c | Memphis, TN | 1977–1985 | 112 | 9.7[c] | 2/112 (1.8%) | 71/112 | (63%) |
| Romero, 1988a | New Haven, CT | 1981–1984 | 58 | 21[a] | N/A | 33/58 | (57%) |
| Sibai, 1993b | Memphis, TN | 1977–1992 | 442 | 20[d] | 4/442 (0.9%) | 185/442 | (42%) |

[a]Among all preeclamptic-eclamptic patients.

[b]Among all live births.

[c]Among severe preeclamptic-eclamptic pregnancies.

[d]Among severe preeclamptic women.

N/A, not available.

T A B L E   **14-12**

Perinatal outcomes in HELLP syndrome

| Series | Location | Years | Cases (n) | Perinatal Mortality | SGA | RDS | Neonatal Thrombo-cytopenia | Neonatal Leukopenia |
|---|---|---|---|---|---|---|---|---|
| MacKenna, 1983 | Greenville, CT | 1978–1982 | 27 | 3/27 (11%) | N/A | 2/24 (8%) | 1/24 (4%) | 1/24 (4%) |
| Weinstein, 1985 | Tucson, AZ | 1980–1984 | 57 | 5/63 (8%) | N/A | 9/58 (16%) | 11/46 (24%) | 17/45 (38%) |
| Sibai, 1986c | Memphis, TN | 1977–1985 | 112 | 38/114 (33%) | 36/114 (32%) |  | 21 (26%) | 11 (14%) |
| Romero, 1988a | New Haven, CT | 1981–1984 | 58 | 4/58 (7%) | 24/58 (41%) | 18/58 (31%) | N/A | N/A |

[a]Among all preeclamptic/eclamptic patients.

[b]Among all live births.

[c]Among severe preeclamptic-eclamptic pregnancies.

SGA, small for gestational age; RDS, respiratory distress syndrome; N/A, not available.

remains controversial. Several investigators recommend immediate delivery, while others reasonably suggest that under certain conditions with marked fetal immaturity, delivery may safely be delayed for a short time (Killam, 1975; Weinstein, 1982; MacKenna, 1983; Thiagarajah, 1984; Goodlin, 1987; Heyborne, 1990). In support of this latter approach, Clark and associates have demonstrated transient improvement in patients with HELLP syndrome following bed rest and/or corticosteroid administration (Clark, 1986a). Following an initial improvement, however, each patient's clinical condition worsened. Similar observations were seen in three of 17 (18%) patients in Sibai's series following steroid administration to enhance fetal pulmonary maturity (Sibai, 1986c). Thus, it appears that in the mother with a very premature fetus and borderline disturbances in platelet count or serum transaminase values, and in the absence of other absolute indications for delivery, careful inhospital observation may at times be appropriate. Certainly, uncontrollable BP, significantly rising liver enzymes, or a serum creatinine would mandate delivery irrespective of gestational age.

The mode of delivery should depend on the state of the cervix and other obstetric indications for cesarean birth. HELLP syndrome, by itself, is not an indication for cesarean delivery. A high percentage of patients with HELLP syndrome, however, will undergo operative delivery (see Table 14-11). A commonly encountered situation involves a mother with a premature fetus, an unfavorable cervix, and a platelet count less than 100,000/$\mu$L. In such patients, cesarean delivery is often preferred to avoid the necessity of later operative delivery for failed induction in the face of more significant thrombocytopenia.

Sullivan and colleagues evaluated 481 women who developed HELLP syndrome at the University of Mississippi Medical Center; 195 subsequent pregnancies occurred in 122 patients (Sullivan, 1994). The incidence of recurrent HELLP syndrome was 19% to 27%, and the recurrence of any form of preeclampsia-eclampsia was 42% to 43%. Sibai and co-workers reviewed 442 pregnancies complicated by HELLP syndrome at the University of Tennessee in Memphis; follow-up data were available in 341 cases (Sibai, 1995). In 192 subsequent pregnancies, obstetric complications were common, including preeclampsia (19%), but only 3% experienced recurrent HELLP syndrome. They attributed the discrepancy in recurrence risk between their study and that of Sullivan (1994) to differences in definitions of the syndrome and patient populations. Blood component therapy is discussed in detail in Chapter 11. Schwartz and co-workers reported the use of exchange plasmapheresis with fresh frozen plasma to treat hemolysis and thrombocytopenia that did not resolve following delivery and standard medical treatment (Schwartz, 1985).

## Liver Rupture

Hepatic infarction may lead to intrahepatic hemorrhage and development of a subcapsular hematoma, which may rupture into the peritoneal space and result in shock and death (Arias, 1976; Rademaker, 1943). Subcapsular hematomas usually develop on the anterior and superior aspects of the liver (Herbert, 1982). The diagnosis of a liver hematoma may be aided by use of ultrasonography, radionuclide scanning, computed tomography (CT), and selective angiography (Herbert, 1982; Henny, 1983).

Henny described a biphasic chronologic sequence of events during rupture of the subcapsular hematoma. The initial presenting symptoms are constant, progressively worsening pain in the epigastrium or right upper quadrant of the abdomen, with or without nausea and vomiting. The second phase is manifested by the development of vascular collapse, shock, and fetal death (Henny, 1983). The maternal and fetal prognoses of liver rupture are poor. Bis and Waxman reported a 59% maternal and 62% fetal mortality rate (Bis, 1976).

Significant or persistent elevations of serum transaminase levels in conjunction with preeclampsia and right-upper-quadrant or epigastric tenderness indicate delivery regardless of gestational age. Especially when such dysfunction occurs in the presence of thrombocytopenia, careful clinical observation during the postpartum period is essential. When the diagnosis of liver hematoma is suspected in severe preeclampsia prior to delivery of the fetus, immediate exploratory laparotomy and cesarean section should be considered in order to prevent rupture of the hematoma secondary to increased abdominal pressure in the second stage of labor, in vomiting, or during eclamptic convulsions (Henny, 1983). Prompt delivery is also mandatory. When the diagnosis of liver hematoma is made in the postpartum period, conservative management with blood transfusion and serial ultrasonography may be reasonable (Henny, 1983; Goodlin, 1985).

Smith and colleagues (1991) reviewed the literature for the years 1976 to 1990 (28 cases) and reported their experience at Baylor College of Medicine for the years 1978 to 1990 (seven new cases) of spontaneous rupture of the liver during pregnancy. The incidence was one per 45,145 live births in the Baylor series. A significant improvement in maternal outcome ($p = 0.006$) was seen among patients who were managed by packing and drainage (82% survival), compared with those managed by hepatic lobectomy (25% survival). This conservative approach is supported by the trauma literature. At Baylor College of Medicine, 1000 consecutive cases of liver injury were evaluated; extensive resection of the liver or lobectomy with selective vascular ligation resulted in a 34% mortality rate, whereas conservative surgery (packing and drainage and/or use of topical hemostatic agents) resulted in a 7% mortality (Feliciano, 1986). Smith and colleagues (1991) proposed an algorithm for antepartum and postpartum management of hepatic hemorrhage in their review.

Liver rupture with intraperitoneal hemorrhage, when suspected, requires laparotomy. Hemostasis may be achieved by compression, simple suture, topical coagulant agents, arterial embolization, omental pedicles, ligation of the hepatic artery, or lobectomy, depending on the extent of the hepatic damage (Lucas, 1976). Temporary control of bleeding may be achieved by packing the rupture site or by application of a gravity suit (Lucas, 1976; Gardner, 1966).

Few cases of pregnancy following hepatic rupture have been reported. There have been several reported cases of nonrecurrence in subsequent pregnancies (Sakala, 1986) and one case of recurrence with survival in a subsequent pregnancy (Greenstein, 1994).

## Neurologic Complications of Preeclampsia

Cerebral hemorrhage, cerebral edema, temporary blindness (amaurosis), and eclamptic seizures are separate but related neurologic conditions that may occur in preeclampsia. Cerebral hemorrhage and cerebral edema are two major causes of maternal mortality in preeclampsia (Hibbard, 1973). Intracranial hemorrhage may result from the combination of severe hypertension and hemostatic compromise (Romero, 1988b).

## Cerebral Edema

*Cerebral edema* is defined as increased water content of one or more of the intracranial fluid compartments of the brain (Bell, 1983). Signs of diffuse cerebral edema may be found in eclamptic women on CT scan (Kirby, 1984) and may develop when the forces affecting the Starling equilibrium are disturbed. The three most important etiologic factors include increased intravascular pressure, damage to vascular endothelium, and reduced plasma COP (Miller, 1979). Miller's classification of cerebral edema includes (1) vasogenic edema with breakdown of the blood-brain barrier, secondary to vascular damage; (2) cytotoxic edema, secondary to damage to the cellular sodium pump; (3) hydrostatic edema from increased intravascular pressure; (4) interstitial edema related to acute obstructive hydrocephalus; and (5) hypoosmotic edema, in which intravascular free water decreases plasma osmolality (Miller, 1979). In the general population, vasogenic edema, which predominantly occurs in the cerebral white matter, is the most common type of cerebral edema (Weiss, 1985).

In PIH, cerebral edema is thought to occur secondary to anoxia associated with eclamptic seizures or secondary to loss of cerebral autoregulation as a result of severe hypertension (Benedetti, 1980b). Cerebral edema is diagnosed on CT scan by the appearance of areas with low density or low radiographic absorption coefficient (Kirby, 1984; Weiss, 1985; Beeson, 1982). Magnetic resonance imaging (MRI) has also been useful in providing an index of water content in select areas of the brain (Weiss, 1985).

General therapeutic principles in the treatment of cerebral edema include correction of hypoxemia and hypercarbia, avoidance of volatile anesthetic agents, control of body temperature, and control of BP (Miller, 1979; Weiss, 1985). Assisted hyperventilation reduces intracranial hypertension and the formation of cerebral edema. Partial pressure of carbon dioxide ($Pco_2$) levels are maintained between 25 mm Hg and 30 mm Hg (Miller, 1979). Hyperbaric oxygenation therapy, considered experimental in the control of cerebral edema, is aimed at maintaining a partial pressure of oxygen ($Po_2$) level of 1000 mm Hg, using an ambient pressure of 2.0 to 2.5 atm to effect cerebral vasoconstriction (Miller, 1979).

The administration of hypertonic solutions such as mannitol increases serum osmolality and draws water from the brain into the vascular compartment, thus reducing brain tissue water and volume. A 20% solution of mannitol is given as a 0.5- to 1.0-g/kg dose over 10 minutes or as a continuous infusion of 5 g/hr. The serum osmolality is maintained in a range between 305 and 315 mosm (Miller, 1979; Weiss, 1985). Steroid therapy (dexamethasone, betamethasone, methylprednisolone) is thought to be most effective in the treatment of focal chronic cerebral edema, which may occur in association with a tumor or abscess. Steroid therapy is less beneficial in cases of diffuse or acute cerebral edema (Miller, 1979). Other pharmacologic agents that have been used to reduce intracranial pressure and cerebral edema include acetazolamide (Diamox), furosemide (Lasix), spironolactone (Aldactone), and ethacrynic acid (Edecrin).

In preeclamptic-eclamptic patients diagnosed with cerebral edema, therapy should be directed at correcting hypoxemia, hypercarbia, hyperthermia, and/or hypertension or hypotension. If assisted ventilation is employed, hyperventilation with controlled hypocapnia should be used. Mannitol may be administered with careful observation of pulmonary, cardiovascular, and renal function. The inciting factor of cerebral edema in preeclampsia and eclampsia, albeit unknown, is eliminated by delivery of the products of conception and, thus, is ultimately treatable in this patient population.

## Temporary Blindness

Temporary blindness may complicate 1% to 3% of cases of preeclampsia-eclampsia (Beeson, 1982; Hill, 1985; Beck, 1980; Beal, 1980; Seidman, 1991) and was recently reported in 15% of women with eclampsia at Parkland Hospital (Cunningham, 1995). Pregnancy-related blindness has been associated with eclampsia, cavernous sinus thrombosis, and hypertensive encephalopathy (Beeson, 1982; Hill, 1985; Beck, 1980; Beal, 1980). Beeson and Duda reported one case associated with eclampsia and occipital lobe edema (Beeson, 1982). Hill and associates noted that recovery of vision correlated with the return of a normal PCWP in severe preeclamptics with amaurosis (Hill, 1985). The injury is usually the result of severe damage to the retinal vasculature or occipital lobe ischemia (Beal, 1980). Cunningham and colleagues evaluated the clinical courses of 15 women with severe preeclampsia or eclampsia who developed cortical blindness over a 14-year period (Cunningham, 1995). Blindness persisted from 4 hours to 8 days but resolved completely in all cases. Ten of the 15 women experienced eclamptic seizures. Based on data from CT imaging and MRI, the Parkland group concluded that cortical blindness resulted from petechial hemorrhages and focal edema in the occipital cortex.

Transient blindness usually resolves spontaneously after delivery of the fetus (Beeson, 1982; Hill, 1985; Beck, 1980). Nevertheless, focal neurologic deficits such as this require ophthalmologic and neurologic consultation and CT or MRI of the brain. Generally, management guidelines are the same as for preeclamptics without this complication (Cunningham, 1995). Associated conditions, such as cerebral edema, should be treated as indicated. Paralysis of the sixth cranial nerve has been reported as a complication of eclampsia (Kinsella, 1994).

## Eclampsia

The precise cause of seizures in preeclampsia remains unknown. Hypertensive encephalopathy, as well as vasospasm, hemorrhage, ischemia, and edema of the cerebral hemispheres, have been proposed as etiologic factors. Thrombotic and hemorrhagic lesions have been identified on autopsy of preeclamptic women (Govan, 1961; Sheehan, 1950). Clark and colleagues noted lower COP associated with eclamptic patients, as opposed to matched severe preeclamptic patients (Clark, 1985b). The importance of low COP in the development of pulmonary dysfunction has been described previously (Benedetti, 1985).

Douglas and Redman (1994) reported that the incidence of eclampsia in the United Kingdom during the year 1992 was 4.9 per 10,000 maternities. During the period 1979 to 1986, the incidence of eclampsia in the United States was 5.6 per 10,000 births (Saftlas, 1990). The eclampsia rate decreased by 36% from 6.8 per 10,000 births during the first half of the series to 4.3 per 10,000 births during the latter half of the series.

Eclamptic seizures usually occur without a preceding aura, although many patients will manifest some form of apprehension, excitability, or hyperreflexia prior to the onset of a seizure. Eclampsia unheralded by hypertension and proteinuria occurred in 38% of cases reported in the United Kingdom (Douglas, 1994). Douglas and Redman conclude that "the term pre-eclampsia is misleading because eclampsia can precede preeclampsia." In a study of 179 cases of eclampsia, approximately one third of patients received obstetric care that met standards for delivery of obstetric services and were thus classified as "unavoidable" cases of eclampsia (Sibai, 1986). Sibai and colleagues recommend magnesium prophylaxis in *all* preeclamptics, regardless of degree, because a significant percentage of eclamptics demonstrated only mild signs and symptoms of preeclampsia prior to the onset of seizures (Sibai, 1986a). Once a seizure occurs, it is usually a forerunner of more convulsions unless anticonvulsant therapy is initiated.

Eclamptic seizures occur prior to the delivery in roughly 80% of patients (Table 14-13). In the remainder, convulsions occur postpartum, and they have been reported up to 23 days following delivery (Sibai, 1980; Brown, 1987). Douglas and Redman observed that most antepartum convulsions (76%) occurred prior to term, while most intrapartum or postpartum convulsions (75%) occurred at term (Douglas, 1994). Late postpartum eclampsia (convulsions more than 48 hours but less than 4 weeks after delivery) constituted 56% of total postpartum eclampsia and 16% of all cases of eclampsia in a series collected at the University of Tennessee, Memphis,

T A B L E   **14-13**

Incidences of eclamptic seizures in relation to delivery

| Series | Location | Years | Eclamptics (n) | Before (%) | After (%) |
|--------|----------|-------|----------------|------------|-----------|
| Bryant, 1940 | Cincinnati, OH | 1930–1940 | 120 | 74/120 (62%) | 46/120 (38%) |
| Bryant, 1962 | Cincinnati, OH | 1940–1960 | 133 | 97/127 (76%) | 30/127 (24%) |
| Zuspan, 1966 | Augusta, GA | 1956–1965 | 69 | 61 (88%) | 8 (12%) |
| Harbert, 1968 | Charlottesville, VA | 1939–1963 | 168 | 131 (78%) | 37 (22%) |
| Pritchard, 1975 | Dallas, TX | 1955–1975 | 154 | 126 (82%) | 28 (18%) |
| Lopez-Llera, 1982 | Mexico City, Mexico | 1963–1979 | 704 | 584 (83%) | 120 (17%) |
| Pritchard, 1984 | Dallas, TX | 1975–1983 | 91 | 83 (91%) | 8 (9%) |
| Adetoro, 1989 | Ilorin, Nigeria | 1972–1987 | 651 | N/A | N/A |
| Sibai, 1992 | Memphis, TN | 1977–1989 | 254 | 181 (71%) | 73 (29%) |
| Douglas, 1994 | United Kingdom | 1992 | 383 | 215 (56%) | 168 (44%) |

N/A, not available

between the years 1977 and 1992 (Lubarsky, 1994). Severe headache or visual disturbances were noted in 83% of patients before the onset of convulsions. When eclampsia occurs more than 24 hours postpartum, however, a thorough search for other potential causes of seizures is mandatory.

A maternal seizure typically results in fetal bradycardia. Although the fetal heart rate pattern usually returns to normal following the seizure, appropriate steps should be taken to enhance maternal-fetal well-being, including maintenance of maternal airway, oxygen administration, and maternal lateral repositioning. Complete maternal recovery following eclampsia usually is expected.

The standard therapy for the management of eclampsia includes (1) magnesium sulfate and (2) delivery of the fetus. We administer 4 to 6 g of magnesium sulfate IV over 20 minutes, and initiate an IV infusion at 2 to 3 g/hr. If control of seizures is not successful after the initial IV bolus, a second 2-g bolus of magnesium sulfate may be cautiously administered. No more than a total of 8 g of magnesium sulfate is recommended at the outset of treatment.

Seizures may recur despite apparently appropriate maintenance-magnesium therapy. The incidence of recurrent seizures ranges from 8% to 13% (Sibai, 1986a). Both IM and IV magnesium sulfate regimens have occasionally been associated with recurrent seizures. Of such patients, one half may have subtherapeutic magnesium levels (Sibai, 1986a). This underscores the importance of individualized therapy to achieve adequate serum magnesium levels and minimize the risk of recurrent seizures. Seizures refractory to standard magnesium sulfate regimens may be treated with a slow 100-mg IV dose of thiopental sodium (Pentothal) or 1 to 10 mg of diazepam. Alternatively, sodium amobarbital (up to 250 mg) may be administered IV. In a clinical study, Lucas and colleagues described a simplified regimen of phenytoin for the treatment of preeclampsia (Lucas, 1994). An IV infusion rate of 16.7 mg/min over 1 hour provided an initial dose of 1000 mg; an additional 500 mg of phenytoin administered orally 10 hours after treatment initiation maintained therapeutic levels for an additional 14 hours.

Eclamptic patients with repetitive seizures despite therapeutic magnesium levels warrant CT evaluation of the brain. Dunn and associates found five of seven such patients to have abnormalities such as cerebral edema, cerebral venous thrombosis, and low-density white matter (Dunn, 1986). However, Sibai et al reported 20 cases of eclamptics with neurologic signs or repetitive seizures who all had normal CT findings (Sibai, 1985a). Their recommendation regarding use of CT scan was restricted to patients with late-onset postpartum preeclampsia or those patients with focal neurologic deficits.

Eclamptic patients require delivery without respect to gestational age (Cunningham, 1994).

Cesarean delivery should be reserved for obstetric indications or deteriorating maternal condition. As demonstrated in Table 14-14, vaginal delivery may be achieved in at least half of eclamptic patients. Pritchard et al reported successful vaginal delivery in 82% of oxytocin-induced patients (Pritchard, 1984).

Maternal mortality rates are increased in patients with eclampsia, but the rates have declined dramatically in recent years (Pritchard, 1984). According to Chesley (1984), the average maternal mortality rate of eclampsia during the mid-nineteenth century (1837–1867) was approximately 30%. In the latter half of the nineteenth century, the average maternal mortality rate was around 24%. During the early twentieth century (1911–1925), the maternal mortality rate was 11% and 22% among women managed conservatively and delivered operatively, respectively. Lazard (1933) reported a 13% gross mortality rate among 225 eclamptics treated in Los Angeles between 1924 and 1932. Eastman and Steptoe (1945) reported a 7.6% maternal mortality and 21.7% fetal mortality rate of eclampsia in Baltimore between the years 1924 and 1943.

Contemporary maternal mortality rates range from 0% to 14% (Table 14-15). In Pritchard's series of 245 eclamptics, one maternal death occurred, which was attributed to magnesium intoxication (Pritchard, 1984). In Sibai's series of 254 eclamptic women, there was one maternal death in a woman who suffered seizures prior to arrival to the hospital and who arrived in a moribund state (Sibai, 1992). In the United Kingdom during 1992, the incidence of eclampsia was 4.9 per 10,000 maternities, with a 1.8% maternal case mortality rate (Douglas, 1994).

At a referral hospital in Mexico City, 704 eclamptic women were managed during a 15-year period (Lopez-Llera, 1982). The maternal mortality rate was 14%, a relatively high rate likely secondary to a high proportion of advanced cases of disease. According to Lopez-Llera, maternal mortality rates are higher in those women with seizures prior to (15%) than after (10%) delivery (Lopez-Llera, 1982). The most common single cause of death in the Mexico City series among 86 fatal cases of antepartum and intrapartum eclampsia was cerebrovascular damage (72%), followed by severe respiratory insufficiency (12%), postpartum hemorrhage (6%), and DIC (4%). Autopsy findings have mirrored these observations (Sheehan, 1950).

Overall, the contemporary perinatal mortality rate among eclamptics ranges from 7% to 16% in the United States and the United Kingdom (see Table 14-15) and is most commonly secondary to placental abruption, prematurity, and perinatal asphyxia. Antenatal deaths accounted for a significant proportion of the overall perinatal

T A B L E   **14-14**

Cesarean delivery rate in eclampsia

| Series | Location | Years | Eclamptics (n) | Cesareans (n) | C/S Rate (%) |
|---|---|---|---|---|---|
| Bryant, 1940 | Cincinnati, OH | 1930–1940 | 120 | 0/120 | 0 |
| Bryant, 1962 | Cincinnati, OH | 1940–1960 | 133 | 10/85 | 12[a] |
| Zuspan, 1966 | Augusta, GA | 1956–1965 | 69 | 1/69 | 1.4[b] |
| Harbert, 1968 | Charlottesville, VA | 1939–1963 | 168 | 10/168 | 6[b] |
| Pritchard, 1975 | Dallas, TX | 1955–1975 | 154 | 29/126 | 23 |
| Lopez-Llera, 1982 | Mexico City, Mexico | 1963–1979 | 704 | 331/584 | 57[a] |
| Pritchard, 1984 | Dallas, TX | 1975–1983 | 91 | 27/83 | 33[a] |
| Adetoro, 1989 | Ilorin, Nigeria | 1972–1987 | 651 | N/A | N/A |
| Sibai, 1992 | Memphis, TN | 1977–1989 | 254 | 124/254 | 49[b] |
| Douglas, 1994 | United Kingdom | 1992 | 383 | 206/383 | 54[b] |

[a]Antepartum and intrapartum cases only.

[b]All cases.

N/A, not available.

T A B L E   **14-15**

Maternal and perinatal mortality in eclampsia

| Series | Location | Years | Eclamptics (n) | Maternal Mortality | Perinatal Mortality |
|--------|----------|-------|----------------|--------------------|--------------------|
| Bryant, 1940 | Cincinnati, OH | 1930–1940 | 120 | 2/120 (1.7%) | 36/125 (29%)[a] |
| Bryant, 1962 | Cincinnati, OH | 1940–1960 | 133 | 2/133 (1.5%) | 71/256 (28%)[b] |
| Zuspan, 1966 | Augusta, GA | 1956–1965 | 69 | 2/69 (2.9%) | 23/73 (32%)[a] |
| Harbert, 1968 | Charlottesville, VA | 1939–1963 | 168 | 8/168 (4.8%) | 37/171 (22%)[a] |
| Pritchard, 1975 | Dallas, TX | 1955–1975 | 154 | 0/154 (0%) | 20/130 (15%)[c] |
| Lopez-Llera, 1982 | Mexico City, Mexico | 1963–1979 | 704 | 98/704 (14%) | 162/604 (27%) |
| Pritchard, 1984 | Dallas, TX | 1975–1983 | 91 | 1/91 (1.1%) | 13/84 (16%)[c] |
| Adetoro, 1989 | Ilorin, Nigeria | 1972–1987 | 651 | 94/651 (14%) | N/A |
| Sibai, 1990 | Memphis, TN | 1977–1989 | 254 | 1/254 (0.4%) | 31/263 (12%)[a] |
| Douglas, 1994 | United Kingdom | 1992 | 383 | 7/383 (1.8%) | 30/411 (7%)[a] |

[a]All cases.

[b]Includes 1930–1940 series.

[c]Antepartum and intrapartum cases only.

N/A, not available.

mortality. Depending on the gestational age and the clinical circumstances, it may be prudent to have a person capable of neonatal resuscitation immediately available at delivery.

Eclamptic patients are at increased risk for developing mild and severe PIH and eclampsia in a subsequent pregnancy (Sibai, 1986b, 1992). Remote mortality is not greater for white primiparous eclamptics but is increased from 2 to 5 times the expected rate for white multiparous eclamptics and all black eclamptics (Chesley, 1976). Moreover, these women appear to be at a greater risk of developing chronic hypertension and diabetes mellitus (Sibai, 1986b; Chesley, 1976, 1978). However, long-term neurologic deficits are rare and long-term anticonvulsant therapy is usually not necessary in the eclamptic woman (Sibai, 1985a).

## Uteroplacental-Fetal Complications of Preeclampsia

The blood flow through the uterus and placenta is significantly decreased in preeclamptic patients (Friedman, 1988; Lunell, 1982, 1984; Browne, 1953; Dixon, 1963). This may lead to IUGR, fetal distress, or fetal death. Hypertensive patients are also at higher risk for abruption. The pathophysiology of placental abruption in preeclamptic patients has been proposed to result from thrombotic lesions in the placental vasculature, leading to decidual necrosis, separation, and hemorrhage. A vicious cycle then continues as the decidual hemorrhage results in further separation. This cycle may be aggravated by coexisting hemostatic compromise. Abdella and colleagues evaluated 265 cases of abruption and estimated an incidence of approximately 1.2% in the total obstetric population; 26.8% were complicated by hypertensive disorder. Preeclamptics, chronic hypertensives, and eclamptics were found to have a 2.3%, 10.0%, and 23.6% incidence of abruption, respectively (Abdella, 1984; Hurd, 1983). Severe preeclamptic patients with chronic hypertension have a significantly increased perinatal mortality rate, abruption rate, and frequency of growth-retarded infants when compared with severe preeclamptics without preexisting hypertension (Sibai, 1984b). Fetal growth retardation appears to occur frequently in multiparous women with preeclampsia, compared with nulliparous women with preeclampsia; the cause of this difference, however, is uncertain (Eskenazi, 1993). Oxygen

---

**IMPLICATIONS OF SEVERE PREECLAMPSIA MANAGEMENT PROTOCOL**

**I.** *Goals of Therapy*

    A. Control of severe hypertension ($> 180–160/110$ mm Hg).
    B. Seizure prophylaxis/therapy.
    C. Delivery of fetus and placenta.
    D. Stabilization and correction of multisystem dysfunction.

**II.** *Management Protocol*

    A. Control of severe hypertension: hydralazine 2.5 to 5.0 mg IV every 20 minutes to maintain BP below above limits.
    B. Seizure prophylaxis therapy: $MgSO_4$ IV loading dose of 4 to 6 g over 20 minutes; then maintenance dose of 2 to 3 g/hr IV.
    C. Delivery of fetus and placenta: induction of labor (artificial rupture of membranes, IV oxytocin infusion, or prostaglandin cervical ripening) or cesarean section (for maternal or fetal indications).
    D. Stabilization and correction of multisystem dysfunction (see text).

**III.** *Clinical Laboratory Tests*

    A. Routine: complete blood count and platelet count, serum creatinine, hepatic transaminase and lactate dehydrogenase, urinalysis.
    B. Additional tests: fibrinogen, PT, PTT, uric acid and BUN, blood type and screen/crossmatch, 24-hour urine for protein and creatinine clearance.

**IV.** *Consultation*

    A. Routine: OB/GYN, Maternal-Fetal Medicine, Anesthesiology, Neonatology
    B. Depending on clinical situation: Critical Care, Neurology, Nephrology, Pathology (Blood Bank).

---

transport and extraction may be negatively affected by preeclampsia. Wheeler (1996) demonstrated a strong negative linear correlation between base deficit and oxygen delivery index and suggested that a base deficit exceeding $-8.0$ mEq/liter consistently predicted fetal acidosis, death, and maternal end-organ ischemic injury (Wheeler, 1996; Belfort, 1995).

**REFERENCES**

Abdella TN, Sibai BM, Hays JM Jr, Anderson GD. Relationship of hypertensive disease to abruptio placentae. Obstet Gynecol 1984;63:365–370.

Abdul-Karim R, Assali NS. Pressor response to angiotensin in pregnant and nonpregnant women. Am J Obstet Gynecol 1961;82:246–251.

Adam K, Kirshon B, Lee W, et al. Acid-base balance in the human fetus during nifedipine therapy. Unpublished.

Adetero OO. A sixteen year survey of maternal mortality associated with eclampsia in Ilorin, Nigeria. Int J Gynecol Obstet 1989;30:117–121.

American College of Obstetricians and Gynecologists. Management of preeclampsia. ACOG Technical Bulletin 1986;91:1–5.

American College of Obstetricians and Gynecologists. Hypertension in pregnancy. ACOG Technical Bulletin 219. Washington, DC: ACOG, 1996.

Arias F, Mancilla-Jimenez R. Hepatic fibrinogen deposits in preeclampsia. N Engl J Med 1976; 295:578–582.

Assali NS, Kaplan S, Oighenstein S, Suyemoto R. Hemodynamic effects of 1-hydrazinophthalazine (Apresoline) in human pregnancy: results of intravenous administration. J Clin Invest 1953;32:922–930.

Atkinson MW, Belfort MA, Saade GR, Moise K. The relation between magnesium sulfate therapy and fetal heart rate variability. Obstet Gynecol 1991;83:967–970.

Atkinson MW, Maher JE, Owen J, et al. The predictive value of umbilical artery Doppler studies for preeclampsia or fetal growth retardation in a preeclampsia prevention trial. Obstet Gynecol 1994;83:609–612.

Baker PN, Hacket GA. The use of urinary albumin-creatinine ratios and calcium-creatinine ratios as screening tests for pregnancy-induced hypertension. Obstet Gynecol 1994;83:745–749.

Balasch J, Mirapeix E, Borche L, et al. Further evidence against preeclampsia as an immune complex disease. Obstet Gynecol 1981;58:435.

Barr M, Cohen M. ACE inhibitor fetopathy and hypocalvaria: the kidney-skull connection. Teratology 1991;44:485–495.

Beal MF, Chapman PH. Cortical blindness and homonymous hemianopia in the postpartum period. JAMA 1980;244:2085–2087.

Beck RW, Gamel JW, Willcourt RJ, Berman G. Acute ischemic optic neuropathy in severe preeclampsia. Am J Ophthalmol 1980;90:342–346.

Beeson JH, Duda EE. Computed axial tomography scan demonstration of cerebral edema in eclampsia preceded by blindness. Obstet Gynecol 1982;60:529–532.

Belfort MA, Saade GR, Moise K, et al. Nimodipine in the management of preeclampsia: maternal and fetal effects. Am J Obstet Gynecol 1994;171:417–424.

Belfort MA, Saade GR, Moise KJ. The effect of magnesium sulfate on maternal retinal blood flow in preeclampsia: A randomized placebo-controlled study. Am J Obstet Gynecol 1992;167:1548–1553.

Belfort MA, Saade GR, Wasserstrum N, et al. Acute volume expansion with colloid increases oxygen delivery and consumption but does not improve the oxygen extraction in severe preeclampsia. J Maternal-Fetal Med 1995;4:57–64.

Belizan JM, Villar J, Gonzalez L, et al. Calcium supplementation to prevent hypertensive disorders of pregnancy. N Engl J Med 1991;325:1399–1405.

Bell BA. A history of the study of cerebral edema. Neurosurgery 1983;13:724–728.

Benedetti TJ, Carlson RW. Studies of colloid osmotic pressure in pregnancy-induced hypertension. Am J Obstet Gynecol 1979;135:308–317.

Benedetti TJ, Cotton DB, Read JC, Miller FC. Hemodynamic observations in severe preeclampsia with a flow-directed pulmonary artery. Am J Obstet Gynecol 1980a;136:465–470.

Benedetti TJ, Quilligan EJ. Cerebral edema in severe pregnancy-induced hypertension. Am J Obstet Gynecol 1980b;137:860–862.

Benedetti TJ, Kates R, Williams V. Hemodynamic observations in severe preeclampsia complicated by pulmonary edema. Am J Obstet Gynecol 1985;152:330–334.

Benigni A, Gregorini G, Frusca T, et al. Effect of low-dose aspirin on fetal and maternal generation of thromboxane by platelets in women at risk for pregnancy-induced hypertension. N Engl J Med 1989;321(6):357–361.

Berg CJ, Atrash HK, Koonin LM, Tucker M. Pregnancy-related mortality in the United States, 1987–1990. Obstet Gynecol 1996;88:161.

Bis KA, Waxman B. Rupture of the liver associated with pregnancy: a review of the literature and report of two cases. Obstet Gynecol Surv 1976;31:763–773.

Bletka M, Hlavaty V, Trnkova M, et al. Volume of whole blood and absolute amount of serum proteins in the early stage of late toxemia of pregnancy. Am J Obstet Gynecol 1970;106:10–13.

Bohman VR, Cotton DB. Supralethal magnesemia with patient survival. Obstet Gynecol 1990; 76(5):984–985.

Borges LF, Gucer G. Effect of magnesium on epileptic foci. Epilepsia 1978;19:81–91.

Branch DW, Andres R, Digre KB, et al. The association of antiphospholipid antibodies with severe preeclampsia. Obstet Gynecol 1989;73:541–545.

Branch DW, Silver RM, Blackwell JL, et al. Outcome of treated pregnancies in women with antiphospholipid syndrome: an update of the Utah experience. Obstet Gynecol 1992;80:614–620.

Brown CEL, Cunningham FG, Pritchard JA. Convulsions in hypertensive proteinuric primiparas more than 24 hours after delivery: eclampsia or some other course. J Reprod Med 1987;32:449–503.

Brown JCM, Veall N. The maternal placental blood flow in normotensive and hypertensive women. J Obstet Gynaecol Br Emp 1953;60:141–147.

Bryant RD, Fleming JG. Veratrum viride in the treatment of eclampsia: II. JAMA 1940;115:1333–1339.

Bryant RD, Fleming JG. Veratrum viride in the treatment of eclampsia: III. Obstet Gynecol 1962; 19(3):372–383.

Burrows RF, Hunter DJS, Andrew M, Kelton JG. A prospective study investigating the mechanism of thrombocytopenia in preeclampsia. Obstet Gynecol 1987;70:334–338.

Chesley LC, Duffus GM. Preeclampsia, posture, and renal function. Obstet Gynecol 1971;38:1–5.

Chesley LC. Plasma and red cell volumes during pregnancy. Am J Obstet Gynecol 1972;112:440–450.

Chesley LC. A short history of eclampsia. Obstet Gynecol 1974;43:599–602.

Chesley LC, Annitto JE, Cosgrove RA. The remote prognosis of eclamptic women. Am J Obstet Gynecol 1976;124:446–459.

Chesley LC. Remote prognosis. In: Chesley LC, ed. Hypertensive disorders in pregnancy. New York: Appleton-Century-Crofts, 1978:421.

Chesley LC. Parenteral magnesium sulfate and the distribution, plasma levels, and excretion of magnesium. Am J Obstet Gynecol 1979;133:1–7.

Chesley LC. History and epidemiology of preeclampsia-eclampsia. Clin Obstet Gynecol 1984; 27:801–820.

Chesley LC. Diagnosis of preeclampsia. Obstet Gynecol 1985;65:423–425.

Clark SL, Horenstein JM, Phelan JP, et al. Experience with the pulmonary artery catheter in obstetrics and gynecology. Am J Obstet Gynecol 1985;152:374–378.

Clark SL, Divon MY, Phelan JP. Preeclampsia/eclampsia: hemodynamic and neurologic correlations. Obstet Gynecol 1985;66:337–340.

Clark SL, Phelan JP, Allen SH, Golde SH. Antepartum reversal of hematologic abnormalities with the HELLP syndrome. J Reprod Med 1986;31:70–72.

Clark SL, Greenspoon JS, Aldahl D, Phelan JP. Severe preeclampsia with persistent oliguria: management of hemodynamic subsets. Am J Obstet Gynecol 1986;154:490–494.

Clark SL, Cotton DB. Clinical indications for pulmonary artery catheterization in the patient with severe preeclampsia. Am J Obstet Gynecol 1988;158:453–458.

Clark SL, Cotton DB, Lee W, et al. Central hemodynamic observations in normal third trimester pregnancy. Am J Obstet Gynecol 1989;161:1439–1442.

CLASP Collaborative Group. A randomized trial of low-dose aspirin for the prevention and treatment of preeclampsia among 9364 pregnant women. Lancet 1994;343:619–629.

Coevoet B, Leuliet J, Comoy E, et al. Labetalol in the treatment of hypertension of pregnancy: clinical effects and interactions with plasma renin and dopamine betahydroxylase activities, and with plasma concentrations of catecholamine. Kidney Int 1980;17:701.

Conde-Agudelo A, Belizan JM, Lede R, Bergel EF. What does an elevated mean arterial pressure in the second half of pregnancy predict—gestational hypertension or preeclampsia? Am J Obstet Gynecol 1993;169:509–514.

Conde-Agudelo A, Lede R, Belizan J. Evaluation of methods used in the prediction of hypertensive disorders of pregnancy. Obstet Gynecol Surv 1994;49:210–222.

Connell H, Dalgleish JG, Downing JW. General anaesthesia in mothers with severe preeclampsia/eclampsia. Br J Anaesth 1987;59:1375–1380.

Cotton DB, Benedetti TJ. Use of the Swan-Ganz catheter in obstetrics and gynecology. Obstet Gynecol 1980;56:641–645.

Cotton DB, Gonik B, Spillman T, Dorman KF. Intrapartum to postpartum changes in colloid osmotic pressure. Am J Obstet Gynecol 1984a; 149:174–177.

Cotton DB, Gonik B, Dorman KR. Cardiovascular alterations in severe pregnancy-induced hypertension: acute effects of intravenous magnesium sulfate. Am J Obstet Gynecol 1984b; 148:162–165.

Cotton DB, Gonik B, Dorman K, Harrist R. Cardiovascular alterations in severe pregnancy-induced hypertension: relationship of central venous pressure to pulmonary capillary wedge pressure. Am J Obstet Gynecol 1985;151:762–764.

Cotton DB, Jones MM, Longmire S, et al. Role of intravenous nitroglycerin in the treatment of severe pregnancy-induced hypertension complicated by pulmonary edema. Am J Obstet Gynecol 1986a;154:91–93.

Cotton DB, Longmire S, Jones MM, et al. Cardiovascular alterations in severe pregnancy-induced hypertension: effects of intravenous nitroglycerin coupled with blood volume expansion. Am J Obstet Gynecol 1986b;154:1053–1059.

Cotton DB, Lee W, Huhta JC, Dorman KF. Hemodynamic profile of severe pregnancy-induced hypertension. Am J Obstet Gynecol 1988;158:523–529.

Cunningham FG, Gant NF. Management of eclampsia. Semin Perinatol 1994;18:103–113.

Cunningham FG, Pritchard JA. Hematologic considerations of pregnancy-induced hypertension. Semin Perinatol 1978;2:29–38.

Cunningham FG, Lowe T, Guss S, Mason R. Erythrocyte morphology in women with severe preeclampsia and eclampsia. Preliminary observations with scanning electron microscopy. Am J Obstet Gynecol 1985;153:358–363.

Cunningham FG, Fernandez CO, Hernandez C. Blindness associated with preeclampsia and eclampsia. Am J Obstet Gynecol 1995;172:1291–1298.

Dadek C, Kefalides A, Sinzinger H, Weber G. Reduced umbilical artery prostacyclin formation in complicated pregnancies. Am J Obstet Gynecol 1982;144:792–795.

Dekker GA, Sibai BM. Low-dose aspirin in the prevention of preeclampsia and fetal growth retardation: rationale, mechanisms, and clinical trials. Am J Obstet Gynecol 1993;168:214–227.

Dieckmann WJ, Michel HL. Vascular-renal effects of posterior pituitary extracts in pregnant women. Am J Obstet Gynecol 1937;33:131–137.

Dildy GA, Cotton DB. Hemodynamic changes in pregnancy and pregnancy complicated by hypertension. Acute Care 1988;89:14–15, 26–46.

Dildy GA, Cotton DB. Management of severe preeclampsia and eclampsia. Crit Care Clin 1991; 7:829–850.

Dixon HG, Brown JCM, Davey DA. Choriodecidual and myometrial blood flow. Lancet 1963;ii: 369–373.

Donaldson JO. The case against magnesium sulfate for eclamptic convulsions. Int J Obstet Anesth 1992;1:159–166.

Dorsett L. The intramuscular injection of magnesium sulphate for the control of convulsions in eclampsia. Am J Obstet Gynecol 1926;11:227–231.

Douglas KA, Redman CWG. Eclampsia in the United Kingdom. Br Med J 1994;309:1395–1399.

Downing I, Shepherd GI, Lewis PJ. Kinetics of prostacyclin synthetase in umbilical artery microsomes from normal and preeclamptic pregnancies. Br J Clin Pharmacol 1982;13:195–198.

Duley L, Johanson R. Magnesium sulphate for preeclampsia and eclampsia: the evidence so far. Br J Obstet Gynaecol 1994;101:565–567.

Dunn R, Lee W, Cotton DB. Evaluation by computerized axial tomography of eclamptic women with seizures refractory to magnesium sulfate therapy. Am J Obstet Gynecol 1986;155:267–268.

Easterling TR, Benedetti TJ. Preeclampsia: a hyperdynamic disease model. Am J Obstet Gynecol 1989;160:1447–1453.

Eastman NJ, Steptoe PP. The management of preeclampsia. Can Med Assoc J 1945;52:562–568.

Eclampsia Trial Collaborative Group. Which anticonvulsant for women with eclampsia? Evidence from the Collaborative Eclampsia Trial. Lancet 1995;345:1455–1463.

Entman SS, Kambam JR, Bradley CA, Cousar JB. Increased levels of carboxyhemoglobin and serum iron as an indicator of increased red cell turnover in preeclampsia. Am J Obstet Gynecol 1987;156:1169–1173.

Eskenazi B, Fenster L, Sidney S, Elkin EP. Fetal growth retardation in infants of multiparous and nulliparous women with preeclampsia. Am J Obstet Gynecol 1993;169:1112–1118.

Fein A, Grossman RF, Jones JG, et al. The value of edema fluid protein measurement in patients with pulmonary edema. Am J Med 1979;67:32–38.

Feliciano DV, Mattox KL, Jordan GL, et al. Management of 1,000 consecutive cases of hepatic trauma (1979–1984). Ann Surg 1986;204:438–445.

Fenakel K, Fenakel G, Appleman ZVI, et al. Nifedipine in the treatment of severe preeclampsia. Obstet Gynecol 1991;77:331–336.

Ferris TF, Weir EK. Effect of captopril on uterine blood flow and prostaglandin E synthesis in the pregnant rabbit. J Clin Invest 1983;71:809–815.

Fisher KA, Luger A, Spargo BH, Lindheimer MD. Hypertension in pregnancy: Clinical-pathological correlations and remote prognosis. Medicine 1981;60:267–276.

Friedman SA. Preeclampsia: a review of the role of prostaglandins. Obstet Gynecol 1988;71:122–137.

Friedman SA, de Groot CJM, Taylor RN, et al. Plasma cellular fibronectin as a measure of endothelial involvement in preeclampsia and intrauterine growth retardation. Am J Obstet Gynecol 1994;170:838–841.

Gallery EDM, Hunyor SN, Gyory AZ. Plasma volume contraction: a significant factor in both pregnancy-associated hypertension (preeclampsia) and chronic hypertension in pregnancy. Q J Med 1979;48:593–602.

Gallery ED, Ross M, Gyory AZ. Urinary red blood cell and cast excretion in normal and hypertensive human pregnancy. Am J Obstet Gynecol 1993;168:67–70.

Gant NF, Daley GL, Chand S, et al. A study of angiotensin II pressor response throughout primigravid pregnancy. J Clin Invest 1973;52:2682–2689.

Gardner WJ, Storer J. The use of the G suit in control of intra-abdominal bleeding. Surg Gynecol 1966;123:792–798.

Gibson B, Hunter D, Neame PB, Kelton JG. Thrombocytopenia in preeclampsia and eclampsia. Semin Thromb Hemost 1982;8:234–247.

Gonik B, Cotton DB. Peripartum colloid osmotic pressure changes: influence of intravenous hydration. Am J Obstet Gynecol 1984;150:90–100.

Goodlin RC. Preeclampsia as the great imposter. Am J Obstet Gynecol 1991;164:1577–1581.

Goodlin RC, Mostello D. Maternal hyponatremia and the syndrome of hemolysis, elevated liver enzymes, and low platelet count. Am J Obstet Gynecol 1987;156:910–911.

Goodlin RC, Anderson JC, Hodgson PE. Conservative treatment of liver hematoma in the postpartum period. A report of two cases. J Reprod Med 1985;30:368–370.

Goodlin RC. Severe preeclampsia: another great imitator. Am J Obstet Gynecol 1976;125:747–753.

Govan ADT. The pathogenesis of eclamptic lesions. Pathol Microbiol (Basel) 1961;24:561–575.

Graham C, Goldstein A. Epidural analgesia and cardiac output in severe preeclamptics. Anaesthesia 1980;35:709–712.

Greenstein D, Henderson JM, Boyer TD. Liver hemorrhage: recurrent episodes during pregnancy complicated by preeclampsia. Gastroenterology 1994;106:1668–1671.

Grimes DA. The morbidity and mortality of pregnancy: still risky business. Am J Obstet Gynecol 1994;170:1489–1494.

Groenendijk R, Trimbos JBMJ, Wallenburg HCS. Hemodynamic measurements in preeclampsia: preliminary observations. Am J Obstet Gynecol 1984;150:232–236.

Grunfeld JP, Pertuiset N. Acute renal failure in pregnancy. Am J Kidney Dis 1987;9:359–362.

Gutsche B. The experts opine: is epidural block for labor and delivery and for cesarean section a safe form of analgesia in severe preeclampsia or eclampsia? Surv Anesth 1986;30:304–311.

Hankins GDV, Wendell GD, Cunningham FG, Leveno KJ. Longitudinal evaluation of hemodynamic changes in eclampsia. Am J Obstet Gynecol 1984;150:506–512.

Hanssens M, Keirse MJ, Vankelecom F, Van Assche FA. Fetal and neonatal effects of treatment with angiotensin-converting enzyme inhibitors in pregnancy. Obstet Gynecol 1991;78:128–135.

Harbert GM, Claiborne HA, McGaughey HS, et al. Convulsive toxemia. Am J Obstet Gynecol 1968;100:336–342.

Hauth JC, Goldenberg RL, Parker R, et al. Low-dose aspirin therapy to prevent preeclampsia. Am J Obstet Gynecol 1993;168:1083–1093.

Hays PM, Cruikshank DP, Dunn LJ. Plasma volume determination in normal and preeclamptic pregnancies. Am J Obstet Gynecol 1985;151:958–966.

Henderson DW, Vilos GA, Milne KJ, Nichol PM. The role of Swan-Ganz catheterization in severe pregnancy-induced hypertension. Am J Obstet Gynecol 1984;148:570–574.

Henny CP, Lim AE, Brummelkamp WH, et al. A review of the importance of acute multidisciplinary treatment following spontaneous rupture of the liver capsule during pregnancy. Surg Gynecol Obstet 1983;156:593–598.

Herbert WNP, Brenner WE. Improving survival with liver rupture complicating pregnancy. Am J Obstet Gynecol 1982;142:530–534.

Herling IM. Intravenous nitroglycerin: clinical pharmacology and therapeutic considerations. Am Heart J 1984;108:141–149.

Heyborne KD, Burke MS, Porreco RP. Prolongation of premature gestation in women with hemolysis, elevated liver enzymes and low platelets: a report of five cases. J Reprod Med 1990; 35(1):53–57.

Hill JA, Devoe LD, Elgammal TA. Central hemodynamic findings associated with cortical blindness in severe preeclampsia. A case report. J Reprod Med 1985;30:435–438.

Hodgkinson R, Husain FJ, Hayashi RH. Systemic and pulmonary blood pressure during cesarean section in parturients with gestational hypertension. Can Anaesth Soc J 1980;27:389–394.

Hurault de Ligny B, Ryckelynck JP, Mintz P, et al. Captopril therapy in preeclampsia. Nephron 1987;46:329–330.

Hurd WW, Miodovnik M, Herzberg V, Lavin JP. Selective management of abruptio placentae: a prospective study. Obstet Gynecol 1983;61:467–473.

Hutt R, Ogunniyi SO, Sullivan MHF, Elder MG. Increased platelet volume and aggregation precede the onset of preeclampsia. Obstet Gynecol 1994;83:146–149.

Hutton JD, James DK, Stirrat GM, et al. Management of severe preeclampsia and eclampsia by UK consultants. Br J Obstet Gynaecol 1992; 99:554–556.

Imperiale TF, Petrulis AS. A meta-analysis of low-dose aspirin for the prevention of pregnancy-induced hypertensive disease. JAMA 1991;266: 261–265.

Jones MM, Longmire S, Cotton DB, et al. Influence of crystalloid versus colloid infusion on peripartum colloid osmotic pressure changes. Obstet Gynecol 1986;68:659–661.

Jouppila P, Jouppila R, Hollman A, Koivula A. Lumbar epidural analgesia to improve intervillous blood flow during labor in severe preeclampsia. Obstet Gynecol 1982;59:158–161.

Jouppila P, Kirkinen P, Koivula A, Ylikorkala O. Effects of dihydralazine infusion on the fetoplacental blood flow and maternal prostanoids. Obstet Gynecol 1985;65:115–118.

Joyce TH, Debnath KS, Baker EA. Preeclampsia—relationship of central venous pressure and epidural anesthesia. Anesthesiology 1979;51:S297.

Kaunitz AM, Hughes JM, Grimes DA, et al. Causes of maternal mortality in the United States. Obstet Gynecol 1985;65:605–612.

Killam AP, Dillard SH, Patton RC, Pederson PR. Pregnancy-induced hypertension complicated by acute liver disease and disseminated intravascular coagulation. Am J Obstet Gynecol 1975;123:823–828.

Kinsella CB, Milner M, McCarthy N, Walshe J. Sixth nerve palsy: an unusual manifestation of preeclampsia. Obstet Gynecol 1994;83:849–851.

Kirby JC, Jaindl JJ. Cerebral CT findings in toxemia of pregnancy. Radiology 1984;154:114.

Kirshon B, Lee W, Mauer MB, Cotton DB. Effects of low-dose dopamine therapy in the oliguric patient with preeclampsia. Am J Obstet Gynecol 1988a;159:604–607.

Kirshon A, Moise KJ Jr, Cotton DB, et al. Role of volume expansion in severe preeclampsia. Surg Gynecol Obstet 1988b;167:367–371.

Kirshon B, Cotton DB. Invasive hemodynamic monitoring in the obstetric patient. Clin Obstet Gynecol 1987;30:579–590.

Klechner HB, Giles HR, Corrigan JJ. The association of maternal and neonatal thrombocytopenia in high risk pregnancies. Am J Obstet Gynecol 1977;128:235–238.

Koch-Weser J. Hydralazine. N Engl J Med 1976; 295:320–323.

Koontz WLL, Reid KH. Effect of parenteral magnesium sulfate on penicillin-induced seizure in foci in anesthetized cats. Am J Obstet Gynecol 1985;153:96–99.

Krane NK. Acute renal failure in pregnancy. Arch Intern Med 1988;148:2347–2357.

Kupferminc MJ, Peaceman AM, Wigton TR, et al. Tumor necrosis factor-α is elevated in plasma and amniotic fluid of patients with severe preeclampsia. Am J Obstet Gynecol 1994;170:1752–1759.

Kuzniar J, Skret A, Piela A, et al. Hemodynamic effects of intravenous hydralazine in pregnant women with severe hypertension. Obstet Gynecol 1985;66:453–458.

Lamming GD, Symonds EM. Use of labetalol and methyldopa in pregnancy-induced hypertension. Br J Clin Pharmacol 1979;8:217S-222S.

Lazard EM. An analysis of 575 cases of eclamptic and pre-eclamptic toxemias treated by intravenous injections of magnesium sulphate. Am J Obstet Gynecol 1933;26:647–656.

Leduc L, Lederer E, Lee W, Cotton DB. Urinary sediment changes in severe preeclampsia. Obstet Gynecol 1991;77:186–189.

Lee W, Gonik B, Cotton DB. Urinary diagnostic indices in preeclampsia-associated oligura: correlation with invasive hemodynamic monitoring. Am J Obstet Gynecol 1987;156:100–103.

Lees MM. Central circulatory response to normotensive and hypertensive pregnancy. Postgrad Med J 1979;55:311–314.

Lewis PJ, Shepherd GI, Ritter J. Prostacyclin and preeclampsia. Lancet 1981;1:559.

Liedholm H, Wahlin-Boll E, Hanson A, et al. Transplacental passage and breast milk concentrations of hydralazine. Eur J Clin Pharmacol 1982;21:417–419.

Lin CC, Lindheimer MD, River P, Moawad AH. Fetal outcome in hypertensive disorders of pregnancy. Am J Obstet Gynecol 1982;142:255–260.

Lindheimer MD, Katz AI. Current concepts. Hypertension in pregnancy. N Engl J Med 1985; 313:675–680.

Lopez-Llera M. Complicated eclampsia—fifteen years experience in a referral medical center. Am J Obstet Gynecol 1982;142:28–35.

Lubarsky SL, Barton JR, Friedman SA, et al. Late postpartum eclampsia revisited. Obstet Gynecol 1994;83:502–505.

Lubbe WF. Hypertension in pregnancy: whom and how to treat. Br J Clin Pharmacol 1987;24:15S–20S.

Lucas CE, Ledgerwood AM. Prospective evaluation of hemostatic techniques for liver injuries. J Trauma 1976;16:442.

Lucas MJ, Leveno KJ, Cunningham FG. A comparison of magnesium sulfate with phenytoin for the prevention of eclampsia. N Engl J Med 1995;333:201–205.

Lucas MJ, DePalma RT, Peters MT, et al. A simplified phenytoin regimen for preeclampsia. Am J Perinatol 1994;11:153–156.

Lund-Johansen P. The haemodynamic pattern in mild and borderline hypertension. Acta Med Scand [Suppl] 1983;686:15.

Lund-Johnson P. Short- and long-term (six year) hemodynamic effects of labetalol in essential hypertension. Am J Med 1983;75:24–31.

Lunell NO, Hjemdahl P, Fredholm BB, et al. Circulatory and metabolic effects of a combined and β-adrenoceptor blocker (labetalol) in hypertension of pregnancy. Br J Clin Pharmacol 1981; 12:345–348.

Lunell NO, Lewander R, Mamoun I, et al. Uteroplacental blood flow in pregnancy-induced hypertension. Scand J Clin Lab Invest [Suppl] 1984;169:28–35.

Lunell NO, Nylung LE, Lewander R, Sabey B. Uteroplacental blood flow in preeclampsia measurements with indium-113m and a computer-linked gamma camera. Clin Exp Hypertens 1982;B1:105–107.

Mabie WC, Gonzalez AR, Sibai BM, Amon E. A comparative trial of labetalol and hydralazine in the acute management of severe hypertension complicating pregnancy. Obstet Gynecol 1987;70: 328–333.

Mabie WC, Ratts TE, Sibai BM. The central hemodynamics of severe preeclampsia. Am J Obstet Gynecol 1989;161:1443–1448.

MacKenna J, Dover NL, Brame RG. Preeclampsia associated with hemolysis, elevated liver enzymes, and low platelets—an obstetric emergency? Obstet Gynecol 1983;62:751–754.

Martin JN, Blake PG, Perry KG, et al. The natural history of HELLP syndrome: patterns of disease progression and regression. Am J Obstet Gynecol 1991;164:1500–1513.

Massé J, Forest JC, Moutquin JM, et al. A prospective study of several potential biologic markers for early prediction of the development of preeclampsia. Am J Obstet Gynecol 1993;169:501–508.

Massobrio M, Benedetto C, Bertini E, et al. Immune complexes in preeclampsia and normal pregnancy. Am J Obstet Gynecol 1985;152:578–583.

Messer RH. Symposium on bleeding disorders in pregnancy: observations on bleeding in pregnancy. Am J Obstet Gynecol 1987;156:1419–1420.

Meyer NL, Mercer BM, Friedman SA, Sibai BM. Urinary dipstick protein: a poor predictor of absent or severe proteinuria. Am J Obstet Gynecol 1994;170:137–141.

Michael CA. Use of labetalol in the treatment of severe hypertension during pregnancy. Br J Clin Pharmacol 1979;8:211S–215S.

Michael CA. The evaluation of labetalol in the treatment of hypertension complicating pregnancy. Br J Clin Pharmacol 1982;13:127S–131S.

Mikhail MS, Anyaegbunam A, Garfinkel D, et al. Preeclampsia and antioxidant nutrients: decreased plasma levels of reduced ascorbic acid, α-tocopherol, and beta-carotene in women with preeclampsia. Am J Obstet Gynecol 1994;171:150–157.

Miller JD. The management of cerebral edema. Br J Hosp Med 1979;21:152–165.

Mitchell SE, Clark RA. Complications of central venous catheterization. AJB 1979;133:467–476.

Morgan MA, Silavin SL, Dormer KJ, et al. Effects of labetalol on uterine blood flow and cardiovascular hemodynamics in the hypertensive gravid baboon. Am J Obstet Gynecol 1993;168:1574–1579.

Morris RH, Vassalli P, Beller PK, McCluskey RT. Immunofluorescent studies of renal biopsies in the diagnosis of toxemia of pregnancy. Obstet Gynecol 1964;24:32–46.

Mroczek WJ, Lee WR, Davidov ME. Effect of magnesium sulfate on cardiovascular hemodynamics. Angiology 1977;28:720–724.

Naden RP, Redman CWG. Antihypertensive drugs in pregnancy. Clin Perinatol 1985;12:521–538.

National High Blood Pressure Education Program Working Group report on high blood pressure in pregnancy. Am J Obstet Gynecol 1990;163: 1689–1712.

Neiger R, Contag SA, Coustan DR. The resolution of preeclampsia-related thrombocytopenia. Obstet Gynecol 1991;77(5):692–695.

Newsome LR, Bramwell RS, Curling PE. Severe preeclampsia: hemodynamic effects of lumbar epidural anesthesia. Anesth Analg 1986;65:31–36.

Oates JA, Wood AJJ. Converting-enzyme inhibitors in the treatment of hypertension. N Engl J Med 1988;319:1517–1525.

Odendaal HJ, Pattinson RC, Bam R, et al. Aggressive or expectant management for patients with severe preeclampsia between 28–34 weeks' gestation: a randomized controlled trial. Obstet Gynecol 1990;76:1070–1074.

Oosterhof H, Voorhoeve PG, Aarnoudse JG. Enhancement of hepatic artery resistance to blood flow in preeclampsia in presence or absence of HELLP syndrome (hemolysis, elevated liver enzymes, and low platelets). Am J Obstet Gynecol 1994;171:526–530.

Pasch T, Schulz V, Hoppelshauser G. Nitroprusside-induced formation of cyanide and its detoxification with thiosulfate during deliberate hypotension. J Cardiovasc Pharmacol 1983;5:77–85.

Phelan JP, Yurth DA. Severe preeclampsia. I. Peripartum hemodynamic observations. Am J Obstet Gynecol 1982;144:17–22.

Pickles CJ, Symonds EM, Pipkin FB. The fetal outcome in a randomized double-blind controlled trial of labetalol versus placebo in pregnancy-induced hypertension. Br J Obstet Gynaecol 1989;96:38–43.

Pritchard JA. The use of magnesium sulfate in preeclampsia-eclampsia. J Reprod Med 1979; 23:107–114.

Pritchard JA. The use of magnesium iron in the management of eclamptogenic toxemias. Surg Gynecol Obstet 1955;100:131–140.

Pritchard JA, Cunningham FG, Mason RA. Coagulation changes in preeclampsia: their frequency and pathogenesis. Am J Obstet Gynecol 1976; 124:855–864.

Pritchard JA, MacDonald PC, Grant NF. Williams obstetrics. 17th ed. Norwalk, CT: Appleton-Century-Crofts, 1985:525.

Pritchard JA, Pritchard SA. Standardized treatment of 154 consecutive cases of eclampsia. Am J Obstet 1975;123:543–552.

Pritchard JA, Weisman R, Ratnoff OD, Vosburgh GJ. Intravascular hemolysis, thrombocytopenia, and other hematologic abnormalities associated with severe toxemia of pregnancy. N Engl J Med 1954;150:89–98.

Pritchard JA, Cunningham FG, Pritchard SA, Mason RA. How often does maternal preeclampsia-eclampsia incite thrombocytopenia in the fetus? Obstet Gynecol 1987;69:292–295.

Pritchard JA, Cunningham FG, Pritchard SA. The Parkland Memorial Hospital protocol for the treatment of eclampsia: evaluation of 245 cases. Am J Obstet Gynecol 1984;148:951–963.

Pruett KM, Krishon B, Cotton DB, et al. The effects of magnesium sulfate therapy on Apgar scores. Am J Obstet Gynecol 1988;159:1047–1048.

Rademaker L. Spontaneous rupture of liver complicating pregnancy. Ann Surg 1943;118:396–401.

Rafferty TD, Berkowitz RL. Hemodynamics in patients with severe toxemia during labor and delivery. Am J Obstet Gynecol 1980;138:263–270.

Ramos-Santos E, Devoe LD, Wakefield ML, Sherline DM, Metheny WP. The effects of epidural anesthesia on the Doppler velocimetry of umbilical and uterine arteries in normal and hypertensive patients during active term labor. Obstet Gynecol 1991;77(1): 20–26.

Redman CWG, Beilin LJ, Bonner J. Renal function in preeclampsia. J Clin Pathol 1976;10:94–96.

Redman CWG. Immunologic factors in the pathogenesis of preeclampsia. Contrib Nephrol 1981;25:120.

Repke JT, Friedman SA, Kaplan PW. Prophylaxis of eclamptic seizures: current controversies. Clin Obstet Gynecol 1992;35:365–374.

Riley AJ. Clinical pharmacology of labetalol in pregnancy. J Cardiovasc Pharmacol 1981;3:S53–S59.

Robillard P, Hulsey TC, Perianin J, et al. Association of pregnancy-induced hypertension with duration of sexual cohabitation before conception. Lancet 1994;344:973–975.

Rodgers GM, Taylor RN, Roberts JM. Preeclampsia is associated with a serum factor cytotoxic to human endothelial cells. Am J Obstet Gynecol 1988;159:908–914.

Romero R, Mazor M, Lockwood CJ, et al. Clinical significance, prevalence, and natural history of thrombocytopenia in pregnancy-induced hypertension. Am J Perinatol 1989;6:32–38.

Romero R, Vizoso J, Emamian M, et al. Clinical significance of liver dysfunction in pregnancy-induced hypertension. Am J Perinatol 1988a; 5:146–151.

Romero R, Lockwood C, Oyarzun E, Hobbins JC. Toxemia: new concepts in an old disease. Semin Perinatol 1988b;12:302–323.

Rote NS, Caudle MR. Circulating immune complexes in pregnancy, preeclampsia, and auto-immune diseases: evaluation of Raji cell enzyme-linked immunosorbent assay and polyethylene glycol precipitation methods. Am J Obstet Gynecol 1983;147:267–273.

Rubin AA, Roth FE, Taylor RM, Rosenkilde H. Pharmacology of diazoxide, an antihypertensive, non-diuretic benzothiadiazine. J Pharmacol Exp Ther 1962;136:344–352.

Saftlas AF, Olson DR, Franks AL, Atrash HK, Pokras R. Epidemiology of preeclampsia and eclampsia in the United States, 1979–1986. Am J Obstet Gynecol 1990;163(2):460–465.

Sakala EP, Moore WD. Successful term delivery after previous pregnancy with ruptured liver. Obstet Gynecol 1986;68:124–126.

Sanchez-Ramos L, Briones DK, Kaunitz AM, et al. Prevention of pregnancy-induced hypertension by calcium supplementation in angiotensin II-sensitive patients. Obstet Gynecol 1994;84:349–353.

Savelieva GM, Efimov VS, Grishin VL, et al. Blood coagulation changes in pregnant women at risk of developing preeclampsia. Int J Gynecol Obstet 1995;48:3–8.

Schubiger G, Flury G, Nussberger J. Enalapril for pregnancy-induced hypertension: acute renal failure in a neonate. Ann Intern Med 1988;108:215–216.

Schwartz ML, Brenner W. Severe preeclampsia with persistent postpartum hemolysis and thrombocytopenia treated by plasmapheresis. Obstet Gynecol 1985;65:53S–55S.

Seidman DS, Serr DM, Ben-Rafael Z. Renal and ocular manifestations of hypertensive diseases of pregnancy. Obstet Gynecol Surv 1991;46:71–76.

Sheehan HL. Pathological lesions in the hypertensive toxemias of pregnancy. In: Hammond J, Browne FJ, Walstenholme GEW, eds. Toxemias of pregnancy, human and veterinary. Philadelphia: Blakiston, 1950:16–22.

Shelley WC, Gutsche BB. Magnesium and seizure control. Am J Obstet Gynecol 1980;136:146–147.

Shukla PK, Sharma D, Mandal RK. Serum lactate dehydrogenase in detecting liver damage associated with preeclampsia. Br J Obstet Gynecol 1978;85:40–42.

Sibai BM. Treatment of hypertension in pregnant women. N Engl J Med 1996;335:257.

Sibai BM, Schneider JM, Morrison JC, et al. The late postpartum eclampsia controversy. Obstet Gynecol 1980;55:74–78.

Sibai BM, Graham JM, McCubbin JH. A comparison of intravenous and intramuscular magnesium sulfate regimens in preeclampsia. Am J Obstet Gynecol 1984a;150:728–733.

Sibai BM, Spinnato JA, Watson DL, et al. Effect of magnesium sulfate on electroencephalographic findings in preeclampsia-eclampsia. Obstet Gynecol 1984b;64:261–266.

Sibai BM, Spinnato JA, Watson DL, et al. Pregnancy outcome in 303 cases with severe preeclampsia. Obstet Gynecol 1984c;64:319–325.

Sibai BM, Sarinoglu C, Mercer BM. Pregnancy outcome after eclampsia and long term prognosis. Am J Obstet Gynecol 1992;166:1757.

Sibai BM, Spinnato JA, Watson DL, et al. Eclampsia. IV. Neurological findings and future outcome. Am J Obstet Gynecol 1985a;152:184–192.

Sibai BM, Saslimi M, Abdella TN, et al. Maternal and perinatal outcome of conservative management of severe preeclampsia in midtrimester. Am J Obstet Gynecol 1985b;152:32–37.

Sibai BM, Abdella TN, Spinnato JA, et al. Eclampsia. V. The incidence of non-preventable eclampsia. Am J Obstet Gynecol 1986a;154:561–566.

Sibai BM, El-Nazer A, Gonzalez-Ruiz A. Severe preeclampsia-eclampsia in young primigravid women: subsequent pregnancy outcome and remote prognosis. Am J Obstet Gynecol 1986b;155:1011–1016.

Sibai BM, Taslimi MM, El-Nazer A, et al. Maternal-perinatal outcome associated with the syndrome of hemolysis, elevated liver enzymes, and low platelets in severe preeclampsia-eclampsia. Am J Obstet Gynecol 1986c;155:501–509.

Sibai BM, Mabie BC, Harvey CJ, Gonzalez AR. Pulmonary edema in severe preeclampsia-eclampsia: analysis of thirty-seven consecutive cases. Am J Obstet Gynecol 1987;156:1174–1179.

Sibai BM. Pitfalls in diagnosis and management of preeclampsia. Am J Obstet Gynecol 1988;159: 1–5.

Sibai BM, Mercer B, Sarinoglu C. Severe preeclampsia in the second trimester: recurrence risk and long-term prognosis. Am J Obstet Gynecol 1991;165:1408–1412.

Sibai BM, Ramadan MK. Acute renal failure in pregnancies complicated by hemolysis, elevated liver enzymes, and low platelets. Am J Obstet Gynecol 1993a;168:1682–1690.

Sibai BM, Ramadan MK, Usta I, et al. Maternal morbidity and mortality in 442 pregnancies with hemolysis, elevated liver enzymes, and low platelets (HELLP syndrome). Am J Obstet Gynecol 1993b;169:1000–1006.

Sibai BM, Caritis SN, Thom E, et al. Prevention of preeclampsia with low-dose aspirin in healthy, nulliparous pregnant women. N Engl J Med 1993c;329:1213–1218.

Sibai BM, Mercer BM, Schiff E, Friedman SA. Aggressive versus expectant management of severe preeclampsia at 28 to 32 weeks' gestation: a randomized controlled trial. Am J Obstet Gynecol 1994;171:818–822.

Sibai BM, Ramadan MK, Chari RS, Friedman SA. Pregnancies complicated by HELLP syndrome (hemolysis, elevated liver enzymes, and low platelets): subsequent pregnancy outcome and long-term prognosis. Am J Obstet Gynecol 1995; 172:125–129.

Smith LG, Moise KJ, Dildy GA, Carpenter RJ. Spontaneous rupture of liver during pregnancy: current therapy. Obstet Gynecol 1991;77(2):171–175.

Sorensen JD, Olsen SF, Pedersen AK, et al. Effects of fish oil supplementation in the third trimester of pregnancy on prostacyclin and thromboxane production. Am J Obstet Gynecol 1993; 168:915–922.

Spinnato JA, Sibai BM, Anderson GD. Fetal distress after hydralazine therapy for severe pregnancy-induced hypertension. South Med J 1986; 79:559–562.

Stone JL, Lockwood CJ, Berkowitz GS, et al. Risk factors for severe preeclampsia. Obstet Gynecol 1994;83:357–361.

Strauss RG, Keefer JR, Burke T, Civetta JM. Hemodynamic monitoring of cardiogenic pulmonary edema complicating toxemia of pregnancy. Obstet Gynecol 1980;55:170–174.

Sullivan CA, Magann EF, Perry KG, et al. The recurrence risk of the syndrome of hemolysis, elevated liver enzymes, and low platelets (HELLP) in subsequent gestations. Am J Obstet Gynecol 1994;171:940–943.

Swan HJC, Ganz W, Forrester JS, et al. Catheterization of the heart in man with the use of flow-directed balloon-tipped catheter. N Engl J Med 1970;283:447–451.

Thein T, Koene RAP, Schijf C, Peters GFFM, et al. Infusion of diazoxide in severe hypertension during pregnancy. Europ J Obstet Gynec Reprod Biol 1980;10(6):367–374.

Thiagarajah S, Bourgeois FJ, Harbert GM, Caudle MR. Thrombocytopenia in preeclampsia: associated abnormalities and management principles. Am J Obstet Gynecol 1984;150:1–7.

Van Dam PA, Reiner M, Baekelandt M, et al. Disseminated intravascular coagulation and the syndrome of hemolysis, elevated liver enzymes, and low platelets in severe preeclampsia. Obstet Gynecol 1989;73:97–102.

Vardi J, Fields GA. Microangiopathic hemolytic anemia in severe preeclampsia. Am J Obstet Gynecol 1974;119:617–622.

Villar MA, Sibai BM. Clinical significance of elevated mean arterial blood pressure in second trimester and threshold increase in systolic or diastolic blood pressure during third trimester. Am J Obstet Gynecol 1989;160:419.

Waisman GD, Mayorga LM, Camera MI, et al. Magnesium plus nifedipine: potentiation of hypotensive effect in preeclampsia? Am J Obstet Gynecol 1988;159:308–309.

Ward K, Hata A, Jeunemaitre X, Helin C, et al. A molecular variant of angiotensinogen associated with preeclampsia. Nature Genetics 1993;4:59–61.

Wasserstrum N, Cotton DB. Hemodynamic monitoring in severe pregnancy-induced hypertension. Clin Perinatol 1986;13:781–799.

Wasserstrum N, Kirshon B, Willis RS, et al. Quantitive hemodynamic effects of acute volume expansion in severe preeclampsia. Obstet Gynecol 1989;73:546–550.

Weil MN, Henning RJ, Puri VK. Colloid osmotic pressure: clinical significance. Crit Care Med 1979; 7:113–116.

Weiner CP, Kwaan HC, Xu C, et al. Antithrombin III activity in women with hypertension during pregnancies. Obstet Gynecol 1985;65:301–306.

Weinstein L. Preeclampsia/eclampsia with hemolysis, elevated liver enzymes, and thrombocytopenia. Obstet Gynecol 1985;66:657–660.

Weinstein L. Syndrome of hemolysis, elevated liver enzymes, and low platelet count: a severe consequence of hypertension in pregnancy. Am J Obstet Gynecol 1982;142:159–167.

Weiss MH. Cerebral edema. Acute Care 1985;11:187–204.

Whalley PJ, Everett RB, Gant NF, et al. Pressor responsiveness to angiotensin II in hospitalized primigravid women with pregnancy-induced hypertension. Am J Obstet Gynecol 1983;145:481–483.

Wheeler TC, Graves CR, Troianon H, Reed GW. Base deficit and oxygen transport in severe preeclampsia. Obstet Gynecol 1996;87:375.

Worley RJ. Pathophysiology of pregnancy-induced hypertension. Clin Obstet Gynecol 1984;27:821–823.

Young BK, Weinstein HM. Effects of magnesium sulfate on toxemic patients in labor. Obstet Gynecol 1977;49:681–685.

Zimmerman JL. Hypertensive crisis: emergencies and urgencies. In: Ayers SM, ed. Textbook of critical care. Philadelphia: WB Saunders, 1995.

Zuspan FP. Treatment of severe preeclampsia and eclampsia. Clin Obstet Gynecol 1966;9:945–972.

Zuspan FP. Problems encountered in the treatment of pregnancy-induced hypertension. Am J Obstet Gynecol 1978;131:591–597.

# CHAPTER 15

# Cardiac Disease

*P*regnancy brings about many significant alterations in the maternal cardiovascular system. The pregnant patient with normal cardiac function accommodates these physiologic changes without difficulty. In the presence of significant cardiac disease, however, pregnancy may be extremely hazardous, resulting in decompensation and even death. Despite advances in the diagnosis and treatment of maternal cardiovascular disease, such conditions continue to account for up to 10% to 25% of maternal mortality (Koonin, 1991; DeSwiet, 1993; Hogberg, 1994; Berg, 1996; Varner, 1997). This chapter focuses on the interaction between cardiac disease and pregnancy.

## Counseling the Pregnant Cardiac Patient

Prior to 1973, the Criteria Committee of the New York Heart Association (NYHA) recommended a classification of cardiac disease based on clinical function (classes I–IV). Such a classification is useful in discussing the pregnant cardiac patient, although even patients who begin pregnancy as functional class I may develop congestive heart failure and pulmonary edema during the course of gestation. Although this functional classification has been replaced by a more complex descriptive system encompassing etiologic, anatomic, and physiologic diagnoses, the functional classification remains most useful when comparing the performance of individuals with relatively uniform etiologic and anatomic defects. In general, women who begin pregnancy as functional class I or II have improved outcome compared with those in classes III and IV (Hsieh, 1993).

Counseling the pregnant cardiac patient regarding her prognosis for successful pregnancy is further complicated by recent advances in medical and surgical therapy, fetal surveillance, and neonatal care. Such advances render invalid many older estimates of maternal mortality and fetal wastage. Table 15-1 represents a synthesis of maternal risk estimates for various types of cardiac disease that was initially developed for the first edition of this text in 1987. Counseling of the pregnant cardiac patient, as well as general management approaches, were based on this classification (Clark, 1987). Category I included conditions that, with proper management, were associated with negligible maternal mortality ( < 1%). Cardiac lesions in category II traditionally carried a 5% to 15% risk of maternal mortality. Patients with cardiac lesions in group III were, and probably remain, subject to a mortality risk exceeding 25%. In all but exceptional cases, this risk is unacceptable, and prevention or interruption of pregnancy is generally recommended.

Although this classification has proven useful in predicting mortality risk in the past, a review of more recent data from the United States and Europe suggests the need to revise these estimates. Currently available data suggest that today maternal mortality is almost exclusively seen

T A B L E   **15-1**

**Maternal risk associated with pregnancy**

*Group I: Minimal Risk of Complications*
Atrial septal defect*
Ventricular septal defect*
Patent ductus arteriosus*
Pulmonic/tricuspid disease
Corrected tetralogy of Fallot
Bioprosthetic valve
Mitral stenosis, New York Heart Association
    (NYHA) classes I and II
Marfan syndrome with normal aorta

*Group II: Moderate Risk of Complications*
Mitral stenosis with atrial fibrillation*
Artificial valve*
Mitral stenosis, NYHA classes III and IV
Aortic stenosis
Coarctation of aorta, uncomplicated
Uncorrected tetralogy of Fallot
Previous myocardial infarction

*Group III: Major Risk of Complications
    or Death*
Pulmonary hypertension
Coarctation of aorta, complicated
Marfan syndrome with aortic involvement

*If anticoagulation with heparin, rather than coumadin, is
    elected.

in patients with pulmonary hypertension, endocarditis, coronary artery disease, cardiomyopathy, and sudden arrhythmia. DeSwiet, reporting on maternal mortality from heart disease in the United Kingdom between 1985 and 1987, stated that all deaths occurred due to endocarditis (22%), pulmonary hypertension (30%), coronary artery disease (39%), and cardiomyopathy or myocarditis (9%) (DeSwiet, 1993). Similarly, a review of maternal mortality in Utah from 1982 to 1994 revealed 13 cardiac deaths, four (31%) due to pulmonary hypertension, four secondary to cardiomyopathy (31%), two due to coronary artery disease (15%), and three (23%) due to sudden arrhythmia (Varner, 1997). In a smaller series of maternal deaths from West Virginia between 1985 and 1989, the two cardiac deaths described were due to cardiomyopathy (Dye, 1992). This is not to imply that the relative risk categories outlined in Table 15-1 are not still valid with respect

to the likelihood of maternal complications or that interruption of pregnancy or cardiac surgery may not be necessary prior to term. The possibility of fetal morbidity and mortality, especially in cases of cyanotic heart disease, also cannot be overlooked. It would appear, however, that with appropriate obstetric care, the presence or absence of the aforementioned secondary complications of cardiomyopathy appear to play a much more important role in determining ultimate maternal outcome, than the primary structural nature of the cardiac lesion itself.

## Physiologic Considerations

The unique problems encountered by the pregnant woman with cardiac disease are secondary to four principal physiologic changes (ACOG, 1992):

1. *A 50% increase in intravascular volume* is seen in normal pregnancy by early to mid-third trimester. In patients whose cardiac output is limited by intrinsic myocardial dysfunction, valvular lesions, or ischemic cardiac disease, volume overload will be poorly tolerated and may lead to congestive failure or worsening ischemia. In patients with an anatomic predisposition, such volume expansion may result in aneurysm formation or dissection (e.g., Marfan syndrome). Even in women with multiple pregnancies, the heart is able to withstand repetitive episodes of volume overload in pregnancy without lasting detrimental structural or functional changes (Sadaniartz, 1996).

2. *Decreased systemic vascular resistance* (SVR) becomes especially important in patients with the potential for right-to-left shunts, which will invariably be increased by falling SVR during pregnancy. Such alterations in cardiac afterload also complicate adaption to pregnancy in patients with some types of valvular disease.

3. *The hypercoagulability associated with pregnancy* heightens the need for adequate anticoagulation in patients at risk for arterial thrombosis (artificial valves and

some subsets of atrial fibrillation) at a time when optimum anticoagulation with coumarin derivatives may have adverse fetal consequences. For women receiving any type of therapeutic anticoagulation, the risk of serious postpartum hemorrhage is also increased.

4. *Marked fluctuations in cardiac output* normally occur in pregnancy, particularly during labor and delivery (van Oppen, 1996). Such changes increase progressively from the first stage of labor, reaching, in some cases, an additional 50% by the late second stage. The potential for further dramatic volume shifts occurs around the time of delivery, both secondary to postpartum hemorrhage and as the result of an "autotransfusion" occurring with release of vena caval obstruction and sustained uterine contraction. Such volume shifts may be poorly tolerated by women whose cardiac output is highly dependent on adequate preload (pulmonary hypertension) or in those with fixed cardiac output (mitral stenosis). Despite these considerations, induction of labor appears safe in patients with most types of cardiac disease (Sau, 1993).

The risk classification presented in Table 15-1 assumes clean delineation of various cardiovascular lesions. Unfortunately, in actual practice this is only rarely the case. Optimal management of a patient with any specific combination of lesions requires a thorough assessment of the anatomic and functional capacity of the heart, followed by an analysis of how the physiologic changes described previously will impact on the specific anatomic or physiologic limitations imposed by the intrinsic disease. Such an analysis will allow a prioritization of often conflicting physiologic demands and greatly assist the clinician in avoiding or managing potential complications.

Certain management principles generally apply to most patients with cardiac disease. These include the judicious use of antepartum bed rest and meticulous prenatal care. Intrapartum management principles include laboring in the lateral position; the use of epidural anesthesia, which will minimize intrapartum fluctuations in cardiac output; the administration of oxygen; and endocarditis prophylaxis. Positional effects on maternal cardiac output during labor with epidural analgesia have recently been detailed by Danilenko-Dixon (1996). Additional management recommendations may vary according to the specific lesion present. For patients with significant cardiac disease, management and delivery in a referral center is mandatory. In many cases, management with peripheral pulse oximetry is replacing invasive hemodynamic monitoring.

## Congenital Cardiac Lesions

The relative frequency of congenital as opposed to acquired heart disease is changing (Ullery, 1954; Szekely, 1973; DeSwiet, 1993; Hsieh, 1993). Rheumatic fever is less common in the United States, and more patients with congenital cardiac disease now survive to reproductive age. In a review in 1954, the ratio of rheumatic to congenital heart disease seen during pregnancy was 16:1; by 1967, this ratio had changed to 3:1 (Ullery, 1954; Szekely, 1973; Niswander, 1967). A more recent report from Taiwan suggested a rheumatic-congenital cardiac ratio of 1:1.5 during pregnancy (Hsieh, 1993). Similarly, in the United Kingdom between 1973 and 1987, the number of deaths from congenital heart disease has doubled, whereas the number of deaths from acquired heart disease has halved (DeSwiet, 1993). In the subsequent discussion of specific cardiac lesions, no attempt will be made to duplicate existing comprehensive texts regarding physical diagnostic, electrocardiographic, and radiographic findings of specific cardiac lesions. (For a comprehensive discussion of diagnostic findings, see Braunwald E, ed. Heart disease: a textbook of cardiovascular medicine. 5th ed. Philadelphia: WB Saunders, 1997.) Rather, the discussion presented here focuses on aspects of cardiac disease that are unique to pregnancy.

### Atrial Septal Defect

Atrial septal defect (ASD) is the most common congenital lesion seen during pregnancy, and, in general, it is asymptomatic (Veran, 1968;

Etheridge, 1971; Rush, 1979). The two significant potential complications seen with ASD are arrhythmias and heart failure. Although atrial arrhythmias are not uncommon in patients with ASD, their onset generally occurs after the fourth decade of life; thus, such arrhythmias are unlikely to be encountered in the pregnant woman. In patients with ASD, atrial fibrillation is the most common arrhythmia encountered; however, supraventricular tachycardia and atrial flutter also may occur. Initial therapy is with digoxin; less commonly, propranolol, quinidine, or even cardioversion may be necessary. The hypervolemia associated with pregnancy results in an increased left-to-right shunt through the ASD, and, thus, a significant burden is imposed on the right ventricle. Although this additional burden is tolerated well by most patients, congestive heart failure and death with ASD have been reported (Schaeffer, 1968; Neilson, 1970; Hibbard, 1975). In contrast to the high-pressure–high-flow state seen with ventricular septal defect (VSD) and patent ductus arteriosus (PDA), ASD is characterized by high pulmonary blood flow associated with normal pulmonary artery pressures. Because pulmonary artery pressures are low, pulmonary hypertension is unusual. The vast majority of patients with ASD tolerate pregnancy, labor, and delivery without complication. Neilson et al (1970) reported 70 pregnancies in 24 patients with ASD; all patients had an uncomplicated ante- and intrapartum course. During labor, avoidance of fluid overload, oxygen administration, labor in the lateral recumbent position, and pain relief with epidural anesthesia, as well as prophylaxis against bacterial endocarditis, are the most important considerations (Table 15-2).

## Ventricular Septal Defect

Ventricular septal defect may occur as an isolated lesion or in conjunction with other congenital cardiac anomalies, including tetralogy of Fallot, transposition of the great vessels, and coarctation of the aorta. The size of the septal defect is the most important determinant of clinical prognosis during pregnancy. Small defects are tolerated well, while larger defects are associated more

T A B L E    **15-2**

### Characteristics of patients at risk for bacterial endocarditis

Prosthetic heart valves (including bioprostheses)
Most congenital cardiac malformations
Surgical systemic-pulmonary shunts
Rheumatic and other acquired valvular dysfunction
Idiopathic hypertrophic subaortic stenosis
Previous history of bacterial endocarditis
Mitral valve prolapse with insufficiency

frequently with congestive failure, arrhythmias, or the development of pulmonary hypertension. In addition, a large VSD often is associated with some degree of aortic regurgitation, which may add to the risk of congestive failure. Pregnancy, labor, and delivery generally are tolerated well by patients with uncomplicated VSD. Schaefer et al (1968) compiled a series of 141 pregnancies in 56 women with VSD. The only two maternal deaths were in women whose VSD was complicated by pulmonary hypertension (Eisenmenger's syndrome). Because of the high risk of death associated with unrecognized pulmonary hypertension, echocardiography or cardiac catheterization is essential in any adult patient in whom persistent VSD is suspected, or in whom the quality or success of the previous repair is uncertain (Gilman, 1991; Jackson, 1993).

Although very rarely indicated, successful primary closures of VSDs during pregnancy have been reported (see Chapter 13). Intrapartum management considerations for patients with uncomplicated VSD or PDA are similar to those outlined for ASD. In general, invasive hemodynamic monitoring is unnecessary.

## Patent Ductus Arteriosus

Although PDA is one of the most common congenital cardiac anomalies, its almost universal detection and closure in the newborn period makes it uncommon during pregnancy (Szekely, 1979). As with uncomplicated ASD and VSD, most patients are asymptomatic, and PDA is generally tolerated well during pregnancy, labor, and delivery. As with a large VSD, however, the high-pressure–high-flow left-to-right shunt associated with a large, uncorrected PDA can lead to pulmonary hypertension. In such cases, the prognosis becomes much worse. In one study of 18 pregnant women who died of congenital heart disease, three had PDA; however, all of these patients had secondary severe pulmonary hypertension (Hibbard, 1975).

## Eisenmenger's Syndrome

Eisenmenger's syndrome develops when, in the presence of congenital left-to-right shunt, progressive pulmonary hypertension leads to shunt reversal or bidirectional shunting. Although this syndrome may occur with ASD, VSD, or PDA, the low-pressure–high-flow shunt seen as ASD is far less likely to result in pulmonary hypertension and shunt reversal than is the condition of high-pressure and high-flow symptoms seen with the VSD and PDA. Whatever the etiology, pulmonary hypertension carries a grave prognosis during pregnancy. During the antepartum period, the decreased SVR associated with pregnancy increases the likelihood or degree of right-to-left shunting. Pulmonary perfusion then decreases; this decrease results in hypoxemia and deterioration of maternal and fetal condition. In such a patient, systemic hypotension leads to decreased right ventricular filling pressures; in the presence of fixed pulmonary hypertension, such decreased right heart pressures may be insufficient to perfuse the pulmonary arterial bed. This insufficiency may result in sudden, profound hypoxemia. Such hypotension can result from hemorrhage or complications of conduction anesthesia and may result in sudden death (Knapp, 1967; Gleicher, 1979; Pirlo, 1979; Sinnenberg, 1980). Avoidance of such hypotension is the principal clinical concern in the intrapartum management of patients with pulmonary hypertension of any etiology.

Maternal mortality in the presence of Eisenmenger's syndrome is reported as 30% to 50% (Gleicher, 1979; Pirlo, 1979; Gilman, 1991; Jackson, 1993). In a review of the subject, Gleicher et al (1979) reported a 34% mortality associated with vaginal delivery and a 75% mortality associated with cesarean section. Eisenmenger's syndrome associated with VSD appears to carry a higher mortality risk than that associated with PDA or ASD. In addition to the previously discussed problems associated with hemorrhage and hypovolemia, thromboembolic phenomena have been associated with up to 43% of all maternal deaths in Eisenmenger's syndrome (Gleicher, 1979). Sudden delayed postpartum death, occurring 4 to 6 weeks after delivery, also has been reported (Gleicher, 1979; Clark, 1985a). Such deaths may involve a rebound worsening of pulmonary hypertension associated with the loss of pregnancy-associated hormones, which leads to decreased pulmonary vascular resistance during gestation (Clark, 1989).

Because of the high mortality associated with continuing pregnancy, abortion is the preferred management of choice for the woman with significant pulmonary hypertension of any etiology. If any question exists regarding the presence of pulmonary hypertension, pulmonary artery catheterization with direct measurement of pulmonary artery pressures may be performed on an outpatient basis in early pregnancy. Where significant pulmonary hypertension exists, pregnancy termination in either the first or second trimester appears to be safer than allowing the pregnancy to progress to term (Elkayam, 1984). Dilation and curettage in the first trimester or dilation and evacuation in the second trimester are the methods of choice. Hypertonic saline and F-series prostaglandins are contraindicated, the latter due to arterial oxygen desaturation seen with the use of this agent (Hankins, 1988). Prostaglandin $E_2$ suppositories appear to be safe under these circumstances.

For the patient with a continuing gestation, hospitalization for the duration of pregnancy is often appropriate. Continuous administration of oxygen, the pulmonary vasodilator of choice, is mandatory and may improve perinatal outcome. In cyanotic heart disease of any etiology, fetal outcome correlates well with maternal hemoglobin, and successful pregnancy is unlikely with a hemoglobin greater than 20 dL (Presbitero, 1994). Maternal $Pao_2$ should be maintained at a level of 70 mm Hg or above (Sobrevilla, 1971).

Third-trimester fetal surveillance with antepartum testing is important because at least 30% of the fetuses will suffer growth restriction (Gleicher, 1979). Overall fetal wastage with Eisenmenger's syndrome is reported to be up to 75%.

Pulmonary artery catheterization is often useful to monitor preload and cardiac output during the intrapartum period, although some clinicians feel the risk of this technique may outweigh its benefits in patients with cyanotic heart disease (Weiss, 1993). During labor, uterine contractions are associated with a decrease in the ratio of pulmonary to systemic blood flow (Qp/Qs) (Midwall, 1978). Pulmonary artery catheterization and serial arterial blood gas determinations allow the clinician to detect and treat early changes in cardiac output, pulmonary artery pressure, and shunt fraction. In some cases, pulse oximetry may assist in the intrapartum management of these patients without the need for invasive monitoring. Because the primary concern in such patients is the avoidance of hypotension, any attempt to preload reduction (i.e., diuresis) must be undertaken with great caution, even in the face of initial fluid overload. We prefer to manage such patients on the "wet" side, maintaining a preload margin of safety against unexpected blood loss, even at the expense of some degree of pulmonary edema.

Anesthesia for patients with pulmonary hypertension is controversial. Theoretically, conduction anesthesia, with its accompanying risk of hypotension, should be avoided. However, there are several reports of its successful use in patients with pulmonary hypertension of different etiologies (Spinnato, 1981; Abboud, 1983). The use of epidural or intrathecal morphine sulfate, a technique devoid of effect on systemic BP, represents perhaps the best approach to anesthetic management of these difficult patients. Laparoscopic tubal ligation under local anesthesia has also been described in a group of women with various types of cyanotic heart disease (Snabes, 1991).

## Ebstein's Anomaly

Ebstein's anomaly is uncommonly encountered in pregnancy, because it accounts for only 1% of all congenital cardiac disease (Waickman, 1984;

Donnelly, 1991; Connolly, 1994). This anomaly consists of apical displacement of the tricuspid valve, with secondary tricuspid regurgitation and enlargement of both right atrium and ventricle. In a review of 111 pregnancies in 44 women, no serious maternal complications were noted. Seventy-six percent of pregnancies ended in live births, with a 6% incidence of congenital heart disease in the offspring of these women (Connolly, 1994).

## Coarctation of the Aorta

Coarctation of the aorta accounts for approximately 10% of all congenital cardiac disease. The most common site of coarctation is the origin of the left subclavian artery. Associated anomalies of the aorta and left heart, including VSD and PDA, are common, as are intracranial aneurysms in the circle of Willis (Taylor, 1960). Coarctation is often asymptomatic. Its presence is suggested by hypertension confined to the upper extremities, although Goodwin (1961) cites data suggesting a generalized increase in peripheral resistance throughout the body. Resting cardiac output may be increased; however, increased left atrial pressure with exercise suggests occult left ventricular dysfunction. Aneurysms also may develop below the coarctation or involve the intercostal arteries and may lead to rupture. In addition, ruptures without prior aneurysm formation have been reported (Barrett, 1982).

Over 400 patients with coarctation have been reported during pregnancy, with maternal morality ranging from 0% to 17% (Schaeffer, 1968; Deal, 1973; Barrett, 1982). In a review of 200 pregnant women with coarctation of the aorta before 1940, Mendelson (1940) reported 14 maternal deaths and recommended routine abortion and sterilization of these patients. Deaths in this series were from aortic dissection and rupture, congestive heart failure, cerebral vascular accidents, and bacterial endocarditis. Six of the 14 deaths occurred in women with associated lesions. In contrast to this dismal prognosis, a more recent series by Deal and Wooley (1973) reported 83 pregnancies in 23 women with uncomplicated coarctation of the aorta. All were NYHA class I or

II prior to pregnancy. In these women, there were no maternal deaths or permanent cardiovascular complications. In one review, aortic rupture was more likely to occur in the third trimester, prior to labor and delivery (Barash, 1975). Thus, it appears that today, patients having coarctation of the aorta uncomplicated by aneurysmal dilation or associated cardiac lesions who enter pregnancy as class I or II have a good prognosis and a minimal risk of complications or death. Even if uncorrected, uncomplicated coarctation has historically carried with it a risk of maternal mortality of only 3% to 4% (Goodwin, 1961). Maternal risk is increased if preeclampsia develops (Shime, 1987). In the presence of aortic or intervertebral aneurysm, known aneurysm of the circle of Willis, or associated cardiac lesions, however, the risk of death may approach 15%; therefore, therapeutic abortion must be strongly considered.

## Tetralogy of Fallot

Tetralogy of Fallot refers to the cyanotic complex of VSD, overriding aorta, right ventricular hypertrophy, and pulmonary stenosis. Most cases of tetralogy of Fallot are corrected during infancy or childhood. Several published reports attest to the relatively good outcome of pregnancy in patients with corrected tetralogy of Fallot (Loh, 1975; Shime, 1987). In a review of 55 pregnancies in 46 patients, there were no maternal deaths among nine patients with correction prior to pregnancy; in patients with an uncorrected lesion, however, maternal mortality has traditionally ranged from 4% to 15%, with a 30% fetal mortality due to hypoxia (Meyer, 1964; Shime, 1987). In patients with uncorrected VSD, the decline in SVR that accompanies pregnancy can lead to worsening of the right-to-left shunt. This condition can be aggravated further by systemic hypotension as a result of peripartum blood loss. A poor prognosis for successful pregnancy has been related to several prepregnancy parameters, including a hemoglobin exceeding 20 dL, a history of syncope or congestive failure, electrocardiographic evidence of right ventricular strain, cardiomegaly, right ventricular pressure in excess of 120 mm Hg, and peripheral oxygen saturation below 85%.

## Transposition of the Great Vessels

Transposition of the great vessels is uncommon in pregnancy. A series of pregnant patients following the Mustad operation, however, reported 12 of 15 live births and no maternal deaths (Clarkson, 1994). In a similar series of seven patients with transposition having undergone the Mustad or Rastelli procedure, no maternal deaths were reported (Lao, 1994). In one case, however, pregnancy termination was necessary due to maternal deterioration.

## Pulmonic Stenosis

Pulmonic stenosis is a common congenital defect. Although obstruction can be valvular, supravalvular, or subvalvular, the degree of obstruction, rather than its site, is the principal determinant of clinical performance. A transvalvular pressure gradient exceeding 80 mm Hg is considered severe and may mandate surgical correction. Maternal well-being is rarely significantly affected by pulmonic stenosis. Even 20 years ago, a compilation (totaling 106 pregnancies) of three series of patients with pulmonic stenosis revealed no maternal deaths (Schaefer, 1968; Nielsen, 1970; Hibbard, 1975). With severe stenosis, right heart failure can occur; fortunately, this is usually less severe clinically than is the left heart failure associated with mitral or aortic valve lesions.

## Fetal Considerations

Perinatal outcome in patients with cyanotic congenital cardiac disease correlates best with hematocrit; successful outcome in patients with a hematocrit exceeding 65% or hemoglobin exceeding 20 dL is unlikely. Presbitero and associates (1994) described outcome in 96 pregnancies complicated by cyanotic congenital heart disease. Patients with Eisenmenger's syndrome were excluded from this analysis. Although only one maternal death was seen (from endocarditis 2 mo postpartum), the pregnancy loss rate was 51%. Functional class III or IV, hemoglobin greater than 20 g/dL, and a prepregnancy oxygen saturation less than 85% all were associated with a high risk of poor pregnancy outcome. Such patients have an increased risk of spontaneous abortion, intrauterine growth retardation, and stillbirth. Maternal $Pao_2$ below 70% results in decreased fetal oxygen saturation; thus, $Pao_2$ should be kept above this level during pregnancy, labor, and delivery. In the presence of maternal cardiovascular disease, the growth-retarded fetus is especially sensitive to intrapartum hypoxia, and fetal decompensation may occur sooner (Block, 1984; Hsieh, 1993). During the antepartum period, serial antepartum sonography for the detection of growth retardation and antepartum fetal heart rate testing are mandatory in any patient with significant cardiac disease. Fetal activity counting also may be of value in patients with severe disease (Simon, 1986). In a series of six patients with cyanotic cardiac disease, every pregnancy was eventually delivered based on fetal, rather than maternal, deterioration (Patton, 1990).

Of equal concern in patients with congenital heart disease is the risk of fetal congenital cardiac anomalies. This risk appears to be on the order of 5%, although one older study suggested that the actual risk may be as high as 10%, or even higher in women whose congenital lesion involves ventricular outflow obstruction (Whittmore, 1982; Driscoll, 1993; Presbitero, 1994) (see Table 15-2). In such patients, fetal echocardiography is indicated for prenatal diagnosis of congenital cardiac defects (Allan, 1994) (Fig 15-1). Of special interest is that affected fetuses appear to be concordant for the maternal lesion in only 50% of cases. The genetics and embryologic development of congenital cardiac defects have been reviewed by Clark (1996). (See Table 15-3.)

## Acquired Cardiac Lesions

Acquired valvular lesions generally are rheumatic in origin, although endocarditis secondary to intravenous drug abuse may occasionally be involved, especially with right heart lesions. During pregnancy, maternal morbidity and mortality with such lesions result from congestive failure with pulmonary edema or arrhythmias. Szekely (1973) found the risk of pulmonary edema in pregnant patients with rheumatic heart disease to increase

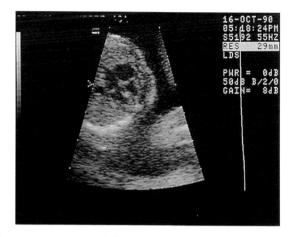

F I G U R E   **15-1**
Echocardiographic image of a fetus at 19 weeks in a mother with a VSD. A similar VSD is demonstrated in this fetus.

with increasing age and with increasing length of gestation. The onset of atrial fibrillation during pregnancy carries with it a higher risk of right and left ventricular failure (63%) than does fibrillation with onset prior to gestation (22%). In addition, the risk of systemic embolization after the onset of atrial fibrillation during pregnancy appears to exceed that associated with onset in the nonpregnant state. In counseling the patient with severe rheumatic cardiac disease on the advisability of initiating or continuing pregnancy, the physician must also consider the long-term prognosis of the underlying disease. Chesley (1980) followed 134 women who had functionally severe rheumatic heart disease and who had completed pregnancy for up to 44 years. He reported a mortality of 6.3% per year but concluded that in patients who survived the gestation, maternal life expectancy was not shortened by pregnancy. Thus, in general, pregnancy has no long-term sequelae for patients who survive the pregnancy (Elkayam, 1984).

Intrapartum management of patients with valvular disease and/or pulmonary hypertension may be facilitated by the use of the pulmonary artery catheter. In determining which patients may benefit from such invasive monitoring, we have found the older NYHA functional classification to be useful. Patients who reach term as class I or II usually tolerate properly managed labor without invasive monitoring. Patients who are or have been class III or IV or those in whom pulmonary hypertension is present or suspected often benefit from pulmonary artery catheterization during the intrapartum period (Clark, 1985a, 1985b).

## Pulmonic and Tricuspid Lesions

Physiologic valvular regurgitation is common in pregnancy, especially with right-sided valves, and the degree of regurgitation progresses as gestation advances (Campos, 1993). An understanding of these changes is essential to the correct interpretation of echocardiograms in the pregnant woman.

Isolated right-sided valvular lesions of rheumatic origin are uncommon; however, such lesions are seen with increased frequency in intravenous drug abusers, where they are secondary to valvular endocarditis. Pregnancy-associated hypervolemia is far less likely to be symptomatic with right-sided lesions than with those involving the mitral or aortic valves. In a review of 77 maternal cardiac deaths, Hibbard (1975) reported none associated with isolated right-sided lesions. In a more recent review, congestive heart failure occurred in only 2.8% of women with pulmonic stenosis (Whittmore, 1982). Even following complete tricuspid valvectomy for endocarditis, pregnancy, labor, and delivery are generally well tolerated. Cautious fluid administration is the mainstay of labor and delivery management in such patients. In general, invasive hemodynamic monitoring during labor and delivery is not necessary. A successful pregnancy has been reported following Fontan repair of congenital tricuspid atresia (Hess, 1991).

## Mitral Stenosis

Mitral stenosis is the most common rheumatic valvular lesion encountered during pregnancy (Clark, 1985a). It can occur as an isolated lesion or in conjunction with aortic or right-sided lesions. The principal hemodynamic aberration involves ventricular diastolic filling obstruction, resulting in a relatively fixed cardiac output. Marked increases in cardiac output accompany normal pregnancy, labor, and delivery. If the pregnant patient is unable to accommodate such volume fluctuations, pulmonary edema may result.

Cardiac output in patients with mitral stenosis is largely dependent on two factors. First, these patients are dependent on adequate diastolic filling time. Thus, while in most patients tachycardia is a clinical sign of underlying hemodynamic instability, in patients with mitral stenosis, the tachycardia itself, regardless of etiology, may contribute significantly to hemodynamic decompensation. During labor, such tachycardia may accompany the exertion of pushing or be secondary to pain or anxiety. Such a patient may exhibit a rapid and dramatic fall in cardiac output and BP in response to tachycardia. This fall compromises maternal as well as fetal well-being. To avoid hazardous tachycardia, the physician should consider oral beta-blocker therapy for any patient with severe mitral stenosis who enters labor with a pulse exceeding 90 to 100 beats per minute. In patients who are not initially tachycardic, acute control of tachycardia with an intravenous beta-blocking agent is only rarely necessary (Clark, 1985a).

A second important consideration in patients with mitral stenosis is left ventricular preload. In the presence of mitral stenosis, pulmonary capillary wedge pressure is not an accurate reflection of left ventricular filling pressures. Such patients often require high-normal or elevated pulmonary capillary wedge pressure in order to maintain adequate ventricular filling pressure and cardiac output. Any preload manipulation (i.e., diuresis), therefore, must be undertaken with extreme caution and careful attention to maintenance of cardiac output.

Potentially dangerous intrapartum fluctuations in cardiac output can be minimized by using epidural anesthesia (Ueland, 1972); however, the most hazardous time for these women appears to be the immediate postpartum period. Such patients often enter the postpartum period already operating at maximum cardiac output and cannot accommodate the volume shifts that follow delivery. In a series of patients with severe mitral stenosis, we found that a postpartum rise in wedge pressure of up to 16 mm Hg could be expected in the immediate postpartum period

(Fig 15-2) (Clark, 1985a). Because frank pulmonary edema generally does not occur with wedge pressures below 28 to 30 mm Hg (Forrester, 1974), it follows that the optimal predelivery wedge pressure for such patients is 14 mm Hg or lower, as indicated by pulmonary artery catheterization (Clark, 1985a). Such a preload may be approached by cautious intrapartum diuresis and with careful attention to the maintenance of adequate cardiac output. Active diuresis is not always necessary in patients who enter labor with evidence of only mild fluid overload. In such patients, simple fluid restriction and the associated sensible and insensible fluid losses that accompany labor can result in a significant fall in wedge pressure prior to delivery.

Previous recommendations for delivery in patients with cardiac disease have included the liberal use of midforceps to shorten the second stage of labor. In cases of severe disease, cesarean section with general anesthesia also has been advocated as the preferred mode of delivery (Ueland, 1970). If intensive monitoring of intrapartum cardiac patients cannot be carried out in the manner described here, such recommendations for elective cesarean delivery may be valid. With the aggressive management scheme presented, however, our experience suggests that vaginal delivery is safe, even in patients with severe disease and pulmonary hypertension. Midforceps deliveries are rarely appropriate in modern obstetrics

(ACOG, 1994) and should be reserved for standard obstetric indications only.

## Mitral Insufficiency

Hemodynamically significant mitral insufficiency is usually rheumatic in origin and most commonly occurs in conjunction with other valvular lesions. This lesion generally is tolerated well during pregnancy, and congestive failure is an unusual occurrence. A more significant risk is the development of atrial enlargement and fibrillation. There is some evidence to suggest that the risk of developing atrial fibrillation may be increased during pregnancy (Szekely, 1973). In Hibbard's review of 28 maternal deaths associated with rheumatic valvular lesions, no patient died with complications of mitral insufficiency unless there was coexisting mitral stenosis (Hibbard, 1975).

## Mitral Valve Prolapse

Congenital mitral valve prolapse is much more common during pregnancy than is rheumatic mitral insufficiency and can occur in up to 17% of young healthy women. This condition is generally asymptomatic (Markiewicz, 1976). The midsystolic click and murmur associated with congenital mitral valve prolapse are characteristic; however, the intensity of this murmur, as well as

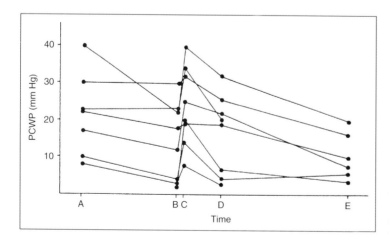

F I G U R E   **15-2**

Intrapartum alterations in pulmonary capillary wedge pressure (PCWP) in eight patients with mitral stenosis. (A) First-stage labor. (B) Second-stage labor, 15 to 30 minutes before delivery. (C) Five to 15 minutes postpartum. (D) Four to 6 hours postpartum. (E) Eighteen to 24 hours postpartum. (Reproduced with permission from Clark SL, Phelan JP, Greenspoon J, et al. Labor and delivery in the presence of mitral stenosis: central hemodynamic observations. Am J Obstet Gynecol 1985b; 152:986.)

that associated with rheumatic mitral insufficiency, may decrease during pregnancy because of decreased SVR (Haas, 1976). Endocarditis prophylaxis during labor and delivery is recommended for rheumatic mitral insufficiency as well as for the more common mitral valve prolapse syndrome, if associated with a regurgitant murmur or evidence of valve insufficiency by echocardiography (Fig 15-3).

## Aortic Stenosis

Aortic stenosis is most commonly of rheumatic origin and usually occurs in conjunction with other lesions. Less often it occurs congenitally and represents 5% of all congenital cardiac lesions. In several series of pregnancies in women with cardiac disease, no maternal deaths due to aortic stenosis have been observed (Shime, 1987; DeSwiet, 1993; Varner, 1997). In contrast to mitral valve stenosis, aortic stenosis generally does not become hemodynamically significant until the orifice has diminished to one third or less of normal. The major problem experienced by patients with valvular aortic stenosis is maintenance of cardiac output. Because of the relative hypervolemia associated with gestation, such patients generally tolerate pregnancy well. With severe disease, however, cardiac output will be relatively fixed, and during exertion it may be inadequate to maintain coronary artery or cerebral perfusion. This inadequacy can result in angina, myocardial infarction, syncope, or sudden death. Thus, marked limitation of physical activity is vital to patients with severe disease. If activity is limited and the mitral valve is competent, pulmonary edema will be rare during pregnancy.

Delivery and pregnancy termination appear to be the times of greatest risk for patients with aortic stenosis (Arias, 1978). The maintenance of cardiac output is crucial; any factor leading to diminished venous return will cause an increase in the valvular gradient and diminished cardiac output. Hypotension resulting from blood loss, ganglionic blockade from epidural anesthesia, or supine vena caval occlusion by the pregnant uterus may result in sudden death. Such problems are similar to those encountered in patients with pulmonary hypertension, discussed previously.

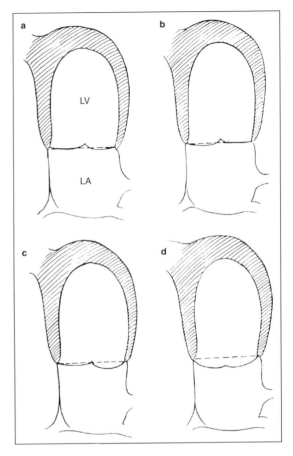

F I G U R E   **15-3**

Echocardiographic apical four-chamber view findings in mitral valve prolapse. Panels a and b represent mild systolic displacement of posterior and anterior valve leaflets superior to the annular plane. Panel c shows moderate displacement with elevation of the coaptation point to the level of the annular plane. Panel d demonstrates marked displacement of valve leaflets and coaptation point. In the absence of additional clinical or sonographic findings, patients with minor to moderate degrees of leaflet displacement without coaptation point displacement should not be considered to have mitral valve prolapse syndrome. LV, left ventricle; LA, left atrium. (Reproduced by permission from Perloff JC, Child JS, Edwards JE. New guidelines for the clinical diagnosis of mitral valve prolapse. Am J Cardiol 1986;57:1127.)

The cardiovascular status of patients with aortic stenosis is complicated further by the frequent coexistence of ischemic heart disease; thus, death associated with aortic stenosis often occurs secondary to myocardial infarction rather than as a direct complication of the valvular lesion itself (Arias, 1978). The overall reported mortality associated with aortic stenosis in pregnancy has been as high as 17%. Today, it would appear that with appropriate care and in the absence of coronary artery disease, however, the risk of death is minimal (DeSwiet, 1993; Varner, 1997). Patients with shunt gradients exceeding 100 mm Hg are at greatest risk. Pulmonary artery catheterization may allow precise hemodynamic assessment and control during labor and delivery. Because hypovolemia is a far greater threat to the patient than is pulmonary edema, the wedge pressure should be maintained in the range of 15–17 mm Hg to maintain a margin of safety against unexpected peripartum blood loss.

A small series of five patients with congenital aortic stenosis demonstrated relatively uncomplicated pregnancies in all, although balloon valvuloplasty was necessary in one woman (Lao, 1993).

## Aortic Insufficiency

Aortic insufficiency is most commonly rheumatic in origin and as such is associated almost invariably with mitral valve disease. The aortic insufficiency generally is tolerated well during pregnancy because the increased heart rate seen with advancing gestation decreases time for regurgitant flow during diastole. In Hibbard's series of 28 maternal rheumatic cardiac deaths, only one was associated with aortic insufficiency in the absence of concurrent mitral stenosis (Hibbard, 1975). Endocarditis prophylaxis during labor and delivery is indicated.

## Peripartum Cardiomyopathy

*Peripartum cardiomyopathy* is defined as cardiomyopathy developing in the last month of pregnancy or the first 6 months postpartum in a woman without previous cardiac disease and after exclusion of other causes of cardiac failure (DeMakis, 1971). It is, therefore, a diagnosis of exclusion that should not be made without a con-

certed effort to identify valvular, metabolic, infectious, or toxic causes of cardiomyopathy. Much of the current controversy surrounding this condition is the result of many older reports in which these causes of cardiomyopathy were not investigated adequately. Other peripartum complications, such as amniotic fluid embolism, severe preeclampsia, and corticosteroid or sympathomimetic-induced pulmonary edema, also must be considered before making the diagnosis of peripartum cardiomyopathy. Sympathomimetic agents also may unmask underlying peripartum cardiomyopathy (Blickstein, 1988).

The incidence of peripartum cardiomyopathy is estimated at between 1 in 1500 and 1 in 4000 deliveries in the United States (Homans, 1985). An incidence as high as 1% has been suggested in women of certain African tribes; however, idiopathic heart failure in these women may be primarily a result of unusual culturally mandated peripartum customs involving excessive sodium intake and may represent, as such, simple fluid overload (Seftel, 1961; Homans, 1985; Veille, 1984). In the United States, the peak incidence of peripartum cardiomyopathy occurs in the second postpartum month, and there appears to be a higher incidence among older, multiparous Black females (Veille, 1984; Witlin, 1997). Other suggested risk factors include twinning and pregnancy-induced hypertension (Veille, 1984; Cunningham, 1986). In some cases, a familial recurrence pattern has been reported. The condition is manifest clinically by the gradual onset of increasing fatigue, dyspnea, and peripheral or pulmonary edema. Physical examination reveals classic evidence of congestive heart failure, including jugular venous distention, rales, and an $S_3$ gallop. Cardiomegaly and pulmonary edema are found on chest x-ray, and the ECG often demonstrates left ventricular and atrial dilatation and diminished ventricular performance. In addition, up to 50% of patients with peripartum cardiomyopathy may manifest evidence of pulmonary or systemic embolic phenomena. Overall mortality ranges from 25% to 50% (Homans, 1985; Veille, 1984).

The histologic picture of peripartum cardiomyopathy involves nonspecific cellular hypertrophy, degeneration, fibrosis, and increased lipid deposition. Although some reports have documented the presence of a diffuse myocarditis, it must be questioned whether such cases represent the same syndrome.

Because of the nonspecific clinical and pathologic nature of peripartum cardiomyopathy, its existence as a distinct entity has been questioned (Cunningham, 1986). Evidence supporting its existence as a distinct entity is supported primarily by epidemiologic evidence suggesting that 80% of cases of idiopathic cardiomyopathy in women of child-bearing age occur in the peripartum period. Such an epidemiologic distribution also could be attributed to an exacerbation of underlying subclinical cardiac disease related to the hemodynamic changes accompanying normal pregnancy. Because such changes are maximal in the third trimester of pregnancy and return to normal within a few weeks postpartum, however, such a pattern does not explain the peak incidence of peripartum cardiomyopathy occurring, in most reports, during the second month postpartum. Nevertheless, the diagnosis of peripartum cardiomyopathy remains primarily a diagnosis of exclusion and cannot be made until underlying conditions, including chronic hypertension, valvular disease, and viral myocarditis, have been excluded.

Although nutritional, hormonal, and autoimmune etiologies have been suggested, substantial backing for any of these theories is lacking. In one case, an autoimmune phenomenon clearly seemed involved due to the documentation of transplacental passage of antibody and subsequent stillbirth (Rand, 1975).

Therapy includes digitalization, diuretics, sodium restriction, and prolonged bed rest. In refractory cases, concomitant afterload reduction with hydralazine or nitrates may be useful. Early endomyocardial biopsy to identify a subgroup of patients who have a histologic picture of inflammatory myocarditis and who may be responsive to immunosuppressive therapy has been suggested.

A notable feature of peripartum cardiomyopathy is its tendency to recur with subsequent pregnancies. Several older reports have suggested that a prognosis for future pregnancies is related to heart size. Patients whose cardiac size returned

to normal within 6 to 12 months had an 11% to 14% mortality in subsequent pregnancies; those patients with persistent cardiomegaly had a 40% to 80% mortality (DeMakis, 1971). Lampert (1997), however, demonstrated persistent decreased contractile reserve even in women who had regained normal resting left ventricular size. Witlin (1997), in a series of 28 patients with peripartum cardiomyopathy, reported that only 7% had regression; in those undertaking subsequent pregnancy, two thirds decompensated earlier than in the index pregnancy. Thus, while pregnancy is absolutely contraindicated in all patients with persistent cardiomegaly, the substantial risk of maternal decompensation with subsequent pregnancy seen in patients with normal heart size would seem, in most cases, to be unacceptable as well.

## Idiopathic Hypertrophic Subaortic Stenosis

Idiopathic hypertrophic subaortic stenosis (IHSS) is an autosomal dominantly inherited condition with variable penetrance. It most commonly becomes clinically manifest in the second or third decade of life; thus, it often may be first manifest during pregnancy. Detailed physical and echocardiographic diagnostic criteria have been described elsewhere. Primarily, IHSS involves left ventricular hypertrophy, typically involving the septum to a greater extent than the free wall. The hypertrophy results in obstruction to left ventricular outflow and secondary mitral regurgitation, the two principal hemodynamic concerns of the clinician (Kolibash, 1975). Although the increased blood volume associated with normal pregnancy should enhance left ventricular filling and improve hemodynamic performance, this positive effect of pregnancy is counterbalanced by the fall in arterial pressure and vena caval obstruction that are found in late pregnancy. In addition, tachycardia resulting from pain or fear in labor diminishes left ventricular filling and aggravates the relative outflow obstruction, an effect also resulting from the second-stage Valsalva maneuver.

The keys to successful management of the peripartum period in patients with IHSS involve avoidance of hypotension (resulting from conduction anesthesia or blood loss) and tachycardia, as well as conducting labor in the left lateral recumbent position. The use of forceps to shorten the second stage also has been recommended. As with most other cardiac disease, cesarean section of IHSS patients should be reserved only for obstetric indications. General management principles for these patients have been reviewed by Spirito (1997).

Despite the potential hazards, maternal and fetal outcomes in IHSS patients are generally good. In a report of 54 pregnancies in 23 patients with IHSS, no maternal or neonatal deaths occurred (Oakley, 1979). Although beta-blocking agents once were used routinely in patients with IHSS, currently they are reserved for patients with angina, recurrent supraventricular tachycardia, or occasional beta-blocker-responsive arrhythmias. Although fetal bradycardia and growth retardation have been reported in patients receiving beta-blockers, a cause-and-effect relationship is not clear; in general, the benefits of such therapy outweigh potential fetal effects. Antibiotic prophylaxis against subacute bacterial endocarditis is recommended.

## Marfan Syndrome

Marfan syndrome is an autosomal dominant disorder characterized by generalized weakness of connective tissue; the weakness results in skeletal, ocular, and cardiovascular abnormalities. The increased risk of maternal mortality during pregnancy stems from aortic root and wall involvement, which may result in aneurysm formation, rupture, or aortic dissection. Fifty percent of aortic aneurysm ruptures in women under age 40 occur more frequently during pregnancy (Barrett, 1982). Rupture of splenic artery aneurysms also occurs more frequently during pregnancy. Sixty percent of patients with Marfan syndrome have associated mitral or aortic regurgitation (Pyeritz, 1979). Although some authors feel pregnancy is contraindicated in any woman with documented Marfan syndrome, prognosis is best individualized and should be based on echocar-

diographic assessment of aortic root diameter and postvalvular dilation. It is important to note that enlargement of the aortic root is not demonstrable by chest x-ray until dilation has become pronounced.

Women with an abnormal aortic valve or aortic dilation may have up to a 50% pregnancy-associated mortality; women without these changes and having an aortic root diameter less than 40 mm have a mortality less than 5% (Pyeritz, 1984). Such patients do not appear to have evidence of aggravated aortic root dilatation over time (Rossiter, 1995). Even in patients meeting these echocardiographic criteria, however, special attention must be given to signs or symptoms of aortic dissection, because even serial echocardiographic assessment is not invariably predictive of complications (Rosenblum, 1983). In counseling women with Marfan syndrome, the genetics of this condition and the shortened maternal life span must be considered, in addition to the immediate maternal risk. The routine use of oral beta-blocking agents to decrease pulsatile pressure on the aortic wall has been recommended (Slater, 1979). If cesarean section is performed, retention sutures should be used because of generalized connective tissue weakness.

## Myocardial Infarction

Coronary artery disease is uncommon in women of reproductive age; therefore, myocardial infarction in conjunction with pregnancy is rare (Hankins, 1985; Sheikh, 1993; Badui, 1994). In a review of 68 reported cases, myocardial infarction during pregnancy was associated with a 35% mortality rate (Hankins, 1985). Only 13% of patients were known to have had coronary artery disease prior to pregnancy. Two thirds of the women suffered infarction in the third trimester; mortality for these women was 45%, as compared with 23% in those suffering infarction in the first or second trimesters. Thus, it appears that the increased hemodynamic burden imposed on the maternal cardiovascular system in late pregnancy may unmask latent coronary artery disease in some women and worsen the prognosis for patients suffering infarction. Fetuses of surviving women appear to have an increased risk of spontaneous abortion and unexplained stillbirth.

Women with class H diabetes mellitus face risks beyond those imposed by their cardiac disease alone. Although successful pregnancy outcome may occur, maternal and fetal risks are considerable. Such considerations, as well as the anticipated shortened life span of these patients, makes special counseling of such women of major importance (Gast, 1985).

Antepartum care of women with prior myocardial infarction includes bed rest to minimize myocardial oxygen demands. Diagnostic radionucleotide cardiac imaging during pregnancy results in a fetal dose of no more than 0.8 rads and, thus, does not carry a significant risk of teratogenesis (Elkayam, 1984). If cardiac catheterization becomes necessary, the simultaneous use of contrast echocardiography may reduce the need for cineangiography and, thus, reduce radiation exposure to the fetus (Elkayam, 1983). In women with angina, nitrates have been used without adverse fetal effects. Schumacher (1997) reported success for treatment of acute myocardial infarction during pregnancy with tissue plasminogen activator. Although minor electrocardiographic changes are often seen in pregnant women, evaluation of the electrocardiogram in women with suspected ischemic heart disease should not vary significantly because of pregnancy (Veille, 1996). The evaluation of chest pain in women has been recently reviewed (Douglas, 1996). Delivery within 2 weeks of infarction is associated with increased mortality; therefore, if possible, attempts should be made to allow adequate convalescence prior to delivery. If the cervix is favorable, cautious induction under controlled circumstances after a period of hemodynamic stabilization is optimal. Labor in the lateral recumbent position, the administration of oxygen pain relief with epidural anesthesia, and, in some cases, hemodynamic monitoring with a pulmonary artery catheter are important management considerations.

In two prospective American studies, having six or more pregnancies was associated with a small but significant increase in the risk of subsequent coronary artery disease (Ness, 1993).

## Anticoagulation

Anticoagulation in the patient with an artificial heart valve and/or atrial fibrillation during pregnancy is controversial (Ginsberg, 1994). The key issue involves our lack of an ideal agent for anticoagulation during pregnancy. Coumadin is relatively contraindicated at all stages of gestation due to its association with fetal warfarin syndrome in weeks 6 to 9 and its relationship to fetal intracranial hemorrhage and secondary scarring at later stages (Hall, 1980; Briggs, 1994). On the other hand, there is some evidence to suggest that for arterial thrombosis with artificial valves (unlike the situation with venous thromboembolic disease), heparin may be less effective than coumadin (Oakley, 1976; Antunes, 1984; Golby, 1992).

In 1984, Salazar et al (1984) described 227 pregnancies in 156 women with cardiac valve prostheses. Women treated with coumadin throughout gestation had a 28% incidence of spontaneous abortion, 7% stillbirths, and 2% neonatal deaths. Eight percent of the fetuses had features of the fetal warfarin syndrome. In contrast, no spontaneous abortions, stillbirths, or neonatal deaths were observed in women receiving heparin before and coumadin after the thirteenth week of gestation. A subsequent series of pregnancies revealed a 30% incidence of fetal warfarin syndrome in patients treated with coumadin throughout gestation, with no cases when heparin was given prior to week 12, coumadin until week 38, and then heparin until delivery. Chang (1984) reported a 43% perinatal mortality in women treated throughout pregnancy with warfarin. In 1986, Lee reported 18 pregnancies in 16 women with artificial valves who received heparin during weeks 6 to 13 and then with coumadin. He observed a 50% stillbirth rate but no fetal anomalies.

One deficiency in these studies is a lack of detailed neonatal neurologic evaluation and follow-up; thus, while the risk of fetal warfarin syndrome when coumarin derivatives are taken between weeks 6 and 9 is between 8% and 30%, the frequency of intracranial hemorrhage in fetuses whose mothers receive warfarin after week 12 is unknown. Several more recent series from outside the United States have reported on the use of coumadin in pregnant patients with prosthetic valves. In patients receiving coumadin, spontaneous abortion rates of 7% to 37% have been reported, with a 2% incidence of embryopathy (Vitali, 1986; Sareli, 1989; Born, 1992; Lee, 1994; Hanania, 1994; Sbarouni, 1994). On the other hand, two series comparing maternal thromboembolic events in patients receiving heparin versus coumadin showed a two- to threefold increase of this potentially devastating complication in the former group (Hanania, 1994; Sbarai, 1994). Thus, a choice between fetal and maternal risks must be made, and neither choice is ever ideal. Two approaches, however, appear to be acceptable. One involves substitution of heparin for coumadin from the time pregnancy is diagnosed until 12 weeks' gestation, followed by coumadin until 38 weeks, at which time heparin is reinstituted until delivery. The second approach involves using adjusted-dose subcutaneous heparin throughout pregnancy (Deviri, 1985; Dahlen, 1986). The patient must be involved in this choice and thoroughly informed of the risks and benefits of either approach (Vongpatanasin, 1996). A patient who requires anticoagulation when not pregnant should be treated during pregnancy, although the medication used may be different. Pregnant women having prosthetic heart valves should be treated with one of the aforementioned regimens from conception until delivery. During the postpartum period, coumarin may be reinstituted.

The adjusted-dose regimen employs sodium heparin given subcutaneously in doses of 8000 to 14,000 units every 8 to 12 hours in a dose sufficient to prolong the activated partial thromboplastin time (aPTT) obtained at 8 to 12 hours after the dose (trough) to 1.5 to 2.0 times control. This heparin regimen should provide plasma heparin levels of 0.2 to 0.4 units/mL if measured by heparin assay.

There have been small series of patients with nonbiologic prosthetic heart valves who have been treated during pregnancy with antiplatelet agents, including aspirin and dipyridamole. Although maternal outcome was good, a high rate of spontaneous abortion was encountered in one study, and the size of these series makes it difficult to draw conclusions about the safety and efficacy of these regimens (Deviri, 1985; Biale, 1980; Nunez, 1983).

Patients with bioprosthetic or xenograft valves usually are not treated with anticoagulants (Vongpatanasin, 1996). This fact makes the bioprosthetic valve the ideal choice of prosthesis for young women of childbearing age (Starr, 1984). Patients with a bioprosthetic valve who are in atrial fibrillation or have evidence of thromboembolism, however, should be anticoagulated. Prosthetic valves and specific anticoagulation regimens have recently been reviewed by Vongpatanasin (1996).

## Prevention of Bacterial Endocarditis in Patients with Artificial Valves

American Heart Association recommendations for endocarditis prophylaxis are outlined in Table 15-4. Controversy persists regarding the need for prophylaxis with vaginal delivery. One approach is to administer the high-risk regimen to patients with systemic-pulmonary shunts, artificial valves, or a history of endocarditis, reserving the low-risk regimen for pregnant patients with other structural abnormalities. There appear to be two major problems with the current suggestion by the American Heart Association that uncomplicated vaginal delivery does not require endocarditis prophylaxis. First, to be most effective, antibiotic administration is recommended from one half to 1 hour prior to the anticipated bacteremia; we have yet to meet the clinician who can reliably predict, one half to 1 hour prior to birth, that the delivery will be "uncomplicated" and not involve vaginal or rectal lacerations or the need for manual exploration of the uterus. Second, as outlined at the beginning of this chapter, a review of recent maternal cardiac deaths in Western countries reveals that postpartum endocarditis is one of the leading causes of mortality. Thus, most clinicians involved in the day-to-day management of pregnant cardiac patients recommend one of the aforementioned regimens for most patients.

T A B L E    **15-3**

Congenital heart defects in 372 offspring of 233 mothers
with congenital cardiac anomalies

| Defect in Infant | Obstruction | | Left-to-Right Shunts | | | Misc. | Cyanotic | | Total |
|---|---|---|---|---|---|---|---|---|---|
| | LHO | RHO | PDA | VSD | ASD | | Cyan. | Rep. | |
| AS | 9* | 1 | 1 | 1 | | | | | 12 |
| PS | | 3* | 1 | | | 2 | 1* | 1* | 8 |
| PS + ASD | | 1* | | | | | | | 1 |
| PPS | 1 | | | | | | | 1* | 2 |
| PDA | 1 | 1 | 3* | 1 | | | 1 | | 7 |
| VSD | 1 | | 3 | 9* | 3 | 1 | 1* | | 18† |
| VSD + PS | | | | 5* | | | | | 5 |
| ASD | | | 1 | 1 | 1* | | | 1 | 4 |
| MVP | | 1 | | | | | | | 1 |
| Complex | | | | | 2 | | | | 2 |
| Total | | | | | | | | | 60 |

*Concordant anomalies.

†Seven ventricular septal defects closed: AS = aortic stenosis; ASD = atrial
    septal defect; LHO = left heart outflow obstruction; MVP = mitral valve
    prolapse; PDA = patient ductus arteriosus; PPS = peripheral pulmo-
    nary valve stenosis; PS = pulmonary stenosis; Rep. = repaired; RHO =
    right heart outflow obstruction; VSD = ventricular septal defect.

Reproduced by permission from Whittemore R, Hobbins JC, Engle MA. Preg-
    nancy and its outcome in women with and without surgical treatment of
    congenital heart disease. Am J Cardiol 1982;50:645.

T A B L E    **15-4**

Bacterial endocarditis prophylaxis

| Drug | Dosage Regimen |
|---|---|
| **Standard Regimen** | |
| Ampicillin, gentami-<br>cin, and amoxicillin | Intravenous or intramuscular administration of ampicillin, 2 g, plus gentamicin, 1.5 mg/kg (not to exceed 120 mg), 30 min before procedure; followed by amoxicillin, 1.0 g, orally 6 hr after initial dose; alternatively, the parenteral regimen (1 g) may be repeated once 6 hr after intial dose. |
| **Ampicillin/Amoxicillin/Penicillin-Allergic Patient Regimen** | |
| Vancomycin and gen-<br>tamicin | Intravenous administration of vancomycin, 1 g over 1 hr plus intravenous or intramuscular administration of gentamicin, 1.5 mg/kg (not to exceed 120 mg), 1 hr before procedure. Complete infusion within 20 min of procedure onset. |
| **Alternate Low-Risk Patient Regimen** | |
| Amoxicillin/Ampicillin | 2 g orally 1 hr before procedure; or Ampicillin 50 mg/kg within 30 min of pro-cedure onset. |

Modified by permission from Dajani AS, Taubert KA, Wilson W, et al. Preven-
    tion of bacterial endocarditis: recommendations of the American Heart
    Association. JAMA 1997;277:1794–1801. Copyright 1990, American Med-
    ical Association.

## Dysrhythmias

While minor ECG changes are commonly seen in pregnancy, significant dysrhythmias are rare (Veille, 1996). The use of antiarrhythmic therapy has been reviewed extensively by Rotmensch et al (1987). Many of these medications have been used to treat fetal dysrhythmias as well (Kleinman, 1985). Digoxin, procainamide, and quinidine may be used for the usual indications and in therapeutic doses have not been shown to be harmful to the fetus. A digoxin-like immunoreactive substance appears in some normal and pre-eclamptic patients during the second trimester and can be identified in many patients during the third trimester (Phelps, 1988). If serum monitoring of digoxin levels is anticipated, a pretreatment level should be obtained to improve interpretation of results.

The use of beta-blockers is appropriate in some tachyarrhythmias, in IHSS, and for the control of hyperthyroid symptoms. In a critical review, Frishman (1988) concluded that beta-blocker therapy is not associated with adverse neonatal outcome. Neonatal hypoglycemia and bradycardia may occur, although they are usually not serious. Intrauterine growth retardation may be a consequence of the disease for which the beta-blockers are prescribed rather than a complication of therapy itself. Beta-blockers such as atenolol and acebutolol have lower degrees of plasma binding and are excreted in breast milk at higher concentrations, sufficient to cause bradycardia, hypotension, and poor perfusion in the infant. Verapamil is a calcium-entry–blocking drug that is effective in the conversion of a supraventricular tachycardia to sinus rhythm. Although there are no reports of its adverse effect on the fetus, there is little experience with it in pregnancy.

Women with life-threatening arrhythmias should have them evaluated prior to conception to determine whether (1) surgical or catheter ablation, (2) an antitachycardia pacemaker, or (3) an automatic implantable cardiovert-defibrillator is appropriate. The issue of anticoagulation for atrial fibrillation in pregnancy has not been addressed specifically. It seems reasonable, however, to anticoagulate a pregnant patient if she meets the criteria described for nonpregnant patients. These include atrial fibrillation with a history of thromboembolic complications, atrial fibrillation in the presence of valvular disease such as mitral stenosis or regurgitation, atrial fibrillation in cardiomyopathy, or atrial fibrillation with thyrotoxic heart disease. Anticoagulation is recommended for 3 weeks prior to cardioversion of atrial fibrillation and for 4 weeks after conversion to sinus rhythm. Anticoagulation should be considered in the patient with atrial fibrillation and congestive heart failure. Patients with this degree of cardiomyopathy, however, should not attempt pregnancy because of their poor prognosis.

Cardioversion appears safe for the fetus (Schroeder, 1971). The presence of an artificial pacemaker, similarly, does not affect the course of pregnancy (Jaffe, 1987).

## Pregnancy After Cardiac Transplantation

The number of pregnant women who have undergone cardiac transplantation is small; nevertheless, from a compilation of 30 case reports, several generalizations can be made (Scott, 1993). First, most such patients are maintained on cyclosporine and azathioprine; often, prednisone is added to the regimen. While theoretic concerns may exist regarding potential teratogenesis of these agents, limited experience with heart transplant patients and more extensive experience with patients having undergone renal transplant suggest that such fears are unfounded (Kossoy, 1988; Key, 1989). Patients should be counseled that these agents appear to pose minimal, if any, risk of adverse fetal effects.

Second, with regard to maternal risk, patients with cardiac transplants who have no evidence of rejection and have normal cardiac function at the onset of pregnancy appear to tolerate pregnancy, labor, and delivery well (Lowenstein, 1988; Key, 1989; Hedon, 1990; Camann, 1991; Scott, 1993). The denervated heart retains normal systolic function and contractile reserve (Borrow, 1985; Greenberg, 1985; Ku-Mie, 1996). Such patients undergo the normal hemodynamic response to pregnancy, as well as the expected intrapartum hemodynamic changes (Key, 1989; Ku-Mie, 1996). To date, no cases exist of maternal death during pregnancy in cardiac transplant recipients. While three cases have been reported of delayed death following pregnancy, in two of these, voluntary withdrawal from the immunosuppresive agents and/or inappropriate medical care was implicated; there is no evidence that the antecedent pregnancy was in any way related to the death of any of these women.

During pregnancy, meticulous prenatal care is essential, as is careful cardiology follow-up with frequent ECGs, cardiac catheterizations, and heart biopsy, as would be indicated in the nonpregnant state. Close attention must be paid to symptoms or signs of transplant rejection, which generally may be successfully managed by adjustments in medication. There appears to be an increased risk of pregnancy-induced hypertension and preterm delivery in these patients, and some have advocated adding low-dose aspirin (80 mg) during pregnancy. Serial sonography for fetal growth and third-trimester antepartum fetal surviellance appears reasonable as well. Several authors have advocated the use of intrapartum pulmonary artery catheterization for these patients, but no convincing evidence exists that management has been altered significantly by the availability of data so derived. Cesarean section and all but outlet instrumental vaginal deliveries should be reserved only for standard obstetric indications.

Central hemodynamic changes associated with pregnancy in a stable cardiac transplant recipient were described by Kim (1996), and were not significantly different than those expected during normal pregnancy.

## REFERENCES

Abboud JK, Raya J, Noueihed R, et al. Intrathecal morphine for relief of labor pain in a parturient with severe pulmonary hypertension. Anesthesiology 1983;59:477.

Allan LD, Sharland GK, Milburn A, et al. Prospective diagnosis of 1006 consecutive cases of congenital heart disease in the fetus. J Am Coll Cardiol 1994;23:1452.

American College of Obstetricians and Gynecologists. Cardiac disease in pregnancy. Technical Bulletin 168, June 1992.

American College of Obstetricians and Gynecologists. Operative vaginal delivery. Technical Bulletin 196, August 1994.

Antunes MJ, Myer IG, Santos LP. Thrombosis of mitral valve prosthesis in pregnancy: management by simultaneous caesarean section and mitral valve replacement. Case report. Br J Obstet Gynaecol 1984;91:716–718.

Arias F, Pineda J. Aortic stenosis and pregnancy. J Reprod Med 1978;20:229.

Badui E, Rangel A, Enciso R. Acute myocardial infarction during pregnancy and puerperium in athletic women. Two case reports. Angiology 1994;45:897.

Barash PG, Hobbins JC, Hook R, et al. Management of coarctation of the aorta during pregnancy. J Thorac Cardiovasc Surg 1975;69:781.

Barrett JM, VanHooydonk JE, Boehm FH. Pregnancy-related rupture of arterial aneurysms. Obstet Gynecol Surv 1982;37:557.

Berg CJ, Atrash HK, Koonin LM, et al. Pregnancy related mortality in the United States, 1987–1990. Obstet Gynecol 1996;88:161.

Biale Y, Cantor A, Lewenthal H, et al. The course of pregnancy in patients treated with artificial heart valves treated with dipyridamole. Int J Gynaecol Obstet 1980;18:128–132.

Blickstein I, Zalel Y, Katz Z, et al. Ritodrine-induced pulmonary edema unmasking underlying peripartum cardiomyopathy. Am J Obstet Gynecol 1988;159:332.

Block BSB, Llanos AJ, Creasy RK. Responses of the growth-retarded fetus to acute hypoxemia. Am J Obstet Gynecol 1984;148:878.

Born D, Martinez EE, Almeida P, et al. Pregnancy in patients with prosthetic heart valves: the effects of anticoagulation on mother, fetus and neonate. Am Heart J 1992;124:413.

Borrow KM, Neumann A, Arensman FW, et al. Left ventricular contractility and contractile reserver in humans after cardiac transplantation. Circulation 1985;71:866.

Briggs GB, Bodendorfer JW, Freeman RK, Yaffe SJ, eds. Drugs in pregnancy and lactation. Baltimore: Williams and Wilkins, 1994.

Camann WR, Goldman GA, Johnson MD, et al. Cesarean delivery in a patient with a transplanted heart. Anesthesiology 1989;71:618.

Camann WR, Jarcho J, Mintz KJ, et al. Uncomplicated vaginal delivery 14 months after cardiac transplantation. Am Heart J 1991;121:939.

Campos O, Andrade JL, Bocanegra J, et al. Physiologic multivalvular regurgitation during pregnancy: a longitudinal Doppler echocardiographic study. Int J Cardiol 1993;40:265.

Chesley LC. Severe rheumatic cardiac disease and pregnancy: the ultimate prognosis. Am J Obstet Gynecol 1980;126:552.

Clark EB. Pathogenic mechanisms of congenital cardiovascular malformations revisited. Semin Perinatol 1996;20:465.

Clark SL, Phelan JP, Greenspoon J, et al. Labor and delivery in the presence of mitral stenosis: central hemodynamic observations. Am J Obstet Gynecol 1985a;152:984.

Clark SL. Structural cardiac disease in pregnancy. In: Clark SL, Cotton DB, Phelan JP, eds. Critical care obstetrics. Oradell, NJ: Medical Economics Books, 1987:92.

Clark SL, Cotton DB, Lee W, et al. Central hemodynamic assessment of normal term pregnancy. Am J Obstet Gynecol 1989;161:1439.

Clark SL, Horenstein JM, Phelan JP, et al. Experience with the pulmonary artery catheter in obstetrics and gynecology. Am J Obstet Gynecol 1985b;151:724.

Clarkson PM, Wilson NJ, Neutze JM, et al. Outcome of pregnancy after the Mustad operation for transposition of the great arteries with intact ventricular septum. J Am Coll Cardiol 1994;24:190.

Connolly HM, Warnes CA. Ebstein's anomaly: outcome of pregnancy. J Am Coll Cardiol 1994;23:1194.

Cunningham FG, Pritchard JA, Hankins GDV, et al. Peripartum heart failure: idiopathic cardiomyopathy or compounding cardiovascular events? Obstet Gynecol 1986;67:157.

Dajani AS, Taubert KA, Wilson W, et al. Prevention of bacterial endocarditis: recommendations of the American Heart Association. JAMA 1997;277:1794.

Dalen E, Hirsh J, co-chairmen. American College of Chest Physicians and the National Heart, Lung, and Blood Institute National Conference on Antithrombotic Therapy. Chest 1986;89 (suppl 2):1S–106S.

Danilenko-Dixon DR, Tefft L, Cohen RA, et al. Positional effects on maternal cardiac output during labor with epidural analgesia. Am J Obstet Gynecol 1996;175:867.

Deal K, Wooley CF. Coarctation of the aorta and pregnancy. Ann Intern Med 1973;78:706.

Demakis JG, Rahimtoola SH, Sutton GC, et al. Natural course of peripartum cardiomyopathy. Circulation 1971;44:1053.

DeSwiet M. Maternal mortality from heart disease in pregnancy. Br Heart J 1993;69:524.

Deviri E, Levinsky L, Yechezkel M, et al. Pregnancy after valve replacement with porcine xenograft prosthesis. Surg Gynecol Obstet 1985;160:437.

Donnolly JE, Brown JM, Radford DJ. Pregnancy outcome and Ebstein's anomaly. Br Heart J 1991;66:368.

Douglas PS, Ginsberg GS. The evaluation of chest pain in women. N Engl J Med 1996;334:1311.

Driscoll DJ, Michels VV, Gesony WM, et al. Occurrence risk for congenital heart defects in relatives of patients with aortic stenosis, pulmonary stenosis, or ventricular septal defect. Circulation 1993;87(suppl 2):I114.

Dye TD, Gordon H, Held B, et al. Retrospective maternal mortality case ascertainment in West Virginia. Obstet Gynecol 1992;167:72.

Elkayam U, Kawanishi D, Reid CL, et al. Contrast echocardiography to reduce ionizing radiation associated with cardiac catheterization during pregnancy. Am J Cardiol 1983;52:213.

Elkayam V, Gleicher N. Cardiac problems in pregnancy, I. Maternal aspects: the approach to the pregnant patient with heart disease. JAMA 1984;251:2838.

Etheridge MJ, Pepperell RJ. Heart disease and pregnancy at the Royal Women's Hospital. Med J Aust 1971;2:277.

Forrester JS, Swan HJC. Acute myocardial infarction: a physiological basis for therapy. Crit Care Med 1974;2:283.

Frishman WH, Chesner M. Beta-adrenergic blockers in pregnancy. Am Heart J 1988;115:147.

Gast MJ, Rigg LA. Class H diabetes and pregnancy. Obstet Gynecol 1985;66:5(s).

Gilman DH. Cesarean section in undiagnosed Eisenmenger's syndrome. Report of a patient with a fatal outcome. Anesthesia 1991;46:371.

Ginsberg JS, Barron WM. Pregnancy and prosthetic heart valves. Lancet 1994;344:1170. Editorial.

Gleicher N, Midwall J, Hochberger D, et al. Eisenmenger's syndrome and pregnancy. Obstet Gynecol Surv 1979;34:721.

Golby AJ, Bush EC, DeRook FA, et al. Failure of high-dose heparin to prevent recurrent cardioembolic strokes in a pregnancy patient with a mechanical heart valve. Neurology 1992;42:2204.

Goodwin JF. Pregnancy and coarctation of the aorta. Clin Obstet Gynecol 1961;4:645.

Greenberg ML, Uretsky BF, Reddy PS, et al. Long-term hemodynamic follow-up of cardiac transplant patients treated with cyclosporin and prednisone. Circulation 1985;71:487.

Haas JM. The effect of pregnancy on the midsystolic click and murmur of the prolapsing posterior leaflet of the mitral valve. Am Heart J 1976;92:407.

Hall JG, Pauli RM, Wilson KM. Maternal and fetal sequelae of anticoagulation during pregnancy. Am J Med 1980;68:122.

Hanania G, Thomas D, Michel PL, et al. Pregnancy and prosthetic heart valves: a French cooperative retrospective study of 155 cases. Eur Heart J 1994;15:1651.

Hankins GDV, Berryman GK, Scott RT, et al. Maternal arterial desaturation with 15 methyl prostaglandin F2 alpha for uterine atony. Obstet Gynecol 1988;72:367.

Hankins GDV, Wendel GD, Leveno KJ, et al. Myocardial infarction during pregnancy: a review. Obstet Gynecol 1985;65:139.

Hedon B, Montoya F, Cabrol A. Twin pregnancy and vaginal birth after heart transplantation. Lancet 1990;335:476.

Hess DB, Hess LW, Heath BJ, et al. Pregnancy after Fontan repair of tricuspid atresia. South Med J 1991;84:532.

Hibbard LT. Maternal mortality due to cardiac disease. Clin Obstet Gynecol 1975;18:27.

Hogberg U, Innala E, Sandstrom S. Maternal mortality in Sweden, 1980–1988. Obstet Gynecol 1994;84:240.

Homans DC. Peripartum cardiomyopathy. N Engl J Med 1985;312:1432.

Hsieh TT, Chen KC, Soong JH. Outcome of pregnancy in patients with organic heart disease in Taiwan. Asia Oceania J Obstet Gynecol 1993;19:21.

Hunt SA. Pregnancy in heart transplant patients: a good idea? J Heart Lung Transplant 1991;10:499.

Jackson GM, Dildy GA, Varner MW, et al. Severe pulmonary hypertension in pregnancy following successful repair of ventricular septal defect in childhood. Obstet Gynecol 1993;82 (suppl):680.

Jaffe R, Gruber A, Fejgin M, et al. Pregnancy with an artificial pacemaker. Obstet Gynecol Surv 1987;42:137–139.

Key TG, Resnik R, Dittrich HC, et al. Successful pregnancy after cardiac transplantation. Am J Obstet Gynecol 1989;160:367.

Kim KM, Sukhani R, Slogoff S, Tomich PG. Central hemodynamic changes associated with pregnancy in a long term cardiac transplant recipient. Am J Obstet Gynecol 1996;174:1651.

Kleinman CS, Copel JA, Weinstein EM, et al. In-utero diagnosis and treatment of fetal supraventricular tachycardia. Semin Perinatol 1985;9:113.

Knapp RC, Arditi LI. Pregnancy complicated by patent ductus arteriosus with reversal of flow. NY J Med 1967;67:573.

Koh KS, Friesen RM, Livingstone RA, et al. Fetal monitoring during maternal cardiac surgery with cardiopulmonary bypass. Can Med Assoc J 1975;112:1102.

Kolibash AJ, Ruiz DE, Lewis RP. Idiopathic hypertrophic subaortic stenosis in pregnancy. Ann Intern Med 1975;82:791.

Koonin LM, Atrash HK, Lawson HW, et al. Maternal mortality surveillance, United States 1979–1986. MMWR 1991;40:SS1.

Kossoy LR, Herbert CM, Wentz AC. Management of heart transplant recipients: guidelines for the obstetrician gynecologist. Am J Obstet Gynecol 1988;159:490.

Ku-Mie K, Sukhani R, Slogoff S, et al. Central hemodynamic changes associated with pregnancy in a long-term cardiac transplant recipient. Am J Obstet Gynecol 1996;174:1651.

Lao TT, Sermer M, MaGee, L et al. Congenital aortic stenosis and pregnancy—a reappraisal. Am J Obstet Gynecol 1993;169:540.

Lao TT, Sermer M, Colman JM. Pregnancy following surgical correction for transposition of the great arteries. Obstet Gynecol 1994;83:665.

Laupert MB, Weinert L, Hibbard J, et al. Contractile reserve in patients with peripartum cardiomyopathy and recovered left ventricular function. Am J Obstet Gynecol 1997;176:189.

Lee CN, Wu CC, Lin PY, et al. Pregnancy following cardiac prosthetic valve replacement. Obstet Gynecol 1994;83:353.

Loh TF, Tan NC. Fallot's tetralogy and pregnancy: a report of a successful pregnancy after complete correction. Med J Aust 1975;2:141.

Lowenstein BR, Vain NW, Perrone SV, et al. Successful pregnancy and vaginal delivery after heart transplantation. Am J Obstet Gynecol 1988; 158:589.

Markiewicz W, Stoner J, London E, et al. Mitral valve prolapse in one hundred previously healthy young females. Circulation 1976;53:464.

Mendelson CL. Pregnancy and coarctation of the aorta. Am J Obstet Gynecol 1940;39:1014.

Meyer EC, Tulsky AS, Sigman P, et al. Pregnancy in the presence of tetralogy of Fallot. Am J Cardiol 1964;14:874.

Midwall J, Jaffin H, Herman MV, et al. Shunt flow and pulmonary hemodynamics during labor and delivery in the Eisenmenger syndrome. Am J Cardiol 1978;42:299.

Neilson G, Galea EG, Blunt A. Congenital heart disease and pregnancy. Med J Aust 1970;30: 1086.

Ness RB, Harris T, Cobb J, et al. Number of pregnancies and the subsequent risk of cardiovascular disease. N Engl J Med 1993;328:1528.

Niswander KR, Berendes H, Dentschberger J, et al. Fetal morbidity following potential anoxigenic obstetric conditions: V. Organic heart disease. Am J Obstet Gynecol 1967;98:871.

Nunez L, Larrea JL, Aguado MG, et al. Pregnancy in 20 patients with bioprosthetic valve replacement. Chest 1983;84:26–28.

Oakley C. Valve prostheses and pregnancy. Br Heart J 1987;58:303–305. Editorial.

Oakley CM, Doherty P. Pregnancy in patients after heart valve replacement. Br Heart J 1976;38: 1140–1148.

Oakley GDG, McGarry K, Limb DG, et al. Management of pregnancy in patients with hypertropic cardiomyopathy. Br Med J 1979;1:1749.

Patton DE, Lee W, Cotton DB, et al. Cyanotic maternal heart disease in pregnancy. Obstet Gynecol Surv 1990;45:594.

Perloff JK, Child JS, Edwards JE. New guidelines for the clinical diagnosis of mitral valve prolapse. Am J Cardiol 1986;57:1127.

Phelps SJ, Cochran EC, Gonzalez-Ruiz A, et al. The influence of gestational age and preeclampsia on the presence and magnitude of serum endogenous digoxin-like immunoreactive substance(s). Am J Obstet Gynecol 1988;158:34–39.

Pirlo A, Herren AL. Eisenmenger's syndrome and pregnancy. Anesth Rev 1979;6:9.

Presbitero P, Somerville J, Stone S. Pregnancy in cyanotic congenital heart disease. Outcome of mother and fetus. Circulation 1994;89:2673.

Pyeritz RE, McKusick VA. The Marfan syndrome: diagnosis and management. N Engl J Med 1979;300:772.

Pyeritz RE. Maternal and fetal complications of pregnancy in the Marfan syndrome. Am J Med 1984;71:784.

Rand RJ, Jenkins DM, Scott DG. Maternal cardiomyopathy of pregnancy causing stillbirth. Br J Obstet Gynecol 1975;82:172.

Rosenblum NG, Grossman AR, Gabbe SG, et al. Failure of serial echocardiographic studies to predict aortic dissection in a pregnant patient with Marfan's syndrome. Am J Obstet Gynecol 1983;146:470.

Rossiter JP, Repke JT, Morales AJ, et al. A prospective, longitudinal evaluation of pregnancy in the Marfan syndrome. Am J Obstet Gynecol 1995; 173:1599.

Rotmensch HH, Rotmensch S, Elkayam U. Management of cardiac arrhythmias during pregnancy: current concepts. Drugs 1987;33:623–633.

Rush RW, Verjans M, Spraklen FH. Incidence of heart disease in pregnancy. S Afr Med J 1979;55:808.

Sadaniantz A, Laurent LS, Parisi AF. Long-term effects of multiple pregnancies on cardiac dimensions and systolic and diastolic function. Am J Obstet Gynecol 1996;174:1061.

Salazar E, Zajarias A, Gutierrez N, Iturbe I. The problem of cardiac valve prostheses, anticoagulants, and pregnant women. Circulation 1984;70 (suppl I):I-169–I-177.

Sareli P, England MJ, Berk MR, et al. Maternal and fetal sequelae of anticoagulation during pregnancy in patients with mechanical heart valve prostheses Am J Cardiol 1989;63:1462.

Sau AK, Vasishta K, Dhar KK, et al. Induction of labour in pregnancy complicated by cardiac disease. Aust NZ J Obstet Gynecol 1993;33:37.

Sbarouni E, Oakley CM. Outcome of pregnancy in women with valve prostheses. Eur Heart J 1994;15:1651.

Schaefer G, Arditi LI, Solomon HA, et al. Congenital heart disease and pregnancy. Clin Obstet Gynecol 1968;11:1048.

Scheikh AU, Harper MA. Myocardial infarction during pregnancy: management and outcome of two pregnancies. Am J Obstet Gynecol 1993;169:279.

Schroeder JS, Harrison DC. Repeated cardioversion during pregnancy. Treatment of refractory paroxysmal atrial tachycardia during three successive pregnancies. Am J Cardiol 1971;27:445.

Schumacher B, Belfort MA, Card RJ. Successful treatment of acute myocardial infarction during pregnancy with tissue plasminogen activator. Am J Obstet Gynecol 1997;176:716.

Scott JR, Wagoner LE, Olsen SL, et al. Pregnancy in heart transplant recipients: management and outcome. Obstet Gynecol 1993;82:324.

Seftel H, Susser M. Maternity and myocardial failure in African women. Br Heart J 1961;23:43.

Shime J, Mocarski EJM, Hastings D, et al. Congenital heart disease in pregnancy: short- and long-term implications. Am J Obstet Gynecol 1987;156:313.

Simon A, Sadovsky E, Aboulatia Y, et al. Fetal activity in pregnancies complicated by rheumatic heart disease. J Perinat Med 1986;14:331.

Sinnenberg RJ. Pulmonary hypertension in pregnancy. South Med J 1980;73:1529.

Slater EE, DeSanctis RW. Dissection of the aorta. Med Clin North Am 1979;63:141.

Snabes MC, Poindexter AN. Laparoscopic tubal sterilization under local anethesia in women with cyanotic heart disease. Obstet Gynecol 1991; 78:437.

Sobrevilla LA, Cassinelli MT, Carcelen A, et al. Human fetal and maternal oxygen tension and acid-base status during delivery at high altitude. Am J Obstet Gynecol 1971;111:1111.

Spinnato JA, Kraynack BJ, Cooper MW. Eisenmenger's syndrome in pregnancy: epidural anesthesia for elective cesarean section. N Engl J Med 1981;304:1215.

Spirito P, Seidman CE, McKenna WJ, Maron BJ. The management of hypertrophic cardiomyopathy. N Engl J Med 1997;336:775.

Starr A, Grunkemeier GL. Selection of a prosthetic valve. JAMA 1984;251:1739–1742.

Szekely P, Turner R, Snaith L. Pregnancy and the changing pattern of rheumatic heart disease. Br Heart J 1973;35:1293.

Szekely P, Julian DG. Heart disease and pregnancy. Curr Probl Cardiol 1979;4:1.

Taylor SH, Donald KW. Circulatory studies at rest and during exercise in coarctation, before and after correction. Br Heart J 1960;22:117.

Ueland K, Akamatsu TJ, Eng M, et al. Maternal cardiovascular dynamics: VI: Cesarean section under epidural anesthesia without epinephrine. Am J Obstet Gynecol 1972;114:775.

Ueland K, Hansen J, Eng M, et al. Maternal cardiovascular dynamics. V. Cesarean section under thiopental, nitrous oxide and succinylcholine anesthesia. Am J Obstet Gynecol 1970;108:615.

Ullery JC. Management of pregnancy complicated by heart disease. Am J Obstet Gynecol 1954; 67:834.

van Oppen ACC, Stigter RH, Bruinse HW. Cardiac output in normal pregnancy: A critical review. Obstet Gynecol 1996;87:310.

Varner MW, Jacob S, Bloebaum L. Maternal mortality in Utah, 1982–1994. West J Med 1997 (in press)

Veille JC. Peripartum cardiomyopathies: a review. Am J Obstet Gynecol 1984;148:805.

Veille JC, Kitzman DW, Bacevice AE. Effects of pregnancy on the electrocardiogram in healthy subjects during strenuous exercise. Am J Obstet Gynecol 1996;175:1360.

Veran FX, Cibes-Hernandez JJ, Pelegrina I. Heart disease in pregnancy. Obstet Gynecol 1968; 34:424.

Vitali E, Donatelli R, Quanini E, et al. Pregnancy in patients with mechanical prosthetic heart valves. J Cardiovasc Surg 1986;27:221.

Vongpatanasin W, Hillis LD, Lange RA. Prosthetic heart valves. N Engl J Med 1996;335:407.

Waickman LA, Skorton DJ, Varner MW, et al. Ebstein's anomaly and pregnancy. Am J Cardiol 1984;53:357.

Weiss BM, Atanassoff PG. Cyanotic congenital heart disease and pregnancy: natural selection, pulmonary hypertension and anesthesia. J Clin Anesth 1993;5:332.

Whittmore R, Hobbins JC, Engle MA. Pregnancy and its outcome in women with and without surgical treatment of congenital heart disease. Am J Cardiol 1982;50:641.

Witlin AG, Mabie WC, Sibai BM. Peripartum cardiomyopathy: An ominous diagnosis. Am J Obstet Gynecol 1997;176:182.

Zitnick RS, Brandenburg RO, Sheldon R, et al. Pregnancy and open heart surgery. Circulation 1969;39:157.

# CHAPTER 16

# Acute Renal Failure

$\mathcal{R}$enal failure is now an uncommon complication of pregnancy, occurring in less than 1% of all pregnancies in developed countries (Pertuiset, 1984). In fact, the incidence of acute renal failure (ARF) requiring dialytic support is not significantly different in pregnant women in Western countries as compared with the general population. Just as the incidence of ARF in pregnancy has sharply declined, so has the mortality rate. Acute renal failure, however, remains a potentially devastating complication, with a substantial number of those affected requiring chronic renal replacement therapy.

In previous decades, rates of ARF as high as 20% to 40% were documented in pregnancy, largely attributed to the high incidence of septic abortion (Lindheimer, 1988; Stratta, 1989; Turney, 1989). In underdeveloped parts of the world, ARF remains a well-recognized complication, secondary to limited prenatal care and the continued frequency of illegal abortion.

## Etiologies of Acute Renal Failure

The approach to the pregnant patient with ARF is similar to that of the nonpregnant patient, although diseases unique to the pregnant state must be considered in the differential as well (Table 16-1) (Thadhani, 1996). Disorders causing ARF in pregnancy include prerenal azotemia, intrinsic renal disease, urinary obstruction, as well as pre-eclampsia, the HELLP (*h*emolysis, *e*levated *l*iver enzymes, *l*ow *p*latelets) syndrome, acute fatty liver of pregnancy (AFLP), and postpartum renal failure (also known as postpartum hemolytic uremic syndrome [HUS]). This latter group of disorders is unique to the differential diagnosis of pregnancy-associated ARF. Bilateral renal cortical necrosis (BRCN) is another consideration in the evaluation of the pregnant woman with ARF, which, though not unique to the pregnant state, is seen overwhelmingly in pregnancy (see Table 16-1).

In the past, a bimodal incidence of ARF was seen in pregnancy, with a peak in the first trimester corresponding to the high incidence of septic abortion, and a second peak in the third trimester corresponding to a number of other disorders uniquely seen in pregnancy. Currently, the majority of ARF is seen in the latter part of gestation. [Rapid acceleration of the renal failure, with accompanying hypertension and proteinuria, is seen in 10% of women entering pregnancy with moderate or severe renal insufficiency (Jones, 1996). Although less common, significant deterioration in renal function may also occur during pregnancy in women with underlying diabetic nephropathy (Gordon, 1996).] Renal biopsy is infrequently performed, because the clinical presentation and the timing of renal failure are usually adequate to establish a diagnosis. In those patients with an unexplained deterioration in renal failure or development of the nephrotic syndrome prior to 32 weeks' gestation, however, renal biopsy can be performed safely (Lindheimer, 1994).

TABLE   **16-1**

Acute renal failure in pregnancy

**Differential Diagnosis**

Prerenal azotemia
Acute tubular necrosis
Acute interstitial nephritis
Acute glomerulonephritis
Obstruction
Preeclampsia
HELLP syndrome
Acute fatty liver of pregnancy
Postpartum renal failure
Pyelonephritis
Bilateral renal cortical necrosis

TABLE   **16-2**

Laboratory evaluation of acute renal failure

|  | **Prerenal Azotemia** | **Acute Tubular Necrosis** |
|---|---|---|
| BUN:creatinine ratio | >20:1 | 10:1 |
| Urine $Na^+$ (mEq/liter) | <20 | >40 |
| Fractional excretion of $Na^+$ ($FENa^+$) | <1% | >2% |
| Urine osmolality (mosm/kg $H_2O$) | >500 | <350 |
| Urine sp gr | >1.020 | 1.010 |
| Urine sediment | Bland | Granular casts, renal tubular epithelial cells |

## Prerenal Azotemia

Prerenal azotemia is the result of decreased renal perfusion, due to either true volume depletion, decreased cardiac output, or altered renal perfusion. The latter can be seen with cirrhosis, the nephrotic syndrome, renal artery stenosis, or the use of nonsteroidal antiinflammatory agents. By definition, prerenal azotemia is readily reversible with restoration of renal perfusion. Early in pregnancy, hyperemesis gravidarum is one of the more common causes of ARF secondary to profound volume depletion resulting from poor oral intake and vomiting. Similarly, any gastrointestinal illness with vomiting or diarrhea, excessive use of cathartics or laxatives, or bulimia may result in prerenal azotemia. Generally, these disorders are easily recognized on the basis of the history and physical examination and can be treated successfully with volume repletion. Laboratory studies that may be of additional benefit in establishing the diagnosis of prerenal azotemia include urine electrolytes and osmolality (Table 16-2). Urine sodium is typically low, as is the fractional excretion of sodium (urine $Na^+$/serum $Na^+$/urine creatinine/serum creatinine) or $FENa^+$, reflecting a sodium avid state, and urine osmolality is high, indicating intact urinary concentrating ability. A low urine chloride may also provide a clue to surreptitious vomiting.

Uterine hemorrhage is an important cause of hypovolemia and subsequent ARF late in preg-

nancy. Hemorrhage may be concealed in patients with placental abruption or may occur in the postpartum period. Hemorrhage with resultant hypotension was a major cause of pregnancy-associated ARF in 7% of patients studied at the Necker Hospital, and was a contributing factor in as many as 79% of cases in other studies (Pertuiset, 1984). Patients with preeclampsia may be particularly susceptible to ARF secondary to hemorrhage, due to preexisting alterations in maternal physiology, including decreased intravascular volume, heightened vascular responsiveness to catecholamines and angiotensin II, and altered prostaglandins (Grunfeld, 1980). To prevent the development of fixed renal tubular injury, prerenal azotemia due to hemorrhage or other causes must be treated aggressively with blood product support and fluid resuscitation.

## Intrinsic Renal Disease

Acute renal failure may result from a variety of intrinsic renal diseases similar to those in the nonpregnant patient. Involvement of the glomeruli may predominate in one of the many primary or secondary glomerulonephritides. The renal tubules and interstitium are the primary areas of injury in acute tubular necrosis (ATN) and acute interstitial nephritis (AIN). Both clinical presentation and examination of the urinary sediment can

T A B L E   **16-3**

Acute renal failure: evaluation of intrinsic renal disease

|  | Acute Tubular Necrosis | Acute Interstitial Nephritis | Acute Glomerulonephritis |
|---|---|---|---|
| Urine sediment | Brown granular casts, renal tubular cells | Hematuria, pyuria, eosinophils, WBC casts | Hematuria, RBC casts, oval fat bodies |
| Proteinuria | $< 2$ g/day | $< 2$ g/day | $> 2$ g/day, possible nephrotic syndrome |
| $FENa^+$ | $> 2\%$ | $> 2\%$ | $< 1\%$ |
| Hypertension | Uncommon | Uncommon | Common |
| Systemic manifestations | Hypotension, sepsis, hemorrhage | Fever, skin rash, new medication | Collagen-vascular disease, infection |

provide valuable clues to the diagnosis, although renal biopsy may eventually be required to distinguish among the many glomerular diseases and to predict prognosis (Table 16-3).

## Acute Glomerulonephritis

The numerous causes of acute glomerulonephritis (GN) include primary glomerular diseases such as poststreptococcal GN, membranoproliferative GN, idiopathic rapidly progressive (or crescentic) GN (RPGN), as well as secondary glomerular diseases such as lupus nephritis, systemic vasculitis, and bacterial endocarditis (Table 16-4). The classic presentation of acute GN is that of hypertension, edema and volume overload, nephrotic range proteinuria, and an active urinary sediment with RBC casts. In those women with preexisting renal disease, these features are often noted in the first two trimesters of gestation, although systemic lupus erythematosus (SLE) may manifest at any time during pregnancy. Serology including serum complement levels, antinuclear antibodies, antistreptolysin-O titers, antineutrophil cytoplasmic antibodies, and other autoantibodies may be helpful in establishing a diagnosis, although in most cases renal biopsy is eventually necessary. Treatment of acute GN is largely supportive, including diuretics, antihypertensive agents, and occasionally dialysis. Depending on the underlying disease, corticosteroids or cytotoxic agents are often employed as well.

## Acute Interstitial Nephritis

The most common cause of AIN is drug exposure, with an extensive list of agents that have been implicated. Among those more commonly noted are the beta-lactam antibiotics such as the semisynthetic penicillins, sulfa-based drugs, histamine H-2 blockers, and nonsteroidal antiinflammatory agents. Acute interstitial nephritis also may occur in association with viral infections, including cytomegalovirus and infectious mononucleosis,

T A B L E   **16-4**

Causes of glomerulonephritis

*Primary*
Minimal change disease
Focal segmental glomerulosclerosis
IgA nephropathy
Membranoproliferative GN
Membranous nephropathy
Poststreptococcal GN

*Secondary*
SLE
Henoch-Schönlein purpura
Cryoglobulinemia
Polyarteritis nodosa
Wegener's granulomatosis
Hypersensitivity vasculitis
Goodpasture's syndrome
Infection-related (i.e., shunt nephritis, endocarditis)

direct bacterial invasion, parasitic infections such as malaria and leptospirosis, and systemic diseases such as SLE and sarcoidosis (Table 16-5). Unlike acute GN, AIN typically presents with modest proteinuria (<2 g/day), pyuria, eosinophiluria, hematuria, and WBC casts on urinalysis. Systemic manifestations may include fever, rash, arthralgias, and other signs of a hypersensitivity reaction in those patients with drug-induced interstitial nephritis. Hypertension and edema are infrequently seen with AIN, except in those cases of severe ARF. When history, physical examination, and laboratory evaluation are inadequate to establish a diagnosis, renal biopsy is often necessary. Withdrawal of the offending agent or treatment of the underlying infection or disease usually results in improvement in renal function. In some cases of drug-induced or idiopathic AIN, steroids have been used with varying degrees of success.

## Acute Tubular Necrosis

Acute tubular necrosis results from a variety of toxic exposures, including aminoglycosides, radiographic contrast, heavy metals, and several of the chemotherapeutic agents. Pigment-induced ATN may occur in cases of rhabdomyolysis or massive hemolysis. More commonly, ATN is ischemic in nature, as a result of a hemodynamic insult with hypotension and impaired renal perfusion. In those patients with preeclampsia who develop ARF, ATN appears to be the underlying renal lesion. Clinically, it may be difficult to distinguish between severe prerenal azotemia and ATN, although urinary indices and urinalysis may be helpful (see Table 16-2). Urinalysis typically reveals muddy brown granular casts and renal tubular epithelial cells. In light of impaired renal tubular function, laboratory evaluation reveals a high urinary sodium excretion and $FENa^+$ and urine that is neither concentrated nor dilute. Acute tubular necrosis may be either oliguric (24-hr urine <400 mL) or non-oliguric (>400 mL/day), depending on the mechanism of injury and the severity. Treatment of ATN is supportive and necessitates optimization of hemodynamics, avoidance of potential nephrotoxin exposure, nutritional support with careful monitoring of fluids and electrolytes, and, occasionally, dialysis. Renal function typically recovers in 7 to 14 days.

## Urinary Obstruction

Although urinary obstruction is a relatively uncommon cause of ARF in pregnancy, it is readily reversible and, therefore, should not be missed. Obstruction may occur at any level of the urinary tract due to a wide variety of causes, the majority of which are not unique to pregnancy (Table 16-6). In addition, ureteral compression by the gravid uterus has been reported (Satin, 1993). Women with an abnormally configured or overdistended uterus, such as those with uterine leiomyomata, polyhydramnios, or multiple gestations, may be particularly susceptible. Renal ultrasound

T A B L E   **16-5**

**Causes of acute interstitial nephritis**

Drug-induced
Infection
   Viral: CMV, infectious mononucleosis, hemorrhagic fever
   Bacterial: streptococcal infections, diphtheria, Legionnaires' disease
   Parasitic: malaria, leptospirosis, toxoplasmosis
Systemic disease
   Sarcoidosis
   SLE
   Sjögren's syndrome
   Transplant rejection
   Leukemic or lymphomatous infiltration
Idiopathic

CMV, cytomegalovirus.

T A B L E   **16-6**

**Causes of urinary obstruction**

| Upper Tract | Lower Tract |
|---|---|
| Stones | Stones |
| Blood clots | Blood clots |
| Tumor | Tumor |
| Sloughed papillae | Neuropathic bladder |
| Ureteral stricture or ligation | Urethral stricture |
| Retroperitoneal fibrosis | |
| Extrinsic compression by tumor, gravid uterus | |

is the first step in the evaluation of possible urinary tract obstruction, although results may be inconclusive due to the physiologic dilatation of the collecting system often seen in pregnancy. Thus, anterograde or retrograde pyelography may be necessary for definitive diagnosis. Relief of obstruction, either by ureteral stent placement or percutaneous nephrostomy, may allow a substantial delay in delivery as well as recovery of renal function.

## Acute Renal Failure Unique to Pregnancy

### Pyelonephritis

As a result of the hormonal and mechanical changes accompanying pregnancy, the urinary collecting system is prone to dilatation and urinary stasis. This results in an increased incidence in both upper and lower tract infections that is estimated at 2% (Gilstrap, 1981). Whalley and colleagues demonstrated a substantial decrease in creatinine clearance among gravidas with pyelonephritis, with a return to normal or near-normal renal function in the majority of women reevaluated following appropriate antibiotic therapy (Whalley, 1975). It has been postulated that this decline in renal function is related to an increased vascular sensitivity to bacterial endotoxin and vasoactive mediator release in pregnancy (Pertuiset, 1984). Although bacterial invasion is not unique to pregnancy, pyelonephritis typically does not result in a significant decline in glomerular filtration rate in nonpregnant patients.

### Preeclampsia

Among those causes of ARF unique to pregnancy, severe preeclampsia or eclampsia accounts for the majority. Between 1957 and 1979, preeclampsia was the apparent cause of ARF in 21% of pregnant women presenting with renal failure to the Necker Hospital (Grunfeld, 1987). However, the diagnosis was not confirmed by renal biopsy, and because the majority of these women were older multigravidas, this study may have overestimated the true incidence. Classically, *preeclampsia* is defined by the development of hypertension, pro-

teinuria, and edema after the twentieth week of gestation. Elevated liver enzymes, coagulation abnormalities, and microangiopathic hemolytic anemia may be seen as well. The diagnosis is established clinically and rarely confirmed by renal biopsy. Pathologically, preeclampsia is characterized by swollen glomerular capillary endothelial cells or glomerular endotheliosis, with resultant capillary obstruction and glomerular ischemia (Antonovych, 1981). Importantly, the extent of the morphologic lesion does not necessarily correspond to the degree of renal functional impairment (Lindheimer, 1988). In addition, the presence of subtle volume depletion and enhanced sensitivity of renal vasculature to vasoconstriction may contribute to superimposed ATN, which many believe to be the lesion associated with significant ARF in preeclampsia. Treatment of severe preeclampsia and the associated renal failure ultimately depend on the termination of pregnancy with delivery of the infant. Spontaneous renal recovery is seen within days to several weeks, without residua. Histologic evaluation in those patients with persistent renal impairment, proteinuria, or hypertension postpartum has revealed evidence of underlying chronic renal disease, presumably unmasked by pregnancy and/or preeclampsia (Stratta, 1989).

### HELLP Syndrome

HELLP is an acronym used to describe a constellation of findings, including hemolysis, elevated liver enzymes, and low platelets. Nausea and epigastric or right upper quadrant pain and tenderness are common at presentation, as are proteinuria and renal failure. Coagulation studies including fibrinogen, prothrombin time, and partial thromboplastin time may be useful in distinguishing this disorder from others associated with disseminated intravascular coagulation, in that they are normal in the vast majority. The HELLP syndrome has been described in 4% to 12% of patients with severe preeclampsia (Martin, 1991) and is considered to represent a variant of severe preeclampsia. In a small study in which patients with the HELLP syndrome underwent renal biopsy, however, less than half had the glomerular endotheliosis classic for preeclampsia

(Krane, 1988). A more recent retrospective review documented 158 cases of HELLP over a 10-year period at one institution (Martin, 1991). Although there was no discussion of renal involvement, hematologic disease activity peaked at 24 to 48 hours following delivery, and 11 of the patients were treated with plasma exchange for ongoing clinical deterioration postpartum. Generally, treatment of the HELLP syndrome consists of expeditious delivery once the diagnosis is established. Rapid recovery of renal function is the rule.

## Acute Fatty Liver of Pregnancy

Acute fatty liver of pregnancy is another uncommon cause of ARF in pregnancy, with an incidence of approximately one in 13,000 deliveries (Kaplan, 1985). The disease usually occurs in primiparas in the last few weeks of gestation, although it has been reported as early as 24 weeks' gestation and as late as 1 day postpartum (Lindheimer, 1988; Usta, 1994). Initial manifestations are nonspecific, including nausea, vomiting, headache, malaise, and abdominal pain. Laboratory evaluation reveals mild elevation of serum transaminase levels, hyperbilirubinemia, and leukocytosis. Renal failure develops in the majority of cases. Left untreated, patients may progress to fulminant hepatic failure with jaundice, encephalopathy, disseminated intravascular coagulopathy, gastrointestinal hemorrhage, and death. Maternal and fetal mortality rates as high as 85% were seen in the past, although with earlier diagnosis and treatment, mortality rates are now closer to 20%.

A report by Usta and colleagues described their experience with 13 patients (14 cases) of AFLP over an 8-year period, all of whom had ARF on presentation (Usta, 1994). They reported 100% maternal survival, with 13% perinatal mortality. Although nine of 14 cases were initially diagnosed as preeclampsia, the diagnosis of AFLP was subsequently confirmed either by liver biopsy (10/14), computed tomography (CT) of the liver (2/14), or clinically. Of note, one patient whose diagnosis was established by CT actually presented on the first postpartum day. Additionally, one patient experienced a recurrence of AFLP in a subsequent pregnancy. Diagnosis of fatty liver may be established by liver biopsy revealing microvesicular fatty infiltration or, alternatively, suggested by CT revealing decreased hepatic attenuation. Although CT revealing hepatic density below the normal range of 50 to 70 Hounsfield units has been reported as suggestive of AFLP, Usta's study demonstrated a high false-negative rate with only two of 10 abnormal scans, including nine biopsy-proven cases (Usta, 1994). Contributing to the diagnostic dilemma in these women is the frequent occurrence of hypertension, edema, and proteinuria suggestive of preeclampsia, although renal pathology has failed to reveal evidence of glomerular endotheliosis. As is the case with severe preeclampsia, expeditious delivery is warranted, with prompt improvement in both hepatic and renal failure noted in most cases (Kaplan, 1985).

## Postpartum Renal Failure

Idiopathic postpartum renal failure, also referred to as postpartum HUS is a unique cause of pregnancy-associated ARF that typically develops in the puerperium following an uncomplicated pregnancy and delivery. Women present from the peripartum period to several months following delivery with severe hypertension, microangiopathic hemolytic anemia, and oliguric renal failure, often with congestive heart failure and CNS manifestations as well. A prodromal flu-like illness, gastrointestinal or respiratory, and initiation of oral contraceptives may be associated with postpartum renal failure as well as with idiopathic HUS, suggesting a toxic or hormonal influence.

Pathologically, the disease is often indistinguishable from the thrombotic microangiopathies, idiopathic HUS and thrombotic thrombocytopenic purpura (TTP), with arteriolar injury, fibrin deposition, and microvascular (arteriolar and glomerular capillary) thrombosis. Unlike TTP, the major pathologic involvement is in the kidney, as opposed to the CNS. The pathogenesis of the thrombotic microangiopathies remains unclear, although intravascular coagulation, disordered platelet aggregation, endothelial damage, and alterations in prostaglandins have been suggested (Hayslett, 1985). Therapies have been chosen in an attempt to intervene in one or more of these processes, including plasma exchange–plasma infusion, antiplatelet agents, and anticoagulants. In addition, acute and long-term dialytic support is often necessary, with approximately 12% to 15% of patients developing end-stage renal disease. The maternal mortality rate is estimated at greater than 55% (Weiner, 1987).

Although treatment guidelines are not well established, plasma exchange is recommended due to an apparent benefit in survival in a small number of patients. Due to the continuum of disease, both HUS and TTP have been considered together in most clinical trials. The Canadian Apheresis Study Group and a group at Johns Hopkins University examined the outcome in TTP and HUS-TTP, respectively (Rock, 1991; Bell, 1991). Both reported the superiority of plasma exchange therapy in terms of clinical response and survival, with mortality rates of 22% and 9%, respectively, in those receiving such treatment. Additional therapeutic interventions varied, including aspirin, dipyridamole, and corticosteroids. Greater than 50% of all patients had evidence of renal dysfunction, although those with severe ARF or anuria were excluded from the Canadian multicenter trial. Nine of the 76 women seen at Johns Hopkins presented in their third trimester of pregnancy, although there was no comment as to degree of renal impairment in this subset of patients. Similarly, Hayward and colleagues described nine pregnant women with TTP-HUS among 67 cases presenting between the first trimester of gestation and 1 month postpartum (Hayward, 1994). Of these eighteen women, all but one survived, and none required renal replacement therapy.

## Bilateral Renal Cortical Necrosis

Acute BRCN is a pathologic entity consisting of partial or complete destruction of the renal cortex, with sparing of the medulla. While not unique to pregnancy, this rare and catastrophic form of ARF occurs most commonly in pregnancy, with obstetric causes accounting for 50% to 70% of cases (Donohoe, 1983). Although BRCN represents less than 2% of cases of ARF in the nonpregnant population, in the past it has accounted for 10% to 38% of obstetric renal failure, perhaps secondary to the hypercoagulable state and altered vascular sensitivity of pregnancy (Krane, 1988). It typically develops between 30 and 35 weeks' gestation in association with profound shock and renal hypoperfusion, such as that seen with abruptio placentae, placenta previa, and other causes of hemorrhage. Early in pregnancy, septic abortion is a common cause of cortical necrosis. Abruptio placentae with either overt or concealed hemorrhage is the most common antecedent event (Donohoe, 1983). Patients with BRCN present with severe and prolonged oliguria or anuria (24-hr urine < 50 mL), flank pain, gross hematuria, urinalysis revealing hematuria, and RBC and granular casts. Diagnosis is established by renal arteriogram demonstrating virtual absence of cortical blood flow (interlobular arteries), despite patency of the renal arteries. More recently, diagnosis has been established by ultrasonography or contrast-enhanced CT demonstrating areas of cortical lucency or by histologic examination. The extent of cortical necrosis is relevant to prognosis because 25% of survivors require maintenance dialysis for end-stage renal disease.

## Management of Acute Renal Failure

Management of ARF in pregnancy is similar to that in the nonpregnant patient, including supportive therapy as well as dialysis. Close attention to fluid balance is critical because superimposed volume depletion or fluid overload may exacerbate ARF or necessitate earlier dialytic intervention. Adequate nutrition also is of utmost importance to promote healing and minimize the risk of infectious complications. Correction of the metabolic acidosis seen with ARF may require bicarbonate therapy or dialysis if it remains refractory to medical therapy or occurs in the setting of congestive heart failure. Prevention of hyperphosphatemia includes dietary phosphate restriction and either aluminum- or calcium-containing phosphate binders given with meals. Dietary potassium restriction also is imperative to avoid potentially life-threatening hyperkalemia. A cation-exchange resin, such as kayexalate, can be used for mild hyperkalemia or until dialysis is available. For hyperkalemia with associated electrocardiographic changes, acute therapy includes intravenous calcium gluconate to stabilize the cardiac membrane, infusion of glucose and insulin or inhaled beta-agonists to transiently shift potassium intracellularly, and acute dialysis (see Chapter 9). Additional conservative measures include avoiding further nephrotoxic exposure and hypotension, BP control, and medication dose adjustment according to the degree of renal impairment.

In those patients with severe metabolic abnormalities that are unresponsive to conservative medical management, volume overload and pulmonary congestion that are unresponsive to diuretics, or signs and symptoms of uremia, including pericarditis and encephalopathy, dialysis is indicated. With regard to dialysis and pregnancy, it is generally accepted that intensive dialysis is indicated to minimize fetal exposure to the azotemic environment. Although there are no data in pregnancy, studies evaluating the role of intensive dialysis in the nonpregnant patient have attempted to maintain levels of urea nitrogen and

creatinine less than 70 mg/dL and 5 mg/dL, respectively (Hou, 1991). Both hemodialysis and peritoneal dialysis have been used successfully in the management of the pregnant patient with acute and chronic renal failure.

## Summary

Evaluation of the pregnant patient with ARF encompasses a broad range of disorders, many of which are not unique to pregnancy. Prerenal azotemia; intrinsic renal disease, including ATN, GN, and interstitial nephritis; and urinary obstruction should be considered based on clinical presentation, urinalysis and urinary diagnostic indices, and in some cases, renal biopsy, similar to evaluation of ARF in the nonpregnant patient. In addition, diseases unique to pregnancy and those more common during pregnancy must be considered, including preeclampsia, the HELLP syndrome, AFLP, postpartum renal failure, and BRCN (Table 16-7). This latter group of diseases is unique in that treatment often necessitates prompt termination of pregnancy and delivery of the infant.

T A B L E   **16-7**
Classification of pregnancy-associated acute renal failure

| Preeclampsia | HELLP Syndrome | Acute Fatty Liver of Pregnancy | Postpartum (HUS) Renal Failure | Pyelonephritis | Bilateral Renal Cortical Necrosis |
|---|---|---|---|---|---|
| Proteinuria Hypertension Edema | RUQ pain Proteinuria Hemolysis Elevated LFTs Thrombocytopenia Normal coags | Elevated LFTs Hyperbilirubinemia Coagulopathy Oliguria Nausea Abdominal pain Leukocytosis | Occurring postpartum MAHA Oliguria Severe HTN Prodromal illness Thrombocytopenia CNS involvement | Positive urine culture Fever | Hemorrhage Hypotension/ shock Oliguria/anuria Flank pain Gross hematuria |

RUQ, right upper quadrant; LFTs, liver function tests; MAHA, microangiopathic hemolytic anemia; HTN, hypertension.

---

## ACUTE RENAL FAILURE

### I. *Goals of Therapy*

A. Avoid volume overload and subsequent cardiopulmonary complications.

B. Maintain metabolic homeostasis; prevent hyperkalemia, hyperphosphatemia, metabolic acidosis, etc.

C. Prevent uremic complications (i.e., encephalopathy, pericarditis, bleeding diatheses, etc.).

D. Control hypertension.

E. Maintain adequate nutrition.

F. Optimize fetal growth and well-being.

### II. *Management Protocol*

A. Volume status

1. Optimize intravascular volume and cardiac filling pressures. Invasive hemodynamic monitoring may be necessary.
2. Limit fluid intake to insensible losses (400–500 mL/day) plus urine output.
3. Attempt to diurese or establish a non-oliguric state:
   a. Loop diuretics such as furosemide can be given in incremental doses from 40 mg to 5 mg/kg IV.
   b. Zaroxolyn (5 mg by mouth) or chlorothiazide (250–500 mg IV) can be used in conjunction with a loop diuretic to augment diuresis.
   c. Continuous infusion of furosemide (40–80 mg/hr) or bumetanide (1–2 mg/hr) can be used if bolus therapy is unsuccessful.
4. Renal-dose dopamine (2–3 μg/kg/min) can be used early in the course of ARF, although it should not be continued if oliguria persists.
5. Dialysis or isolated ultrafiltration is indicated for congestive failure unresponsive to diuretics.

B. Metabolic status

1. Hyperkalemia
   a. Check ECG for acute changes.
   b. If ECG changes are present, give 10 mL of a 10% calcium gluconate IV to stabilize the cardiac membrane, in addition to the following measures, including dialysis.
   c. For $K^+$ < 6 mEq/liter:
      (1) Diuretics to augment urinary excretion
      (2) Kayexalate in sorbitol 30 g by mouth or per rectum every 3 to 4 hours
   d. For $K^+$ ≥ 6 mEq/liter or in the setting of oliguric ARF or ECG changes:
      (1) Inhaled beta-agonists
      (2) $NaHCO_3$ 1 mEq/kg
      (3) Glucose 50 g with regular insulin 10 units IV
      (4) Consider dialysis
2. Hyperphosphatemia
   a. Calcium acetate or calcium carbonate 3 to 4 times a day by mouth with meals to maintain normal phosphate.

## ACUTE RENAL FAILURE *CONTINUED*

        b. Aluminum-containing antacids can be used instead when the calcium $\times$ phosphate double product reaches 60 to 70.

   3. Acidosis

        a. Maintain pH $>7.2$.

        b. Calculate the $Hco_3$ deficit to partially correct serum $Hco_3$ to 18 to 20 mEq/liter:

          (1) $Hco_3$ deficit $=$ ($Hco_3$ desired $-$ measured $Hco_3$) $\times$ (0.6 $\times$ weight, kg)

        c. Rule out concurrent ketoacidosis in diabetics.

        d. Consider dialysis for severe metabolic acidosis in the setting of volume overload.

C. Nutritional support

   1. Daily protein intake of 0.8 g/kg/day $+$ 10 g, or up to 1.0 to 1.5 g/kg/day in ARF requiring dialysis.

   2. Caloric needs per the Harris-Benedict equation, or 30 to 35 kcal/kg/day in ARF requiring dialysis.

        a. BEE $=$ 655 $+$ (9.6 $\times$ weight, kg) $+$ (1.7 $\times$ height, cm) $-$ (4.7 $\times$ age) $+$ 250 kcal

   3. Potassium restriction 1 mEq/kg/day.

   4. Sodium restriction 2 to 4 g/day.

   5. Iron supplement 30 mg/day elemental iron.

   6. Calcium intake 1200 mg/day.

   7. Folate intake 400 $\mu$g/day.

   8. Phosphate restriction 1 g/day.

D. Indications for dialysis

   1. Uremic encephalopathy

   2. Uremic pericarditis

   3. Uremic platelet dysfunction and bleeding abnormalities

   4. Refractory volume overload

   5. Refractory metabolic acidosis, hyperkalemia, or other severe metabolic abnormalities

   6. Uremic symptoms including nausea/vomiting, sleep-wake reversal, pruritus, dysgeusia, etc.

   7. Moderate levels of azotemia:

        a. BUN $>60$ to 70 mg/dL

        b. Creatinine $>6$ to 7 mg/dL

**REFERENCES**

Antonovych TT, Mostofi FK. Atlas of kidney biopsies. Washington, DC: Armed Forces Institute of Pathology, 1981:266–275.

Bell WR, Braine HG, Ness PM, Kickler TS. Improved survival in thrombotic thrombocytopenic purpura-hemolytic uremic syndrome. N Engl J Med 1991;325:398–403.

Donohoe JF. Acute bilateral cortical necrosis. In: Brenner BM, Lazarus JM, eds. Acute renal failure. 1st ed. Philadelphia: WB Saunders, 1983: 252–269.

Gilstrap LC, Cunningham FG, Whalley PJ. Acute pyelonephritis during pregnancy: an anterospective study. Obstet Gynecol 1981;57:409–413.

Gordon M, Candon MB, Samuels P, et al. Perinatal outcome and long-term follow-up associated with modern management of diabetic nephropathy. Obstet Gynecol 1996;87:401.

Grunfeld JP, Pertuiset N. Acute renal failure in pregnancy. Am J Kidney Dis 1987;9:359–362.

Grunfeld JP, Ganeval D, Bournerias F. Acute renal failure in pregnancy. Kidney Int 1980;18:179–191.

Hayslett JP. Postpartum renal failure. N Engl J Med 1985;312:1556–1559.

Hayward CPM, Sutton DMC, Carter WH, et al. Treatment outcomes in patients with adult thrombotic thrombocytopenic purpura-hemolytic uremic syndrome. Arch Intern Med 1994;154:982–987.

Hou S. Acute and chronic renal failure in pregnancy. In: Clark SL, Cotton DB, Hankins GDV, Phelan JP, eds. Critical care obstetrics. Boston: Blackwell Scientific, 1991:429–463.

Jones DC, Hayslett JP. Outcome of pregnancy in women with moderate or severe renal insufficiency. N Engl J Med 1996;335:226.

Kaplan MM. Acute fatty liver of pregnancy. N Engl J Med 1985;313:367–370.

Krane NK. Acute renal failure in pregnancy. Arch Intern Med 1988;148:2347–2357.

Lindheimer MD, Cunningham FG. Renal diseases complicating pregnancy. In: Cunningham FG, MacDonald PC, Gant NF, et al, eds. Williams obstetrics. 19th ed. suppl 6. Norwalk, CT: Appleton & Lang, 1994.

Lindheimer MD, Katz AI, Ganeval D, et al. Acute renal failure in pregnancy. In: Brenner BN, Lazarus JM, eds. Acute renal failure. New York: Churchill Livingstone, 1988:597–620.

Martin JN, Blake PG, Perry KG, et al. The natural history of HELLP syndrome: patterns of disease progression and regression. Am J Obstet Gynecol 1991;164:1500–1513.

Pertuiset N, Ganeval D, Grunfeld JP. Acute renal failure in pregnancy: an update. Semin Nephrol 1984;3:232–239.

Rock GA, Shumak KH, Buskard NA, et al. Comparison of plasma exchange with plasma infusion in the treatment of thrombotic thrombocytopenic purpura. N Engl J Med 1991;325:393–397.

Satin AJ, Seiken GL, Cunningham FG. Reversible hypertension in pregnancy caused by obstructive obstetric uropathy. Obstet Gynecol 1993;81:823–825.

Stratta P, Canavese C, Dogliani M, et al. Pregnancy-related acute renal failure. Clin Nephrol 1989;32:14–20.

Thadhani R, Pascual M, Bonventre JV. Acute renal failure. N Engl J Med 1996;335:1448.

Turney JH, Ellis CM, Parsons FM. Obstetric acute renal failure 1956–1987. Br J Obstet Gynaecol 1989;96:679–687.

Usta IM, Barton JR, Amon EA, et al. Acute fatty liver of pregnancy: an experience in the diagnosis and management of fourteen cases. Am J Obstet Gynecol 1994;171:142–147.

Weiner CP. Thrombotic microangiopathy in pregnancy and the postpartum period. Semin Hematol 1987;24:119–129.

Whalley PJ, Cunningham FG, Martin FG. Transient renal dysfunction associated with acute pyelonephritis of pregnancy. Obstet Gynecol 1975;46:174–177.

The opinions or assertions contained herein are the private views of the author and are not to be construed as official or as reflecting the views of the Department of the Army or the Department of Defense.

# CHAPTER 17

# Severe Acute Asthma

*A* search of the Medline database (1991–1996) shows that since the last edition of this text, asthma has been the subject of more than 8500 medical journal articles, with more than 800 of these pertaining to severe asthma. Old therapies have become obsolete, new ones have been developed, and still, deaths due to asthma continue to increase (Arrighi, 1995). In 1992, using data from the National Center for Health Statistics, Weiss and colleagues (1992) reported that health-care costs for asthma in the United States exceeded $6.2 billion per year. Despite this enormous expenditure on asthma and the large volume of material available on the subject, the continued increase in asthma-associated mortality is disturbing. Spevetz and associates (1992) audited the medical records of asthma patients from a university teaching center. These authors found that, in general, the clinicians whose records were audited do not document the severity of illness, do not use objective measures to assess the disease, do not use appropriate medications, do not monitor the response to medications, and do not practice according to the current state of knowledge reflected in the literature.

The National Asthma Education Program (NAEP) of the National Heart, Lung, and Blood Institute (NHLBI) constitutes a significant step toward resolving some of this problem. This section of the National Institutes of Health has issued expert panel consensus reports concerning the management of asthma in adults and children and is taking great steps to disseminate the information. The report of the Working Group on Asthma and Pregnancy of the NAEP was published in 1993. While not meant as an official regulatory document, the report represents a broad consensus of obstetricians, reproductive toxicologists, pediatric and adult pharmacologists, allergists, maternal-fetal medicine specialists, and pulmonologists. The report is in the public domain and is available from the NHLBI Information Center online at *http://www.nhlbi.nih.gov/nhlbi/nhlbi.htm* or by calling 301-251-1222. Relying on the NAEP report and other recent publications, the specific purpose of this chapter is to review the current management of acute, life-threatening asthma in pregnancy.

## Definitions

In an attempt to consolidate the many diverse clinical definitions of *asthma*, the American Thoracic Society's Joint Committee on Pulmonary Nomenclature (1975) has defined *asthma* as "a disease characterized by an increased responsiveness of the airways to various stimuli, manifested by slowing of forced expiration, which changes in severity either spontaneously or as a result of therapy." The definition may be modified by including words indicating the etiology, such as *cold*, *exercise*, or *allergen-induced asthma. Status asthmaticus*, on the other hand, denotes severe asthma of any type not responding after a 30- to 60-minute period of intensive therapy (Summer, 1985; Koch-Weser, 1977). More recently, the terms *potentially fatal asthma*, *near-fatal asthma*, and *life-threatening asthma* have been used to denote particularly worrisome features that may be predictive of asthma mortality. Criteria for potentially fatal asthma include intubation for respiratory failure or respiratory arrest, respiratory acidosis without intubation, two or more hospitalizations despite oral corticosteroids, and two or more episodes of pneumothorax or pneumomediastinum associated with status asthmaticus (Miller, 1992). Life-threatening features include a peak expiratory flow rate (PEFR) less than 33% of predicted or personal best, silent chest, cyanosis, feeble respiratory effort, bradycardia, hypotension, exhaustion, confusion, and coma (Guidelines, 1993).

## Effect of Pregnancy on Asthma

Pregnancy may or may not affect the course of asthma in any individual patient. Turner et al (1980), summarizing the large retrospective studies published to date, reported that 22% of patients experienced improvement in their asthma, while 40% remained unchanged and another 20% noted worsening disease. In a prospective study of 366 pregnancies complicated by asthma, Schatz and colleagues (1988) tracked both symptoms and spirometry throughout gestation and the postpartum period. Of their subjects, 28% improved, 33% remained unchanged, 35% clearly worsened, and 4% demonstrated equivocal changes. In a subsequent prospective study with 198 pregnancies reported by Stenius-Aariala et al (1988), over 40% required additional therapy at some time during gestation.

Although predicting which gravida will experience exacerbations is generally not possible, several historic factors may be of help. Gluck and Gluck (1976) found that patients beginning pregnancy with severe disease were more likely to worsen than were those beginning with mild disease. Others have shown that the natural history of asthma during one pregnancy tends to be repeated in subsequent gestations (Schatz, 1988). Finally, these same authors have shown that approximately 10% of pregnant women with asthma will experience exacerbations during labor and delivery.

## Effect of Asthma on Perinatal Outcome

Asthma, especially when severe or uncontrolled, can substantially alter pregnancy outcome. Several authors have noted significant increases in rates of abortion, preterm labor, low birth weight, and neonatal hypoxia (Schaefer, 1961; Bahna, 1972; Sims, 1976). Reporting on 277 patients with asthma in the Collaborative Study of Cerebral Palsy, Mental Retardation, and Other Allied Neurological Diseases, Gordon et al (1970) found a perinatal mortality rate double that of controls without asthma. Furthermore, they found that in 16 patients with severe asthma (repetitive attacks, persistent symptoms, or status asthmaticus), the perinatal mortality rate was 28%. Greenberger and colleagues (Fitsimons, 1986; Greenberger, 1988) have shown that among women with asthma, those whose pregnancy is complicated by status asthmaticus have significantly smaller infants and a greater frequency of intrauterine growth retardation. Conversely, Shatz and coauthors (1995) reported that when asthma during pregnancy is controlled with step therapy, adverse perinatal outcomes are not increased over those in the general population. Despite reports that aggressive management can reduce perinatal morbidity and mortality, fetal deaths secondary to maternal asthma are described (Topilski, 1974; Sachs, 1987). Postulating a common smooth-muscle dysfunction, Lehrer and colleagues (1993) reported an association between pregnancy-induced hypertension and maternal asthma.

In addition to its implications for fetal outcome, severe asthma during pregnancy is associated with a small but definite risk to the life of the mother. Gordon et al (1970) reported four deaths among the 16 patients with severe disease from the Collaborative Group. Shaefer et al (1961), Schatz et al (1995), and Jewett (1973) have also described maternal status asthmaticus refractory to all therapy short of interrupting the pregnancy. When asthma becomes this severe, complications that directly threaten the life of the mother may include pneumothorax, pneumomediastinum, acute cor pulmonale, arrhythmias, and respiratory muscle fatigue. Levine and associates (1995) confirmed reversible severe myocardial depression with left ventricular ejection fractions between 11% and 34%. The gravity of these morbid complications is emphasized by a mortality rate over 40% when asthma has progressed to the point of requiring mechanical ventilation (Scoggin, 1977). Tragically, studies analyzing the causes of death in severe asthma have shown that most occur outside of a hospital and that the severity of the disease usually was not appreciated by the patient or the physician (Woolcock, 1988). Considering this, and that modern management of the severely asthmatic gravida can often avert fetal and maternal catastrophes, it is imperative that the obstetrician thoroughly evaluate and aggressively manage any pregnant woman presenting with reactive airway disease.

## Pathophysiology

Pathologic examination of the lung from patients who have died of status asthmaticus discloses several characteristic features. These include persistent hyperinflation, mucus plugging, detached bronchial epithelium, damage to extensive areas of the bronchial epithelium with exposed basal cells, infiltration with eosinophils, collagen deposition beneath the basement membrane, edema and vascular congestion, bronchial smooth-muscle hyperplasia, and goblet-cell hyperplasia (Beasely, 1993). Even patients with mild asthma show eosinophilic infiltrates throughout the bronchial wall; an increase in mast cells in the bronchial lamina propria, with evidence of degranulation; and collagen deposition beneath the bronchial epithelium (Beasely, 1993). This information confirms that asthma is not just a disease of intermittent acute airway narrowing, but is, more importantly, a chronic inflammatory process with increased bronchial reactivity.

Important biochemical mediators of asthma are listed in Table 17-1. Primary mediators are those released from lung tissue immediately upon challenge with an appropriate allergen, and they include histamine, slow-reacting substance of ana-phylaxis, eosinophil chemotactic factor (ECF), and platelet-activating factor (PAF) (Beasely, 1993; Austen, 1975). Histamine, released predominantly from macrophages, causes increased vasodilation, leaking venules, and direct bronchial smooth muscle contraction, which results in increased airway resistance and decreased compliance (Austen, 1975; Greenberger, 1985a). The eosinophil-rich mucus in the airways and eosinophilic infiltration of the airway walls are a tropic response to mast-cell release of ECF (Woolcock, 1988; Austen, 1975). Eosinophils produce several tissue-damaging proteins, including cationic proteins, peroxidase, and major basic protein, the ground substance found in the tenacious mucus of asthmatics (Kay, 1987). Slow-reacting substance of anaphylaxis, formed immediately before release by mast cells, causes increased vascular permeability and decreased lung compliance; simultaneously, PAF, produced by both mast cells and basophils, mediates platelet aggregation, which, in turn, may modulate production of the secondary mediators of asthma. Secondary mediators are the products of arachidonic acid metabolism and include the prostaglandins ($PGF_2$, $PGD_2$, $PGE_2$, $PGI_2$, and thromboxane $A_2$) and the leukotrienes ($LTC_4$, $LTD_4$, $LTB_4$, and $LTE_4$). $PGF_2$, $PGD_2$, thromboxane $A_2$, and $LTC_4$, $LTD_4$, and $LTE_4$ are all known to cause bronchoconstriction (Woolcock, 1988; Greenberger, 1985a; Weinberger, 1980).

Bronchial smooth-muscle hyperactivity and mediator release are thought to be influenced by intracellular levels of the nucleotides cAMP and cGMP (Koch-Weser, 1977; Fishburne, 1979). Beta-receptor stimulation of bronchial smooth muscle activates adenylate cyclase, raises the level of cAMP, and thus promotes relaxation and decreased mediator release (Koch-Weser, 1977; Austen, 1975). Vagally mediated cholinergic stimulation causes increased intracellular cGMP, which results in increased contractility and further release of the biochemical mediators (Koch-Weser, 1977; Austen, 1975). Beta-adrenergic receptors are found throughout the bronchial tree on smooth muscle and epithelial, alveolar, and circulating cells (Woolcock, 1988). Similarly, cholinergic nerves supply most of the bronchial tree, with receptors concentrated in smooth-muscle and mucus-producing cells (Woolcock, 1988).

T A B L E   **17-1**

Biochemical mediators of asthma

|  | Source | Actions |
|---|---|---|
| *Primary Mediators* | | |
| Histamine | Mast cells, macrophages | Vasodilation, leaking venules, bronchial smooth-muscle contraction |
| Slow-reacting substance of anaphylaxis | Mast cells, basophils, peripheral leukocytes | Bronchial smooth-muscle contraction, increased vascular permeability |
| Eosinophil chemotactic factor | Basophils, mast cells | Recruitment of eosinophils, release of tissue-damaging peroxidase, cationic and major base protein |
| Platelet-activating factor | Mast cells, basophils | Aggregation and degranulation of platelets, increased secondary mediators |
| *Secondary Mediators* | | |
| Prostaglandins: $PGF_2$, $PGE_2$, $PGD_2$, $PGI_2$, thromboxane | Phospholipid membrane substrate | Alterations in bronchial smooth-muscle tone, alteration in pulmonary vascular resistance |
| Leukotrienes: $LTC_4$, $LTD_4$, $LTE_4$ | Phospholipid membranes | Bronchoconstriction chemotaxis of neutrophils and eosinophils |

Bronchospasm and mediator release may be precipitated by a number of different stimuli. *Extrinsic asthma* is the result of immunoglobulin E (IgE)-mediated mast-cell recognition of a specific allergen (Woolcock, 1988). Cross-bridging of IgE molecules alters cell membrane permeability to calcium ions, whose influx promotes the activity of $Ca^{++}$-dependent enzymes and eventually alters the relative amounts of the cyclic nucleotides. *Intrinsic asthma* occurs in a patient without evidence of atopy. Bronchospasm may be precipitated by numerous other stimuli, including cold, exercise, or occupational agents. Finally, infection, especially viral syndromes, may cause bronchospasm. Several authors have noted decreased leukocyte responses to beta-adrenergic stimulation during viral illnesses (Safko, 1981).

## Clinical Course

The functional result of bronchospasm is airway obstruction with a concomitant decrease in airflow. As airways constrict, the work of breathing increases and patients then present with chest tightness, wheezing, or breathlessness. Subsequent alterations in oxygenation are primarily the result of ventilation/perfusion (V/Q) mismatching, because the distribution of airway narrowing during an acute attack is uneven (Rodriguez-Roisin, 1989). With mild disease, initial hypoxia is well compensated, as reflected by a normal arterial oxygen tension and decreased carbon dioxide, with resultant respiratory alkalosis. As airway narrowing worsens, V/Q defects increase, and hypoxemia ensues. With severe obstruction, ventilation becomes impaired enough to result in early carbon dioxide retention. Superimposed on hyperventilation, this may only be seen as an arterial carbon dioxide tension returning to the normal range. Finally, with critical obstruction, respiratory failure follows, characterized by hypoxemia, hypercarbia, and acidemia. At this extreme, oxygen consumption and cardiac work are increased, and the magnitude of pulmonary hypertension is frequently severe (Rodriguez-Roisin, 1989; Kingston, 1984). The clinical stages of asthma are presented in Table 17-2.

T A B L E    **17-2**

Clinical stages of asthma

| Stage | Arterial Blood Gases | | | FEV$_1$, Peak Flow % Predicted | Comment |
|---|---|---|---|---|---|
| | Po$_2$ | Pco$_2$ | pH | | |
| I | Normal | ↓ | ↑ | 65–80 | Mild respiratory alkalosis |
| II | ↓ | ↓ | ↑ | 50–64 | Respiratory alkalosis |
| III | ↓ | Normal | Normal | 35–49 | Danger zone |
| IV | ↓ | ↑ | ↓ | 35– | Respiratory acidosis |

Au: Range?

Po$_2$, pressure of oxygen; Pco$_2$, pressure of carbon dioxide; FEV$_1$, forced expiratory volume (1 second).

While such changes in pulmonary function are generally reversible and well tolerated in the healthy nonpregnant individual, even the early stages of asthma may pose grave risk to the gravida and her fetus. Maternal factors responsible for this include (1) increased basal metabolic rate and oxygen consumption, (2) a decreased diffusing capacity, (3) decreased available buffer, and (4) pregnancy-induced alterations in lung volumes (Sachs, 1987; Weinberger, 1980; Fishburne, 1979; Greenberger, 1985b; Cugell, 1953). Most importantly, as pregnancy progresses, functional residual capacity (FRC) decreases 10% to 25% and frequently falls below the critical closing volume, a phenomenon much more likely to occur during the advanced stages of pregnancy (Garrard, 1978; Awe, 1979). The smaller FRC and the increased effective shunt thus render the gravida more rapidly susceptible to the effects of hypoxia. Clinically, only 30 seconds of apnea are needed to drop maternal arterial oxygen tension to less than 60 mm Hg (Levinson, 1987). As the mother increases ventilation to maintain oxygen tension, respiratory alkalosis develops.

Data from both sheep and human studies have shown that maternal alkalosis may cause dangerous hypoxemia in the fetus before maternal oxygenation is compromised (Moya, 1965; Rolston, 1974). Mechanisms proposed to explain this include decreased uterine blood flow, de-creased maternal venous return, and an alkaline-induced leftward shift of the hemoglobin-oxygen dissociation curve (Rolston, 1974; Wulf, 1972; Bartels, 1962). The latter mechanism, known as the Bohr effect, appears to become clinically significant when the maternal carbon dioxide tension and hypoxemia develops; the fetus responds with decreased umbilical blood flow, increased systemic and pulmonary vascular resistance, and ultimately decreased cardiac output (Brinkman, 1970). Because the fetus may be in jeopardy before maternal disease becomes severe, it is again emphasized that the obstetrician should take an aggressive approach to the management of any pregnant woman presenting with asthma.

## Differential Diagnosis

While over 60% of pregnant women experience a physiologic dyspnea of pregnancy, severe shortness of breath and wheezing are clearly abnormal (Weinberger, 1980; Cugell, 1953). Although a careful history and physical examination can usually assure the diagnosis, other life-threatening entities that must be excluded include severe allergic reactions, aspiration pneumonitis, pulmonary edema, pulmonary emboli, amniotic fluid embolus, left heart failure, and mitral stenosis (Weinberger, 1980; Cugell, 1953). Large airway obstruction from either a foreign body or an endobronchial tumor also should be considered. Mettam and colleagues (1992) have reported a case in which life-threatening acute respiratory distress in late pregnancy was caused by an enlarged thyroid and resultant external airway compression.

## Clinical Management

Although several authors have proposed the use of clinical scoring systems to predict the severity of asthma, its response to therapy, or the need for hospitalization, the prospective application of these formulas has shown them to be frequently misleading (Baker, 1988). Furthermore, their use has not been applied to or tested in a pregnant population. Recalling that fetal oxygenation may be jeopardized even with early stages of asthma, and that pregnant women are poorly tolerant of rapid ventilatory derangements, prompt and thorough evaluation and treatment of any pregnant woman with acute asthma is imperative.

The NAEP Working Group on Asthma and Pregnancy (1993) lists the essential components of effective management of asthma for pregnant women as (1) objective measures for assessment and monitoring maternal lung function and fetal well-being in order to make appropriate therapeutic recommendations, (2) avoiding or controlling asthma triggers in the patient's environment, (3) pharmacologic therapy, and (4) patient education. For guidance in the management of chronic mild, moderate, and severe asthma and home management of acute asthma, the reader is referred to the text and charts contained in the report from this working group. Importantly, the authors of the report stress that patients attempting home therapy of an acute exacerbation "should not delay in seeking medical help if therapy does not provide rapid improvement, if the improvement is not sustained, if there is further deterioration, if the asthma exacerbation is severe, or if the fetal kick count decreases." This chapter concentrates on the management of pregnant women who present with acute severe asthma or life-threatening asthma.

## History and Physical Examination

A patient's subjective impression of the severity of her asthma frequently does not accurately reflect objective measures of airway function or ventilation. McFadden and colleagues (1973), in a classic work correlating subjective complaints with measures of lung mechanics, have shown that when patients thought their asthma had resolved, mean 1-second forced expiratory volume ($FEV_1$) and mid-expiratory flow rates were still only 20% and 22% of predicted values, respectively. Although others have confirmed a poor correlation between dyspnea and objective assessment of airway obstruction, Rees et al (1967) have shown that when dyspnea is so severe as to interfere with normal speech, the $FEV_1$ is consistently less than 0.45/1 min. Several historic factors should warn the physician of the possibility of rapid progression and potentially fatal airway obstruction. These include prior intubation for asthma, two or more hospitalizations for asthma in the past year, three or more emergency care visits for asthma in the past year, hospitalization or an emergency care visit for asthma within the past month, current use of systemic corticosteroids or recent withdrawal from systemic corticosteroids, history of syncope or hypoxic seizure due to asthma, prior admission for asthma to a hospital-base intensive care unit, and serious psychiatric disease or psychosocial problems (Working Group, 1993; Miller, 1992). Miller and associates (1992) have demonstrated that major psychiatric diagnoses and noncompliance are significantly related to cases of potentially fatal asthma, emphasizing the importance of increased vigilance when caring for these patients.

Physical examination of the patient with asthma, while helpful in establishing the diagnosis, is also an inaccurate predictor of the severity of airway disease. Several authors have shown that expiratory wheezing correlates with neither objective measures of airflow nor derangements in arterial blood gas analysis (McFadden, 1973; Corre, 1985). Indeed, an increase in auscultated wheezing may indicate an increase in airflow, while the absence of wheezing may indicate critical airway narrowing and absent flow (Corre,

1985). Physical signs that should warn the clinician of life-threatening or severe asthma include labored breathing, tachycardia, pulsus paradoxus of greater than 10 mm Hg, prolonged expiration, and use of accessory muscles of respiration. Signs that may warn of a potentially fatal attack include difficulty speaking, central cyanosis, and altered consciousness.

## Pulmonary Function Tests

Clinical management is most appropriately guided by the use of pulmonary function tests. Measurement of either the $FEV_1$ or the PEFR can help to assess the severity of obstruction and to monitor the response to therapy. A classic work by Sims et al (1976) has shown that pulmonary function tests in stable asthmatics, active asthmatics, and non-asthmatic controls are not altered by pregnancy. Brancazio (1997) reported mean peak expiratory flow rates in normal pregnant women of 430–450 liter/min, with valves not changing significantly as pregnancy progresses. Unfortunately, complex bedside spirometry equipment is not commonly available. Peak flow rates, however, may now be measured with simple, hand-held devices that are operated entirely by the patient (Mini-Wright, Armstrong Medical Industries, Lincoln, IL). Predicted values based on age, height, and gender have been published in nomogram form but, in general, range between 380 and 550 liters/min for women (Gregg, 1989). Summarizing several large studies that recorded peak flow rates in acute asthma, Corre et al (1985) concluded that values less than 100 liters/min correlate well with severe obstruction. Rather than relying on predicted normal values, Clark and the NAEP Working Group (1993) recommend that pregnant women should establish their own personal best PEFR after a period of monitoring when the asthma has been well controlled. Whether one uses a percent of predicted normal or personal best, pulmonary function tests should not be used to the exclusion of arterial blood gas assessment for pregnant women. Tai and Road (1967) have demonstrated a $PaO_2$ less than 60 mm Hg in over 16% of acute asthmatics whose $FEV_1$ was 1.0 li-

ters or more. Because a maternal $PaO_2$ of less than 60 mm Hg is associated with a rapid decline in fetal oxygenation, relying solely on reassuring pulmonary function tests could prove detrimental to an already stressed fetus. Pulmonary function test results that identify life-threatening or potentially fatal asthma for the mother include a peak flow less than 100 liters/min, an $FEV_1$ less than 25% of predicted, or less than a 10% improvement in peak flow or $FEV_1$ with treatment in the emergency department (NAEP Working Group, 1993).

## Arterial Blood Gases

While clinical signs and symptoms with acute asthma may prove misleading, arterial blood gas analysis allows direct assessment of maternal oxygenation, ventilation, and acid-base status. With this information, the clinician can correctly assess the severity of an acute attack (see Table 17-2). Care must be taken, however, to interpret the results in light of normal values for pregnancy. A normal maternal $PaO_2$ varies from 101 to 108 mm Hg early in pregnancy and falls to 90 to 100 mm Hg near term secondary to an increased critical closing volume, as previously discussed (Weinberger, 1980; Noble, 1988). These changes are responsible for the widened alveolar-arterial oxygen gradient $[P(A-a)O_2]$, which averages 20 mm Hg in the third trimester (Awe, 1979). The normal physiologic increase in minute ventilation during pregnancy is reflected by a $PaCO_2$ of 27 to 32 mm Hg and an increase in pH from 7.40 to 7.45 (Noble, 1988; Hankins, 1996). Consequently, a $PaCO_2$ greater than 35 mm Hg, with a pH less than 7.35 in the presence of a falling $PaO_2$, should be considered respiratory failure in a pregnant asthmatic.

As discussed, arterial blood gas assessment should be used liberally in the management of pregnant women presenting with an acute exacerbation of asthma. Guidance from the NAEP Working Group (1993) suggests that arterial blood gases must be assessed when patients present with obvious hypoventilation, cyanosis, or severe distress after initial therapy, or if the peak flow is less than 200 liters/min or the $FEV_1$ remains less than 40% of predicted. Finally, initiation of therapy for acute asthma in pregnancy should not be delayed while performing or awaiting the results of pulmonary function tests or arterial blood gas analysis.

## Other Laboratory Tests

When patients without an established history of asthma present with wheezing and respiratory distress, clinicians should consider an initial ECG, because these may be the signs of a more serious cardiac disease. The ECG in acute asthma may show right bundle branch block, acute enlargement of the right atrium, and ventricular ectopy (Kingston, 1984). Additionally, institution of a bronchodilator may precipitate or worsen such arrhythmias (Koch-Weser, 1977). Pulse oximetry should be employed to monitor maternal oxygenation to ensure maintenance of an oxygen saturation greater than 95% (NAEP Working Group, 1993). If the patient is febrile or in severe distress, a chest x-ray should be obtained to rule out pneumonia or one of the severe complications of asthma, such as pneumothorax or pneumomediastinum. A Gram stain and microscopic examination of the sputum should be done to rule out a contribution from bacterial pneumonia or bronchitis (Woolcock, 1988). When the diagnosis of asthma is in question, demonstration of eosinophils on microscopic examination of the sputum may help narrow the differential (NAEP Working Group, 1993). Finally, when patients present with asthma exacerbations in the third trimester, intensive continuous electronic fetal monitoring should be considered. As mentioned previously, significant fetal hypoxemia can occur prior to significant maternal compromise. Decreased fetal movement and hypoxic decelerations on the monitor may alert the clinician to significant fetal distress not otherwise apparent. In a similar manner, persistent evidence of fetal hypoxia, such as diminished variability or repetitive late decelerations, may suggest the need for increased hydration or oxygenation, even in the nominally stable mother.

## Treatment

Ultimate goals in the treatment of severe acute asthma in pregnancy are the prevention of maternal and fetal mortality and morbidity. Therapy should be directed toward correcting maternal hypoxia, relieving bronchospasm, assuring adequate ventilation, and optimizing uteroplacental function. Recommendations on treatment setting vary. Whether evaluated and treated in the emergency department, labor and delivery, or an observation unit, the location is not as important as the unit's capabilities. Monitoring and resuscitative equipment should be readily available (including electronic fetal heart rate monitoring if in the third trimester), and if a severe exacerbation or life-threatening asthma is suspected, provisions for intubation and ventilation should be accessible, preferably in an intensive care unit. Guidelines from both the American College of Obstetricians and Gynecologists (1996) and the NAEP Working Group on Asthma and Pregnancy (1993), suggest that in patients who respond rapidly (an $FEV_1$ or PEFR $> 70\%$ of predicted) to bronchodilator therapy, follow-up may be continued on an outpatient basis. As discussed previously, however, clinicians caring for a pregnant woman and her fetus should have a low threshold for admission to the hospital. Clinicians should be especially liberal with admission to the hospital if the patient presents in the evening, has had the recent onset of nocturnal symptoms, has had previous episodes of severe exacerbations, or if there are concerns about social circumstances or the relatives' ability to respond if the condition should worsen (Guidelines, 1993).

The first step in treatment is administration of supplemental oxygen to the mother, with a goal of maintaining a $Pao_2$ greater than 65 mm Hg or an oxygen saturation of 95% on oxygen ($Fio_2$) of 35% to 60%, without causing hypercarbia. The patient should be placed in a near-sitting position, with leftward tilt, especially if in the third trimester. Awe and colleagues (1979) have shown that in the third trimester, more than 25% of normal pregnant women will develop moderate hypoxia in the supine position. In their series, simply sitting the patient up in bed changed the mean $P(A-a)o_2$ from 20 to 14 mm Hg.

Intravenous (IV) access should be achieved, both for administration of medications and for careful rehydration. Patients presenting in extremis are frequently volume depleted if they have been too breathless to maintain oral intake at a time when insensible losses are high (Fish, 1982). In such circumstances, rehydration may help prevent inspissation of mucus plugs and may aid in expectoration (Summer, 1985; Sawicka, 1987).

## Adrenergic Agents

The first-line pharmacologic therapy of acute severe asthma in pregnancy should consist of an inhaled beta$_2$-adrenergic agonist (NAEP Working Group, 1993; Guidelines, 1993; Clark, 1993). These agents, when used alone, produce a greater degree of bronchodilation than either methylxanthines or anticholinergic drugs (Chaieb, 1989). Evidence now suggests that there is no clear advantage to the use of parenteral rather than inhaled beta$_2$-agonists in patients with asthma

(Leatherman, 1994). Although ingrained in clinical practice, administration of these agents via a wet nebulizer offers no advantage over the supervised use of a metered-dose inhaler plus a holding chamber, and it is significantly more expensive (Idris, 1993; Calocone, 1993; Newhouse, 1993). Furthermore, in severe cases (FEV$_1$ < 30% of predicted), Idris and colleagues (1993) noted a trend toward faster improvement with a metered-dose inhaler plus holding chamber. If, for some reason, patients cannot effectively use a metered-dose inhaler or wet nebulizer, beta$_2$-agonists can be administered subcutaneously. Table 17-3 includes the more common adrenergic agents, their dosages, and their possible routes of administration.

Recent epidemiologic studies have demonstrated an association between the regular use of beta-agonists and an increased risk of death due to asthma (Crane, 1989; Spitzer, 1992). As emphasized by Burrows and Lebowitz (1992) in a *New England Journal of Medicine* editorial, however, this "should not be interpreted as an

T A B L E   **17-3**

**Medications used in the treatment of acute severe asthma**

| | **Drug** | **Route of Administration and Dosage** |
|---|---|---|
| Inhaled beta-agonists | Albuterol | Nebulizer; 2.5–5.0 mg (0.5–1.0 mL of a 5% solution, diluted with 2–3 mL normal saline)<br>MDI with a holding chamber (90 μg/puff given as 4 puffs over 4 min) |
| | Metaproterenol | Nebulizer; 15 mg (0.3 mL of a 5% solution, diluted with 2–3 mL normal saline) |
| Subcutaneous beta-agonists | Epinephrine | 0.3 mg subcutaneously |
| | Terbutaline | 0.25 mg subcutaneously |
| Corticosteroids | Methylprednisolone | 60–80 mg IV bolus every 6–8 hr or 125 mg IV bolus followed by above or oral steroids, depending on response |
| | Hydrocortisone | 2.0 mg/kg IV bolus every 4 hr or<br>2.0 mg/kg IV bolus then 0.5 mg/kg/hr continuous infusion |
| Anticholinergics | Ipratropium bromide | Nebulizer; 0.5 mg (one vial 0.02% solution)<br>MDI; 18 μg/puff, 2–3 puffs |
| | Glycopyrrolate | Nebulizer; 0.8–2.0 mg |
| Magnesium sulfate | | 2-g IV bolus over 2 min (followed immediately by inhaled beta$_2$-agonist) |
| Methylxanthine | Aminophylline | Loading dose of 6 mg/kg actual body weight, followed by continuous IV infusion at 0.4–0.6 mg/kg/hr (must follow serum theophylline levels with a goal of 8–12 μg/mL during pregnancy) |

MDI, metered-dose inhaler; IV, intravenous.

indication that inhaled beta-agonists are themselves harmful or that patients should stop taking them altogether." Whether the chronic use of beta-agonists causes an increased risk of death or is just a marker of more severe disease, the regular use of beta-agonists alone in chronic asthma is no longer recommended (Burrows, 1992). On the other hand, these drugs remain the agents of choice for severe acute asthma and life-threatening asthma.

Beta-agonists act in concert with specific cell-surface receptors to activate the membrane-associated enzyme, adenyl cyclase. Adenyl cyclase then promotes the conversion of adenosine triphosphate to cyclic adenosine-3′,5′-monophosphate (cAMP). Increased intracellular cAMP then mediates relaxation of bronchial smooth muscle, prevents further contraction, increases clearance of mucus, and prevents mediator release, as described earlier (Koch-Weser, 1977). Beta$_2$-adrenergic receptors are located primarily in the bronchia, blood vessels, pancreas, and uterus, while beta$_1$ receptors are confined largely to the heart (Koch-Weser, 1977). Nonbronchodilator effects of beta$_2$-agonists that may play a role in asthma include the following: (1) increased mucociliary clearance, (2) inhibition of cholinergic neurotransmission, (3) enhancement of vascular integrity, and (4) inhibition of mediator release from mast cells, basophils, and other cells (Nelson, 1995).

One side effect of beta-agonists that is observed when they are used specifically for severe asthma is a paradoxical decrease in $PaO_2$ and oxygen saturation soon after initiation of therapy (Koch-Weser, 1977; Nelson, 1995). This is a transient phenomenon secondary to the beta$_1$-mediated increase in cardiac output that occurs before effective bronchodilation and possible relief of compensatory hypoxic pulmonary vasoconstriction. Contraindications to beta-adrenergic therapy include coronary artery disease, cardiac asthma, and cerebrovascular disease (Koch-Weser, 1977). While these are rare in the reproductive age group, cases of symptomatic cerebral ischemia following beta-adrenergic therapy have been reported in pregnant women with a history of severe migraines (Oserne, 1982). Nonetheless, Shatz and colleagues (1988) have demonstrated

the safety of beta$_2$-agonists for asthma during pregnancy in a large prospective study. Comparing 259 pregnant asthmatics using beta-agonists with 101 using other bronchodilators, the authors found no difference in rates of intrauterine growth retardation, congenital anomalies, or perinatal mortality.

## Corticosteroids

For patients not responding immediately to bronchodilators and for those already taking regular oral corticosteroids, systemic steroids should be administered (NAEP Working Group, 1993; ACOG, 1996). Specifically, corticosteroids should also be started immediately for patients with a peak flow rate less than 200 liters/min or an $FEV_1$ less than or equal to 40% of predicted after an initial hour of beta$_2$-agonist therapy (NAEP Working Group, 1993). Systemic corticosteroids should be given immediately to any patient presenting with signs or symptoms of life-threatening or potentially fatal asthma (Leatherman, 1994).

Glucocorticoids enter the cell by diffusion, bind to a specific cytoplasmic receptor, and are rapidly transported to the nucleus. There, nuclear gene expression is altered, messenger RNA is formed, and proteins subsequently produced then mediate specific pharmacologic effects (Morris, 1985a, 1985b). Additionally, corticosteroids have a more immediate action, altering calcium entry into cells and affecting calcium-dependent enzyme systems such as the phospholipases (Morris, 1985b). Pharmacologic effects thought to play a role in acute asthma include (1) direct bronchial smooth-muscle relaxation; (2) constriction of the bronchial microvasculature, with reduced capillary permeability and reduced edema formation; (3) decreased activity and number of circulating inflammatory cells; (4) increased prostaglandin formation; and, perhaps most importantly, (5) increased responsiveness to beta-adrenergic stimulation (Beasely, 1993; Morris, 1985a, 1985b; Spector, 1985). This potentiation of beta-adrenergic therapy is seen within 1 to 2 hours of steroid administration (Ellul-Micallef, 1975). Finally, corticosteroids have been noted to improve V/Q mismatching in status asthmaticus, possibly as a result of altered prostaglandin metabolism and pulmonary perfusion (Pierson, 1974; Winfield, 1980).

Two separate studies have established the efficacy of early administration of parenteral corticosteroids in acute severe asthma. In a randomized, prospective, double-blind study using hydrocortisone for the treatment of acute asthma, Fanta and colleagues (1983) found an increase in both the rate and the magnitude of improvement in $FEV_1$ when compared with controls. In a similar study, Littenberg and Gluck (1986) found that early administration of a 125-mg IV bolus of methylprednisolone helped to terminate the acute attack, alleviate symptoms, and decrease the need for hospitalization. Not all clinical trials have demonstrated a benefit to the early administration of corticosteroids. A randomized, double-blind clinical trial conducted by Rodrigo and Rodrigo (1994) was unable to detect a difference in the duration of bronchodilator therapy, hospital admission rates, or length of stay when early administration of 500 mg of IV hydrocortisone was compared with placebo in patients receiving aggressive beta$_2$-agonist therapy. In a similar trial, McNamara and Rubin (1993) demonstrated that early administration does decrease subsequent relapse rates in patients presenting with acute asthma exacerbations. Wendel (1996) prospectively studied 84 pregnant women with asthma, and demonstrated a clear superiority of corticosteroids over aminophylline in the treatment of asthma exacerbation.

In the setting of acute severe asthma, corticosteroids should be administered parenterally. Although inhaled corticosteroids (beclomethasone dipropionate) are now available, they have little systemic action and do not affect the lung parenchyma. Even though beclomethasone has been reported safe for severe asthma during pregnancy, it does not have a role in the acute management of women with status asthmaticus (Greenberger, 1983). Inhaled corticosteroids or a nonsteroidal antiinflammatory drug such as nedocromil or cromolyn sodium, however, should be used regularly by patients with chronic moderate and severe asthma or by those thought to be at high risk. Recommendations for dosing systemic corticosteroids in acute severe asthma are included in Table 17-3.

Maternal side effects from corticosteroids are largely limited to long-term use. The two potential effects from short-term use are salt retention and possible suppression of the hypothalamic-pituitary-adrenal axis. If sodium retention is thought to be a concern, methylprednisolone should be used in lieu of hydrocortisone. Finally, if follow-up on oral therapy is used, 40 mg of prednisone per day for 10 days is sufficient, and tapering the dose is not necessary (O'Driscoll, 1993). The sum of animal and human toxicologic data regarding short-term use of systemic corticosteroids does not support an increase in adverse fetal effects (NAEP Working Group, 1993). In fact, Fitzsimons and colleagues (1986) have noted that adverse fetal outcomes were more likely when maternal asthma was poorly controlled or complicated by status asthmaticus.

## Anticholinergic Agents

Although they are less potent bronchodilators than the beta-agonists, anticholinergic agents may have a role in the management of acute severe asthma that is not responding to usual therapy (Leatherman, 1994; Chapman, 1996). Parasympathetic or cholinergic stimulation increases the activity of guanylate cyclase, which raises intracellular cGMP, causing mediator release and bronchial smooth-muscle contraction (Woolcock, 1988). Currently available anticholinergic agents include atropine, glycopyrrolate, and ipratropium bromide. Published experience with these agents varies. Reporting the results of a randomized clinical trial that compared 1.5 mg of atropine versus 15 mg of metaproterenol via nebulizer in patients not responding to standard therapy, Young and Freitas (1991) concluded that atropine was of no benefit. Two clinical trials using nebulized glycopyrrolate also failed to demonstrate significant improvements in bronchodilation when compared with beta$_2$-agonists (Gilman, 1990; Cydulka, 1994). Data on the efficacy of ipratropium bromide, a synthetic derivative of atropine, are more convincing. Rebuck and associates (1987) randomized patients with asthma to nebulized fenoterol (a beta$_2$-agonist), fenoterol and ipratropium, and ipratropium alone. These authors demonstrated better improvement in the $FEV_1$ at 45 and 90 minutes with combined therapy when compared with either therapy used alone. In a smaller study, O'Driscoll and colleagues (1989) randomized patients with asthma to salbutamol versus salbutamol plus ipratropium and found that the improvement in PEFR at 1 hour was greater with the combined therapy (31% vs. 77%). Most authors now suggest that ipratropium bromide may benefit some patients and that its use should be considered when the initial response to beta₂-agonists is suboptimal (Leatherman, 1994; Chapman, 1996). Dosages and routes of administration of the anticholinergic medications that may be used in acute severe asthma are listed in Table 17-3. Again, the sum of animal and human toxicology studies suggests that anticholinergic therapy is not associated with adverse fetal effects (NAEP Working Group, 1993).

## Theophylline

Theophylline is a methylxanthine that, in large concentrations, inhibits the action of phosphodiesterase and results in intracellular accumulation of cAMP (Koch-Weser, 1977). Although this has long been thought to be the major mechanism of action involved in bronchodilation, concentrations of theophylline that relax bronchial smooth muscle do not inhibit phosphodiesterase (Rossing, 1989; Berstrand, 1980). Other mechanisms of action established for theophylline that may play a role in the management of acute severe asthma include decreased fatigue in diaphragmatic muscles, increased mucociliary clearance, decreased microvascular leakage of plasma in airways, and a CNS effect that blocks the decrease in ventilation that occurs with sustained hypoxia (Weinberger, 1996). Long-term use appears to have immunomodulatory, antiinflammatory, and bronchoprotective effects (Weinberger, 1996).

Theophylline is available for clinical use in the form of aminophylline, an ethylenediamine salt constituting 80% theophylline by weight. For the patient not currently taking a theophylline preparation, dosing should begin with an initial 6-mg/kg IV bolus over 20 minutes. Because the volume of distribution is increased in pregnancy, doses should be based on actual body weight (NAEP Working Group, 1993). The loading dose should be followed by an IV infusion of 0.5 to 0.7 mg/kg/hr. Theophylline clearance in the third trimester falls between 20% and 50% (Gardner, 1987; Carter, 1986). Maternal toxic effects may include nausea and vomiting, abdominal pain, insomnia, irritability, agitation, seizures, and ventricular arrhythmias (Koch-Weser, 1977). Case reports of minor neonatal toxicity have been recorded when maternal levels at delivery were therapeutic (Yeh, 1977; Arwood, 1979). Consequently, even though no major fetal toxic effects have been seen, the NAEP Working Group currently recommends a therapeutic range for pregnancy between 8 μg/mL and 12 μg/mL (NAEP Working Group, 1993).

The efficacy of aminophylline in the modern management of status asthmaticus remains controversial. Most clinical trials have failed to show any added benefit when aminophylline was used to augment beta-adrenergic therapy of acute severe asthma (Fanta, 1982; Siegel, 1985; Josephson, 1979; Strauss, 1994; Murphy, 1993). Considering its lack of proven benefit, narrow therapeutic range, and frequent side effects, as well as the availability of more effective agents, theophylline is not the first choice of therapy for status asthmaticus. To conclude that theophylline plays no role in life-threatening or potentially fatal asthma, however, would be premature. Noting that patients with respiratory failure were excluded from most of the clinical trials for ethical reasons, Weinberger and Hendeles (1996) suggest that "the addition of theophylline to drug therapy may be justified for patients with severe acute symptoms that do not respond to other measures." Current guidelines from the NAEP Expert Panel Report (NHLBI, NIH) (1991) continue to list theophylline in the text and flow charts for patients failing to respond to standard therapy and for those with impending respiratory failure.

## Magnesium Sulfate

While more familiar to obstetricians as a tocolytic agent or as an effective drug for seizure prophylaxis in preeclampsia, IV magnesium sulfate may play a role in acute severe asthma. Several case reports and small case series suggest that IV magnesium sulfate is an effective bronchodilator, especially in cases not responding to more conventional therapy with beta$_2$-agonists and corticosteroids (Noppen, 1990; Okayama, 1991; Kuitert, 1991; Sydow, 1993). Clinical trials using magnesium sulfate in acute asthma have produced mixed results. Tiffany and colleagues (1993) randomized patients with acute asthma to one of three groups: (1) a 2-g IV infusion over 20 minutes followed by an infusion of 2 g over 4 hours, (2) a 2-g infusion over 20 minutes plus a placebo infusion, and (3) a placebo bolus and placebo infusion. While these authors noted no significant improvements in measures of expiratory flow with magnesium, they did note a trend toward improvement in female patients. Green and Rothrock (1992) were unable to demonstrate a difference in the required duration of treatment, need for hospitalization, or peak flows in patients with acute asthma when a 2-g infusion over 20 minutes was added to conventional therapy soon after presentation to the emergency department. Conversely, among 38 patients not responding to conventional therapy with beta$_2$-agonists, Skobeloff and colleagues (1989) demonstrated significant improvement in PEFR and a lower hospital admission rate among patients randomized to IV magnesium sulfate when compared with placebo. One explanation for the mixed results seen in clinical trials may be the varied rates of administration of the initial magnesium bolus. Noting that a 2-g IV bolus given rapidly over 2 minutes seemed to avert the impending need for intubation in patients progressing to respiratory failure, Shiermeyer and Finkelstein (1994) suggested that the hot flushes and the slight drop in BP were markers for immediate smooth-muscle relaxation associated with the rapid bolus. Noting that such rapid boluses of 4 to 6 g are safely administered in obstetric patients for other reasons, these authors suggested that the immediate and short-lived bronchodilator effect may allow a window of opportunity to more effectively deliver nebulized beta$_2$-agonists to the target tissues. In summary, this experience suggests that clinicians should consider the administration of a rapid bolus of magnesium sulfate for patients who

are not responding to conventional therapy and who are approaching respiratory failure and the need for intubation.

## Refractory Status Asthmaticus and Respiratory Failure

Pregnant women with severe asthma and impending respiratory failure ($P_{ACO_2} \geq 35$ mm Hg or measured expiratory flow less than 25% of predicted) should be managed in an intensive care unit (NAEP Working Group, 1993; Clark, 1993). Indications for intubation of the gravida with status asthmaticus include (1) inability to maintain a $P_{AO_2}$ of greater than 60 mm Hg with 90% hemoglobin saturation despite supplemental oxygen, (2) inability to maintain a $P_{CO_2}$ less than 40 mm Hg, (3) evidence of maternal exhaustion, (4) worsening acidosis despite intensive bronchodilator therapy (pH < 7.2–25), and (5) altered maternal consciousness (NAEP Working Group, 1993; Nolde, 1988; Leatherman, 1994; Hankins, 1987). Importantly, individualization and clinical judgment must play a role in the decision to perform endotracheal intubation. Neither hypercapnia nor respiratory acidosis without cardiorespiratory arrest or altered consciousness are in every case an indication for intubation before intensive bronchodilator therapy (Leatherman, 1994).

Intubation may be accomplished either orally or via a nasotracheal tube. Conventional guidance has been to use the oral route with the largest possible caliber tube to minimize airflow resistance (O'Donnell, 1995). The clinical importance of this step, however, may have been overrated, and some authorities now recommend nasotracheal intubation for the alert, spontaneously breathing patient (Leatherman, 1994). Regardless of the route, tracheal intubation in the asthmatic patient should be preceded by 1 to 2 mg of nebulized atropine (or 0.5 mg subcutaneously) to prevent airway spasm and worsening airway obstruction (Leatherman, 1994).

Management of the pregnant patient with asthma-related respiratory failure requiring endotracheal intubation should be supervised by clinicians with special training and expertise in mechanical ventilation of patients with life-threatening asthma. Alterations in respiratory mechanics associated with severe asthma include increased resistance to inspiratory and expiratory flow, with resultant gas trapping or dynamic hyperinflation (DHI) (Maltais, 1994). Also referred to as intrinsic positive end-expiratory pressure, or auto-PEEP, the magnitude of DHI in mechanically ventilated patients is determined largely by tidal volume, expiratory time, and the degree of resistance to expiratory flow. When DHI becomes severe, the resulting cardiovascular sequelae may include decreased venous return, hypotension, decreased cardiac output, hypercapnia, and, in extreme cases, cardiac arrest and electromechanical dissociation (Leatherman, 1994; O'Donnell, 1995). Alveolar rupture and pneumothorax are more related to the degree of DHI than to measured peak airway pressures (Leatherman, 1994). To minimize DHI, initial ventilator settings for the patient with asthma should include a tidal volume of 8 to 10 mL/kg, an inspiratory flow rate of 80 to 100 liters/min, and a respiratory rate of 11 to 14 breaths per minute (Leatherman, 1994; O'Donnell, 1995). This intentional hypoventilation, or permissive hypercapnia, must be balanced with other measures to minimize DHI. These include the use of a square wave of inspiratory flow, low-compliance ventilator tubing, and maneuvers that prolong the expiratory time (decreased respiratory rate, increased inspiratory flow rate) (Leatherman, 1994). Extrinsic PEEP should be avoided in patients with severe asthma, because it may contribute to hyperinflation.

Complications associated with the need for mechanical ventilation in patients with severe asthma include hypotension (25%), pneumothorax (13%), and death (13%) (Williams, 1992). Hypotension that develops in a ventilated asthmatic patient should be assumed secondary to DHI until proven otherwise. Leatherman (1994) recommends that when hypotension develops, the clinician should respond with a diagnostic trial of apnea and intravascular volume expansion. If the patient's pressure responds, the diagnosis of DHI is made, and the respiratory rate can be decreased and IV fluids increased. If there is no response, one should consider the possibility of a pneumothorax. Short-term neuromuscular blockade may

be required for some patients in order to achieve an adequate level of ventilation at low peak airway pressures. Published series have documented the development of acute myopathy in patients receiving steroidal muscle relaxants and concurrent corticosteroids for severe asthma requiring mechanical ventilation (Griffin, 1992; Hirano, 1992). Although the myopathy always resolves, some patients required months of rehabilitative therapy before they could walk independently. Griffin and colleagues (1992) suggested that serum creatine phosphokinase levels should be assessed for patients treated with both corticosteroids and steroidal muscle relaxants to facilitate early detection. Alternatives to neuromuscular blockade include inhalational anesthesia or IV thiopental. Two series demonstrate that both may improve ventilation and respiratory mechanics in patients requiring mechanical ventilation for status asthmaticus (Maltais; 1994; Grunberg, 1991).

When traditional mechanical ventilation fails to improve maternal respiratory status, several additional modalities have been reported with anecdotal success. Fiberoptically directed bronchoalveolar lavage with normal saline, dilute metaproterenol, and the mucolytic, acetylcysteine, have all been successful in the critically ill asthmatic when mucus plugging was a major factor (Schreier, 1989; Munakata, 1987; Henke, 1994). Artificial surfactant therapy, high-frequency ventilation, extracorporeal membrane oxygenation, and controlled hypothermia have also been reported with anecdotal success (Kurashima, 1991; Raphael, 1993; Tajimi, 1988; Shapiro, 1993; Browning, 1992).

## Other Therapeutic Modalities

Certain medications commonly used for the management of asthma either have no role in acute therapy or are relatively contraindicated in pregnancy. Cromolyn sodium, which stabilizes mast-cell membranes, has only a preventive effect and does nothing to reverse bronchospasm (Koch-Weser, 1977). Immunotherapy or desensitization therapy, although safe in pregnancy, likewise has no acute effects (Metzger, 1978). Antihistamines have an inconsistent action, and they may actually decrease pulmonary function in asthmatics (Schuller, 1986). Finally, without evidence of infection, empiric antibiotics have demonstrated no proven benefit in acute asthma.

Medications with adverse fetal effects include iodides and sodium bicarbonate. Long-term in utero exposure to iodides given as expectorants for asthma has clearly been associated with neonatal hypothyroidism, goiter, and critical upper airway obstruction (Yaffe, 1976; Hassan, 1968). Sodium bicarbonate therapy has been advocated by some when the maternal pH falls to less than 7.30 (Nolan, 1988). However, such therapy should be used with caution, because the administration of sodium bicarbonate will diminish the transfer of carbon dioxide from the fetus to the mother and may result in maternal alkalosis, with its aforementioned adverse effects (Moya, 1965).

## Considerations for Labor and Delivery

Attention to the gravida with a recent history of severe asthma will avoid several pitfalls during labor, delivery, and the puerperium. Any long-term medications for the control of asthma should be continued. Women with symptoms and those whose expiratory flow is less than 80% of their personal best should be treated with inhaled beta$_2$-agonists (NAEP Working Group, 1993). Stress-dose steroids should be administered to women who have taken systemic steroids within the past 9 months. This can be accomplished with IV hydrocortisone at a dose of 100 mg every 8 hours, continued until 24 hours postpartum. When choosing a sedative for labor, one of the nonhistamine-releasing narcotics, such as fentanyl, would be preferable to others, such as morphine and meperidine (NAEP Working Group, 1993; Hermens, 1985). Oxytocin is the drug of choice for induction of labor. Prostaglandin can safely be used in the patient with asthma for therapeutic abortion or labor induction with a dead fetus (Towers, 1991). In the second trimes-

ter, higher-dose oxytocin is equally effective for termination or induction for a dead fetus (Winkler, 1991). Because endotracheal intubation has been associated with severe bronchospasm, consideration should be given to the early placement of epidural anesthesia or access (Kingston, 1984). Finally, in the event of postpartum hemorrhage, PGE$_2$ and other uterotonics should be used in lieu of PGF$_2$. In two reports, PGF$_2$ has been associated with clinically diminished pulmonary function. Kreisman et al (1975) documented significant bronchospasm in asthmatics receiving PGF$_2$ for midtrimester abortion, while Hankins et al (1988) noted dangerous oxygen desaturation following 15-methyl PGF$_2$ given for postpartum hemorrhage.

## Summary

Severe acute asthma in pregnancy poses a serious threat to both maternal and fetal health. Physiologic alterations in pulmonary function render the pregnant woman rapidly susceptible to acute derangements in ventilation. Similarly, fetal health may be jeopardized, even with early stages of maternal asthma. For these reasons, the obstetrician must take an aggressive approach to the management of severe asthma complicating pregnancy.

Evaluation of the pregnant asthmatic should be objective and interpreted in light of pregnancy-induced changes. Treatment must be aggressive, with the goals of (1) correcting maternal hypoxia, (2) relieving bronchospasm, (3) ensuring adequate ventilation, and (4) optimizing uteroplacental exchange. Initial therapy should consist of supplemental oxygen and inhaled beta$_2$-agonists. Parenteral corticosteroids should be given early in the course of therapy. Ipratropium bromide and high-dose IV magnesium sulfate should be considered for patients not responding to initial therapy and who are progressing toward respiratory failure. Finally, should maternal ventilation worsen despite pharmacologic therapy, early consideration should be given to intubation and mechanical ventilation.

## SEVERE ACUTE ASTHMA

### I. *Goals of Therapy*
A. To correct hypoxia
B. To alleviate bronchospasm and optimize airflow
C. To avoid maternal exhaustion and progression to respiratory failure
D. To prevent hypoxic fetal morbidity and mortality

### II. *Management Protocol*
A. Administer supplemental oxygen.
B. Begin bronchodilator therapy with inhaled albuterol (metered-dose inhaler with a holding chamber device or via wet nebulizer).
C. Assess $FEV_1$/PEFR; if greater than 75% of predicted or personal best and no symptoms or wheezing, can discharge to follow-up in clinic.
D. If there is no rapid or sustained relief after 30 to 60 minutes, or if there are signs or symptoms of life-threatening asthma, draw arterial blood gases and begin parenteral corticosteroids (2.0 mg/kg hydrocortisone IV bolus or equivalent, followed by 2.0 mg/kg every 4 hr).
E. If airflow or oxygenation is still severely compromised, add ipratropium bromide 0.5 mg via nebulizer.
F. If still progressing to respiratory failure and intubation appears imminent, give 2-g IV bolus of magnesium sulfate over 2 minutes, followed immediately by inhaled albuterol and ipratropium.
G. Endotracheal intubation should be performed when, despite maximal pharmacologic therapy, the following exists or occurs:
  1. Inability to maintain a $PaO_2$ of greater than 60 mm Hg with 90% hemoglobin saturation despite supplemental oxygen
  2. Inability to maintain a $PcO_2$ less than 40 mm Hg
  3. Evidence of maternal exhaustion
  4. Worsening acidosis despite intensive bronchodilator therapy (pH < 7.2–25)
  5. Altered maternal consciousness

### III. *Critical Laboratory Tests*
A. Arterial blood gases
B. $FEV_1$
C. PEFR, chest x-ray, sputum Gram stain

### IV. *Consultation*
Respiratory therapy, pulmonary medicine, and intensive care medicine

**REFERENCES**

American College of Obstetricians and Gynecologists. Pulmonary disease in pregnancy. Technical Bulletin Number 224, June 1996.

Arrighi HM. U.S. asthma mortality 1941–89. Ann Allerg Asthma Immunol 1995;74:321–326.

Arwood LL, Dasta JF, Friedman C. Placental transfer of theophylline: two case reports. Pediatrics 1979;63:844–846.

Austen KF, Orange RP. Bronchial asthma: the possible role of chemical mediators of immediate hypersensitivity in the pathogenesis of subacute chronic disease. Am Rev Respir Dis 1975; 112:423–435.

Awe RJ, Nicotra MB, Newsom TD, Viles R. Arterial oxygenation and alveolar-arterial gradients in term pregnancy. Obstet Gynecol 1979;53:182–186.

Bahna SL, Bjerkedal T. The course and outcome of pregnancy in women with bronchial asthma. Acta Allerg 1972;27:397–406.

Baker MD. Pitfalls in the use of clinical asthma scoring. Am J Dis Child 1988;142:183–185.

Bartels H, Moll W, Metcalfe J. Physiology of gas exchange in the human placenta. Am J Obstet Gynecol 1962;84:1714–1730.

Beasely R, Burgess C, Crane J, et al. Pathology of asthma and its clinical implications. J Allergy Clin Immunol 1993;92:148–154.

Berstrand H. Phosphodiesterase inhibition and theophylline. Eur J Respir Dis 1980;61:(suppl 109):37–44.

Brancazio LR, Laifer SA, Schwartz T. Peak expiratory flow rate in normal pregnancy. Obstet Gynecol 1997;89:383.

Brinkman CR, Weston P, Kirschbaum TH, Assali NS. Effects of maternal hypoxia on fetal cardiovascular hemodynamics. Am J Obstet Gynecol 1970;198:288–301.

Browning D, Goodrum DT. Treatment of acute severe asthma assisted by hypothermia. Anaesthesia 1992;47:223–225.

Burrows B, Huang N, Hughes R, et al. Pulmonary terms and symbols: a report of the ACCP-ATS Joint Committee on Pulmonary Nomenclature. Chest 1975;67:583–593.

Burrows B, Lebowitz MD. The beta-agonist dilemma. N Engl J Med 1992;326:560–561. Editorial.

Calocone A, Afilalo M, Wolkove N, Kreisman H. A comparison of albuterol administered by metered-dose inhaler (and holding chamber) or wet nebulizer in acute asthma. Chest 1993; 104:835–841.

Carter BL, Driscoll CE, Smith GD. Theophylline clearance during pregnancy. Obstet Gynecol 1986; 68:555–559.

Chaieb J, Belcher N, Rees PJ. Maximum achievable bronchodilation in asthma. Respir Med 1989; 83:497–502.

Chapman KR. An international perspective on anticholinergic therapy. Am J Med 1996;100(suppl 1A):2S–4S.

Clark SL, and the National Asthma Education Program Working Group on Asthma and Pregnancy, National Institutes of Health, National Heart, Lung, and Blood Institute. Asthma in pregnancy. Obstet Gynecol 1993;82:1036–1040.

Corre KA, Rothstein RJ. Assess severity of adult asthma and need for hospitalization. Ann Emerg Med 1985;14:45–52.

Crane J, Pearce N, Flatt A, et al. Prescribed fenoterol and death from asthma in New Zealand, 1981–1983: case-control study. Lancet 1989;1:917.

Cugell DW, Frank NR, Gaensler EA, Badger TL. Pulmonary function in pregnancy. Am Rev Tuber 1953;67:568–597.

Cydulka RK, Emerman CL. The effects of combined treatment with glycopyrrolate and albuterol in acute exacerbation of asthma. Ann Emerg Med 1994;23:270–274.

Ellul-Micallef R, Fenech FF. Effect of intravenous prednisolone in asthmatics with diminished adrenergic responsiveness. Lancet 1975;2:1269.

Fanta CH, Rossing TH, McFadden ER. Emergency room treatment of asthma: relationships among therapeutic combinations, severity of obstruction and time course of response. Am J Med 1982;72:416–422.

Fanta CH, Rossing TH, McFadden ER. Glucocorticoids in acute asthma; a critical contolled trial. Am J Med 1983;74:845–851.

Fish JE, Summer WR. Acute lower airway obstruction: asthma. In: Moser KM, Spragg RG, eds. Respiratory emergencies. 2nd ed. St. Louis: Mosby, 1982:144–165.

Fishburne JI. Physiology and disease of the respiratory system in pregnancy: a review. J Reprod Med 1979;22:177–189.

Fitsimons R, Greenberger PA, Patterson R. Outcome of pregnancy in women requiring corticosteroids for severe asthma. J Allergy Clin Immunol 1986;78:349–353.

Gardner MJ, Schatz M, Coursins L, et al. Longitudinal effects of pregnancy on the pharmacokinetics of theophylline. Eur J Clin Pharmacol 1987;31:289–295.

Garrard GS, Littler WA, Redman CWG. Closing volume during normal pregnancy. Thorax 1978; 33:488–492.

Gilman MJ, Meyer L, Carter J, Slovis C. Comparison of aerosolized glycopyrrolate and metaproterenol in acute asthma. Chest 1990;98:1095–1098.

Gluck JC, Gluck PA. The effects of pregnancy on asthma: a prospective study. Ann Allergy 1976;37:164–168.

Gordon M, Niswander KR, Berendes H, Kantor AG. Fetal morbidity following potentially anoxigenic obstetric conditions: bronchial asthma. Am J Obstet Gynecol 1970;106:421–429.

Green S, Rothrock S. Intravenous magnesium sulfate for acute asthma: failure to decrease emergency treatment duration or need for hospitalization. Ann Emerg Med 1992;21:260–265.

Greenberger PA. Asthma in pregnancy. Clin Perinatol 1985a;17:571–584.

Greenberger PA, Patterson R. Management of asthma during pregnancy: current concepts. N Engl J Med 1985b;312:897–902.

Greenberger PA, Patterson R. Beclomethasone dipropionate for severe asthma during pregnancy. Ann Intern Med 1983;98:498.

Greenberger PA, Patterson R. The outcome of pregnancy complicated by severe asthma. Allergy Proc 1988;9:539–543.

Gregg I, Nunn AJ. New regression equations for predicting peak expiratory flow in adults. Br Med J 1989;298:1068–1070.

Griffin D, Fairman N, Coursin D, et al. Acute myopathy during treatment of status asthmaticus with corticosteroids and steroidal muscle relaxants. Chest 1992;102:510–514.

Grunberg G, Cohen JD, Keslin J, Gassner S. Facilitation of mechanical ventilation in status asthmaticus with continuous intravenous thiopental. Chest 1991;99:1216–1219.

Guidelines on the management of asthma. Statement by the British Thoracic Society, the British Paediatric Association, the Research Unit of the Royal College of Physicians of London, the King's Fund Centre, the National Asthma Campaign, the Royal College of General Practitioners, the General Practitioners in Asthma Group, the British Association of Accident and Emergency Medicine, and the British Paediatric Respiratory Group. Acute severe asthma in adults and children. Thorax 1993;48:S1–S24.

Hankins GDV. Acute pulmonary injury and respiratory failure during pregnancy. In: Clark SL, Phelan JP, Cotton DB, eds. Critical care obstetrics. Oradell, NJ: Medical Economics Books, 1987: 290–314.

Hankins GDV, Berryman GK, Scott RT Jr, Hood D. Maternal arterial desaturation with 15-methyl prostaglandin F2 alpha for uterine atony. Obstet Gynecol 1988;72:367–370.

Hankins GDV, Clark SL, Harvey CJ, et al. Third-trimester arterial blood gas and acid base values in normal pregnancy at moderate altitude. Obstet Gynecol 1996;88:347.

Hassan AI, Aref GH, Kassem AS. Congenital iodide-induced goiter with hypothyroidism. Arch Dis Child 1968;43:702–704.

Henke CA, Hertz M, Gustafson P. Combined bronchoscopy and mucolytic therapy for patients with severe refractory status asthmaticus on mechanical ventilation: a case report and review of the literature. Crit Care Med 1994;22:1880–1883.

Hermens JM, Ebertz JM, Hannfin JM, et al. Comparison of histamine release in human skin mast cells induced by morphine, fentanyl, and oxymorphone. Anesthesiology 1985;62:124.

Hirano M, Ott BR, Raps EC, et al. Acute quadriplegic myopathy: a complication of treatment with steroids, nondepolarizing blocking agents, or both. Neurology 1992;42:2082–2087.

Idris AH, McDermott MF, Raucci JC, et al. Emergency department treatment of severe asthma:

metered-dose inhaler plus holding chamber is equivalent in effectiveness to nebulizer. Chest 1993;103:665–672.

Jewett JF. Asthma, emboli and cardiac arrest. N Engl J Med 1973;288:265–266.

Josephson GW, Mackenzie EJ, Leitman PS, et al. Emergency treatment of asthma: a comparison of two treatment regimens. JAMA 1979;242:639–643.

Kay AB. Eosinophils in immunologic reactions. Clin Allergy 1987;17:251–258.

Kingston HCG, Hirshman CA. Perioperative management of the patient with asthma. Anesth Analg 1984;63:844–855.

Koch-Weser J, Webb-Johnson DC, Andrews JL. Bronchodilator therapy. Part one. N Engl J Med 1977;297:476–482. Part 2. N Engl J Med 1977;297:758–764.

Kreisman H, deWrel WV, Mitchell CA. Respiratory function during prostaglandin-induced labor. Am Rev Respir Dis 1975;111:564–566.

Kuitert LM, Kletchko SL. Intravenous magnesium sulfate in acute, life-threatening asthma. Ann Emerg Med 1991;20:1243–1245.

Kurashima K, Ogawa H, Ohka T, et al. A pilot study of surfactant inhalation in the treatment of asthma attack. Arerugi 1991;40:160–163.

Leatherman J. Life-threatening asthma. Clin Chest Med 1994;15:453–479.

Lehrer S, Stone J, Lapinski R, et al. Association between pregnancy induced hypertension and asthma during pregnancy. Am J Obstet Gynecol 1993;168:1435–1436.

Levine GN, Posell C, Bernard SA, et al. Acute, reversible left ventricular dysfunction in status asthmaticus. Chest 1995;107:1469–1473.

Levinson G, Shnider SM. Anesthesia for surgery during pregnancy. In: Shnider SM, Levinson G, eds. Anesthesia for obstetrics. 2nd ed. Baltimore: Williams and Wilkins, 1987:188–205.

Littenberg B, Gluck EH. A controlled trial of methylprednisolone in the emergency treatment of acute asthma. N Engl J Med 1986;314:150–152.

Maltais F, Sovilj M, Goldberg P, Gottfried SB. Respiratory mechanics in status asthmaticus: effects of inhalational anesthesia. Chest 1994;106: 1401–1406.

McFadden ER, Kiser R, de Groot WJ. Acute bronchial asthma: relations between clinical and physiologic manifestations. N Engl J Med 1973; 288:221–225.

McNamarra RM, Rubin JM. Intramuscular methylprednisolone acetate for the prevention of relapse in acute asthma. Ann Emerg Med 1993; 22:1829–1835.

Mettam IM, Reddy TR, Evans FE. Life-threatening acute respiratory distress in late pregnancy. Br J Anaesth 1992;69:420–421.

Metzger WJ, Turner E, Patterson R. The safety of immunotherapy during pregnancy. J Allergy Clin Immunol 1978;61:268–272.

Miller TP, Greenberger PA, Patterson R. The diagnosis of potentially fatal asthma in hospitalized adults: patient characteristics and increased severity of asthma. Chest 1992;102:516–518.

Morris HG. Mechanisims of action and therapeutic role of corticosteroids in asthma. J Allergy Clin Immunol 1985a;75:1–12.

Morris HG. Mechanisms of glucocorticoid action in pulmonary disease. Chest 1985b;88:133s–140s.

Moya F, Morishima HO, Shnider SM, James LS. Influence of maternal hyperventilation on the newborn infant. Am J Obstet Gynecol 1965; 91:76–84.

Munakata M, Abe S, Fujimoto S, Kawakami Y. Bronchoalveolar lavage during third-trimester pregnancy in patients with status asthmaticus: a case report. Respiration 1987;51:252–255.

Murphy DG, McDermott MF, Rydman RJ, et al. Aminophylline in the treatment of acute asthma when beta 2-adrenergics and steroids are provided. Arch Intern Med 1993;153:1784–1788.

National Asthma Education Program, Anonymous. Guidelines for the diagnosis and management of asthma. National Heart, Lung, and Blood Institute. National Asthma Education Program. Expert Panel Report. J Allergy Clin Immunol 1991;88:425–534.

National Asthma Education Program Working Group. Management of asthma during pregnancy: report of the working group on asthma and pregnancy. National Asthma Education Program, National Heart, Lung, and Blood Institute, National Institutes of Health. Public Health Service, U.S. Department of Health and Human Services. NIH Publication No. 93-3279. September 1993.

Nelson HS. Beta-adrenergic bronchodilators. N Engl J Med 1995;333:499–506.

Newhouse MT. Emergency department management of life-threatening asthma: are nebulizers obsolete? Chest 1993;103:661–662.

Noble PW, Lavee AE, Jacobs MM. Respiratory diseases in pregnancy. Obstet Gynecol Clin North Am 1988;15:391–428.

Nolan TE, Hess LW, Hess DB, Morrison JC. Severe medical illness complication cesarean section. Obstet Gynecol Clin North Am 1988;15:697–717.

Noppen M, Vanmaele L, Impens N, Schandevyl W. Bronchodilating effect of intravenous magnesium sulfate in acute severe bronchial asthma. Chest 1990;97:373–376.

O'Donnell WJ, Drazen JM. Life-threatening asthma. In: Ayers AM, Grenvik A, Holbrook PR, Shoemaker WC, eds. Textbook of critical care. 3rd ed. Philadelphia: WB Saunders, 1995:750–756.

O'Driscoll BR, Kalra S, Wilson M, et al. Double-blind trial of steroid tapering in acute asthma. Lancet 1993;341:324–327.

O'Driscoll BR, Taylor RJ, Horsley MG. Nebulized salbutamol with and without ipratropium bromide in acute airflow obstruction. Lancet 1989; 1:1418–1420.

Okayama H, Okayama M, Aidawa T, et al. Treatment of status asthmaticus with intravenous magnesium sulfate. J Asthma 1991;28:11–17.

Oserne KA, Featherstone JH, Benedetti TJ. Cerebral ischemia associated with parenteral terbutaline use in pregnant migraine patients. Am J Obstet Gynecol 1982;143:405–407.

Pierson WE, Bierman CW, Kelley VC. A double-blind trial of corticosteroid therapy in status asthmaticus. Pediatrics 1974;54:782.

Raphael JH, Bexton MD. Combined high frequency ventilation in the management of respiratory failure in late pregnancy. Anaesthesia 1993; 48:596–598.

Rebuck AS, Chapman KR, Abboud R, et al. Nebulized anticholinergic and sympathomimetic treatment of asthma and chronic obstructive airways disease in the emergency room. Am J Med 1987;82:59–64.

Rees HA, Millar JS, Donald KW. A study of the clinical course and arterial blood gas tensions of patients in status asthmaticus. Q J Med 1967; 37:541–561.

Rodrigo C, Rodrigo G. Early administration of hydrocortisone in the emergency room treatment of acute asthma; a controlled clinical trial. Resp Med 1994;88:755–761.

Rodriguez-Roisin R, Ballester E, Roca J, et al. Mechanisms of hypoxemia in patients with status asthmaticus requiring mechanical ventilation. Am Rev Respir Dis 1989;139:732–739.

Rolston DH, Shnider SM, de Lorimer AA. Uterine blood flow and fetal acid-base changes after bicarbonate administration to the pregnant ewe. Anesthesiology 1974;40:348–353.

Rossing TH. Methylxanthines in 1989. Ann Intern Med 1989;110:502–504.

Sachs BP, Brown RS, Yeh J, et al. Is maternal alkalosis harmful to the fetus? Int J Gynaecol Obstet 1987;25:65–68.

Safko MJ, Chan SC, Cooper KD, Hanifin JM. Heterologous desensitization of leukocytes: a possible mechanism of beta adrenergic blockage in atopic dermatitis. J Allergy Clin Immunol 1981;68:218–225.

Sawicka EH, Branthwaithe MA. Severe acute asthma. In: Sawicka EH, Branthwaithe MA, eds. Respiratory emergencies. London: Butterworths, 1987: 23–31.

Schaefer G, Silverman F. Pregnancy complicated by asthma. Am J Obstet Gynecol 1961;82:182–191.

Schatz M, Harden K, Forsythe A, et al. The course of asthma during pregnancy, post partum, and with successive pregnancies: a prospective analysis. J Allergy Clin Immunol 1988;81:509–517.

Schatz M, Zeiger RS, Harden KM, et al. The safety of inhaled beta-agonist bronchodilators during pregnancy. J Allergy Clin Immunol 1988;82:686–695.

Schatz M, Zeiger RS, Hoffman CP, et al. Perinatal outcomes in the pregnancies of asthmatic women; a prospective controlled analysis. Am J Respir Crit Care Med 1995;151:1170–1174.

Schiermeyer RP, Finkelstein JA. Rapid infusion of magnesium sulfate obviates need for intubation in status asthmaticus. Am J Emerg Med 1994;12:164–166.

Schreier L, Cutler RM, Saigal V. Respiratory failure in asthma during the third trimester: report of two cases. Am J Obstet Gynecol 1989;160:80–81.

Schuller DE, Turkewitz D. Adverse effects of antihistamines. Postgrad Med 1986;79:75–86.

Scoggin CH, Sahn S, Petty TL. Status asthmaticus. JAMA 1977;238:1158.

Shapiro MB, Kleaveland AC, Bartlett RH. Extracorporal life support for status asthmaticus. Chest 1993;103:1651–1654.

Siegel D, Sheppard D, Gelb A, et al. Aminophylline increases the toxicity but not the efficacy of inhaled beta-adrenergic agonists in the treatment of acute exacerbations of asthma. Am Rev Respir Dis 1985;132:283.

Sims CD, Chamberlain GVP, De Swret M. Lung function tests in bronchial asthma during and after pregnancy. Br J Obstet Gynaecol 1976;83:434–437.

Skobeloff EM, Spivey WH, McNamara RM, Greenspon L. Intravenous magnesium sulfate for the treatment of acute asthma in the emergency department. JAMA 1989;262:1210–1213.

Spector SL. The use of corticosteroids in the treatment of asthma. Chest 1985;87:73s–79s.

Spevetz A, Barter T, Dubois J, Pratter MR. Inpatient management of status asthmaticus. Chest 1992;102:1392–1396.

Spitzer WO, Suissa S, Ernst P, et al. The use of beta-agonists and the risk of death and near death from asthma. N Engl J Med 1992;326:501–506.

Stenius-Aarniala B, Pririla P, Teramo K. Asthma and pregnancy: a prospective study of 198 pregnancies. Thorax 1988;43:12–18.

Strauss RE, Wertheim DL, Bonagura VR, Valacer DJ. Aminophylline therapy does not improve outcome and increases adverse effects in children hospitalized with acute asthma exacerbations. Pediatrics 1994;93:205–210.

Summer WR. Status asthmaticus. Chest 1985;87:87s–94s.

Sydow M, Crozier TA, Zielman S, et al. High-dose intravenous magnesium sulfate in the management of life-threatening status asthmaticus. Intensive Care Med 1993;19:467–471.

Tai E, Road J. Blood-gas tensions in bronchial asthma. Lancet 1967;1:644–646.

Tajimi K, Kasai T, Nakatimi T, Kobayashi K. Extracorporal lung assist for patients with hypercapnia due to status asthmaticus. Intensive Care Med 1988;14:588–589.

Tiffany BR, Berk WA, Todd IK, White SR. Magnesium bolus or infusion fails to improve expiratory flow in acute asthma exacerbations. Chest 1993;104:831–834.

Topilski M, Levo Y, Spitzer SA, et al. Status asthmaticus in pregnancy: a case report. Ann Allergy 1974;32:151–153.

Towers CV, Rojas JA, Lewis DF, et al. Usage of prostaglandin E2 (PGE$_2$) in patients with asthma. Am J Obstet Gynecol 1991;164:295.

Turner ES, Greenberger PA, Patterson R. Management of the pregnant asthmatic. Ann Intern Med 1980;6:905–918.

Weinberger M, Hendeles L. Theophylline in asthma. N Engl J Med 1996;334:1380–1388.

Weinberger SE, Weiss ST, Cohen WR, et al. Pregnancy and the lung. Am Rev Respir Dis 1980;121:559–581.

Weiss KB, Gergen PJ, Hodgson TA. An economic evaluation of asthma in the United States. N Engl J Med 1992;326:862–866.

Wendel PJ, Ramin SM, Barnett-Hamm C, et al. Asthma treatment in pregnancy: A randomized controlled study. Am J Obstet Gynecol 1996;175:150.

Williams TJ, Tuxen DV, Scheinkestel CD. Risk factors for morbidity in mechanically ventilated patients with acute severe asthma. Am Rev Respir Dis 1992;146:607–615.

Winfield CR, McAllister WAC, Collins JV. Changes in effective pulmonary blood flow with prednisolone. Thorax 1980;35:238.

Winkler CL, Gray SE, Hauth JC, et al. Mid-second-trimester labor induction: concentrated oxytocin compared with prostaglandin E2 vaginal suppositories. Obstet Gynecol 1991;77:297–300.

Woolcock AJ. Asthma. In: Murray JF, Nadel JA, eds. Textbook of respiratory medicine. Philadelphia: WB Saunders, 1988:1030–1068.

Wulf KH, Kunze LW, Lehman V. Clinical aspects of placental gas exchange. In: Respiratory gas exchange and blood flow in the placenta. Bethesda, MD: National Institutes of Health, Public Health Service, 1972:505–521.

Yaffe SJ, Bierman CW, Cann HM, et al. Adverse reactions to iodide therapy of asthmas and other pulmonary diseases. Pediatrics 1976;57:272–274.

Yeh TF, Pildes RS. Transplacental aminophylline toxicity in a neonate. Lancet 1977;1:910.

Young GP, Freitas P. A randomized comparison of atropine and metaproterenol inhalational therapies for refractory status asthmaticus. Ann Emerg Med 1991;20:513–519.

# CHAPTER 18

# Acute Respiratory Distress Syndrome

*A*cute respiratory failure may be caused by a variety of clinical conditions, including pulmonary embolus, congestive heart failure, pneumonia, or the clinical entity referred to as the acute respiratory distress syndrome (ARDS). This chapter focuses on the pathophysiologic and clinical treatment aspects of ARDS as they relate to women in pregnancy and the immediate postpartum period.

Acute respiratory distress syndrome is an acute lung injury that may result in diffuse infiltrates radiographically, severe decreases in lung compliance, and profound intrapulmonic shunting. There are a variety of insults that may lead to this final common pathway of lung injury. Some of these insults may occur in any patient, and several are unique to pregnancy. It is essential that these conditions be identified early and treated aggressively to optimize outcome. The outcome is strongly correlated to the extent of the initial lung injury, the success of early resuscitation efforts, and the avoidance of further lung injury and complications. Although it has been almost 30 years since the original description of the "acute respiratory distress syndrome" by Ashbaugh and associates, there is still very little obstetric literature available on this devastating condition. Consequently, much of the information contained herein is derived from the medical and critical care literature, with inferences made to pregnant patients as appropriate.

## Definition and Diagnosis

The term *ARDS* is derived from the title of its first description in the literature by Ashbaugh et al, in which they used the term *acute respiratory distress in adults* to differentiate this condition from the respiratory distress found in premature newborns (Ashbaugh, 1967). *Acute respiratory distress syndrome* refers to an acute lung injury associated with bilateral infiltration in the frontal chest radiograph and a pulmonary capillary wedge pressure (PCWP) of 18 mm Hg or less. It is a clinical disorder and should not be confused with the pathologic condition, permeability pulmonary edema. Although increased vascular permeability leading to pulmonary edema is always present in the initial phases of ARDS, the clinical constellation of ARDS includes many other significant structural and functional abnormalities of the lung, and ARDS has a vastly different prognosis and treatment than simple pulmonary edema. In the later stages of ARDS, pulmonary vascular permeability may even return to normal as the condition progresses to its chronic stage, which is marked by significant fibrosis and a honeycomb architecture of the lungs (Tomashefski, 1990).

Acute respiratory distress syndrome may occur in patients of any age (Faix, 1989). It is important to distinguish ARDS from related conditions with some similar features because of differences in treatment and prognosis (Marinelli, 1994). The progression is extremely rapid, and patients usually develop respiratory failure within 48 hours of the initial injury (Fowler, 1983). The radiographic appearance is variable. It is never focal, as is the case with lobar pneumonia, but is always bilateral and extensive. While cardiogenic pulmonary edema is often present in cases of severe ARDS, PCWPs should be restored to normal ($\leq 18$ mm Hg in pregnant women) with no improvement in the lung infiltrates for at least 24 hours before the diagnosis of ARDS is definitively made. Lung mechanics and gas exchange are severely disrupted in ARDS (Zimmerman, 1982). In general, patients with ARDS require administration of oxygen concentrations exceeding $Fio_2$ of 0.5, and most will require mechanical ventilation. Although physiologic disturbance criteria have been proposed as a basis for diagnosing ARDS, none has been accepted universally (Murray, 1988) (Table 18-1).

## Pathophysiology

Whatever the precipitating factors, ARDS tends to follow a predictable pathophysiologic course, which can be divided into three phases: the acute or exudative phase, the chronic or proliferation fibrosis phase, and finally, the repair and recovery phase. Not every patient with ARDS will progress through all of the phases, and patients may expire or recover at any point along the progression.

T A B L E **18-1**

Physiologic criteria for the diagnosis of acute respiratory distress syndrome

$po_2$ < 50 with $Fio_2$ > 0.6
Pulmonary capillary wedge pressure $\leq 12$ mm Hg
Total respiratory compliance < 50 mL/cm (usually 20–30 mL/cm)
Functional residual capacity reduced
Shunt ($Q_S/Q_T$) > 30%
Dead space ($V_D/V_T$) > 60%
Alveolar-arterial gradient on 100% oxygen $\geq 350$ mm Hg

$po_2$, partial pressure of oxygen; $Fio_2$, fraction of inspired oxygen; $Q_S$, blood flow to nonventilated areas; $Q_T$, total blood flow to both ventilated and nonventilated areas; $V_D$, dead space volume; $V_T$, tidal volume.

## Acute or Exudative Phase

In this first phase of ARDS, the capillary membranes of the lungs are injured. Pulmonary edema follows due to the increased permeability of the capillary membrane and acute inflammatory changes. Microscopically, there is widespread injury to both the endothelial and epithelial cells of the lungs, typically involving large cytoplasmic vacuoles, disrupted mitochondria, pyknotic nuclei, and localized swelling of the cytoplasm (Katzenstein, 1986). The damaged capillaries recover relatively quickly as the surviving endothelial cells spread out to close the gaps in the surface. The epithelial surface of the alveolus, on the other hand, usually shows a much more widespread and persistent level of damage. The type I epithelial cells necrose and sluff away, leaving large areas of exposed basement membrane. It often takes several days for the type II epithelial cells to proliferate and close these gaps (Bachofen, 1982). The alveolar walls become distended with edema fluid as the damaged endothelial and epithelial surfaces allow protein-rich fluid to leak into the extravascular space in the lung (Pratt, 1979). Some of the alveoli are compressed by the increased pressure in the interstitial space, others collapse due to changes in the surface tension within them, while others simply fill with edema fluid. This phase is marked by the presence of hyaline membranes, which differentiates ARDS from simple cardiogenic pulmonary edema. Alveolar macrophages begin to release cytokines, such as tumor necrosis factor, which further exacerbate the inflammation (Rinaldo, 1993). Leukocytes begin to congregate and migrate across the endothelium in response to chemoattractants emitted by the macrophages. These neutrophils release oxygen-free radicals as well as a variety of enzymes, which cause extensive damage to the lung tissue (Dorinsky, 1986). These events occur very early in the course of the disease, and neutrophils can be recovered on bronchioalveolar lavage within 48 hours of the initial lung injury (Fowler, 1987).

In addition to these events within the alveolus, microthrombi begin to form in the pulmonary circulation. These occlusions further exacerbate intrapulmonic shunt and probably contribute to the thrombocytopenia, which is frequently a feature of this phase of ARDS (Tomashefski, 1983). In some instances, macrothrombi also form, which can lead to hemorrhagic infarcts in the lung (Jones, 1985).

## Proliferation and Fibrosis Phase

The early proliferative changes begin in the small blood vessels of the lung as well as the alveoli. New connective tissue is deposited in the intima and media of the pulmonary arterioles by the replicating mesenchymal cells. Unfortunately, this proliferation and fibrosis tends to narrow the vessels, making them susceptible to thrombosis within the lumen (Marinelli, 1990). During this same period, which begins as early as 3 days after the initial injury, gaps in the alveolar epithelial surface are created by the death and sloughing of the type I pneumocytes, which are filled in by the spread of type II pneumocytes along the alveolar wall. These migrating type II cells subsequently differentiate into type I cells and restore the surface of the alveolar wall. Fibroblasts migrate to the adjacent interstitium as well as the alveolar spaces and proliferate, forming granulation tissue (Fukuda, 1987). At this point, the patient may begin to recover if these events are regulated and structure and function is restored. If, on the other hand, the proliferation continues unchecked, the granulation tissue in the alveoli begins to remodel, and fibrosis of the alveolar and capillary membranes ensues (Kuhn, 1991). As the pulmonary vasculature becomes thickened and distorted by progressive fibrosis, the alveoli begin to collapse or merge into larger air spaces, giving rise to the classic honeycomb appearance seen on biopsy specimens. This level of fibrotic change is usually fully developed by 3 weeks from the time of injury, but may begin to appear as early as 10 days after the onset of respiratory failure (Kuhn, 1991).

## Repair and Recovery Phase

Those patients who have not recovered at an earlier phase of ARDS and who are fortunate enough to have survived the proliferation and fibrosis phase enter the repair and recovery phase

of the disease. Obviously, few tissue specimens are taken during this time of recovery, and thus, surprisingly little is known about the actual histopathology of this phase (Bachofen, 1982; Bitterman, 1991, 1994). Patients fortunate enough to survive the earlier phases will begin to recover normal function in their lungs over 6 to 12 months in spite of profound fibrosis (Elliott, 1990). Unfortunately, nearly three fourths of the patients who recover from severe ARDS are left with a clinically detectable decrease in pulmonary function, and some suffer severe chronic debilitating lung disease (Ghio, 1989; Peters, 1989). The degree and nature of the residual lung injuries vary from pulmonary hypertension to new-onset reactive airway disease (Simpson, 1978; Hudson, 1994). In patients who fail to recover after a number of months, a correctable cause, such as tracheal stenosis from an endotracheal tube site, should be sought.

## Radiographic Manifestations

As with other lung injuries, radiographic changes in the early phase of ARDS often lag behind the pathologic changes and may be absent when the patient first develops respiratory distress (Aberle, 1990). Initial changes may be nothing more than a minimal ground-glass infiltrate (Fig 18-1). However, by 48 hours, most chest radiographs will show either widespread consolidation or diffuse, patchy dense infiltrates. There may be a paradoxical "clearing" of these infiltrates with the initiation of positive end-expiratory pressure (PEEP) ventilation as some of the atelectatic air spaces are re-expanded and edema fluid is driven into the interstitial space from the alveoli (Malo, 1984).

As computerized tomography scans have become more available to these patients, the belief that ARDS is a homogeneous insult affecting all areas of the lung equally has been replaced with the concept that, particularly in this early phase, areas of damage and consolidation may be patchy (Maunder, 1986; Gattinoni, 1988). Often the apical areas of the lung are well expanded, while the more dependent portions show areas of consolidation. This pattern changes rapidly as the area of the lung that is dependent changes. These observations have led some practitioners to believe

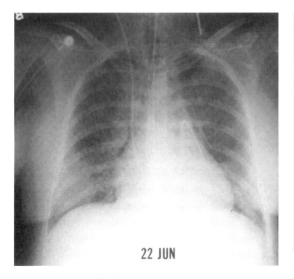

22 JUN

FIGURE **18-1**

Chest radiograph of a 20-year-old woman at 32 weeks' estimated gestational age with varicella pneumonia. Arterial partial pressure of oxygen ($po_2$) was 79 mm Hg with 20 cm $H_2O$ of positive end-expiratory pressure. The patient was on 100% oxygen.

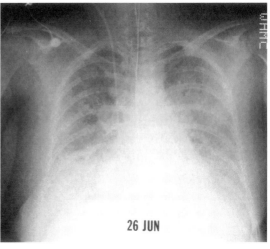

26 JUN

FIGURE **18-2**

Chest radiograph on seventh day of varicella pneumonia. Bilateral lung injury is characterized by a ground-glass appearance. Lung expansion and oxygenation at this point were maintained with 20 to 23 cm $H_2O$ of PEEP. (Reproduced with permission from Hankins GDV, Gilstrap LC, Patterson AR. Acyclovir treatment of varicella pneumonia in pregnancy. Crit Care Med 1987;15:336. Copyright © 1987, Williams & Wilkins Co.)

that changing the patient's position frequently from supine to prone to lateral may improve the clinical course by varying the areas of the lung that are over- or under-ventilated.

As the disease progresses into the chronic, or proliferation and fibrosis phase, the radiographic appearance begins to evolve (Fig 18-2). Alveolar infiltrates become less dense and are replaced by reticular infiltrates interspersed with ground-glass opacities (Greene, 1987). As the lungs become more fibrotic, chest radiographs develop the "honeycomb," which typifies the x-ray pattern of the disease in this late fibrotic phase. It is important to obtain chest x-rays frequently in these patients, particularly in this phase, because of the significantly increased risk of pulmonary barotrauma. In addition to the dramatic and clinically apparent tension pneumothoraces, x-ray can detect more subtle findings such as pulmonary interstitial emphysema and loculated pneumothoraces.

During the repair and recovery phase, the fibrous tissue in the lungs is slowly reabsorbed and/or remodeled. This is apparent on repeated chest x-rays, which show a gradual but progressive clearing of the dense reticular infiltrates. Chest radiographs may return completely to normal or may show residual changes such as scattered linear densities or slightly obscured diaphragmatic and heart borders (Unger, 1989).

## Clinical Manifestations

### Hypoxemia

One of the earliest clinical manifestations in the initial phases of ARDS is a rapidly progressive hypoxia (Table 18-1). The hypoxemia is frequently resistant, even to high concentrations of inspired oxygen. This is due to the relatively large amount of blood that is shunted from right to left through the nonventilated lung segments (Dantzger, 1979, 1982). Simply increasing the fraction of inspired oxygen ($Fio_2$) will not improve hypoxemia significantly, but the addition of PEEP in appropriate amounts can help recruit collapsed alveolar segments and decrease the shunt fraction. If a pulmonary artery (PA) catheter is in place, shunt fraction can be determined directly by measuring mixed venous and arterial partial pressures of oxygen simultaneously (Shapiro, 1977). Alternatively, shunt fraction can be estimated by measuring the alveolar-arterial gradient and dividing by 20, with the patient on 100% oxygen. A value of 50, for example, corresponds to a shunt fraction of approximately 50% (assuming a normal cardiac output). A shunt fraction that is greater than 50% is an ominous sign, and, in such cases, central hemodynamic monitoring should be considered to guide management. With invasive cardiac monitoring, shunt fraction can be accurately determined and corrective measures more accurately assessed for efficacy (Marini, 1990).

## Decreased Pulmonary Compliance

Some decrease in lung compliance is present in every case of ARDS, and as a result, higher inspiratory pressures are required to inflate the stiff lungs (Shapiro, 1977). It was formerly believed that this decrease in compliance was simply a function of the diffuse edema and fibrosis causing a decrease in lung elasticity. It is now known that the lung injury is not homogenous and that areas of atelectasis are intermingled with areas of normal lung. Consequently, the normal areas remain normally elastic, while the collapsed areas do not participate in ventilation. This results in a net loss of compliance in the lung due to a decrease in the total lung volume participating in ventilation, not because the injured lung is more inelastic (Marini, 1988). This has profound implications on the use of mechanical ventilation and particularly PEEP in patients with ARDS. If this theory is correct, too much PEEP can be as deleterious as too little PEEP. Increasing PEEP (in an effort to recruit the consolidated areas) will overdistend the normally elastic segments on which the patient is relying for most of her ventilation.

Static compliance is the amount of pressure necessary to expand the entire thorax to a given volume, including lungs, chest wall, and diaphragm. Practically, serial measurements of static thoracic compliance can serve as a useful measure of clinical improvement or deterioration in ARDS as well as of the benefit of therapeutic interventions. The compliance of a healthy thorax, for example, is generally 100 mL of volume expansion for every centimeter of water pressure exerted on the airway at a tidal volume of 8 mL/kg of the patient's nonpregnant, basal, ideal body weight. By contrast, in severe ARDS, compliance may be as low as 10 mL/cm of water pressure. If a patient is mechanically ventilated on a full-assist mode and is either deeply sedated or paralyzed such that she makes no breathing effort, static compliance can be estimated easily. One simply adjusts the ventilator to temporarily introduce a pause of approximately 0.4 seconds at the end of inspiration. This is known as plateau airway pressure, which is measured during each breath as stepwise increases in tidal volume are delivered, usually in 200-mL increments. A pressure volume curve is then drawn by plotting these end-inspiratory plateau pressures less PEEP on the x-axis versus tidal volume on the y-axis. The slope of the resulting curve (i.e., tidal volume ÷ [plateau pressure − PEEP]) gives the static compliance of the thorax (Bone, 1976).

## Increased Airway Resistance

It is generally held that airway resistance increases in ARDS because the disease process leads to functionally small lungs due to widespread consolidation with overall resistance to flow proportionally increasing with the number of airways that do not participate in ventilation (Marini, 1990). This effect is compounded if there is further narrowing of the airways from secretions or bronchospasm. In patients on mechanical ventilators, it is difficult to directly assess airway resistance using standard equipment. Expiratory airway resistance, however, can be assessed qualitatively by noting the total time required for passive expiration. The longer the expiratory time, the greater the expiratory resistance. Total expiratory resistance of the airways can be estimated by measuring the difference between the peak airway pressure at end-inspiration and the plateau pressure. The larger this pressure difference, the greater the total inspiratory resistance of the airways. The increased airway resistance seen in

ARDS has several implications for the clinical management of these patients. First, the increase in expiratory resistance necessitates a longer exhalation time, which may lead to air-trapping at the end of expiration, sometimes referred to as auto-PEEP. This may become problematic in patients requiring high respiratory rates due to severe disease. Another unfortunate effect of the increased airway resistance of ARDS is that higher airway pressures are needed to overcome the airway resistance and inflate the lungs. This greatly increases the risk of barotrauma in these patients. During the recovery phase, these patients may be more difficult to wean from mechanical ventilation because of the increased work of breathing from high-resistance airways.

## Increased Physiologic Dead Space

Paradoxically, as a patient with ARDS improves and hypoxemia begins to resolve, the physiologic dead space actually may increase (Shimada, 1979). This may be due to the fact that, as the injured lung begins to repair itself, poorly perfused alveoli begin to have ventilation restored to them. Thus, the dead space–tidal volume ratio of the lung increases. In normal individuals, the dead space fraction is usually less than 0.35. In ARDS, on the other hand, the dead space fraction is often greater than 0.6. The clinical effect of this is that unless minute ventilation increases dramatically, the partial pressure of carbon dioxide will begin to rise. In the past, extraordinary measures were sometimes undertaken to maintain a normal $Paco_2$. Today, however, many clinicians feel that the increased morbidity from these extremely high ventilatory rates outweighs the relatively insignificant risks of elevations in the partial pressure of carbon dioxide, a technique sometimes referred to as permissive hypercapnia.

## Pulmonary Hypertension

Mild-to-moderate pulmonary hypertension occurs frequently in ARDS. During the initial phase, it is believed that the perivascular edema and vasoconstriction, in addition to microthrombi in the pulmonary capillaries, are responsible. Later in the course of the disease, the increase in pulmo-

nary vascular resistance is thought to be due to fibrosis of the pulmonary capillary vascular beds. While some patients may develop right-sided heart failure, this is relatively rare, and in most cases the pulmonary hypertension reverses as the ARDS resolves (Brunet, 1988).

## Precipitators

Acute respiratory distress syndrome is, by definition, not a disease but a clinical syndrome. As such, a wide variety of disease processes may lead to this final common pathway of lung injury and pathophysiologic response. Some potential precipitators of ARDS in pregnant women include aspiration, exposure to tocolytic agents, preeclampsia and eclampsia, pyelonephritis, chorioamnionitis, endometritis, septic abortion, thromboembolism, amniotic fluid embolism, air embolism, bacterial and viral pneumonia, drug overdose, and severe hemorrhage (Eriksen, 1990).

Although large series of ARDS in pregnancy are limited, the most common causes of ARDS in pregnancy, in order of frequency, are infection, preeclampsia and eclampsia, and hemorrhage (Smith, 1990). By far the most common precipitator of ARDS in pregnancy is infection, particularly infection that leads to a septic syndrome. Because sepsis is the most frequent precipitator of ARDS in obstetric patients, it should be suspected in any case of ARDS in which the etiology is unknown, particularly if the patient is hypotensive and/or febrile. While gram-negative septicemia has been associated traditionally with ARDS, any number of infectious agents can cause ARDS, including fungi and viruses (Meduri, 1993; Niederman, 1990). In the gravida, infectious pneumonia is a common cause of ARDS and may be the most common cause of nonhospital-acquired ARDS (Baumann, 1986). Acute respiratory distress syndrome that develops in the hospital is often attributable to pneumonia as well.

If a primary pulmonic source is not identified in a patient suspected of having sepsis-induced ARDS, another common source or location of the primary infection is the abdomen, particularly in the postoperative patient (Montgomery, 1985; Bell, 1983). Shock, profound malnutrition, or any other severe injury or illness can interrupt the intestine-blood barrier and allow for translocation of bacteria from the intestinal lumen (Poole, 1992; Deitch, 1990; Runcie, 1990).

In the population at large, aspiration is a significant precipitator of ARDS. It is estimated that up to 30% of patients who experience a documented episode of aspiration will go on to develop ARDS (Bynum, 1976; Mendelson, 1946). Pregnant women are at a greatly increased risk of aspiration of gastric contents, particularly during labor and operative procedures. Unfortunately, alkalization of the gastric secretions does not protect completely against this form of lung injury. It is likely that particulate matter and gastric enzymes may be sufficiently damaging to the lung to precipitate an episode of ARDS (Wynne, 1982).

Labor and delivery also place the pregnant patient at greatly increased risk of severe hemorrhage and hypotension. It is now recognized that these events can lead to a sepsis-like syndrome sometimes referred to as the systemic inflammatory response syndrome, even when infection is not present (Demling, 1990). Aggressive treatment of blood loss with transfusions also has been implicated in precipitating acute lung injury due to rare but catastrophic leukoagglutinin reactions. These unusual reactions should be suspected in the patient who develops evidence of acute lung injury following transfusion. The diagnosis is confirmed by testing for antibodies in the transfused blood that are directed against the patient's WBCs (Maggart, 1987; Vermeji, 1991). Other rare and unusual causes of ARDS include high therapeutic doses of opiates used during labor, which can cause ARDS in susceptible individuals (Lusk, 1988). Likewise, venous air emboli from large transected uterine veins during cesarean section, as well as neurogenic pulmonary edema following eclamptic seizures, are other potential precipitators of ARDS in the gravida (Colice, 1984).

## Management

### General Goals of Management

Three principal challenges must be met in patients with ARDS. First, the immediate problem is achieving appropriate pulmonary gas exchange. The second is the careful weaning of the patient from mechanical ventilation. The management plan must incorporate a wide variety of clinical details, including identifying and treating the underlying cause of injury when possible, treatment of secondary infections and other developing complications, keeping the patient adequately nourished and hydrated, and limiting iatrogenic injuries. A third major challenge in dealing with the ARDS patient is the ability to provide realistic evaluation of the patient's condition and to accurately determine prognosis. Given present mortality rates for this disease, a number of patients will come to a point in therapy at which assisted life-prolonging measures are no longer appropriate.

To meet these challenges, care is best delivered with a multidisciplinary approach and must be individualized (Surratt, 1994). Still, certain basic elements are common to most patients with ARDS, and an appropriate treatment plan should include the following elements. First, an effort should be made to identify and eliminate any precipitators of the syndrome. Second, in the pregnant woman, one should use the minimal $FiO_2$ necessary to support the partial pressure of oxygen at between 60 and 80 mm Hg (which corresponds to an oxygen saturation of approximately 90%). Oxygen may be toxic in any patient, but there is a suggestion that there is enhanced oxygen toxicity in ARDS. Every effort should be made to optimize the delivery of oxygen ($Do_2$) by maintaining an optimal cardiac output and a hemoglobin of approximately 10 g/dL. In many cases, mechanical ventilation will become required, and supraphysiologic levels of PEEP may be required to maintain adequate oxygenation. One must constantly keep in mind that the desired endpoint is not a given partial pressure of oxygen in the arterial blood but an optimal oxygen delivery. To this end, invasive monitoring with PA catheter may help to not only exclude cardiogenic pulmonary edema, but also optimize PEEP. The optimal level of PEEP is that level which is associated with the highest oxygen delivery, not necessarily that which provides the highest $Pao_2$. Third, sources of sepsis should be actively sought and aggressively treated. As a rule of thumb, where sepsis is thought to be the cause of the ARDS, the source is often abdominal. On the other hand, if the sepsis occurs after the onset of ARDS, the source is frequently pulmonic. Fourth, it is best to keep the patient at a volume status, which provides the lowest PCWP compatible with adequate oxygen delivery. In this way, optimal cardiac output and, thus, optimal $Do_2$ is achieved, but the risk of increasing the hydrostatic pressures that may lead to pulmonary edema is minimized. There are few effective direct and specific therapies for ARDS. Consequently, the emphasis is on minimizing further injury and providing adequate supportive care until the lungs can repair themselves.

## Specific Approaches

### Exudative Phase

**Oxygen** In the initial phase of ARDS, the first line of therapy is supplemental oxygen to prevent pulmonary morbidity and mortality due to extreme hypoxemia. In pregnant women, ample oxygen therapy should be given to keep the $Pao_2$ at or above 60 mm Hg, which corresponds roughly to an oxygen saturation of 90%. Ever-increasing levels of oxygen must be provided as ARDS begins to worsen. In some cases, the patients' symptoms will resolve, and endotracheal intubation might be avoided simply by providing adequate fractions of inspired oxygen with a face mask. Some authors advocate using positive-pressure aviator-type masks, which can deliver high $Fio_2$ and PEEP (Venus, 1979). This method for attempting to avoid intubation may be less desirable in the gravida (particularly in the late third trimester and during labor and delivery) because of the theoretical increased risk for aspiration. Unfortunately, the hypoxemia of ARDS tends to be resistant to supplemental oxygen alone, a function of the increased right-to-left shunt past collapsed or flooded alveoli. At higher $Fio_2$ concentrations, oxygen toxicity may become problematic. It is believed that any level of inspired oxygen greater than 21% has some level of toxicity and that this toxicity is enhanced in the ARDS patient. At least one study suggests that exposing a patient with ARDS for greater than 24 hours to an $Fio_2$ level

greater than 0.6 may cause permanent lung damage (Elliot, 1987).

Of greater biologic significance than $Pao_2$ or oxygen saturation is oxygen delivery. Oxygen delivery is a function of oxygen content and cardiac output. Oxygen content is in turn a function of hemoglobin concentration and saturation (Tables 18-2, 18-3). Given the nature of these relationships, much greater increases in oxygen delivery can be obtained by raising hemoglobin concentrations to appropriate levels and appropriately raising cardiac output than can be achieved by increasing $Fio_2$ (Table 18-3). Furthermore, these increases in oxygen delivery can be made without the potentially toxic effects to the lung caused by increasing oxygen concentration (Clark, 1974; Davis, 1983).

**Positive End-Expiratory Pressure** To avoid the problems of oxygen toxicity and to more directly address the underlying pathophysiology of the right-to-left shunt, PEEP is frequently used in the treatment of ARDS. When a patient requires more than 48 hours of high-dose oxygen therapy

T A B L E   **18-2**

**Formulas for derivation of cardiopulmonary parameters**

*Oxygen Content: Arterial or Mixed Venous*
(Hb-g%) (1.39) (%Sat) + ($Pao_2$ × .0031)

*Oxygen Delivery*
Cardiac output [(Hb-g%) (1.39) (%Sat) + ($Pao_2$ × .0031)]

*Lung Compliance*

$$\text{Static} = \frac{\text{Tidal volume}}{\text{Plateau inspiratory pressure}}$$

$$\text{Dynamic} = \frac{\text{Tidal volume}}{\text{Peak inspiratory pressure}}$$

*Shunt*

$$Q_S/Q_T = \frac{Cco_2 - Cao_2}{Cco_2 - Cvo_2}$$

*Alveolar-Arterial Oxygen Difference or Gradient*

$(A\text{-}aDo_2) = (713 × Fio_2 - 1.25 × Paco_2) - Pao_2$

Hb-g%, hemoglobin, gram percentage; % Sat, percentage of saturation; $Pao_2$, arterial pressure of oxygen; $Q_S/Q_T$, shunt; $Cco_2$, end-capillary blood oxygen content; $Cao_2$, arterial blood oxygen content; $Cvo_2$, mixed venous blood oxygen content; $Paco_2$, partial arterial pressure of carbon dioxide; A, alveolar; a, arterial.

T A B L E   **18-3**

Effects of hemoglobin concentration and of the partial pressure
of oxygen on arterial blood oxygen content

| | | Room Air $Pao_2$ 100 mm Hg* | 100% $O_2$ $Pao_2$ 650 mm Hg |
|---|---|---|---|
| Hemoglobin (15 g) | $Hbo_2$ | 19.60 mL | 20.10 mL |
| | $O_2$ dissolved | 0.30 mL | 1.95 mL |
| | Total | 19.90 mL | 22.05 mL |
| Hemoglobin (10 g) | $Hbo_2$ | 13.00 mL | 13.40 mL |
| | $O_2$ dissolved | 0.30 mL | 1.95 mL |
| | Total | 13.30 mL | 15.35 mL |
| Hemoglobin (5 g) | $Hbo_2$ | 6.50 mL | 6.70 mL |
| | $O_2$ dissolved | 0.30 mL | 1.95 mL |
| | Total | 6.80 mL | 8.65 mL |

*Assuming 97% saturation of hemoglobin with oxygen.

$Hbo_2$, hemoglobin oxygen content; $O_2$, oxygen; $Pao_2$, arterial pressure of
oxygen.

at $Fio_2$ levels approaching 0.9, strong consideration should be given to endotracheal intubation and the initiation of mechanical ventilation with PEEP. Positive end-expiratory pressure helps to reduce the right-to-left shunt across the lungs by helping to restore the functional residual capacity of the lungs (Ranieri, 1991). Positive end-expiratory pressure prevents small-airway collapse during expiration, which improves the ventilation-perfusion ratio. It also may favorably affect the compliance of the lung by a redistribution of water into the interstitial space from the intra-alveolar space, and finally, the recruitment of some alveoli that may otherwise not be ventilated. Care must be taken not to use excessive PEEP, which has been shown to overdistend lung regions with normal alveoli and to cause acute lung injury (Dreyfuss, 1988; Kolobow, 1987; Suter, 1975).

There is no question that PEEP can increase $Pao_2$ in ARDS, and, as a result, patients may survive longer. An increase in overall survival, however, has never been rigorously demonstrated via use of PEEP in prospective controlled, randomized clinical trials. This may be due to several factors. First, PEEP is not without risks and has significant side effects, such as barotrauma, over-distension of alveoli, and decreased cardiac out-

put with subsequent decrease in oxygen delivery. Second, most deaths due to ARDS are not due directly to hypoxemia (Montgomery, 1985; Bell, 1983).

Effects on venous return and cardiac output of PEEP can be profound. With PEEP there is a dose-related decrease in venous return to the thorax due to the increase in the pleural pressure. This increased pressure compresses the walls of the great veins and the right side of the heart, both of which are quite compliant. As a result, stroke volume is decreased, leading to a decrease in cardiac output and, ultimately, hypotension. At pressures greater than 15 cm of water, PEEP actually may have a direct, negative inotropic effect on the left ventricle (Jardin, 1981). It also decreases cardiac output by increasing right ventricular afterload.

In determining the appropriate level of PEEP to apply to a given patient, one must keep in mind the therapeutic goals of PEEP. Initially, the desired endpoint is the effective restoration of an acceptable $Pao_2$ with a nontoxic $Fio_2$ level. Once this has been established, there is time to determine the patient's optimal or "best PEEP." Until noninvasive methods are available, this is best accomplished using a PA catheter (Belfort, 1994). If a PA catheter is not in place, one approach is to increase PEEP until $Pao_2$ is acceptable or there is a clinically significant fall in BP. If $Fio_2$ levels are still at a toxic level and hypoxemia remains a problem, the decreased cardiac output and BP may be dealt with through the use of inotropes and vasopressors such as dobutamine and norepinephrine. Once the cardiac performance is restored, PEEP may be increased until nontoxic levels of oxygen and simultaneous acceptable oxygenation levels are achieved. If, on the other hand, a PA catheter is available, a PEEP trial may be undertaken, in which PEEP is incrementally increased while the $Fio_2$ is held constant at 0.6 or less. The optimal PEEP is determined by that level of PEEP that provides the highest oxygen delivery ($Do_2$). The highest oxygen delivery is a product of oxygen concentration and cardiac output, and, thus, is the best index of appropriate tissue oxygenation (Suter, 1975). Alternatively, a higher initial $Fio_2$ may be chosen, the optimal level of PEEP determined by a PEEP trial, and then PEEP held constant while tapering the patient's inspired oxygen concentration down to nontoxic levels. Once a nontoxic range is achieved ($Fio_2 \leq 0.6$), an effort is made to lower PEEP as the patient's $Pao_2$ allows. This is frequently a slow process and must be done carefully, because an overly aggressive withdrawal of PEEP may cause adverse effects on oxygenation, which may take many hours to fully correct, even when the previous level of PEEP is reinstituted (Lamy, 1976).

**Contemporary Approaches to Mechanical Ventilation** Several important goals should be met in the mechanical ventilation of patients with ARDS. First, in contrast to previous thinking, large tidal volumes should not be used. Second, one should avoid the overdistension of the alveoli. Third, pressure should be slightly greater than that necessary to distend the alveolar units (Cole, 1995). The simplest clinical measure of the pressure needed to hold open the alveolar units is the mean airway pressure. In the gravida with ARDS, increasing $Pao_2$ generally requires increasing mean airway pressure, regardless of the method used to increase that pressure (i.e., PEEP, tidal volume, etc.) (Marini, 1992). The adverse affects of mechanical ventilation also correlate closely with mean airway pressures (Cournand,

1948). Thus, the higher the mean airway pressure, the more likely the woman is to suffer from increased lung water, barotrauma, and decreased cardiac performance. Mean airway pressure may be altered by increasing minute ventilation, extending the inspiratory time, changing the inspiratory peak pressure, altering the pressure waveform, and, of course, increasing PEEP. Because of its correlation with respiratory complications, the minimal amount of mean airway pressure needed to maintain appropriate oxygen delivery should be used.

Because of potential complications of volutrauma, high tidal volumes are rarely the method of choice for increasing mean airway pressure and, thus, arterial oxygenation. Likewise, increasing inspiratory frequency excessively can lead to complications of air trapping within the bronchioles (auto-PEEP). Thus, at higher minute ventilations, increases in mean airway pressure, for the purpose of increasing oxygenation, are usually accomplished either by increasing end-expiration (PEEP) or by extending the inspiratory time (increase I:E ratio). Small increases in inspiratory time (in contrast to PEEP) do not tend to adversely affect the driving pressure needed for ventilation, provided that the patient does not require extremely high minute ventilations and that the I:E ratio does not exceed 2:1 (Pesenti, 1985).

Historically, volume-cycled ventilators replaced negative pressure units such as the iron lung, principally because of their ability to guarantee a given minute ventilation, which could be controlled by the operator. In disease processes such as ARDS, as the resistance to flow increases, these modes allow airway pressures to increase to overcome this resistance. Because we now know these increased pressures can lead to lung damage, there is an increase in the use of pressure-controlled, timed-cycled ventilators (Shapiro, 1995; Morris, 1994). Pressure-controlled ventilation allows the operator to select and control mean airway pressure as well as peak airway pressure while tidal volumes become variable. When the operator presets the maximal airway pressure, the tidal volume that is ultimately delivered depends on the compliance of the respiratory system, the time available for inspiration, and the resistance to air flow. If the operator elects to add PEEP (or if there is auto-PEEP present), this is subtracted from the total pressure, and it is the difference between total pressure minus end-expiratory pressures that determines the pressure difference available to ventilate the lung. This mode of ventilation has a strong theoretical advantage over volume-cycled modes for avoiding lung trauma, namely mean, peak, and end-expiratory alveolar pressure can be controlled and specifically limited (Marini, 1994). This is very useful in restrictive lung diseases such as ARDS, where low compliance can lead to dangerously high airway pressures (Benito, 1990).

Inverse inspiratory-to-expiratory ratio ventilation is another tool that can be used in particularly refractory cases of low $Pao_2$. Although some authors feel that inverse ratio ventilation adds little benefit and can be dangerous, others are using this method and reporting significant success (Kacmarek, 1990; Duncan, 1987). Unfortunately, there is a paucity of randomized controlled trials in the literature and none that specifically address pregnant women (Tharatt, 1988; Gurevitch, 1986). Although details of the mechanism have not been fully investigated, there is experimental evidence in both animal and human lung injury models of small but significant improvements in ventilatory efficiency and $Pao_2$, which is most likely due to increased average lung volume through the respiratory cycle (Marini, 1992). One of the principal risks of inverse ratio ventilation is barotrauma, if inappropriate peak alveolar pressures are chosen. Much of the negative experience with this complication stems from studies in which larger tidal volumes were used, producing peak airway pressures greater than those that are currently considered safe (Tharatt, 1988; Gurevitch, 1986). To avoid these possibly catastrophic complications, smaller tidal volumes and higher partial pressures of carbon dioxide may be allowed. Furthermore, peak airway pressure should be kept below 33 mm Hg, and I:E ratios of greater than 3:1 should be avoided until more experience is gained with this technique, even though considerably higher ratios have been successfully employed (Marcy, 1991; Cole, 1984).

As noted, one of the most important factors in reducing the risk of exacerbating lung injury is the reduction of mean airway pressure and minute ventilation. At minute ventilations, which may allow for an adequate $Pao_2$, $Paco_2$ may be significantly elevated. Increased arterial carbon dioxide, in and of itself, is relatively benign. The ill effects of an elevated $Paco_2$ are primarily referable to the rate and degree of change in intracellular pH. If these pH changes are attenuated by buffering with bicarbonate or permitting a very gradual increase in $Paco_2$, the potential ill effects of decreased intracellular pH, such as muscular weakness, increased pulmonary vascular resistance, and CNS dysfunction, can usually be avoided. This strategy of reducing minute ventilation and slowly allowing $Paco_2$ to reach relatively high levels is referred to as permissive hypercapnia. There is clinical evidence to suggest that mortality rates can be favorably affected using low tidal volume permissive hypercapnia in patients with ARDS (Lewandowski, 1992; Hickling, 1990). Other, more extreme methods for reducing airway pressures and minute ventilation involve the extrapulmonic removal of carbon dioxide from the blood. Although successful in some cases, these methods suffer from being expensive, invasive, and relatively experimental (Mortensen, 1991; Gattinoni, 1986). For these reasons the simple, inexpensive, and relatively safe permissive hypercapnia approach has enjoyed considerably more clinical popularity.

Another strategy for minimizing barotrauma, keeping peak airway pressures and tidal volumes small without sacrificing oxygenation, is high frequency ventilation. A conventional volume-control ventilator can be used at high rates ($>50$ breaths per minute) with low tidal volumes of approximately 5 mL/kg and, thus, be run at lower airway pressures. The term *high-frequency ventilation*, however, usually refers to extremely high ventilation rates, often exceeding 100 breaths per minute, with even smaller tidal volumes (Slusky, 1988). This mode of ventilation has been shown to provide adequate oxygenation while keeping tidal volumes and peak airway pressures low, but carbon dioxide removal may be limited, and an alternative form of its removal may be needed. The usual indication for this type of ventilation has been in cases of bronchopleural fistula. High-frequency, or jet, ventilation seems to work well in patients without underlying lung disease (Carlon, 1982; Turnbull, 1981). Unfortunately, in patients with ARDS who developed fistulas, the results are poor, and, in many cases, air-leak actually increased as a result of high-frequency ventilation (Bishop, 1987; Ritz, 1984). Consequently, this form of ventilation should be employed with extreme caution, if at all, in these patients.

**Nosocomial Infection** The presence of a new, persistent, or recurring fever in the patient with ARDS provides a significant diagnostic dilemma for the practitioner. If the fever is coupled with an infiltrate on chest radiographs, the chance that it is in response to pneumonia is greatly increased. However, there are a variety of other clinical conditions in these patients that can lead to the presence of a fever and an infiltrate, such as fibroproliferation in the late phase of ARDS, chemical aspirations, atelectases, or pulmonary embolism. To further complicate this issue, two separate coexisting causes of fever and infiltrate might be present, for example, an extrapulmonary infection with a plural effusion, a drug reaction in the presence of congestive heart failure, or a blood transfusion reaction coexisting with pulmonary hemorrhage. In addition, the full spectrum of traditional clinical findings for pneumonia, such as new pulmonary infiltrate, fever, sputum production, cough, and leukocytosis, may not be present in the severely compromised patient with a nosocomial pneumonia. In clinical studies testing the utility of clinical parameters in predicting nosocomial pneumonia, the results have been extremely disappointing. Using purely clinical assessments, one study showed a 10% false-positive rate and a 62% false-negative rate for the detection of pneumonia when compared with histologic evaluation (Johanson, 1972). Another study comparing 16 clinical variables, such as leukocytosis, hypoxia, fever, and so on, found no combinations that were useful in determining which patients had bacterial pneumonia (Chastre, 1988). In the chronically ventilated patient, the addition of microscopic evaluation of tracheal secretions often adds little to the diagnostic accuracy, given the high rate of colonization with potential pulmonary pathogens in these patients, even when deep pulmonic pressure is not present (Hill,

1976). The unfortunate results of this reliance on clinical signs and symptoms for the diagnosis of nosocomial pneumonia are several. First, some patients with nosocomial pneumonias may not be recognized clinically due to an atypical presentation. Next (and probably more commonly), a great many patients are treated with antibiotics for "pneumonia" in which no bacterial infection is present. As a result, there is a delay in the diagnosis of the actual etiology of the infiltrate and fever and exposure to unnecessary drugs for both mother and fetus, as well as the risk of superinfection with highly resistant strains of hospital-acquired bacteria. Furthermore, even if the diagnosis of a nosocomial bacterial pneumonia is accurately made, a reliance on blind, broad-spectrum coverage or treating culture results from tracheal aspirates (which may not reflect the actual pathogens) does not allow for optimum therapy.

A variety of techniques have been proposed to deal with this dilemma. The most promising of these center on the use of flexible fiberoptic bronchoscopy to direct sampling of the lower pulmonary tract. One of the best of these techniques is a modified bronchoalveolar lavage method that utilizes a protected transbronchoscopic balloon-tipped catheter, which avoids exposing the instilled and aspirated bronchoalveolar lavage solution to contaminants. Results with this technique have been extremely favorable, providing diagnostic sensitivities of up to 97% and specificities of up to 92% (George, 1992). Other advantages of this technique are that it allows sampling of a sizable area of the lower respiratory tract, allows for the collection of suitable material for a culture, and can provide an immediate result based on microscopic analysis and Gram stain (Trouillet, 1990).

Potential concerns about this strategy for rapidly and accurately diagnosing nosocomial infections include cost, the need for appropriate equipment and expertise, and potential risks of the procedure in critically ill patients. Although the procedure does require some expertise and incurs some additional cost, these are probably far outweighed by the ability to make a precise and timely diagnosis of potentially devastating illnesses. Furthermore, using current techniques, the relative risk of bronchoscopy is extremely small.

Whatever protocol is followed, it should be based on sound principles of accurate diagnosis, targeted therapy, and timely intervention. If the expertise or resources are not available or if a patient's condition precludes use of a protocol, it may not be possible to employ the most precise diagnostic techniques. When using empiric antibiotic therapy, care should be taken to appropriately cover the most likely pathogens.

### Proliferative/Fibrosis Phase

The pathologic features that differentiate the exudative and proliferative phases of ARDS have been discussed previously. The differences in these pathologic characteristics also give rise to differences in clinical features that necessitate some differences in therapeutic approach. Much of the supportive care in the early and late phases of ARDS is identical. Two areas that differ somewhat, however, are the approach to the evaluation and treatment of fever and the use of PEEP.

Unlike the exudative phase, in the proliferative and fibrosis phase, a large number of alveoli are completely obliterated by fibroproliferative changes. Consequently, increasing PEEP does little or nothing to improve gas exchange because it is impossible to recruit these obliterated alveoli! Indeed, increasing PEEP often not only fails to improve oxygenation, but also may actually reduce oxygen delivery by decreasing preload and, thus, reducing cardiac output (Kiiski, 1992; Klose, 1981).

Fever is an extremely important physical finding in late ARDS. Fibroproliferation itself can cause fever, even in the absence of infection, probably mediated by the elaboration of inflammatory cytokines within the pulmonic tissue (Meduri, 1991; Kohler, 1993). Fibroproliferative fever without any other source of infection may account for up to 25% of the febrile morbidity seen in the proliferative phase of ARDS (Belenchia, 1991). Unfortunately, sepsis is such a serious complication of ARDS that fever cannot simply be attributed to fibroproliferation without an exhaustive search for a site of infection.

As discussed previously, there are many potential sources of infection. Ventilator-associated pneumonia is the most commonly identified primary source of infection in advanced ARDS, and pulmonary superinfection is the leading cause of death in patients who survive the initial phase of ARDS (Seidenfeld, 1986). Other regularly identified sites include catheter-related infections, sinusitis, urinary tract infections, intra-abdominal infections, wound infections, empyema, and primary candidemia. This wide range of types and locations of infections underscores the importance of accurately identifying and precisely treating the source of fever in the patient with ARDS. When possible, empiric therapy should be avoided (Meduri, 1993).

## Extrapulmonic Gas Exchange Techniques

This unique approach to avoid exacerbating lung injury seeks to relieve the lungs of part or all of their gas exchange responsibility. Several methods of accomplishing this have been used with varying degrees of success. One such method is extracorporeal membrane oxygenation (ECMO), which has been used successfully in pregnancy (Plotkin, 1994). This method has been employed in patients who have severe life-threatening hypoxemia despite $FiO_2$ levels of 1.0 and maximal mechanical ventilation. In these cases, the lung injury is so severe that the intrinsic ability of the lung to oxygenate blood is impaired to a point that is incompatible with life. In these extreme circumstances, an artificial "auxiliary lung" may be placed in a vascular circuit and allowed to supplant or supplement pulmonary oxygenation. Some investigators have even suggested that this might become a first-line therapy once the technique is improved, because it allows the lung to repair itself under a situation of complete rest while using alternative means of supporting gas exchange. The "lung rest" hypothesis has not been proven, but it is known that in some cases, hyaline membrane formation may be prevented and renal function and hemodynamics improved when the stresses on the lung are minimized (Pesenti, 1982; Gattinoni, 1980a,b; Dorrington, 1989). Despite its theoretic appeal, this technique has been plagued with technical problems, such as hemolysis, bleeding, and infection. Extracorporeal membrane oxygenation has been compared with conventional ventilation in a formal controlled, prospective, multicenter study of ARDS (Zapol, 1979). The results of this study have been questioned on a variety of grounds. For instance, there was a much higher incidence of viral pneumonia in this study than in other series, nonvalidated entry criteria were used, and a much higher mortality rate in both the control and ECMO groups was reported relative to other series. In this series, mortality was nearly 90%, compared with an average 60% mortality in most clinical experiences. Nonetheless, this study failed to show any advantage in the use of ECMO over conventional techniques.

In an attempt to overcome some of the drawbacks of ECMO, the emphasis in extracorporeal gas exchange has shifted from oxygenation to the removal of carbon dioxide via a technique known as $ECCO_2R$, or extracorporeal lung assist (Cottongham, 1995). While some oxygenation is provided across the artificial membrane, thus avoiding oxygen toxicity to the lungs, the primary goal is the removal of carbon dioxide to reduce minute ventilation and prevent alveolar damage. Unlike ECMO, $ECCO_2R$ utilizes a lower pressure, lower flow, venous-to-venous system (Gattinoni, 1986). Although results are preliminary, $ECCO_2R$ seems to have greater success and fewer complications than ECMO. Still, early results in controlled trials do not show a significant advantage over conventional therapy. Nonetheless, several institutions, located principally in Europe, have begun to use this method as standard therapy for severe ARDS in patients who fail to respond to PEEP. When the European register becomes available and the United States' experience becomes more extensive, clinicians will have a better concept of if and when to apply this expensive technology; until the safety and utility of this technique is better defined, its use is best regarded as investigational.

## Specific Therapy

The historic failure of some specific therapies may, in part, be due to an incomplete understanding of the precise mechanisms involved in ARDS as well as the closely related multiorgan system failure (Bernard, 1994). Contemporary opinion on the cause of ARDS centers on lung injury secondary to sepsis-induced organ dysfunction, mediated by endotoxin or like substances that stimulate the release of the host's own cytokines and lipid mediators. These lipid mediators may damage the lung directly but also may act indirectly by increasing the production of oxygen free radicals (Brigham, 1987; Ogletree, 1987; Vercelloti, 1988). New approaches to specific therapy in ARDS are being directed toward the modification or interruption of these events.

## Corticosteroids

The clinical application of corticosteroids to both ARDS and multiorgan system failure has, in general, been disappointing. This is somewhat surprising because corticosteroids have significant theoretical benefits, such as the ability to decrease the production of arachidonic acid metabolites, inhibit neutrophil aggregation, and decrease the production of tumor necrosis factor.

High-dose corticosteroids have been shown to be relatively ineffective in improving the outcome of patients with ARDS when examined in a rigorous, randomized, double-blind clinical trial (Bernard, 1987). In another study, corticosteroids did not prevent the development of ARDS or change overall outcome in patients with septic shock when administered prophylactically prior to the development of clinical symptoms of ARDS (Luce, 1988). Such findings tend to suggest that corticosteroids should not be used except in a very limited and defined subset of patients with ARDS, as mentioned in an earlier section of this chapter. Clearly, more effective agents with fewer side effects are needed.

## Surfactant

Acute respiratory distress syndrome was originally called adult respiratory distress syndrome because of its clinical similarity to the neonatal respiratory distress syndrome, which has been shown to be the result of a lack of surfactant in the immature neonatal lung. While the principal lesion of ARDS is due to increased capillary-alveolar permeability, there is also a decrease in functional surfactant, which could contribute to alveolar instability and worsening hypoxemia. Theoretically, by restoring normal levels of surfactant activity within the damaged alveoli, some improvement in oxygenation and lung compliance might be realized. This could help to reduce the need for more aggressive mechanical ventilation, which can lead to alveolar overdistension and damage. Unfortunately, a limited initial study of artificial surfactant instillation failed to show any sustained clinical improvement (Haslam, 1994). Apparent therapeutic benefits may not have been seen in part due to the fact that an optimal ratio of phosphatidylcholine to phosphatidylglycerol was not achieved. Additional studies are needed before any benefit of surfactant replacement can be determined accurately.

## Nitric Oxide

Nitric oxide is a potent endothelial-dependent relaxing agent that can selectively dilate the pulmonary vasculature when the gas is inhaled. As noted previously, the premature lung in ARDS is often associated with some degree of pulmonary hypertension. As a result, there is an element of intrapulmonary shunt as blood passes by damaged and poorly vented lung segments. Theoretically, if nitric oxide were inhaled, it would travel only to the well-ventilated lung units and cause local vasodilation. It would not travel to the unventilated regions, and, therefore, they would not experience the same degree of vasodilation and increased perfusion as the well-ventilated units. This would lead to a redistribution of blood flow from the poorly ventilated to the well-ventilated lung units, which could reduce intrapulmonary shunting and improve systemic oxygenation. Because of its extremely short half-life, nitric oxide could accomplish this without decreasing systemic arterial pressure (Rossaint, 1993). Several clinical reports have demonstrated that $Pao_2$ can be influenced favorably by the inhalation of very low concentrations of nitric oxide (Grover, 1993; Zapol, 1993). Interestingly, the degree of vasodilation appears to correlate directly to the degree of vasoconstriction present in a given vascular bed; the greater the degree of pulmonary hypertension, the better the response to nitric oxide inhalation (Rich, 1993; Bigatello, 1993). This may

add some level of safety in the clinical application of this agent, because normally perfused lung segments may not become overdilated. Tachyphylaxis has not been seen, even with extended periods of exposure to nitric oxide (Rossaint, 1993). Unfortunately, the beneficial effects of nitric oxide disappear very quickly after the agent is discontinued and can lead to rebound pulmonary vasoconstriction (Bigatello, 1993). Enthusiasm for these beneficial effects of nitric oxide must be tempered with concern over its potential toxicity; both short-term exposure at a high level of nitric oxide and long-term exposure at a low level have demonstrated toxicity. The relative risks and benefits of this therapy in patients with ARDS remain to be determined. Until these issues are better defined clinically, the use of inhaled nitric oxide in treating ARDS remains investigational (Rossaint, 1994).

## Immunotherapy

Neutrophil response may be part of the common pathway of both ARDS and multiorgan failure. The initiating insult may be either exogenous, such as the presence of bacterial endotoxin, or some other failure of endogenous mediation of neutrophil response (Weiss, 1989). Consequently, if therapy could be developed that would counteract the effect of endotoxin or mediate the overreaction of endogenous host defenses, this might prove effective, not only for ARDS but also for the multiorgan system failure syndrome as well.

Monoclonal antibody therapy directed against endotoxin has enjoyed some limited success in decreasing mortality in certain subsets of patients with gram-negative sepsis. Unfortunately, the improved survival in these select patients was not associated with a decrease in the occurrence of ARDS. Because two of the major factors in the mortality of ARDS are concomitant sepsis and multisystem organ failure, these therapies may yet prove to be beneficial in overall survival.

Research is progressing rapidly toward the development of agents that may successfully block other steps in the pathway of neutrophil expression. One of the initiating steps in neutrophil-mediated organ injury is the binding of neutrophils to the endothelial cells themselves. This

## ACUTE RESPIRATORY DISTRESS

I. *Goals of Therapy*

    A.  To identify and eliminate the casual agent

    B.  To achieve

        1.  $Pa_{O_2}$ >60 mm Hg or 90% hemoglobin saturation

        2.  $Pv_{O_2}$ >30 mm Hg

        3.  $Pa_{CO_2}$ >35 to 45 mm Hg

II. *Management Protocol*

    A.  Identify that a lung injury has been sustained and eliminate the casual agent.

    B.  Assess pulmonary function:

        1.  $Pa_{O_2} \div Fi_{O_2}$.

            a.  >3 = good function.

            b.  <3 = suspect injury.

        2.  100% oxygen × 2 minutes.

            a.  $Pa_{O_2}$ 400 mm Hg: probably hypoventilation; aggressive pulmonary toilet and/or incentive spirometry.

            b.  $Pa_{O_2}$ 300 to 400 mm Hg: possible early ARDS; aggressive pulmonary toilet; supplemental mask oxygen; monitor with pulse oximetry. Reevaluate immediately if there is any clinical, laboratory deterioration.

            c.  $Pa_{O_2}$ 300 mm Hg: probable ARDS; intubate and ventilate.

    C.  Maximize oxygen delivery to tissue. Correct anemia, hypothermia, and alkalosis. Optimize cardiac output via pulmonary artery catheter-guided hemodynamic manipulation.

    D.  Avoid therapeutic pitfalls:

        1.  Fluid overload: Use daily weights, intake and output balance, invasive hemodynamic monitoring

        2.  Oxygen toxicity: Use minimum $Fi_{O_2}$ required to achieve a $Pa_{O_2}$ of 60 mm Hg or a 90% hemoglobin saturation.

        3.  Barotrauma: Limit by use of "best" PEEP.

        4.  Nosocomial infections: Sinus infections in intubated patients, urinary tract infections resulting from indwelling catheter, and phlebitis from peripheral and central lines should be identified. Central and peripheral intravenous lines should be changed every 72 hours.

III. *Critical Laboratory Tests*

    A.  Arterial blood gases, mixed venous blood gases, complete blood count, electrolytes, and chest x-ray

    B.  Critical monitoring

        1.  Pulse oximetry

        2.  Pulmonary artery catheter

        3.  Arterial lines

        4.  Foley catheter

IV. *Consultation*

    A.  Respiratory therapy, pulmonary medicine, intensivists, and infectious disease.

involves linking molecules such as CD11b. By blocking CD11b with anti-CD11b antibodies, it may be possible to temporarily inhibit this element of the host defenses and, thus, limit tissue injury (Wortel, 1993). These investigations need to be confirmed by appropriate clinical trials but are very appealing on theoretical grounds.

### Lipid Mediator Antagonists

The inflammatory response relies on a number of lipid mediators, including various metabolites of arachidonic acid and platelet-activating factors. Some of these mediators appear to be associated with the initial inflammatory phase of ARDS. It has been demonstrated that there are large quantities of both prostacyclin and thromboxane in patients who are septic (Bernard, 1991b). In a prospective, double-blind, randomized, clinical trial, the effect of the prostaglandin inhibitor, ibuprofen, was studied in patients with sepsis. There was a significant reduction in prostaglandins as well as a significant improvement in clinical factors such as BP, arterial blood gases, body temperature, peak airway pressure, and minute ventilation (Bernard, 1991b).

When platelet-activating factors are administered to experimental animals, many of the pathologic stigmata of ARDS can be produced (Christman, 1988). In one prospective, double-blind, randomized clinical trial, the effects of an anti-platelet-activating factor agent were investigated. Although there was no significant difference in overall mortality between the treatment and control groups, there was a significant decrease in the mortality of the subset of patients who had documented gram-negative sepsis and received the anti-platelet-activating factor (Tenaillon, 1993). Although these results are very preliminary, they are encouraging.

### Antioxidants

One of the mechanisms of injury due to neutrophil and macrophage activation is mediated by oxygen-free radicals and hydrogen peroxide. The release of these highly cytotoxic agents has been associated with diffuse capillary injury of the type seen in ARDS. These findings led to the suspicion

that providing antioxidants to patients with ARDS might limit the severity of the injury. In one randomized, double-blind, controlled clinical trial, patients with ARDS were given either the antioxidant N-acetylcysteine or placebo. The treatment group showed significant improvement in chest radiograph appearance and cardiac output and a transient improvement in thoracic compliance (Bernard, 1991a). While not definitive, such findings suggest that antioxidants may have a future role in the treatment of ARDS.

## Conclusion

As our understanding of the complex pathophysiology of ARDS increases, so does our ability to effectively and selectively influence the factors that contribute to this devastating condition. In addition to improved, specific therapies, supportive management has improved over the past decade (Temmesfeld-Wollbruck, 1995; Demling, 1993). There is evidence that overall survival has improved somewhat in recent years (Kollef, 1995). To continue this trend toward improving clinical outcome, it is essential to evaluate new therapies for ARDS carefully and objectively. Their use should be incorporated only after careful evaluation and outcomes-based research. This rigor and caution will help to minimize the unnecessary costs and excessive risks that are often incurred with the overzealous clinical application of unproven therapies.

**R E F E R E N C E S**

Aberle DR, Brown K. Radiologic considerations in the adult respiratory distress syndrome. Clin Chest Med 1990;11:737.

Ashbaugh DG, Bigelow DB, Petty TL, et al. Adult respiratory distress in adults. Lancet 1967;2:319.

Bachofen M, Weibel ER. Structural alterations of lung parenchyma in the adult respiratory distress syndrome. Clin Chest Med 1982;3:35.

Baumann WR, Jung RC, Koss M, et al. Incidence and mortality of adult respiratory distress syndrome:

a prospective analysis from a large metropolitan hospital. Crit Care Med 1986;14:1.

Belenchia JM, Meduri GI, Massey JD, et al. Sources of fever in the ventilated patient. Diagnostic value of gallium-67 citrate scan. Chest 1991; 100:145S.

Belfort MA, Saade GR. Oxygen delivery and consumption in critically ill pregnant patients: association with ophthalmic artery diastolic velocity. Am J Obstet Gynecol 1994;171:211.

Bell RC, Coalson J, Smith JD, et al. Multiple organ failure and infection in adult respiratory distress syndrome. Ann Intern Med 1983;99:293.

Benito S, Lemaire F. Pulmonary pressure-volume relationship in acute respiratory distress syndrome in adults: role of positive end-expiratory pressure. J Crit Care 1990;5:27.

Bernard GR. N-acetylcysteine in experimental and clinical acute lung injury. Am J Med 1991a;91:54.

Bernard GR, Reines HD, Halushka PV, et al. Prostacyclin and thromboxane A$_2$ formation is increased in human sepsis syndrome: effects of cyclooxygenase inhibition. Am Rev Respir Dis 1991b;144:1095.

Bernard GR, Artigas A, Brigham KL, et al. The American-European Consensus Conference on ARDS. Definitions, mechanisms, relevant outcomes, and clinical trial coordinations. Am J Respir Crit Care Med 1994;149:818.

Bernard GR, Luce JM, Sprung CL, et al. High-dose corticosteroid in patients with the adult respiratory distress syndrome. N Engl J Med 1987;317:1565.

Bigatello LM, Hurford WE, Kacmarek RM, et al. The hemodynamic and respiratory response of ARDS patients to prolonged nitric oxide inhalation. Am Rev Respir Dis 1993;147:A720.

Bishop MJ, Benson MS, Sato P, et al. Comparison of high-frequency jet ventilation with conventional mechanical ventilation for bronchopleural fistula. Anesth Analg 1987;66:833.

Bitterman PB, Henke CA. Fibroproliferative disorders. Chest 1991;99:81S.

Bitterman PB, Polunovsky VA, Ingbar DH. Repair after acute lung injury. Chest 1994;105:118S.

Bone RC. Diagnosis of causes for acute respiratory distress by pressure-volume curves. Chest 1976;70:740.

Brigham KL, Meyrick B, Berry LJ, et al. Antioxidants protect cultured bovine lung endothelial cells from injury by endotoxin. J Appl Physiol 1987;63:840.

Brunet F, Dhainaut JF, Devaux JY, et al. Right ventricular performance in patients with acute respiratory failure. Intensive Care Med 1988;14:474.

Bynum LJ, Pierce AK. Pulmonary aspiration of gastric contents. Am Rev Respir Dis 1976;114:1129.

Carlon GC, Ray C, Pierri MK, et al. High frequency jet ventilation: theoretical considerations and clinical observations. Chest 1982;32:468.

Chastre J, Fagon JY, Soler P, et al. Diagnosis of nosocomial bacterial pneumonia in intubated patients undergoing ventilation: comparison of the usefulness of bronchoalveolar lavage and the protected specimen brush. Am J Med 1988; 85:499.

Christman BW, Lefferts PL, King GA, et al. Role of circulating platelets and granulocytes in PAF-induced pulmonary dysfunction in awake sheep. J Appl Physiol 1988;64:2033.

Clark JM. The toxicity of oxygen. Am Rev Respir Dis 1974;110:40.

Cole AGH, Weller SF, Sykes MK. Inverse ratio ventilation compared with PEEP in adult respiratory failure. Intensive Care Med 1984;10:227.

Cole FJ Jr, Shouse BA. Alternative modalities of ventilation in acute respiratory failure. Surg Annu 1995;27:55.

Colice GL, Matthay MA, Bass E, et al. Neurogenic pulmonary edema. Am Rev Respir Dis 1984; 130:941.

Cottongham CA, Habashi NM. Extracorporeal lung assist in the adult trauma patient. AACN Clin Issues 1995;6:229.

Cournand A, Motley HL, Werko L, et al. Physiologic studies of the effects of intermittent positive pressure breathing on cardiac output in man. Am J Physiol 1948;152:162.

Dantzger DR. Gas exchange in the adult respiratory distress syndrome. Clin Chest Med 1982;3:57.

Dantzger DR, Brook CJ, Dehart P, et al. Ventilation-perfusion distributions in the adult respiratory distress syndrome. Am Rev Respir Dis 1979; 120:1039.

Davis WB, Rennard WI, Bitterman PB, et al. Early reversible changes in human alveolar structures induced by hypoxia. N Engl J Med 1983;309:878.

Deitch EA, Ma WJ, Ma L, et al. Protein malnutrition predisposes to inflammatory-induced gut-origin septic states. Ann Surg 1990;211:560.

Demling RH. Adult respiratory distress syndrome: current concepts. New Horiz 1993;1:388.

Demling RH. Current concepts on the adult respiratory distress syndrome. Circ Shock 1990;30:297.

Dorinsky PM, Gadek JE. Lung neutrophils in the adult respiratory distress syndrome: clinical and pathophysiological significance. Am Rev Respir Dis 1986;133:218.

Dorrington KL, McRae KM, Gardaz JP, et al. A randomized comparison of total extracorporeal $CO_2$ removal with conventional mechanical ventilation in experimental hyaline membrane disease. Intensive Care Med 1989;15:184.

Dreyfuss D, Soler P, Basset G, et al. High inflation pressure pulmonary edema: respective effects of high airway pressure, high tidal volume and positive end-expiratory pressure (PEEP). Am Rev Respir Dis 1988;137:1159.

Duncan SR, Rizk NW, Raffin TA. Inverse ratio ventilation. PEEP in disguise? Chest 1987;92:390.

Elliot CG. Pulmonary sequelae in survivors of ARDS. Clin Chest Med 1990;11:789.

Elliot CG, Rasmusson BY, Crapo RO, et al. Prediction of pulmonary function abnormalities after adult respiratory distress syndrome (ARDS). Am Rev Respir Dis 1987;135:634.

Eriksen NL, Parisi VM. Adult respiratory distress syndrome and pregnancy. Semin Perinatol 1990; 14:68.

Faix R, Viscardi RM, DiPietro MA, et al. Adult respiratory distress syndrome in full-term newborns. Pediatrics 1989;83:971.

Fowler AA, Hamman RF, Good JT, et al. Adult respiratory distress syndrome: risk with common predispositions. Ann Intern Med 1983;98:593.

Fowler AA, Hyers TM, Fisher BJ, et al. The adult respiratory distress syndrome: cell populations and soluble mediators in the airspaces of patients at high risk. Am Rev Respir Dis 1987;136:1225.

Fukuda Y, Ishizaki M, Masuda Y, et al. The role of intra-alveolar fibrosis in the process of pulmonary structural remodeling in patients with diffuse alveolar damage. Am J Pathol 1987;126:171.

Gattinoni L, Agostoni A, Damia G, et al. Hemodynamics and renal function during low frequency positive pressure ventilation with extracorporeal $CO_2$ removal. Intensive Care Med 1980a;6:155.

Gattinoni L, Agostoni A, Pesenti A, et al. Treatment of acute respiratory failure with low frequency positive pressure ventilation and extracorporeal removal of $CO_2$. Lancet 1980b;ii:292.

Gattinoni L, Pesenti A, Bombino M, et al. Relationships between lung computed tomographic density, gas exchange, and PEEP in acute respiratory failure. Anesthesiology 1988;69:812.

Gattinoni L, Pesenti A, Mascheroni D, et al. Low frequency positive pressure ventilation with extracorporeal $CO_2$ removal in severe acute respiratory failure. JAMA 1986;256:881.

George DL, Falk PS, Meduri GU, et al. The epidemiology of nosocomial pneumonia in medical intensive care unit (MICU) patients: a prospective study based on bronchoscopic sampling. Infect Control Hosp Epidemiol 1992;21:496.

Ghio AJ, Elliott CG, Crapo RO, et al. Impairment after adult respiratory distress syndrome. Am Rev Respir Dis 1989;139:1158.

Greene R. Adult respiratory distress syndrome: acute alveolar damage. Radiology 1987;163:57.

Grover R, Smithies M, Bihari D. A dose profile of the physiological effects of inhaled nitric oxide in acute lung injury. Am Rev Respir Dis 1993; 147:A350.

Gurevitch MJ, Van Dyke J, Young ES, et al. Improved oxygenation and lower peak airway pressure in severe adult respiratory distress syndrome: treatment with inverse ratio ventilation. Chest 1986;89:211.

Haslam PL, Hughes DA, MacNaughton PD, et al. Surfactant replacement therapy in late-stage adult respiratory distress syndrome. Lancet 1994;343:1009.

Hickling KG, Henderson SJ, Jackson R. Low mortality associated with permissive hypercapnia in severe adult respiratory distress syndrome. Intensive Care Med 1990;16:372.

Hill JD, Ratliff JL, Parrott JCW, et al. Pulmonary pathology in acute respiratory insufficiency: lung biopsy as a diagnostic tool. J Thorac Cardiovasc Surg 1976;71:64.

Hudson LD. What happens to survivors of the adult respiratory distress syndrome? Chest 1994;105:123S.

Jardin F, Farcot JC, Boisante L, et al. Influence of positive end-expiratory pressure on left ventricular performance. N Engl J Med 1981;304:387.

Johanson WG Jr, Pierce AK, Sanford JP, et al. Nosocomial respiratory infections with Gram-negative bacilli: the significance of colonization of the respiratory tract. Ann Intern Med 1972;77:701.

Jones R, Reid LM, Zapol WM, et al. Pulmonary vascular pathology: human and experimental studies. In: Zapol WM, Falke KJ, eds. Acute respiratory failure. New York: Marcel Dekker, 1985:23.

Kacmarek RM, Hess D. Panacea or auto-PEEP? Respir Care 1990;35:945.

Katzenstein AA, Myers JL, Mazur MT. Acute interstitial pneumonia: a clinicopathologic, ultrastructural, and cell kinetic study. Am J Surg Pathol 1986;10:256.

Kiiski R, Takala J, Kari A, et al. Effect of tidal volume on gas exchange and oxygen transport in the adult respiratory distress syndrome. Am Rev Respir Dis 1992;146:1131.

Klose R, Osswald PM. Effects of PEEP on pulmonary mechanics and oxygen transport in the late stages of acute pulmonary failure. Intensive Care Med 1981;7:165.

Kohler G, Medur GU, Stentz F, et al. Inflammatory cytokines in the BAL of ARDS. Chest 1993;104:151S.

Kollef MH, Schuster DP. The acute respiratory distress syndrome. N Engl J Med 1995;332:27.

Kolobow R, Moretti MP, Gumagalli R, et al. Severe impairment in lung function induced by high

peak airway pressure during mechanical ventilation. An experimental study. Am Rev Respir Dis 1987;135:312.

Kuhn C. Patterns of lung repair: a morphologist's view. Chest 1991;99:11S.

Lamy M, Fallat RJ, Koeniger E, et al. Pathologic features and mechanisms of hypoxemia in adult respiratory distress syndrome. Am Rev Respir Dis 1976;114:267.

Lewandowski K, Slama K, Falke KJ. Approaches to improve survival in severe ARDS. In: Vincent JL, ed. Update in intensive care and emergency medicine. Berlin: Springer, 1992:372–377.

Luce JM, Montgomery AB, Marks JD, et al. Ineffectiveness of high-dose methylprednisolone in preventing parenchymal lung injury and improving mortality in patients with septic shock. Am Rev Respir Dis 1988;138:62.

Lusk JA, Maloney PA. Morphine-induced pulmonary edema. Am J Med 1988;84:367.

Maggart M, Stewart S. The mechanisms and management of noncardiogenic pulmonary edema following cardiopulmonary bypass. Ann Thorac Surg 1987;43:231.

Malo J, Jameel A, Wood LDH. How does positive end-expiratory pressure reduce intrapulmonary shunt in canine pulmonary edema? J Appl Physiol 1984;57:1002.

Marcy TW, Marini JJ. Inverse ratio ventilation in ARDS: rationale and implementation. Chest 1991;100:9.

Marinelli WA, Henke CA, Harmon KR, et al. Mechanisms of alveolar fibrosis after acute lung injury. Clin Chest Med 1990;11:657.

Marinelli WA, Ingbar DH. Diagnosis and management of acute lung injury. Clin Chest Med 1994;15:517.

Marini JJ. Pressure-targeted, lung-protective ventilatory support in acute lung injury. Chest 1994;105:109S.

Marini JJ. Monitoring during mechanical ventilation. Clin Chest Med 1988;9:73.

Marini JJ. Lung mechanics in ARDS. Clin Chest Med 1990;11:673.

Marini JJ, Ravenscraft SA. Mean airway pressure: physiologic determinants and clinical importance: Part 1 and 2. Crit Care Med 1992;20:1461–1462, 1604–1616.

Maunder RJ, Shuman WP, McHugh JW, et al. Preservation of normal lung regions in the adult respiratory distress syndrome. JAMA 1986;255:2463.

Meduri GU. Diagnosis of ventilator-associated pneumonia. Infect Dis Clin North Am 1993;7:295.

Meduri GU, Belenchia JM, Estes RJ, et al. Fibroproliferative phase of ARDS. Clinical findings and effects of corticosteroids. Chest 1991;100:943.

Mendelson CL. The aspiration of stomach contents into the lungs during obstetric anesthesia. Am J Obstet Gynecol 1946;52:191.

Montgomery AB, Stager MA, Carrico J, et al. Causes of mortality in patients with the adult respiratory distress syndrome. Am Rev Respir Dis 1985;132:485.

Morris AH. Adult respiratory distress syndrome and new modes of mechanical ventilation: reducing the complications of high volume and high pressure. New Horiz 1994;2:19.

Mortensen JD. Augmentation of blood gas transfer by means of an intravascular blood gas exchanger (IVOX). In: Marini JJ, Roussos C, eds. Ventilatory failure. New York: Springer, 1991:318–346.

Murray JF, Mathay MA, Luce J, et al. An expanded definition of the adult respiratory distress syndrome. Am Rev Respir Dis 1988;138:720.

Niederman MS, Fein AM. Sepsis syndrome, the adult respiratory distress syndrome and nosocomial pneumonia. Clin Chest Med 1990;11:633.

Ogletree ML, Snapper JR, Brigham KL. Direct and indirect effects of leukotriene $D_4$ on the lungs of unanesthetized sheep. Respiration 1987;51:256.

Pesenti A, Kolobow T, Buckhold DK, et al. Prevention of hyaline membrane disease in premature lambs by apneic oxygenation and extracorporeal carbon dioxide removal. Intensive Care Med 1982;8:11.

Pesenti A, Marcolin R, Prato P, et al. Mean airway pressure vs. positive end-expiratory pressure during mechanical ventilation. Crit Care Med 1985;13:34.

Peters JI, Bell RC, Prihoda TJ, et al. Clinical determinants of abnormalities in pulmonary function in survivors of the adult respiratory distress syndrome. Am Rev Respir Dis 1989;139:1163.

Plotkin JS, Shah JB, Lofland GK, et al. Extracorporeal membrane oxygenation in the successful treatment of traumatic adult respiratory distress syndrome: case report and review. J Trauma 1994;37:127.

Poole GV, Muakkassa FF, Griswold JA. Pneumonia, selective decontamination and multiple organ failure. Surgery 1992;111:1.

Pratt PC, Vollmer RT, Shelburne JD, et al. Pulmonary morphology in a multihospital collaborative extracorporeal membrane oxygenation project: I. Light microscopy. Am J Pathol 1979;95:191.

Ranieri VM, Eissa NT, Corbeil C, et al. Effects of positive end-expiratory pressure on alveolar recruitment and gas exchange in patients with the adult respiratory distress syndrome. Am Rev Respir Dis 1991;144:544.

Rich GF, Murphy GD, Roos CM, et al. Inhaled nitric oxide: selective pulmonary vasodilation in cardiac surgical patients. Anesthesiology 1993;78:1028.

Rinaldo JE, Christman JW. Mechanisms and mediators of ARDS. Clin Chest Med 1990;11:621.

Ritz R, Benson M, Bishop MJ. Measuring gas leakage from bronchopleural fistulas during high-frequency jet ventilation. Crit Care Med 1984;12:836.

Rossaint R, Gerlach H, Falke KJ. Inhalation of nitric oxide—a new approach in severe ARDS. Eur J Anaesthesiol 1994;11:43.

Rossaint R, Falke KF, Lopez F, et al. Inhaled nitric oxide for the adult respiratory distress syndrome. N Engl J Med 1993;328:399.

Runcie C, Ramsay G. Intra-abdominal infection: pulmonary failure. World J Surg 1990;14:196.

Seidenfeld JJ, Pohl DF, Bell RC, et al. Incidence, site, and outcome of infections in patients with the adult respiratory distress syndrome. Am Rev Respir Dis 1986;134:12.

Shapiro VA, Peruzzi WT. Changing practices in ventilator management: a review of the literature and suggested clinical correlations. Surgery 1995;117:121.

Shapiro AR, Peters RM. A nomogram for planning respiratory therapy. Chest 1977;72:197.

Shimada Y, Yoshiya I, Tanaka K, et al. Evaluation of the progress and prognosis in the adult respiratory distress syndrome. Chest 1979;76:180.

Simpson DL, Goodman M, Spector SL, et al. Long-term follow-up and bronchial reactivity testing in survivors of the adult respiratory distress syndrome. Am Rev Respir Dis 1978;117:449.

Slusky AS. Nonconventional methods of ventilation. Am Rev Respir Dis 1988;138:175.

Smith JL, Thomas F, Orme JF, et al. Adult respiratory syndrome during pregnancy and immediately postpartum. West J Med 1990;153:508.

Surratt N, Troiano NH. Adult respiratory distress in pregnancy: critical care issues. J Obstet Gynecol Neonatal Nurs 1994;23:773.

Suter PM, Fairley HB, Isenberg MD. Optimum end-expiratory airway pressure in patients with acute pulmonary failure. N Engl J Med 1975;292:284.

Temmesfeld-Wollbruck B, Walmrath D, Grimminger F, et al. Prevention and therapy of the adult respiratory distress syndrome. Lung 1995;173:139.

Tenaillon A, Dhainaut JF, Letulzo Y, et al. Efficacy of P.A.F. antagonist (BN 52021) in reducing mortality of patients with severe Gram-negative sepsis. Am Rev Respir Dis 1993;147:A196.

Tharatt RS, Allen RP, Albertson TE. Pressure controlled inverse ratio ventilation in severe adult respiratory failure. Chest 1988;94:755.

Tomashefski JF. Pulmonary pathology of the adult respiratory distress syndrome. Clin Chest Med 1990;11:593.

Tomashefski JF, Davies P, Boggis L, et al. The pulmonary vascular lesions of the adult respiratory distress syndrome. Am J Pathol 1983;112:112.

Trouillet JL, Guiguet M, Gilbert C, et al. Fiberoptic bronchoscopy in ventilated patients. Evaluation of cardiopulmonary risk under midazolam sedation. Chest 1990;97:927.

Turnbull AD, Carlon GC, Howland WS, et al. High-frequency jet ventilation in major airway or pulmonary disruption. Ann Thorac Surg 1981;32:468.

Unger JM, England DM, Bogust GA. Interstitial emphysema in adults: recognition and prognostic implications. J Thorac Imaging 1989;4:86.

Venus B, Jacobs HK, Lim L. Treatment of the adult respiratory distress syndrome with continuous positive airway pressure. Chest 1979;76:257.

Vercelloti GM, Yin HQ, Gustafson KS, et al. Platelet-activating factor primes neutrophil responses to agonists: role in promoting neutrophil endothelial damage. Blood 1988;71:100.

Vermeji CG, Feenstra BWA, Adrichem WJ, et al. Independent oxygen uptake and oxygen delivery in septic and postoperative patients. Chest 1991;99:1438.

Weiss SJ. Tissue destruction by neutrophils. N Engl J Med 1989;320:365.

Wortel CH, Doerschuk CM. Neutrophils and neutrophil-endothelial cell adhesion in adult respiratory distress syndrome. New Horiz 1993;1:631.

Wynne JW. Aspiration pneumonitis: correlation of experimental models with clinical disease. Clin Chest Med 1982;3:25.

Zapol WM, Falke KJ, Roissant R. Inhaled nitric oxide for the adult respiratory distress syndrome. N Engl J Med 1993;329:207.

Zapol WM, Snider MT, Hill JD, et al. Extracorporeal membrane oxygenation in severe acute respiratory failure. A randomized prospective study. JAMA 1979;242:2193.

Zimmerman GA, Morris AH, Cengiz M. Cardiovascular alterations in the acute respiratory distress syndrome. Am J Med 1982;73:25.

# CHAPTER 19

# Thromboembolic Disease

*P*ulmonary embolism (PE) is the leading cause of maternal mortality in Western countries (Gabel, 1987; Kaunitz, 1985; McLean, 1979; Moses, 1987; Rochat, 1988; Rutherford, 1991a; Sachs, 1987, 1988; Worthington, 1989). The actual incidences of deep venous thrombosis (DVT) and PE during pregnancy are unknown. This is probably due in part to the inadequacies of clinical and objective techniques to detect these disorders and also to the pathophysiology of venous thrombosis, in which the location and size of clots and degree of vessel obstruction are highly variable. Approximately 75% of patients who present with suspected thromboembolic disease do not have this condition (Ginsberg, 1996). When DVT has been diagnosed and heparin treatment instituted, the incidence of pulmonary embolus and maternal mortality have declined 3.2- and 18-fold. The goal of this review is to facilitate the recognition of the clinical signs and symptoms of thromboembolic disorders and describe a rational approach to the use of various diagnostic and treatment modalities.

## Incidence

Although many studies of maternal mortality with "pulmonary embolism" as the leading cause of death do not distinguish venous thromboembolism from amniotic fluid or air embolism (Rochat, 1988; Franks, 1990; Lawson, 1990), half or more of these deaths are due to thrombotic embolism (Gabel, 1987; Kaunitz, 1985; McLean, 1979; Sachs, 1987; Franks, 1990; Barbour, 1995a). Using the years 1980 to 1985 as a base period, the maternal mortality rate in the United States was 14.1 of 100,000 live births. Of these, 14.3% were due to embolism (Rochat, 1988). From 1970 to 1985, maternal mortality rates from PE declined by 50% (Franks, 1990) (Fig 19-1).

Ethnic background and age are important risk factors for PE. For example, the overall mortality rate for Black women was 3.2 times higher than for white women. In addition, older women (40 yr or older) were at a 10 times greater risk than women under 25 for both ethnic groups (Franks, 1990) (Fig 19-2).

Deep venous thrombosis occurs in 0.018% to 0.29% of all deliveries (Toglia, 1996; Rutherford, 1991; Barbour, 1995a; Anderson, 1982; Basu, 1972; Bergqvist, 1983). The traditional view has been that the greatest maternal risk for venous thrombosis and embolism was in the immediate postpartum period, especially following cesarean delivery. Postpartum DVT has been reported to occur 3 to 5 times more often than antepartum DVT, and 3 to 16 times more frequently after cesarean as opposed to vaginal delivery (Bergqvist, 1983; Letsky, 1985). In contrast, Rutherford and associates (1991) found that the highest incidence of DVT/PE was not in the puerperium but in the first trimester of pregnancy (Fig 19-3). These authors also found that the risk of DVT

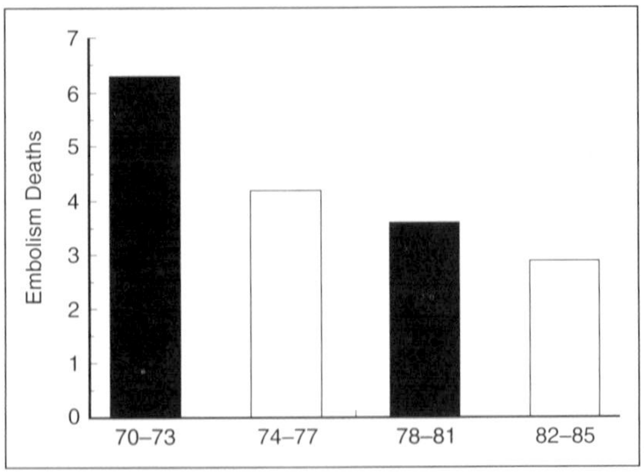


FIGURE 19-1

**The declining incidence of maternal deaths per 100,000 births due to pulmonary embolus from 1970 to 1985.** (From Franks AL, Atrash HK, Lawson HW, et al. Obstetrical pulmonary embolism mortality, United States, 1970–1985. Am J Public Health 1990;80:720–722.)

did not increase with advancing gestational age but stayed relatively constant (Fig 19-4). In contrast, the risk of PE (Fig 19-3) was almost twice as likely to occur in the postpartum patient (Rutherford, 1991a) and appears to be related to the route of delivery (Fig 19-5).

FIGURE 19-2

**Incidence of maternal deaths per 100,000 births by maternal age and race.** (From Franks AL, Atrash HK, Lawson HW, et al. Obstetrical pulmonary embolism mortality, United States, 1970–1985. Am J Public Health 1990;80:720–722; and reproduced by permission from Rutherford SE, Phelan JP. Clinical management of thromboembolic disorders in pregnancy. Crit Care Clin 1991;7:809–828.)

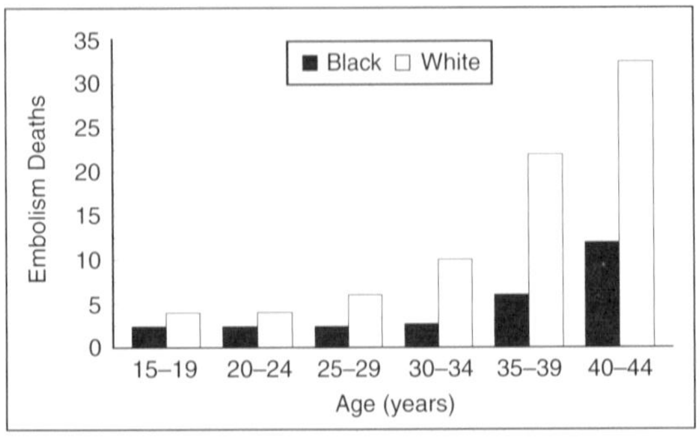


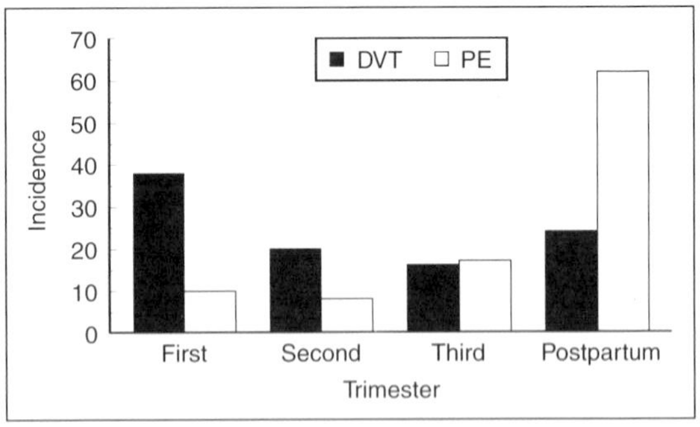


FIGURE 19-3

**Frequency of deep venous thrombosis (DVT) and pulmonary embolus (PE) during each trimester of pregnancy and the postpartum period.** (From Rutherford SE, Montoro M, McGehee W, et al. Thromboembolic disease associated with pregnancy: an 11-year review. Am J Obstet Gynecol 1991;164:286.)

In summary, a pregnant woman's risk of DVT/PE will vary and will depend not only on the trimester of pregnancy, but also on additional clinical factors such as a prior history of a thromboembolism (Rutherford, 1991a; Tengborn, 1989), an operative delivery, prolonged immobilization, and inherited deficiencies in the natural inhibitors of coagulation such as antithrombin III (AT III), protein S, protein C, or factor V Leiden mutation (Table 19-1). Additional risks include

FIGURE 19-4

**The frequency of deep venous thrombosis by trimester.** (From Rutherford SE, Montoro M, McGehee, et al. Thromboembolic disease associated with pregnancy: an 11-year review. Am J Obstet Gynecol 1991;164:286.)

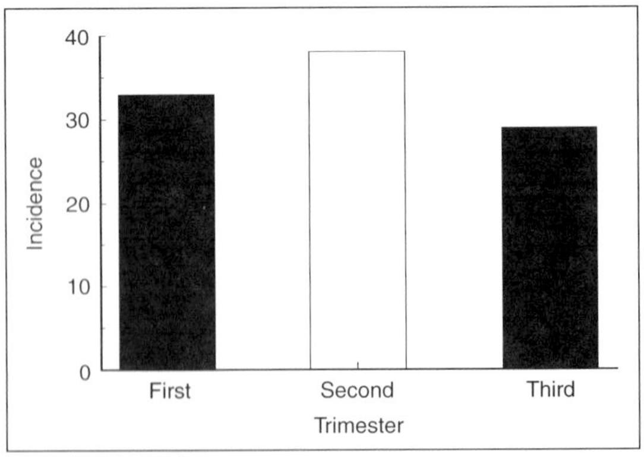

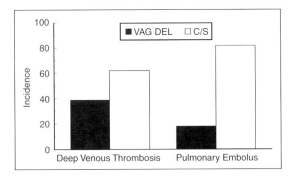

F I G U R E  **19-5**

**The frequency of postpartum deep venous thrombosis and pulmonary embolus separated by the route of delivery.** VAG DEL, vaginal delivery; C/S, cesarean delivery. (From Rutherford SE, Montoro M, McGehee W, et al. Thromboembolic disease associated with pregnancy: an 11-year review. Am J Obstet Gynecol 1991;164:286.)

extremity or pelvic trauma, ethnic background, and higher parity.

## Normal Hemostasis

Few systems are more complex than that designed to maintain normal blood flow within the vasculature tree. Interactions among the vessel wall, platelets, and soluble molecules in the vicinity of an injury work to seal a vessel defect without sacrificing nearby vessel patency. The key processes are (1) vasoconstriction, (2) formation of a platelet plug, (3) formation of a stable "seal" by coagulation factors, (4) prevention of spread of the clot along the vessel wall, (5) when possible,

T A B L E  **19-1**

**Factors associated with a higher risk of pulmonary embolus**

Maternal age
Ethnic background
Operative delivery
Prior thromboembolus
Prolonged immobilization
Inherited coagulation disorders
Trauma

prevention of occlusion of the vessel by clot, and (6) remodeling and gradual degradation of the clot after it is no longer needed.

The maintenance of normal blood flow requires intact, patent blood vessels. After an injury, the hemostatic and fibrinolytic systems work together to protect vascular integrity and assist in repair. Vessel wall integrity, platelet aggregation, normal function of the coagulation cascade, and fibrinolysis are all vital to this process. The initial response to injury is vasoconstriction, which reduces local blood flow and limits the size of the thrombus needed to seal a defect (Stead, 1985). After platelets begin to adhere to the exposed vessel wall, they change shape and secrete their granule contents; this action leads to further platelet accumulation or aggregation. This results in the formation of a platelet plug.

The numerous substances released by the platelets include thromboxane $A_2$ ($TxA_2$), a potent vasoconstrictor and preaggregatory agent (Needleman, 1976; Thompson, 1983); serotonin, a vasoconstrictor (Thompson, 1983); and adenosine diphosphate (ADP), which enhances platelet aggregation. Platelets also produce vascular permeability factor and platelet growth factor, which stimulate fibroblasts and vascular smooth muscle (Letsky, 1985; Stead, 1985). Released platelet factor 4 ($PF_4$) and beta-thromboglobulin are used as markers of platelet activity (Files, 1981; Kaplan, 1981). The platelet contractile protein, thrombasthenin, enables secretion of these substances and also enhances clot retraction (Letsky, 1985). A platelet surface phospholipoprotein, platelet factor 3 ($PF_3$), becomes available to bind factor V, which catalyzes the formation of thrombin. Thrombin, in turn, potentiates platelet aggregation (Kaplan, 1981).

Whereas $TxA_2$ is the result of platelet arachidonic acid metabolism, arachidonic acid in endothelial cells is synthesized to prostacyclin ($PGI_2$). Prostacyclin inhibits aggregation and stimulates vasodilation and, thus, acts in opposition to $TxA_2$ by increasing cAMP monophosphate (AMP) (Stead, 1985). Because $PGI_2$ is concentrated within the vessel wall, the greater the distance from the lumen, the lower the concentration of $PGI_2$ and the higher the concentration of proaggretory substances.

As platelets begin to seal a vascular defect, the coagulation cascade produces fibrin, which is polymerized as clot and incorporated into the platelet plug. Proteolytic cleavage or conformational changes activate the circulating clotting factors at the site of injury.

Factors II, VII, IX, and X require a vitamin K–dependent reaction in the liver in which gamma-carboxyglutamic acid residues are attached to the protein structure. This action provides a location to form a complex with calcium ion and phospholipid receptors on the platelet or endothelial cell membranes. Subsequent steps in the clotting cascade occur at those sites and include the formation of thrombin. Once formed, this is released into the fluid phase.

Two pathways, the intrinsic and extrinsic, lead to the final common clotting pathway. Both pathways are activated by components of the vessel wall and lead to activation of progressively greater amounts of subsequent factors (see Chapter 29).

In the intrinsic pathway, high-molecular-weight kininogen and kallikrein are cofactors for the initial step of the process. This is the activation of factor XII. By catalyzing the formation of kallikrein from prekallikreins, factor XIIa also helps to initiate fibrinolysis, to activate the complement, and to produce kinins (Stead, 1985). Factor XI is activated by XIIa and then cleaves factor IX to form IXa.

The extrinsic pathway is so named because this path relies on tissue thromboplastin as a cofactor. Tissue thromboplastin is released to the circulation following membrane damage or proteolysis (Stead, 1985). Factor VII is then activated to VIIa, which, with tissue thromboplastin, can activate factors IX or X.

The common pathway begins with activation of factor X by either VIIa or IXa, in combination with the protein cofactor VIII:C (the antihemophilic factor) and the calcium ion on the platelet surface (to form PF$_3$) (see Chapter 29). Factor Xa, assisted by cofactor Va, enzymatically divides prothrombin into thrombin and a peptide activation fragment, F$_{1+2}$. Separation from this fragment liberates thrombin into the fluid phase. Thrombin catalyzes the formation of fibrin monomers from fibrogen and, thus, releases fibrinopeptides A and B and facilitates activation of V, VIII:C, and XIII.

A fibrin gel is created by the hydrophobic and electrostatic interactions of the fibrin alpha and gamma chains. Subsequently, factor XIIIa forms covalent bonds linking nearby alpha and gamma chains to form a stable polymerized fibrin clot into which water also is incorporated.

Trapped within the clot are proteins that contribute to the enzymatic digestion of the fibrin matrix: plasminogen and plasminogen activators. A variety of substances can activate plasminogen. Plasma plasminogen activator is activated by factor XIIa. Release of tissue activators (tissue plasminogen activator) from blood vessel epithelium (especially venous) is stimulated by exercise, emotional stress, trauma, surgery, hypotensive shock, pharmacologic agents, and activated protein C (Letsky, 1985; Stead, 1985; Comp, 1981). The fibrinolytic enzymes streptokinase and urokinase also activate plasminogen (Robbins, 1982).

Having been activated from plasminogen, plasmin cleaves arginyl-lysine bonds in many substrates, including fibrinogen, fibrin, factor VIII, and complement (Robbins, 1982; Bonnar, 1970). The result of plasmin action on fibrin and fibrinogen is release of protein fragments, referred to as fibrin degradation products (or fibrin split products). The larger fragments, which may have slow clotting activity, are further divided by plasmin. These fragments have anticoagulant activity, in that they inhibit the formation and cross-linking of fibrin (Stead, 1985). Measurement of fibrin degradation products provides an indirect measurement of fibrinolysis.

Alpha-2 antiplasmin, a specific plasmin inhibitor that binds to fibrin and fibrinogen, is found in serum, platelets, and within the clot, along with other inhibitors of plasmin or plasminogen activity (Robbins, 1982).

As a potent inhibitor of thrombin, AT III is important in the regulation of hemostasis. To lesser degrees, AT III binds and inactivates factors IXa, Xa, XIa, and XIIa. Antithrombin III acts as a substrate for these serine proteases but forms stable intermediate bonds with the active portion and, thus, neutralizes the enzyme (Brandt, 1985). Heparin binds to AT III and induces a conformational change that increases the affinity of AT III for thrombin. The otherwise slow inactivation of thrombin by AT III is accelerated greatly by even small amounts of heparin. After a stable thrombin-antithrombin complex is formed, heparin is released and available for repetitive catalysis.

Excess amounts of AT III are circulating, and some are bound to endothelial cell membranes via heparan, a sulfated mucopolysaccharide with a function similar to heparin. The presence of heparan on intact endothelial cell surfaces and its binding of AT III, which neutralizes the thrombin, help to prevent local extension of thrombus beyond the sites of vessel injury (Comp, 1985). Deficiency of AT III leads to a higher incidence of thrombotic events (Megha, 1990).

Proteins C and S together are another important anticoagulant system. Like certain clotting factors, their synthesis depends on vitamin K and involves addition of gamma-carboxyglutamic acid residues that enable binding, via calcium ions, to cell surfaces. Protein C is attached to endothelial cells, and protein S is attached to endothelial and platelet membranes. Endothelial cell surfaces also have a specific protein receptor for thrombin, called thrombomodulin. Binding of thrombin to thrombomodulin changes its activity from procoagulant to activation of protein C, opposing coagulation. Complexes of protein Ca and adjacently bound protein S cofactor proteolyze the phospholipid-bound factors VIII:Ca and Va. This action results in a second mechanism to prevent extension of thrombus beyond the area of vessel injury (Comp, 1985). Heterozygous defects in the protein C or S genes can be associated with an increase in thromboembolic events (Comp, 1985; Broekmans, 1985). Homozygosity of protein C deficiency leads to the often fatal neonatal purpura fulminans (Malciniak, 1985).

## Changes in Hemostasis in Pregnancy

Pregnancy is a hypercoagulable state in which there exists an increased potential for coagulation and thrombosis. Although these coagulation alterations have been studied extensively, there is no reliable test to determine one's "state of hypercoagulability" (i.e., a test to determine which pregnant patient is at risk for a DVT). While there may be an ongoing increase in activation

of coagulation during pregnancy, compensatory mechanisms such as a concomitant rise in fibrinolytic activity help to maintain coagulation equilibrium (Woodhams, 1989). As pregnancy progresses, a low-grade chronic intravascular coagulation results in fibrin deposition in the spiral arteries of the placental bed. This gradually replaces the internal elastic lamina and smooth muscle (Hathaway, 1978). Within an hour of delivery, this fibrinolytic potential decreases and returns to normal. These changes are believed to contribute to the hypercoagulability of pregnancy and the puerperium (Rutherford, 1991a). Increased fibrin split products and D-dimers during this period suggest ongoing fibrinolytic activity (Hathaway, 1978).

The hypercoagulable state is due primarily to changes in clotting factors (Table 19-2); levels of factors V, VII, VIII, IX, X, XII, and fibrinogen increase during pregnancy. The fibrinogen level undergoes the most marked increase, as the total circulating amount approximately doubles. In contrast, the levels of factors XI and XIII decrease. Plasma fibrinolytic activity decreases as a result of placental inhibitors but can return to normal within 1 hour after delivery (Bonnar, 1969). When the placenta separates, tissue thromboplastin is released into the circulation, increasing the chance of thrombosis (Bonnar, 1981). The increased tendency toward coagulation may be balanced partially by a pregnancy-specific protein, PAPP-A, which, like heparin, facilitates neutralization of thrombin by AT III (Brandt, 1985). Platelet

T A B L E   **19-2**

Hemostatic changes that occur during pregnancy

*Hemostatic Changes Promoting Thrombosis*
Increased factor levels V, VII, VIII, IX, X, XII, fibrinogen
Placental inhibitors of fibrinolysis
Tissue thromboplastin released into the circulation at placental separation
Venous stasis of the lower extremities
Endothelial damage associated with parturition

*Hemostatic Changes Discouraging Thrombosis*
Decreased factor levels XI, XIII
Pregnancy-specific protein neutralizing AT III

counts appear to remain in the normal range during pregnancy.

The net effect of hemostasis during pregnancy is an increased potential for thrombosis resulting from increased levels of coagulation factors and decreased fibrinolysis. This change is most marked at term and in the immediate puerperium and serves to control blood loss after placental separation.

## Deep Venous Thrombosis

### Clinical Diagnosis

In the pregnant patient, DVT appears to begin more often in the deep proximal veins and has a predilection for the left leg (Barbour, 1995a; Dahlman, 1989). The clinical diagnosis of DVT (Barnes, 1975) is difficult and requires objective testing: In many instances, PE may occur in the absence of clinical symptoms (Dorfman, 1987; Hull, 1983). When clinical symptoms and signs do occur, they are sufficiently reliable to arouse suspicion but insufficient to establish a diagnosis. Of patients suspected of a DVT, half will not have it objectively confirmed. Moreover, it is clinically impossible to determine which DVT will result in a PE.

Symptoms and signs of DVT are illustrated in Table 19-3. Swelling is considered whenever there is at least a 2-cm measured difference in circumference between the affected and normal limbs. Homan's sign is present when passive dorsiflexion of the foot in a relaxed leg leads to pain, presumably in the calf or popliteal areas. The Lowenberg test is positive if pain occurs distal to a BP cuff rapidly inflated to 180 mm Hg. The

T A B L E   **19-3**

**Clinical symptoms and signs of deep venous thrombosis of the legs**

Unilateral pain, swelling, tenderness, and/or
  edema
Limb color changes
Palpable cord
Positive Homan's sign
Positive Lowenberg test
Limb-size difference > 2 cm

presence of marked swelling, cyanosis or paleness, a cold extremity, or diminished pulses signals the rare obstructive iliofemoral vein thrombosis. To cloud the issue clinically, years after a severe obstructive DVT, patients may experience postphlebitic syndrome (skin stasis dermatitis or ulcers). An investigation of 104 women with a median postthrombosis interval of 11 years revealed that 4% had ulceration, and only 22% were without complaints (Bergqvist, 1990). Finally, it is important to remember that pregnant patients commonly complain of swelling and leg discomfort and, as such, do not require objective testing in every instance.

The first sign of deep venous disease may be the occurrence of a pulmonary embolus. In a similar manner, silent DVT has been found in 70% of patients with angiographically proven PE (Hull, 1983).

### Diagnostic Studies

#### Ultrasound

Noninvasive testing is the first step in confirming the diagnosis of DVT. Real-time ultrasonographic imaging, including duplex Doppler, is a valuable addition to continuous-wave Doppler. Experience is required for accurate interpretation with both modalities, and the affected leg should be compared with the asymptomatic one. Doppler studies allow one to detect alterations in blood flow but do not determine the cause of the alteration. Real-time imaging with high-frequency transducers, on the other hand, does allow visualization of deep vessels and surrounding tissue.

Maneuvers such as Valsalva (which distends the vein and slows the proximal flow), release of pressure over a distal vein (which causes a rapid proximal flow of blood), and squeezing of the muscles all cause changes in Doppler shift. Thrombi that completely occlude proximal veins, causing an absence of blood flow sound, and those not large enough to obstruct blood flow may escape detection with continuous-wave Doppler. Real-time imaging in the presence of DVT may detect a mass in the vessel lumen, a failure of the lumen diameter to increase with Valsalva, or a failure of the vein to compress with pressure (Raghavendra, 1984). Alternatively, imaging may identify a hematoma, popliteal cyst, or other pathology to explain the patient's symptoms.

Duplex Doppler may be used to detect the absence of either spontaneous flow or normal variation with respiration. Imaging is most useful for the distal iliac, femoral, and popliteal veins. Doppler also is useful for proximal iliac DVT. The sensitivity and specificity for proximal veins is 90% (PIOPED Investigators, 1990). At least 50% of small calf thrombi are missed due to collateral venous channels (PIOPED Investigators, 1990). The combination of continuous-wave Doppler and real-time imaging results in 98% detection proximal DVT with 95% specificity compared with venography (Elias, 1987; Killwich, 1989). Experience again must be emphasized because the choice of parameters used to reach a diagnosis affects the sensitivity and specificity (Killwich, 1989). Repeating the examination after 2 to 3 days also may reveal a clot not previously seen.

During pregnancy, the iliac vessels are especially difficult to image. This is due to pressure from the gravid uterus on the inferior vena cava. As a result, Doppler results must be interpreted cautiously. In the puerperal patient, imaging may visualize a clot in the iliac vessels as in pelvic thrombophlebitis, or ovarian vein thrombosis. The use of computerized tomography or magnetic resonance imaging, however, may be more helpful in these latter conditions (Spritzer, 1995).

### Ascending Venography

Venography is the diagnostic gold standard of DVT in pregnancy. With the patient at an approx-imately 40-degree incline and bearing weight on her unaffected leg, radiographic contrast dye is injected into a dorsal vein of the involved foot. This position allows for the gradual and complete filling of the leg veins without layering of the dye and reduces the likelihood of a false-positive test. Nonetheless, false-positive tests may result from poor technique, poor choice of injection site, contraction of the leg muscles, or extravascular pathology such as a Baker's (popliteal) cyst, hematoma, cellulitis, edema, or muscle rupture. In addition, the larger diameter of the deep femoral and iliac veins can lead to incomplete filling with the dye and unreliable results. Positive identification of a thrombus requires visualization of a well-defined filling defect in more than one radiographic view (Fig 19-6). Suggestive signs of a DVT include abrupt termination of a vessel, absence of opacification, or diversion of blood flow.

Unlike ultrasonography and Doppler procedures, venography is associated with significant side effects. Twenty-four percent of patients will experience minor side effects of muscle pain, leg swelling, tenderness, or erythema (Bettman, 1977). These side effects can be reduced 70% by lowering the concentration of contrast medium (PIOPED Investigators, 1990). Using a heparinized saline flush after dye injection and the concomitant use of corticosteroids can minimize the risks of phlebitis and clot formation. Radiation exposure to the fetus has been estimated at 0.0314 rad for unilateral venography including fluoroscopy and spot films without an abdominal shield (Ginsberg, 1989). This is well below

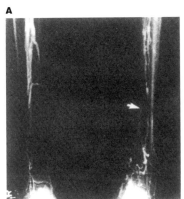
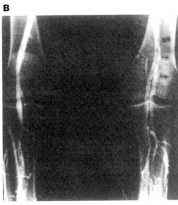

A

B

F I G U R E  **19-6**

A contrast venogram shows each of two legs: (A) A cut-off sign in the posterior tibial vein and filling defects in the popliteal vein in one leg. (B) A normal study in the other leg.

the minimum level of radiation exposure considered teratogenic (ACOG, 1997).

## Impedance Plethysmography

Impedance plethysmography (IPG) uses changes in electrical resistance to measure changes in blood volume in a limb. It is highly sensitive to proximal thrombosis but frequently fails to detect those below the knee. With inflation of a thigh cuff, blood is retained in the leg. In the absence of venous obstruction, sudden deflation results in immediate outflow of blood and a concomitant sudden increase in electrical resistance. A much slower change is associated with impaired outflow, which indirectly implies venous thrombosis (Markisz, 1985). Because DVT confined to the calf rarely results in PE, anticoagulation for such DVT is not mandatory; in patients with suspected calf vein thrombosis, IPG may allow the clinician to avoid anticoagulation or venography by excluding extension of the clot above the knee over 2 weeks while the presumed calf thrombosis is treated with heat and elevation (Mohr, 1988; Huisman, 1986; Kohn, 1987; Moser, 1981; Monreal, 1987). In pregnancy, compression of the inferior vena cava by the gravid uterus can yield falsely positive results (Nicholas, 1985), and confirmation of DVT by venography may be necessary.

## Thermography

Though infrequently used, thermography detects DVT by an increase in skin temperature. Infrared radiation emission is increased when blood flow is diverted to superficial collaterals or when inflammation is present. Changes are more likely to occur with extensive disease. False-negative results can occur with early or limited thrombosis.

## Iodine 125 Fibrinogen Scanning

This technique is contraindicated during pregnancy because unbound iodine 125 ([125]I) crosses the placental barrier to enter the fetal circulation, where it can collect in the fetal thyroid (Kakkar,

1972; Bentley, 1979). Unbound [125]I also enters breast milk. In both instances, [125]I can be concentrated in the fetal or neonatal thyroid and produce goiter. Because [125]I has a half-life of 60.2 days (PIOPED Investigators, 1990), temporary interruption of lactation is impractical. Thus, the preferred approach, if this radiographic technique is medically necessary, is to avoid breast-feeding. To avoid the small risk of hypothyroidism, non-radioactive iodine should be administered orally from 24 hours prior to and for 2 weeks after the procedure.

In nonlactating postpartum patients, [125]I-labeled fibrinogen can be used to identify DVT. Iodine 125 has a longer half-life and gives a smaller radiation dose than the previously used [131]I. After intravenous (IV) injection, [125]I is incorporated like normal fibrinogen into developing thrombi. Sequential scintillation scanning is performed at any time between 4 hours and 7 days later but usually at 24, 48, and 72 hours. With each scan, radioactivity is compared with background precordial values in the search for a hot spot. For the lower thigh and calf, accuracy can be as high as 92% (Kakkar, 1972). Higher background counts in the femoral artery, the bladder, and the overlying muscle mass make detection of thrombi in the common femoral and pelvic chins difficult. False-positives can be due to hematoma, inflammation, or surgical wound uptake. Alternatively, if an old thrombus is no longer taking up fibrinogen or forms after the [125]I has been cleared from the circulation, a false-negative study may result.

## Radionuclide Venography

Radionuclide venography using technetium 99m ([99m]Tc) particles is of low risk to the fetus and can be used to obtain leg studies as well as perfusion lung scans. When performed with a rapid-sequence gamma camera, which may not be available in many institutions, this technique is more than 90% accurate for DVT above the knee (Kakkar, 1972; Bentley, 1979). Sequential, staged imaging using BP cuffs on the legs to delay flow is an alternative. Correlations with conventional venography of 95% thigh and 100% pelvis have been reported (Bentley, 1979).

## Pulmonary Embolus

### Clinical Diagnosis

The sudden onset of unexplained dyspnea and tachypnea are the most common clinical findings that suggest a pulmonary embolus (Table 19-4) (Leclerc, 1994; Rosenow, 1981; Kohn, 1987). Other symptoms include cough, pleuritic chest pain, apprehension, atelectatic rales, hemoptysis, fever, diaphoresis, friction rub, cyanosis, and changes in the heart sounds (accentuated second heart sound, gallop, or murmur). The clinical manifestations of pulmonary embolus are influenced primarily by the number, size, and location of the emboli. Preexisting health problems, such as pneumonia, congestive heart failure, or cancer, may also confuse the clinical interpretation. If an infarction of the lung occurs after a PE, the patient will typically complain of pleuritic chest pain and hemoptysis and will have a friction rub. It is also important to remember that patients with a DVT can experience an occult PE (Dorfman, 1987).

T A B L E   **19-4**

**Clinical symptoms and signs associated with pulmonary thromboembolus**

*Symptoms*

| | |
|---|---|
| Tachypnea | 90% |
| Tachycardia | 40% |
| Less common | Hemoptysis |
| | Diaphoresis |
| | Fever |
| | Rales |
| | Wheezing |
| | Syncope |

*Signs*

| | |
|---|---|
| Dyspnea | 80% |
| Pleuritic chest pain | 70% |
| Apprehension | 60% |
| Nonproductive cough | 50% |

Sources: Leclerc JR. Pulmonary embolism. In: Rakel RE, ed. Conn's current therapy—1994. Philadelphia: WB Saunders, 1994:199–205; Rosenow EC III, Osmundson PJ, Brown ML. Pulmonary embolism. Mayo Clin Proc 1981;56:161–178; and Kohn H, Konig B, Mostbeck A. Incidence and clinical feature of pulmonary embolism in patients with deep venous thrombosis. A prospective study. Eur J Nucl Med 1987;13:S11–S13.

Signs of right-sided heart failure, such as jugular venous distention, liver enlargement, left parasternal heave, and fixed splitting of the second heart sound, can be seen in instances in which at least 50% of the pulmonary circulation has been obstructed. This may be caused by large emboli or multiple small ones and is termed *massive pulmonary embolism* (Bell, 1977). Of note, while multiple small pulmonary emboli can mimic massive pulmonary emboli, they can cause no symptoms at all or resemble common pregnancy discomforts.

Less commonly, pulmonary embolus can manifest clinically as hypotension, syncope, or convulsions. Clinical findings may also resemble myocardial infarction. Cortical blindness has been reported as the presenting symptom for a massive pulmonary embolus (Stiller, 1990). If one encounters pulmonary hypertension or an inability to obtain a wedge pressure during pulmonary artery catheterization for other presumed causes of shock, occlusive PE should be suspected (Traeger, 1985).

### Relationship to Deep Venous Thrombosis

Not only does silent DVT sometimes lead to symptomatic PE, but some patients with clinical DVT can develop silent PE. For example, in a group of 105 patients with objectively confirmed DVT, 60 (57%) were felt to have PE by lung scanning; 59% of these were asymptomatic (Kohn, 1987). In another study, 49 patients had proximal DVT and no symptoms of PE; 35% had high-probability lung scans (Dorfman, 1987). Thus, although noninvasive tests for DVT have been proposed as screening tools for PE, sensitivity and negative predictive values are poor (38% and 53%, respectively) (Schiff, 1987). Doppler and IPG results should not be used to rule out PE. The occurrence of silent PE is of little clinical import, because after DVT is diagnosed, the treatment in pregnancy is similar.

### Diagnostic Studies

#### Laboratory Studies

In addition to a clinical examination, an arterial blood gas reading obtained on room air is the first step in confirming the diagnosis. An arterial $Pao_2$ greater than 85 mm Hg is reassuring but does not exclude PE. In one study (Robin, 1977), 14% of 43 patients with angiographically proven PE had a $Pao_2$ greater than or equal to 85 mm Hg. If the $Pao_2$ is low and PE is suspected, anticoagulation should be considered while definite diagnostic tests are performed. Other laboratory tests include WBC count, erythrocyte sedimentation rate, lactic dehydrogenase, creatinine phosphokinase, SGOT, and fibrin split products. Although these tests provide information regarding the patient and her status, they do not help to distinguish a PE from other disease processes and are generally not helpful (Table 19-5).

## Electrocardiogram

The most common ECG finding is tachycardia. Unfortunately, this sign is often transient and may not be observed. In cases of massive PE, the ECG signs of acute cor pulmonale may be seen. These include a right axis shift with an S1 Q3 T3 pattern and nonspecific T-wave inversion. The "classic" S1 Q3 T3 pattern is encountered in only 10% of patients with confirmed PE (Leclerc, 1994). Here, two-dimensional echocardiography may be helpful to visualize a large clot, right atrial enlargement, or right ventricular dilation with poor contractility.

## Chest X-Ray

Chest radiographs are abnormal in 70% of patients with a pulmonary embolus (Rosenow, 1981). Elevation of the hemidiaphragm, atelectasis, and pleural effusion are the most common

TABLE **19-5**

**Commonly used laboratory and radiographic techniques for assisting in the diagnosis of pulmonary embolus**

| | |
|---|---|
| Arterial blood gas | $Pao_2$ <85 mm Hg |
| Electrocardiogram | Sinus tachycardia |
| | Right axis shift |
| | S1 Q3 T3 pattern |
| Chest x-ray | Focal oligemia |
| | Atelectasis |
| | Pleural effusion |
| | Hemidiaphragm elevation |

radiographic abnormalities. Focal oligemia (an area of increased radiolucency and decreased vascular markings) is seen in 2% of cases (Moses, 1974). Massive PE can lead to a change in cardiac size or shape, increased filling of a pulmonary artery, or a sudden termination of a vessel. Infiltrates or plural effusion are later signs of pulmonary infarction. In summary, the primary role of the chest radiograph is to eliminate other causes of the patient's symptoms and to assist in the interpretation of the lung scans.

## Pulmonary Artery Catheterization

During pulmonary artery catheterization, several findings can suggest pulmonary embolism. Failure to wedge or the inability to obtain the appropriate waveform can occur in the case of completely occlusive embolism distal to the catheter tip. If the failure to wedge is combined with pulmonary hypertension, further investigation to rule out PE is warranted (Traeger, 1985). Bedside fluoroscopy using a minimal amount of contrast material can be useful. Occlusion of the distal port of the catheter (Fairfax, 1984) or inability to measure cardiac output because of embedding of the tip in clot (Lewis, 1982) also can be clues to the occurrence of PE. Elevated central venous pressures (>10 mm Hg) may suggest massive PE (Dalen, 1969).

## Ventilation-Perfusion Lung Scan

Regardless of clinical suspicion, arterial blood gas, ECG, or chest x-ray findings, any patient with suspected PE should undergo a lung scan. Perfusion lung scans are highly sensitive and provide definitive information on the presence or absence of a pulmonary embolus. A perfusion lung scan is performed by the IV injection of $^{99m}$Tc-labeled albumin microspheres or macroaggregates. These particles are trapped within the pulmonary precapillary arteriolar bed and occlude less than 0.2% of the vessels (Gold, 1966). Pulmonary function does not change, except in patients with severe pulmonary hypertension (Mills, 1980; Vincent, 1968). Injection is performed with the patient supine, to increase apical perfusion; imaging is performed with the patient upright, to better visualize the lung base. The following views should be obtained: anterior, posterior, right and left lateral, and right and left posterior oblique.

Perfusion lung scans are highly sensitive, and a normal study virtually excludes PE (Kipper, 1982; Rutherford, 1991b). Altered pulmonary perfusion from any source, such as pneumonia, tumor, atelectasis, or effusion, can result in a false-positive scan. For example, separate investigations revealed normal pulmonary arteriograms in 38% of patients with segmental perfusion defects (Markisz, 1985) and in 83% of those with a high probability of PE by perfusion lung scan (Urokinase Pulmonary Embolism Trial, 1973).

Ventilation scans complement perfusion scans and increase specificity. Using both ventilation and perfusion scans, with or without noninvasive studies for DVT, the reliability of diagnosis of PE is approximately 90% (Alderson, 1987). Scans are interpreted as normal, as indeterminate, or as having a low, moderate, or high probability of PE. When chest x-ray opacification corresponds with perfusion defects, the scan is considered nondiagnostic. Subsequent angiography has shown that the likelihood of PE is low with isolated subsegmental defects or matching ventilation/perfusion defects and high in the presence of ventilation/perfusion (V/Q) mismatching or multiple defects (Fig 19-7). Chronic obstructive pulmonary disease is the most common confounding factor in evaluation of the scans; in such cases, arteriography often is recommended.

No adverse fetal effects of xenon 133 ($^{133}$Xe) or $^{99m}$Tc lung scanning have been reported, and the exposure dose has been estimated to be significantly less than that received with pulmonary arteriography (Henkin, 1982). The absorbed radiation dose to the lung is approximately 50 to 75 mrad with $^{99m}$Tc aerosol versus 300 mrad with $^{133}$Xe (the highest dose of the ventilation agents mentioned) (Alderson, 1987). Even if both V/Q scanning and pulmonary angiography are performed, the total dose will be far less than the lowest dose associated with a teratogenic effect in the human fetus (National Council on Radiation Protection and Measurement, 1977).

Oxygen-15 ($^{15}$O)-labeled carbon dioxide inhalation may, in the future, be useful in pregnancy, due to the low radiation dose. The $^{15}$O is incorporated rapidly into $H_2^{15}O$, which fails to clear the pulmonary circulation in areas of underperfusion. Resulting hot spots are visualized scintigraphically. The major disadvantage is the requirement for a cyclotron in order to produce the $^{15}$O, which has a half-life of 2.1 minutes (Nichols, 1980).

## Pulmonary Arteriography

Pulmonary arteriography is the definitive technique for confirming the diagnosis of PE, but it occasionally may be indeterminate. Injection of contrast medium selectively into lobar or segmental branches of the pulmonary artery yields clear visualization of vessels greater than 2.5 mm (Hull, 1983). A clot may be seen as a filling defect that does not obstruct flow or as an abruptly terminated vessel, possibly with a trailing edge of dye where the clot incompletely fills the lumen (Fig 19-8).

Multiple views may be essential to exclude PE. Risks are related to the use of catheterization

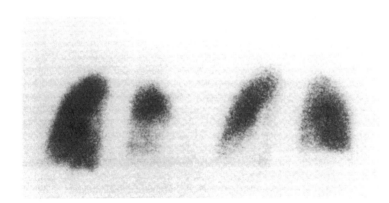

F I G U R E   **19-7**

In these posterior views, the perfusion lung scan (left) reveals segmental defects, which are not "matched" in the normal ventilation scan (right). This is consistent with a high probability of PE.

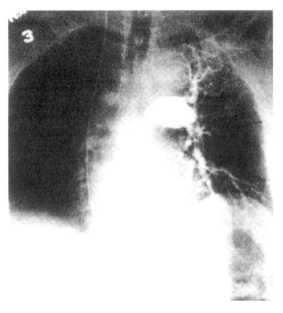

F I G U R E    **19-8**

Arteriogram of the left pulmonary artery shows filling defects (illustrated by arrows) and an unperfused segment of lung as shown by the absence of contrast dye (outlined by broken line).

and contrast dye. With pulmonary arteriography, morbidity has been reported as 4% to 5% and mortality as 0.2% to 0.3% (Mills, 1980; Dalen, 1979). Most series' complications, however, occur in patients with underlying pulmonary hypertension and right ventricular end-diastolic pressure exceeding 20 mm Hg (Mills, 1980).

Pulmonary arteriography is advised when lung scanning is indeterminate, does not correlate with clinical suspicion, or indicates moderate probability of PE; the physician should take into account corresponding V/Q defects and/or chest x-ray findings (PIOPED Investigators, 1996). The risks of thrombolytic therapy (e.g., streptokinase) or surgical interruption of the vena cava necessitate angiographic confirmation prior to consideration of these measures.

### Digital Subtraction Pulmonary Angiography

This relatively noninvasive tool involves the injection of a contrast medium into a peripheral vein and computerized subtraction of the preinjection chest x-ray from the postinjection film. Theoretically, an image of the pulmonary arterial vasculature, as exemplified by contrast filling, is obtained; however, poor imaging often results from respiratory and cardiac motion, and resolution is not as good as with conventional arteriography. In addition, it is difficult to obtain multiple projection views, and nonselective filling can cause vessel overlap. Digital subtraction angiography holds promise, given continued technologic improvement.

### Indium 111 Platelet Imaging

This technique is not yet available for widespread clinical use but shows promise in the diagnosis and management of patients with thromboembolic disease. Platelets are extracted from venous blood, labeled, and reinjected into the donor. The platelets then accumulate at sites of active thrombosis. Heparin blocks the incorporation of these platelets into an established nonexpanding thrombus. Images are obtained with gamma-camera scintigraphy. For DVT, sensitivity is 90% to 95%, and specificity is 95% to 100% (Ezekowitz, 1985). Hematomas, wound infection, and prostheses can cause false-positive results. Few data are available regarding the usefulness of this technique in PE. As long as thrombosis is active, uptake of platelets can be visualized and, thus, allow anticoagulation to be monitored.

## Anticoagulant Therapy

### Heparin

Heparin (Hirsch, 1991) is a heterogeneous acidic mucopolysaccharide with a high molecular weight, which prevents it from crossing the placenta (Table 19-6). The molecular weights in commercial preparations range from 4000 to 40,000 daltons, and biologic activities of the different fractions also vary. Recent reports have suggested that the separation and use of the lower-molecular-weight molecules (4000–6000) may provide a preparation of higher, more uniform activity (Bratt, 1985; Gillis, 1992; Fejgin, 1994;

T A B L E   **19-6**

The distinguishing pharmacologic features of the
anticoagulants heparin and warfarin

|  | **Heparin** | **Warfarin** |
|---|---|---|
| Molecular weight (daltons)* | 12,000–15,000 | 1000 |
| Mechanism of action | Binds AT III | Vitamin K–dependent factors |
| Administration | Intravenous, subcutaneous | Oral |
| Half-life | 1.0–2.5 hr | 2.5 days |
| Anticoagulant effect | Immediate | 36–72 hr |
| Laboratory monitoring | Heparin levels, aPTT antifactor Xa | Prothrombin time, INR |
| Reversal | Protamine sulfate | Vitamin K |
| Placental transfer | None | Crosses |

*Mean molecular weight.

INR, international normalized ratio.

Lensing, 1995; Sturridge, 1994; Rasmussen, 1994; Ginsberg, 1995; Samama, 1986; Levine, 1996; Koopman, 1996). Low-molecular-weight heparin (LMWH) differs slightly in its anticoagulant activity from standard heparin, and it has been shown to have greater bioavailability and longer antifactor Xa activity (Samama, 1986; Levine, 1996; Koopman, 1996).

Heparin exerts its anticoagulant activity by binding to plasma AT III. Once bound, the configuration of AT III is changed. This facilitates its binding to and neutralization of, primarily, factor Xa and thrombin and, to a lesser extent, factors IXa, XIa, and XIIa. Its antifactor Xa activity is inversely proportional to the molecular weight of the heparin fragment (Fejgin, 1994). Then, heparin is released and leaves stable complexes. Once released, heparin can then interact similarly with other molecules of AT III. Small amounts of heparin can inhibit the initial steps of the clotting cascade. After a thrombus has been formed, however, much more heparin is needed to neutralize the larger amounts of already formed thrombin and prevent extension of the clot (White, 1979). As thrombin production diminishes, heparin requirements may decrease.

A disadvantage of heparin is the need for parenteral administration via IV or subcutaneous routes. Heparin is not absorbed via the gastrointestinal tract, and intramuscular injections result in erratic absorption and carry a risk of hematoma formation. The half-life of heparin varies with the dose, the type of heparin, and the extent of active thrombosis. For example, higher doses result in both a higher peak and a longer half-life (DeSwart, 1982). Half-lives of less than 1 hour to more than 2.5 hours have been found. Moreover, heparin levels may become abnormally elevated in hepatic or renal failure (Perry, 1974). Continuous IV infusion has been shown to result in more consistent levels and fewer hemorrhagic events than does administration via intermittent IV bolus. Subcutaneous administration also gives a steadier effect, but slower absorption results in a 2- to 4-hour delay in peak levels.

Another difficulty associated with heparin is adequate monitoring of the bioeffect of heparin to ensure an adequate yet safe dose. Laboratories vary in the type of tests they can offer, partly because the procedures are technique-sensitive, and skill is required for consistent results. The activated partial thromboplastin time (aPTT) is the most commonly available test. Prolongation of the aPTT to 1.5 to 2.5 times (Hyers, 1986; Basu, 1972) the control value has been shown to be useful in monitoring patients. There is a significant increase in clot extension with aPTT levels below 1.5, but no increase in bleeding complications as 2.5 is approached. Thus, anticoagulation in the upper range of 1.5 to 2.5 times control appears to be ideal.

Although no single laboratory test appears clearly superior in predicting bleeding, heparin assay may be the most helpful (Holm, 1985). Heparin levels are measured indirectly, using the protamine sulfate neutralization test, in which the amount of protamine sulfate needed to reverse the effects of heparin on the thrombin clotting time is measured. Plasma heparin levels of 0.2 to 0.4 IU/mL are desirable. In some institutions, measurement of inhibition of factor Xa has been developed as a monitoring tool for heparin anticoagulation. In general, however, the aPTT is used.

## Low-Molecular-Weight Heparin

Low-molecular-weight heparin is distinguishable pharmacologically from standard unfractionated heparin (S-Heparin) by its preferential inactivation of factor Xa (Table 19-7). Here, antifactor Xa activity is inversely related to the molecular weight of the fragment. This means that LMWH has a greater anti-Xa activity. While any heparin will inactivate factor Xa by binding to AT III, S-Heparin, by virtue of its longer saccharide chain and pentasaccharide sequence, also inactivates thrombin by forming a ternary complex with AT III and thrombin. In this way, S-Heparin inhibits the activity of both factor Xa and thrombin. Because LMWH lacks the longer saccharide chains, this

agent does not inhibit thrombin, and its associated potential for bleeding is, therefore, less.

Low-molecular-weight heparin offers additional advantages over S-Heparin (Fejgin, 1994; Lensing, 1995). For example, LMWH has a plasma half-life 2 to 4 times longer and a more predictable anticoagulant response than S-Heparin. Second, LMWH has less pronounced effects on platelet function and vascular permeability (with significantly less risk of heparin-induced thrombocytopenia). Third, unlike S-Heparin, LMWH can resist inhibition by $PF_4$.

Low-molecular-weight heparin and S-Heparin are similar in that neither crosses the placenta and both are administered either IV or subcutaneously. Protamine sulfate is used to reverse both heparins, although LMWH is less affected by the action of protamine sulfate (Fejgin, 1994). Further LMWH is administered as a weight-dependent dose, and because of its predictable effect, no monitoring of levels is necessary.

Low-molecular-weight heparin has been shown to be effective when administered on an outpatient basis for the treatment of DVT. Thus, the higher initial cost of the drug may be outweighed by the absence of need for hospitalization. Numerous studies demonstrate equivalence

T A B L E   **19-7**

The distinguishing pharmacologic features of standard (unfractionated) heparin (S-Heparin) and low-molecular-weight heparin (L-Heparin)

|  | **S-Heparin** | **L-Heparin** |
|---|---|---|
| Molecular weight (daltons)* | 12,000–15,000 | 4000–6000 |
| Mechanism of action | Binds AT III | Binds AT III |
| Inhibitory activity | Factor Xa | Factor Xa |
|  | Thrombin |  |
| Administration | IV | IV |
|  | SQ | SQ |
| Half-life (hr) |  |  |
|   IV | 1 | 4 |
|   SQ | 3 | 4 |
| Laboratory monitoring | aPTT | None needed; may be measured by antifactor Xa |
|  | Heparin levels |  |
|  | Antifactor Xa |  |
| Reversal | Protamine sulfate | Protamine sulfate |
| Placental transfer | None | None |

*Mean molecular weight.

IV, intravenous; SQ, subcutaneous.

or superiority of LMWH to S-Heparin for a variety of prophylactic and therapeutic indications (Levine, 1996; Koopman, 1996; McMahon, 1996; Berquist, 1996; Clagett, 1995; Geertz, 1996; Levine, 1996). Although not yet approved for therapeutic anticoagulation, this agent is increasingly prescribed for this indication, and most authorities believe LMWH will soon completely replace S-Heparin for the prophylaxis and treatment of thromboembolic disorders. Although ideal dosage for the pregnant patient has not been established, standard doses in nonpregnant women are enoxaprin 1 mg/kg subcutaneously twice a day (therapeutic) and 30 mg subcutaneously twice a day (prophylactic).

## Heparin Side Effects

The primary risk of heparin anticoagulation (Table 19-8) is bleeding, which occurs in approximately 5% to 10% of patients (Bonnar, 1981; Hall, 1978; Walker, 1980) but can affect as many as one third (Holm, 1985). Prior to initiating anticoagulation, the physician should request a baseline clotting profile to identify those patients with an underlying coagulation defect and possibly to prevent hemorrhagic complications. The number of bleeding episodes appears to relate to the total daily dose of heparin and the prolongation of the aPTT. Unlike continuous infusion or subcutaneous injection, bolus infusion is associated with a higher total dose of heparin and a much greater risk of bleeding. Rapid reversal of heparinization in the case of overdose or to prevent bleeding at the time of emergency surgery can be accomplished, if necessary, with protamine sulfate.

Because the primary hemostatic defense in heparinized patients is platelet aggregation, drugs such as nonsteroidal antiinflammatory agents or

dextran, which interfere with platelet number or function, may induce bleeding. For example, patients receiving aspirin have twice the risk of bleeding (Walker, 1980). Because heparin is an acidic molecule and incompatible with many solutions containing medications (e.g., aminoglycosides), heparin activity may be affected. When such drugs are administered at separate sites, however, there is no loss of heparin activity (Hirsch, 1991).

A second side effect of heparin therapy is thrombocytopenia. Estimates of the incidence of thrombocytopenia for S-Heparin vary from 1% to 30% (Barbour, 1995a; Chang, 1982) and for LMWH, around 2% (Fejgin, 1994). Thrombocytopenia typically occurs, if at all, within 2 to 15 days after the initiation of full-dose heparin therapy (Barbour, 1995a; Hirsch, 1991). Clinically, the thrombocytopenia may be mild (platelet count > 100,000 per cubic millimeter) or severe (platelet count < 100,000 per cubic millimeter). With the mild form, treatment can be continued without an undue risk of bleeding. The severe form, however, requires discontinuation of heparin therapy and is reversible. In this latter circumstance, heparinoids have been found to be 93% efficacious (Magnani, 1993). To follow a patient on heparin therapy, maternal platelet counts are only medically necessary for the first 2 to 3 weeks of therapy. Thereafter, platelet counts are probably superfluous (Barbour, 1995a).

The mechanism involved in the thrombocytopenia is incompletely understood but appears to involve platelet clumping and sequestration, immune-mediated destruction, and consumption through low-grade disseminated intravascular coagulation. While heparin-associated thrombocytopenia is most frequently encountered in patients receiving high-dose heparin, patients on prophylactic low-dose heparin have a lower risk of this condition (Galle, 1978; Phillipps, 1983; Hirsch, 1992), and those on LMWH (Ginsberg, 1995) also occasionally been noted to experience thrombocytopenia. Heparin derived from bovine lung rather than porcine gut is more often associated with thrombocytopenia (Rao, 1989). Hypersensitivity to heparin therapy can result in chills, fever, and urticaria. Rarely, anaphylactic reactions to heparin have occurred.

T A B L E  **19-8**

Side effects of heparin anticoagulation

| Side Effect | Incidence (%) |
|---|---|
| Bleeding | 5–10 |
| Thrombocytopenia | 5–10 |
| Osteoporotic changes | 2–17 |
| Anaphylaxis | Rare |

Osteoporosis and symptomatic fractures are a third side effect from prolonged heparin therapy (Griffith, 1965; deSwiet, 1983; Zimran, 1986; Dahlman, 1990, 1993, 1994). These changes in bone density have ranged from demineralization changes observed in the spine, hip, and femur radiographs to overt fractures (deSwiet, 1983; Dahlman, 1990, 1993, 1994) and occur in patients who receive both S-Heparin and LMWH. Doses found in patients with symptomatic vertebral fractures were as little as 15,000 units/day for 7 weeks, with a mean dose of 25,000 to 30,000 units/day (Dahlman, 1993). Radiographic changes have been observed in up to one third of women receiving heparin therapy for longer than a month (Ginsberg, 1995). Reversal after discontinuing therapy can be slow (deSwiet, 1983; Zimran, 1986), but there is reassuring evidence that reversal of osteopenia does occur and that treatment in consecutive pregnancies may not increase a woman's risk of this complication (Dahlman, 1990).

The careful administration of subcutaneous heparin prevents erratic absorption and local bruising. Preferably, the subcutaneous fat of the anterior flank (lateral abdominal wall) should be used rather than sites in the arms and legs. These latter sites are more painful and are subject to rapid absorption of heparin associated with movement. A small needle is fully inserted vertically into a raised fold of skin and withdrawn atraumatically after injection. Patients should be advised against massaging the injection sites as this increases absorption.

Heparin is safe for use in pregnancy; the perinatal outcome among heparin users is comparable to nonheparin users (Ginsberg, 1988).

## Warfarin

Warfarin, a coumarin derivative, is the most commonly used oral anticoagulant (see Table 19-6). It inhibits regeneration of active vitamin K in the liver. Vitamin K is required to carboxylate the glutamic acid residues on factors II, VII, IX, and X and protein C. These factors are otherwise inactive and are unable to complex normally with calcium and phospholipid receptors.

Except in the rare situation in which heparin cannot or should not be used, warfarin is contraindicated in pregnancy (Table 19-9). With a molecular weight of 1000 daltons, warfarin easily crosses the placenta. Administration in the first 6 to 9 weeks of gestation is associated with warfarin embryopathy, a syndrome that may include nasal hypoplasia, depression of the bridge of the nose, and epiphyseal stippling, such as is seen in Conradi-Hunermann chondrodysplasia punctata (Hall, 1978; Ginsberg, 1989; Ginsberg, 1992; Colvin, 1992). Exposure during the second and third trimesters is associated with a variety of CNS and ophthalmologic abnormalities. It is suspected that some of these abnormalities are related to fetal hemorrhage and scar tissue formation. From a retrospective review of published reports, it appears that 13% of pregnancies in which warfarin or related substances were used resulted in abnormal live-born infants. Approximately 4% resulted in infants with warfarin embryopathy. Of patients with warfarin embryopathy, approximately 30% may be developmentally retarded (Hall, 1978). In those infants with CNS abnormalities, dorsal midline dysplasia (e.g., agenesis of the corpus callosum), Dandy-Walker malformation, midline cerebellar atrophy and ventral midline dysplasia (e.g., optic atrophy) have been described (Stevenson, 1980). Such literature reviews, however, may be skewed in favor of abnormal outcomes. A review of 22 children of mothers who took warfarin during pregnancy revealed no significant difference when compared with controls; this outcome suggests that the incidence of abnormalities may be lower than previously reported (Chang, 1984). Because of the anticoagulant effect in the fetus, there is also a

T A B L E    **19-9**

**Maternal and fetal side effects of warfarin therapy during pregnancy**

| Maternal | Bleeding |
|---|---|
| | Skin necrosis/gangrene |
| | Purple toes syndrome |
| | Hypersensitivity |
| Fetal | Hemorrhage |
| | Warfarin embryopathy |
| | CNS abnormalities |
| | Optic atrophy |
| | Mental retardation |

higher risk of fetal hemorrhage at delivery. Thus, women who are treated with coumarin derivatives and contemplate pregnancy should be switched to heparin prior to conception. In select patients with cardiac disease at risk for arterial thromboembolic events, the apparent increased effectiveness of warfarin may justify the associated fetal risks (see Chapter 15). There appears, however, to be little justification for the use of coumarin derivatives in the treatment or prophylaxis of venous thromboembolism.

The major maternal complication (see Table 19-9) of warfarin use is bleeding, which occurs more often with warfarin than with subcutaneous heparin (Hull, 1982). Warfarin anticoagulation is also more sensitive to fluctuations in clotting factors and plasma volume and requires more frequent monitoring and adjustments of dose. Numerous medications (Standing Advisory Committee, 1982), including some antibiotics, will augment or inhibit warfarin (coumarin derivative) activity (Table 19-10).

Less common side effects of warfarin therapy are skin necrosis and gangrene (Horn, 1981). Once an underlying disease is excluded as a cause of such dermatologic changes, warfarin therapy should be discontinued and appropriate medical and/or surgical therapy instituted. The purple toes syndrome (Lebsack, 1982; Park, 1993), an infrequent complication of warfarin therapy, is characterized by dark, purplish, mottled toes and occurs 3 to 10 weeks after the initiation of therapy. In most instances, this condition is reversible, but a few patients will progress to necrosis or gangrene. In rare circumstances, amputation may be necessary.

Measurement of the prothrombin time (PT) is used to monitor the anticoagulant effect of warfarin. Therapeutic levels can be reached after 3 to 5 days and should yield a PT of 1.5 to 2.5 times control (international normalized ratio [INR]) (Hirsch, 1988a). In a study of 266 nonpregnant patients with PE, early treatment with warfarin (begun during days 1–3) was found to be as effective as continuous IV heparin in preventing recurrences, with similar rates of bleeding complications. The major advantage with couwarfarin was a 30% decrease in hospital time (Gallus, 1986).

Reversal of anticoagulation depends on regeneration of clotting factors and is slow. Administration of parenteral vitamin K can lead to reversal in 6 to 12 hours. In an acute situation, fresh frozen plasma can be given to provide clotting factors.

T A B L E   **19-10**

Selected drugs that interact with coumarin derivative anticoagulants

| Potentiate Oral Anticoagulants | May Antagonize Oral Anticoagulants |
|---|---|
| Alcohol, dose-dependent | Antacids |
| Chlorpromazine | Antihistamines |
| Cimetidine | Barbiturates |
| Danocrine | Carbamazepine |
| Metronidazole | Corticosteroids |
| Neomycin | Oral contraceptives |
| Nonsteroidal antiinflammatory drugs | |
| Salicylates, large doses | Primidone |
| Thyroxine | Rifampin |
| Trimethoprim | Vitamin K |
| Phenytoin | |

Source: Standing Advisory Committee for Haematology of the Royal College of Pathologists. Drug interaction with coumarin derivative anticoagulants. Br Med J 1982;185:274–275.

## Antepartum Management

Suspicion of thromboembolism must be weighed against risk factors for severe hemorrhage with anticoagulation. Except for [125]I fibrinogen scanning (Mant, 1981), heparin does not interfere with performance or interpretation of diagnostic procedures. If the patient's clinical picture strongly suggests PE or obstructive proximal DVT, anticoagulation with heparin should be considered prior to diagnostic studies to minimize the risk of an embolic event during the time from clinical suspicion until the diagnosis is confirmed radiographically.

After obtaining a baseline clotting profile, the physician can most easily achieve rapid anticoagulation by using an initial IV bolus of 70 to 100 units/kg or 5000 to 10,000 units (Hirsch, 1991). For massive PE, an initial bolus as high as 15,000 units has been recommended (Moser, 1983). Initial continuous infusion rates can be calculated at 15 to 20 units/kg/hr. Therapeutic doses are con-

sidered those that prolong the aPTT 1.5 to 2.5 times normal or give a plasma heparin level of 0.2 to 0.4 units/mL. Adequate and rapid initial anticoagulation is essential to minimize the risk of PE. The heparin dose is ideally adjusted every 4 hours until adequate anticoagulation has been achieved. Excessive doses that prolong the aPTT beyond 2.5 times normal or give heparin levels above 0.5 units/mL are associated with a greater likelihood of maternal bleeding (Bonnar, 1969; Hirsch, 1991). In pregnancy, the required dose is related more closely to the maternal circulating blood volume than to maternal body weight (Ellison, 1989). To assure accurate results, blood samples should be drawn remote from the site of heparin infusion. After initial adjustment and stabilization of the heparin dose, daily laboratory testing is adequate. The infusion dose required may change as active thrombosis is halted. A useful protocol for the adjustment of the dose of IV heparin is presented in Table 19-11 (Toglia, 1996).

T A B L E    **19-11**

Protocol for adjustment of the dose of intravenous heparin[a]

| Activated Partial Thromboplastin Time (sec)[b] | Repeat Bolus? | Stop Infusion? | New Rate of Infusion | Repeat Measurement of Activated Partial Thromboplastin Time |
|---|---|---|---|---|
| <50 | Yes (5000 IU) | No | +3 mL/hr (+2880 IU/24 hr) | 6 hr |
| 50–59 | No | No | +3 mL/hr (+2880 IU/24 hr) | 6 hr |
| 60–85[c] | No | No | Unchanged | Next morning |
| 86–95 | No | No | −2 mL/hr (−1920 IU/24 hr) | Next morning |
| 96–120 | No | Yes (for 30 min) | −2 mL/hr (−1920 IU/24 hr) | 6 hr |
| >120 | No | Yes (for 60 min) | −4 mL/hr (−3840 IU/24 hr) | 6 hr |

[a]A starting dose of 5000 IU is given as an intravenous bolus, followed by 31,000 IU per 24 hours, given as a continuous infusion in a concentration of 40 IU per milliliter. The activated partial thromboplastin time is first measured 6 hours after the bolus injection, adjustments are made according to the protocol, and the activated partial thromboplastin time is measured again as indicated. Adapted from Hirsch J. Heparin. N Engl J Med 1991;324:1565.

[b]The normal range, measured with the Dade-Actin-FS reagent, is 27 to 35 seconds.

[c]The therapeutic range of 60 to 85 seconds is equivalent to a heparin level of 0.2 to 0.4 IU per milliliter by protamine titration or 0.35 to 0.7 IU per milliliter according to the level of inhibition of factor Xa. The therapeutic range varies with the responsiveness of the reagent used to measure the activated partial thromboplastin time to heparin.

Reproduced by permission from Toglia MR, Weg JG. Venous thromboembolism during pregnancy. N Engl J Med 1996;335:108.

There is no difference between patients with DVT and PE as to the amount of heparin required to achieve therapeutic anticoagulation (Tenero, 1989). However, recommendations for duration of IV infusion vary. A *minimum* of 2 days with DVT and 5 days with PE are suggested (Letsky, 1985; Bonnar, 1981). Most authors recommend IV therapy for 5 to 7 days. Historically, the goal was to continue IV heparin until (1) active thrombosis had stopped, (2) thrombi were firmly attached to the vessel wall, and (3) organization had begun (Letsky, 1985; Bonnar, 1981).

The period of continuous IV infusion is followed in pregnancy by therapeutic subcutaneous heparin for the duration of the pregnancy (Anderson, 1982). Postpartum anticoagulation will need to be continued for 8 to 12 weeks in most patients. According to Schulman and associates (1995), 6 months, not 6 weeks, of prophylactic anticoagulation after a first episode of venous thromboembolism may be required to lower the recurrence rate. In contrast, Hirsch (1995) suggests that prolonged anticoagulant therapy depends on whether the patient has a reversible risk factor for DVT, such as DVT after surgery or trauma or a permanent risk factor such as idiopathic DVT (the absence of any risk factors). With the Hirsh classification (Barbour, 1995b), prolonged anticoagulant therapy would be 6 weeks for the reversible group and 6 months for idiopathic DVT.

Monitoring of therapy in patients receiving adjusted-dose (therapeutic) subcutaneous heparin is more complex than with the IV route. With respect to the timing of aPTT in relationship to intermittent injection, some authorities recommend monitoring the mid-dose aPTT (i.e., draw at 6 hr for patients receiving a 12-hr injection), while an increasing number of physicians favor adjusting the heparin dose to achieve a level near 2.5 times control just prior to the next dose. Data to document the superiority of the approach are lacking; it is hoped that the use of L-Heparin will, in the near future, make such discussion moot.

The dosage and timing are also affected by the type of heparin used. Both sodium and calcium salts are available. Sodium heparin is less expensive, achieves higher levels, has a longer duration of action, and generally is preferred over calcium heparin. In contrast, the use of calcium heparin necessitates higher and more frequent doses. In this chapter, the dosages suggested are for sodium heparin.

Reported alternatives to long-term intermittent injections in pregnancy have included continuous infusions of heparin via a Hickman catheter (Nelson, 1984) or subcutaneous pump (Barss, 1985). In one series, six patients received continuous subcutaneous infusion to reach therapeutic PTTs of 1.5 to 2.0 times controls. Although there were no recurrences of thrombosis, five of the patients experienced major or minor bleeding complications (Barss, 1985).

## Intrapartum Management

For anticoagulated patients delivering vaginally, the risk of significant hemorrhage is small, as long as the platelet count and function are normal and uterine atony is avoided. Regional anesthetics (epidural and spinal), however, are not recommended because of the potential risk of epidural or spinal cord hematoma formation. Such patients do have an increased risk of vaginal hematomas. For patients requiring cesarean section, therapeutics become more complex. On admission to labor and delivery, a clotting profile and hematocrit should be drawn. There are three basic choices in the approach to anticoagulant management:

1. *Administer continued therapeutic anticoagulation:* This approach is recommended for particularly high-risk patients, such as those with recent PE, iliofemoral thrombosis, or mechanical heart valve prostheses. Because a more uniform therapeutic heparin level is desirable, the patient may be changed from subcutaneous injection to continuous IV infusion. A heparin level of 0.4 units/mL or a low therapeutic aPTT (close to 1.5 times normal) may be desirable in these surgical patients.

2. *Reduce the subcutaneous heparin dose:* In patients at lower risk of thromboembolism, the heparin dose can be reduced to a prophylactic level; this dose (5000 units/12 hr) is not associated with increased surgical bleeding.

**3.** *Stop or withhold heparin administration:* For patients at increased risk for operative bleeding (i.e., suspected placenta accreta) and at relatively low risk of clot propagation, heparin may be withheld or its effects reversed with protamine sulfate. Nonpharmacologic prophylaxis (e.g., pneumatic compression stockings) may be substituted during the intraoperative period.

With patients who are anticoagulated and in whom rapid reversal is deemed essential, protamine sulfate can be used to reverse heparinization. One milligram of protamine sulfate neutralizes 100 units of heparin. To determine the proper dose of protamine, several approaches are available. One is to calculate the amount of circulating heparin by estimating plasma volume at 50 mL/kg of body weight and multiplying the plasma volume by the heparin concentration (Letsky, 1985). In many institutions, however, this procedure may not be technically feasible.

If protamine sulfate is necessary, the amount should be underestimated or slowly titrated to the whole-blood clotting time because of the short half-life (rapid metabolism) of heparin and the irreversible anticoagulant effect of excess protamine. No single dose should exceed 50 mg. A 50-mg dose would rarely be needed because it would neutralize 5000 units of circulating heparin, an amount of heparin highly unlikely ever to be present. Protamine sulfate should be administered IV over 20 to 30 minutes to prevent hypotension. In patients receiving adjusted-dose subcutaneous heparin, a dose of 5 to 10 mg of protamine sulfate is often sufficient; further doses may be given, depending on the aPTT value. *Note:* It should be emphasized that for vaginal delivery, even significantly prolonged aPTT values rarely result in clinical hemorrhage and, thus, do not require protamine sulfate therapy.

Patients who present for delivery on warfarin anticoagulant are at heightened risk for bleeding with either vaginal or operative delivery. Parenteral vitamin K can help to regenerate the clotting factors within 12 hours. If there is little time, or reversal is not adequate, fresh frozen plasma can be given to supply clotting factors. Regardless, the pregnant woman should be stabilized and sufficiently able to clot before operative delivery is initiated.

## Postpartum Management

Conversion from heparin to warfarin anticoagulation should be initiated postpartum in the hospital to minimize the maternal risk of complications. Therefore, once the patient has delivered and is sufficiently stable, resume full heparin anticoagulation. Then, begin oral warfarin therapy with 10 to 15 mg orally per day for 2 to 4 days, followed by 2 to 15 mg per day as indicated by the INR or PT (Hirsch, 1991). One way to approach this is to give the warfarin sodium at 6 PM, then draw an INR or PT at 6 AM the following day, adjusting the order for the subsequent day's Coumadin dose according to that morning's results. Once the patient is therapeutically anticoagulated, heparin is discontinued.

Postpartum suppression of lactation with estrogen is associated with a much higher incidence of thromboembolic complications and is contraindicated (Daniel, 1967; Jeffcoate, 1968).

## Prophylaxis of Thromboembolism

Patients at high risk for thromboembolic disease require consideration for anticoagulant therapy or prophylaxis during pregnancy and the puerperium. Such patients are those with histories of PE, DVT, artificial heart valves, and primary hypercoagulable disorders such as AT III deficiency. Individuals with other risk factors (e.g., age, higher parity, obesity, operative delivery, and prolonged immobilization) may, in selected circumstances, require antepartum or intrapartum prophylaxis. Prolonged bed rest associated with prevention of preterm birth, due to preeclampsia, or due to preterm premature rupture of membranes has not yet been identified specifically as a risk factor for venous thromboembolism. In some instances, however, such immobilized patients may benefit from prophylactic heparin.

Prophylaxis or therapeutic anticoagulation throughout pregnancy should be considered for a patient with a thrombotic or embolic event during an earlier pregnancy. If while taking oral contraceptives the thromboembolism occurred as a result of trauma or taking oral contraceptives, authors vary as to their recommendations for prophylaxis during pregnancy (Barbour, 1995a). Recently, the American College of Obstetricians and Gynecologists has published guidelines for prophylaxis in a variety of situations (ACOG, 1996).

Prophylaxis against recurrent DVT and/or PE has consisted of subcutaneous heparin injections every 12 hours, but this approach may be inadequate. The primary reason is that uteroplacental coagulation and platelet activity increase during pregnancy. This, in turn, leads to progressive neutralization of heparin. As such, the dose or the frequency of injections needs to be adjusted to reflect these coagulation changes. An increase from 5000 units to 7500 to 10,000 units in the third trimester (Bonnar, 1981) is often recommended (Howell, 1983). Others have suggested 5000 units every 8 hours. Except for doses exceeding 8000 units, laboratory monitoring is not usually required (Bonnar, 1981). Caution should be used in the patient with diminished renal function, which may elevate heparin levels.

Employing only perioperative (cesarean) prophylaxis may be considered for certain additional patients, such as those with obesity or unusually reduced ambulation. Conservative mechanical methods, such as intermittent pneumatic compression boots or graduated elastic compression stockings, also may be helpful. Early postoperative ambulation also is important in preventing thromboembolism. Low-dose heparin is accepted as prophylaxis for a variety of surgical procedures (Collins, 1988). Although heparin combined with dihydroergotamine is felt in some general surgical or orthopedic patients to be more effective than heparin alone (Salzman, 1987; Kakkar, 1979), its use in pregnant or parturient women has not been studied. Thus, its use cannot be recommended. The combination of mechanical methods, especially pneumatic compression, and low-dose heparin may be the optimum approach for high-risk patients (Stringer, 1989; Clark-Pearson, 1993). Low-molecular-weight heparin has been found useful in abdominal surgery; one dose is given preoperatively, followed by doses once every 24 hours, as a result of its longer antifactor Xa

activity (European Fraxiparin Study Group, 1988; Hirsch, 1988b).

Therapeutic anticoagulation is necessary as prophylaxis during pregnancy for those patients with mechanical heart valves (Salazar, 1984) or inherited deficiency of a natural anticoagulant such as AT III (Nelson, 1985). Successful pregnancy outcome has been achieved with the use of subcutaneous and IV heparinization, accompanied by infusion of AT III concentrate at the time of abortion or delivery (Nelson, 1985). Without such therapy, maternal morbidity or mortality and fetal loss are extremely high. Deficiencies of proteins C and S also are associated with thrombotic tendency (DeStefano, 1988). Screening of patients with significant unexplained thromboembolic histories can reveal these hereditary disorders.

Antiplatelet agents such as aspirin and dipyridamole may be helpful in preventing thrombosis in the arterial circulation or with some prosthetic heart valves. There is no known role for these agents in the prevention of pregnancy-associated thromboembolic disease. Perioperative prophylaxis with dextran appears beneficial in some surgical patients, but the risk of bleeding is higher than with heparin, and dextran's usefulness in pregnant patients has not been established (Salzman, 1987).

A potential but yet unproven approach in pregnancy for intrapartum prophylaxis in patients without an active thrombotic process is ultra-low-dose IV heparin (Negus, 1980). In a randomized study to prevent postoperative DVT in nonpregnant patients, a dose of 1 IU/kg/hr reduced the incidence of DVT from 22% to 4%.

## Thrombolytic Therapy

Defibrinating agents may be indicated in cases of life-threatening thromboembolism (Urokinase-Streptokinase Pulmonary Embolism Trial, 1974; Moran, 1989; Sharma, 1985; Turrentine, 1995). Streptokinase, urokinase, and tissue plasminogen activator activate plasminogen, which sets in motion the body's natural fibrinolytic system. Although helpful in the early management of massive PE, thrombolysis plus heparin may not yield improved mortality over heparin alone (Urokinase-Streptokinase, 1974). Because of the potential risk of bleeding, thrombolytic therapy has not been recommended until 10 days after surgery or parturition (Moran, 1989). Recommended treatment schedules vary, but all consist of an IV loading dose followed by continuous infusion for 12 to 72 hours, depending on the clinical situation (Sharma, 1985). Thrombolytic therapy is followed by anticoagulant therapy to prevent recurrence. A review by Turrentine et al (1995) of 172 patients who received thrombolytic therapy during pregnancy demonstrated that thrombolytic therapy could be used relatively safely during pregnancy in selected clinical situations (Table 19-12) and that these agents were partially or completely successful in 86% to 90% of recipients. Nonetheless, the authors suggested that traditional therapies be used first, and, if unsuccessful, thrombolytic agents could be used with the understanding of the increased risk of bleeding complications.

Ancrod, derived from Malayan pit viper venom, is contraindicated in pregnancy. Animal studies have shown a high incidence of fetal death. Postpartum hemorrhage from the placental site also occurs at a greater frequency.

## Surgical Intervention

With pregnancy, surgical intervention may be indicated in some clinical situations, such as replacement of a thrombosed cardiac valve prosthesis, thrombectomy for acute iliofemoral thrombosis, embolectomy of a life-threatening

T A B L E  **19-12**

Maternal and perinatal outcome for 172 patients who received thrombolytic therapy during pregnancy

|  | N | (%) |
|---|---|---|
| Hemorrhage | 14 | (8) |
| Preterm birth | 10 | (6) |
| Perinatal deaths | 10 | (6) |
| Maternal deaths | 2 | (1) |

Source: Turrentine MA, Braems G, Ramirez MM. Use of thrombolytics for the treatment of thromboembolic disease during pregnancy. Obstet Gynecol Surv 1995;50:534–541.

massive PE, or vena cava interruption for recurrent venous emboli despite adequate anticoagulation or when anticoagulation is absolutely contraindicated. Embolectomy is an heroic measure, which may occasionally be life-saving. Transvenous catheter embolectomy has been performed successfully for expeditious management of massive PE with cardiovascular collapse (Kramer, 1986). There are a variety of methods for interruption of the vena cava. These methods include complete ligation, Teflon clips, and devices inserted transvenously, such as the umbrella filter or the Greenfield filter (Hux, 1986).

## Special Considerations

### Antithrombin III Deficiency

The first evidence of an inherited AT III defect is not infrequently a thromboembolic event (Megha, 1990). Pregnant patients with inherited AT III deficiency often require therapeutic anticoagulation throughout the pregnancy and the puerperium (De Stefano, 1988; Nelson, 1985; Hellgren, 1982; Conrad, 1990; Schwartz, 1989; Brandt, 1981; Samson, 1984; Leclerc, 1986). In addition to heparin therapy throughout pregnancy (Conrad, 1990; Brandt, 1981; Samson, 1984; Leclerc, 1986), IV administration of AT III concentrate may be necessary (De Stefano, 1988; Nelson, 1985) to minimize the patient's risk of a thromboembolism. This can be accomplished with fresh-frozen plasma, but AT III concentrate is preferable (Brandt, 1981; Samson, 1984; Leclerc, 1986). The loading dose of AT III is 50 to 70 units/kg. This is followed by 20 to 30 units/kg/day to maintain an AT III level of 80% of normal (Hellgren, 1982). Remember, the higher the AT III level, the less heparin will be required for therapeutic anticoagulation. In the untreated gravida, maternal morbidity and mortality and perinatal mortality are significantly increased. If these patients remain untreated during pregnancy, 68% will develop thromboembolism (Nelson, 1985; Hellgren, 1982; Conrad, 1990; Schwartz, 1989). In patients who require high doses of heparin to achieve anticoagulation, prophylactic biweekly doses of AT III concentrate have been necessary (Schwartz,

---

## PULMONARY EMBOLISM IN PREGNANCY

### I. *Goals of Therapy*

    A.  Maintenance of oxygenation and cardiac output

    B.  Promotion of thrombus resolution

    C.  Prevention of thrombus extension and recurrence

### II. *Management Protocol**

    A.  Immediately begin therapy, based on strong clinical suspicion, pending complete diagnostic work-up.

    B.  Administer oxygen via mask, 6 liters/min.

    C.  Administer heparin, 5000 to 10,000 units IV, followed by 1000 to 2000 units/hr via infusion pump.

    D.  Adjust heparin infusion to achieve aPTT 1.5 to 2.5 times that of control.

    E.  Maintain full anticoagulation for 7 to 10 days.

    F.  Continue anticoagulation with adjusted-dose subcutaneous heparin, initially 8000 to 12,000 units twice or three times daily (antepartum or postpartum) or oral anticoagulation (only if postpartum) until 6 weeks postpartum.

    G.  Implement bed rest, elastic hose, and extremity elevation if the source of embolus is the leg.

### III. *Critical Laboratory Tests*

    A.  ABG, aPTT, complete blood count with platelet count, chest x-ray, ECG, invasive or noninvasive diagnostic tests, as indicated.

### IV. *Consultation*

    A.  Pulmonary medicine, hematology

*Applies to management of DVT, except that oxygen may be omitted and an initial heparin dose of 5000 units is more appropriate.

---

1989). Many patients require lifelong anticoagulation, which is best served by oral anticoagulants when not pregnant and heparin throughout pregnancy.

## Protein C or S Deficiencies

In contrast to patients with AT III deficiency, patients with protein C or S deficiency carry a lower risk of antepartum thrombosis (Comp, 1985; Broekmans, 1985; Malciniak, 1985; Conrad, 1990; Goodwin, 1995; Malm, 1988; Lao, 1989, 1990; Faught, 1995; Rose, 1986; Tharakan, 1993). The incidence depends on whether the patient has protein C or protein S deficiency; the incidence of antepartum thrombosis in the untreated patient with protein C and protein S deficiency in one series was 17% and 0%, respectively. The postpartum risks, however, were similar (Conrad, 1990). While there is a split of opinion regarding heparin prophylaxis during pregnancy, there is uniform agreement that anticoagulant therapy is warranted in the puerperium (Comp, 1985; Broekman, 1985; Malciniak, 1985; Conrad, 1990; Goodwin, 1995; Malm, 1988; Lao, 1989, 1990; Faught, 1995; Rose, 1986; Tharakan, 1993). For patients with recurrent thromboembolism or a family history of these deficiencies, prenatal screening for AT III, protein C, and protein S would appear reasonable. A mutation in the gene for coagulation factor V (factor V Leiden), resulting in resistance to activated protein C, may be the most common genetic factor predisposing to thromboembolism (Simioni, 1997). Additional controversies in the management of thromboembolic disease during pregnancy have been reviewed by Barbour and Pickard (1995a) and Toglia and Weg (1996).

## REFERENCES

Alderson PO. Scintigraphic evaluation of pulmonary embolism. Eur J Nucl Med 1987;13:S6–S10.

American College of Obstetricians and Gynecologists Education Bulletin #233 Teratology. Washington, D.C., Feb. 1997.

American College of Obstetricians and Gynecologists Education Bulletin #234 Thromboembolism in Pregnancy. Washington, D.C., March 1997.

Anderson G, Fagrell B, Holmgren K, et al. Subcutaneous administration of heparin: a randomized comparison with intravenous administration of heparin to patients with deep-vein thrombosis. Thromb Res 1982;27:631–639.

Barbour LA, Pickard J. Controversies in thromboembolic disease during pregnancy: a critical review. Obstet Gynecol 1995a;86:621–633.

Barbour LA, Smith JM, Marar RA. Heparin levels to guide thromboembolism prophylaxis during pregnancy. Am J Obstet Gynecol 1995b;173: 1869–1873.

Barnes RW, Wu KK, Hoak JC. Fallibility of the clinical diagnosis of venous thrombosis. JAMA 1975;234:605–608.

Barss VA, Schwartz PA, Greene MF, et al. Use of the subcutaneous heparin pump during pregnancy. J Reprod Med 1985;30:899–901.

Basu D, Gallus A, Hirsh J, et al. A prospective study of the value of monitoring heparin treatment with the activated partial thromboplastin time. N Engl J Med 1972;287:324–327.

Bell WR, Simon TL, DeMets DL. The clinical features of submassive and massive pulmonary emboli. Am J Med 1977;62:355–360.

Bentley PG, Kakkar VV. Radionuclide venography for the demonstration of the proximal deep venous system. Br J Surg 1979;66:687–690.

Bergqvist D, Benoni G, Bjorgell O, et al. Low-molecular-weight heparin as prophylaxis against venous thromboembolism after total hip replacement. N Engl J Med 1996;335:696.

Bergqvist A, Bergqvist D, Hallbook T. Acute deep vein thrombosis (DVT) after cesarean section. Acta Obstet Gynecol (Scand) 1983;62:473–477.

Bergqvist A, Bergqvist D, Lindhagen A, et al. Late symptoms after pregnancy-related deep vein thrombosis. Br J Obstet Gynaecol 1990;97:338–344.

Bettman MA, Paulin S. Leg phlebography: the incidence, nature and modification of undesirable side effects. Radiology 1977;122:101–108.

Bonnar J. Venous thromboembolism and pregnancy. Clin Obstet Gynecol 1981;8:445–473.

Bonnar J, McNichol GP, Douglas AS. Fibrinolytic enzyme system and pregnancy. Br Med J 1969;3:387–389.

Bonnar J, McNichol GP, Douglas AS. Coagulation mechanisms during and after normal childbirth. Br Med J 1970;2:200–203.

Brandt JT. Current concepts of coagulation. Clin Obstet Gynecol 1985;28:3–14.

Brandt P. Observations during the treatment of antithrombin III deficient women with heparin and antithrombin concentrate during pregnancy, parturition, and abortion. Thromb Res 1981;22:15–24.

Bratt G, Tornebohm E, Lockner D, et al. A human pharmacological study comparing conventional heparin and a low molecular weight heparin fragment. Thromb Haemost 1985;53:208–211.

Broekmans AW, Bertina RM, Reinalda-Poot J, et al. Hereditary protein-S deficiency and venous thromboembolism. Thromb Haemost 1985;53: 273–277.

Chang MKB, Harvey D, deSwiet M. Follow-up study of children whose mothers were treated with warfarin during pregnancy. Br J Obstet Gynaecol 1984;91:70–73.

Chang BH, Pitney WR, Castaldi PA. Heparin-induced thrombocytopenia: association of thrombotic complications with heparin-dependent IgG antibody that induces thromboxane synthesis and platelet aggregation. Lancet 1982;2:1246–1249.

Clagett GP, Anderson FA, Heit J, et al. Prevention of venous thromboembolism. Chest 1995;108 (suppl):312.

Clark-Pearson DL, Synan IS, Dodge R, et al. A randomized trial of low-dose heparin and intermittent pneumatic calf compression for the prevention of deep venous thrombosis after gynecologic oncology surgery. Am J Obstet Gynecol 1993;168:1146–1154.

Collins R, Scrimgeour A, Peto R. Reduction in fatal pulmonary embolism and venous thrombosis by perioperative administration of subcutaneous heparin. N Engl J Med 1988;318:1162–1173.

Colvin BT, Barrowcliff TW. The British Society for Haematology guidelines on the use and monitoring of heparin 1992: second revision. J Clin Pathol 1993;46:97–103.

Comp PC, Clouse L. Plasma proteins C and S: the function and assay of two natural anticoagulants. Lab Management 1985;23:29–32.

Comp PC, Esman CT. Generation of fibrinolytic activity by infusion of activated protein C in dogs. J Clin Invest 1981;68:1221–1228.

Conrad J, Horellou MH, Van Dredan P, et al. Thrombosis and pregnancy in congenital deficiencies in antithrombin III, protein C or protein S: study of 78 women. Thromb Haemost 1990;63:319–320.

Dahlman TC. Osteoporotic fractures and the recurrence of thromboembolism during pregnancy and the puerperium in 184 women undergoing thromboprophylaxis with heparin. Am J Obstet Gynecol 1993;168:1265–1270.

Dahlman TC, Hellgren M, Blomback M. Thrombosis prophylaxis in pregnancy with use of subcutaneous heparin adjusted by monitoring heparin concentration in plasma. Am J Obstet Gynecol 1989;161:420–425.

Dahlman T, Lindvall N, Hellgren M. Osteopenia in pregnancy during long-term heparin treatment: a radiologic study postpartum. Br J Ostet Gynaecol 1990;97:221–224.

Dahlman TC, Sjoberg HE, Ringertz H. Bone mineral density during long-term prophylaxis with heparin in pregnancy. Am J Obstet Gynecol 1994;170:1315–1320.

Dalen JE, Banas JS, Brooks HC, et al. Resolution rate of acute pulmonary embolism in man. N Engl J Med 1969;280:1194–1198.

Dalen JE, Brooks HL, Johnson LW, et al. Pulmonary angiography in acute pulmonary embolism: indications, techniques, and results in 367 patients. Am Heart J 1979;81:175–185.

Daniel DG, Campbell H, Turnbull AC. Puerperal thromboembolism and suppression of lactation. Lancet 1967;2:287.

De Stefano V, Leone G, De Carolis S, et al. Management of pregnancy in women with antithrombin III congenital defect: report of four cases. Thromb Haemost 1988;59:193–196.

DeSwart CAM, Nijmeter B, Roelofs JMM, et al. Kinetics of intravenously administered heparin in normal humans. Blood 1982;60:1251–1258.

deSwiet M, Ward PD, Fidler J, et al. Prolonged heparin therapy in pregnancy causes bone demineralization. Br J Obstet Gynaecol 1983;90:1129–1134.

Dorfman GS, Cronan JJ, Tupper TB, et al. Occult pulmonary embolism: a common occurrence in deep venous thrombosis. AJR 1987;148:263–267.

Elias A, LeCorff G, Boucier JL, et al. Value of real time B mode ultrasound imaging in the diagnosis of deep vein thrombosis of the lower limbs. Int Angiol 1987;6:175–177.

Ellison MJ, Sawyer WT, Mills TC. Calculation of heparin dosage in a morbidly obese woman. Clin Pharm 1989;8:65–68.

European Fraxiparin Study (EFS) Group. Comparison of a low molecular weight heparin and unfractionated heparin for the prevention of deep vein thrombosis in patients undergoing abdominal surgery. Br J Surg 1988;75:1058–1063.

Ezekowitz MD, Pope CF, Smith EO. Indium-111 platelet imaging. In: Goldhaber SE, ed. Pulmonary embolism and deep venous thrombosis. Philadelphia: WB Saunders, 1985:261–267.

Fairfax WR, Thomas F, Orme JF. Pulmonary artery catheter occlusion as an indication of pulmonary embolism. Chest 1984;86:270–272.

Faught W, Garner P, Jones G, Ivey B. Changes in protein C and protein S levels in normal pregnancy. Am J Obstet Gynecol 1995;172:147–150.

Fejgin MD, Lourwood DL. Low molecular weight heparins and their use in obstetrics and gynecology. Obstet Gynecol Surv 1994;49:424–431.

Files JC, Malpass TW, Yee EK, et al. Studies of human platelet alpha-granule release in vivo. Blood 1981;58:607–618.

Franks AL, Atrash HK, Lawson HW, et al. Obstetrical pulmonary embolism mortality, United States, 1970–85. Am J Public Health 1990;80:720–722.

Gabel HD. Maternal mortality in South Carolina from 1970 to 1984: an analysis. Obstet Gynecol 1987; 69:307–311.

Galle PC, Muss HB, McGrath KM, et al. Thrombocytopenia in two patients treated with low-dose heparin. Obstet Gynecol 1978;52(suppl):95–115.

Gallus A, Jackaman J, Tillet J, et al. Safety and efficacy of warfarin started early after submassive venous thrombosis or pulmonary embolism. Lancet 1986;2:1293–1296.

Gerts WH, Jay RM, Code K, et al. A comparison of low-dose heparin with low-molecular-weight heparin as prophylaxis against venous thromboembolism after major trauma. N Engl J Med 1996;335:701.

Gillis S, Shushan A, Eldor A. Use of low molecular weight heparin for prophylaxis and treatment of thromboembolism in pregnancy. Int J Gynecol Obstet 1992;39:297–301.

Ginsberg JS. Management of venous thromboembolism. N Engl J Med 1996;334:1816.

Ginsberg JS, Hirsh J. Use of antithrombotic agents during pregnancy. Chest 1992;315:1109–1114.

Ginsberg JS, Hirsh J. Use of antithrombotic agents during pregnancy. Chest 1995;108:3055–3115.

Ginsberg JSA, Hirsh J, Rainbow AJ, et al. Risks to the fetus of radiologic procedures used in the diagnosis of maternal venous thromboembolic disease. Thromb Haemost 1989a;61:189–196.

Ginsberg JS, Hirsh J, Tuner C, et al. Risks to the fetus of anticoagulant therapy during pregnancy. Thromb Haemost 1989b;61:197–203.

Ginsberg JS, Kowalchick G, Brill-Edwards P, et al. Heparin therapy in pregnancy: effects on the fetus. Clin Res 1988;36:A410.

Gold WM, McCormack KR. Pulmonary function response to radioisotope scanning of the lungs. JAMA 1966;197:146–148.

Goodwin TM, Gazit G, Gordon EM. Heterozygous protein C deficiency presenting as severe protein C deficiency and peripartum thrombosis: successful treatment with protein C concentrate. Obstet Gynecol 1995;86:662–664.

Griffith GC. Heparin osteoporosis. JAMA 1965;143: 85–88.

Hall JG, Pauli RM, Wilson KM. Maternal and fetal sequelae of anticoagulation during pregnancy. Am J Med 1978:122–140.

Hathaway WE, Bonnar J. Perinatal coagulation. New York: Grune & Stratten, 1978.

Hellgren M, Tengborn L, Abildgaard U. Pregnancy in women with congenital antithrombin III deficiency: experience of treatment with heparin and antithrombin. Obstet Gynecol Invest 1982; 14:127–130.

Henkin RE. Radionuclide detection of thromboembolic diseases. In: Kwaan HC, Bowie EJW, eds. Thrombosis. Philadelphia: WB Saunders, 1982: 236–252.

Hirsch J. Heparin. N Engl J Med 1991;324:1565.

Hirsch J. The optimal duration of anticoagulant therapy for venous thrombosis. N Engl J Med 1995;332:1710–1711.

Hirsch J. The treatment of venous thromboembolism. Nouv Rev Fr Hematol 1988a;30:149–153.

Hirsch J, Barrowcliffe TW. Standardization and clinical use of LMW heparin. Thromb Haemost 1988b;59:333–337.

Hirsch J, Dalen JE, Deykin D, Poller L. Heparin: mechanisms of action, dosing considerations, monitoring, efficacy, and safety. Chest 1992;102:337–350.

Holm HA, Abildgaard U, Kalvenes S. Heparin assays and bleeding complications in treatment of deep venous thrombosis with particular reference to retroperitoneal bleeding. Thromb Haemost 1985;53:278–281.

Horn JR, Danzinger LH, Davis RJ. Warfarin-induced skin necrosis: report of four cases. Am J Hosp Pharm 1981;38:1763–1768.

Howell R, Fidler J, Letsky E, deSwiet M. The risks of antenatal subcutaneous heparin prophylaxis: a controlled trial. Br J Obstet Gynecol 1983;90:1124–1128.

Huisman MV, Buller HR, ten Cate JW, Vreeken JR. Serial impedance plethysmography for suspected deep venous thrombosis in outpatients: the Amsterdam General Practitioners Study. N Engl J Med 1986;314:823–882.

Hull R, Delmore T, Carter C, et al. Adjusted subcutaneous heparin versus warfarin sodium in the long-term treatment of venous thrombosis. N Engl J Med 1982;306:189–194.

Hull RD, Hirsh J, Carter CJ, et al. Pulmonary angiography, ventilation lung scanning, and venography for clinically suspected pulmonary embolism with abnormal perfusion lung scan. Ann Intern Med 1983;98:891–899.

Hux CH, Wagner R, Rattan P, et al. Surgical treatment of thromboembolic disease in pregnancy. Proceedings of the Society of Perinatal Obstetricians, January 30–February 1, 1986:62. Abstract.

Hyers TM, Hull RD, Weg JG. Antithrombotic therapy for venous thromboembolic disease. Chest 1986;89:265–355.

Jeffcoate TNA, Miller J, Roos RF, Tindall VR. Puerperal thromboembolism in relation to the inhibition of lactation by oestrogen therapy. Br Med J 1968;4:19–22.

Kakkar V. The diagnosis of deep vein thrombosis using the $^{125}$I fibrinogen test. Arch Surg 1972;104:152–159.

Kakkar VV, Stamatakis JD, Bentley PG, et al. Prophylaxis for postoperative deep-vein thrombosis: synergistic effect of heparin and dihydroergotamine. JAMA 1979;241:39–42.

Kaplan KL, Owen J. Plasma levels of B-thromboglobulin and platelet factor 4 and indices of platelet activation in vivo. Blood 1981;57:199–202.

Kaunitz AM, Hughes JM, Grimes DA, et al. Causes of maternal mortality in the United States. Obstet Gynecol 1985;65:605–612.

Killwich LA, Bedford GR, Beach KW, et al. Diagnosis of deep venous thrombosis: a prospective study comparing duplex scanning to contrast venography. Circulation 1989;79:810–812.

Kipper MS, Moser KM, Kortman KE, et al. Long-term follow-up of patients with suspected pulmonary embolism and a normal lung scan. Perfusion scans in embolic subjects. Chest 1982;82:411–415.

Kohn H, Konig B, Mostbeck A. Incidence and clinical feature of pulmonary embolism in patients with deep venous thrombosis: a prospective study. Eur J Nucl Med 1987;13:S11–S13.

Koopman MMW, Prandoni P, Piovella F. Treatment of venous thrombosis with intravenous unfractionated heparin administered in the hospital as compared with subcutaneous low-molecular-weight heparin administered at home. N Engl J Med 1996;334:682–687.

Kramer FL, Teitelbaum G, Merli GJ. Panvenography and pulmonary angiography in the diagnosis of deep venous thrombosis and pulmonary thromboembolism. Radiol Clin North Am 1986;24:397–418.

Lao TT, Yin JA, Ng WK, Yuen PMP. Relationship between maternal antithrombin III and protein C/protein S levels before, during, and after delivery. Gynecol Obstet Invest 1990;30:87–90.

Lao TT, Yuen PMP, Yin JA. Protein S and protein C levels in Chinese women during pregnancy, delivery, and the puerperium. Br J Obstet Gynaecol 1989;96:167–170.

Lawson HW, Atrash HK, Franks AL. Fatal pulmonary embolism during legal induced abortion in the United States from 1972 to 1985. Am J Obstet Gynecol 1990;162:986–990.

Lebsack CS, Weibert RT. "Purple toes" syndrome. Postgrad Med 1982;71:81–84.

Leclerc JR. Pulmonary embolism. In: Rakel RE, ed. Conn's current therapy—1994. Philadelphia: WB Saunders, 1994:199–205.

Leclerc JR, Geerts W, Panju A, et al. Management of antithrombin III deficiency during pregnancy without administration of antithrombin III. Thromb Res 1986;41:567–573.

Lensing AW, Prins MH, Davison BE, et al. Treatment of deep-venous thrombosis with low molecular weight heparins: a meta-analysis. Arch Intern Med 1995;155:601.

Letsky EA. Coagulation problems during pregnancy. In: Lind T, ed. Current review in obstetrics and gynecology. Edinburgh: Churchill Livingstone, 1985.

Levine M, Gent M, Hirsh J, et al. A comparison of low-molecular-weight heparin administered primarily at home with unfractionated heparin administered in the hospital for proximal deep-vein thrombosis. New Engl J Med 1996;334:677–681.

Lewis JF, Anderson TW, Fennel WH, et al. A clue to pulmonary embolism obtained during Swan-Ganz catheterization. Chest 1982;81:527–529.

Magnani HN. Heparin induced thrombocytopenia (HIT): an overview of 230 patients treated with orgaran (Org 10172). Thromb Haemost 1993; 70:554–561.

Malciniak E, Wilson HD, Marlar RA. Neonatal purpura fulminans: a genetic disorder related to the absence of protein C in blood. Blood 1985;65:15–20.

Malm J, Laurell M, Dahlbeck B. Changes in the plasma levels of vitamin K dependent protein C and S and of C4b-binding protein during pregnancy and oral contraception. Br J Haematol 1988;68:437–443.

Mant MJ, O'Brien BD, Russell DB. Diagnostic leg scanning for deep venous thrombosis in the recently heparinized patient. Arch Intern Med 1981;141:1757–1760.

Markisz JA. Radiologic and nuclear medicine diagnosis. In: Goldhaber SZ, ed. Pulmonary embolism and deep venous thrombosis. Philadelphia: WB Saunders, 1985:41–72.

McLean R, Mattison ET, Cochrane NE. Maternal mortality study annual report 1970–1976. NY State J Med 1979;79:39–43.

Megha A, Finzi G, Poli T, et al. Pregnancy, antithrombin III deficiency and venous thrombosis: report of another case. Acta Haematol 1990;83: 111–114.

Mills SR, Jackson DC, Older RA, et al. The incidence, etiologies and avoidance of complications of pulmonary angiography in a large series. Radiology 1980;136:295–299.

Mohr DN, Ryu JH, Litin SC, Rosenow EC III. Recent advances in the management of venous thromboembolism. Mayo Clin Proc 1988;63:281–290.

Monreal M, Salvador R, Ruiz J. Below-knee deep venous thrombosis and pulmonary embolism. AJR 1987;149:860. Letter.

Moran KT, Jewell ER, Persson AV. The role of thrombolytic therapy in surgical practice. Br J Surg 1989;76:298–304.

Moser KM, Fedullo PF. Venous thromboembolism: three simple decisions (part 2). Chest 1983; 83:256–260.

Moser KM, LeMoine JR. Is embolic risk conditioned by location of deep venous thrombosis? Ann Intern Med 1981;94:439–444.

Moses DC, Silver TM, Bookstein JJ. The complementary roles of chest radiography, lung scanning and selective pulmonary angiography in the diagnosis of pulmonary embolism. Circulation 1974;44:179–185.

Moses V, DePersio SR, Lorenz D, et al. A thirty-year review of maternal mortality in Oklahoma, 1950 through 1979. Am J Obstet Gynecol 1987;157: 1189–1194.

Needleman P, Minkes M, Raz A. Thromboxanes: selected biosynthesis and distinct biological properties. Science 1976;193:163–165.

Negus D, Friedgood A, Cox SJ, et al. Ultra-low dose intravenous heparin in the prevention of postoperative deep-vein thrombosis. Lancet 1980; 1:891–894.

Nelson DM, Stempel LE, Brandt JT. Hereditary antithrombin III deficiency and pregnancy: report of two cases and review of the literature. Obstet Gynecol 1985;65:848–853.

Nelson DM, Stempel LE, Fabri PJ, et al. Hickman catheter use in a pregnant patient requiring therapeutic heparin anticoagulation. Am J Obstet Gynecol 1984;149:461–462.

Nicholas GG, Lorenz RP, Botti JJ, et al. The frequent occurrence of false-positive results in phleborrheography during pregnancy. Surg Gynecol Obstet 1985;161:133–136.

Nichols AB, Beller GA, Cochari S, et al. Detection of pulmonary embolism by positron imaging of inhaled $^{15}$O-labeled carbon dioxide. Semin Nucl Med 1980;10:252–258.

Park S, Schroeter AL, Park YS, Fortson J. Purple toes and livido reticularis in a patient with cardiovascular disease taking coumadin. Arch Dermatol 1993;129:775–780.

Perry PJ, Herron GR, King JC. Heparin half-life in normal and impaired renal function. Clin Pharmacol Res 1974;16:514–519.

Phillipps YY, Copley JB, Stor RA. Thrombocytopenia and low dose heparin. South Med J 1983;76:526–528.

PIOPED Investigators. Valve of the ventilation 1 perfusion scan in acute pulmonary embolism: results of the prospective investigation of pulmonary embolism diagnosis (PIOPED). JAMA 1990;263:2753.

Raghavendra BN, Rosen RJ, Lam S, et al. Deep venous thrombosis: detection by high-resolution real-time ultrasonography. Radiology 1984;152:789–792.

Rao AK, White GC, Sherman L, et al. Low incidence of thrombocytopenia with porcine mucosal heparin. A prospective multicenter study. Arch Intern Med 1989;149:1285–1288.

Rasmussen C, Wadt J, Jacobsen B. Thromboembolic prophylaxis with low molecular weight heparin during pregnancy. Int J Obstet Gynecol 1994;47:121–125.

Robbins KC. The plasminogen-plasmin enzyme system. In: Colman RW, Hirsh J, Marder VJ, et al, eds. Hemostasis and thrombosis. Philadelphia: JB Lippincott, 1982.

Robin ED. Overdiagnosis and overtreatment of pulmonary embolism: the emperor may have no clothes. Ann Intern Med 1977;87:775–776.

Rochat RW, Koonin LM, Atrash HK, et al. Maternal mortality in the United States: report from the Maternal Mortality Collaborative. Obstet Gynecol 1988;72:91–97.

Rose PG, de Moerloose PA, Bounameaux H. Protein S deficiency in pregnancy. Am J Obstet Gynecol 1986;155:140–141.

Rosenow EC III, Osmundson PJ, Brown ML. Pulmonary embolism. Mayo Clin Proc 1981;56:161–178.

Rutherford SE, Montoro M, McGehee W, et al. Thromboembolic disease associated with pregnancy: an 11-year review, SPO Abstract 139. Am J Obstet Gynecol 1991a;164:286.

Rutherford SE, Phelan JP. Deep venous thrombosis and pulmonary embolism in pregnancy. Obstet Gynecol Clin North Am 1991b;18:345–370.

Sachs BP, Brown DAJ, Driscoll SG, et al. Maternal mortality in Massachusetts. N Engl J Med 1987;316:667–672.

Sachs BP, Yeh J, Acker D, et al. Cesarean section-related maternal mortality in Massachusetts, 1954–1985. Obstet Gynecol 1988;71:385–388.

Salazar E, Zajarias A, Gutierrez N, et al. The problem of cardiac valve prostheses, anticoagulants, and pregnancy. Circulation 1984;70(suppl I):169–177.

Salzman EW, Hirsh J. Prevention of venous thromboembolism. In: Colman RW, Hirsh J, Marder VJ, Salzman EW, eds. Hemostasis and thrombosis: basic principles and clinical practice. 2nd ed. Philadelphia: JB Lippincott, 1987:1252–1264.

Samama M. [The new heparins]. Presse Med 1986;15:1631–1635.

Samson D, Stirling Y, Woolf L, et al. Management of planned pregnancy in a patient with congenital antithrombin III deficiency. Br J Haematol 1984;56:243–249.

Schiff MJ, Feinberg AW, Naidich JB. Noninvasive venous examinations as a screening test for pulmonary embolism. Arch Intern Med 1987;147:505–507.

Schulman S, Rhedin A, Lindmarker P, et al. A comparison of six weeks with six months of oral anticoagulant therapy after a first episode of venous thromboembolism. N Engl J Med 1995;332:1661–1665.

Schwartz RS, Bauer KA, Rosenberg RD, et al. Clinical experience with antithrombin III concentrate in treatment of congenital and acquired deficiency of antithrombin. Am J Med 1989;87(suppl 3B):53S–60S.

Sharma GVRK, Cella G, Parisi AF, et al. Thrombolytic therapy. N Engl J Med 1985;306:1268–1276.

Simioni P, Prandoni P, Lensing AWA. The risk of recurrent venous thromboembolism in patients with an Arg[506] → Gln mutation in the gene for factor V (factor V Leiden). N Engl J Med 1997;336:399.

Spritzer CE, Evans AC, Kay HH. Magnetic resonance imaging of deep venous thrombosis in pregnant women with lower extremity edema. Obstet Gynecol 1995;85:603–607.

Standing Advisory Committee for Haematology of the Royal College of Pathologists. Drug interaction with coumarin derivative anticoagulants. Br Med J 1982;185:274–275.

Stead RB. Regulation of hemostasis. In: Goldhaber SZ, ed. Pulmonary embolism and deep venous thrombosis. Philadelphia: WB Saunders, 1985: 27–40.

Stevenson RE, Burton OM, Ferlauto GJ, Taylor HA. Hazards of oral anticoagulants during pregnancy. JAMA 1980;243:1549–1551.

Stiller RJ, Leone-Tomaschoff S, Cuteri J, et al. Postpartum pulmonary embolus as an unusual cause of cortical blindness. Am J Obstet Gynecol 1990;162:696–697.

Stringer MD, Kakkar VV. Prevention of venous thromboembolism. Herz 1989;14:135–147.

Sturridge F, Letsky E. The use of low molecular weight heparin for thrombophylaxis in pregnancy. Br J Obstet Gynecol 1994;101:69–71.

Tenero DM, Bell HE, Deitz PA, Bertino JS Jr. Comparative dosage and toxicity of heparin sodium in the treatment of patients with pulmonary embolism versus deep-vein thrombosis. Clin Pharm 1989;8:40–43.

Tengborn L, Bergqvist D, Matzsch T, et al. Recurrent thromboembolism in pregnancy and puerperium: is there a need for thromboprophylaxis? Am J Obstet Gynecol 1989;160:90–94.

Tharakan T, Baxi LV, Dinguid D. Protein S deficiency in pregnancy. A case report. Am J Obstet Gynecol 1993;168:141–142.

Thompson AR, Harker CA. Manual of thrombosis and hemostasis. Philadelphia: FA Davis, 1983.

Toglia MR, Weg JG. Venous thromboembolism during pregnancy. N Engl J Med 1996;335:108.

Traeger SM. Failure to wedge and pulmonary hypertension during pulmonary artery catheterization: a sign of totally occlusive pulmonary embolism. Crit Care Med 1985;13:544–547.

Turrentine MA, Braems G, Ramirez MM. Use of thrombolytics for the treatment of thromboembolic disease during pregnancy. Obstet Gynecol Surv 1995;50:534–541.

Urokinase Pulmonary Embolism Trial. A national cooperative study. Circulation 1973;43(suppl II): 47.

Urokinase-Streptokinase Pulmonary Embolism Trial. Phase 2 results. A cooperative study. JAMA 1974; 229:1606–1613.

Vincent WR, Goldberg SJ, Desilets D. Fatality immediately following rapid infusion of macroaggregates of [99m]Tc albumin (MAA) for lung scan. Radiology 1968;91:1181–1184.

Walker AM, Jick H. Predictors of bleeding during heparin therapy. JAMA 1980;244:1209–1212.

White TM, Bernene JL, Marino AM. Continuous heparin infusion requirements: diagnostic and therapeutic implications. JAMA 1979;241:2717–2720.

Woodhams BJ, Candotti G, Shaw R, et al. Changes in coagulation and fibrinolysis during pregnancy: evidence of activation of coagulation preceding spontaneous abortion. Thromb Res 1989;55: 99–102.

Worthington D. Maternal mortality in Wisconsin: embolism. Wisconsin Med J 1989;88:26–30.

Zimran A, Shilo S, Fisher D, et al. Histomorphometric evaluation of reversible heparin-induced osteoporosis in pregnancy. Arch Intern Med 1986;146:386–388.

# CHAPTER 20

# Anaphylactoid Syndrome of Pregnancy (Amniotic Fluid Embolism)

*A* mniotic fluid embolism (AFE) is an uncommon obstetric disorder with a mortality of 60% to 70% and is a leading cause of maternal mortality in Western industrialized countries (Morgan, 1979; Kaunitz, 1985; Hogberg, 1994; Grimes, 1994; Clark, 1995). It is classically characterized by hypoxia, hypotension or hemodynamic collapse, and coagulopathy. Despite numerous attempts to develop an animal model, AFE remains incompletely understood. Nevertheless, during the past decade, there have been several significant advances in our understanding of this enigmatic condition.

## Historic Considerations

The earliest description of AFE was by Meyer in 1926. The condition was not widely recognized, however, until the report of Steiner and Luschbaugh in 1941. These investigators described autopsy findings in eight pregnant women with sudden shock and pulmonary edema during labor. In all cases, squamous cells or mucin, presumably of fetal origin, were found in the pulmonary vasculature. In a follow-up report in 1969 by Liban and Raz, cellular debris was also observed in the kidneys, liver, spleen, pancreas, and brain of several such patients. Squamous cells also were identified in uterine veins of several control patients in this series, a finding confirmed in a report of Thompson and Budd in a patient without AFE (Thompson, 1963). It should be noted, how-

ever, that in the initial description of Steiner and Luschbaugh (1941), seven of the eight patients carried clinical diagnoses other than AFE (including sepsis and unrecognized uterine rupture) that were not materially different from the diagnoses of their control patients without these specific histologic findings. Only one of the eight patients in the classic AFE group died of "obstetric shock" without an additional clinical diagnosis. Thus, the relevance of this original report to patients presently dying of AFE after the exclusion of other diagnoses is questionable.

Since the initial descriptions of AFE, more than 300 case reports have appeared in the literature. Although most cases were reported during labor, sudden death in pregnancy has been attributed to AFE under many widely varying circumstances, including cases of first- and second-trimester abortion (Resnik, 1976; Guidotti, 1981; Meier, 1983; Cromley, 1983). In 1948, Eastman, in an editorial review, stated, "Let us be careful not to make [the diagnosis of AFE] a waste basket for cases of unexplained death in labor." Fortunately, increased understanding of the syndrome of AFE makes such errors highly unlikely today.

## Experimental Models

The first animal model of AFE was that of Steiner and Luschbaugh, who showed that rabbits and dogs could be killed by the intravenous injection of heterologous amniotic fluid and meconium

T A B L E    **20-1**

Animal models of amniotic fluid embolism

| Investigator | Year | Animal | Anesthetized | Pregnant | Filtered AF | Pathology with Whole/Concentrated AF |
|---|---|---|---|---|---|---|
| Steiner and Luschbaugh | 1941 | Rabbit/dog | No | No | No | Yes |
| Cron | 1952 | Rabbit | No | No | NE | Yes |
| Schneider | 1953 | Dog | No | No | NE | Yes |
| Jaques | 1960 | Dog | Yes | No | NE | Yes |
| Halmagyi | 1962 | Sheep | Yes | No | No | Yes |
| Attwood | 1965 | Dog | Yes | No | Yes (mild) | Yes |
| Stolte | 1967 | Monkey | Yes | Yes | No | No |
| Macmillan | 1968 | Rabbit | No | No | No | Yes |
| Reis | 1969 | Sheep | Yes | Yes | Yes | Yes |
| Dutta | 1970 | Rabbit | Yes | No | NE | Yes |
| Adamsons | 1971 | Monkey | Yes | Yes | NE | No |
| Kitzmiller | 1972 | Cat | Yes | No | No | Yes |
| Spence | 1974 | Rabbit | No | Yes | No | No |
| Reeves | 1974 | Calf | No | No | NE | Yes |
| Azegami | 1986 | Rabbit | No | No | No | Yes |
| Richards | 1988 | Rat* | Yes | No | Yes | NE |
| Hankins | 1993 | Goat | Yes | Yes | Yes | Yes |

*Isolated heart preparation.

AF, amniotic fluid; BP, blood pressure; CO, cardiac output; CVP, central venous pressure; LAP, left atrial pressure; NE, not examined; Nl, normal; P, pulse; PAP, pulmonary artery pressure; PCWP, pulmonary capillary wedge pressure; PVR, pulmonary vascular resistance; RR, respiratory rate; SVR, systemic vascular resistance.

(Steiner, 1941). Several subsequent reports of AFE in experimental animals have yielded conflicting results (Table 20-1) (Steiner, 1941; Cron, 1952; Schneider, 1955; Jaques, 1960; Halmagyi, 1962; Attwood, 1965; Stolte, 1967; MacMillan, 1968; Reis, 1965; Dutta, 1970; Adamsons, 1971; Kitzmiller, 1972; Spence, 1974; Reeves, 1974; Richards, 1988; Azegami, 1986; Hankins, 1993). In most series, experimental injection of amniotic fluid had adverse effects, ranging from transient alterations

| AF Species | Injection Arterial | Pathologic Venous | Hemodynamic Changes | Coagu- lopathy | Autopsy |
|---|---|---|---|---|---|
| Human | NE | Yes | NE (death) | No | Debris in pulmonary artery |
| Human | No | Yes | NE (death) | No | Debris in pulmonary artery |
| Human | NE | Yes | NE (death) | 5 of 8 | Debris in pulmonary artery |
| Human/ dog | NE | Yes | ↑ PAP, Nl BP | Fibrinogen 12 of 13 | Debris in pulmonary artery |
| Human | NE | Yes | ↑ PAP, Nl SVR, Nl CO | No | NE |
| Human | Yes | Yes | ↑ PAP, ↑ PVR, ↓ SVR, Nl to ↑ LAP, BP | 4 of 12 | NE |
| Human/ monkey | No | No | Nl BP, Nl P | 1 of 12 | NE |
| Human | Yes | Yes | NE (death) | 2 of 12 | Minimal debris, hemorrhage |
| Sheep | Yes | Yes | ↑ PAP, ↑ PVR, ↓ SVR, ↓ BP, Nl LAP, Nl PCWP | No | Normal |
| Human | NE | Yes | NE (death) | No | Minimal debris, massive infarction |
| Monkey | NE | No | Nl BP, Nl P, Nl RR | No | NE |
| Human | NE | Yes | ↓ BP, ↑ P, ↑ CVP | No | NE |
| Rabbit | NE | No | Nl BP, Nl P, Nl RR | No | NE |
| Calf | NE | Yes | ↓ BP, ↑ PAP, Nl CO, Nl PCWP | | |
| Human | NE | Yes | NE (death) | No | Pulmonary edema, debris in pulmonary vessels |
| Human | NE | Yes | Coronary flow | | |
| Goat | NE | Yes | SVR, ↑↓ PVR, ↑↓ MAP, ↑↓ | No | NE |

in systemic and pulmonary artery pressures in dogs, sheep, cats, and calves to sudden death in rabbits. Only two of these studies, however, involved pregnant animals, and in most, heterologous amniotic fluid was used. In several studies, the effects of whole or meconium-enriched amniotic fluid were contrasted with those of filtered amniotic fluid. A pathologic response was obtained only in particulate rich amniotic fluid in four such studies, whereas, three reports demonstrated physiologic changes with filtered amniotic fluid as well. Data produced with the models involving particulate-enriched amniotic fluid may have little relevance to the human model, because the concentration of particulate matter injected has been many times greater than that present in human amniotic fluid, even in the presence of meconium. In the four studies in which injections of amniotic fluid into the arterial and venous systems were compared, three showed toxic effects with both arterial and venous injection, implying a pathologic humoral substance or response. In studies in which autopsy was performed, pulmonary findings ranged from massive vascular plugging with fetal debris (after embolization with particulate-enriched amniotic fluid) to normal.

In contrast, the only two studies carried out in primates showed the intravenous injection of amniotic fluid to be entirely innocuous without effects on BP, pulse, or respiratory rate (Stolte, 1967; Adamsons, 1971). In one study, the volume of amniotic fluid infused would, in the human, represent 80% of the total amniotic fluid volume. More recently, a carefully controlled study in the goat model using homologous amniotic fluid demonstrated hemodynamic and clinical findings similar to that seen in humans, including an initial transient rise in pulmonary and systemic vascular resistance and myocardial depression (Hankins, 1993). These findings were especially prominent when the injectate included meconium. Importantly, the initial phase of pulmonary hypertension in all animal models studied has been transient and in survivors has resolved within 30 minutes (Clark, 1990). Because most attempts at the development of an animal model of AFE have involved the injection of tissue from a foreign species, the resultant physiologic effects may have limited clinical relevance to the human condition and must be interpreted with caution.

## Hemodynamic Alterations

In humans, an initial, transient phase of hemodynamic change involving both systemic and pulmonary vasospasm leads to a more often recognized secondary phase involving principally hypotension and depressed ventricular function (Clark, 1985a, 1988, 1995; Girard, 1986).

Figure 20-1 demonstrates in a graphic manner the depression of left ventricular function seen in five patients with pulmonary artery catheterization. The mechanism of left ventricular failure is uncertain. Work in the rat model by Richards and co-workers suggests the presence of possible

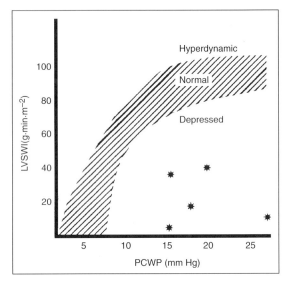

F I G U R E **20-1**

**Modified Starling curve, demonstrating depressed left ventricular function in five patients with AFE.** PCWP, pulmonary capillary wedge pressure; LVSWI, left ventricular stroke work index.

coronary artery spasm and myocardial ischemia in animal AFE (Richards, 1988). On the other hand, the global hypoxia commonly seen in patients with AFE could account for left ventricular dysfunction. The in vitro observation of decreased myometrial contractility in the presence of amniotic fluid also suggests the possibility of a similar effect of amniotic fluid on myocardium (Courtney, 1970).

## Pulmonary Manifestations

Patients suffering AFE typically develop rapid and often profound hypoxia, which may result in permanent neurologic impairment in survivors of this condition. This hypoxia is likely due to a combination of initial pulmonary vasospasm and ventricular dysfunction. In both animal models and human experience, however, this initial hypoxia is often transient. Table 20-2 details arterial blood gas findings in a group of patients with AFE for whom paired data are available. Initial profound shunting and rapid recovery are seen. In survivors, primary lung injury often leads to acute respiratory distress syndrome and secondary oxygenation defects.

T A B L E    **20-2**

Resolution of hypoxia after amniotic fluid embolism

| Patient No. | Initial Po₂ (mm Hg) | Time from Amniotic Fluid Embolism (min) | Next Po₂ (mm Hg) | Time from Amniotic Fluid Embolism (min) |
|---|---|---|---|---|
| 2 | 34 | 11 | 242 | 62 |
| 4 | 19 | 20 | 587 | 40 |
| 12 | 98 | 21 | 388 | 45 |
| 22 | 24 | 60 | 128 | 75 |
| 25 | 12 | 37 | 484 | 96 |

Reproduced by permission from Clark SL, Hankins GVD, Dudley DA, et al.
Amniotic fluid embolism: analysis of the national registry. Am J Obstet
Gynecol 1995;172:1158–1169.

## Coagulopathy

Patients surviving the initial hemodynamic insult may succumb to a secondary coagulopathy (Clark, 1995; Porter, 1996). The exact incidence of the coagulopathy is unknown. Coagulopathy was an entry criterion for inclusion in the initial analysis of the National AFE Registry; however, several patients submitted to the registry who clearly had AFE did not have clinical evidence of coagulopathy (Clark, 1995). In a similar manner, a number of patients have been observed who developed an acute obstetric coagulopathy alone in the absence of placental abruptio and suffered fatal exsanguination without any evidence of primary hemodynamic or pulmonary insult (Porter, 1996).

As with experimental investigations into hemodynamic alterations associated with AFE, investigations of this coagulopathy has yielded contradictory results. In in vitro studies, amniotic fluid has been shown to shorten whole blood clotting time, to have a thromboplastin-like effect, to induce platelet aggregation and release of platelet factor III, and to activate the compliment cascade (Ratnoff, 1952; Beller, 1963). In addition, Courtney and Allington showed that amniotic fluid contains a direct factor X activating factor (Courtney, 1972). Although confirming the factor X activating properties of amniotic fluid, Phillips and Davidson concluded that the amount of procoagulant in clear amniotic fluid is insufficient to cause significant intervascular coagulation, a finding disputed by the more recent studies of Lockwood and colleagues (1991) and Phillips et al (1972).

In the experimental animal models discussed previously, coagulopathy has likewise been an inconsistent finding. Thus, the exact nature of the consumptive coagulopathy demonstrated in humans with AFE is yet to be satisfactorily explained. The powerful thromboplastin effects of trophoblast are well established. The coagulopathy associated with severe placental abruption and that seen with AFE are probably similar in origin and represent an activation of the coagulation cascade following exposure of the maternal circulation to a variety of fetal antigens with varying thromboplastin-like effects (Clark, 1995).

## Pathophysiology

In an analysis of the National AFE Registry, a marked similarity was noted between the clinical, hemodynamic, and hematologic manifestations of AFE and both septic and anaphylactic shock (Clark, 1995). Clearly, the clinical manifestations of this condition are not identical; fever is unique to septic shock, and cutaneous manifestations are more common in anaphylaxis. Nevertheless, the marked similarities of these conditions suggest similar pathophysiologic mechanisms.

Detailed discussions of the pathophysiologic features of septic shock and anaphylactic shock are presented in Chapters 22 and 23, respectively. Both of these conditions involve the entrance of a foreign substance (bacterial endotoxin or specific antigens) into the circulation, which then result in the release of various primary and

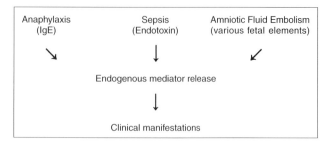

F I G U R E   **20-2**

**Proposed pathophysiologic relation between AFE, septic shock, and anaphylactic shock. Each syndrome also may have specific direct physiologic effects.** Reproduced by permission from Clark SL, Hankins GVD, Dudley DA, et al. Amniotic fluid embolism: analysis of the national registry. Am J Obstet Gynecol 1995;172:1158–1169.)

secondary endogenous mediators (Fig 20-2). Similar pathophysiology has also been proposed in nonpregnant patients with pulmonary fat embolism. It is the release of these mediators that results in the principal physiologic derangements characterizing these syndromes. These include profound myocardial depression and decreased cardiac output, described in both animals and humans; pulmonary hypertension, demonstrated in lower primate models of anaphylaxis; and disseminated intervascular coagulation, described in both human anaphylactic reactions and septic shock (Raper, 1988; Smedegard, 1981; Parillo, 1993; Enjeti, 1983; Smith, 1980; Kapin, 1985; Wong, 1990; Silverman, 1984; Lee, 1988; Parker, 1980). Further, the temporal sequence of hemodynamic decompensation and recovery seen in experimental AFE is virtually identical to that described in canine anaphylaxis (Kapin, 1985). An *anaphylactoid* response is also well described in humans and involves the nonimmunologic release of similar mediators (Parker, 1980). It is also intriguing that, on admission to the hospital, 41% of patients in the AFE registry gave a history of either drug allergy or atopy (Clark, 1995).

The ability of arachidonic acid metabolites to cause the same physiologic and hemodynamic changes observed in human AFE has been noted (Clark, 1985). Further, in the rabbit model of AFE, pretreatment with an inhibitor of leukotriene synthesis has been shown to prevent death (Aze-

gami, 1986). These experimental observations further support the clinical conclusions of the National AFE Registry analysis that this condition involves the anaphylactoid release of endogenous mediators, including arachidonic acid metabolites, which result in the devastating pathophysiologic sequence seen in clinical AFE (Clark, 1995).

Earlier anecdotal reports suggested a possible relationship between hypertonic uterine contractions or oxytocin use and AFE. Although disputed on statistical grounds by Morgan in 1979, this misconception persisted in some writings until recently (Morgan, 1979). The historic anecdotal association between hypertonic uterine contractions and the onset of symptoms in AFE was made clear by the analysis of the National Registry (Clark, 1995). These data demonstrated that the hypertonic contractions commonly seen in association with AFE appear to be a result of the release of catecholamines into the circulation as part of the initial human hemodynamic response to any massive physiologic insult. Under these circumstances, norepinephrine, in particular, acts as a potent uterotonic agent (Paul, 1978; Clark, 1995). Thus, while the association of hypertonic contractions and AFE appears to be valid, it is the physiologic response to AFE that causes the hypertonic uterine activity rather than the converse. Indeed, there is a complete cessation of uterine blood flow in the presence of even moderate uterine contractions; thus, a tetanic contraction is the least likely time during an entire labor process for any exchange between maternal and fetal compartments (Towell, 1976). Oxytocin is not used with increased frequency in patients suffering AFE compared with the general population, nor does oxytocin-induced hyperstimulation commonly precede this condition (Clark, 1995). Thus, several authorities, including the American College of Obstetricians and Gynecologists, have concluded that oxytocin use has no relationship to the occurrence of AFE (Morgan, 1979; ACOG, 1993; Clark, 1995).

The syndrome of AFE appears to be initiated after maternal intervascular exposure to various types of fetal tissue. Such exposure may occur during the course of normal labor and delivery; after potentially minor traumatic events, such as intrauterine pressure catheter placement; or during cesarean section. Because fetal-to-maternal tissue transfer is virtually universal during the labor and delivery process, actions by health-care providers, such as intrauterine manipulation or cesarean delivery, may effect the timing of the exposure; no evidence exists, however, to suggest that exposure itself can be avoided by altering clinical management. Simple exposure of the maternal circulatory system to even small amounts of amniotic fluid or other fetal tissue may, under the right circumstances, initiate the syndrome of AFE. This understanding explains the well-documented occurrence of fatal AFE during first-trimester pregnancy termination at a time when neither the volume of fluid nor positive intrauterine pressure could be contributing factors (Guidotti, 1981). Whereas much has been written about the importance to the fetus of an immunologic barrier between the mother and the antigenically different products of conception, little attention has been paid to the potential importance of this barrier to maternal well-being. The observations of the National Registry as well as cumulative data for the past several decades suggest that breaches of this barrier may, under certain circumstances and in susceptible maternal-fetal pairs, be of immense significance to the mother as well (Clark, 1995).

Previous experimental evidence in animals and humans unequivocally demonstrates that the intravenous administration of even large amounts of amniotic fluid per se is innocuous (Sparr, 1958; Stolte, 1967; Adamsons, 1971). Further, the clinical findings described in the National Registry are not consistent with an embolic event as commonly understood (Table 20-3). Thus, the term *amniotic fluid embolism* itself appears to be a misnomer. In the National Registry analysis, the authors suggested that the term *amniotic fluid embolism* be discarded and the syndrome of acute peripartum hypoxia hemodynamic collapse and coagulopathy should be designated in a more descriptive manner, as *anaphylactoid syndrome of pregnancy.*

## Clinical Presentation

Clinical signs and symptoms noted in patients with AFE are described in Table 20-3. In a typical

T A B L E    **20-3**

Signs and symptoms noted in patients with amniotic fluid embolism

| Sign or Symptom | No. of Patients | % |
|---|---|---|
| Hypotension | 43 | 100 |
| Fetal distress[a] | 30 | 100 |
| Pulmonary edema or adult respiratory distress syndrome[b] | 28 | 93 |
| Cardiopulmonary arrest | 40 | 87 |
| Cyanosis | 38 | 83 |
| Coagulopathy[c] | 38 | 83 |
| Dyspnea[d] | 22 | 49 |
| Seizure | 22 | 48 |
| Atony | 11 | 23 |
| Bronchospasm[e] | 7 | 15 |
| Transient hypertension | 5 | 11 |
| Cough | 3 | 7 |
| Headache | 3 | 7 |
| Chest pain | 1 | 2 |

[a]$n = 30$. Includes all live fetuses in utero at time of event.

[b]$n = 30$. Eighteen patients did not survive long enough for these diagnoses to be confirmed.

[c]$n = 38$. Eight patients did not survive long enough for this diagnosis to be confirmed.

[d]$n = 45$. One patient was intubated at the time of the event and could not be assessed.

[e]Difficult ventilation was noted during cardiac arrest in six patients, and wheezes were auscultated in one patient.

Reproduced by permission from Clark SL, Hankins GVD, Dudley DA. Amniotic fluid embolism: analysis of a national registry. Am J Obstet Gynecol 1995;172: 1158–1169.

case, a patient laboring, having just undergone cesarean delivery or immediately following vaginal delivery or pregnancy termination, suffers the acute onset of profound hypoxia and hypotension followed by cardiopulmonary arrest. The initial episode often is complicated by the development of a consumptive coagulopathy, which may lead to exsanguination, even if attempts to restore hemodynamic and respiratory function are successful. It must be emphasized, however, that in any individual patient, any of the three principal phases (hypoxia, hypotension, or coagulopathy) may either dominate or be entirely absent (Clark, 1995; Porter, 1996). Clinical

T A B L E   **20-4**

Cardiac arrest-to-delivery interval
and neonatal outcome

| Interval (min) | Survival (no.) | Intact Survival (no.) |
|---|---|---|
| <5 | 3/3 | 2/3 (67%) |
| 5–15 | 3/3 | 2/3 (67%) |
| 16–25 | 2/5 | 2/5 (40%) |
| 26–35 | 3/4 | 1/4 (25%) |
| 36–54 | 0/1 | 0/1 (0%) |

Reproduced by permission from Clark SL, Hankins GVD, Dudley DA. Amniotic fluid embolism: analysis of the national registry. Am J Obstet Gynecol 1995;172: 1158–1169.

variations in this syndrome appear to be related to variations in both antigenic exposure and maternal response.

Maternal outcome is dismal in patients with AFE syndrome. The overall maternal mortality rate appears to be 60% to 80% (Clark, 1990, 1995). Only 15% of patients, however, survive neurologically intact. In a number of cases, following successful hemodynamic resuscitation and reversal of disseminated intravascular coagulation, life-support systems were withdrawn because of brain death resulting from the initial profound hypoxia. In patients progressing to cardiac arrest, only 8% survive neurologically intact (Clark, 1995). In the National Registry data, no form of therapy appeared to be consistently associated with improved outcome.

Neonatal outcome is similarly poor. Among fetuses in utero at the time of onset of maternal symptoms, the survival rate is approximately 80%; only half of these fetuses survive neurologically intact (Clark, 1995). Fetuses surviving to delivery generally demonstrate profound respiratory acidemia. Although at the present time no form of therapy appears to be associated with improved maternal outcome, there is a clear relationship between neonatal outcome and event to delivery interval in those women suffering cardiac arrest (Table 20-4) (Clark, 1995). Similar findings were reported by Katz et al in patients suffering cardiac arrest in a number of different clinical situations (Katz, 1986).

## Diagnosis

In the past, histologic confirmation of the clinical syndrome of AFE was often sought by the detection of cellular debris of presumed fetal origin either in the distal port of a pulmonary artery catheterization or at autopsy (Clark, 1990). Several studies of the past decade, however, suggest that such findings are commonly encountered, even in normal pregnant women (Fig 20-3) (Plauche, 1983; Covone, 1984; Clark, 1986; Lee, 1986). In the analysis of the National AFE Registry, fetal elements were found in roughly 50% of cases in which pulmonary artery catheter aspirate was analyzed and in roughly 75% of patients who went to autopsy (Clark, 1995). The frequency with which such findings are encountered varies with the number of histologic sections obtained. In addition, multiple special stains often are required to document such debris (Clark, 1990). Thus, the diagnosis of AFE remains a clinical one; histologic findings are neither sensitive nor specific. It is interesting to note that similar conclusions have been drawn regarding the diagnostic

F I G U R E   **20-3**

**Squamous cells recovered from the pulmonary arterial circulation of a pregnant patient with class IV rheumatic mitral stenosis**. (Magnification, 1000×.)

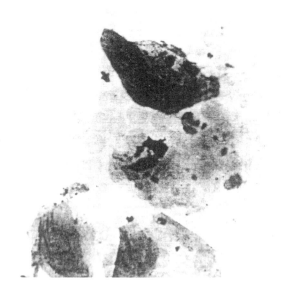

significance of histologic findings in patients with pulmonary fat embolism (Gitin, 1993).

## Treatment

Treatment remains disappointing, with an overall mortality rate of 60% to 80%. In the National Registry, we found no difference in survival among patients suffering initial cardiac arrest in small rural hospitals attended by family practitioners when compared with those suffering identical clinical signs and symptoms in tertiary-level centers attended by board-certified anesthesiologists, cardiologists, and maternal fetal medicine specialists. Nevertheless, several generalizations can be drawn:

1. The initial treatment for AFE is supportive. Cardiopulmonary resuscitation is performed if the patient is suffering from a lethal dysrhythmia. Oxygen should be provided at high concentrations.
2. In the patient who survives the initial cardiopulmonary insult, it should be remembered that left ventricular failure is commonly seen. Thus, volume expansion to optimize ventricular preload is performed, and if the patient remains significantly hypotensive, the addition of an inotropic agent such as dopamine seems most appropriate. In patients who remain unstable following the initial resuscitative efforts, pulmonary artery catheterization may be of benefit to guide hemodynamic manipulation.
3. Although no evidence exists to document the benefit of corticosteroids in patients with AFE, the similar pathophysiologies proposed in the National Registry suggest that the administration of high doses of corticosteroids would be a consideration. In the absence of any data to suggest the benefit of this, however, such steroid treatment is not mandated by standard of care.
4. In patients suffering AFE with the fetus still in utero, careful attention must be paid to the fetal condition. In a mother who is hemodynamically unstable but has not

yet undergone cardiorespiratory arrest, maternal considerations must be weighed carefully against those of the fetus. The decision to subject such an unstable mother to a major abdominal operation (cesarean section) is a difficult one, and each case must be individualized. However, it is axiomatic in these situations that where a choice must be made, maternal well-being must take precedence over that of the fetus.
5. In mothers who have progressed to frank cardiac arrest, the situation is different. Under these circumstances, maternal survival is extremely unlikely, regardless of the therapy rendered. In such women, it is highly unlikely that the imposition of cesarean section would significantly alter the maternal outcome. Even properly performed cardiopulmonary resuscitation (difficult at best in a pregnant woman) provides only a maximum of 30% of normal cardiac output. Under these circumstances, it is fair to assume that the proportion of blood shunted to the uterus and other areas in the splanchnic bed approaches zero. Thus, the fetus will be, for practical purposes, anoxic at all times following maternal cardiac arrest, even during ideal performance of cardiopulmonary resuscitation. Because the interval from maternal arrest to delivery is directly correlated with newborn outcome, perimortum cesarean section should be initiated immediately on the diagnosis of maternal cardiac arrest in patients with AFE, assuming sufficient personnel are available to continue to provide care to the mother and deliver the baby (Katz, 1986; Clark, 1995). For the pregnant patient, the standard ABCs of cardiopulmonary resuscitation should be modified to include a fourth category, D: delivery.

Despite many advances in the understanding of this condition, AFE or anaphylactoid syndrome of pregnancy remains enigmatic and in most cases is associated with dismal maternal and fetal outcomes, regardless of the quality of care

---

## AMNIOTIC FLUID EMBOLISM

### I. *Goals of Therapy*

    A.  To maintain systolic BP $>90$ mm Hg, urine output $>25$ mL/hr, and arterial $po_2$ $>60$ mm Hg

    B.  To correct coagulation abnormalities

### II. *Management Protocol*

    A.  Initiate cardiopulmonary resuscitation if indicated.

    B.  Administer oxygen at high concentrations. If the patient is not breathing, she should be intubated and ventilated with 100% $Fio_2$.

    C.  Amniotic fluid embolism is often associated with and, in fact, may be heralded by fetal distress. Therefore, the fetal heart rate should be monitored carefully if gestational age is sufficient to warrant intervention for fetal distress.

    D.  Hypotension is usually secondary to cardiogenic shock. Treatment involves optimization of cardiac preload by rapid volume infusion. Subsequent dopamine infusion would be appropriate if the patient remains hypotensive.

    E.  Pulmonary artery catheterization may be helpful in guiding hemodynamic management.

    F.  After correction of hypotension, fluid therapy should be restricted to maintenance levels to minimize pulmonary edema due to developing acute respiratory distress syndrome. Hemodynamic assessment with the pulmonary artery catheter may be of tremendous value in judging appropriate fluid therapy.

    G.  Administer fresh whole blood or packed RBCs and fresh-frozen plasma to treat bleeding secondary to disseminated intravascular coagulation. Such component replacement is often successful.

    H.  Consider hydrocortisone 500 mg IV every 6 hours (two doses).

### III. *Critical Laboratory Tests*

    A.  Arterial blood gas, complete blood count, platelet count, fibrinogen, fibrin split products, prothrombin time, and partial thromboplastin time.

### IV. *Consultation*

    A.  Pulmonary medicine, hematology

---

rendered. Thus, AFE remains unpredictable, unpreventable, and, for the most part, untreatable. It is anticipated that the new directions in pathophysiology suggested by the analysis of the registry data may allow future advances in the treatment of this condition.

**REFERENCES**

Adamsons K, Mueller-Heubach E, Myer RE. The innocuousness of amniotic fluid infusion in the pregnant rhesus monkey. Am J Obstet Gynecol 1971;109:977.

American College of Obstetricians and Gynecologists. Prologue. Amniotic fluid embolism syndrome. In: Obstetrics. 3rd ed. Washington, DC: American College of Obstetricians and Gynecologists, 1993:94–95.

Attwood HD, Downing SE. Experimental amniotic fluid embolism. Surg Gynecol Obstet 1965;120:255.

Azegami M, Mori N. Amniotic fluid embolism and leukotrienes. Am J Obstet Gynecol 1986;155:1119–1123.

Beller FK, Douglas GW, Debrovner CH, et al. The fibrinolytic system in amniotic fluid embolism. Am J Obstet Gynecol 1963;87:48.

Clark SL, Montz FJ, Phelan JP. Hemodynamic alterations in amniotic fluid embolism: a reappraisal. Am J Obstet Gynecol 1985a;151:617.

Clark SL. Arachidonic acid metabolites and the pathophysiology of amniotic fluid embolism. Semin Reprod Endocrinol 1985b;3:253.

Clark SL, Pavlova Z, Horenstein J, et al. Squamous cells in the maternal pulmonary circulation. Am J Obstet Gynecol 1986;154:104–106.

Clark SL, Cotton DB, Gonik B, et al. Central hemodynamic alterations in amniotic fluid embolism. Am J Obstet Gynecol 1988;158:1124–1126.

Clark SL. New concepts of amniotic fluid embolism: a review. Obstet Gynecol Surv 1990;45:360–368.

Clark SL, Hankins GDV, Dudley DA, et al. Amniotic fluid embolism: analysis of a national registry. Am J Obstet Gynecol 1995;172:1158–1169.

Covone AE, Johnson PM, Mutton D, et al. Trophoblast cells in peripheral blood from pregnant women. Lancet 1984;1:841.

Cromley MG, Taylor PJ, Cummings DC. Probable amniotic fluid embolism after first trimester pregnancy termination. J Reprod Med 1983;28:209–210.

Cron RS, Kilkenny GS, Wirthwein C, et al. Amniotic fluid embolism. Am J Obstet Gynecol 1952;64:1360.

Courtney LD. Coagulation failure in pregnancy. Br Med J 1970;1:691.

Courtney LD, Allington LM. Effect of amniotic fluid on blood coagulation. Br J Haematol 1972;113:911.

Dutta D, Bhargava KC, Chakravarti RN, et al. Therapeutic studies in experimental amniotic fluid embolism in rabbits. Am J Obstet Gynecol 1970;106:1201.

Eastman NJ. Editorial comment. Obstet Gynecol Surv 1948;3:35.

Enjeti S, Bleecker ER, Smith PL, et al. Hemodynamic mechanisms in anaphylaxis. Circ Shock 1983;11:297–307.

Girard P, Mal H, Laine JF, et al. Left heart failure in amniotic fluid embolism. Anesthesiology 1986;64:262.

Gitin TA, Seidel T, Cera PJ, et al. Pulmonary microvascular fat: the significance? Crit Care Med 1993;21:664.

Grimes DA. The morbidity and mortality of pregnancy: still a risky business. Am J Obstet Gynecol 1994;170:1489.

Guidotti RJ, Grimes DA, Cates W. Fatal amniotic fluid embolism during legally induced abortion in the United States, 1972–1978. Am J Obstet Gynecol 1981;141:257–348.

Halmagyi DFJ, Starzecki B, Shearman RP. Experimental amniotic fluid embolism: mechanism and treatment. Am J Obstet Gynecol 1962;84:251.

Hankins GDV, Snyder RR, Clark SL, et al. Acute hemodynamic and respiratory effects of amniotic fluid embolism in the pregnant goat model. Am J Obstet Gynecol 1993;168:1113–1129.

Hogberg U, Innala E, Sandstrom A. Maternal mortality in Sweden, 1980–1988. Obstet Gynecol 1994;84:240.

Jacques WE, Hampton JW, Bird RM, et al. Pulmonary hypertension and plasma thromboplastin antecedent deficiency in dogs. Arch Pathol 1960;69:248.

Kapin MA, Ferguson JL. Hemodynamic and regional circulatory alterations in dog during anaphylactic challenge. Am J Physiol 1985;249:H430–H437.

Katz VJ, Dotters DJ, Droegemueller W. Perimortem cesarean delivery. Obstet Gynecol 1986;68:571–576.

Kaunitz AM, Hughes JM, Grimes DA. Causes of maternal mortality in the United States. Obstet Gynecol 1985;65:605.

Kitzmiller JL, Lucas WE. Studies on a model of amniotic fluid embolism. Obstet Gynecol 1972;39:626.

Lee W, Ginsburg KA, Cotton DB, Kaufman RH. Squamous and trophoblastic cells in the maternal pulmonary circulation identified by invasive hemodynamic monitoring during the peripartum period. Am J Obstet Gynecol 1986;155:999–1001.

Lee WP, Clark SL, Cotton DB, et al. Septic shock during pregnancy. Am J Obstet Gynecol 1988;159:410–416.

Liban E, Raz S. A clinicopathologic study of fourteen cases of amniotic fluid embolism. Am J Clin Pathol 1969;51:477–481.

Lockwood CJ, Bach R, Guha A, et al. Amniotic fluid contains tissue factor, a potent initiator of coagulation. Am J Obstet Gynecol 1991;165:1335–1341.

MacMillan D. Experimental amniotic fluid embolism. J Obstet Gynaecol Br Comwlth 1968;75:8.

Meier PR, Bowes WA. Amniotic fluid embolus-like syndrome presenting in the second trimester of pregnancy. Obstet Gynecol 1983;61(suppl):31–33.

Meyer JR. Bras/Med 1926;2:301–303.

Morgan M. Amniotic fluid embolism. Anaesthesia 1979;34:29.

Parker CW. In: Clinical immunology. Philadelphia: WB Saunders, 1980:1208–1218.

Parrillo JE. Pathogenic mechanisms of septic shock. N Engl J Med 1993;328:1471–1477.

Paul RH, Koh BS, Bernstein SG. Changes in fetal heart rate: uterine contraction patterns associated with eclampsia. Am J Obstet Gynecol 1978;130:165–169.

Phillips LL, Davidson EC. Procoagulant properties of amniotic fluid. Am J Obstet Gynecol 1972;113:911.

Plauche WC. Amniotic fluid embolism. Am J Obstet Gynecol 1983;147:982–983.

Porter TF, Clark SL, Dildy GA, Hankins GDV. Isolated disseminated intravascular coagulation and amniotic fluid embolism. Society of Perinatal Obstetricians 16th Annual Meeting, Poster Presentation, Kona, Hawaii, January 1996.

Raper RF, Fisher MM. Profound reversible myocardial depression after anaphylaxis. Lancet 1988;1:386–388.

Ratnoff OD, Vosbugh GJ. Observations of the clotting defect in amniotic fluid embolism. N Engl J Med 1952;247:970.

Reeves JT, Daoud FS, Estridge M, et al. Pulmonary pressor effects of small amounts of bovine amniotic fluid. Respir Physiol 1974;20:231.

Reis RL, Pierce WS, Behrendt DM. Hemodynamic effects of amniotic fluid embolism. Surg Gynecol Obstet 1965;129:45.

Resnik R, Schwartz WH, Plumer MH, et al. Obstet Gynecol 1976;47:295.

Richards DS, Carter LS, Corke B, et al. The effect of human amniotic fluid on the isolated perfused rat heart. Am J Obstet Gynecol 1988;158:210.

Schneider CL. Coagulation defects in obstetric shock: meconium embolism and defibrination. Am J Obstet Gynecol 1955;69:748.

Silverman HJ, Van Hook C, Haponik EF. Hemodynamic changes in human anaphylaxis. Am J Med 1984;77:341–344.

Smedegard G, Revenas B, Lundberg C, Arfors KE. Anaphylactic shock in monkeys passively sensitized with human reaginic serum. I. Hemodynamics and cardiac performances. Acta Physiol Scand 1981;111:239–247.

Smith PL, Kagey-Sobotka A, Bleecker ER, et al. Physiologic manifestations of human anaphylaxis. J Clin Invest 1980;66:1072–1080.

Sparr RA, Pritchard JA. Studies to detect the escape of amniotic fluid into the maternal circulation during parturition. Surg Gynecol Obstet 1958;107:550–564.

Spence MR, Mason KG. Experimental amniotic fluid embolism in rabbits. Am J Obstet Gynecol 1974;119:1073.

Steiner PE, Luschbaugh CC. Maternal pulmonary embolism by amniotic fluid. JAMA 1941;117:1245–1253.

Stolte L, van Kessel H, Seelen J, et al. Failure to produce the syndrome of amniotic fluid embolism by infusion of amniotic fluid and meconium into monkeys. Am J Obstet Gynecol 1967;98:694.

Thompson WB, Budd JW. Erroneous diagnosis of amniotic fluid embolism. Am J Obstet Gynecol 1963;91:606–617.

Towell ME. Fetal acid-base physiology and intrauterine asphyxia. In: Goodwin JW, Godden JO, Chance GW, eds. Perinatal medicine. Baltimore: Williams and Wilkins, 1976:200.

Wong S, Dykewicz MS, Patterson R. Idiopathic anaphylaxis—a clinical summary of 175 patients. Arch Intern Med 1990;150:1323–1328.

# CHAPTER *21*

# Hypovolemic Shock

*D*espite the availability of modern blood-banking techniques, hemorrhage remains one of the leading causes of maternal death both in affluent Western nations and poorer countries (Fig 21-1) (Koonin, 1991; Hogberg, 1994; Ayhan, 1994; Kochanek, 1995; Varner, 1997). Between 1987 and 1990, hemorrhage was the leading cause of maternal death in the United States (Berg, 1996). Most of these deaths were due to ectopic pregnancy. Hypovolemic shock is also responsible for a number of serious nonfatal complications, including acute tubular necrosis (see Chapter 16), acute respiratory distress syndrome (ARDS) (see Chapter 18), and, more rarely, postpartum pituitary necrosis. The pregnant woman undergoes important physiologic alterations in preparation for blood loss at the time of parturition; however, complications unique to the pregnant state can lead to blood loss exceeding that anticipated and can quickly result in shock. The obstetric health-care provider must be prepared to act swiftly and decisively in managing hypovolemic shock resulting from obstetric hemorrhage.

## Shock in Pregnancy

*Shock* is perhaps best defined as reduced tissue oxygenation resulting from poor perfusion (Shoemaker, 1995). A common factor in all types of shock syndrome is a reduction in cellular oxygen consumption. Such oxygen deficits are commonly due to either reduced or uneven blood flow. In hemorrhagic shock, the disparity is a result of blood loss that leads to both compensatory neurohormonal activation as well as the release of various endogenous mediators, which may aggravate the primary physiologic effects of hypovolemia (Pullicino, 1990; Abraham, 1991; Hoch, 1993). These processes, if not corrected, lead rapidly to hypotension, decreased tissue perfusion, cellular hypoxia, organ damage, and death.

Blood flow to the capillary beds of various organs is controlled by arterioles, resistance vessels that in turn are controlled by the CNS. On the other hand, 70% of the total blood volume is contained in venules, capacitance vessels controlled by humoral factors. Hypovolemic shock evolves through several pathophysiologic stages as body mechanisms combat the acute blood volume loss.

Early in the course of massive hemorrhage, there are decreases in mean arterial pressure (MAP), cardiac output (CO), central venous pressure (CVP) and pulmonary capillary wedge pressure (PCWP), stroke volume and work, mixed venous oxygen saturation, and oxygen consumption. Increases are seen in systemic vascular resistance (SVR) and arteriovenous oxygen content differences. These latter changes serve to improve tissue oxygenation when blood flow is reduced (Bassin, 1971). Catecholamine release also causes a generalized increase in venular tone, resulting in an autotransfusion from the capacitance reservoir. These changes are accompanied by

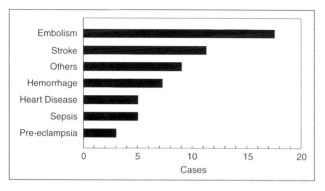

F I G U R E  **21-1**

**Causes of maternal mortality in Sweden, 1980–1988, according to cause of death (n = 58).** (Reprinted with permission from the American College of Obstetricians and Gynecologists [Obstetrics and Gynecology, 1994, vol. 84, page 240].)

compensatory increases in heart rate, SVR and pulmonary vascular resistance, and myocardial contractility. Nonsurvivors tend to have greater initial reduction in MAP, CO, oxygen delivery ($Do_2$), and oxygen consumption ($Vo_2$) with the initial hemorrhage, and less complete return of these factors to normal within the first 24 hours after resuscitation (Bishop, 1991, 1993). In addition, redistribution of CO and blood volume occurs via selective arteriolar constriction mediated by the CNS. This results in diminished perfusion to the kidneys, gut, skin, and uterus, with relative maintenance of blood flow to the heart, brain, and adrenal glands. In the pregnant patient, such redistribution may result in fetal hypoxia and distress, even before the mother becomes overtly hypotensive; in such situations, the uterus has, from a teleologic viewpoint, become relatively unimportant. Regardless of the absolute maternal BP, significant maternal shock is highly unlikely in the absence of fetal distress (Clark, 1990).

Although initial oxygen extraction by maternal tissue is increased, continued maldistribution of blood flow results in local tissue hypoxia and metabolic acidosis. If not corrected promptly, such shunting of blood from the renal and splanchnic beds may result in acute tubular necrosis and contribute to pulmonary capillary endothelial damage and ARDS, even if resusci-

tation is eventually successful. As the blood volume deficit approaches 25%, such compensatory mechanisms become inadequate to maintain CO and arterial pressure. At this point, small additional losses of blood result in rapid clinical deterioration, producing a vicious cycle of cellular death and vasoconstriction, leading to organ ischemia, loss of capillary membrane integrity, and additional loss of intravascular fluid volume into the extravascular space (Shoemaker, 1973; Slater, 1973).

Increased platelet aggregation also is found in hypovolemic shock. Aggregated platelets release vasoactive substances; the vasoactive substance release causes small vessel occlusion and impaired microcirculatory perfusion. These platelet aggregates can embolize to the lungs and be a factor contributing to respiratory failure, which is seen often following prolonged shock.

## Physiologic Changes in Preparation for Pregnancy Blood Loss

The pregnant woman undergoes profound physiologic changes to prepare for the blood loss that will occur at the time of parturition. By the end of the second trimester of pregnancy, the maternal blood volume has increased by 1000 to 2000 mL (Pritchard, 1965). The maternal CO increases by 40% to 45% while total peripheral resistance decreases (Clark, 1989). This decreased peripheral resistance results from hormonal factors (progesterone, prostaglandin metabolites, or other factors) that decrease overall vasomotor tone as well as the development of a low-resistance arteriovenous shunt of the placenta. The decreased peripheral resistance is maximal in the second trimester. About 20% to 25% of the maternal CO goes to the placental shunt to yield a blood flow there of 500 mL per minute. Placental blood flow is directly proportional to the uterine perfusion pressure, which in turn is proportional to systemic BP. Any decrease in maternal CO results in a proportionate decrease in placental perfusion. The uterine arterioles are very sensitive to exogenous vasopressor substances (Greiss, 1966), but, because of an incompletely understood pregnancy-related stimulus of the renin-angiotensin system, the vasopressor effect of the elevated angiotensin levels appears to be blunted during pregnancy.

Thus, during her pregnancy, the mother has been prepared for a blood volume loss of up to 1000 mL. Following a normal spontaneous vaginal delivery, a first-day postpartum hematocrit usually is not altered significantly from the admission hematocrit. In the past, the usual estimated blood loss at delivery has often been underestimated. Actual measurements show that the average blood loss after normal spontaneous vaginal delivery is over 600 mL. With a postpartum blood loss of less than 1000 mL, the parturient's vital signs may not reflect acute blood loss (i.e., hypotension and tachycardia).

During the antepartum period, the obstetrician must be concerned with both of the patients. Fetal oxygenation decreases in proportion to the decrease in maternal CO. The catecholamine output from the mother's adrenal medulla may preferentially increase arteriolar resistance of the spiral arterioles of the placental bed, thus further decreasing fetal oxygenation. Under such circumstances, the fetus may be in jeopardy, even though compensatory mechanisms maintain stable maternal vital signs. Thus, even in the absence of overt hypotension, for the well-being of the fetus, the health-care team must act quickly to expand the intravascular volume of an antepartum patient who has lost blood.

Although all vital organs receive increased blood flow during pregnancy, three (other than the placenta) are particularly susceptible to damage when perfusion pressure decreases as a result of hemorrhagic shock. These organs are the anterior pituitary gland, the kidneys, and the lungs. During pregnancy, the anterior pituitary enlarges and receives an increased blood flow. Under the condition of shock, blood flow is shunted away from the anterior pituitary gland, which may undergo ischemic necrosis. Sheehan and Murdoch first described the syndrome of hypopituitarism secondary to postpartum hypotension as result of hemorrhage (Sheehan, 1938). This condition is now a rare complication in modern obstetrics. The clinical presentation can vary, but secondary amenorrhea resulting from loss of pituitary gonadotrophs is usually present. In severe cases, thyrotropic and adrenotropic pituitary

hormones also may be deficient. The diagnosis of atypical or partial deficiency syndromes of these hormones requires a high index of suspicion.

Hypovolemia from any cause leads to reduced renal perfusion, which can result in acute tubular necrosis. In one older series, hemorrhage and hypovolemia were precipitating factors in 75% of obstetric patients with acute renal failure (Smith, 1968). Prompt blood and fluid replacement is essential, because such sequelae are to be avoided. Lung injury resulting from hypovolemic shock is discussed in detail in Chapter 18. In the nonpregnant state, a critical cardiac output exists below which oxygen extraction becomes impaired. Evans (1996) presented evidence that in the pregnant sheep model, such a critical cardiac output does not exist.

## Causes of Obstetric Hemorrhage

Any disruption in the integrity of the maternal vascular system during pregnancy has the potential for devastating blood loss. In the first half of gestation, ectopic pregnancy is the leading cause of life-threatening obstetric hemorrhage (Koonin, 1991). Beyond the first trimester, antepartum obstetric hemorrhage usually results from a disruption of the placental attachment site (involving either a normally implanted placenta or placenta previa) or uterine rupture (spontaneous or trauma related). During the intrapartum period, the likelihood of clinical shock is enhanced in patients with pregnancy-induced hypertension. Because of the intravascular volume depletion associated with this condition, even the usual blood loss associated with delivery may result in clinical instability. Another pathophysiologic change often associated with pregnancy-induced hypertension is thrombocytopenia, which when severe, may contribute to postpartum blood loss (see Chapter 14).

Most serious obstetric hemorrhage occurs in the postpartum period. The most common cause is uterine atony following placental separation. Under normal conditions, shortening myometrial fibers act as physiologic ligatures around the arterioles of the placental bed. Thus, uterine atony results in arterial hemorrhage. Factors that predispose a patient to uterine atony include either precipitous or prolonged labor, oxytocin augmentation, magnesium sulfate infusion, chorioamnionitis, enlarged uterus resulting from increased intrauterine contents, and operative deliveries (Clark, 1984; Naef, 1994). Obstetric trauma is another common cause of postpartum hemorrhage. Cervical and vaginal lacerations are more common with midpelvic operative deliveries and as a consequence of an extension of a uterine incision for cesarean birth. Other causes of postpartum hemorrhage include uterine inversion, placenta accreta, amniotic fluid embolism, retroperitoneal bleeding from either birth trauma or episiotomy, and coagulopathies of various causes (Clark, 1990; Zelop, 1993; Naef, 1994) (Table 21-1).

## Management of Hypovolemic Shock in Pregnancy

Perhaps the most important aspect of treating shock of any etiology is to recognize that physiologic manifestations such as hypotension and oliguria are *secondary* problems; all too often they are approached by the administration of vasopressors or diuretics, which, while effecting a temporary improvement in vital signs and urine output, may actually aggravate the underlying physiologic derangements and hasten the development of secondary organ damage and death. It also must be emphasized that in the initial resuscitation of the patient in hypovolemic shock, time is of the essence in restoring hemodynamic and oxygenation parameters to normal if survival is to be optimized (Bishop, 1991, 1993; Shoemaker, 1995).

T A B L E  **21-1**

Common causes of obstetric hemorrhage

| Antepartum and Intrapartum | Postpartum |
| --- | --- |
| Placental abruption | Retained placenta |
| Uterine rupture | Uterine atony |
| Placenta previa | Uterine rupture |
| | Genital tract trauma |
| | Coagulopathy |

## Oxygenation

The most frequent cause of death of a patient in shock is inadequate respiratory exchange leading to multiple organ failure (Shoemaker, 1992). The duration of relative tissue hypoxia is important in the accumulation of by-products of anaerobic metabolism. Thus, increasing the partial pressure of oxygen across the pulmonary capillary membrane by giving 8 to 10 liters of oxygen per minute by tight-fitting mask may forestall the onset of tissue hypoxia and is a logical first priority. Also, in a pregnant patient, increasing the partial pressure of oxygen in maternal blood will increase the amount of oxygen carried to fetal tissue (Dildy, 1995). If the airway is not patent or the tidal volume is inadequate, the clinician should not hesitate to perform endotracheal intubation and institute positive-pressure ventilation to achieve adequate oxygenation. In patients who do not respond promptly to simple resuscitative measures, assessment of $Do_2$ and $Vo_2$ and aggressive efforts to restore these values to normal or supranormal are essential. A therapeutic goal of achieving $Do_2$ greater than 800 mL/mm.m$^2$ and $Vo_2$ greater than 180 mL/mm.m$^2$ has been suggested in the nonpregnant patient (Shoemaker, 1988a). Two prospective, randomized trials, however, found no benefit to normalization of $Svo_2$, or to supraphysiologic goals of hemodynamic manipulation (Hays, 1994; Gattinoni, 1995).

## Volume Replacement

Protracted shock appears to cause secondary changes in the microcirculation; these changes affect circulating blood volume. In early shock, there is a tendency to draw fluid from the interstitial space and into the capillary bed. As the shock state progresses, however, damage to the capillary endothelium occurs and is manifested by an increase in capillary permeability, which further accentuates the loss of intravascular volume. This deficit is reflected clinically by the disproportionately large volume of fluid necessary to resuscitate patients in severe shock; sometimes, the amount of fluid required for resuscitation is twice the amount indicated by calculation of blood loss volume. Prolonged hemorrhagic shock also alters active transport of ions at the cellular level, and intracellular water decreases. Thus, replacement of intracellular fluid with crystalloid or colloid solutions may be considered the primary therapeutic goal.

The two most common crystalloid fluids used for resuscitation are 0.9% sodium chloride and lactated Ringer's solution. Both have equal plasma volume–expanding effects. The large volumes of crystalloids required can diminish markedly the colloid osmotic pressure (Fig 21-2). Because albumin is integral to the maintenance of plasma colloid oncotic pressure (COP), a 5% or 25% albumin solution also can be used to resuscitate patients with acute hypovolemia. The intravascular effect of infused albumin lasts approximately 24 hours, much longer than that of infused crystalloids (Hauser, 1980). For a given infusion volume, colloids expand the plasma to a greater extent than do crystalloids. A randomized prospective clinical trial comparing 5% albumin, 5% hetastarch, and 0.9% saline for resuscitation of patients in hypovolemic or septic shock found that 2 to 4 times the volume of saline, compared with that of the albumin or hetastarch, was re-

FIGURE **21-2**

**Relationship between serum albumin and colloid oncotic pressure. The regression equation is calculated as follows: Colloid oncotic pressure (mm Hg) = 8.1 (serum albumin [g/dL]) − 8.2.** (Reprinted with permission from the American College of Obstetricians and Gynecologists [Obstetrics and Gynecology, 1986, vol. 68, page 807].)

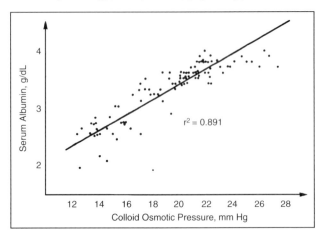

quired to reach the same hemodynamic endpoint and that saline decreased the COP by 34% (Rackow, 1983). Albumin and the hetastarch significantly increased the COP compared with baseline throughout the study period. In one report, only 20% of crystalloids remains in the intravascular space after 1 hour, and by 2 hours, virtually all of the infused fluid is interstitial (Shoemaker, 1991). In studies including critically ill patients, 500 mL of 5% albumin persisted in the intravascular space for approximately 4 hours, compared with 5 to 6 hours for a similar volume of hetastarch and 40 minutes for crystalloid (Hauser, 1980; Appel, 1981). Fluid resuscitation in young, previously healthy patients can be accomplished safely with modest volumes of either colloid or crystalloid fluid and with little risk of pulmonary edema. The enormous volumes of crystalloids necessary to adequately resuscitate profound hypovolemic shock, however, will reduce the gradient between the COP and the PCWP and may contribute to the pathogenesis of pulmonary edema (Harms, 1981). This concept, however, remains unproven in actual clinical practice, and the use of crystalloid versus colloid solutions for initial resuscitation of patients in hypovolemic shock remains controversial. The clinician must understand the effects and potential risk of such fluid therapy and must choose either or both for rapid repletion of intravascular volume and restoration of hemodynamic stability (Carey, 1970).

Modern blood transfusion practice emphasizes the use of cell components rather than whole blood (see Chapter 11). Red blood cells are administered to improve oxygen delivery in patients with decreased red-cell mass resulting in hemorrhage. A National Institutes of Health (NIH) consensus conference concluded that transfusion of fresh-frozen plasma (FFP) was inappropriate for volume replacement or as a nutritional supplement (Consensus Conference, 1985). In the past, up to 90% of FFP use was for volume replacement. The other 10% was for the following conditions approved by the NIH consensus conference: replacement of isolated coagulation factor deficiencies, reversal of coumarin effect, antithrombin III deficiency, immunodeficiency syndromes, and treatment of thrombotic thrombocytopenic purpura. The current concern for excessive use of FFP is at least threefold. First, the current importance of cost containment has caused blood banks to reevaluate use of blood products and the time involved in their preparation. Second, the routine use of FFP compromises the availability of raw material for preparation of factor VIII concentrates for hemophiliacs. Third, with regard to recipient safety, the risk of FFP includes disease transmission, anaphylactoid reactions, alloimmunization, and excessive intravascular volume (Oberman, 1985) (see Chapter 11).

*Massive blood replacement* is defined as transfusion of at least one total blood volume within 24 hours. The NIH consensus conference report noted that pathologic hemorrhage in the patient receiving massive transfusions is caused more frequently by thrombocytopenia than by depletion of coagulation factors. This finding was demonstrated in a prospective study of 27 massively transfused patients in whom levels of factors V, VII, and IX and fibrinogen could not be correlated with the number of units of whole blood transfused (Counts, 1979). A study of combat casualties suggested the thrombocytopenia was more important than depletion of coagulation factors as cause of bleeding in massively transfused patients (Miller, 1971). In this report, restoration of the prothrombin times (PT) and partial thromboplastin times (PTT) to normal with FFP had little effect on abnormal bleeding; however, platelet transfusions were effective. There is no evidence that routine administration of FFP per a given number of units of RBCs decreases transfusion requirements in patients who are receiving multiple transfusion and who do not have documented coagulation defects (Mannucci, 1982). Thus, during massive blood replacement, correction of specific coagulation defects (fibrinogen levels < 100 dL) and thrombocytopenia (< 30,000/mL) will minimize further transfusion requirements. In acute hemorrhagic shock, CVP or PCWP are accurate reflectors of intravascular volume status and may be useful in guiding fluid therapy. In the critically ill patient, however, CVP may be a less reliable indicator of volume status due to compliance changes in vein walls (Shippy, 1984). Fortunately, in obstetrics, rapid recovery is the rule following prompt and adequate resuscitative measures, and such considerations are of less practical importance.

## Pharmacologic Agents

During the antepartum and intrapartum periods, only correction of maternal hypovolemia will maintain placental perfusion and prevent fetal compromise. Although vasopressors may temporarily correct hypotension, they do so at the expense of uteroplacental perfusion. Thus, vasopressors are not used in the treatment of obstetric hemorrhagic shock except as a last resort, because the uterine spiral arterioles are especially sensitive to these agents. In situations of acute circulatory failure, inotropic drugs such as dopamine may have a beneficial effect on hemodynamic function. Dopamine, however, has been demonstrated to decrease uterine blood flow in healthy and hypotensive pregnant sheep (Callender 1978; Rolbin, 1979) (Fig 21-3). In hypovolemic shock, vasopressors or inotropic agents are rarely indicated and should never be given until intravascular preload (PCWP) has been optimized. When given in equivalent doses to patients in shock, the vasopressor dopamine results in greater increases in MAP and PCWP. However, cardiac index, $Vo_2$, and $Do_2$ are improved to a much greater extent with dobutamine (Fig 21-4). For this reason, the latter agent is preferred by some critical care specialists (Shoemaker, 1988b).

F I G U R E **21-3**

**Uterine artery response to vasopressors.** (Courtesy of Dr. Renee Bobrowski.)

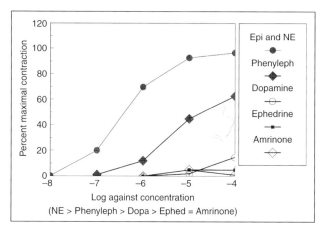

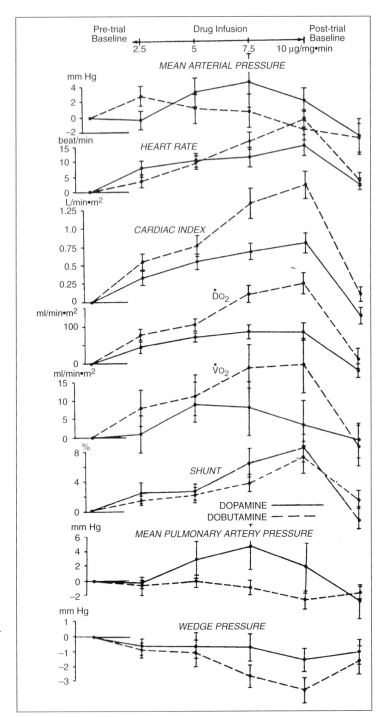

FIGURE **21-4**

Hemodynamic and oxygen transport effects of dobutamine (dashed line) and dopamine (solid line) in high-risk postoperative patients. (Reproduced by permission from Shoemaker WC. Diagnosis and treatment of the shock syndrome. In: Ayers SM, Grenvik A, Holbrook PR, Shoemaker WC, eds. Textbook of critical care. Philadelphia: WB Saunders, 1995.)

---

**HYPOVOLEMIC SHOCK**

**I. *Goals of Therapy***

    A.  Maintain the following:
        1.  Systolic pressure $\geq$ 90 mm Hg
        2.  Urine output $\geq$ 0.5 mL/kg/hr
        3.  Normal mental status
    B.  Eliminate the source of hemorrhage.
    C.  Avoid overzealous volume replacement that may contribute to pulmonary edema.

**II. *Management Protocol***

    A.  Establish two large-bore intravenous lines.
    B.  Place patients in the Trendelenburg position.
    C.  Rapidly infuse 5% dextrose in lactated Ringer's solution while blood products are obtained.
    D.  Infuse fresh whole blood or packed RBCs, as available.
    E.  Infuse platelets and FFP only as indicated by documented deficiencies in platelets ( < 30,000/mL) or clotting parameters (fibrinogen, PT, PTT).
    F.  Search for and eliminate the source of hemorrhage.
    G.  Use invasive hemodynamic monitoring if patients fail to respond to clinically adequate volume replacement.

**III. *Critical Laboratory Tests***

    A.  Complete blood count, platelet count, fibrinogen, PT, PTT, and arterial blood gases.

---

## Further Evaluation

After the patient's oxygenation and expansion of intravascular volume have been accomplished and her condition is beginning to stabilize, it is essential for the health-care team to evaluate the patient's response to therapy, to diagnose the basic condition that resulted in circulatory shock, and to consider the fetal condition. Serial evaluation of vital signs, urine output, acid-base status, blood chemistry, and coagulation status aid in this assessment. In select cases, placement of a pulmonary artery catheter should be considered to assist in the assessment of cardiac function and oxygen transport variables. In general, however, such central hemodynamic monitoring is not necessary in simple hypovolemic shock.

Evaluation of the fetal cardiotocograph may indicate fetal distress; only after the maternal condition is stabilized, however, can the clinician consider delivery of a fetus in jeopardy. It is important to realize that as the maternal hypoxia, acidosis, and underperfusion of the uteroplacental unit are being corrected, the fetus may recover. Serial evaluation of the fetal status and in utero resuscitation are preferable to delivery of a depressed infant.

## Hemostasis

In certain situations, such as uterine rupture with intraperitoneal bleeding, definitive surgical therapy may need to be given before stabilization is achieved fully. With postpartum hemorrhage resulting from uterine atony that has not responded to the conventional methods of uterine compression and dilute intravenous oxytocin, the physician should consider intramyometrial or systemic injection of 15 methyl prostaglandin $F_{2a}$.

---

## POSTPARTUM HEMORRHAGE

I. *Management Protocol*
   *(To be undertaken simultaneously with management of hypovolemic shock)*

   A.  Examine the uterus to rule out atony.
   B.  Examine the vagina and cervix to rule out lacerations; repair if present.
   C.  Explore the uterus and perform curettage to rule out retained placenta.
   D.  For uterine atony:
      1.  Firm bimanual compression
      2.  Oxytocin infusion, 40 units in 1 liter of $D_5RL$
      3.  15-methyl prostaglandin $F_{2a}$, 0.25 to 0.50 mg intramuscularly; may be repeated
      4.  Methergine 0.2 mg IM, $PGE_1$ 200 mg, or $PGE_2$ 20 mg are second line drugs in appropriate patients
      5.  Bilateral uterine artery ligation
      6.  Bilateral hypogastric artery ligation (if patient is clinically stable and future childbearing is of great importance)
      7.  Hysterectomy

---

A 0.25- to 0.50-mg intramuscular or intramyometrial injection is used, and it may be repeated if necessary.

If hemorrhage persists, a careful exploration of the vagina, cervix, and uterus is performed. The clinician looks for retained products of conception or lacerations. For hemorrhage resulting from uterine atony that has failed to respond to the previously described conservative measures, as well as in cases of extensive placenta accreta or uterine rupture not amenable to simple closure, a total or subtotal hysterectomy can be performed, depending on the patient's clinical condition and her desire for future fertility. If the patient does desire future fertility and is clinically stable, uterine and, rarely, hypogastric artery ligation may be considered. Balloon occlusion and embolization of the internal iliac arteries have also been described in cases of placenta percreta (Dubois, 1997). These surgical techniques, as well as a more comprehensive discussion of techniques for achieving medical and surgical hemostasis in patients with postpartum bleeding have been described elsewhere (Hankins, 1995).

It should be emphasized that preventable surgical death in obstetrics often represents an error in judgment and a reluctance to proceed with laparotomy or hysterectomy, rather than deficiencies in knowledge or surgical technique. Proper management of serious hemorrhage requires crisp medical and surgical decision making as well as meticulous attention to the aforementioned principles of blood and volume replacement.

### REFERENCES

Abraham E. Physiologic stress and cellular ischemia. Crit Care Med 1991;19:613.

Appel PL, Shoemaker WC. Fluid therapy in adult respiratory failure. Crit Care Med 1981;9:862.

Ayhan A, Bilgin F, Tuncer ZS, et al. Trends in maternal mortality at a university hospital in Turkey. Int J Obstet Gynecol 1994;44:223.

Bassin R, Vladik B, Kim SI, et al. Comparison of hemodynamic responses of two experimental shock models with clinical hemorrhage. Surgery 1971;69:722.

Berg CJ, Atrash HK, Koonin LM, et al. Pregnancy-related mortality in the United States, 1987–1990. Obstet Gynecol 1996;88:161.

Bishop MH, Shoemaker WC, Fleming AW, et al. Relationship between ARDS, hemodynamics, fluid balance and pulmonary infiltration in critically ill surgical patients. Am Surg 1991;57:785.

Bishop MH, Shoemaker WC, Appel PL, et al. Influence of time and optimal circulatory resuscitation in high-risk trauma. Crit Care Med 1993; 221:56.

Callender K, Levinson G, Shnider SM, et al. Dopamine administration in the normotensive pregnant ewe. Obstet Gynecol 1978;51:586.

Carey JS, Scharschmidt BF, Culliford AF, et al. Hemodynamic effectiveness of colloid and electrolyte solutions for replacement of simulated operative blood loss. Surg Gynecol Obstet 1970; 131:679.

Clark SL, Cotton DB, Lee W, et al. Central hemodynamic assessment of normal term pregnancy. Am J Obstet Gynecol 1989;161:1439.

Clark SL. Shock in the pregnant patient. Semin Perinatol 1990;14:52.

Consensus Conference. Fresh frozen plasma. JAMA 1985;253:551.

Counts RB, Haisch C, Simon TL, et al. Hemostasis in massively transfused trauma patients. Ann Surg 1979;190:91.

Dildy GA, Clark SL, Loucks CA. Intrapartum fetal pulse oximetry: the effects of maternal hyperoxia on fetal arterial oxygen saturation. Am J Obstet Gynecol 1995;172:158.

Dubois J, Burel L, Brignon A, et al. Placenta percreta: Balloon occlusion and embolization of the internal iliac arteries to reduce intraoperative blood loss. Am J Obstet Gynecol 1997; 176:723.

Gattinoni L, Brazzi L, Pelosi P, et al. A trial of goal-oriented hemodynamic therapy in critically ill patients. N Engl J Med 1995;333:1025.

Hankins GDV, Clark SL, Cunningham FG, Gilstrap LC, eds. Operative obstetrics. East Norwalk, CT: Appleton & Lange, 1995.

Harms BA, Kramer GC, Bodai BI, et al. The effect of hypoproteinemia and pulmonary and soft tissue edema formation. Crit Care Med 1981;9:503.

Hauser CJ, Shoemaker WC, Turpin I, et al. Hemodynamic and oxygen transport responses to body water shifts produced by colloids and crystalloids in critically ill patients. Surg Gynecol Obstet 1980;150:811.

Hays MA, Timmins AC, Yau EHS, et al. Evaluation of systemic oxygen delivery in the treatment of critically ill patients. N Engl J Med 1994; 330:1717.

Hoch RC, Rodriquez R, Manning T, et al. Effects of accidental trauma on cytokine and endotoxin production. Crit Care Med 1993;21:839.

Hogberg U, Innala E, Sandstrom A. Maternal mortality in Sweden, 1980–1988. Obstet Gynecol 1994; 84:240.

Kochanek KD, Hudson BL. Advance report of final mortality statistics, 1992. Monthly Vital Stat Rep 1995;43(suppl)6.

Koonin LM, Atrash HK, Lawson HW, et al. Maternal mortality surveillance, United States 1979–1986. MMWR 1991;40:551.

Mannucci PM, Federici AB, Sirchia G. Hemostasis testing during massive blood replacement: a study of 172 cases. Vox Sang 1982;42:113.

Miller RD, Robbins TO, Tong MJ, et al. Coagulation defects associated with massive blood transfusions. Ann Surg 1971;174:794.

Naef RW, Chauhan SP, Chevalier SP, et al. Prediction of hemorrhage at cesarean delivery. Obstet Gynecol 1994;83:923.

Nguyen HN, Clark SL, Greenspoon J, et al. Peripartum colloid osmotic pressure: correlation with serum proteins. Obstet Gynecol 1986;68:807.

Oberman HA. Uses and abuses of fresh frozen plasma. In: Garrity A, ed. Current concepts in transfusion therapy. Arlington, VA: American Association of Blood Banks, 1985.

Pritchard JA. Changes in the blood volume during pregnancy and delivery. Anesthesiology 1965; 26:393.

Pullicino EA, Carli F, Poole S, et al. The relationship between circulating concentrations of interleukin-6, tumor necrosis factor, and the acute phase response to elective surgery and accidental injury. Lymphokine Res 1990;9:231.

Rackow EC, Falk JL, Fein IA. Fluid resuscitation in circulatory shock: a comparison of the cardiorespiratory effects of albumin, hetastarch and saline solutions in patients with hypovolemic and septic shock. Crit Care Med 1983;11:839.

Rolbin SH, Levinson G, Shnider SM, et al. Dopamine treatment of spinal hypotension decreases uterine blood flow in pregnant ewes. Anesthesiology 1979;31:36.

Sheehan HL, Murdoch R. Postpartum necrosis of the anterior pituitary: pathologic and clinical aspects. Br J Obstet Gynaecol 1938;45:456.

Shippy CR, Appel PL, Shoemaker WC. Reliability of clinical monitoring to assess blood volume in critically ill patients. Crit Care Med 1984;12:107.

Shoemaker WC. Diagnosis and treatment of the shock syndromes. In: Ayers SM, Grenvik A, Holbrook PR, Shoemaker WC, eds. Textbook of critical care, 3rd ed. Philadelphia: WB Saunders, 1995.

Shoemaker WC. Pathophysiologic basis for therapy for shock and trauma syndromes. Semin Drug Treat 1973;3:211.

Shoemaker WC, Kram HB. Comparison of the effects of crystalloids and colloids on hemodynamic oxygen transport, mortality and morbidity. In: Simmon RS, Udeko AJ, eds. Debates in General Surgery. Chicago: Year Book Medical, 1991.

Shoemaker WC, Appel PL, Kram HB, et al. Prospective trial of supranormal values of survivors as therapeutic goals in high risk surgical patients. Chest 1988a;94:1176.

Shoemaker WC, Appel PL, Kram HB. Comparison of dobutamine and dopamine in prospective crossover clinical trials in critically ill postoperative patients. Chest 1988b;96:120.

Shoemaker WC, Appel PL, Kram HB, et al. Role of oxygen debt in the development of organ failure, sepsis and death in high-risk surgical patients. Chest 1992;102:208.

Slater G, Vladek BA, Bassin R, et al. Sequential changes in the distribution of cardiac output in various stages of experimental hemorrhagic shock. Surgery 1973;73:714.

Smith K, Browne JCM, Shackman R, et al. Renal failure of obstetric origin. Br Med Bull 1968;24:49.

Varner MW, Jacob S, Bloebaum L. Maternal mortality in Utah, 1982–1994. Obstet Gynecol 1997 (in press).

Zelop CM, Harlow BL, Frigoletto FD, et al. Emergency peripartum hysterectomy. Am J Obstet Gynecol 1993;168:1443.

# CHAPTER 22

# Septic Shock

*S* *epsis* is a clinical syndrome that en- compasses a variety of host re- sponses to systemic infection. *Shock* is a morbid condition in which the functional intravascular volume adequately fills the patient's vascular bed, resulting in hypotension and inadequate tissue perfusion. If the course of this pathologic pro- cess is left unaltered, cellular hypoxia, organ dys- function, and death ensue (Bone, 1992a). *Septic shock* describes the constellation of clinical find- ings marked by alteration of the ability of the host to maintain vascular integrity and homeostasis, resulting in inadequate tissue oxygenation and circulatory failure, which results from the systemic inflammatory response to an infectious insult. The spectrum of host response ranges from simple sepsis to septic shock with multiple-organ sys- tem dysfunction and death.

Septic shock accounts for approximately 10% of admissions to noncoronary intensive care units (ICUs) and is the thirteenth leading cause of death in the United States. Its incidence appears to be increasing (CDCP, 1993). After correcting for the increased age of the population, the rate of sep- tic shock reported by the Centers for Disease Control (CDC) between 1979 and 1987 more than doubled. This increased rate of septic shock was observed regardless of age group or geographic area (Progress in Chronic Disease Progression, 1990). Despite optimal ICU care, the mortality rate from septic shock remains 40% to 50% in most series (Brun-Buisson, 1995). Although sep- tic shock remains an uncommon event in the

obstetric population, factors that contribute to the increased rate of sepsis in the general popu- lation are also more common in women of repro- ductive age. Additionally, because maternal mor- tality is so uncommon, sepsis will remain an important overall cause of maternal mortality (Gibbs, 1976).

## Systemic Inflammatory Response Syndrome

The systemic inflammatory response syndrome (SIRS) is a recently popularized method that de- scribes the general inflammatory response to a variety of insults. Its etiology is not limited to infection, because burns, trauma, and pancreati- tis can illicit a similar clinical picture. It is charac- terized by two or more of the following: (1) body temperature less than 36°C or more than 38°C, (2) pulse greater than 90 beats per minute, (3) tachypnea manifested as respiratory rate exceed- ing 20 per minute or $Paco_2$ less than 32 mm Hg, (4) leukocyte count less than 4000 μL, greater than 12,000/μL, or more than 10% immature forms in the differential count. When SIRS is the result of documented infection, it is termed *sepsis*.

*Severe sepsis* is diagnosed when SIRS is asso- ciated with organ dysfunction, hypoperfusion, or hypotension. Useful indicators of hypoperfusion include lactic acidosis, oliguria, or acute alter- ations in mental status. If abnormalities of BP and perfusion persist despite adequate fluid resuscitation, *septic shock* is present. Hypotension is not necessary for the diagnosis if the patient requires vasopressor support. Multiple-organ system dysfunction syndrome (MODS) is the terminal phase of this spectrum, represented by the progressive physiologic deterioration of interdependent organ systems such that homeostasis cannot be maintained without active intervention. Commonly affected organ systems include pulmonary and renal dysfunction with acute respiratory distress syndrome (ARDS) and acute renal failure, respectively (Bone, 1992a).

## Clinical Presentation

The observed clinical spectrum of sepsis represents increasing severity of the host response to infection rather than increasing severity of infection (Bone, 1991). Although various risk factors have been identified and scoring systems developed, no effective way to predict which patients will progress from bacteremia to septic shock and MODS has been identified (Bone, 1992b). This classification scheme has proven useful, however, in prognosticating the prevalence of infection as well as the risk of mortality. More severe inflammatory responses are accompanied by progressively greater mortality rates (Rangel-Frausto, 1995). Because experimentally infused endogenous inflammatory mediators such as interleukins 1 and 2 (IL-1, IL-2) and tumor necrosis factor-alpha (TFN-α) reproduce this syndrome, an exaggerated host inflammatory response is felt to be central to its pathophysiology (Tracey, 1987; Okusawa, 1988; Sculier, 1988).

The clinical manifestations of septic shock fall into three broad categories, which correlate with progressive physiologic derangement. *Early (warm) shock* is characterized by a hyperdynamic circulation and decreased systemic vascular resistance (SVR). The hallmark of *late (cold) shock* is abnormal perfusion and oxygenation secondary to regional (peripheral) vasoconstriction and myocardial dysfunction. *Secondary (irreversible) shock* is frequently a terminal condition associated with multiple-organ system dysfunction (Table 22-1). Each phase represents a continued downward progression in the course of this disease process.

T A B L E   **22-1**

## Presenting features of septic shock

*Early (Warm) Shock*
Altered mental status
Peripheral vasodilation (warm skin, flushing)
Tachypnea or shortness of breath
Tachycardia
Temperature instability
Hypotension
Increased cardiac output and decreased peripheral resistance

*Late (Cold) Shock*
Peripheral vasoconstriction (cool, clammy skin)
Oliguria
Cyanosis
ARDS
Decreased cardiac output and decreased peripheral resistance

*Secondary (Irreversible) Shock*
Obtundation
Anuria
Hypoglycemia
Disseminated intravascular coagulation
Decreased cardiac output and decreased peripheral resistance
Myocardial failure

In the early phase of septic shock, bacteremia is heralded typically by shaking chills, sudden rise in temperature, tachycardia, and warm extremities. Although the patient may appear ill, the diagnosis of septic shock may be elusive until hypotension is documented. In addition, patients may present initially with nonspecific complaints such as malaise, nausea, vomiting, and at times, profuse diarrhea. Abrupt alterations in mental status also may herald the onset of septic shock; these behavior alterations have been attributed to the reductions in cerebral blood flow. Tachypnea or dyspnea, may be present with minimal findings on physical examination. These findings may represent the endotoxin's direct effect on the respiratory center and may immediately precede the clinical development of ARDS.

Laboratory findings are quite variable during the early stages of septic shock. The WBC count may be depressed at first; soon afterward, a marked leukocytosis is usually evident. Although there is a transient increase in blood glucose level secondary to catecholamine release and tissue underutilization, hypoglycemia may prevail later when a reduction in gluconeogenesis occurs secondary to hepatic dysfunction. Early evidence of disseminated intravascular coagulation (DIC) may be represented by a decreased platelet count, decreased fibrinogen, elevated fibrin split products, and elevated thrombin time. Initial arterial blood gases may show a transient respiratory alkalosis secondary to tachypnea. These parameters later reflect an increasing metabolic acidosis, because tissue hypoxia and lactic acid levels increase.

Later clinical manifestations of untreated shock include cold extremities, oliguria, and peripheral cyanosis. As suggested previously, myocardial depression becomes a prominent feature of severe septic shock, with marked reductions in cardiac output and SVR (Parker, 1983). Overt evidence of prolonged cellular hypoxia and dysfunction include profound metabolic acidosis, electrolyte imbalances, and DIC. If these symptoms are left unabated, rapid progression to irreversible shock is the rule.

Progressive cardiac dysfunction features prominently in the clinical presentation of septic shock. Cardiac output and cardiac index (CI) are initially increased due to increased heart rate and the profound decreases in SVR. The increased cardiac output, however, is inadequate to meet the patient's metabolic needs. Both the left and right ventricles dilate, and the ejection fractions decrease (Porembka, 1993). The limitation in cardiac performance and ejection fraction is greater than that seen in equally ill nonseptic patients (Parker, 1984). Ventricular compliance is also affected, as evidenced by a decrease in the ability to increase contractility in response to increase in preload (Ognibene, 1988).

Parker and Parillo (1983) studied 20 patients in septic shock. By conventional criteria, 95% of the patients would have been classified as hyperdynamic, but 10 of the 20 had abnormally depressed ejection fractions. These alterations in ejection fraction were not accounted for by differences in preload, afterload, or positive end-expiratory pressure (PEEP). In the acute phase of septic shock, the ability to dilate the left ventricle to maintain cardiac output in the face of declining ejection fraction appears to represent an adap-

tive response that confers a survival advantage (Parker, 1984). Two subsets of patients have been identified based on response to volume loading: those who respond with ventricular dilation and those who respond with increased pulmonary capillary wedge pressure (PCWP) rather than an increased cardiac output (Parrillo, 1985a). Cardiac depression of similar magnitude and frequency has been reported in obstetric patients with septic shock managed with pulmonary artery (PA) catheters (Lee, 1988).

Extensive study in humans and animal models points to a circulating myocardial depressant factor rather than alterations in coronary flow or myocardial oxygenation as the etiology for myocardial dysfunction (Marksad, 1979). Alterations in ejection fraction observed with structural heart disease, in postinfarction patients, or in critically ill nonseptic patients are not associated with a similar circulating factor (Parrillo, 1985b). Endotoxin infusion in humans produces comparable left ventricular dilation and decreases in performance (Porembka, 1993), suggesting that endotoxin plays some role in stimulating the production of this myocardial depressant factor.

## Predisposing Factors in Obstetrics

Pregnancy is often considered an immunocompromised state, although little objective evidence exists comparing the ability of pregnant and nonpregnant individuals to process bacterial antigens and elicit an appropriate immune response. Pregnant women remain at risk for common medical and surgical illnesses such as pneumonia and appendicitis, as well as conditions unique to pregnancy, all of which may result in sepsis (Table 22-2). Although genital tract infections are common on an obstetric service (Balk, 1989; Duff, 1986; Gibbs, 1978), septic shock in this same population tends to be an uncommon event. When an obstetric patient has clinical evidence of local infection, the incidence of bacteremia is approximately 8% to 10% (Blanco, 1981; Ledger, 1975; Reimer, 1984; Monif, 1976; Bryan, 1984). Overall, rates of bacteremia of 7.5 per 1000 admissions to the obstetrics and gynecology services at two large teaching hospitals have been reported (Blanco,

T A B L E   22-2

Bacterial infections associated with septic shock
and found in the obstetric patient

| | Incidence (%) |
|---|---|
| Chorioamnionitis | 0.5–1.0 |
| Postpartum endometritis | |
|    Cesarean section | 0.5–85.0 |
|    Vaginal delivery | < 10 |
| Urinary tract infections | 1–4 |
| Pyelonephritis | 1–4 |
| Septic abortion | 1–2 |
| Necrotizing fasciitis<br>   (postoperative) | < 1 |
| Toxic shock syndrome | < 1 |

1981; Ledger, 1975). More striking is that patients with bacteremia rarely progress to develop more significant complications, such as septic shock. Ledger and colleagues (1975) identified only a 4% rate of shock in pregnant patients with bacteremia. This value agrees with that of other investigators, who have reported a 0% to 12% incidence of septic shock in bacteremic obstetric and gynecologic patients (Blanco, 1981; Ledger, 1975; Reimer, 1984; Monif, 1976; Bryan, 1984; Chow, 1974). Obstetric conditions that have been identified as predisposing to the development of septic shock are listed in Table 22-2 (Blanco, 1981; Cavanagh, 1982; Marione, 1980; Lowthian, 1980; Duff, 1984; Lloyd, 1983; Chow, 1984).

The physiologic changes that accompany pregnancy may place the gravida at greater risk for morbidity than her nonpregnant counterpart. Elevation of the diaphragm by the gravid uterus, delayed gastric emptying, and the emergent nature of many intubations in obstetrics dramatically increase the risk of aspiration pneumonitis. Although the pregnant patient has been previously identified as being at increased risk of pulmonary sequelae from systemic infection such as pyelonephritis, the pathophysiologic mechanisms have been known only for the past decade (Cunningham, 1987). Hemodynamic investigation in normal women using flow-directed PA catheters has quantified the physiologic alterations that place the patient at increased risk for pulmonary injury. Pregnancy decreases the gradient between colloid oncotic pressure and PCWP (Clark, 1989). This increases the propensity for pulmonary edema if pulmonary capillary permeability changes or the PCWP increases. In the critically ill, nonpregnant patient, decreases in the COP-PCWP gradient predict an increased propensity for pulmonary edema (Rackow, 1977, 1982; Weil, 1978a), and that gradient is already decreased by normal pregnancy. The intrapulmonary shunt fraction (QS/QT) is also increased (Hankins, 1996), which may increase the risk of pulmonary morbidity.

Fortunately, mortality from septic shock, which is extremely high in the face of bacteremia in other medical and surgical specialties, tends to be an infrequent event in obstetrics and gynecology. The incidence of death from sepsis is estimated at 0% to 3% in obstetric patients, as compared with 10% to 81% in nonobstetric patients (Blanco, 1981; Ledger, 1975; Cavanagh, 1982; Wernstein, 1983). Suggested reasons for these more favorable outcomes in the parturient include (1) younger age group, (2) transient nature of the bacteremia, (3) type of organisms involved, (4) primary site of infection (pelvis) more amenable to both surgical and medical intervention, and (5) lack of associated medical diseases that could adversely impact the prognosis for recovery. This fifth factor is supported by Fried and Vosti (1968), who reported increased mortality in patients with underlying disease in addition to sepsis.

## Pathophysiology of Septic Shock

The clinical manifestations of septic shock can be categorized as either systemic responses, including tachycardia, tachypnea, and hypotension, or end-organ dysfunction, such as ARDS and acute renal failure (Parrillo, 1993). The severity of the clinical presentation is felt to be determined by the vigor of the host inflammatory response rather than the virulence of the inciting infection (Lynn, 1995). Once septic shock is established, the physiologic derangements induced by systemic activation of inflammatory mediators are more important than the microbial milieu in prognosticating outcome. In those patients who succumb, death is predominantly a function of the host response to the initiating insult (Brun-Buisson, 1995).

For the most part, gram-negative sepsis has been the model used to study this phenomenon in experimental animals. Endotoxin, a complex lipopolysaccharide present in the cell wall of aerobic gram-negative bacteria, appears to be the critical factor in producing the pathophysiologic derangements associated with septic shock (Gibbs, 1976). Endotoxin is released from the bacterium at the time of the organism's death. In patients with gram-positive sepsis, shock can also develop and appears to be closely related to the release of an exotoxin (Kwan, 1969). Cleary et al (1992) demonstrated the production of exotoxin A by isolates of *Streptococcus pyogenes* associated with septic shock, whereas isolates from patients not in septic shock were unable to produce the exotoxin. From a clinical perspective, the overt physiologic alterations induced by either lipopolysaccharide endotoxins or exotoxins are the same.

Some investigators have suggested that differences may exist at the cellular level with regard to various gram-positive bacterial toxins (Kwan, 1969). Superantigenic toxins elaborated by some *Staphylococcus* and *Streptococcus* species, for example, can directly activate large numbers of T-lymphocytes without the need for intermediate antigen processing cells such as macrophages (Webb, 1994). This abbreviated mechanism of lymphocyte activation may explain the rapidly progressive and particularly fulminant clinical course observed with some gram-positive bacterial infections.

The ability of both gram-positive and gram-negative organisms to systematically activate the inflammatory cascade has particular relevance in the obstetric patient, in whom mixed polymicrobial infections are commonly identified (Monif, 1976). Although gram-negative coliforms make up a significant portion of the organisms recovered in bacteremic obstetric patients, other organisms, including aerobic and anaerobic streptococci, *Bacteroides fragilis*, and *Gardnerella vaginalis*, are found frequently. Septic shock in pregnancy associated with legionella pneumonia has also been described (Tewari, 1997). As in other areas of medicine, cases of obstetric sepsis

associated with group A streptococcus appear to be increasing (Holm, 1996).

The series of events initiated by endotoxin is presented schematically in Figure 22-1. Local activation of the immune system and its effector cells is important at the site of infection. The inflammatory process is normally tightly regulated and functions to locally confine the spread of infection. If the ability to regulate this response is lost, systemic activation of effector cells results in the elaboration of proinflammatory cytokines with widespread systemic effects (Pinsky, 1989). The syndrome of septic shock represents the culmination of overzealous activation of normal body defense mechanisms in an attempt to eradicate the invading pathogen (Sugerman, 1981).

Preliminary evidence suggests that an initial insult may cause simultaneous subclinical injury to multiple organ systems. It is theorized that this initial insult primes the immune system for a disproportionate response to any subsequent insult (Moore, 1992; Van Bebber, 1989; Daryani, 1990; Poggetti, 1992). The immune system, as one of the affected organ systems, responds to a second insult with an outpouring of inflammatory mediators (Demling, 1994). Activation of the complement cascade also plays a central role in activation of the immune system (Fearon, 1975) and can produce the hemodynamic changes characteristic of sepsis in animal models (Schirmer, 1988).

A wide variety of proinflammatory mediators have been implicated in the pathogenesis of septic shock. Several lines of experimental evidence in both humans and animal models support the central role of lipopolysaccharide-induced secretion of the cytokine TNF-α in the pathophysiology of the sepsis syndrome (Tracey, 1988). Large amounts of TNF-α are produced in response to endotoxin administration in healthy human subjects (Hesse, 1988; Michie, 1988a), and the administration of either endotoxin or TNF-α provokes similar physiologic derangements (Michie, 1988b). Elevated levels of TNF-α in animals are associated with shock and lethality (Tracey, 1987a; Mayoral, 1990). The infusion of TNF-α into experimental animals produces the pulmonary, renal, and gastrointestinal (GI) histopathology observed at autopsy in septic patients (Tracey, 1986;

F I G U R E **22-1**

Pathophysiology of septic shock.

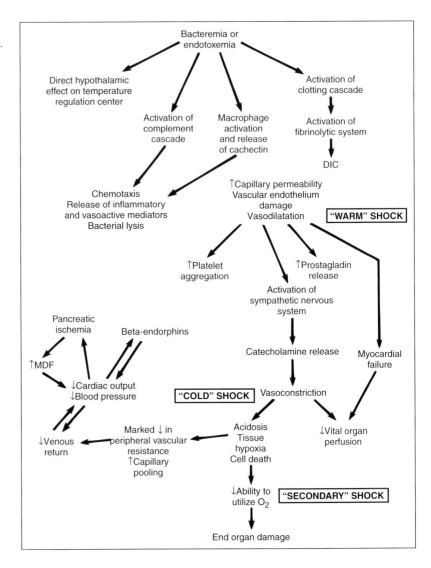

Remick, 1987). In similar models, antibodies directed against TNF-α provide protection and decrease mortality if given early enough to provide adequate tissue levels (Beutler, 1985; Tracey, 1987b). At the cellular level, lipopolysaccharide bound to a carrier protein interacts with the CD14 receptor on cells of the monocyte line. The resulting monocyte activation leads to production of TNF-α and IL-1, either simultaneously or in parallel. Lipopolysaccharide also binds to soluble CD14 to facilitate interaction with tissues lacking the CD14 receptor, such as vascular endothelium (Lynn, 1992). The production of TNF-α stimulates the secretion of interleukins, prostaglandins,

leukotrienes, and other inflammatory mediators. These inflammatory products cause the clinical symptoms associated with sepsis as well as capillary leak, hypotension, and activation of the coagulation system (Hageman, 1995).

Vascular endothelium is a metabolically active tissue that exerts a pivotal role in the regulation of underlying vascular smooth muscle and maintenance of vessel integrity and the fluidity of blood, and in the regulation of leukocyte adhesion. Maintenance of vascular homeostasis is regulated in large part by production of nitric oxide (endothelium-derived relaxing factor) (Hollenberg, 1994). Tumor necrosis factor-α stimulation of macrophages causes a sustained increase in nitrous oxide production, resulting in profound effects on vascular tone and permeability. Cyclooxygenase is also activated, and the elaboration of prostaglandins contributes to the maldistribution of blood flow (Dinerman, 1993).

Disruption of endothelial and vascular smooth muscle is a well-recognized component of septic shock, as is the blunting of response to vasoactive drugs. Because these effects are blocked in experimental models by treatment with nitric oxide synthesis inhibitors, alterations in nitrous oxide metabolism are felt to play a role in the development of refractoriness to endogenous catecholamines and exogenous vasopressors (Siegel, 1967). The elaboration of inflammatory mediators may also affect sympathetic vasomotor tone, resulting in impaired vasoconstriction to sympathetic stimulation. The combination of a leaky vasculature and loss of smooth muscle tone results in refractory hypotension (Siegel, 1991; Sibbald, 1991).

Tumor necrosis factor-α and activated complement fragments attract neutrophils whose products exacerbate endothelial injury (Sriskandan, 1995). This results in altered ability of the host to maintain tissue perfusion by regulating BP, cardiac output, and SVR (Parrillo, 1993). The production of IL-1β by macrophages has the added effect of producing procoagulant activity, which results in fibrin deposition in the microvasculature, leading to further perturbations of organ perfusion (Jacobs, 1989; Bonney, 1984; Goetzl, 1984). Activation of the microvasculature endothelium by TNF-α and IL-1β produces capillary leak and increased leukocyte receptor expression.

Leukocyte migration and activation result in release of vasoactive substances such as histamine, serotonin, and bradykinin. These substances, in turn, increase capillary permeability, induce endothelial damage, and promote vasodilation (Sugerman, 1981). A respiratory burst is stimulated by neutrophil activation, with increased production and release of lysosomal enzymes and toxic oxygen species such as superoxide, hydroxyl, and peroxide radicals. This has deleterious effects on the vasculature as well as other organs and is especially detrimental in the lung, where it is felt to play a key role in the

pathogenesis of ARDS (Hollenberg, 1994). Stimulation of neutrophils by activated complement fragments also leads to leukotriene secretion, further affecting capillary permeability and blood flow distribution (Jacobs, 1989). At the same time, the damage to the vascular endothelium stimulates platelet aggregation. Complement activation ensues, with microthrombus formation and fibrin deposition leading to further derangements of perfusion (Lee, 1989).

Intact reflex responses to what are initially local events, via sympathetic activation, may produce profound vasoconstriction in some organ systems; this vasoconstriction results in reductions in tissue perfusion (Sugerman, 1981). The local loss of control of vascular tone can also result in failure of arterioles and metaarterioles to dilate in response to physiologic vasodilating substances such as histamine and bradykinin (Altura, 1985). Further capillary leak continues and leads to increased intravascular fluid loss. In addition, cellular hypoxia and acidosis disrupt the ability of individual cells to utilize available oxygen (Duff, 1969). Marked reductions in peripheral vascular resistance now appear with extensive capillary pooling of blood.

In a rabbit model of IL-1β–induced hypotension, the lung is the primary organ that is injured. Although TNF-α produces more injury than IL-1β, pulmonary injury is massive when sublethal doses of both TNF-α and IL-1β are administered. The investigators concluded that TNF-α and IL-1 may act synergistically to disrupt vascular endothelium (Okusawa, 1988). Additional evidence of the role for cytokine mediation of lung injury in ARDS includes the increased production of IL-1 and TNF-α by lung macrophages in response to endotoxin administration (Tabor, 1988) and the in vivo observation that alveolar macrophages from ARDS patients produce increased amounts of IL-1 (Jacobs, 1988). Direct effects of bacterial immunologic complexes are also thought to play an important role in tissue injury (Knuppel, 1984). Immune complex precipitants have been identified within the lung vasculature, and they are thought to contribute to the development of ARDS. Likewise, focal areas of acute tubular necrosis seen in the kidney have been associated with the deposition of inflammatory infiltrates.

Disseminated intravascular coagulation frequently complicates septic shock. Disseminated intravascular coagulation involves activation of the coagulation cascade as well as fibrinolysis, with depletion of circulating coagulation factors. Tissue factor is released by TNF-$\alpha$ stimulation of monocytes and by exposure of subendothelially located tissue factor following injury to the vascular endothelium with activation of the extrinsic pathway. Microvasculature fibrin deposition compromises end-organ perfusion. At the same time, TNF-$\alpha$ also inhibits the production and action of regulatory proteins such as protein C, amplifying the procoagulant state. Although its role in DIC is not significant, activation of the intrinsic pathway provides a powerful stimulus to the production of kinins, such as bradykinin, contributing to the hypotension and disruption of vascular homeostasis. Derangements in the coagulation system are magnified by endotoxin's rapid activation and then suppression of fibrinolysis, which again appears to be mediated by TNF-$\alpha$ (Levi, 1993).

## Pregnancy and Septic Shock

The peripartum host may be different from the traditional septic shock host in ways other than the presence of different microbiologic pathogens. Physiologic adaptations to pregnancy designed to promote favorable maternal and fetal outcome occur in almost every organ system (Table 22-3) (Clark, 1989; Hankins, 1996; Metcalfe, 1974; Pritchard, 1985; Fletcher, 1979). Some of these changes, such as a dramatic increase in pelvic vascularity, promote maternal survival after infection. They also can influence the presentation and course of septic shock in the gravida, although such potential differences have received little attention in the literature. On the other hand, other physiologic adaptations to pregnancy (e.g., ureteral dilatation) may predispose the gravid female to more significant infectious morbidity than her nonpregnant counterpart.

In an animal model of endotoxin-induced septic shock, Beller and co-workers (1985) compared pregnant and nonpregnant responses with fixed doses of lipopolysaccharide. The pregnant animals had a much more pronounced respiratory and metabolic acidosis than did the controls, and they died secondary to cardiovascular collapse substantially faster than did nonpregnant controls. Although the increased susceptibility to endotoxin observed in pregnant animals agreed with the findings of other investigators (Beller, 1985; Morishima, 1978; Bech-Jansen, 1972), different animal species appear to succumb to different physiologic aberrations; thus, caution is warranted in applying the results of animal studies to critically ill pregnant women.

It is interesting to note that in the experimental model, the fetus and the neonate are

T A B L E **22-3**

Hemodynamic and ventilatory parameters in pregnancy

|  | Nonpregnant | Pregnant | Relative Change (%) |
|---|---|---|---|
| Cardiac output (liters/min) | 4.3 | 6.2 | 43 |
| Heart rate (beats per minute) | 71 | 83 | 17 |
| Systemic vascular resistance (dyne·sec·cm$^{-5}$) | 1530 | 1210 | 21 |
| Pulmonary vascular resistance (dyne·sec·cm$^{-5}$) | 119 | 78 | 34 |
| COP (mm Hg) | 20.8 | 18.0 | 14 |
| COP-PCWP gradient (mm Hg) | 14.5 | 10.5 | 18 |
| Mean arterial pressure (mm Hg) | 86.4 | 90.3 | No change |
| Central venous pressure (mm Hg) | 3.7 | 3.6 | No change |
| PCWP (mm Hg) | 6.3 | 7.5 | No change |
| Left ventricular stroke work index (g/m/m$^{-2}$) | 41 | 48 | No change |

Source: Clark SL, Cotton DB, Lee W, et al. Central hemodynamic assessment of normal term pregnancy. Am J Obstet Gynecol 1989;161:1439–1442.

much more resistant to the direct deleterious effects of endotoxin than is the mother. Bech-Jansen et al (1972) demonstrated that although blood flow to the uterus declined out of proportion to maternal hypotension, the fetus and the neonate were capable of tolerating endotoxin doses 10 times those proving to be lethal to the adult pregnant sheep. The fetal circulation was not affected until the adult's condition was terminal. The investigators hypothesize that these altered effects are related to the immature status of the fetal and neonatal vascular responsiveness. Morishima et al (1978) administered endotoxin to pregnant baboons. They observed profound asphyxia and severe maternal and fetal acidemia with rapid deterioration in the fetus, evidenced by late decelerations and fetal death in utero during maternal circulatory collapse. These effects were thought to result primarily from maternal factors such as hypotension and increased myometrial activity, both of which contribute to a reduction in placental perfusion. Although the pathophysiologic basis for the increased susceptibility during gestation to endotoxin remains speculative, the results suggest that the gravida should be considered a compromised host. The response of the gravid female to infectious stimuli probably represents the combined effects of alterations in her physiology as well as enhanced responsiveness to the effects of endotoxin.

As would be expected in an uncommon condition, the available human data regarding septic shock in human pregnancy are limited. The data describing contemporary ICU management including invasive hemodynamic monitoring in the septic obstetric patient are even more limited. The patient populations studied tend to be small and heterogenous and suffer from a variety of preexisting medical conditions, as well as some degree of ascertainment bias. A multi-institution review of women with sepsis in pregnancy whose management was guided by a PA catheter characterized the hemodynamic alterations seen in this patient population (Lee, 1988). In this series, maternal morbidity was 20%. Similar to the nonpregnant patient, septic shock was accompanied by an overall decrease in peripheral SVR. The range of values for this hemodynamic variable was quite wide and was dependent on the stage

of shock at which the PA catheter was initially inserted. At presentation, normal to increased cardiac output and decreased SVR were observed. Those patients who ultimately survived had increases in mean arterial pressure (MAP), SVR, and left ventricular stroke work index (LVSWI) during therapy. Left ventricular stroke work index appeared to be the best measure of cardiac function and predictor of outcome (Fig 22-2). Longitudinal measurements of SVR also proved to be useful in monitoring the progress of therapy. Response to intervention was reflected in normalization of the SVR to intermediate values (Fig 22-3) (Lee, 1984). These findings are consistent with physiologic patterns observed in nonpregnant septic shock patients (Shoemaker, 1973).

## Treatment of Septic Shock

The resuscitation goals for the patient in septic shock have been directed toward the aggressive use of volume replacement and inotropes to treat hypotension. Contemporary management has modified these therapeutic goals and emphasizes oxygen delivery and organ perfusion as endpoints

F I G U R E  **22-2**

Systemic vascular resistance (SVR) index values measured serially in gravidas with septic shock.

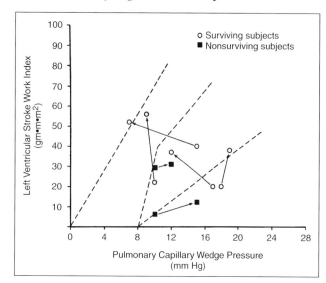

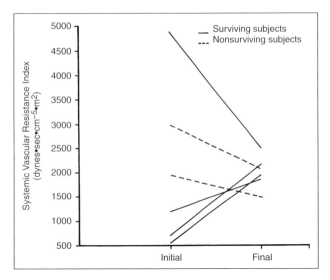

F I G U R E   **22-3**
**Serial ventricular function determinations in gravidas with septic shock.**

for hemodynamic intervention. Similar manipulation will probably be included in future management algorithms with the addition of efforts to mediate or neutralize the effects of inflammatory mediators (Lindeborg, 1993).

Initial intervention should be directed at the following general goals: (1) improvement in functional circulating intravascular volume, (2) establishment and maintenance of an adequate airway to facilitate management of respiratory failure, (3) assurance of adequate tissue perfusion and oxygenation, (4) initiation of diagnostic evaluations to determine the septic focus, and (5) institution of empiric antimicrobial therapy to eradicate the most likely pathogens.

If the patient is pregnant, priorities should be directed toward maternal well-being first, even in the face of the potential deleterious effects of septic shock on the fetus. Because fetal compromise results primarily from maternal cardiovascular decompensation, improvements in the maternal status should have positive effects on the fetal condition. Furthermore, attempts at delivery of the fetus in a hemodynamically compromised mother may lead to increased risks of fetal distress and the need for more aggressive obstetric intervention. In a mother who is not adequately

resuscitated or is unstable, further decreases in intravascular volume associated with blood loss at abdominal delivery may result in irrecoverable decompensation in maternal hemodynamic status. Maternal interests should take precedence, especially early in the course of resuscitation. This, of course, presumes that the fetal compartment is not the source of sepsis. Under such circumstances, therapy includes initiating delivery while stabilizing the mother.

## Volume Expansion

The mainstay of the acute management of septic shock involves volume expansion and correction of absolute or relative hypovolemia (Knuppel, 1984; Rackow, 1983; Packman, 1983; Kaufman, 1984; Hawkins, 1980; Roberts, 1971). Such therapy is always needed and correlates closely with improvement in cardiac output, oxygen delivery, and survival (Weil, 1978b). At times, considerable quantities of fluid are needed because of profound vasodilation, increased capillary permeability, and extravasation of fluid into the extravascular space. Blood pressure, heart rate, urine output, and hematocrit are conventionally used to assess the adequacy of intravascular volume. While these criteria are adequate for the initiation of volume resuscitation, they are unreliable in guiding optimal fluid and inotrope management in the patient with septic shock or multiple-organ system dysfunction (Shippy, 1984). The best means of monitoring this critical therapy is with the use of a flow-directed PA catheter (Swan, 1970; Shoemaker, 1990). Although central venous pressure (CVP) monitoring has been suggested as an alternative, available evidence suggesting erroneous information obtained with CVP monitoring supports the use of a flow-directed PA catheter (Cotton, 1985). In addition, PA catheterization allows determination of cardiac output and the calculation of variables related to oxygen delivery and utilization. These determinants cannot be made with standard CVP systems. Use of a PA catheter to optimize oxygen delivery and allow earlier intervention in the event of decompensation has been shown to decrease morbidity and mortality in high-risk surgical ICU patients (Lindeborg, 1993; Shoemaker, 1990).

A common endpoint for volume replacement is a PCWP of 14 to 16 mm Hg, a point at which, according to Starling's law, ventricular performance is optimal. Starling forces and ventricular performance are altered by sepsis, however, and a specific numerical value should not be chosen as an endpoint. Titration of therapy to optimize cardiopulmonary performance is preferable (Porembka, 1993; Packman, 1983; Rackow, 1987). Pulmonary capillary wedge pressure is used as an indicator of left ventricular end-diastolic pressure (LVEDP), and left ventricular end-diastolic volume (LVEDV) and circulating intravascular volume are inferred from PCWP. For a given volume, LVEDP will vary with left ventricular compliance, which is influenced by a multitude of factors in the septic patient (Packman, 1983; Lewis, 1980). Fluid resuscitation is a dynamic process, not an endpoint, and the value for PCWP that optimizes preload varies by patient. Therapy is optimized for the individual patient by sequentially expanding intravascular volume until a plateau is reached where further volume challenge produces no incremental increase in cardiac output (Porembka, 1993). An elevated PCWP may reflect an overexpanded intravascular space or a reduction in left ventricular function or both. The LVSWI can be used to differentiate between these two possibilities and select appropriate intervention. Information obtained from the PA catheter should be interpreted based on norms established for pregnancy rather than those derived from a nonpregnant population.

Apparently insurmountable controversy surrounds the debate about the optimal type of fluid to be used for volume expansion. Although isotonic crystalloid solutions such as normal saline are advocated most often, some investigators have recommended the use of colloid solutions (e.g., 5% normal human albumin) to maintain a normal COP-PCWP gradient (Haupt, 1982). Rackow et al (1983) have suggested that maintenance of this relationship reduces the risk of pulmonary edema. Various colloid and crystalloid solutions have been studied. In one series, both were able to restore cardiac function and hemodynamic stability, but the use of crystalloid required 2 to 4 times as much volume to achieve the same hemodynamic endpoint. Crystalloids significantly decrease the

COP and the COP-PCWP gradient with a potential commensurate increase in the incidence of pulmonary edema (Rackow, 1983). These findings are supported by the results of other series that found, in addition, that the risk of pulmonary edema was lower in younger patients (Rackow, 1977; Weil, 1978a). These authors concluded that younger, healthier patients are more able to tolerate crystalloid resuscitation. Colloids also have been shown to increase oxygen delivery and extraction (Shoemaker, 1991). Coupled with the decrease in COP and increased risk of pulmonary edema with massive infusion of crystalloids, further study in a homogenous group of patients is warranted. In clinical trials comparing crystalloid and colloid resuscitation, different endpoints and methodologies have been used, and the study groups are heterogenous, making them difficult to compare (Wagner, 1993). No consensus is currently available, and with appropriate caution, the use of either crystalloid or colloid solutions for volume resuscitation in septic shock is appropriate.

## Vasoactive Drug Therapy

At times, fluid resuscitation proves inadequate in restoring optimal cardiovascular performance. *After* restoration of adequate intravascular volume guided by a PA catheter, the use of vasoactive agents is indicated. The most commonly used agent in this regard is dopamine hydrochloride. Dopamine is a drug with dose-dependent effects on dopaminergic, alpha-, and beta-adrenergic receptors (Rao, 1982). In very low doses (<5 μg/kg/min), a selective dopaminergic increase in mesenteric and renal blow flow occurs. As the dosage is increased, the predominant effect is to increase myocardial contractility and cardiac output without increasing myocardial oxygen consumption. With doses exceeding 20 μg/kg/min, alpha effects predominate, with marked vasoconstriction and a further reduction in tissue perfusion. Dopamine is administered as a continuous infusion, starting at 2 to 5 μg/kg/min and titrated according to clinical and hemodynamic responses (Goldberg, 1974).

Dobutamine is an inotropic agent with fewer chronotropic effects than dopamine. It increases

CI and oxygen delivery and decreases SVR, improving perfusion (Bollaert, 1990). It is commonly combined with low-dose dopamine to improve myocardial performance and maintain renal perfusion in the ICU setting. Other vasoconstrictive drugs, including both norepinephrine (Desjars, 1987; Meadows, 1988) and epinephrine (Lindeborg, 1993; Bollaert, 1990; MacKenzie, 1991; Moran; 1993), have been suggested as alternatives in dopamine-resistant shock. Epinephrine increases CI, oxygen delivery, BP, and contractility. Oxygen debt is increased, possibly reflecting decreased tissue oxygenation, but hypotension is reversed by a balanced effect on both SVR and cardiac output (Bollaert, 1990). These hemodynamic improvements come at the expense of increased myocardial work and oxygen requirement (Lindeborg, 1993), which has limited the use of epinephrine. Significant vasoconstriction and end-organ hypoperfusion are also concerns.

Early experience using norepinephrine as a primary agent for inotropic support in septic shock was disappointing. Fears of excessive vasoconstriction and reversal of hypotension at the expense of organ perfusion limited its use. As newer catecholamines, such as dopamine, became available with more "favorable" side-effect profiles, they were used as first-line agents (Martin, 1993). Some now argue that norepinephrine's poor initial response related to inadequate monitoring and suboptimal volume replacement. This led to the subsequent need for excessively large vasopressor doses and development of hypoperfusion (Lucas, 1994). As a second-line drug reserved for cases of dopamine-resistant or refractory shock, additional adverse outcomes were reported (Desjars, 1987; Meadows, 1988).

Until the past few years, little attempt was made to compare the effects of dopamine and norepinephrine on hemodynamic parameters and oxygen delivery in septic shock in a randomized, controlled fashion. In one such study, Martin et al (1993) demonstrated that norepinephrine more reliably reversed hypotension and oliguria than did dopamine. Likewise, oxygen delivery and consumption were more favorably improved with norepinephrine. Additionally, norepinephrine effectively reversed shock in those patients who failed dopamine therapy. Dopamine has also been demonstrated to adversely affect the balance between splanchnic oxygen delivery and utilization when compared with norepinephrine. Both agents comparably increased MAP, but dopamine decreased gastric intramucosal pH (pHi), suggesting detrimental effects on splanchnic perfusion (Marik, 1994).

Unfortunately, microvascular shunting and hypoperfusion associated with any vasoactive agent are at times difficult to recognize and only become apparent with deterioration of the patient's overall condition or with increased serum lactic acid concentrations (Porembka, 1993). Despite well-described limitations to this biochemical test, serially following lactic acid levels may be useful as an indicator of end-organ perfusion. Changes in calculated oxygen delivery and extraction are also helpful in assessing adequacy of tissue perfusion and response to therapy. Of note is the demonstration by Rolbin et al (1979) that dopamine decreased uterine blood flow in hypotensive pregnant sheep. Therefore, dopamine (and the other vasoactive agents) may compromise fetal status while improving the maternal condition, a situation analogous to other sites of decreased end-organ perfusion. This latter example suggests the need for continuous heart rate monitoring as a "marker" for end-organ perfusion in the gestationally viable fetus during resuscitation attempts with vasopressor therapy.

The ability to spontaneously generate a hyperdynamic state in response to sepsis is associated with lower mortality (Parker, 1983; Moore, 1992; Shoemaker, 1973; Shippy, 1984). It is unclear whether the beneficial effect on mortality reflects the impact of therapeutic intervention or better underlying cardiovascular function in a host who is more responsive to intervention. Survivors are clearly more responsive to inotropic therapy (Shoemaker, 1991), but this may simply reflect underlying hemodynamic differences in survivors versus nonsurvivors.

The observation that better cardiovascular performance was associated with survival has prompted many intensivists to conclude that titration of inotropic support to supranormal values should improve outcome (Shoemaker, 1988, 1992; Tuchschmidt, 1992; Boyd, 1993; Bishop, 1995; Yu, 1993). The desired hemodynamic profile usually includes a CI greater than 4.5 liters/min/m$^2$ and a $Do_2$ greater than 600 mL/min/m$^2$. These values are not prospectively derived; rather, they represent median values for survivors. This approach to management is controversial and has been criticized by two large prospective series. The controversy surrounding endpoints for inotropic support is in part attributable to differences in the populations studied and indication for ICU admission. This approach was initially evaluated as prophylaxis in high-risk surgical patients. The more recent work, which questions this management scheme, randomized patients after shock and organ failure were established. These prospective, randomized series found no benefits to normalization of $Svo_2$ or supraphysiologic goals for hemodynamic manipulation. Hayes et al (1994) were unable to demonstrate a decrease in mortality as long as volume replacement was adequate and perfusion pressure was maintained. A large multicenter European trial also found that the targeted parameters were difficult to achieve, and the propensity to achieve them was a function of the patient's age. No decrease in mortality was found in patients who achieved supraphysiologic levels of cardiovascular performance regardless of group or reason for ICU admission (Gattinoni, 1995).

These series should not be interpreted as advocating a conservative approach to hemodynamic therapy in septic shock. The apparently contradictory findings may be viewed as complementary. In susceptible patients, oxygen delivery, intravascular volume, and perfusion should be optimized to prevent progression to organ failure. In patients who develop shock, inotropic therapy should be directed toward maintenance of adequate cardiac output and BP with inotropes to maintain perfusion and oxygenation (Hinds, 1995). Responsiveness to inotropic support and the ability to spontaneously generate a hyperdynamic state may allow some prognostication regarding outcome.

## Oxygenation

Although oxygenation at the lungs can be assessed easily by arterial blood gas determinations, oxygen consumption or utilization is a more difficult parameter to evaluate. The use of a PA catheter allows direct measurement and calculation of parameters relevant to oxygen delivery and consumption. Early in the course of shock, BP may actually be normal due to peripheral vasoconstriction, because perfusion is disproportionately diverted from the renal and splanchnic circulations to maintain central BP. Impairment of splanchnic perfusion permits translocation of bacteria and toxins across the GI mucosa, worsening septic shock (Demling, 1994; Fiddian-Green, 1993). Oxygen delivery and tissue extraction are decreased in all forms of shock. Untreated, anaerobic metabolism and progressive oxygen debt develop and result in lactic acidemia, organ dysfunction, and death (Shoemaker, 1992).

Septic patients have increased metabolic needs for oxygen and, at the same time, a decreased ability to extract the oxygen that is delivered (Tuchschmidt, 1991). Peripheral tissue utilization of oxygen is frequently reduced, resulting in tissue hypoxia (Duff, 1969). Two possible mechanisms play a pivotal role in this phenomenon. First, there is evidence to suggest that cellular dysfunction during later stages of septic shock can lead to underextraction of delivered oxygen. Mitochondrial and cellular dysfunction decrease the ability to utilize oxygen (Rackow, 1988; Dantzker, 1989; Gutierrez, 1989). Second, microvascular shunting and loss of autoregulation of blood flow may decrease local availability of oxygen (Duff, 1969; Siegel, 1967). Additionally, hypophosphatemia, alkalosis, and multiple blood transfusions all shift the oxyhemoglobin dissociation curve to the left, resulting in a decrease in peripheral availability of oxygen.

Decreased tissue extraction can be measured indirectly by elevations in mixed-venous oxygen saturation ($Svo_2$) or by the determination of a reduced arteriovenous oxygen content difference (Tuchschmidt, 1991). Actual peripheral oxygen consumption can be calculated by using the Fick equation; the normal indexed nonpregnant range is 120 to 140 mlO$_2$/min/m$^2$ (Shoemaker, 1983). Oxygen consumption is normally independent of oxygen delivery, because delivery far exceeds consumption. In the septic patient, oxygen delivery should be increased until lactic acid concentrations return to normal (Lindeborg, 1993; Shoemaker, 1991). Even in the absence of lactic acidosis, it is prudent to maintain excess oxygen delivery to avoid local reduction in tissue perfusion and subsequent organ dysfunction (Demling, 1994). The gut, for example, demonstrates anaerobic metabolism (implying inadequate perfusion) in an animal model of sepsis with supranormal cardiac output and oxygen delivery adequate for the rest of the body (Pinsky, 1989).

## Acute Respiratory Distress Syndrome

The diagnosis of ARDS is made on the basis of progressive hypoxemia, with a normal PCWP, diffuse infiltrates on chest x-ray, or decreased pulmonary compliance (Sugerman, 1981). These findings are consistent with a pathophysiological state in which increased capillary permeability leads to extravasation of fluid into interstitial spaces, with the development of progressive oxygen debt that contributes to multiple-organ system dysfunction and death.

The development of pulmonary hypertension increases the rate at which extravascular interstitial fluid collects and contributes to the progressive hypoxemia observed clinically. Pulmonary hypertension develops initially in response to neurohormonal mechanisms. Later, structural changes develop in the pulmonary microvasculature and parenchyma, probably in response to inflammatory by-products in the lung parenchyma (Bersten, 1989). During this later inflammatory fibrotic phase, ARDS is commonly associated with fever, leukocytosis, and decreased SVR, making it exceedingly difficult to distinguish from pneumonia and worsening sepsis (Meduri, 1991; Ashbaugh, 1985).

The cornerstone of the treatment of ARDS involves intubation and ventilatory support to maintain adequate gas exchange at nontoxic levels of inspired oxygen. Positive end-expiratory pressure is often necessary to accomplish this goal, and serial monitoring of arterial blood gases is essential. The clinician must remember that even in the face of overt pulmonary capillary leakage, intravenous hydration should be continued and adequate intravascular volume maintained to promote systemic perfusion. Positive end-expiratory pressure generates increased intrathoracic pressure and may decrease venous return and consequently cardiac output, depending on volume status and amount of PEEP. The clinician must keep in mind that PEEP can artificially increase PCWP measurements when interpreting hemodynamic readings and assessing intravascular volume status.

## Antimicrobial Therapy

In concert with attempts at restoring normal cardiovascular function and tissue oxygenation, an aggressive investigation into the underlying etiology of sepsis should be initiated. Because the course of septic shock can be short and fulminant, such a work-up must be carried out without delay, and empiric antimicrobial therapy should be started. At times, the cause of sepsis in the parturient is obvious (e.g., chorioamnionitis or pyelonephritis). At other times, the etiology can be elusive (e.g., postpartum toxic shock syndrome, necrotizing fasciitis, septic pelvic thrombophlebitis). The diagnostic work-up may include the microbiologic evaluation of specimens from blood, urine, sputum, and wound. Because mixed flora are usually identified in transvaginal cultures, a careful sampling of the endometrial cavity is seldom clinically useful (Duff, 1983). In patients thought to have chorioamnionitis, transabdominal amniocentesis or cultures taken from a free-flowing internal pressure transducer catheter have been described, but are also of limited clinical utility (Gibbs, 1982).

Empiric therapy in the obstetric patient should include coverage for a wide variety of both aerobic and anaerobic gram-negative and gram-positive bacteria. Institution-specific sensitivities of common nosocomial pathogens and specific patient factors should be considered in the choice of empiric therapy until culture results are available. Parenteral therapy that includes a combination of ampicillin (2 g/6 hr), an aminoglycoside appropriately dosed for patient weight and renal function, and clindamycin phosphate (900 mg/8 hr) is generally recommended. Other treatment regimens are acceptable, and each clinician must be familiar with the administration and potential toxic effects of these drugs.

In patients who previously received cephalosporin therapy, additional coverage specifically directed against enterococci may be warranted. In addition, if *Staphylococcus aureus* is a suspected pathogen, a semisynthetic penicillin may be substituted for ampicillin. Because nephrotoxicity is a well-established complication of aminoglycoside usage and these patients may already have renal compromise, monitoring of peak and trough aminoglycoside levels is imperative to achieve therapeutic levels while minimizing potential toxicity. When available, culture results and organism sensitivities should be used to more selectively guide subsequent antimicrobial therapy.

The critically ill patient is at high risk for developing sources of infection not commonly encountered by obstetricians, and careful physical examination and selected imaging studies are important in excluding uncommon sources. Sinusitis may develop secondary to prolonged intubation or nasogastric suction, for example. Nosocomial pneumonia commonly develops in patients admitted to the ICU and is independently associated with increased risk of mortality (Fagon, 1996). When broad-spectrum antibiotics are utilized, careful surveillance for resistant organisms and fungal infection is imperative.

## Surgical Therapy

Most clinicians agree that in a life-threatening condition such as septic shock, surgical extirpation of infected tissues (if possible) is important to ensure survival. In patients with suspected septic abortion, evacuation of the uterus should begin promptly after initiating antibiotics and stabilizing the patient. Septic shock in association with chorioamnionitis in a viable fetus is treated by delivery; this can be accomplished vaginally if maternal hemodynamic parameters are stable and delivery is imminent. Under certain circumstances, after initial maternal resuscitation, cesarean section may be appropriate, given the increased chance of survival of the fetus and the

uncertain risks to the mother if the nidus for infection is not removed rapidly. In the postpartum patient, hysterectomy may be indicated if microabscess formation is identified within myometrial tissues or if there is clinical evidence of deterioration in the patient's condition despite appropriate antibiotic therapy. When the diagnosis of septic pelvic thrombophlebitis is entertained, treatment with heparin in combination with broad-spectrum antibiotics is appropriate. If this proves unsuccessful, surgical evaluation may be necessary (Collins, 1970).

## Coagulation System

Disseminated intravascular coagulation frequently complicates septic shock. Severe bleeding may result from the depletion of coagulation factors after activation of the coagulation system. Unless the patient has clinical evidence of bleeding or surgical or invasive procedures are anticipated, aggressive attempts at correcting these laboratory defects should not be undertaken. The best treatment for DIC is treatment of the underlying condition, and spontaneous improvement will occur when the overall clinical picture improves. An exception to this approach is when platelets fall below 5000 to 10,000 per milliliter; platelet transfusion to prevent spontaneous hemorrhage may be indicated at this point.

Whenever thrombocytopenia occurs in the septic patient, the effect of heparin must be considered in the differential diagnosis. The use of heparin in the ICU is common, and it can cause thrombocytopenia via two mechanisms. The first, generally seen within 2 to 5 days after initiation of therapy, is usually mild and of little clinical significance. Immune-mediated heparin-induced thrombocytopenia is less common but of considerably more importance and may cause profound thrombocytopenia. This phenomena occurs 7 to 15 days after initiation of therapy and is independent of dose or route (Mei, 1993). Rather than transfusing platelets, all sources of heparin must be eliminated, including subcutaneous injections for deep venous thrombosis prophylaxis, flushing indwelling lines, and total parenteral nutrition (TPN) solutions.

## Renal Function

Renal function is best monitored with an indwelling catheter and serial creatinine and BUN determinations. Although acute tubular necrosis most often presents with oliguria, it may present occasionally as a high-output state. Regardless, tests of tubular function will demonstrate increased fractional excretion of sodium and impaired concentrating ability, evidenced by a urinary sodium greater than 40 mEq/liter and urine osmolality less than 400 mosm/kg $H_2O$, respectively. Serum creatinine concentrations also rise at a rate of 0.5 to 1.5 mg/dL/day (Miller, 1978). Provided irreversible acute tubular necrosis has not occurred, correction of the hemodynamic and perfusion deficits should result in restoration of renal function. Table 22-4 lists various prognostic indicators of poor outcome in addition to renal parameters in patients with septic shock (Sugerman, 1981; Shoemaker, 1973, 1983; Kaufman, 1984; Weil, 1978b; Hardaway, 1981).

## Gastrointestinal Tract and Nutrition

Although often overlooked, the GI tract can be a reservoir of infection and a source of considerable morbidity to the ICU patient. Three interrelated areas requiring attention include provision for adequate nutrition, preventing or minimizing the effect of translocation of bacteria from the gut to the systemic circulation, and stress ulcer prophylaxis. All three relate directly to efforts to

T A B L E 22-4

**Prognostic indicators of poor outcome in septic shock**

Delay in initial diagnosis
Underlying debilitation disease process
Poor response to intravenous fluid resuscitation
Depressed cardiac output
Reduced oxygen extraction
Presence of ARDS or renal failure
High serum lactate (>4 mmol/liter)
Reduced COP (<15 mm Hg)

maintain adequate splanchnic circulation and the integrity of the GI mucosa.

Sepsis provokes a catabolic state, the effects of which are especially pronounced in skeletal muscle, loose connective tissue, and intestinal viscera (Pinsky, 1989). Metabolic alterations provoked by sepsis differ from starvation in that the compensatory mechanisms to preserve lean body mass in starvation are absent in sepsis (Wojnar, 1995). Provision for adequate nutrition early in the patient's ICU course is vital. In addition to providing adequate calories, carbohydrates, lipids, protein, vitamins, and trace elements to prevent catabolism, restoration of adequate nutritional support has other beneficial effects. Inadequate nutrition is associated with significant immune impairment, with suppression of both cellular and humoral immunity. The potential for alterations in immune function emphasizes the importance of providing adequate nutrition early in the course of sepsis. There is good animal evidence and preliminary human data to suggest that specific nutrients such as glutamine, arginine, and omega-3 fatty acids may have significant immunomodulatory functions (Mainous, 1994).

Malnutrition has additional deleterious effects. It alters gut mucosal integrity and promotes increases in endogenous gut flora. By itself, malnutrition does not promote translocation of bacteria and bacterial toxins into the circulation (Deitch, 1987). Sepsis increases the permeability of GI mucosa, and permeability increases with increasing severity of infection, an effect probably mediated by endotoxin (Deitch, 1987; Ziegler, 1988). When endotoxin is administered in the face of starvation or malnutrition, an increase in translocation of bacteria across the mucosa is observed that correlates with the duration of malnutrition (Deitch, 1987).

The mucosa is highly susceptible to injury from hypotension and reperfusion because of its high metabolic rate. It is affected early when perfusion is redirected away from the gut to maintain CNS and cardiac perfusion. Ischemia interferes with mucosal function to prevent bacterial translocation into the systemic circulation (Pinsky, 1989; Riddington, 1996). Several investigators have suggested that gastric tonometry be used to follow intramucosal pH (pHi) as an indicator of GI and splanchnic perfusion. pH has been correlated with perfusion, the propensity for mucosal injury and transmural migration of gut flora, and clinical outcome (Fiddian-Green, 1993; Gys, 1988; Doglio, 1991; Sauve, 1993). Clinical improvement in the patient's condition should be reflected in normalization of mucosal pH and no further increases in oxygen consumption with increased delivery.

When selecting the route to provide nutritional supplementation, the adage, "If the gut works, use it," should be borne in mind. Even in the face of nutritionally adequate replenishment, TPN is associated with impairment of host defenses and intrinsic gut immunity. Excluding complications associated with central access and line sepsis, infectious complications are increased with TPN (Mainous, 1994). The enteral route slows atrophy and maintains integrity of the mucosal barrier, especially if glutamine is provided. If adequate caloric replacement cannot be provided enterally, even small-volume feedings with the remaining nutrition provided by TPN are better than TPN alone in promoting mucosal integrity and preventing atrophy (Wojnar, 1995). Enteral nutrition can be provided to the intubated patient either through a needle catheter jejunostomy or through a small nasogastric tube advanced well into the duodenum.

Alterations in splanchnic perfusion, the patient response to stress, and drugs administered to ICU patients can all promote ulceration and upper GI bleeding. Prophylaxis is commonly provided in the form of either regular administration of antacids, $H_2$-receptor antagonists, or cytoprotective agents such as sucralfate. More than 50 trials have been performed with various endpoints and have found a comparable protective effect regardless of which type of prophylaxis is used. A relative disadvantage of antacids and $H_2$-receptor antagonists is that they increase gastric pH, promoting overgrowth of the normally sterile stomach with gram-negative enteric pathogens. The risk of aspiration and nosocomial pneumonia is increased significantly by their use and has led some to recommend sucralfate over antacids or $H_2$ blockers (Sauve, 1993; Cannon, 1987; Craven, 1986; Driks, 1987; Bresalier, 1987; Tryba, 1987; Cook, 1996). Although sucralfate is associated with reductions in nosocomial pneumonias in intubated patients, adequate trials have not been conducted to demonstrate conclusively a reduction in mortality with sucralfate. Potential advantages of sucralfate in the gravid patient include poor GI absorption and lack of the potential systemic effects associated with $H_2$ blockers. It has no effect on fertility, does not cross the placenta, and is not teratogenic (Briggs, 1995). It should be considered a viable alternative for prophylaxis in the pregnant ICU patient who can tolerate nasogastric medications.

Additional measures that require the meticulous attention of the clinician include management of electrolyte imbalances, correction of metabolic acidosis, stabilization of coagulation defects, prophylaxis for deep venous thrombosis with subcutaneous heparin or sequential compression boots, and monitoring of renal function. Patients in septic shock may have either hypokalemia secondary to losses from the alimentary canal or hyperkalemia resulting from either acute cation shifts in the face of acidosis or from renal failure. Lactic acidosis from anaerobic metabolism should be monitored serially and treated aggressively by increasing oxygen delivery and perfusion to peripheral tissues. Half-normal saline infusions with one to two ampules of sodium bicarbonate can be administered periodically to help correct severe acidosis. Serum glucose levels may be elevated, normal, or depressed. If the serum glucose levels are depressed, some clinicians advocate the administration of glucose in combination with insulin to improve tissue uptake of the substrate.

## Controversial Treatment Modalities

Historically, the most controversial modality in the treatment of septic shock was the use of high-dose steroids. Their use is theoretically appealing, with potential benefits including stabilization of lysosomal membranes, inhibition of complement-induced inflammatory changes, and attenuation of the effects of cytokines and other inflammatory mediators. In an early trial, Sprung and co-workers (1984) reported reversal of shock when steroids were given early in the course of sepsis. Although there was some short-term improvement, no change in ultimate inhospital mortality or reversal of shock was observed. Significantly, more than 25% of patients treated with steroids developed superinfections. Two large randomized, placebo-controlled, prospective studies subsequently demonstrated neither benefit of early administration of corticosteroids in the treatment of severe sepsis and septic shock nor prophylactic value of steroids in preventing clinical evolution to septic shock (Bone, 1987; VA Systemic Sepsis Cooperative Study Group, 1987). Currently, there is no compelling reason to use corticosteroids in the therapy of septic shock; their use should be reserved for those patients with documented adrenal insufficiency.

Other potential roles for steroids in the management of the septic gravida may include their use in the late fibroproliferative phase of ARDS to prevent lung injury from evolving to fibrosis. Several small series have suggested that although progression from lung injury to ARDS is not prevented, steroids may be of some benefit in the prevention of pulmonary fibrosis and may accelerate recovery in this subgroup of patients (Meduri, 1991; Ashbaugh, 1985; Hooper, 1990; Weigelt, 1985). Transient suppression of maternal immune function has been described following betamethasone therapy for fetal pulmonary maturation (Cunningham, 1991). This effect is inconsequential and probably poses no maternal risk (Crowley, 1995).

Prostaglandins have long been thought to play a central role in septic shock. Oettinger and colleagues (1983) demonstrated increased production and decreased degradation of prostaglandin $F_2$ in severe sepsis. Other researchers have suggested that these alterations are associated with known endotoxin-induced pulmonary vascular changes (Vada, 1984). Cefalo et al (1980) used prostaglandin synthetase inhibitors to blunt these pathophysiologic responses in sheep. These same beneficial effects could be observed in other organ systems when experimental animals were pretreated with prostaglandin synthetase inhibitors prior to exposure to endotoxin (Makabali, 1983; O'Brien, 1981; Rao, 1981). Further clinical trials using adjunctive antiprostaglandin therapy are needed prior to endorsing their clinical use.

Lachman et al (1984) administered antilipopolysaccharide immunoglobulin to obstetric and gynecologic patients in septic shock. In treated patients, a reduction in both morbidity and mortality was observed. Despite this initial enthusiasm, antiendotoxin and anticytokine therapies are of questionable benefit in the therapy of septic shock. Preliminary studies showed that antibodies specifically directed against endotoxin or inflammatory mediators such as TNF-α reduced mortality in animal models and human septic shock patients (Beutler, 1985). Clinical trials have, unfortunately, produced inconsistent results. Although initially promising, the clinical experience has not been as good as expected (Natanson, 1994; Greenman, 1991; Ziegler, 1991; Warren, 1992; Wenzel, 1991). Circulating natural inhibitors of proinflammatory cytokines have been described. In animal models, these circulating inhibitors decrease mortality in endotoxic shock. The interactions between these circulating antagonists and the proinflammatory cytokines on the molecular level and their impact on the clinical course of sepsis are only beginning to be investigated. Their presence may explain the inconsistent results observed in clinical trials of exogenously administered inflammatory mediators (Goldie, 1995).

Beta-endorphins are a group of polypeptides present in the CNS. They are derived from the precursor molecule proopiomelanocortin, which is produced in response to stress. There may be a release of this opiate-like substance in the presence of septic shock. After release, this peptide is thought to produce a profound BP reduction, which can be reversed by using narcotic antagonists such as naloxone (Holaday, 1978). Several anecdotal reports in the literature support these preliminary observations. It is interesting to note that beta-endorphin levels have been shown to increase progressively throughout gestation (Genazzani, 1981). This specific pregnancy-related effect on septic shock remains to be elucidated.

---

**SEPTIC SHOCK**

**I.** *Goals of Therapy*

  A.  Systolic BP $>90$ mm Hg
  B.  Urine output $>30$ mL/hr
  C.  Arterial $po_2$ $>60$ mm Hg
  D.  Normal mental status
  E.  Normalization of tissue oxygenation and perfusion
  F.  Eradication of source of infection

**II.** *Management Protocol*

  A.  Rapid volume expansion with D5LR (1000 mL), followed by 150 to 200 mL/hr.
  B.  Administer oxygen to maintain $po_2$ $>60$ mm Hg.
  C.  Initiate empiric antibiotic therapy:
    1.  Ampicillin 2 g IV every 6 hours
    2.  Gentamicin 1.5 mg/kg, then 1 mg/kg IV every 8 hours
    3.  Clindamycin 900 mg every 8 hours IV
  D.  Search for an infectious source amenable to surgical correction (abscess, appendicitis, etc.).
  E.  If there is no clinical response to volume loading, place a PA catheter to guide fluid and vasopressor therapy. Optimize preload to maximize cardiac output.
  F.  After optimal preload is reached, begin norepinephrine if necessary (starting dose 0.5–1.0 μg/min). Titrate to hemodynamic and clinical response.
  G.  Consider digitalization of other inotropic support if invasive monitoring parameters (LVSWI) indicate myocardial failure.
  H.  Control overt hyperthermia with acetaminophen or a cooling blanket.

**III.** *Critical Laboratory Tests*

  A.  Complete blood count with platelet count, urinalysis, fibrinogen, prothrombin time, partial thromboplastin time, fibrin split products, D-dimer, electrolytes, BUN, creatinine, SGPT, SGOT, arterial blood gas, urine, sputum, wound and other clinically indicated cultures, serum lactate, chest x-ray, pelvic-abdominal computed tomography scan or magnetic resonance imaging if abscess is suspected. Monitor mixed venous oxygen saturation or arterial-venous oxygen difference.

**IV.** *Consultations*

  A.  Infectious disease, critical care medicine.

**REFERENCES**

Altura BM, Gebrewold A, Burton RW. Failure of microscopic metaarterioles to elicit vasodilator responses to acetylcholine, bradykinin, histamine and substance P after ischemic shock, endothelial cells. Microcirc Endothelium Lymphatics 1985;2:121.

Ashbaugh DG, Maier RV. Idiopathic pulmonary fibrosis in adult respiratory distress syndrome: diagnosis and treatment. Arch Surg 1985;120:530.

Balk RA, Bone RC. The septic syndrome: definition and clinical implications. Crit Care Clin 1989;5:1.

Bech-Jansen P, Brinkman CR, Johnson GH, et al. Circulatory shock in pregnant sheep. Am J Obstet Gynecol 1972;112:1084.

Beller JF, Schmidt EH, Holzgreve W, et al. Septicemia during pregnancy: a study in different species of experimental animals. Am J Obstet Gynecol 1985;151:967.

Bersten A, Sibbald WJ. Acute lung injury in septic shock. Crit Care Clin 1989;5:49.

Beutler B, Milsark IW, Cerami AC. Passive immunization against cachectin/tumor necrosis factor protects mice from lethal effect of endotoxin. Science 1985;229:869.

Bishop MH, Shoemaker WC, Appel PL, et al. Prospective, randomized trial of survivor values of cardiac index, oxygen delivery, and oxygen consumption as resuscitation endpoints in severe trauma. J Trauma 1995;38:780.

Blanco JD, Gibbs RS, Castaneda YS. Bacteremia in obstetrics: clinic course. Obstet Gynecol 1981;58:621.

Bollaert PE, Bauer P, Audibert G, et al. Effects of epinephrine on hemodynamics and oxygen metabolism in dopamine-resistant septic shock. Chest 1990;98:949.

Bone RC. Sepsis syndrome: new insights into its pathogenesis and treatment. Infect Dis Clin North Am 1991;5:793.

Bone RC, Balk RA, Cerra FB, et al. Definitions for sepsis and organ failure and guidelines for the use of innovative therapies in sepsis. Chest 1992a;101:1644.

Bone RC, Sibbald WJ, Sprung CL. The ACCP-SCCM consensus conference on sepsis and organ failure. Chest 1992b;101:1481.

Bone RC, Fisher CJ Jr, Clemmer TP, et al. A controlled clinical trial of high-dose methylprednisolone in the treatment of severe sepsis and septic shock. N Engl J Med 1987;317:653.

Bonney RJ, Humes JL. Physiological and pharmacological regulation of prostaglandin and leukotriene production by macrophages. J Leukoc Biol 1984;35:1.

Boyd O, Grounds RM, Bennett ED. A randomized clinical trial of the effect of deliberate perioperative increase of oxygen delivery on mortality in high-risk surgical patients. JAMA 1993;270:2699.

Bresalier RS, Grendell JH, Cello JP, et al. Sucralfate suspension versus titrated antacid for the prevention of acute stress-related gastrointestinal hemorrhage in critically ill patients. Am J Med 1987;83:110.

Briggs GG, Freeman RK, Yaffe SJ, eds. Sucralfate: gastrointestinal agent. In: A reference guide to fetal and neonatal risk: drugs in pregnancy and lactation. 4th ed. Baltimore: Williams and Wilkins, 1995:792–793.

Brun-Buisson C, Doyon F, Carlet J, et al. Incidence, risk factors, and outcome of severe sepsis and septic shock in adults. A multicenter prospective study in intensive care units. JAMA 1995;274:968.

Bryan CS, Reynolds KL, Moore EE. Bacteremia in obstetrics and gynecology. Obstet Gynecol 1984;64:155.

Cannon LA, Heiselman D, Gardner W, et al. Prophylaxis of upper gastrointestinal tract bleeding in mechanically ventilated patients. Arch Intern Med 1987;147:2101.

Cavanagh D, Knuppel RA, Shepherd JH, et al. Septic shock and the obstetrician/gynecologist. South Med J 1982;75:809.

Cefalo RC, Lewis PE, O'Brien WF, et al. The role of prostaglandins in endotoxemia: comparisons in response in the nonpregnant, maternal, and fetal model. Am J Obstet Gynecol 1980;137:53.

Centers for Disease Control and Prevention. National Center for Health Statistics Mortality Patterns—United States, 1990. Monthly Vital Stat Rep 1993;41:5.

Chow AW, Guze LB. Bacteroidaceae bacteremia: clinical experience with 112 patients. Medicine 1974;53:93.

Chow AW, Wittman BK, Bartlett KH, et al. Variant postpartum toxic shock syndrome with probable intrapartum transmission to the neonate. Am J Obstet Gynecol 1984;148:1074.

Clark SL, Cotton DB, Lee W, et al. Central hemodynamic assessment of normal term pregnancy. Am J Obstet Gynecol 1989;161:1439.

Cleary PP, Kaplan EL, Handley JP, et al. Clonal basis for resurgence of serious *Streptococcus pyogenes* disease in the 1980s. Lancet 1992;339:518.

Collins CG. Suppurative pelvic thrombophlebitis. Am J Obstet Gynecol 1970;108:681.

Cook DJ, Reeve BK, Guyatt GH, et al. Stress ulcer prophylaxis in critically ill patients: resolving discordant meta-analyses. JAMA 1996;275:308.

Cotton DB, Gonik B, Dorman K, et al. Cardiovascular alterations in severe pregnancy-induced hypertension: relationship of central venous pressure to pulmonary capillary wedge pressure. Am J Obstet Gynecol 1985;151:762.

Craven DE, Kunches LM, Kilinshy V, et al. Risk factors for pneumonia and fatality in patients receiving continuous mechanical ventilation. Am Rev Respir Dis 1986;133:792.

Crowley PA. Antenatal corticosteroid therapy: a meta-analysis of the randomized trials, 1972 to 1994. Am J Obstet Gynecol 1995;173:322.

Cunningham DS, Evan EE. The effects of betamethasone on maternal cellular resistance to infection. Am J Obstet Gynecol 1991;165:610.

Cunningham FG, Lucas MJ, Hankins GDV. Pulmonary injury complicating antepartum pyelonephritis. Am J Obstet Gynecol 1987;156:797.

Dantzker D. Oxygen delivery and utilization in sepsis. Crit Care Clin 1989;5:81.

Daryani R, Lalonde C, Zhu D, et al. Effect of endotoxin and a burn injury on lung and liver lipid peroxidation and catalase activity. J Trauma 1990;30:1330.

Deitch EA, Winterton J, Li M, et al. The gut as a portal of entry for bacteremia: role of protein malnutrition. Ann Surg 1987;195:681.

Demling RH, Lalonde C, Ikegami K. Physiologic support of the septic patient. Surg Clin North Am 1994;74:637.

Desjars P, Pinaud M, Poptel G, et al. A reappraisal of norepinephrine therapy in human septic shock. Crit Care Med 1987;15:134.

Dinerman JL, Lowenstein CJ, Snyder SH. Molecular mechanisms of nitric oxide regulation: potential relevance to cardiovascular disease. Circ Res 1993;73:217.

Doglio GR, Pusajo JF, Egurrola MA, et al. Gastric mucosal pH as a prognostic index of mortality in critically ill patients. Crit Care Med 1991;19:1037.

Driks MR, Craven DE, Celli BR, et al. Nosocomial pneumonia in intubated patients given sucralfate as compared with antacids or histamine type 2 blockers. N Engl J Med 1987;317:1376.

Duff JH, Groves AC, McLean LPH, et al. Defective oxygen consumption in septic shock. Surg Gynecol Obstet 1969;128:1051.

Duff P. Pyelonephritis in pregnancy. Clin Obstet Gynecol 1984;27:17.

Duff P. Pathophysiology and management of postcesarean endomyometritis. Obstet Gynecol 1986;67:269.

Duff P, Gibbs RS, Blanco JD, et al. Endometrial culture techniques in puerperal patients. Obstet Gynecol 1983;61:217.

Fagon JY, Chastre J, Vuagnat A, et al. Nosocomial pneumonia and mortality among patients in intensive care units. JAMA 1996;275:866.

Fearon DT, Ruddy S, Schur PH, et al. Activation of the properdin pathway of complement in patients with gram-negative bacteremia. N Engl J Med 1975;292:937.

Fiddian-Green RG, Haglund U, Gutierrez G, et al. Goals for the resuscitation of shock. Crit Care Med 1993;21:S25.

Fletcher AP, Alkjaersig NK, Burstein R. The influence of pregnancy upon blood coagulation and plasma fibrinolytic enzyme function. Am J Obstet Gynecol 1979;134:743.

Freid MA, Vosti KL. The importance of underlying disease in patients with gram-negative bacteremia. Arch Intern Med 1968;121:418.

Gattinoni L, Brazzi L, Pelosi P, et al. A trial of goal-oriented hemodynamic therapy in critically ill patients. N Engl J Med 1995;333:1025.

Genazzani AR, Facchinetti F, Parrini D. β-lipotrophin and β-endorphin plasma levels during pregnancy. Clin Endocrinol 1981;14:409.

Gibbs CE, Locke WE. Maternal deaths in Texas, 1969 to 1973. Am J Obstet Gynecol 1976;126:687.

Gibbs RS, Blanco JD, Hrilica VS. Quantitative bacteriology of amniotic fluid. J Infect Dis 1982;145:1.

Gibbs RS, Jones PM, Wilder CJ. Antibiotic therapy of endometritis following cesarean section: treatment successes and failures. Obstet Gynecol 1978;52:31.

Goetzl EJ, Payan DG, Goldman DW. Immunopathogenic roles of leukotrienes in human diseases. J Clin Immunol 1984;4:79.

Goldberg LI. Dopamine: clinical uses of an endogenous catecholamine. N Engl J Med 1974;291:707.

Goldie AS, Fearon KCH, Ross JA, et al. Natural cytokine antagonists and endogenous antiendotoxin core antibodies in sepsis syndrome. JAMA 1995;274:172.

Greenman RL, Schein RMH, Martin MA, et al. A controlled clinical trial of E5 murine monoclonal IgM antibody to endotoxin in the treatment of gram-negative sepsis. JAMA 1991;266:1097.

Gutierrez G, Lund N, Bryan-Brown CW. Cellular oxygen utilization during multiple organ failure. Crit Care Clin 1989;5:271.

Gys T, Hubens A, Neels H, et al. Prognostic value of gastric intramural pH in surgical intensive care patients. Crit Care Med 1988;16:1222.

Hageman JR, Caplan MS. An introduction to the structure and function of inflammatory mediators for clinicians. Clin Perinatol 1995;22:251.

Hankins G, Clark S, Uckan E. Intrapulmonary shunt (QS/QT) and position in healthy third-trimester pregnancy. Am J Obstet Gynecol 1996;174:322A.

Hardaway RM. Prediction of survival or death of patients in a state of severe shock. Surg Gynecol Obstet 1981;152:200.

Haupt MT, Rackow EC. Colloid osmotic pressure and fluid resuscitation with hetastarch, albumin, and saline solutions. Crit Care Med 1982;10:159.

Hawkins DF. Management and treatment of obstetric bacteremia shock. J Clin Pathol 1980;33:895.

Hayes MA, Timmins AC, Yau EHS, et al. Elevation of systemic oxygen delivery in the treatment of critically ill patients. N Engl J Med 1994;330:1717.

Hesse DG, Tracey KJ, Fong Y, et al. Cytokine appearance in human endotoxemia and primate bacteremia. Surg Gynecol Obstet 1988;166:147.

Hinds C, Watson D. Manipulating hemodynamic and oxygen transport in critically ill patients. N Engl J Med 1995;333:1074.

Holaday JW, Faden AI. Naloxone reversal of endotoxin hypotension suggests role of endorphins in shock. Nature 1978;275:450.

Hollenberg SM, Cunnion RE. Endothelial and vascular smooth muscle function in sepsis. J Crit Care 1994;9:262.

Holm SE. Invasive group A streptococcal infections. N Engl J Med 1996;335:590.

Hooper RG, Kearl RA. Established ARDS treatment with a sustained course of adrenocortical steroids. Chest 1990;97:138.

Jacobs RF, Tabor DR. Immune cellular interactions during sepsis and septic injury. Crit Care Clin 1989;5:9.

Jacobs RF, Tabor DR, Lary CH, et al. Interleukin-1 production by alveolar macrophages and monocytes from ARDS and pneumonia patients compared to controls. Am Rev Respir Dis 1988;137:228.

Kaufman BS, Rackow EC, Falk JL. The relationship between oxygen delivery and consumption during fluid resuscitation of hypovolemic and septic shock. Chest 1984;85:33.

Knuppel RA, Papineni SR, Cavanagh D. Septic shock in obstetrics. Clin Obstet Gynecol 1984;27:3.

Kwaan HM, Weil MH. Differences in the mechanism of shock caused by infections. Surg Gynecol Obstet 1969;128:37.

Lachman E, Pitsoe SB, Gaffin SL. Antilipopolysaccharide immunotherapy in management of septic shock of obstetric and gynaecologic origin. Lancet 1984;1:981.

Ledger WJ, Norman M, Gee C, et al. Bacteremia on an obstetric-gynecologic service. Am J Obstet Gynecol 1975;121:205.

Lee W, Clark SL, Cotton DB, et al. Septic shock during pregnancy. Am J Obstet Gynecol 1988;159:410.

Lee W, Clark SL, Cotton DB, et al. Septic shock during pregnancy. Obstet Gynecol 1984;159:410.

Lee W, Cotton DB, Hankins GDV, et al. Management of septic shock complicating pregnancy. Obstet Gynecol Surv 1989;16:431.

Levi M, ten Cate H, van der Poll T, et al. Pathogenesis of disseminated intravascular coagulation in sepsis. JAMA 1993;270:975.

Lewis BS, Gotsman MS. Current concepts of left ventricular relaxation and compliance. Am Heart J 1980;99:101.

Lindeborg DM, Pearl RG. Recent advances in critical care medicine: inotropic therapy in the critically ill patient. Int Anesthesiol Clin 1993;31:49.

Lloyd T, Dougherty J, Karlen J. Infected intrauterine pregnancy presenting as septic shock. Ann Emerg Med 1983;12:707.

Lowthian JT, Gillard LJ. Postpartum necrotizing faciitis. Obstet Gynecol 1980;56:661.

Lucas CE. A new look at dopamine and norepinephrine for hyperdynamic septic shock. Chest 1994;105:7.

Lynn WA, Cohen J. Science and clinical practice: management of septic shock. J Infect 1995;30:207.

Lynn WA, Golenbock DT. Lipopolysaccharide antagonists. Immunol Today 1992;13:271.

MacKenzie SJ, Kapadia F, Nimmo GR, et al. Adrenaline in treatment of septic shock: effects on hemodynamics and oxygen transport. Intensive Care Med 1991;17:36.

Mainous MR, Deitch EA. Nutrition and infection. Surg Clin North Am 1994;74:659.

Makabali GL, Mandal AK, Morris JA. An assessment of the participatory role of prostaglandins and serotonin in the pathophysiology of endotoxic shock. Am J Obstet Gynecol 1983;145:439.

Marik PE, Mohedin M. The contrasting effects of dopamine and norepinephrine on systemic and splanchnic oxygen utilization in hyperdynamic sepsis. JAMA 1994;272:1354.

Marione FG, Ismail MA. Clostridium perfringens septicemia following cesarean section. Obstet Gynecol 1980;56:518.

Marksad AK, Ona CJ, Stuart RC, et al. Myocardial depression in septic shock: physiologic and metabolic effect of a plasma factor on an isolated heart. Circ Shock 1979;1(suppl):35.

Martin C, Papazian L, Perrin G, et al. Norepinephrine or dopamine for the treatment of hyperdynamic septic shock? Chest 1993;103:1826.

Mayoral JL, Schweich CJ, Dunn DL. Decreased tumor necrosis factor production during the initial stages of infection correlates with survival during murine gram-negative sepsis. Arch Surg 1990;125:24.

Meadows D, Edwards JD, Wilkins RG, et al. Reversal of intractable septic shock with norepinephrine therapy. Crit Care Med 1988;16:663.

Meduri GU, Belenchia JM, Estes RJ, et al. Fibroproliferative phase of ARDS: clinical findings and effects of corticosteroids. Chest 1991;100:943.

Mei CT, Feeley TW. Coagulopathies and the intensive care setting. Int Anesthesiol Clin 1993;31:97.

Metcalfe J, Ueland K. Maternal cardiovascular adjustments to pregnancy. Prog Cardiovasc Dis 1974;16:363.

Michie HR, Manogue KR, Spriggs DR, et al. Detection of circulating tumor necrosis factor after endotoxin administrations. N Engl J Med 1988a;318:1481.

Michie HR, Spriggs DR, Manogue KB, et al. Tumor necrosis factor and endotoxin induce similar metabolic responses in human beings. Surgery 1988b;104:280.

Miller TR, Anderson RJ, Linas SL, et al. Urinary diagnostic indices in acute renal failure. Ann Intern Med 1978;89:47.

Monif GRG, Baer H. Polymicrobial bacteremia in obstetric patients. Obstet Gynecol 1976;48:167.

Moore FA, Haenel JB, Moore EE, et al. Incommensurate oxygen consumption in response to maximal oxygen availability predicts postinjury multiple organ failure. J Trauma 1992;33:58.

Moran JL, O'Fathartaign MS, Peisach AR, et al. Epinephrine as an inotropic agent in septic shock: a dose-profile analysis. Crit Care Med 1993; 21:70.

Morishima HO, Niemann WH, James LS. Effects of endotoxin on the pregnant baboon and fetus. Am J Obstet Gynecol 1978;131:899.

Natanson C, Hoffman WD, Suffredini AF, et al. Selected treatment strategies for shock based on proposed mechanisms of pathogenesis. Ann Intern Med 1994;120:771.

O'Brien WF, Cefalo RC, Lewis PE, et al. The role of prostaglandins in endotoxemia and comparisons in response in the nonpregnancy, maternal, and fetal models. Am J Obstet Gynecol 1981;139:535.

Oettinger WKE, Walter GO, Jensen UM, et al. Endogenous prostaglandin $F_2$ in the hyperdynamic state of severe sepsis in man. Br J Surg 1983; 70:237.

Ognibene FP, Parker MM, Natanson C, et al. Depressed left ventricular performance: response to volume infusion in patients with sepsis and septic shock. Chest 1988;93:903.

Okusawa S, Gelfand JA, Ikejima T, et al. Interleukin 1 induces a shock-like state in rabbits: synergism with tumor necrosis factor and the effect of cyclooxygenase inhibition. J Clin Invest 1988;81:1162.

Packman MI, Rackow EC. Optimum left heart filling pressure during fluid resuscitation of patients with hypovolemic and septic shock. Crit Care Med 1983;11:165.

Parker MM, Parillo JE. Septic shock: hemodynamics and pathogenesis. JAMA 1983;250:3324.

Parker MM, Shelhamer JH, Bacharach SL, et al. Profound but reversible myocardial depression in patients with septic shock. Ann Intern Med 1984;100:483.

Parrillo JE. Mechanisms of disease: pathogenetic mechanisms of septic shock. N Engl J Med 1993;328:1471.

Parrillo JE. Cardiovascular dysfunction in septic shock: new insights into a deadly disease. Int J Cardiol 1985a;7:314.

Parrillo JE, Burch C, Shelhamer JH, et al. A circulating myocardial depressant substance in humans with septic shock: septic shock patients with a reduced ejection fraction have a circulating factor that depresses in vitro myocardial cell performance. J Clin Invest 1985b;76:1539.

Pinsky MR, Matuschak GM. Multiple systems organ failure: failure of host defense homeostasis. Crit Care Clin 1989;5:199.

Poggetti RS, Moore FA, Moore EE, et al. Liver injury is a reversible neutrophil-mediated event following gut ischemia. Arch Surg 1992;127:175.

Porembka DT. Cardiovascular abnormalities in sepsis. New Horiz 1993;2:324.

Pritchard JA, MacDonald PC, Gant NF, eds. Maternal adaption to pregnancy. In: Williams obstetrics. 20th ed. Norwalk, CT: Appleton-Century-Crofts, 1997.

Progress in Chronic Disease Prevention. Chronic disease reports: deaths from nine types of chronic disease—United States, 1986. MMWR 1990;39:30.

Rackow EC, Astiz ME, Weil MH. Cellular oxygen metabolism during sepsis and shock: the relationship of oxygen consumption to oxygen delivery. JAMA 1988;259:1989.

Rackow EC, Falk JL, Fein IA, et al. Fluid resuscitation in circulatory shock: a comparison of the cardiorespiratory effects of albumin, hetastarch, and saline solutions in patients with hypovolemic and septic shock. Crit Care Med 1983;11:839.

Rackow EC, Fein IA, Leppo J. Colloid osmotic pressure as a prognostic indicator of pulmonary edema and mortality in the critically ill. Chest 1977;72:709.

Rackow EC, Fein IA, Siegel J. The relationship of the colloid osmotic–pulmonary artery wedge pressure gradient to pulmonary edema and mortality in critically ill patients. Chest 1982;82:433.

Rackow EC, Kaufman BS, Falk JL, et al. Hemodynamic response to fluid repletion in patients with septic shock: evidence for early depression of cardiac performance. Circ Shock 1987; 22:11.

Rackow EC, Weil MK. Recent trends in diagnosis and management of septic shock. Curr Surg 1983;40:181.

Rangel-Frausto MS, Pittet D, Costigan M, et al. The natural history of the systemic inflammatory response syndrome (SIRS). JAMA 1995;273:117.

Rao PS, Cavanagh D. Endotoxic shock in the premate: some effects of dopamine administration. Am J Obstet Gynecol 1982;144:61.

Rao PS, Cavanagh D, Gaston LW. Endotoxic shock in the primate: effects of aspirin and dipyridamole administration. Am J Obstet Gynecol 1981;140:914.

Reimer LG, Reller LB. Gardnerella vaginalis bacteremia: a review of thirty cases. Obstet Gynecol 1984;64:170.

Remick DG, Kunkel RG, Larrick JW, et al. Acute *in vivo* effects of human recombinant tumor necrosis factor. Lab Invest 1987;56:583.

Riddington DW, Venkatesh B, Boivin CM, et al. Intestinal permeability, gastric intramucosal pH, and systemic endotoxemia in patients undergoing cardiopulmonary bypass. JAMA 1996; 275:1007.

Roberts JM, Laros RK. Hemorrhagic and endotoxic shock: a pathophysiologic approach to diagnosis and management. Am J Obstet Gynecol 1971;110:1041.

Rolbin SH, Levinson G, Shnider DM, et al. Dopamine treatment of spinal hypotension decreases uterine blood flow in the pregnant ewe. Anesthesiology 1979;51:36.

Sauve JS, Cook DJ. Gastrointestinal hemorrhage and ischemia: prevention and treatment. Int Anesthesiol Clin 1993;31:169.

Schirmer WJ, Schirmer JM, Naff GB, et al. Systemic complement activation produces hemodynamic changes characteristic of sepsis. Arch Surg 1988;123:316.

Sculier JP, Bron D, Verboven N, et al. Multiple organ failure during interleukin-2 and LAK cell infusion. Intensive Care Med 1988;14:666.

Shippy CR, Appel PL, Shoemaker WC. Reliability of clinical monitoring to assess blood volume in critically ill patients. Crit Care Med 1984;12:107.

Shoemaker WC, Appel PL, Bland R, et al. Clinical trial of an algorithm for outcome prediction in acute circulatory failure. Crit Care Med 1983; 11:165.

Shoemaker WC, Appel PL, Kram HB. Oxygen transport measurements to evaluate tissue perfusion and titrate therapy: dobutamine and dopamine effects. Crit Care Med 1991;19:672.

Shoemaker WC, Appel PL, Kram HB. Role of oxygen debt in the development of organ failure sepsis, and death in high-risk surgical patients. Chest 1992;102:208.

Shoemaker WC, Appel PL, Kram HB, et al. Prospective trial of supranormal values of survivors as therapeutic goals in high-risk surgical patients. Chest 1988;94:1176.

Shoemaker WC, Kram HB, Appel PL, et al. The efficacy of central venous and pulmonary artery catheters and therapy based upon them in reducing mortality and morbidity. Arch Surg 1990;125:1332.

Shoemaker WC, Montgomery ES, Kaplan E, et al. Physiologic patterns in surviving and nonsurviving shock patients. Arch Surg 1973;106:630.

Sibbald WJ, Fox G, Martin C. Abnormalities of vascular reactivity in the sepsis syndrome. Chest 1991;100:155S.

Siegel JH, Greenspan M, Del Guercio LRM. Abnormal vascular tone, defective oxygen transport and myocardial failure in human septic shock. Ann Surg 1967;165:504.

Sprung CL, Caralis PV, Marcial EH, et al. The effects of high-dose corticosteroids in patients with septic shock. N Engl J Med 1984;311:1137.

Sriskandan S, Cohen J. Science and clinical practice: the pathogenesis of septic shock. J Infect 1995; 30:201.

Sugerman HJ, Peyton JWR, Greenfield LJ. Gram-negative sepsis. Curr Probl Surg 1981.

Swan HJ, Ganz W, Forrester J, et al. Catheterization of the heart in man with use of a flow-directed balloon-tipped catheter. N Engl J Med 1970; 283:447.

Tabor DR, Burchett SK, Jacobs RF. Enhanced production of monokines by canine alveolar macrophages in response to endotoxin-induced shock (42681). Proc Soc Exp Biol Med 1988;187:408.

Tewari K, Wold SM, Asrat T. Septic shock in pregnancy associated with legionella pneumonia: Case report. Am J Obstet Gynecol 1997;176:706.

The Veterans Administration Systemic Sepsis Cooperative Study Group. Effect of high-dose glucocorticoid therapy on mortality in patients with clinical signs of systemic sepsis. N Engl J Med 1987;317:659.

Tracey KJ, Beutler B, Lowry SF, et al. Shock and tissue injury induced by recombinant human cachectin. Science 1986;234:470.

Tracey KJ, Lowry SF, Fahey TJ III, et al. Cachectin/ tumor necrosis factor induces lethal shock and stress hormone responses in the dog. Surg Gynecol Obstet 1987a;164:415.

Tracey KJ, Fong Y, Hesse DG, et al. Anti-cachectin/ TNF monoclonal antibodies prevent septic shock during lethal bacteriaemia. Nature 1987b; 330:662.

Tracey KJ, Lowry SF, Cerami A. The pathophysiologic role of cachectin/TNF in septic shock and cachexia. Ann Institut Pasteur 1988;139:311.

Tryba M. Risk of acute stress bleeding and nosocomial pneumonia in ventilated intensive care unit patients: sucralfate versus antacids. Am J Med 1987;83:117.

Tuchschmidt J, Fried J, Astiz M, et al. Elevation of cardiac output and oxygen delivery improves outcome in septic shock. Chest 1992;102:216.

Tuchschmidt J, Oblitas D, Fried JC. Oxygen consumption in sepsis and septic shock. Crit Care Med 1991;19:664.

Vada P. Elevated plasma phospholipase $A_2$ levels: correlation with the hemodynamic and pulmonary changes in gram-negative septic shock. J Lab Clin Med 1984;104:873.

Van Bebber PT, Boekholz WKF, Goris RJA, et al. Neutrophil function and lipid peroxidation in a rat model of multiple organ failure. J Surg Res 1989;47:471.

Wagner BKJ, D'Amelio LF. Pharmacologic and clinical considerations in selecting crystalloid, colloidal, and oxygen-carrying resuscitation fluids, part 2. Clin Pharm 1993;12:415.

Warren HS, Danner RL, Munford RS. Anti-endotoxin monoclonal antibodies. N Engl J Med 1992; 326:1153.

Webb SR, Gascoigne NRJ. T-cell activation by superantigens. Curr Opin Immunol 1994;6:467.

Weigelt JA, Norcross JF, Borman KR, et al. Early steroid therapy for respiratory failure. Arch Surg 1985;120:536.

Weil MH, Henning RJ, Morissette M, et al. Relationship between colloid osmotic pressure and pulmonary artery wedge pressure in patients with acute cardiorespiratory failure. Am J Med 1978a;64:643.

Weil MN, Nishijima H. Cardiac output in bacterial shock. Am J Med 1978b;64:920.

Wenzel RP. Monoclonal antibodies and the treatment of gram-negative bacteremia and shock. N Engl J Med 1991;324:486.

Wernstein MP, Murphy JR, Retter LB, et al. The clinical significance of positive blood cultures: a comparative analysis of 500 episodes of bacteremia and fungemia in adults. Rev Infect Dis 1983;5:54.

Wojnar MM, Hawkins WG, Lang CH. Nutritional support of the septic patient. Crit Care Clin 1995;11:717.

Yu M, Levy MM, Smith P, et al. Effect of maximizing oxygen delivery on morbidity and mortality rates in critically ill patients: a prospective, randomized, controlled study. Crit Care Med 1993; 21:830.

Ziegler EJ, Fisher CJ Jr, Sprung CL, et al. Treatment of gram-negative bacteremia and septic shock with HA-1A human monoclonal antibody against endotoxin. N Engl J Med 1991;324:429.

Ziegler TR, Smith RJ, O'Dwyer ST, et al. Increased intestinal permeability associated with infection in burn patients. Arch Surg 1988;123:1313.

# CHAPTER *23*

# Anaphylactic Shock

*H*istorically, the first description of anaphylaxis, the sudden death of an Egyptian pharaoh after a wasp sting, may have been recorded in the hieroglyphics, circa 2640 B.C. (Fig 23-1). The term *anaphylaxis* was first introduced in 1902 (Portier and Richet, 1902) and was used initially to denote a paradoxical effect that occurred with a particular experimental protocol. Attempting to induce improved tolerance or resistance to a toxin derived from the sea anemone, they repeatedly injected large but sublethal doses into dogs. After several weeks had passed, they observed unexpectedly that when reinjected with much smaller doses of the toxin, some dogs died within minutes. This dramatic and unexpected fatal response was the opposite (*ana* from Greek, meaning "back, backwards") of protection (*phylax*' from Greek, meaning "guard"). Later, Richet was awarded the Nobel prize in medicine and physiology for his innovating work in the area.

Although anaphylaxis is a rare event, this dramatic syndrome may occur during a number of

FIGURE **23-1**

Egyptian hieroglyphic describing the death of a pharaoh following a reaction to the sting of a wasp.

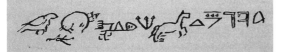

common obstetric procedures and treatments. Therefore, the obstetrician should be well versed in the diagnosis and management of this life-threatening condition.

## Classification

*Hypersensitivity* is the term applied when an adaptive immune response occurs in an exaggerated or inappropriate form, causing cellular destruction and tissue damage. Four types of hypersensitivity reactions have been described (Roitt, 1985). Because these reactions are normal immune responses occurring in an exaggerated form, each type does not necessarily occur at the exclusion of another. Type I, or immediate hypersensitivity, occurs when antigen binds and cross-links immunoglobulin E (IgE)-sensitized mast cells and basophils, resulting in release of pharmacologic mediators such as histamine, serine proteases, and cytokines. Type II, or antibody-dependent cytotoxic hypersensitivity, develops when antibody binds to antigen on cells, leading to phagocytosis, killer-cell activity, or complement-mediated lysis. Type III, or immune complex–mediated hypersensitivity, occurs when immune complexes are deposited in tissues, promoting complement activation and resulting in tissue damage. Finally, type IV, or delayed hypersensitivity, is produced when antigen-sensitized

T cells release lymphokines following a secondary contact with the same antigen, producing an exaggerated immune response.

Anaphylaxis is the cascade of events that occurs in a sensitized individual on subsequent exposure to the sensitizing antigen. The spectrum of events ranges from a localized response to a catastrophic and life-threatening systemic reaction. Anaphylaxis most commonly refers to IgE-mediated, type I hypersensitivity response, produced by antigen-stimulated mast-cell mediator release. A clinically indistinguishable syndrome, anaphylactoid reaction, may occur, involving similar mediators but not requiring IgE antibody or previous exposure to the inciting substance. Anaphylaxis and anaphylactoid reactions have been classified further based on etiology. These classifications include IgE-mediated reactions, complement-mediated reactions, nonimmunologic mast-cell activation, exposure to modulators of arachidonic metabolism or sulfiting agents, exercise-induced anaphylaxis, catamenial anaphylaxis, and idiopathic recurrent anaphylaxis (Atkinson, 1992).

## IgE-Mediated Anaphylaxis

Common sources of antigens triggering IgE-mediated anaphylaxis include antibiotics, insulin, *Hymenoptera* venom, foods, seminal plasma, and latex proteins. IgE-mediated anaphylaxis represents a type I hypersensitivity reaction. Necessary components of this reaction include a sensitizing antigen; an IgE-class antibody reaction, resulting in the systemic sensitization of mast cells and basophils; reintroduction of the sensitizing antigen; and mediator release from mast cells and basophils (Atkinson, 1992). Either antigens or haptens may elicit IgE antibody production. Haptens are molecules too small to initiate an immune response independently. However, they may bind to other endogenous proteins and become antigenic. Penicillin and related antibiotics are probably the most important of all haptens. Typically, penicillin is metabolized to a major determinant, benzylpenicilloyl, and an additional series of minor determinants, including penicilloate, penilloate, penicilloyl-amine, and penicillin itself.

These haptens elicit penicillin-specific IgE antibodies and may be found in 4% to 10% of persons who have received penicillin therapy.

## Complement-Mediated Reactions

Various frequently administered blood products, including whole blood, serum, plasma, fractionated serum products, and immunoglobulins, are the inciting agents of other anaphylactic responses. A type III hypersensitive reaction with complement-mediated cellular destruction is one of the mechanisms causing these reactions. Complement activation with the generation of the anaphylatoxins, C3a, C4a, and C5a cause mast-cell degranulation, mediator release and generation, and the subsequent systemic reactions, including an increased vascular permeability and smooth muscle contraction. A cytotoxic antibody-mediated reaction, or type II hypersensitivity, with subsequent complement activation can also cause anaphylaxis in this setting. Mismatched blood transfusion may promote lysis of RBCs and mast-cell degranulation and result in a similar life-threatening reaction (see Chapter 11).

## Nonimmunologic Mast-Cell Activators (Anaphylactoid Reactions)

A myriad of agents, including radiocontrast media, narcotics, depolarizing agents, and dextrans, may directly cause mast-cell mediator release and anaphylactoid reactions. Radiocontrast media has long been recognized as a cause of anaphylactoid reaction (Bush, 1990, 1991; Lieberman, 1986, 1991a, 1991b; Weese, 1993; Keizur, 1994). Mild reactions occur in approximately 5% of individuals receiving radiocontrast dyes; fatal reactions are much less common (Grammar, 1986; Lieberman, 1986). Two types of reactions to radiographic contrast have been described, including a dose-independent, unpredictable anaphylactoid reaction and a dose-dependent, predictable physicochemical reaction (Wittbrodt, 1994). The use of a lower-osmolar contrast media is associated with a lower incidence of reactions. Wittbrodt and Spinler recommend a lower osmolar contrast, pretreatment with a corticosteroid and an H$_1$-antagonist, and preparation for an anaphylactoid response in high-risk patients requiring a procedure with radiocontrast media. A *high-risk patient* was defined as one having a history of previous anaphylactoid reaction to radiographic contrast, asthma, and reaction to skin allergens or penicillin. More recently, Clark et al (1995) documented the clinically anaphylactoid nature of amniotic fluid embolism.

Both immune- and non-immune-mediated anaphylaxis involves the release of primary and secondary mediators. Those derived from mast cells and basophils are termed *primary mediators,* and include histamine; prostaglandins D2, E2, and F2 alpha; leukotrienes C4, D4, and E4 (formerly known as slow-reacting substance of anaphylaxis); platelet-activating factor, and eosinophil and neutrophil chemotactic factors. Physiologic effects of these primary mediators include altered vascular tone, increased vascular permeability, bronchial smooth-muscle contraction, increased heart rate and contractility, and platelet aggregation. The effects of PGD2 on vascular tone may be especially pronounced (Austen, 1994). These primary mediators also set into effect the cascading release of secondary mediators of anaphylaxis. These include components of the complement system, leading to further membrane injury, increased vascular permeability, and smooth-muscle contraction, as well as activation of the kinin system and intrinsic clotting cascade, the latter leading to disseminated intravascular coagulation. Myocardial depression is also seen in association with such mediator release; the marked coronary artery constriction seen with experimental administration of the cysteinyl leukotrienes may be involved in this process (Raper, 1988; Austen, 1994).

## Hemodynamic Changes

Because the onset of anaphylactic shock has been observed in the setting of intense medical supervision, the hemodynamic evolution of this syndrome has been well delineated (Moss, 1981; Nicolas, 1984). Two phases have been observed: a hyperkinetic phase followed by a hypokinetic phase. The hyperkinetic phase lasts 2 to 3 minutes and involves a fall in systemic vascular resistance and hypotension. However, the combination of tachycardia and an increase in the systolic ejection volume results in a rapid rise in cardiac output. Central venous pressure and pulmonary capillary pressure initially remain stable. This is followed by a hypokinetic phase characterized by continued histamine-mediated vasodilation, hypotension, and tachycardia. The central venous pressure and pulmonary capillary wedge pressure decline. Due to capillary stasis resulting from vasodilation, a rise in hydrostatic pressure in the capillary is seen, favoring interstitial fluid accumulation. This loss of intravascular fluid is superimposed on a relative hypovolemia resulting from vasodilatation, and cardiac output eventually falls. These hemodynamic changes may be complicated further by the development of myocardial depression and disseminated intravascular coagulation (Kapin, 1985; Wong, 1990; Silverman, 1984; Austen, 1994).

## Obstetric Antecedents to Anaphylaxis

More than 50 case reports describing the occurrence of anaphylaxis in association with common obstetric procedures and therapeutic regimens have been described. Anaphylaxis may occur at any time during gestation. Intravenous (IV) antibiotics, oxytocin, anesthetic agents, and blood products are some of the more common causes of anaphylaxis in pregnancy. A rare case of anaphylaxis to laminaria used for a therapeutic abortion has even been described (Nguyen, 1995).

## Antibiotics

Due to the rapid increase and diversification of antibiotic agents, there has been a concordant increase in the recommendations for the usage of antibiotics for both prophylaxis and treatment of obstetric infections. Penicillin and its derivatives are the most common causes of drug reactions. From 0.6% to 10.0% of patients exhibit some form of hypersensitivity to penicillin. Fortunately, most reactions are mild; the incidence of anaphylaxis is reported as only 0.04% to 0.2% of patients receiving these drugs (Mandell, 1990). Approximately 0.001% of patients so treated die of anaphylaxis. Of those who experience fatal reactions, 15% have a history of other types of allergy. Seventy percent of patients with fatal reactions have received penicillin previously—two thirds of these without a reaction. Disturbingly, one third of patients succumbing to penicillin anaphyaxis have a history of prior reaction to these agents (Idsoe, 1968). Anaphylaxis may be seen following IV, oral, or subcutaneous administration of penicillin.

Up to 20% of patients with known penicillin allergy show immunologic cross-reactivity to cephalosporins (Levine, 1973), but only about 1% show actual clinical reaction to this class of drugs (Saxon, 1987). Such clinical cross-reactivity cannot be predicted on the basis of skin tests (Mandell, 1990). As a general rule, patients with a history of minor reactions to penicillin may be given cephalosporins when clinically indicated. In patients with a history of anaphylaxis, however, cephalosporin administration should be withheld unless no acceptable alternative antibiotic is available (Anderson, 1986).

The incidence of penicillin-induced anaphylaxis has been reported to be 10 to 50 per 100,000 injections (Rudolph, 1973; Idsoe, 1968). Fatal cases of penicillin-induced anaphylaxis have been estimated at 100 to 500 annually in the United States (Parker, 1963). There is no convincing evidence of risk factors such as age, sex, race, occupation, or geographic location for identifying individuals who are at increased risk. Most studies conclude that atopy does not predispose individuals to anaphylaxis from penicillin therapy or venom of a stinging insect (Austen, 1994).

Penicillin remains the treatment of choice for syphilis during pregnancy. If skin testing confirms the risk of IgE-mediated allergic reaction to penicillin, then penicillin desensitization is recommended and is followed by benzathine penicillin G treatment (Wendel, 1985). Selective prophylactic antibiotic usage for the prevention of neonatal group B streptococcal sepsis (ACOG, 1992) and for the prevention of endomyometritis after cesarean section (DePalma, 1982) is now

common. Gallaghen (1988) reported a case of anaphylaxis in response to IV ampicillin for treatment of chorioamnionitis. Anaphylaxis secondary to IV cefotetan administered as surgical prophylaxis for cesarean section and transabdominal hysterectomy has also been described (Bloomberg, 1988). As the use of antibiotics for an increasing number of obstetric indications becomes standard, the frequency of antibiotic-induced anaphylaxis may be encountered more commonly.

## Oxytocic Agents

Syntocinon contains the active ingredient oxytocin and the inactive ingredients sodium acetate, chlorobutanol, ethanol, and acetic acid. Chlorobutanol is widely used for its bacteriostatic properties as a preservative for injectables such as oxytocin. Three cases of anaphylactic shock from chlorobutanol-preserved oxytocin have been described (Slater, 1985; Hoffman, 1986; Maycock, 1993; Morriss, 1994). Hoffman et al reported a case of anaphylactic shock that occurred after injection of oxytocin-containing chlorobutanol during an elective termination of pregnancy. Subsequent scratch testing on the forearm with both oxytocin and chlorobutanol yielded a positive reaction to chlorobutanol and no reaction to oxytocin. Maycock and Russell (1993) described a gravida who required an emergency cesarean section for fetal distress. Immediately after delivery of the infant, 5 units of Syntocinon were given. This was followed by profound hypotension and laryngeal edema. Subsequent skin testing revealed chlorobutanol to be responsible for the reaction. A third case, reported by Morriss et al (1994), detailed the occurrence of anaphylaxis during an elective cesarean for breech presentation. Anaphylactoid reaction due solely to oxytocin during cesarean was described by Kawarabayashi et al (1988). In this case, an elective cesarean section under epidural anesthesia with mepivacaine was performed. Following delivery of the baby, 5 units of oxytocin were injected directly into the myometrium and another 5 units were added to the infusion bottle. Within minutes, the patient developed numbness, perioral and periorbital erythema, and edema. Severe and prolonged hypotension that failed to respond to 500 mg of hydrocortisone and 20 mg of ephedrine, but finally improved with 0.05 mg of epinephrine, was observed. Later, intradermal testing with 0.02 mL of oxytocin (5 units/mL) showed a markedly positive reaction at 15 and 30 minutes. Although reactions to Syntocinon and oxytocin are rare, this possibility should always be kept in mind by the practicing obstetrician.

## Methotrexate

Methotrexate is sometimes used for the treatment of ectopic pregnancies in women who want to preserve fertility. In addition, methotrexate is the first line of therapy for persistent gestational trophoblastic disease. Systemic anaphylaxis from low-dose methotrexate has been reported (Cohn, 1993). These authors describe the acute onset of symptoms consisting of burning in the mouth followed by diffuse cutaneous erythema, dyspnea, cyanosis, hypotension, and respiratory arrest following the IV infusion of methotrexate as adjuvant chemotherapy for breast cancer. The patient required endotracheal intubation during the acute episode and subsequently recovered. Intradermal injection testing with methotrexate was done, which supported methotrexate as the offending agent. With this in mind, it seems of paramount importance to be familiar with the diagnosis and management of anaphylaxis when using this chemotherapeutic agent.

## Latex

The combination of latex allergy and overt anaphylaxis is being reported with increasing frequency (ACAAI, 1995). Both delayed (type IV) hypersensitivity and immediate (type I) hypersensitivity reactions have been attributed to latex exposure (Tomazic, 1992). Nutter initially described latex-induced allergic reactions in 1979. Since that time, more severe reactions to latex gloves, Foley catheters, and endotracheal tubes have been reported (Zenarola, 1989; Gerber, 1990; Moneret-Vautrin, 1990; Swartz, 1990). Several cases reports exist of anaphylaxis after latex contact during vaginal or cesarean delivery (Tur-

janmaa, 1988; Fisher, 1992). Laurent (1992) detailed a patient who developed an anaphylactic reaction following manual extraction of a placenta. This patient underwent a number of tests, including skin prick tests, intradermal tests, and IgE levels, which all confirmed latex contact as the triggering event. Infants with spina bifida are at increased risk for severe, systemic reactions to latex and should be delivered and handled by medical personnel wearing and using nonlatex gloves and supplies (Ledger, 1992; Kelly, 1994; Lu, 1995; Nieto, 1996).

## Colloid Solutions

The most commonly used colloid solutions, including human serum albumin, dextran, gelatin, and hydroxyethyl starch, may evoke anaphylactoid reactions (Guharoy, 1991; Ring, 1991; Stafford, 1988). In addition, dextran solutions are known for their antithrombotic effect. A number of case reports emphasize fetal morbidity due to anaphylactoid reactions associated with dextran (Berg, 1991; Barbier, 1992). Barbier and colleagues describe a mother who fainted, developed urticaria, and had mild respiratory distress following dextran infusion. Hypotension was not observed. The infusion was stopped, and a dead neonate was delivered. Berg et al (1991) described three severe cases of dextran-induced anaphylactoid reactions despite immunoprophylaxis with dextran-I hapten. In one of the cases, a patient was given dextran-70 prior to cesarean section and had a mild reaction, but, unfortunately, she gave birth to a child with serious brain damage. Of note in both of these cases was the observation that, despite apparently mild maternal reactions without hypotension, the fetuses were affected severely. Such observations are seen commonly in maternal shock of any etiology and reflect preferential maternal shunting of blood away from the splanchnic bed (including uterus) to maintain central pressure in shock states. Paull (1987) performed a prospective study of dextran-induced anaphylactoid reactions in 5745 gynecologic and obstetric patients who received IV dextran-70 solution. In this study, an incidence of 1:383 reactions per patient treated was observed, and concluded that the risks of dextran-70 treatment exceeded the risks of thromboembolism in this patient population.

## Modulators of Arachidonic Acid Metabolism

The "aspirin triad" includes chronic sinusitis, nasal polyposis, and asthma. Approximately 5% to 10% of patients with this condition will develop a reaction, which may include vasomotor collapse in response to nonsteroidal antiinflammatory drugs. This appears to be a non-IgE-mediated anaphylactoid reaction similar to that seen with contrast medium.

## Sulfiting Agents and Food Allergy

Sulfiting agents are used commonly as preservatives to prevent food discoloration. These preservatives are added to leafy green salads, fruits, wine, beer, dehydrated soups, and fish. Intake of these agents may cause asthma and anaphylaxis in susceptible persons (Nicklas, 1989). Similar reactions may occur in susceptible women following ingestion of peanuts or shellfish (Fig 23-2).

## Exercise-Induced Anaphylaxis

Exercise-induced anaphylaxis is a well-recognized syndrome (Sheffer, 1983, 1984, 1985; Songsiridej, 1983; Kobayashi, 1991; Briner, 1992; Nichols, 1992; Hough, 1994) and has been diagnosed with increasing frequency during the past 20 years. The pathophysiology is somewhat controversial, but the most likely explanation is a combination of heat and water loss leading to endogenous mediator release. Smith (1985) described an interesting case of delivery as a cause of exercise-induced anaphylactoid reaction. This patient was a previously healthy 29-year-old woman whose medical history was significant for a severe anaphylactoid reaction following an intramuscular (IM) injection of 500 μg of ergometrine during her first delivery. During her second delivery, it was emphasized that "no drugs whatsoever were given." A few minutes after delivery of the placenta, the patient developed symptoms similar

to her first episode of anaphylaxis. An extensive work-up, including testing for immune complexes, IgE levels, serum complement studies, and an estimation of C1 esterase inhibitor, failed to unmask the etiology. From a more in-depth history, it was revealed that as a teenager she had puffy eyes and urticaria most often associated with exercise. Of note, these episodes were not cyclical with menses, and it was concluded that the exertion of labor triggered the sequence of events.

## Clinical Presentation

Early recognition of symptoms and prompt treatment of an anaphylactic reaction are the cornerstone for proper management. There are no risk factors in addition to a previous history of anaphylaxis that can assist in early identification of individuals who may manifest the clinical spectrum of anaphylaxis. Organs primarily involved in humans include those of the cutaneous, gastrointestinal, respiratory, and cardiovascular systems (Table 23-1). Anaphylactic reactions have been classified according to severity of symptoms (Table 23-2). The hallmark of the anaphylactic reaction is the onset of some manifestation within seconds to minutes after introduction (either injection or ingestion) of the antigen substance. The patient may report a sense of impending doom that is coincident with flushing, tachycardia, and often pruritus. These symptoms may progress to signs that include urticaria, angioedema, rhinorrhea, bronchorrhea, nasal congestion, asthma, laryngeal edema, abdominal bloating, nausea, vomiting, cramps, arrhythmias, faintness, syncope, cardiovascular collapse, and ultimately, death.

The clinical presentation of anaphylactic and anaphylactoid reactions has been reviewed (Moneret-Vautrin, 1991). Mucocutaneous signs are often the first warning signs. Pruritus, burning, tingling, and numbness are commonly sensed by the patient. A maculopapular erythematous rash on the face and upper trunk may progress rapidly to generalized urticaria. Periorbital and perioral edema may accompany the rash. Associated symptoms include runny eyes, rhinorrhea, and conjunctival hyperemia. Gastrointestinal

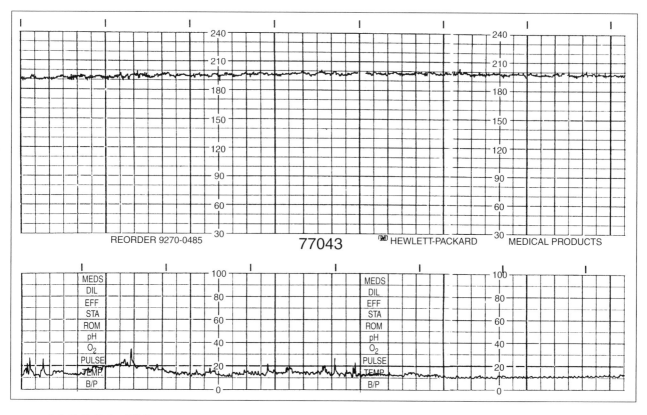

F I G U R E   **23-2**

Fetal heart rate tracing just prior to intrauterine death in a mother
suffering an anaphylactic reaction to a peanut.

T A B L E   **23-1**

Symptoms produced by organ system involved in anaphylactic/
anaphylactoid reactions

| Organ System Involved | Symptoms Produced | Signs Elicited |
|---|---|---|
| Cutaneous | Itching, burning, tingling, numbness, flushing | Rash, swelling, hives |
| Cardiovascular | Faintness, malaise, weakness palpitations, chest discomfort, collapse | Tachycardia, hypotension, arrhythmia, cardiac arrest |
| Respiratory | Congestion, dyspnea, choking, gasping, cough, hoarseness, lump in throat, difficulty swallowing or talking | Tachypnea, rhonchi, laryngeal swelling, pulmonary edema, respiratory arrest |
| Gastrointestinal | Abdominal bloating, cramps, nausea, vomiting, diarrhea, incontinence | Abdominal pain, metallic taste in mouth |
| Fetal | Decreased fetal movement | Late decelerations, tachycardia, diminished variability, bradycardia |

T A B L E 23-2

Severity scale for quantification of intensity of anaphylactic reaction

| Grade | Symptom |
| --- | --- |
| I | Skin symptoms and/or mild fever reaction |
| II | Measurable but not life-threatening cardiovascular reaction (tachycardia, hypotension)<br>Gastrointestinal disturbance<br>Respiratory disturbance |
| III | Shock, life-threatening spasm of smooth muscle, such as bronchi or uterus |
| IV | Cardiac or respiratory arrest |

Source: Modified from Ring J, Messmer K. Incidence and severity of anaphylactoid reactions to colloid volume substitutes. Lancet 1997;i:466.

disturbances consist of nausea, vomiting, diarrhea, and abdominal pains. A tendency for hypothermia (between 35°C and 36°C) is seen, and rarely, hyperpyrexia (38°C to 39°C) may be manifest. Respiratory signs often present in the form of a dry cough, tachypnea, and wheezing secondary to bronchospasm. Laryngeal edema may make intubation difficult. Diffuse pulmonary edema causing severe respiratory distress hampers effective mechanical ventilation. Despite aggressive treatment, cardiovascular collapse is common. Hypotension and tachycardia are the rule. Rhythm and conduction disturbances are frequent and occur early. Cardiac arrest is most often of anoxic origin from irreversible bronchospasm or prolonged shock.

## Management

In addition to anaphylactic shock, the differential diagnosis includes amniotic fluid embolism, myocardial infarction, congestive heart failure, and pulmonary embolism. Initially, the source of the antigen should be removed. When possible, apply a tourniquet to obstruct the draining blood flow from the source of the antigen or inciting medication. Release the tourniquet approximately every 15 minutes. Provide oxygen, place the patient in the recumbent position, and keep her warm. Aqueous epinephrine 1:1000, 0.3 to 0.5 mL injected subcutaneously, is a mainstay of ther-

apy. $H_1$ and $H_2$ antihistamines, diphenhydramine (25–50 mg IM), and cimetidine (300 mg) or ranitidine (50 mg) (given in a slow IV) over 3–5 minutes (3–5 min) should be given. Establish and maintain an airway. Aggressive use of IV fluids for maintaining BP is recommended. A pressor agent such as dopamine hydrochloride (2–10 µg/kg/min) also may be necessary after intravascular preload has been optimized. If wheezing is present and is unresponsive to epinephrine, aminophylline (5–6 mg/kg) may be given over 20 minutes, followed by a maintenance dose of 0.9 mg/kg/hr. Hydrocortisone (100 mg) or its equivalent should be administered every 6 hours. Epinephrine may be repeated every 20 minutes.

While treating the pregnant woman with anaphylaxis, fetal well-being also must be kept in mind. For reasons outlined previously, fetal hypoxia, manifest by an abnormal fetal heart rate pattern, will virtually always accompany maternal shock or hypoxia of any etiology. Further, maternal BP may be maintained at the expense of uterine (as well as other splanchnic) blood flow (Clark, 1990). Thus, the fetal heart rate should be monitored carefully in patients in anaphylactic shock. Heart rate abnormalities are often a sign of insufficient maternal oxygenation or relative hypovolemia and may be valuable clues to the underlying maternal condition (see Fig 23-2). Cesarean section is rarely, if ever, indicated in such cases, and in fact may be detrimental to an unstable mother. Rather, abnormal fetal heart rate patterns can generally be alleviated by maternal position change, maternal volume expansion, and increasing levels of oxygen administration in the borderline or frankly hypoxic mother.

Concern has been raised regarding the use of epinephrine in pregnancy. During embryogenesis, epinephrine was associated with an increased risk of umbilical hernia in the Collaborative Perinatal Project; however, it is difficult to distinguish potential drug effects from those of the condition for which epinephrine was administered (Briggs, 1994). Later in pregnancy, epinephrine may potentially decrease uterine blood flow. Terbutaline sulfate (0.25 mg subcutaneously), an agent devoid of such effects, has been advanced as an alternative agent in patients with asthma or anaphylaxis. In mild cases of anaphylaxis or

---

**ANAPHYLAXIS**

**I.** *Goals of Therapy*

    A.  Prompt recognition of symptoms and signs of anaphylaxis
    B.  Maintenance of oxygenation and BP
    C.  Identification and elimination of inciting agent
    D.  Careful monitoring of fetal condition

**II.** *Management Protocol*

    A.  Discontinue administration of the possible offending agent, including anesthetic agents. If appropriate, use a tourniquet.
    B.  Measure and record vital signs. A flow sheet may be helpful.
    C.  Maintain airway and administer 100% oxygen, as necessary.
    D.  Establish IV access and begin pulse oximetry.
    E.  Begin rapid intravascular volume expansion (2–4 liters of crystalloid).
    F.  Epinephrine aqueous 1:1000, 0.3 to 0.5 mL subcutaneously, or 1:10,000, 3–5 mL subcutaneously; repeat every 20 minutes × 3. In patients with severe hypotension, inject epinephrine 1:1000, 0.1 to 0.2 mL 1:1000 mixed in 10 mL saline, slowly IV.
    G.  Diphenhydramine, 25 to 50 mg IM or IV.
    H.  Cimetidine, 300 mg IV.
    I.  Epinephrine 1:1000 by nebulizer if laryngeal edema is present.
    J.  Maintain BP with IV fluids and dopamine hydrochloride, 2 to 10 µg/kg/min.
    K.  In the presence of continued wheezing, consider aminophylline, 5 to 6 mg/kg, over 20 minutes, with a maintenance dose of 0.9 mg/kg/hr thereafter, with monitoring of serum theophylline levels.
    L.  Hydrocortisone 100 mg IV every 6 hours (or the equivalent).
    M.  Continuous electronic fetal monitoring (at appropriate fetal age).

**III.** *Critical Laboratory Tests*

    A.  Arterial blood gas, complete blood count, platelet count, fibrinogen, fibrin split products, prothrombin time, and partial thromboplastin time. If the diagnosis is in doubt, consider plasma histamine, urine methylhistamine, and serum tryptase levels. After full recovery, appropriate immunologic testing may be performed for future counseling.

---

asthma, a trial of terbutaline may be acceptable. In cases of life-threatening reactions or when terbutaline is not readily available, however, these theoretical disadvantages of epinephrine are far outweighed by its longstanding documented efficacy in combating maternal hemodynamic instability and respiratory compromise.

A variety of serum specimens may be obtained to further investigate the clinical presentation of anaphylaxis and search for a definite cause.

An excellent review of markers and mechanisms of anaphylaxis was presented by Watkins (1992). In the past, several samples taken over a 20-minute period after the onset of the reaction and subsequent measurement of histamine levels were recommended. Histamine, however, has an extremely short half-life (2 min), and such an approach seems impractical. In contrast, the analysis of the histamine metabolite, methylhistamine, is of value, particularly when measured in the urine (Watkins, 1990). Another simpler analytical technique is to measure plasma tryptase release in serum or plasma samples taken sequentially during the immediate 24-hour period following the reaction (Watkins, 1989; Matsson, 1991). This serine protease is long-lived (approximately 2 hr) and is released exclusively from the mast cell in parallel with histamine. A radioimmunoassay based on the ELISA procedures is available. The knowledge of these markers may help confirm an anaphylactic reaction and assist future counseling.

## REFERENCES

American College of Allergy, Asthma and Immunology. Position statement: latex allergy—an emerging healthcare problem. Ann Allergy Asthma Immunol 1995;75:2.

American College of Obstetricians and Gynecologists. Group B streptococcal infections in pregnancy. Technical Bulletin no. 170, July 1992.

Anderson JA. Cross-sensitivity to cephalosporins in patients allergic to penicillin. Pediatr Infect Dis 1986;5:557.

Atkinson TP, Kaliner MA. Anaphylaxis. Clin Allergy 1992;76:841.

Austen KF. Diseases of immediate hypersensitivity. In: Petersdorf, Adams, Braunwald, et al, eds. Harrison's principles of internal medicine. 13th ed. New York: McGraw-Hill, 1994.

Barbier P, Jonville AP, Autret E. Fetal risks with dextrans during delivery. Drug Saf 1992;7:71.

Berg EM, Fasting S, Sellevold OFM. Serious complications with dextran-70 despite hapten prophylaxis. Anaesthesia 1991;46:1033.

Blanloeil Y, Pinaud M, Villers D, Nicolas F. Anaphylactic shock after infusion of a modified gelatin solution. Hemodynamic study (letter). Nouv Presse Med 1982;11:2847.

Bloomberg RJ. Cefotetan-induced anaphylaxis. Am J Obstet Gynecol 1988;159:125.

Briggs GE, Freeman RK, Yaffe SJ. Drugs in pregnancy and lactation. 4th ed. Baltimore: Williams and Wilkins, 1994.

Briner WW, Sheffer AL. Exercise-induced anaphylaxis. Med Sci Sports Exerc 1992;92:849.

Bush WH. Treatment of systemic reactions to contrast media. Urology 1990;35:145.

Bush WH, Swanson DP. Acute reactions to intravascular contrast media: types, risk factors, recognition, and specific treatment. AJR 1991;157:1153.

Clark SL. Shock in the pregnant patient. Semin Perinatol 1990;14:52.

Clark SL, Hankins GDV, Dudley DA, et al. Amniotic fluid embolism: analysis of a national registry. Am J Obstet Gynecol 1995;172:158–169.

Cohn JR, Cohn JB, Fellin R, Cantor R. Systemic anaphylaxis from low dose methotrexate. Ann Allergy 1993;70:384.

DePalma RT, Cunningham FG, Leveno KJ, Roark ML. Continuous investigation of women at high risk for infection following cesarean delivery: the three-dose perioperative antimicrobial therapy. Obstet Gynecol 1982;60:53.

Fisher A. Iatrogenic (intraoperative) rubber glove allergy and anaphylaxis. Cutis 1992;49:17.

Gallaghen JS. Anaphylaxis in pregnancy. Obstet Gynecol 1988;71:491.

Gerber AC, Jorg W, Zbindon S, et al. Severe intraoperative anaphylaxis to surgical gloves: latex allergy, an unfamiliar condition. Anesthesiology 1990;73:556.

Grammar LC, Patterson R. Adverse reactions to radiographic contrast material. Clin Dermatol 1986;4:149.

Guharoy SR, Barajas M. Probable anaphylactic reaction to corn-derived dextrose solution. Vot Hum Toxicol 1991;33:609.

Hoffman H, Goerz G, Plewig G. Anaphylactic shock from chlorobutanol-preserved oxytocin. Contact Dermatitis 1986;15:241.

Hough DO, Dec KL. Exercise-induced asthma and anaphylaxis. Sports Med 1994;18:162.

Idsoe O, Guthe T, Wilcox RR, eds. Nature and extent of penicillin reactions with particular reference to fatalities from anaphylactic shock. WHO 1968;38:159.

Kapin MA, Ferguson JL. Hemodynamic and regional circulatory alterations in dog during anaphylactic challenge. Am J Physiol 1985;249:H430.

Kawarabayashi T, Narisawa Y, Nakamura K, et al. Anaphylactoid reaction to oxytocin during cesarean section. Gynecol Obstet Invest 1988;25: 272.

Keizur JJ, Das S. Current perspectives on intravascular contrast agents for radiological imaging. J Urol 1994;151:1470.

Kelly KJ, Pearson ML, Kurup VP, et al. A cluster of anaphylactic reactions in children with spina bifida during general anesthesia. Epidemiologic features, risk factors and latex hypersensitivity. J Allergy Clin Immunol 1994;94:53.

Kobayashi RH, Mellion MB. Exercise-induced asthma, anaphylaxis, and urticaria. Sports Med 1991;18: 809.

Laurent J, Malet R, Smiejan JM, et al. Latex hypersensitivity after natural delivery. J Allergy Clin Immunol 1992;89:779.

Ledger R, Meripole A. Children at risk: latex allergies and spina bifida. J Pediatr Nurs 1992;7:371.

Lieberman P, Siegle RL, Treadwell G. Radiocontrast reactions. Clin Rev Allergy 1986;4:229.

Lieberman P. Anaphylactoid reactions to radiocontrast. Ann Allergy 1991a;67:91.

Lieberman P. Anaphylactoid reactions to radiocontrast material. Clin Rev Allergy 1991b;9:319.

Levine BB. Antigenicity and cross reactivity of penicillins and cephalosporins. J Infect Dis 1973;128 (suppl):364.

Lu LJ, Kurup VP, Hoffman DR, et al. Characterization of a major latex allergen associated with hypersensitivity in spina bifida patients. J Immunol 1995;155:2721.

Mandell GL, Sande MA. Antimicrobial agents penicillins, cephalosporins and other beta lactam antibiotics. In: Gilman AG, Rall TW, Nies AS, Taylor P, eds. Goodman, The pharmacologic basis of therapeutics. New York: Permagon Press, 1990.

Matsson P, Enander I, Anderson AS, et al. Evaluation of mast cell activation (tryptase) in two patients suffering drug induced hypotensoid reactions. Agents Actions 1991;33:218.

Maycock EJ, Russell WC. Anaphylactoid reaction to syntocinon. Anaesth Intensive Care 1993;21:211.

Moneret-Vautrin DA, Laxenaire MC, Bavoux F. Allergic shock to latex and ethylene oxide during surgery for spina bifida. Anesthesiology 1990;73: 556.

Moneret-Vautrin DA, Laxenaire MC. Anaphylactic and anaphylactoid reactions. Clin Rev Allergy 1991;91:249.

Morriss WW, Lavies NG, Anderson SK, Southgate HJ: Acute respiratory distress during cesarean section under spinal anaesthesia. Anaesthesia 1994;49:41.

Moss J, Fahmy NR, Sunder N, Beaven MA. Hormonal and hemodynamic profile of an anaphylactic reaction in man. Circulation 1981;63:210.

Nguyen MT, Hoffman DR. Anaphylaxis to laminaria. J Allergy Clin Immunol 1995;95:138.

Nichols AW. Exercise-induced anaphylaxis and urticaria. Clin Sports Med 1992;11:303.

Nicklas RA. Sulfites: a review with emphasis on biochemistry and clinical application. Allergy Asthma Proc 1989;10:349.

Nicolas R, Villers D, Blanloeil Y. Hemodynamic pattern in anaphylactic shock with cardiac arrest. Crit Care Med 1984;12:144.

Nieto A, Estornell F, Mazoon A, et al. Allergy to latex in spina bifida: a multivariate study of associated factors. J Allergy Clin Immunol 1996; 98:501.

Nutter AF. Contact urticaria to rubber. Br J Dermatol 1979;101:587.

Parker CW. Penicillin allergy. Ann Intern Med 1963; 34:747.

Paull J. A prospective study of dextran-induced anaphylactoid reactions in 5745 patients. Anaesth Intensive Care 1987;15:163.

Portier P, Richet C. De l'action anaphylactique de certains venins. Crit Rev Soc Biol 1902;6:170.

Raper RF, Fisher MM. Profound reversible myocardial depression after anaphylaxis. Lancet 1988;ii: 386.

Ring J. Anaphylactoid reactions to intravenous solutions used for volume substitution. Clin Rev Allergy 1991;9:397.

Ring J, Messmer K. Incidence and severity of anaphylactoid reactions to colloid volume substitutes. Lancet 1977;1:466.

Roitt IM, Brostoff J, Male DK, eds. Immunology. St. Louis: Mosby, 1985:

Rudolph AH, Price EV. Penicillin reactions among patients in venereal disease clinics: a national survey. JAMA 1973;223:499.

Saxon A, Hassner A, Swab EA, et al. Immediate hypersensitivity reaction to beta lactam antibiotics. Ann Intern Med 1987;107:204.

Sheffer AL, Soter NA, McFadden ER. Exercise induced anaphylaxis: a distinct form of physical allergy. JAMA 1983;250:2049.

Sheffer AL, Austen KF. Exercise-induced anaphylaxis. Allergy Clin Immunol 1984;73:699.

Sheffer AL, Tong AKF, Murphy GF. Exercise-induced anaphylaxis: a serious form of physical allergy associated with mast cell degranulation. J Allergy Clin Immunol 1985;75:479.

Silverman HJ, Van Hook C, Haponik EF. Hemodynamic changes in human anaphylaxis. Am J Med 1984;77:341.

Slater RM, Bowles BJM, Pumphrey RSH. Anaphylactoid reaction to oxytocin in pregnancy. Anaesthesia 1985;40:655.

Smith HS. Delivery as a cause of exercise-induced anaphylactoid reaction: case report. Br J Obstet Gynaecol 1985;92:1196.

Songsiridej V, Busse WW. Exercise-induced anaphylaxis. Clin Allergy 1983;13:312.

Stafford CT, Label SA, Fruge BC, et al. Anaphylaxis to human serum albumin. Ann Allergy 1988;61:85.

Swartz JS, Gold M, Braude BM, et al. Intraoperative anaphylaxis to latex: an identifiable population at risk. Can J Anaesth 1990;37:S131.

Tomazic VJ, Withrow TJ, Fisher BR, Dillard SF. Latex-associated allergies and anaphylactic reactions. Clin Immunol Immunopathol 1992;64:89.

Turjanmaa K, Reunala T, Tuimala R, Karkkainen T. Allergy to latex gloves: unusual complication during delivery. Br Med J 1988;297:1029.

Watkins J. Heuristic decision-making in diagnosis and management of adverse drug reactions in anaesthesia and surgery: the case of muscle relaxants. Theor Surg 1989;4:212.

Watkins J, Wild G. Problems of mediator measurement for a national advisory service to UK anesthetists. Agents Actions 1990;30:247.

Watkins J. Markers and mechanisms of anaphylactoid reactions. Clin Basic Aspects Monogr Allergy 1992;30:108.

Weese DL, Greenberg HM, Zimmern PE. Contrast media reactions during voiding cystourethrography or retrograde pyelography. Urology 1993; 41:81.

Wendel GD, Stark RJ, Jamison RR, et al. Penicillin allergy and desensitization in serious infections during pregnancy. N Engl J Med 1985;312:1229.

Wittbrodt ET, Spinler SA. Prevention of anaphylactoid reactions in high-risk patients receiving radiographic contrast media. Ann Pharmacother 1994;28:236.

Wong S, Dykewicz MS, Patterson R. Idiopathic anaphylaxis—a clinical summary of 175 patients. Arch Intern Med 1990;150:1323.

Zenarola P. Rubber latex allergy: unusual complications during surgery. Contact Dermatitis 1989; 21:197.

# CHAPTER 24

# Acute Fatty Liver

*A*cute fatty liver of pregnancy (AFLP) is a rare yet potentially serious complication of the third trimester of pregnancy, characterized by jaundice, coagulopathy, microvesicular fatty infiltration of the liver, and encephalopathy. Although usually confined to the liver, complications of AFLP may involve every organ system in the body. Acute fatty liver of pregnancy was not recognized as a distinct clinical syndrome until 1940 in a series of cases by Sheehan (Sheehan, 1940). Since that time, the reported incidence has ranged from 1 in 1,000,000 in 1966 (Haemmeili, 1966) to 1 in 7000 in 1996 (Castro, 1996). The increased frequency in recent years probably reflects a greater awareness of this syndrome, particularly of milder and nonfatal cases.

Acute fatty liver of pregnancy results in significant maternal and perinatal mortality; prior to 1980, mortality was as high as 75% and 85%, respectively (Kaplan, 1985; Bairn, 1983; Sherlock, 1983; Pockros, 1984). With prompt diagnosis and immediate institution of treatment, however, the maternal and perinatal prognosis can be greatly improved. One series of 14 cases reported no maternal deaths and a perinatal mortality rate of 6.6% (Usta, 1994). This chapter reviews the current information regarding the pathophysiology, the clinical and laboratory manifestations, diagnosis, and treatment of AFLP.

## Etiology

Acute fatty liver of pregnancy remains a clinical syndrome of unknown etiology. Although there is no apparent racial predilection, it is seen more commonly in primigravidas, patients with multiple gestation, and in pregnancies with male fetuses (Burroughs, 1982). There have been no reported familial cases to suggest genetic factors. While some have suggested that the disorder may result from nutritional deficiencies, this has not been confirmed by either animal or clinical studies.

Viral infection has been suggested as a possible factor in AFLP. Patients with AFLP, however, do not exhibit the characteristic serologic changes of viral infection, nor have viral particles been demonstrated in biopsy or necropsy material. Furthermore, evaluation of liver biopsies has failed to demonstrate a progression from acute fatty liver to the marked necrosis and inflammation characteristic of severe viral hepatitis.

Tetracycline and other drugs may induce hepatic changes that are indistinguishable on biopsy from women with AFLP. Such women, however, generally have a history of exposure to a drug or toxin (Snyder, 1986).

It has also been suggested that AFLP may be an adult variant of Reye's syndrome (Kaplan, 1985). Reye's syndrome, however, is associated with a preceding viral syndrome, whereas this association has not been found with AFLP. In addition, differentiation between the two disorders is possible by detailed microscopic examination of biopsy specimens.

Finally, it has been suggested that AFLP may be part of the spectrum of preeclampsia. Investigators have reported histologic hepatic changes in cases of preeclampsia that are similar to those associated with AFLP (Minakami, 1988). Furthermore, approximately 40% of patients with acute fatty liver have associated clinical findings consistent with the diagnosis of preeclampsia. Careful evaluation of liver histology, however, suggests that the two diseases are separate entities and that preeclampsia probably should be viewed as a complication of the primary hepatic disorder (Latham, 1992).

## Pathophysiology

Acute fatty liver of pregnancy is associated with progressive accumulation of lipids within hepatocytes. Case reports of survivors demonstrate markedly reduced mitochondrial urea cycle enzyme activity that corresponds with the clinical severity of disease (Weber, 1979). Several studies suggest that the intramitochondrial β-oxidation of fatty acids is impaired in patients with AFLP (Grimbert, 1993; Treem, 1994; Sims, 1995). There is also increasing evidence that the offspring of women with AFLP may be affected by a similar inborn error of metabolism (Schoeman, 1991). If these findings are confirmed, currently available genetic and/or medical testing methods may improve our ability to predict, or even prevent, this serious pregnancy complication.

## Clinical Manifestations

Acute fatty liver of pregnancy is most commonly characterized by nausea, vomiting, abdominal pain, and jaundice, beginning late in the third trimester of pregnancy and in the postpartum period (Table 24-1). These may be preceded by prodromal symptoms of malaise, anorexia, lethargy, tachycardia, and sometimes fever. Nausea and vomiting are typically the most common presenting complaints (Usta, 1994; Reyes, 1994). When abdominal pain is present, it may be vari-

able in nature: sometimes epigastric, right upper quadrant, dyspeptic, or radiating to the back (Kaplan, 1985). Neurologic manifestations may include restlessness, confusion, disorientation, asterixis, seizures, psychosis, and ultimately, coma (Usta, 1994; Reyes, 1994).

Physical examination often reveals a jaundiced, ill-appearing patient. Hypertension, edema, and ascites may be present. The liver is usually small and nonpalpable. Intrauterine demise is not uncommon.

Additional systemic clinical manifestations may include generalized edema, pruritus, spider hemangiomas and palmar erythema, gastrointestinal hemorrhage secondary to ulceration, disseminated intravascular coagulation (DIC), ascites, pleural effusion, and renal insufficiency. Respiratory failure requiring assisted ventilation is reported frequently (Usta, 1994). Transient diabetes insipidus commonly accompanies AFLP (Kennedy, 1994; Tucker, 1993). This probably results from fat accumulation in the proximal renal tubules with AFLP, resulting in decreased sensitivity to endogenous vasopressin. It is important to note that while many patients will present with the aforementioned signs and symptoms, milder forms of the disease also occur.

TABLE 24-1

**Signs and symptoms of acute fatty liver of pregnancy**

| *Symptoms* | |
|---|---|
| Nausea, vomiting | Almost always |
| Malaise | Always |
| Abdominal pain | Almost always; may be variable in position, severity |
| *Signs* | |
| Hypertension | Almost always |
| Edema | Almost always |
| Proteinuria | Variable |
| Jaundice | Always |
| Elevated liver transaminases | Always |
| Hypoglycemia | In severe cases |
| Coagulopathy | Common |
| Diabetes insipidus | Common |
| Encephalopathy | Common; may correlate with ammonia levels |

## Laboratory Abnormalities

The complete blood count typically reveals a normochromic, normocytic anemia, often with schistocytes. More severe anemia may occur secondary to gastrointestinal bleeding. The white blood count is variable but is usually elevated to a range of 20,000 to 30,000/μL. Toxic granulation may be present. The platelet count is usually decreased.

When acute hepatic failure is present, synthesis of coagulation factors is impaired and coagulation tests such as the prothrombin time (PT) and partial thromboplastin time (PTT) are prolonged. Disseminated intravascular coagulation also may occur in AFLP by itself or in conjunction with abruptio placentae (Lauersen, 1983; Usta, 1994). Hypofibrinogenemia, thrombocytopenia, and high levels of fibrin degradation products result. The coagulopathy may persist long after delivery and even worsen in the postpartum period, often secondary to low antithrombin III levels (Liebman, 1983). Factor VII levels most accurately reflect the extent of coagulopathy due to liver dysfunction. While these levels are not predictive of ultimate clinical outcome, their return toward normal does identify those patients who are most likely to recover.

A hepatic profile will reveal serum transaminase concentrations that are increased between 100 and 1000 units/liter and are lower than the elevations generally seen in acute viral hepatitis. Bilirubin is variable but usually exceeds 5 mg/dL. Alkaline phosphatase is elevated. Serum albumin is usually low. Ammonia levels are very elevated, suggesting decreased ammonia utilization by urea cycle liver enzymes; such levels correlate with the degree of altered sensorium. Amylase and lipase levels may be elevated because of concomitant pancreatitis (Lauersen, 1983). In women who survive the acute phase of their illness, liver function tests usually return to normal within 4 to 8 weeks after delivery (Kaplan, 1985).

Renal dysfunction is associated frequently with hepatic failure (Davies, 1980; Usta, 1994; Reyes, 1994). Urine volume and creatinine clearance are decreased. Serum concentration of uric acid and BUN are increased. With the onset of jaundice, urobilinogen usually is present in the urine. In addition, serum electrolytes may show a low bicarbonate level secondary to metabolic acidosis. Plasma glucose is often below 60 mg/dL, suggesting reduced hepatic glycogenolysis. This may persist for some time after delivery (Purdie, 1988). Urinalysis may reveal ketones.

## Imaging Studies

Noninvasive imaging studies have been used in AFLP in an effort to avoid potentially dangerous liver biopsies in patients with coagulopathy. Ultrasound has been suggested as a potential diagnostic modality because it is noninvasive, safe, and capable of assessing overall patterns of fat distribution. Unfortunately, sonography has a very high false-negative rate (Usta, 1994). Ultrasound of the biliary tract, however, can distinguish subcapsular hematoma, cholecystitis, and/or cholangitis as potential confounding diagnoses.

Computerized tomography (CT) of the liver also has been reported to be of value in the diagnosis of AFLP (Clements, 1990). Because the liver in AFLP has an increased fat content, an abnormally low density may be seen on CT. Critical evaluation, however, has suggested a relatively high false-negative rate with this technique as well (80% in one study) (Usta, 1994; Van Le, 1990).

Magnetic resonance imaging also has been used in an attempt to diagnose AFLP (Farine, 1990), but the sensitivity and specificity of this procedure is unknown.

## Pathology

The liver in AFLP is typically small and weighs approximately 1000 to 1500 g. Its appearance is a uniform pale yellow. The capsule is thin, transparent, and wrinkled. Subcapsular hemorrhages may be apparent on gross examination, although the lobular structure usually is well preserved (Sheehan, 1940; Pockros, 1984; Kaplan, 1985; Duma, 1965).

Histologic examination should be performed on fresh specimens stained with special fat stains, most commonly oil red O. Microscopically, the hepatocellular cytoplasm is distended by numerous fine vacuoles, giving the cells a distinct foamy

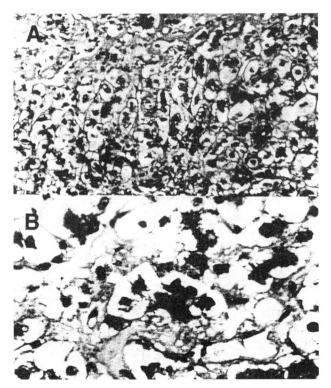

**(A)** Acute fatty liver of pregnancy (H&E stain). Note diffuse fatty infiltration and absence of necrosis and inflammation. (Photomicrograph courtesy of Dr. Patricia Latham, University of Maryland Hospital.) (Magnification, 200×). **(B) Higher magnification demonstrates the fine cytoplasmic vacuoles and centrally placed nuclei (H&E stain).** (Photomicrograph courtesy of Dr. Patricia Latham, University of Maryland Hospital.) (Magnification, 1000×)

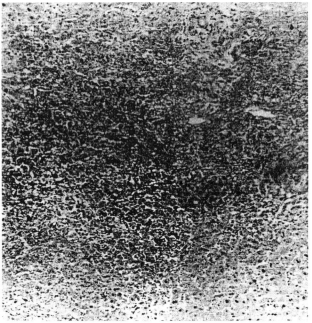

F I G U R E  **24-2**

Liver section from a patient who died of complications of preeclampsia (H&E stain). Note extensive hepatocellular inflammation and necrosis. (Courtesy of Dr. James Kelley, Madigan AMC.) (Magnification 40×)

appearance (Fig 24-1). The fat deposits are primarily free fatty acids rather than triglycerides, which distinguishes them from other syndromes of hepatic microvesicular fat infiltration (Reye's syndrome, defects of hepatic intramitochondrial β-oxidation pathway, and alcoholic cirrhosis). The myriad of tiny vacuoles are separated from each other by thin eosinophilic cytoplasmic strands and do not coalesce to form a single large vacuole. In contrast to the cytoplasm, the cell nucleus is located centrally and is normal in size and appearance.

Histologic changes usually are most prominent in the central portion of the lobule, with a thin rim of normal hepatocytes at the periphery. The lobular architecture usually is preserved, and, with rare exceptions, necrosis and inflammation are absent. This is distinct from the periportal fibrin deposition and hemorrhagic necrosis reported in preeclampsia (Fig 24-2).

Serial liver biopsies in affected patients have confirmed that, even over time, the characteristic lesions do not progress to a stage of necrosis (Duma, 1965). Characteristic histologic changes may be present up to 3 weeks after the onset of jaundice. In addition to these findings, fatty vacuolization of proximal renal tubular cells, pancreatic cells, and CNS neurons may occur (Sheehan, 1940; Pockros, 1984; Latham, 1992).

## Diagnosis

The clinical diagnosis of AFLP can be proven only by liver biopsy. This may be clinically difficult, however, if coagulopathy is present. The correct interpretation of laboratory tests and imaging studies correlated with clinical manifestations often can allow the diagnosis without an invasive procedure. The differential diagnosis includes any cause of jaundice and acute hepatic dysfunction in late pregnancy. The three most common alternative clinical considerations are viral hepatitis, cholestasis of pregnancy, and preeclampsia (Table 24-2) (Knox, 1996).

Perhaps the most important differential consideration for the obstetrician is an atypical presentation of preeclampsia. Women with either AFLP or preeclampsia may have elevated serum transaminases, thrombocytopenia, and coagulation defects. Women with preeclampsia, however, are rarely clinically jaundiced and do not develop hypoglycemia or clinically apparent liver failure. As described earlier, liver biopsy is helpful because AFLP and preeclampsia have distinct histologic appearances (see Fig 24-2) (Douvas, 1983). Unfortunately, patients with AFLP often develop severe preeclampsia secondarily, thus compounding the difficulty in diagnosis. In both cases, however, treatment includes prompt delivery.

Acute hepatitis also is a common differential consideration but does not have a predilection for the third trimester of pregnancy. A history of hepatitis exposure, drug ingestion, and heavy alcohol intake is often present. Moreover, on the basis of specific serologic tests, the diagnoses of hepatitis A and B can be established quickly and with reasonable certainty. Acute hepatitis of any etiology may present with fulminant hepatic failure. Serum transaminase levels usually are elevated well beyond those normally seen in acute fatty liver. Patients with hepatitis do not have signs or symptoms of preeclampsia (e.g., hypertension) that may be present in women with AFLP. If coagulopathy is not present, liver biopsy may be required to establish the diagnosis. In contrast to AFLP, specimens of patients with acute hepatitis show marked hepatocellular disarray and extensive inflammation and necrosis (Fig 24-3).

The third common differential of AFLP is cholestasis of pregnancy (Alsulyman, 1996). Serum bilirubin and alkaline phosphatase concentrations are typically elevated, and transaminase concentrations may be increased. Transaminase concentrations, however, are lower than those

T A B L E   **24-2**

Differential diagnosis of acute fatty liver of pregnancy

|  | **Acute Fatty Liver of Pregnancy** | **Acute Hepatitis** | **Cholestasis of Pregnancy** | **Severe Preeclampsia** |
|---|---|---|---|---|
| Trimester | Third | Variable | Third | Third |
| Clinical manifestations | Nausea, vomiting, malaise, encephalopathy, abdominal pain, coagulopathy | Malaise, nausea, vomiting, jaundice, anorexia, encephalopathy | Pruritus, jaundice | Hypertension, edema, proteinuria, oliguria, CNS hyperexcitability |
| Bilirubin | Elevated | Elevated | Elevated | Normal or elevated |
| Transaminases | Moderately elevated | Markedly elevated | Minimally to moderately elevated | Normal or minimally to moderately increased |
| Alkaline phosphatase | Usually normal for pregnancy | Minimally elevated | Moderately elevated | Normal for pregnancy |
| Histology | Fatty infiltration, no inflammation or necrosis | Marked inflammation and necrosis | Biliary stasis, no inflammation | Inflammation, necrosis, fibrin deposition |
| Recurrence | Reported | No | Yes | Yes |

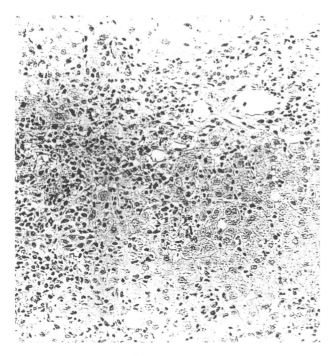

FIGURE 24-3

Liver biopsy from a patient with acute viral hepatitis (H&E stain). Individual hepatocytes are swollen, and there is marked hepatocellular disarray and extensive inflammation and necrosis. (Courtesy of Dr. James Kelley, Madigan AMC.) (Magnification 100×)

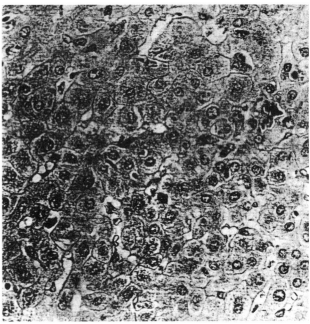

FIGURE 24-4

Liver biopsy demonstrates characteristic features of cholestasis. Bile thrombi are prominent (H&E stain). Fatty infiltration is not present, and hepatic architecture is preserved. (Courtesy of Dr. James Kelley, Madigan AMC.) (Magnification 400×)

seen in AFLP or acute hepatitis. The predominant feature seen on biopsy is biliary stasis (Fig 24-4). Hepatocellular injury and fatty infiltration are not characteristic of cholestasis of pregnancy.

## Treatment

Treatment for patients with AFLP is comprised of two parts: (1) prompt delivery and (2) supportive care. The patient should be hospitalized in an intensive care setting where comprehensive care can be given and where preparations for delivery can be made.

## Delivery

There is no place for expectant care in the management of these patients, regardless of gestational age. Prompt delivery appears to result in improved maternal and perinatal outcome (Kaplan, 1985; Reyes, 1994). One study reported that half of all patients had improvement in laboratory findings by the second day following delivery (Usta, 1994). While delivery is clearly mandatory, there is no clear consensus on the optimum route. Immediate cesarean section provides no clear advantage over induction and vaginal delivery as long as adequate supportive care is given. Long marathon inductions in critical circumstances, however, are potentially dangerous to the mother and the fetus. The decision regarding the method of delivery should be based on assessment of maternal and fetal conditions and the favorability of the cervix for induction of labor. Fetal compromise or intolerance of labor is common, and abdominal delivery is often necessary. There are no reported cases in which patients have recovered prior to delivery.

Anesthetic options in patients with AFLP are limited. General anesthesia can further damage an already compromised liver, and regional anesthesia poses a risk of hemorrhage when coagulopathy is present. If general anesthesia must be used, inhalation agents with potential hepatotoxicity (e.g., halothane) should be avoided. Isoflurane is a logical choice because it has little or no hepatotoxicity and may preserve liver blood flow (Goldfarb, 1990). Epidural anesthesia is the optimal choice because it preserves liver blood flow with no hepatotoxic effects (Antognini, 1991). However, recognition and treatment of thrombocytopenia and deficient clotting factors are essential prior to administration of spinal or epidural anesthesia.

## Supportive Care

Supportive care of patients with AFLP should include careful monitoring for evidence of progressive hepatic failure, hypoglycemia, and coagulopathy. These women are at risk for death from sepsis, aspiration, renal failure, circulatory collapse, gastrointestinal bleeding, pancreatitis, and embolism (Snyder, 1986).

As in any critical care situation, steps should be taken to ensure that the woman with liver failure and hepatic coma has a patent airway and that effective ventilation and oxygenation are maintained. Optimal nutrition should prevent hypoglycemia and reduce the endogenous production of nitrogenous wastes. This can be accomplished by providing approximately 2000 to 2500 calories per day, primarily in the form of glucose. Twenty percent to 25% glucose solutions should be administered by nasogastric tube or by intravenous infusion. Protein intake should be excluded in the acute phase of the illness and restored gradually to the diet when the patient begins to show clinical improvement.

Colonic emptying should be facilitated through the use of enemas and/or magnesium citrate. Neomycin, 6 to 12 g orally per day, is of value in decreasing production of ammonia by intestinal bacteria. With rare exceptions, any drug that requires hepatic metabolism should be withheld from the patient.

Correction of coagulation abnormalities is imperative. Disseminated intravascular coagulation may be present with or without concomitant abruptio placentae and may persist for days after delivery. Correction should be accomplished by administration of vitamin K, platelets and fresh-frozen plasma, as indicated by laboratory evaluation.

Acutely ill patients in an intensive care unit are at particular risk for infection. Frequent cultures should be performed as part of careful surveillance for nosocomial infection. Urosepsis may develop because of prolonged use of an indwelling bladder catheter. Bacteremia also may develop as a complication of extended use of intravenous catheters. Appropriate antibiotics should be administered if infection exists.

The risk of gastrointestinal hemorrhage in patients with AFLP is high. Correction of coagulation abnormalities is the most important preventive measure. Administration of antacid solutions and $H_2$ blocking agents also may be indicated.

In patients who deteriorate despite adequate supportive care, several forms of experimental therapy may be considered. Acute fatty liver of pregnancy has been treated successfully with liver transplantation in at least two patients who did not recover after delivery (Ockner, 1990; Amon, 1991). In addition, exchange transfusion, hemodialysis, plasmapheresis, extracorporeal perfusion, and corticosteroids have been tried in patients with fulminant hepatic failure (Katelaris, 1989). There is no reliable information, however, concerning the actual efficacy of these measures in women with AFLP.

## Prognosis

Maternal and perinatal mortality have decreased significantly since 1980, with maternal survival over 90% and perinatal mortality as low as 6.6% (Usta, 1994). One recent study, however, reported fetal mortality of 58.3% (Reyes, 1994). It is probable that early recognition and treatment with prompt delivery and adequate supportive care in combination with recognition of milder forms of disease have been responsible for the favorable prognoses.

Surviving infants do not show evidence of liver disease. Historically, the literature has suggested

---

### ACUTE FATTY LIVER

#### I. *Goals of Therapy*

    A. To normalize liver function tests, electrolytes, clotting profile, and serum ammonia
    B. To prevent renal failure
    C. To maintain serum glucose >60 dL
    D. To return patient to normal mental status
    E. To deliver the fetus

#### II. *Management Protocol*

    A. Hospitalize in intensive care unit.
    B. If the patient is comatose, provide a secure airway and maintain effective ventilation and oxygenation.
    C. Provide optimal nutrition. Administer 2000 to 2500 calories per 24 hours. Administer most of the calories in the form of concentrated glucose solutions.
    D. Decrease endogenous ammonia production. Restrict protein intake during the acute phase of illness. Evacuate colonic contents by administering magnesium citrate orally or by instilling Fleet enema solutions via the rectum. Administer oral neomycin, 6 to 12 g/24 hr, to decrease production of ammonia by intestinal bacteria.
    E. Avoid use of medications that require hepatic metabolism.
    F. Correct electrolyte and metabolic derangements.
    G. Identify and correct coagulation abnormalities. Administer vitamin K, fresh-frozen plasma, or platelets as indicated.
    H. Maintain surveillance for nosocomial infection, especially pneumonia, urosepsis, or bacteremia.
    I. Prevent gastrointestinal hemorrhage.
    J. Deliver the patient promptly after the diagnosis is established.

#### III. *Critical Laboratory Tests*

    A. Complete blood count, platelet count, partial thromboplastin time, prothrombin time, fibrinogen, fibrin split products, SGPT, SGOT, alkaline phosphatase, total and direct bilirubin, BUN, creatinine, serum electrolytes, serum ammonia, liver biopsy (if coagulopathy is not present)

#### IV. *Consultation*

    A. Internal medicine, gastroenterology

---

that infants who survive without significant insult secondary to prematurity and intrapartum asphyxia can expect normal long-term prognoses. Some reports, however, indicate that these infants are at increased risk for metabolic defects in their hepatic intramitochondrial β-oxidation pathway (Treem, 1994; Wilcken, 1993; Schoeman, 1991). Therefore, infants born to women with AFLP should be screened for fatty acid oxidation disorders.

The maternal prognosis in women who survive AFLP is good, with complete recovery of hepatic, renal, and neurologic function (Breen, 1972; Usta, 1994; Reyes, 1994). Although the actual risk of disease recurrence is unknown, there have been at least three well-documented cases of recurrent AFLP in subsequent pregnancies reported in the literature (Barton, 1990; MacLean, 1994; Schoeman, 1991).

## REFERENCES

Alsulyman OM, Ouzounian JG, Ames-Castro M, Goodwin TM. Intrahepatic cholestasis of pregnancy: Perinatal outcome associated with expectant management. Am J Obstet Gynecol 1996;175:957.

Amon E, Allen SR, Petrie RH, Belew JE. Acute fatty liver or pregnancy associated with preeclampsia: management of hepatic failure with postpartum live transplantation. Am J Perinatol 1991; 8:278–279.

Antognini JF, Andrews S. Anaesthesia for caesarean section in a patient with acute fatty liver of pregnancy. Can J Anaesth 1991;38:904–907.

Bairn J, Degott C, Novel O, et al. Nonfatal acute fatty liver of pregnancy. Gut 1983;24:340.

Barton JR, Sibai BM, Mabie WC, Shanklin DR. Recurrent acute fatty liver of pregnancy. Am J Obstet Gynecol 1990;163:534–538.

Bernau J, Degott C, Novel O, et al. Nonfatal acute fatty liver of pregnancy. Gut 1983;24:340.

Breen KJ, Perkins KW, Schenker S, et al. Uncomplicated subsequent pregnancy after idiopathic fatty liver of pregnancy. Obstet Gynecol 1972; 40:813.

Burroughs AK, Seong NG J, Dojcinov DM, et al. Idiopathic acute fatty liver of pregnancy in twelve patients. Q J Med 1982;204:481.

Castro MA, Goodwin TM, Shaw KJ, et al. Disseminated intravascular coagulation and antithrombin III depression in acute fatty liver of pregnancy. Am J Obstet Gynecol 1996;174:211.

Clements D, Young WT, Thornton JG, et al. Imaging in acute fatty liver of pregnancy. Case report. Br J Obstet Gynaecol 1990;97:631–633.

Davies MH, Wilkinson SP, Hanid MA, et al. Acute liver disease with encephalopathy and renal failure in late pregnancy and the early puerperium: a study of 14 patients. Br J Obstet Gynaecol 1980;87:1005.

Douvas SG, Meeks R, Phillips O, et al. Liver disease in pregnancy. Obstet Gynecol Surv 1983;38:531.

Duma RJ, Dowling EA, Alexander HC, et al. Acute fatty liver of pregnancy: report of a surviving patient with serial liver biopsies. Ann Intern Med 1965;63:851.

Farine D, Newhouse J, Owen J, Fox HE. Magnetic resonance imaging and computed tomography scan for the diagnosis of acute fatty liver of pregnancy. Am J Perinatol 1990;4:316.

Goldfarb G, Debaene B, Ang ET, et al. Hepatic blood flow in humans during isoflurane $N_2O$ and halothane-$N_2O$ anesthesia. Anesth Analg 1990; 71:349–353

Grimbert S, Fromenty B, Fisch C, et al. Decreased mitochondrial oxidation of fatty acids in pregnant mice: possible relevance to development of acute fatty liver of pregnancy. Hepatology 1993;17:628–637.

Haemmeili UP. Jaundice during pregnancy: with special emphasis on recurrent jaundice during pregnancy and its differential diagnosis. Acta Med Scand [Suppl] 1966;444:1–111.

Kaplan MM. Acute fatty liver of pregnancy. N Engl J Med 1985;313:367.

Katelaris PH, Jones DB. Fulminant hepatic failure. Med Clin North Am 1989;73:955–970.

Kennedy SK, Hall PM, Seymore AE, Hague WM. Transient diabetes insipidus and acute fatty liver of pregnancy. Br J Obstet Gynaecol 1994;101:387–391.

Knox TA, Olans LB. Liver disease in pregnancy. N Engl J Med 1996;335:569.

Latham PS. Liver diseases of pregnancy. In: Gleicher N, ed. Principles and practice of medical therapy in pregnancy. Norwalk, CT: Appleton and Lange, 1992.

Lauersen B, Frost B, Mortensen JZ. Acute fatty liver of pregnancy with complicating disseminated intravascular coagulation. Acta Obstet Gynecol Scand 1983;62:403.

Liebman HA, McGhee WG, Patch MJ, Feinstein DI. Severe depression of antithrombin III associated with disseminated intravascular coagulation in women with fatty liver of pregnancy. Ann Intern Med 1983;98:330–333.

MacLean MA, Cameron AD, Cumming GP, et al. Recurrence of acute fatty liver of pregnancy. Br J Obstet Gynaecol 1994;101:453–454.

Minakami H, Oka N, Sato T, et al. Preeclampsia: a microvesicular fat disease of the liver? Am J Obstet Gynecol 1988;159:1043–1047.

Ockner SA, Brunt E, Cohn SM, et al. Fulminant hepatic failure caused by acute fatty liver of pregnancy by orthotopic liver transplantation. Hepatology 1990;11:59–64.

Pockros PJ, Peters RL, Reynolds TB. Idiopathic fatty liver of pregnancy: findings in ten cases. Medicine 1984;63:1.

Purdie JM, Waters BNJ. Acute fatty liver of pregnancy. Clinical features and diagnosis. Aust NZ J Obstet Gynaecol 1988;28:62–67.

Reyes H, Sandoval L, Wainstein A, et al. Acute fatty liver of pregnancy: a clinical study of 12 episodes in 11 patients. Gut 1994;35:101–106

Schoeman MN, Batey RG, Wilcken B. Recurrent acute fatty liver of pregnancy associated with a fatty-acid oxidation defect in the offspring. Gastroenterology 1991;100:544–548.

Sheehan HL. The pathology of acute yellow atrophy and delayed chloroform poisoning. J Obstet Gynaecol Br Emp 1940;47:49.

Sherlock S. Acute fatty liver of pregnancy and the microvesicular fat diseases. Gut 1983;24:265.

Sims HF, Brackett JC, Powell CK, et al. The molecular basis of pediatric long chain 3-hydroxyacyl-CoA dehydrogenase deficiency associated with maternal acute fatty liver of pregnancy. Proc Natl Acad Sci 1995;92:841–845.

Snyder RR, Hawkins GDV. Etiology and treatment of acute fatty liver of pregnancy. Clin Perinatol 1986;13:813.

Treem WR, Rinaldo P, Hale DE, et al. Acute fatty liver of pregnancy and long-chain 3-hydroxyacyl-coenzyme A dehydrogenase deficiency. Hepatology 1994;19:339–345.

Tucker ED, Calhoun BC, Thorneycroft IH, Edwards MS. Diabetes insipidus and acute fatty liver: a case report. J Reprod Med 1993;38:835–838.

Usta IM, Barton JR, Amon EA, et al. Acute fatty liver of pregnancy: an experience in the diagnosis and management of fourteen cases. Am J Obstet Gynecol 1994;171:1342–1347.

Van Le L, Podrasky A. Computed tomographic and ultrasonographic findings in women with acute fatty liver of pregnancy. J Reprod Med 1990;35:815–817.

Weber FL, Snodgrass PJ, Powell DE, et al. Abnormalities of hepatic mitochondrial urea-cycle enzyme activities and hepatic ultrastructure in acute fatty liver of pregnancy. J Lab Clin Med 1979;94:27.

Wilcken B, Leung KC, Hammond J, et al. Pregnancy and fetal long-chain 3-hydroxyacyl coenzyme A dehydrogenase deficiency. Lancet 1993;341:407–408.

# CHAPTER 25

# Acute Pancreatitis

*P*ancreatitis occurring during pregnancy is a substantial threat to both maternal and fetal well-being, with significant morbidity and mortality frequently cited. A clearer understanding of the natural history of this disease as it exists in the gravid woman has evolved over the past two decades. As with all abdominal processes, the diagnosis of pancreatitis during pregnancy may be challenging; maternal outcome, however, does not appear to be altered by the concurrent state of pregnancy. Indeed, reports of maternal mortality range from 0% to 3.4%, comparing favorably with an overall mortality of 9% in the general population (Swisher, 1994; Block, 1989; Ramin, 1995; Klein, 1986; Steinberg, 1994). Fetal and neonatal outcomes, however, are often adversely affected by this disease, with prematurity accounting for a substantial portion of morbidity (Ramin, 1995). However, earlier reports of mortality rates as high as 35% have been tempered by studies demonstrating fetal loss directly attributable to pancreatitis of 0% to 11% (Swisher, 1994; Ramin, 1995; Cortlett, 1972; Jouppila, 1974; Wilkinson, 1973; Block, 1989).

Pancreatitis spans the clinical spectrum from mild disease to multisystem organ failure. This chapter focuses on the epidemiology, clinical course, diagnosis, prognostic indicators, and management of pancreatitis occurring in pregnancy.

## Epidemiology

The reported incidence of pancreatitis complicating pregnancy varies widely, with studies demonstrating rates as frequent as 1 in 459 and as uncommon as 1 in 4350 (Herfort, 1981; Langmade, 1951). Many retrospective studies have been generated from tertiary care hospitals evaluating the frequency of pancreatitis within individual institutions. Compiling data from seven such reports, the estimated incidence of pancreatitis is equal to one case per 2000 deliveries (Langmade, 1951; Cortlett, 1972; Wilkinson, 1973; Jouppila, 1974; Herfort, 1981; Swisher, 1994; Ramin, 1995). In a review of cholecystectomies performed for gallstone pancreatitis, Block and Kelly (1989) found that among 152 female patients, 21 (13.8%) were either pregnant at the time of surgery or within 6 weeks postpartum.

Many studies have shown an increasing incidence of pancreatitis with advancing gestational age, although first trimester pancreatitis is well described (Legro, 1995). While pancreatitis may occur throughout pregnancy and the puerperium, as many as 35% to 50% of cases occur during the third trimester. Approximately 70% to 80% of patients are multigravidas, correlating with the overall distribution within the general obstetric population. Parity, therefore, does not appear to influence the development of pancreatitis. Increased risk among ethnic groups has not been demonstrated within the obstetric population. Incidence rates, however, do correlate with the prevalence of etiologic factors such as cholelithiasis and alcohol abuse, which are known to vary among populations.

Early reports of phenomenally high maternal mortality led to a long-held belief that pancreatitis in pregnancy gravely endangered maternal well-being. It is now accepted that previous maternal mortality figures approaching 35% to 50% of patients considerably overestimated the lethality of the disease (Langmade, 1951; Wilkinson, 1973). Klein collected data from five single institution series and found only three maternal deaths among 87 cases of pancreatitis, for a mortality rate of 3.4%. Other studies also have corroborated this finding, with no deaths occurring among 94 cumulative cases (Swisher, 1994; Block, 1989; Ramin, 1995). Biased reporting of more severe cases, as well as confounding concurrent disease, such as fatty liver of pregnancy, may have contributed to the higher mortality reported in earlier studies. Additionally, two drugs previously used more liberally in pregnancy, thiazide diuretics and tetracycline, have been linked to pancreatitis (Steinberg, 1994; Greenberger, 1991; Gorelick, 1995). The course of pancreatitis associated with these drugs may have incited a more frequently fulminant disease process. Conversely, improvements in laboratory assays and radiologic modalities may now enable detection of a greater number of mild cases. Regardless of the underlying cause of this discrepancy, current maternal mortality from pancreatitis is only a tenth of previously reported rates.

## Etiology

Acute pancreatitis is caused by many different factors. While the list of etiologies is extensive (Table 25-1), approximately 80% of cases are attributable to either biliary tract disease or alcohol abuse in the general population (Steinberg, 1994; Steer, 1995). Gallstones are the most common cause of pancreatitis in the United States, Western Europe, and Asia, accounting for 45% of cases

(Steinberg, 1994). Alcoholism accounts for another 35%, roughly 10% are idiopathic, and the remainder are divided among miscellaneous causes.

Among pregnant patients, causes of pancreatitis parallel those of the general population. Physiologic changes in biliary function, however, appear to influence the incidence of cholelithiasis, although not necessarily gallstone pancreatitis, during pregnancy. Behavioral changes secondary to teratogenic concerns also may decrease the relative proportion of alcohol-induced pancreatitis. This section focuses on those causes most commonly seen in pregnancy: gallstones, hypertriglyceridemia, and drug-associated pancreatitis.

## Biliary Disease in Pregnancy

Cholelithiasis is the most common etiology of pancreatitis in pregnancy, representing a larger percentage of cases than in the nonpregnant population. Biliary disease has been identified in 68% to 100% of pregnant patients with pancreatitis (Ramin, 1995; Swisher, 1994; Block, 1989). The increased proportion of gallstone-induced pancreatitis may be attributable to the direct effects of pregnancy on gallstone formation, rather than a decreased incidence of other etiologies, and remains an area of active investigation.

Physiology of the biliary system during gestation appears to promote the incidence of gallstone formation through changes in both gallbladder function and bile composition. Using direct observation, intravenous contrast, and, most recently, serial ultrasound evaluation, residual gallbladder volume has been shown to increase throughout pregnancy (Potter, 1936; Gerdes,

T A B L E    **25-1**

**Causes of acute pancreatitis in pregnancy**

Obstruction (cholelithiasis)
Drugs (ethanol, thiazides, azathioprine, valproic acid)
Hyperlipidemia
Abdominal trauma
Hypercalcemia
Infection (viral, parasitic)
Vascular disease (systemic lupus erythematosis)
Miscellaneous (Crohn's disease, perforating ulcer, cystic fibrosis)

1938; Braverman, 1980). Braverman et al also demonstrated a slower rate of gallbladder emptying in the latter part of pregnancy. It is felt that these functional changes result in bile stasis, thereby facilitating gallstone formation. Furthermore, studies of bile composition have demonstrated an increase in the lithogenic index of bile, as well as increased bile acid pool size, increased cholesterol secretion, and decreased enterohepatic circulation (Kern, 1981; Scott, 1992). The functional changes that contribute to bile stasis act in concert with physiologic changes that increase the lithogenicity of bile constituents, leading to gallstone formation during pregnancy. In a study of gallstones in Chilean women, Valdivieso et al (1993) demonstrated the effect of pregnancy on the incidence of gallstone formation, noting gallstones in 12.2% of puerperal women, compared with 1.3% in age-matched controls.

The mechanism by which gallstones initiate pancreatitis remains poorly understood. In 1901, Opie proposed the "common channel theory," by which stone impaction at the ampulla of Vater occludes the biliopancreatic duct, creating a channel that allows bile to reflux into the pancreatic duct. Another theory suggests that the pancreatic duct itself becomes blocked, obstructing the outflow of pancreatic secretions, which, in turn, damage the pancreatic acini. While further investigations have challenged these theories, the actual sequence of events remains elusive. Regardless of the mechanism by which stone passage initiates pancreatitis, it is clear that passage is temporally related to the onset of symptoms. Recovery of stones from stool collections has been reported as high as 85% (Gorelick, 1995).

## Hypertriglyceridemia

Elevation of plasma triglycerides is a well-established cause of pancreatitis. The physiologic changes of pregnancy can exacerbate and unmask an underlying familial disorder and can compound the effects of other secondary causes of hypertriglyceridemia. The mechanism by which hyperlipidemia causes pancreatitis is not fully understood. Local injury to the pancreatic acini, however, is felt to occur through the release of free fatty acids by the action of lipases on the excessive

triglycerides (Klein, 1986; DeChalain, 1988). Patients with triglyceride levels exceeding 1000 mg/dL are at greatest risk for pancreatitis, especially those with type V hyperlipidemia (Klein, 1986).

Pregnancy alters lipid metabolism by several mechanisms. An increase in triglyceride production and very low density lipoprotein (VLDL) secretion, as well as a decrease in lipolysis, result in a 50% increase in cholesterol and a threefold increase in triglycerides, with the peak effect seen in the third trimester (Klein, 1986; DeChalain, 1988; Montes, 1984). Superimposed on a familial hyperlipidemia, the metabolic changes of pregnancy can lead to markedly elevated serum levels and greatly increase the risk of pancreatitis. Postpartum total cholesterol and VLDL fall to baseline by 6 weeks (Montes, 1984).

Several features of a patient's medical and family history may suggest an underlying lipid disorder. A history of pancreatitis, recurrent (unexplained) abdominal pain, and known familial disorders can suggest the presence of inherited hyperlipidemia. Chronic renal failure, poorly controlled diabetes mellitus, hypothyroidism, alcohol use, and drugs such as glucocorticoids and beta-blockers can lead to elevated lipid levels (Stone, 1994). In the presence of such conditions in a patient with a familial lipid disorder, the superimposition of pregnancy may result in fulminant pancreatitis (Stone, 1994). Intravenous fat emulsions administered to patients receiving parenteral nutrition are also a rare cause of pancreatitis.

## Drugs

Numerous drugs may occasionally cause pancreatitis. Among these, the immunosuppressants 6-mercaptopurine and azathioprine and the common AIDS therapies pentamidine and 2′,3′-dideoxyinosine have been strongly associated with this condition (Gorelick, 1995). Antibiotics, including erythromycin and sulfonamides, also have been implicated.

More pertinent to the pregnant population, thiazide diuretics and tetracycline historically accounted for a significant portion of pancreatitis during pregnancy. When these agents were used more commonly in the treatment of preeclampsia, thiazides were associated with 8% of cases of pancreatitis in pregnancy (Wilkinson, 1973). In the same review, tetracycline accounted for nearly 28% of cases and was also commonly associated with acute fatty liver of pregnancy. With subsequent elucidation of the teratogenic effects of tetracycline, this agent should no longer cause pancreatitis in pregnancy. Similarly, use of thiazide diuretics has little or no role in the modern management of preeclampsia.

## Pathology and Pathophysiology

The pancreas secretes approximately 20 enzymes in 2000 to 3000 mL of alkaline fluid each day. The fluid is rich in bicarbonate, which serves to neutralize gastric acid and provide the correct pH within the intestinal tract for activation of the pancreatic enzymes. Under hormonal and neural control, amylolytic, lipolytic, and proteolytic enzymes are released into the duodenum. The pancreas is normally protected from autodigestion by the presence of protease inhibitors and storage of proteases as precursors (zymogens).

Pancreatitis can be classified based on its chronicity and severity. Acute pancreatitis implies return of normal pancreatic function, while chronic disease represents residual damage to the gland. The acute form can be further classified as either mild (interstitial or edematous) or severe (necrotizing or hemorrhagic) pancreatitis. Edematous pancreatitis represents roughly 75% to 90% of cases and is typically self-limiting in its course (Reynaert, 1990; Steinberg, 1994). Morphologically, pancreatic interstitial edema and fat necrosis are present, but pancreatic necrosis is absent. In severe cases, the parenchyma of the gland undergoes necrosis and can lead to parenchymal and extrapancreatic hemorrhage.

Multiple diverse etiologies appear to trigger a sequence of events that ultimately leads to parenchymal inflammation and premature activation of pancreatic enzymes. Zymogen activation results in local damage by direct action on the acinar cells and pancreatic blood vessels. Systemic effects occur when complement and kallikrein activation induce disseminated intravascular coagulation and cardiovascular compromise. Degradation of surfactant by activated phospholipase A2 has been implicated as a possible mechanism of pulmonary injury in acute pancreatitis (Buchler, 1989).

## Clinical Manifestations

Symptoms of acute pancreatitis may develop abruptly or intensify over several hours. Present in nearly 100% of patients, epigastric or umbilical pain is constant and noncolicky in nature and often radiates to the back (Swisher, 1994). The pain is variable in severity, often peaking in a matter of hours but frequently continuing for many days. In some patients, the pain is worse in the supine position and relieved partially by sitting and leaning forward. Nausea and vomiting affect 80% of patients, but vomiting does not usually relieve the pain (Gorelick, 1995; Swisher, 1994).

Examination of the patient generally reveals anxious and restless behavior as the patient strives to attain a comfortable position. Fever is present in as many as 60% of patients. Tachycardia and hypotension may result from hemorrhage, vasodilation, increased vascular permeability, or sequestration of fluids in the retroperitoneum or peritoneal cavity (ascites). Pulmonary findings are present in a minority of patients, ranging from decreased breath sounds secondary to effusions (more often left-sided) to severe respiratory distress. Evaluation of the abdomen reveals areas of tenderness, both epigastric and generalized. Voluntary and involuntary guarding is frequently present. Pancreatic pseudocysts may be palpable. The abdomen is commonly distended, and bowel sounds are diminished or absent. Bluish discoloration around the umbilicus (Cullen's sign) or at the flanks (Grey Turner's sign) occurs in less than 1% of patients but represents the ominous development of hemorrhagic pancreatitis with retroperitoneal dissection.

## Complications

Severe cases of pancreatitis can lead to both local and systemic complications (Table 25-2). Locally, pancreatic necrosis and infection may occur early

T A B L E   **25-2**

Complications of acute pancreatitis
in pregnancy

Hypovolemic shock (third-space sequestration)
Disseminated intravascular coagulation
Acute respiratory distress syndrome
Acute tubular necrosis
Hypocalcemia, hyperglycemia
Pseudocyst formation
Pancreatic abscess
Upper gastrointestinal hemorrhage
Premature labor and delivery

in the course of disease, often within the first 2 weeks. Necrosis of greater than 50% of the pancreas is associated with high rates of infection. Increased abdominal tenderness, fever, and elevated WBC counts signal the onset of infection. Late complications include pseudocyst and abscess formation. Pseudocysts are collections of pancreatic secretions that lack epithelial linings and develop in 1% to 8% of cases of acute pancreatitis (Gorelick, 1995; Steinberg, 1994). They usually occur 2 to 3 weeks after the onset of illness. Patients frequently complain of upper abdominal pain and may develop symptoms related to growth and pressure on adjacent structures. Abscesses differ from pseudocysts by the presence of a capsule surrounding a purulent fluid collection. Abscesses complicate 1% to 4% of cases and are most often diagnosed 3 to 4 weeks after the onset of pancreatitis (Steinberg, 1994).

Systemic complications arising in severe cases of pancreatitis are often manifest within the first week of illness and are potentially life-threatening. Multisystem organ failure may involve the pulmonary, cardiovascular, and renal systems, contributing to a mortality rate of nearly 9% (Steinberg, 1994). Pulmonary involvement ranges from pleural effusions and pneumonia to acute respiratory distress syndrome (ARDS). The frequency of ARDS as a cause of death has previously been underestimated. In a review of 405 autopsy cases, 60% of deaths occurred in the first week of illness; among these patients, pulmonary failure was the most common cause of death (Renner, 1985). The exact mechanism of pulmonary injury has not been elucidated. As mentioned earlier, how-

ever, patients with pancreatitis-associated pulmonary complications have been noted to have higher phospholipase A and phospholipase A2 catalytic activity (Buchler, 1989).

Various other organ systems are at risk in severe pancreatitis. Cardiovascular compromise may occur secondary to several mechanisms. Hemorrhage (intra- or retroperitoneal), fluid sequestration, and activation of vasoactive substances can lead to profound, refractory hypotension. Renal failure may develop following hypotensive episodes and acute tubular necrosis. Overwhelming sepsis is the most common cause of death after the first week of illness (Buchler, 1989).

Uncommon complications also may occur during severe cases of pancreatitis. Stress ulcers leading to gastrointestinal hemorrhage, pancreatic pseudoaneurysms, or colonic obstruction or fistulas may develop. Sudden blindness rarely has been reported (Purtscher's angiopathic retinopathy), with funduscopy revealing cotton-wool spots and flame-shaped hemorrhages found solely at the optic disk and macula.

## Diagnosis

### Laboratory Evaluation

While serum amylase has been the cornerstone of diagnosis for many decades, a variety of biochemical indicators have been identified as markers of pancreatitis. Amylase isoenzymes, serum lipase, and the amylase-creatinine clearance ratio also may be used to increase the diagnostic accuracy of more standard serum assays. Several factors influence the accuracy of these tests. For example, amylase levels may be falsely elevated by nonpancreatic production, impaired renal clearance, or acidemia, as in diabetic ketoacidosis (pH < 7.33). Furthermore, concurrent conditions, such as hypertriglyceridemia, can falsely lower measured values.

Serum amylase is a rapidly performed, readily available serum marker of pancreatic enzyme levels. Many organs contribute to total amylase values. The pancreas contributes roughly 40%, while salivary glands contribute 60%, as measured by the P-isoenzyme and S-isoenzyme levels, respectively. Other tissues, such as the lung and fallopian tubes, also produce S-isoamylase. Isoenzyme measurement can improve the sensitivity of amylase testing. However, it is not as widely available. Amylase rises in the first few hours of disease onset and falls rapidly, returning to normal in 24 to 72 hours. It is, therefore, not an accurate test for patients presenting more than several days after the onset of symptoms. Overall, serum amylase has a sensitivity of 95% to 100% and a specificity of 70% (Agarwal, 1990).

In contrast, serum lipase rises in a fashion parallel to amylase but remains elevated for a longer period (as many as 7 to 14 days). Serum lipase, therefore, has greater sensitivity in the subset of patients with late presentation. It is also unaffected by diabetic ketoacidosis. Lipase is produced mainly by the pancreas but is produced by other gastrointestinal sources as well, namely, liver, intestine, biliary tract, and salivary glands. The effect of nonpancreatic production on serum lipase levels, however, is unclear. It is generally regarded that lipase is more specific (99%) and as sensitive (99%–100%) as serum amylase and merits wider use in the evaluation of pancreatitis (Agarwal, 1990).

The effect of pregnancy on amylase and lipase levels has been investigated. Strickland et al (1984) studied 413 asymptomatic women of varying gestational ages. In contrast to earlier studies reporting higher levels in pregnancy that vary through gestation, they concluded that mean amylase activities did not significantly differ among gestational age groups, nor compared with women 6 weeks' postpartum (Kaiser, 1975; Strickland, 1984). Amylase levels measured as high as 150 IU/liter. Ordorica et al (1991) corroborated these findings, noting no difference in amylase activity related to pregnancy. Lipase levels were also studied, and no significant difference was found between gestational age groups or compared with nonpregnant controls. Mean values of lipase in 175 women were approximately 12 IU/liter, with none exceeding 30 IU/liter.

The ratio of amylase to creatinine clearance (Cam/Ccr%) has also been evaluated for its diagnostic usefulness. This ratio is determined by the equation

$$\text{Cam/Ccr}\% = \frac{\text{(Amylase) urine} \times \text{(Creatinine) serum}}{\text{(Amylase) serum} \times \text{(Creatinine) urine}} \times 100$$

This ratio's role in the diagnosis of pancreatitis relies on the increased urinary clearance of amylase secondary to the decreased renal absorption of this enzyme that occurs in pancreatitis. An elevated ratio was felt initially to be a sensitive test for acute pancreatitis (Warshaw, 1975). Subsequent studies, however, have shown this to be of limited utility secondary to poor specificity and sensitivity (Leavitt, 1978; Lankisch, 1977; Levine, 1975).

## Radiologic Evaluation

Radiologic tests aid in the diagnosis of acute pancreatitis and can be used to monitor the development and progression of complications. A plain film of the abdomen may show dilatation of an isolated loop of intestine (sentinel loop) adjacent to the pancreas. Pleural effusions may be detected on chest x-ray. While overlying bowel gas patterns may obscure imaging, ultrasound is very useful in evaluating the biliary tree and for ruling out other differential diagnoses. Free peritoneal fluid, abscess or pseudocyst formation, and morphologic changes of the pancreas can be visualized ultrasonographically. Computed tomography (CT scan) is superior in evaluating the severity of pancreatitis. Unhindered by bowel gas patterns, CT scans can demonstrate pancreatic necrosis and pseudocysts and provide guidance for directed sampling of abscess cavities (Figs 25-1, 25-2).

## Differential Diagnosis

Abdominal complaints in pregnancy present unique diagnostic challenges (Table 25-3). Nonobstetric conditions include cholecystitis, duodenal ulcer, appendicitis, splenic rupture, perinephric abscess, mesenteric vascular occlusion, pneumonia, and diabetic ketoacidosis. In the pregnant patient, preeclampsia, hyperemesis gravidarum, and ruptured ectopic pregnancy must be added to the differential diagnosis.

Preeclampsia may mimic pancreatitis with upper abdominal pain, nausea, and vomiting. Concomitant hypertension, proteinuria, and edema,

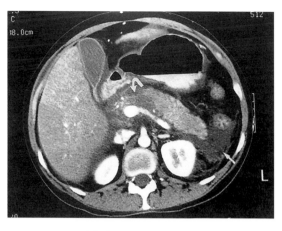

F I G U R E **25-1**
Computed tomography scan demonstrating necrosis in the head of the pancreas (*curved arrow*) and free fluid in the anterior pararenal space (*straight arrow*). (Courtesy of Dr. Paula Woodward.)

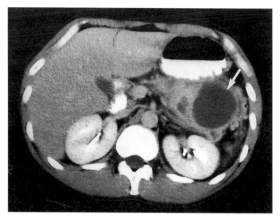

F I G U R E **25-2**
Computed tomography scan demonstrating pseudocyst in the tail of the pancreas (*arrow*). (Courtesy of Dr. Paula Woodward.)

T A B L E **25-3**
Differential diagnosis of acute pancreatitis

*Non-obstetric Conditions*

| | |
|---|---|
| Acute cholecystitis | Perinephric abscess |
| Appendicitis | Pneumonia |
| Duodenal ulcer | Pulmonary embolus |
| Splenic rupture | Myocardial infarction |
| Mesenteric vascular occlusion | Diabetic ketoacidosis |

*Obstetric Conditions*

| | |
|---|---|
| Preeclampsia | Hyperemesis |
| Ruptured ectopic pregnancy | gravidarum |

however, will usually be present. Hyperemesis gravidarum most often affects patients in the first trimester, without a significant component of pain. Ruptured ectopic pregnancy may produce symptoms similar to those seen in acute pancreatitis. Hemoperitoneum can occur with either and will often require laparotomy for diagnosis.

## Prognostic Indicators

Several methods utilizing clinical and laboratory data have been developed to indicate the severity of acute pancreatitis and allow refinement of

prognosis (Ranson, 1974, 1979; Imrie, 1978). The most widely used criteria were developed by Ranson for gallstone pancreatitis (Table 25-4). The number of criteria met correlates with the mortality risk for the individual. For nongallstone pancreatitis, patients with fewer than three signs have rates of mortality less than 3% and morbidity less than 5%. Patients with three or more positive signs carry a 62% mortality rate and a 90% morbidity rate. Utilizing a modified set of criteria for gallstone pancreatitis, individuals with fewer than three signs have a 1.5% mortality rate, while those with three or more signs demonstrate a 29% mortality rate. Critics of this system cite poor specificity, delayed assessment (due to the labs required at 48 hours), and inability to perform repeated assessments as major deterrants to its usefulness.

Another method of clinically evaluating the severity of several types of critical illnesses, including pancreatitis is the Acute Physiology and Chronic Health Evaluation (APACHE) III criteria (Table 25-5) (Knaus, 1991). Unlike Ranson's criteria, the APACHE assessment can be updated and the patient's course monitored on a continuing basis. This system evaluates several variables, both biochemical and physiologic, and calculates scores based on deviation from normal values. A 5-point increase in score is independently associated with

TABLE    25-4

Clinical indicators of poor prognosis: Ranson's criteria

*Nongallstone Pancreatitis*
On admission
    Age >55 yr
    WBC >16,000/μL
    Glucose >200 mg/dL
    LDH >350 IU/liter
    AST >250 IU/liter
Within 48 hr
    Decrease in hematocrit >10%
    Increase in BUN >5 mg/dL
    Calcium <8 mg/dL
    Pao$_2$ <60 mm Hg
    Base deficit >4 mmol/liter
    Fluid deficit >6 liters

*Gallstone Pancreatitis*
On admission
    Age >70 yr
    WBC >18,000/μL
    Glucose >220 mg/dL
    LDH >400 IU/liter
    AST >250 IU/liter
Within 48 hr
    Decrease in hematocrit >10%
    Increase in BUN >2 mg/dL
    Calcium <8 mg/dL
    Base deficit >5 mmol/liter
    Fluid deficit >4 liters

LDH, lactic dehydrogenase; AST, aspartate amino transferase.

TABLE    25-5

Acute Physiology and Chronic Health Evaluation (APACHE) III prognostic system for critically ill adults

| | |
|---|---|
| Temperature | Serum sodium |
| Mean BP | Serum glucose |
| Heart rate | Serum creatinine |
| Respiratory rate | BUN |
| Pao$_2$ | Bilirubin |
| A-aDo$_2$ | Albumin |
| Arterial pH | Hematocrit |
| Urine output | Leukocyte count |

Age, comorbidities, and neurologic state also are scored. A numerical value is assigned to each category (total score 0–299) and weighted by its deviation from the normal range.

Source: Gorelick FS. Acute pancreatitis. In: Yamada T, Alpers DH, Power DW, et al, eds. Textbook of Gastroenterology. 2nd ed. Philadelphia: JB Lippincott, 1995:2064–2091.

a statistically significant increase in the relative risk of hospital death within a specific disease category. Within 24 hours of admission, 95% of patients admitted to the intensive care unit could be given a risk estimate for death within 3% of that actually observed (Knaus, 1991). Although more complex and computer-dependent, the APACHE scoring system appears more accurate than Ranson's criteria in predicting morbidity (Larvin, 1989).

Several single prognostic indicators have been investigated in order to achieve early identification of pancreatic necrosis. Paracentesis can be performed, with return of dark, prune-colored fluid being characteristic of necrotizing pancreatitis. Utilizing color charts, Mayer and McMahon (1985) identified 90% of the patients who subse-

quently died and 72% of patients with severe morbidity. Other biochemical indicators include C-reactive protein, alpha-2 macroglobulin, and leukocyte elastase. While these tests appear promising, further study is needed and availability is limited.

Compared with scoring systems and laboratory markers, contrast-enhanced CT scans offer broader information regarding intra-abdominal anatomy. Areas of necrosis and their extent are identified and can be serially evaluated (see Fig 25-1). Infection within pseudocysts can be suggested by evidence of gas production. This test, however, is limited in its availability and is difficult to obtain in severely ill patients.

## Management

The initial treatment of acute pancreatitis is supportive medical management. Because most cases are mild and self-limiting, this approach is largely successful. Avoidance or cessation of exacerbating factors, such as alcohol or drugs, is a basic principle to be observed. Assessment of prognostic indicators, as discussed earlier, permits appropriate surveillance. Patients with more severe disease should be transferred to an intensive care unit for continuous monitoring, because shock and pulmonary failure often present early in the course of disease and require prompt recognition and management.

Medical therapy is comprised of fluid and electrolyte management, adequate analgesia, and elimination of oral intake. Intravenous fluid resuscitation is a vital component of treatment in both mild and severe cases. Restoration of intravascular volume and avoidance of hypotension is important for cardiovascular stability and renal perfusion. Electrolyte abnormalities are common, including hypokalemia and metabolic alkalosis from severe vomiting and hypocalcemia from fat saponification. Serial assessment of electrolytes and appropriate replacement are essential. Parenteral analgesia is frequently necessary; morphine compounds, however, should be avoided secondary to their actions on the sphincter of Oddi. Oral intake is withheld for the duration of illness. Parenteral nutrition should be implemented early in the hospital course.

Nasogastric suction may be appropriate in a subset of patients with acute pancreatitis. Nasogastric suction, however, does not appear to influence duration of disease or its symptoms. Several studies have investigated the role of nasogastric suction in mild-to-moderate pancreatitis and found no difference in duration of abdominal pain, tenderness, nausea, and elevated pancreatic enzymes or time to resumption of oral feeding (Naeije, 1978; Levant, 1974; Loiudice, 1984). Therefore, nasogastric suction should be utilized on an elective basis for symptomatic relief for those patients with severe emesis or ileus.

Prophylactic antibiotics also have been advocated in an effort to prevent the development of infectious complications. Mild cases of pancreatitis do not appear to benefit from antibiotic prophylaxis, although studies are few (Howes, 1975; Finch, 1976). In contrast, severe cases with pancreatic necrosis have a high rate (40%) of bacterial contamination and represent a subset of patients that might benefit from antibiotic administration (Berger, 1986). A study of 74 patients with acute necrotizing pancreatitis treated with imipenem prophylactically demonstrated a significantly decreased incidence of pancreatic sepsis (12% vs. 30%) in treated versus untreated patients (Pederzoli, 1993). Similar results were observed by Sainio (1995). While further studies are needed to better define both patient and antibiotic selection, antibiotic prophylaxis appears to be indicated in patients at high risk for septic complications.

Antienzyme and hormonal therapies have been designed to reduce the severity of disease by halting the production of pancreatic enzymes and the subsequent cascade activation of the complement, kallikrein-kinin, fibrinolytic, and coagulation systems. Studies evaluating atropine, calcitonin, glucagon, somatostatin, and the enzyme inhibitors, aprotinin and gabexate, however, have not shown improved morbidity or mortality in severe acute pancreatitis (Reynaert, 1990; Steinberg, 1994).

## Surgical Therapy

Although supportive measures are the mainstay of therapy, surgical intervention also has a place in the management of acute pancreatitis. The exact role, timing, and form of surgery remain a matter of debate. The one clear indication for surgery is for diagnosis in patients with an acute abdomen. An uncertain diagnosis mandates exploration for possible surgically correctable conditions. Two other situations also may require surgery: gallstone pancreatitis and select anatomic or infectious complications.

The goals of biliary surgery in cases of gallstone pancreatitis are to prevent recurrence and to decrease morbidity and mortality by removing the instigating agent. Cholecystectomy and bile duct exploration are not performed, however, during the acute episode. Because nearly 95% of stones pass during the first week of illness, the utility of surgery early in the illness does not weigh heavily against the high mortality rates that have been reported for early biliary surgery (Osborne, 1981). While not indicated in the acute phase of illness, biliary surgery should be performed after the acute pancreatitis subsides, prior to discharge from the hospital.

An alternative to open surgical removal of bile duct stones has been developed. Endoscopic retrograde cholangiopancreatography with endoscopic sphincterotomy offers the potential advantages of use in the critically ill patient and lower morbidity and mortality rates than laparotomy. If performed within the first 72 hours of illness, this procedure has been shown to decrease morbidity and length of hospital stay in patients with severe pancreatitis (Neoptolemos, 1988). It has been applied in a small number of pregnant patients without complications and avoids the potential risks of major surgery during pregnancy (Uomo, 1994; Baillie, 1990; Buchner, 1988).

Pancreatic surgery for early and late complications of pancreatitis has also been the subject of controversy. A few situations appear to be clear indications for surgical intervention, such as acute, life-threatening hemorrhage. However, the timing and type of surgical procedures for later complications, such as sterile necrosis, pseudocysts, and abscesses, are less straightforward.

Arterial hemorrhage occurs in 2% of patients with severe pancreatitis. Necrosis and erosion into surrounding arteries of the gastrointestinal tract result in massive intraabdominal or retroperitoneal hemorrhage. Arteriographic embolization followed by surgical debridement and artery ligation improved survival from 0% to 40% (Waltman, 1986). In contrast, the development of sterile pancreatic necrosis is not an automatic indication for surgery, because up to 70% of cases will resolve spontaneously. While few studies have been performed, no benefit for early debridement has been demonstrated (Bradley, 1991; Karimigani, 1992).

The formation of pseudocysts may mandate surgical debridement based on clinical characteristics. Occurring in as many as 10% to 20% of patients with severe acute pancreatitis, pseudocysts resolve in approximately 50% (Raynaert, 1990). Surgery is performed if symptoms of hemorrhage, infection, or compression develop or if the pseudocyst either exceeds 5 to 6 cm or persists longer than 6 weeks. Internal drainage represents the superior surgical approach, although percutaneous drainage may temporize a critically ill patient. Fluid should be collected for culture to rule out infection.

Finally, pancreatic abscess formation occurs in 2% to 4% of patients with severe pancreatitis and is 100% lethal if left undrained. Although percutaneous drainage may be temporizing, the catheter often becomes occluded secondary to the thick purulent effluent. With early and aggressive surgical debridement, mortality is reduced to 5% (Warshaw, 1985). Either transperitoneal or retroperitoneal approaches may be appropriate. Postoperatively, 20% will require reoperation for incomplete drainage, ongoing infection, fistulas, or hemorrhage (Warshaw, 1985).

## Considerations in Pregnancy

Treatment of pancreatitis does not differ in the pregnant patient. Supportive measures are identical to those of the nonpregnant patient, and severe complications are managed aggressively. Two situations, however, merit special consideration in pregnancy: the treatment of biliary disease and hypertriglyceridemia.

The management of biliary disease in pregnancy raises the issue of timing of surgery during gestation. On resolution of acute pancreatitis, cholecystectomy is typically performed in a nonpregnant patient prior to discharge from the hospital. Some advocate continued conservative management in pregnancy to avoid operative complications and fetal morbidity. A high relapse rate (72%), however, is often encountered (Swisher, 1994). For patients presenting in the first trimester, this may be as high as 88%. Surgical intervention decreases the incidence of relapse and the risk of systemic complications.

Several studies support the use of second-trimester cholecystectomy for cholecystitis or pancreatitis (Swisher, 1994; Block, 1989; Ramin, 1995). The second trimester appears optimal in order to avoid both organogenesis and a possible increased rate of spontaneous abortion in the first trimester (vida infra). Third-trimester patients are best managed conservatively because they are close to the postpartum period when operative risks are reduced. Cholecystectomy may be performed by laparotomy or open laparoscopy. The open technique for the laparoscopic approach is often best, to avoid puncturing the gravid uterus with blind trocar insertion.

Fetal loss following cholecystectomy was once reported to be as high as 15% (Green, 1963). Many earlier reports, however, included patients undergoing surgery in the first trimester suffering spontaneous abortion many weeks postoperatively. Because at least 15% of all pregnancies

---

## ACUTE PANCREATITIS

### I. *Goals of Therapy*

    A. Supportive medical management, relief of symptoms
    B. Avoidance of exacerbating factors: alcohol, drugs
    C. Assessment of prognostic factors

### II. *Management Protocol*

    A. Nothing by mouth for the duration of the illness, parenteral nutrition if prolonged.
    B. Adequate analgesia: often parenteral; avoid morphine compounds.
    C. Intravenous fluid resuscitation; avoid hypotension.
    D. Serial electrolyte determinations; supplement as needed.
    E. Consider nasogastric suction for symptom relief: severe emesis, prolonged ileus.
    F. Broad-spectrum antibiotics in severe cases (imipenem).
    G. Transfer severe cases to the intensive care unit.
    H. Consider surgery for gallstone pancreatitis, pseudocyst formation.
    I. Surgery mandatory for pancreatic abscess, hemorrhage, or acute abdomen.

### III. *Critical Laboratory Tests*

    A. Lipase, amylase, complete blood count with differential, electrolytes, calcium, lactic dehydrogenase, arterial blood gas, liver function tests; consider lipid profile; chest x-ray, gallbladder ultrasound, CT scan.

### IV. *Consultation*

    A. General surgery, intensivist

---

are now known to end in spontaneous abortion, and preterm labor is seen in up to 10% of all continuing pregnancies, it would appear that the actual rate of complications related to surgery probably approaches nil, a figure confirmed by several recent studies (Swisher, 1994; Kort, 1993; McKellar, 1992). A review of studies from 1963 to 1987, evaluating fetal loss in patients undergoing cholecystectomy, revealed an 8% spontaneous abortion rate and 7.7% rate of premature labor (McKellar, 1992). In a similar manner, laparoscopic cholecystectomy in the second trimester has been reported in a small number of patients, with no increase in fetal or maternal morbidity or mortality (Morrell, 1992; Elerding, 1993).

Treatment of hypertriglyceridemia in pregnancy is aimed primarily at prevention of pancreatitis. Fats should be limited to fewer than 20 g/day. This restrictive diet, however, is not palatable and is difficult for patients to maintain. Sanderson et al (1991) reported successful management of hypertrigliceridemia during an episode of pancreatitis and the remainder of gestation by utilizing intravenous fluid therapy to provide calories in the form of 5% dextrose and restricting oral intake to clear liquids. Total parenteral nutrition offers another therapeutic approach when dietary adjustments are inadequate to prevent excessive triglyceride elevations (see Chapter 10). Plasma exchange and immunospecific apheresis also have been investigated and have suggested that long-term extracorporeal elimination of lipoproteins may offer a safe and effective method of prevention and treatment of hypertriglyceridemic pancreatitis in pregnancy (Swoboda, 1993).

## REFERENCES

Agarwal N, Pitchumoni CS, Sivaprasad AV. Evaluating tests for acute pancreatitis. Am J Gastroenterol 1990;85:356–366.

Baillie J, Cairns SR, Putnam WS, Cotton PB. Endoscopic management of choledocholithiasis during pregnancy. Surg Gynecol Obstet 1990;171:1–4.

Berger HG, Bittner R, Block S, Buchler M. Bacterial contamination of pancreatic necrosis: a prospective clinical study. Gastroenterology 1986;91:433–438.

Block P, Kelly TR. Management of gallstone pancreatitis. Surg Gynecol Obstet 1989;168:426–428.

Bradley EL, Allen K. A prospective longitudinal study of observation versus surgical intervention in the management of necrotizing pancreatitis. Am J Surg 1991;16:19–25.

Braverman DZ, Johnson ML, Kern F Jr. Effects of pregnancy and contraceptive steroids on gallbladder function. N Engl J Med 1980;302:363.

Buchler M, Malfertheiner P, Schadlich H, et al. Role of phospholipase A2 in human acute pancreatitis. Gastroenterology 1989;97:1521–1526.

Buchner WF, Stoltenberg PH, Kirtley DW. Endoscopic management of severe gallstone pancreatitis during pregnancy. Am J Gastroenterol 1988;83:1073.

Corlett RC, Mishell DR. Pancreatitis in pregnancy. Am J Obstet Gynecol 1972;113:281–290.

DeChalain TMB, Michell WL, Berger GMB. Hyperlipidemia, pregnancy and pancreatitis. Surg Gynecol Obstet 1988;167:469–473.

Elerding SC. Laparoscopic cholecystectomy in pregnancy. Am J Surg 1993;165:625–627.

Finch WT, Sawyers JL, Schenker S. A prospective study to determine the efficacy of antibiotics in acute pancreatitis. Ann Surg 1976;183:667–671.

Gerdes M, Boyden EA. The rate of emptying of the human gallbladder in pregnancy. Surg Gynecol Obstet 1938;66:145.

Gorelick FS. Acute pancreatitis. In: Yamada T, et al, eds. Textbook of gastroenterology. 2nd ed. Philadelphia: JB Lippincott, 1995:2064–2091.

Green J, Rogers A, Rubin L. Fetal loss after cholecystectomy during pregnancy. Canad Med Assoc J 1963;88:576–577.

Greenberger NJ, Toskes PP, Isselbacher KJ. Acute and chronic pancreatitis. In: Wilson JD, et al, eds. Harrison's principles of internal medicine. 12th ed. New York: McGraw-Hill, 1991:1372–1378.

Herfort K, Fialova V, Srp B. Acute pancreatitis in pregnancy. Mater Med Pol 1981;13:15.

Howes R, Zuidema GD, Cameron JL. Evaluation of prophylactic antibiotics in acute pancreatitis. J Surg Res 1975;18:197–200.

Imrie CW, Benjamin IS, Ferguson JC. A single-centre double-blind trial of Trasylol therapy in primary acute pancreatitis. Br J Surg 1978;65:337–341.

Jouppila P, Mokka R, Larmi TK. Acute pancreatitis in pregnancy. Surg Gynecol Obstet 1974;139:879–882.

Kaiser R, Berk JE, Fridhandler L. Serum amylase changes during pregnancy. Am J Obstet Gynecol 1975;122:283–286.

Karimigani I, Porter KA, Langevin RE, Banks P. Prognostic factors in sterile pancreatic necrosis. Gastroenterology 1992;103:1636–1640.

Kern F Jr, Everson FT, Demark B, et al. Biliary lipids, bile acids, and gallbladder function in the human female. J Clin Invest 1981;68:1229.

Klein KB. Pancreatitis in pregnancy. In: Rustgi VK, Cooper JN, eds. Gastrointestinal and hepatic complications in pregnancy. New York: Wiley, 1986.

Knaus WA, Wagner DP, Draper EA, et al. The APACHE III prognostic system. Risk prediction of hospital mortality for critically ill hospitalized adults. Chest 1991;100:1619.

Kort B, Katz VL, Watson WJ. The effect of nonobstetric operation during pregnancy. Surg Gynecol Obstet 1993;177:371–376.

Langmade CF, Edmondson HA. Acute pancreatitis during pregnancy and the postpartum period: a report of nine cases. Surg Gynecol Obstet 1951;92:43–46.

Lankisch PG, Koop H, Otto J, et al. Specificity of increased amylase to creatinine clearance ratio in acute pancreatitis. Digestion 1977;16:160–164.

Larvin M, McMahon MJ. APACHE-II score for assessment and monitoring of acute pancreatitis. Lancet 1989;2:201–205.

Legro RS, Laifer SA. First trimester pancreatitis: Maternal and neonatal outcome. J Reprod Med 1995;40:689.

Levant JA, Secrist DM, Resin HR, et al. Nasogastric suction in the treatment of alcoholic pancreatitis. JAMA 1974;229:51–52.

Levine RJ, Glauser FL, Berk JE. Enhancement of the amylase-creatinine clearance ratio in disorders other than acute pancreatitis. N Engl J Med 1975;292:329–332.

Levitt MD, Johnson SG. Is the C Am/C Cr ratio of value for the diagnosis of pancreatitis? Gastroenterology 1978;75:118–119.

Loiudice TA, Lang J, Mehta H, Banta L. Treatment of acute alcoholic pancreatitis: the roles of cimetidine and nasogastric suction. Am J Gastroenterol 1984;79:553–558.

Mayer DA, McMahon MJ. The diagnostic and prognostic value of peritoneal lavage in patients with acute pancreatitis. Surg Gynecol Obstet 1985; 160:507–512.

McKellar DP, Anderson CT, Boynton CJ. Cholecystectomy during pregnancy without fetal loss. Surg Gynecol Obstet 1992;174:465–468.

Montes A, Walden CE, Knopp RH, et al. Physiologic and supraphysiologic increases in lipoprotein lipids and apoproteins in late pregnancy and postpartum. Arteriosclerosis 1984;4:407–417.

Morrell DG, Mullins JR, Harrison PB. Laparoscopic cholecystectomy during pregnancy in symptomatic patients. Surg 1992;112:856–859.

Naeije R, Salingret E, Clumeck N, et al. Is nasogastric suction necessary in acute pancreatitis? Br Med J 1978;2:659–660.

Neoptolemos JP, Carr-Locke DL, London NJ, et al. Controlled trial of urgent endoscopic retrograde cholangiopancreatography and endoscopic sphincterotomy versus conservative treatment for acute pancreatitis due to gallstones. Lancet 1988;2:979–983.

Opie EL. The relation of cholelithiasis to disease of the pancreas and to fat necrosis. Am J Med Surg 1901;12:27–43.

Ordorica SA, Frieden FJ, Marks F, et al. Pancreatic enzyme activity in pregnancy. J Reprod Med 1991;36:359–362.

Osborne DH, Imrie CW, Carter DC. Biliary surgery in the same admission for gallstone-associated acute pancreatitis. Br J Surg 1981;68:758–761.

Pederzoli P, Bassi C, Vesentini S, Campedelli A. A randomized multicenter clinical trial of antibiotic prophylaxis of septic complications in acute necrotizing pancreatitis with imipenem. Surg Gynecol Obstet 1993;176:480–483.

Potter MG. Observations of the gallbladder and bile during pregnancy at term. JAMA 1936;106:1070.

Ramin KD, Ramin SM, Richey SD, Cunningham FG. Acute pancreatitis in pregnancy. Am J Obstet Gynecol 1995;173:187–191.

Ranson JHC, Rifkind KM, Roses DF, et al. Prognostic signs and the role of operative management in acute pancreatitis. Surg Gynecol Obstet 1974; 139:69–81.

Ranson JC. The timing of biliary surgery in acute pancreatitis. Ann Surg 1979;189:654–663.

Renner IG, Savage WT, Pantoja JL, Renner VJ. Death due to acute pancreatitis. Dig Dis Sci 1985;30: 1005–1018.

Reynaert MS, Dugernier T, Kestens PJ. Current therapeutic strategies in severe acute pancreatitis. Intensive Care Med 1990;16:352–362.

Sainio V, Kemppainen E, Puolakkainen P, et al. Early antibiotic treatment in acute necrotizing pancreatitis. Lancet 1995;346:663.

Sanderson SL, Iverius P, Wilson DE. Successful hyperlipemic pregnancy. JAMA 1991;265:1858–1860.

Scott LD. Gallstone disease and pancreatitis in pregnancy. Gastroenterol Clin North Am 1992;21: 803.

Steer ML. Acute pancreatitis. In: Ayres SM, Gronvik A, Holbrook PR, Shoemaker WC, eds. Textbook of critical care. 3rd ed. Philadelphia: WB Saunders, 1995.

Steinberg W, Tenner S. Acute pancreatitis. N Engl J Med 1994;330:1198–1210.

Stone NJ. Secondary causes of hyperlipidemia. Med Clin North Am 1994;78:117–141.

Strickland DM, Hauth JC, Widish J, et al. Amylase and isoamylase activities in serum of pregnant women. Obstet Gynecol 1984;64:389–391.

Swisher SG, Hunt KK, Schmit PJ, et al. Management of pancreatitis complicating pregnancy. Am Surg 1994;60:759–762.

Swoboda K, Derfler K, Koppensteiner R, et al. Extracorporeal lipid elimination for treatment of gestational hyperlipidemic pancreatitis. Gastroenterology 1993;104:1527–1531.

Uomo G, Manes G, Picciotto FO, Rabitti PG. Endoscopic treatment of acute biliary pancreatitis in pregnancy. J Clin Gastroenterol 1994;18:250–252.

Valdivieso V, Covarrubias C, Siegel F, Cruz F. Pregnancy and cholelithiasis: pathogenesis and natural course of gallstones diagnosed in early puerperium. Hepatology 1993;17:1–4.

Waltman AC, Luers PR, Athanasoulis CA, Warshaw AL. Massive arterial hemorrhage in patients with pancreatitis. Arch Surg 1986;121:439–443.

Warshaw AL, Fuller AF Jr. Specificity of increased renal clearance of amylase in diagnosis of acute pancreatitis. N Engl J Med 1975;292:325–328.

Warshaw AL, Gongliang J. Improved survival in 45 patients with pancreatic abscess. Ann Surg 1985;202:408–417.

Wilkinson EJ. Acute pancreatitis in pregnancy: a review of 98 cases and a report of 8 new cases. Obstet Gynecol Surv 1973;28:281–303.

# CHAPTER *26*

# Systemic Lupus Erythematosus

*S* ystemic lupus erythematosus (SLE) and antiphospholipid syndrome (APS) are among the most commonly encountered autoimmune diseases in women of reproductive age. Pregnancy may influence the expression SLE and APS in women, and occasionally, catastrophic exacerbations of these conditions threaten the mother's life. Both conditions may pose serious risk to the fetus. The management of SLE and APS in pregnancy often requires special medical treatments and careful fetal assessment with appropriate timing of delivery. In some cases, the physician may be required to consider experimental therapies with uncertain risk-benefit profiles. For these reasons, obstetricians should be familiar with SLE and APS, how they influence and are influenced by pregnancy, and what special medical risks may be in store for mother or the fetus.

An *autoimmune disease*, such as SLE or APS, is diagnosed when a state of *autoimmunity* (i.e., evidence of an immune response to self-constituents) is associated with a recognized pattern of clinical signs and symptoms. The state of autoimmunity is usually confirmed by the detection of characteristic *autoantibodies* in the patient's circulation. For some autoimmune diseases, such as autoimmune thyroid disease, there is substantial evidence linking the activity of the autoantibody(ies) or autoimmune effector cells to the disease state. For other conditions, such as SLE, there is less evidence that the clinical manifesta-

tions of the disease are actually caused by detectable autoantibodies or other effector mechanisms.

There are two major theories regarding the fundamental immunologic disturbance that leads to a state of autoimmunity. The earliest of these held that autoimmunity resulted from a failure in the normal deletion of lymphocytes that recognized self-antigens (Burnet, 1959). More recently, authorities have suggested that autoimmunity results from a failure of the normal regulation of the immune system, which contains many immune mechanisms that recognize self-antigens but are normally suppressed. In this construct, autoimmunity may be regarded as a failure to maintain tolerance of self. Regardless of fundamental cause, authorities agree that the full expression of an autoimmune disease requires a combination of environmental, genetic, and host factors.

Most autoimmune diseases have a higher prevalence among women than among men, and sex steroids have been implicated as one factor involved in this disparity. In one mouse model of SLE, females develop autoantibodies, clinical disease, and eventually die of their disease earlier than males (Roubinian, 1978; Steinberg, 1979). Murine experiments also have shown that the onset of disease is accelerated by estrogens, and both the onset and course of disease are retarded by androgens (Roubinian, 1977, 1978, 1979). In humans, an influence of sex steroids on the expression of SLE is suggested by observations that testosterone levels are reduced in males with SLE (Mackworth-Young, 1983), and individuals with Klinefelter's syndrome have a relatively high rate of the disease (Stern, 1977). Finally, estradiol metabolism in both males and females with SLE is abnormal, leading to increased estrogen activity (Lahita, 1979, 1982).

## Systemic Lupus Erythematosus

Systemic lupus erythematosus is an idiopathic chronic inflammatory disease characterized by periods of remission and relapse. It may affect the skin, joints, kidneys, lungs, serous membranes, nervous system, liver, and other organs of the body. The most common presenting complaints and symptoms of exacerbation are extreme fatigue, fever, weight loss, myalgias, and arthralgias (Table 26-1). The reported prevalence of SLE ranges from 15 to 50 cases per 100,000 individuals, and the reported incidence ranges from 2 to 8 cases per 100,000 individuals per year (Seigel, 1973; Fessel, 1974; Michet, 1985). The disease is 5 to 10 times more common among adult women

T A B L E   **26-1**

Approximate frequency of clinical symptoms in systemic lupus erythematosus

| Symptoms | Percent of Patients |
| --- | --- |
| Fatigue | 80–100 |
| Fever | 80–100 |
| Arthralgia, arthritis | 95 |
| Myalgia | 70 |
| Weight loss | >60 |
| Skin | |
|   Photosensitivity | 60 |
|   Malar rash | 50 |
|   Mucous membrane lesions | 35 |
| Renal involvement | 50 |
| Pulmonary | |
|   Pleurisy | 50 |
|   Effusion | 25 |
|   Pneumonitis | 5–10 |
| Cardiac (pericarditis) | 10–50 |
| Lymphadenopathy | 50 |
| CNS | |
|   Seizures | 15–20 |
|   Psychosis | <25 |

than adult men. Certain populations have higher prevalence rates. For example, the prevalence of SLE is 3 times greater among black women than among white women (Seigel, 1973; Fessel, 1974). A genetic predisposition to SLE is strongly implicated by several observations. Systemic lupus erythematosus occurs in approximately 4% to 12% of relatives of patients with SLE (Arnett, 1984; Lawrence, 1987). The concordance rate for SLE among monozygotic twins may be over 50% (Block, 1975), though others have found rates of approximately 25% in same-sex identical twins (Deapen, 1986). A number of genetic markers occur more frequently in SLE patients than in controls. These include HLA-DR2 and HLA-DR3 in white patients and HLA-DR7 in certain other ethnic groups (Howard, 1986; Welsh, 1988; Hartung, 1989). Systemic lupus erythematosus patients also have a higher frequency of homozygous deficiencies of the early complement proteins C2 and C4 (Howard, 1986; Glass, 1976). These products are coded by genes adjacent to the major histocompatibility complex on chromosome 6; hence, whether these complement deficiencies independently contribute to SLE or are merely fellow travelers with HLA-DR associations remains uncertain.

It is crucial for physicians, especially those not experienced in rheumatologic diseases, to understand that the diagnosis of SLE is primarily a clinical one, based on an appreciation of signs and symptoms of the disease and the tendency for more than one or two features to be present in the typical case. Autoantibodies, considered a hallmark of SLE and other autoimmune diseases, are best considered as laboratory markers that may confirm or refute the suspected diagnosis. In 1971, the American Rheumatism Association introduced criteria for SLE as a framework for comparing studies of patients with SLE (Cohen, 1971). These were revised in 1982 (Tan, 1982), changed by the elimination of Raynaud's phenomenon and alopecia and by the addition of a positive test for antinuclear antibodies, antibodies to DNA, and antibodies to the Sm antigen (Table 26-2). To be classified as having definite SLE, an individual must have at least four of the 11 criteria at one time or serially. These criteria are very sensitive and specific for SLE, but the

T A B L E  **26-2**

Revised American Rheumatism Association classification criteria for systemic lupus erythematosus

Malar rash
Discoid rash
Photosensitivity
Oral ulcers
Arthritis (nondeforming polyarthritis)
Serositis (pleuritis and/or pericarditis)
Renal disorder (proteinuria >0.5 g/day or cellular casts)
Neurologic disorder (psychosis and/or seizures)
Hematological disorder (leukopenia or lymphopenia/hemolytic anemia/thrombocytopenia)
Immunologic disorder (anti-DNA/anti-Sm/LE cell/ false-positive STS)
Antinuclear antibody

To be classified as having SLE, one must have at least four of the 11 criteria at one time or serially.

Source: Tan EM, Cohen AS, Fries JF, et al. The 1982 revised criteria for the classification of systemic lupus erythematosus. Arthritis Rheum 1982;25:1271.

practitioner should recognize that they were never intended to form the sine qua non for the diagnosis of SLE. Exclusion of patients with an autoimmune diathesis from the diagnosis of SLE by the dogmatic use of strict diagnostic criteria may result in patients being confused and frustrated. Reasonable and sympathetic medical care and counseling are required as much for patients with "borderline" SLE as for those with definite SLE.

The diagnosis of SLE, suspected by the clinical presentation, is confirmed by demonstrating the presence of circulating autoantibodies. A number of categories of autoantibodies are now recognized to be associated with SLE. The best studied are those directed against nuclear antigens, generally referred to as ANAs. Of these, the first to be described was the serum factor that caused the lupus erythematosus (LE) cell phenomenon (Hargraves, 1948), an autoantibody now known to be directed against nucleoprotein (DNA-histone) (Reichlin, 1989). The LE cell phenomenon is no longer necessary for the diagnosis of SLE. It has been replaced by assays for ANA, which now serve as the screening test in the initial diagnostic evaluation of a patient with suspected SLE.

A positive ANA can be interpreted to some degree according to the pattern of the binding, even though specific antigen-antibody reactions are much more informative. The four basic patterns of binding are homogenous, peripheral, speckled, and nucleolar. The homogenous pattern is found in about 65% of patients with SLE, but the peripheral pattern is the most specific for SLE, even if it is not very sensitive. The speckled and nucleolar patterns are more specific for other autoimmune diseases.

Antinuclear antibody assays are fairly sensitive for SLE, though not highly specific; thus, they serve well as screening tests. Individuals with negative ANA tests are quite unlikely to have SLE, especially when the clinical suspicion of SLE is no more than modest. Those with positive ANA tests may have any one of a number of conditions other than SLE, and additional autoantibody assays should be performed to secure (or refute) the diagnosis of SLE. Antibodies to double-stranded DNA (anti-dsDNA) are the most specific for SLE and are found in 80% to 90% of untreated patients at the time of presentation. The presence and titer of anti-dsDNA may be related to the disease activity (Koffler, 1971; Schur, 1986). Among the several different types of anti-dsDNA assays, the Farr assay, utilizing calf thymus DNA, is probably the most sensitive for the detection of high-affinity immunoglobulin G (IgG) antibodies specific for SLE. At the other end of the spectrum, the *Crithidiae luciliae* assay is less sensitive but even more specific. Antibodies to single-stranded DNA (anti-ssDNA) are also found in a very high percentage of untreated SLE patients, but anti-ssDNA is less specific for SLE than anti-dsDNA. Systemic lupus erythematosus patients may also have antibodies to RNA-protein conjugates, often referred to as soluble or extractable antigens, because they can be separated from tissue extracts. These antigens include the Sm antigen, nuclear ribonucleoprotein (nRNP), the Ro/SSA antigen, and the La/SSB antigen. The Sm and nRNP antigens are nuclear in origin. The presence of anti-Sm, found in about 30% to 40% of patients with SLE, is highly specific for the disease. Anti-Ro/SS-A and La/SS-B, found in the sera of SLE patients and patients with Sjögren's syndrome, are of particular importance to obstetricians because these antibodies are associated with neonatal lupus.

## Complications of Systemic Lupus Erythematosus and Pregnancy

The study of Garenstein et al (1962) is characteristic of a number of studies of the relationship between SLE and pregnancy published from the early 1950s through the early 1970s, suggesting that women with SLE were at substantial risk for severe morbidity or mortality during pregnancy. In this retrospective study of 33 pregnancies in 21 women with SLE, the investigators found that SLE exacerbations were 3 times more frequent in the first 20 weeks of pregnancy and 6 times more frequent in the first 8 weeks postpartum than in the 32 weeks prior to conception. The authors concluded that pregnancy was associated with an increased rate of exacerbation in women with SLE. Moreover, some investigators reported maternal deaths due to SLE in association with pregnancy (Friedman, 1956; Garenstein, 1962), further bolstering the concern that pregnancy increases the rate of serious exacerbation. Finally, several early studies suggested that the rate of pregnancy loss among women with SLE was relatively high (Friedman, 1956; Estes, 1965; McGee, 1970). Taken together, these concerns led many practitioners to the opinion that SLE patients should not become pregnant.

It is now clear that the conclusions reached in these early studies should not be applied to clinical decision making today. All studies prior to the 1980s were retrospective and relatively small. There were no generally agreed on criteria for the classification of SLE, predisposing to the inclusion of a disproportionate number of more severe cases. Also, there were no generally accepted or validated diagnostic criteria for SLE exacerbation. This may have allowed certain events of pregnancy, such as preeclampsia or increasing proteinuria, to be diagnosed incorrectly as SLE exacerbation. The introduction of classification criteria in 1971 and the development of more sophisticated autoantibody assays have led to a more uniform patient selection and inclusion of more typical, usually less severely affected pa-

tients. In addition, treatment of SLE and SLE exacerbations has changed, as has the survival rate of premature and extremely premature newborns. For these reasons, only studies of SLE and pregnancy published since the mid-1970s will be used in making the significant points in this chapter.

### Exacerbation of Systemic Lupus Erythematosus

Both the patient and the physician should understand that between 15% and 60% of women with SLE will experience an exacerbation (flare) of their autoimmune disease during pregnancy (Zurier, 1978; Tozman, 1980; Lockshin, 1984, 1989a; Meehan, 1987; Mintz, 1986; Wong, 1991; Petri, 1991; Le Thi Huong, 1994). The important question is whether pregnancy per se predisposes to exacerbation of SLE. Several studies have done much to clarify the relationship of pregnancy to the rate and nature of SLE exacerbations (Table 26-3), though more investigations are needed. Lockshin et al (1984) matched nonpregnant SLE patients with 28 SLE patients undertaking 33 pregnancies and used a previously published scoring system to define SLE exacerbations. There was no difference in the flare score between the cases and controls, and a similar number in either group required a change in their medication. The same investigators have now followed 80 consecutive pregnancies in women with SLE (Lockshin, 1989) and conclude that exacerbations occur in less than 25% of cases and that most are mild in nature. If only signs or symptoms specific for SLE are included, exacerbations occurred in only 13% of cases. Meehan and Dorsey (1987) performed a similar study, matching pregnant and nonpregnant patients. They also found no difference in the rate of flares between the two groups.

Mintz et al (1986) prospectively studied 92 pregnancies in women with SLE and compared them with a control group comprised of a "similar group" of nonpregnant SLE patients on oral contraceptives derived from a previous study. Exacerbations were defined by specific, acceptable criteria but were different than those used by Lockshin et al (1984) or Petri et al (1991). As a matter of policy, all women were treated during pregnancy with 10 mg of prednisone daily. The

T A B L E    **26-3**

Rates of exacerbations of systemic lupus erythematosus
in pregnancy

| | Pregnant Patients | | | Controls | | |
|---|---|---|---|---|---|---|
| **Author, Year** | **No. of Patients** | **No. of Pregnancies** | **Flares** | **No. of Patients** | **Flares** | **Nature of Control Patients** |
| Lockshin, 1984[a] | 28 | 33 | 7 (21%) | 33 | 6 (18%) | Matched, nonpregnant |
| Mintz, 1986 | NA | 92 | 55 (60%) 0.0605[b] | NA | NA 0.0406[b] | "Similar group of young females" using proges- terone oral contracep- tives |
| Meehan, 1987 | 18 | 22 | 10 (45%) | 22 | 12 (54%) | Matched, nonpregnant |
| Petri, 1991[d] | 36 | 39 | 23 (59%) 1.6337[c] ± 0.30 | 185 | NA 0.6518[c] ± 0.05 | Not matched, non- pregnant |
| | | | | 39 | NA 0.6392[c] ± 0.15 | Same patients after delivery |

Only the study by Petri et al (1991) demonstrated a significant difference
between pregnant and nonpregnant controls.

[a]Figures in table derived from flares, as defined by the requirement for an
increase in medication. Flares were also analyzed using a scoring system
(see reference for definition), and there was no difference between
pregnant patients and nonpregnant controls.

[b]Flares per month at risk.

[c]Flare rate per person years (mean ± SEM). See reference for definition of
flare rate.

[d]Two control groups used.

rate of SLE flares per month was similar in pregnant and control patients. As in Lockshin's studies, most of the exacerbations tended to be
managed easily with low-to-moderate doses of
glucocorticoids, but seven patients (8%) had severe exacerbations requiring more aggressive
therapies. Interestingly, the majority (54%) of the
exacerbations occurred in the first trimester.

The findings of Petri et al (1991) run counter
to those of the other prospective analyses. Using
criteria for SLE flare that differed from those in
other studies, the investigators found SLE flares
to be significantly more common in pregnant
women than in the same women after delivery
and in nonpregnant SLE patients. The study was
prospective, but the control patients were not
matched to the pregnant patients with regard to
disease or organ system involvement. Although
over 80% of the flares were mild to moderate
in nature, severe disease was seen in a few

patients. Differences in the populations of lupus
patients studied by Petri and colleagues, compared with those studied by the other investigators, probably underlies the differences in
findings with regard to exacerbations during
pregnancy.

A case control study of SLE exacerbation in
pregnancy has been published (Urowitz, 1993).
The study included 46 patients having 79 pregnancies. The investigators matched controls according to disease activity and used an established
scoring system for determination of exacerbations. Additionally, the investigators analyzed exacerbations according to the patients' disease activity at the time of pregnancy onset. There was
no difference in the rate of flares in pregnant
patients versus controls.

In summary, the issue of whether pregnancy
predisposes to SLE exacerbation is not yet set-
tled. At most, however, the predisposition to SLE

flare during pregnancy is modest, and most SLE exacerbations are treated easily with low-to-moderate doses of glucocorticoids. The routine use of glucocorticoids in all pregnant SLE patients, as suggested by Mintz et al (1986), seems unwarranted in view of the excellent results achieved by others without the routine use of steroids.

Three studies describe the patients' status during pregnancy in terms of whether the SLE were active or in remission prior to conception (Hayslett, 1980; Jungers, 1982; Bobrie, 1987). In all three, the rate of SLE exacerbation was lower among pregnancies in which the patient was in remission prior to conception. Hayslett and Lynn (1980) and Bobrie et al (1987) also found that the rate of renal deterioration was somewhat lower among pregnancies in which the patient was in remission prior to conception. A more recent case control study of unselected SLE patients confirms that patients with inactive disease at the time of conception have a lower rate of exacerbation than those with active disease at conception (Urowitz, 1993). Thus, it seems reasonable and prudent to recommend that SLE patients achieve remission before considering pregnancy.

A number of investigators believe that serial serologic evaluation of complement components or their activation products allows for the timely detection of an SLE exacerbation during pregnancy. Devoe and colleagues found that SLE exacerbation was "signaled" by a decline of C3 and C4 into the subnormal range (Devoe, 1979, 1984). More recently, Buyon et al (1986) found that a lack of the usual rise in C3 and C4 levels during pregnancy was associated with SLE exacerbation. An earlier study by the same group also found evidence for a classical pathway activation in patients with SLE exacerbation (Hopkins, 1984). Others have questioned the predictive value of serologic determinations in lupus pregnancy. Lockshin and colleagues (1986) found that the concentration of the C1s-C1 inhibitor complex, which should be increased in the face of classical pathway complement activation, was normal in most pregnant patients with hypocomplementemia. The authors suggested that pregnant SLE patients may actually have relatively poor synthesis (rather than consumption) of some complement components. In a prospective study of 19

continuing SLE pregnancies, neither ANA, C3, nor C4 levels predicted which of the nine patients were going to have a flare (Wong, 1991). Finally, there are several studies that show that hypocomplementemia may occur in pregnant patients without SLE and does not predict a poor pregnancy outcome (Tedder, 1975; Adelsberg, 1983). Thus, the utility of serial determinations of complement components or their activation products for the timely detection of SLE exacerbations or poor pregnancy outcome is at best controversial. There is currently no evidence to show that serial serologic studies are better for the timely diagnosis of SLE exacerbation than relatively frequent, thorough clinical assessment of the patient.

### Active Lupus Nephritis Versus Preeclampsia

Distinguishing between an exacerbation of SLE involving active nephritis and preeclampsia may pose an especially difficult problem, because each may present with proteinuria, hypertension, and evidence of multiorgan dysfunction. In the typical troublesome case, the patient develops hypertension and begins to excrete increasing amounts of urinary protein in the latter half of pregnancy. Several laboratory tests may be helpful. Elevated levels of anti-DNA weigh in favor of active SLE. Normal or slightly elevated levels of classical pathway complement components weigh against active SLE, but decreased levels are less helpful, because complement activation or low levels of complement may be seen in preeclampsia (Haeger, 1989, 1990; Hofmeyer, 1991). Buyon et al (1989) found that frank lupus activity in pregnancy was associated with elevated levels of Ba or Bb, fragments of protein B activation in the alternative pathway of complement activation. The terminal attack complex, Sc5b-9, also was elevated in the patients with active SLE. While elevated concentrations of Ba, Bb, and Sc5b-9 were also found in some patients with preeclampsia, the combination of these with a decreased CH50 strongly suggested SLE flare.

A number of laboratory tests have been proposed as being specific for preeclampsia, and may be helpful in distinguishing preeclampsia from SLE nephritis. These include decreased levels of antithrombin-III (Weiner, 1985), increased levels of total plasma or cellular fibronectin (Ballegeer, 1989; Lockwood, 1990), hypocalciuria (Taufield, 1987), and elevated levels of serum thrombomodulin (Hsu, 1995). Unfortunately, none of these has been specifically tested as a marker for preeclampsia in patients with SLE.

Two tests would appear to be particularly helpful in distinguishing between active nephritis and preeclampsia. An active urinary sediment strongly suggests lupus nephritis. Cellular casts, aseptic pyuria, and/or hematuria are usually present in diffuse proliferative glomerulonephrosis and often present in focal proliferative glomerulonephrosis, the two conditions most likely to be confused with preeclampsia. The second test of immense benefit is the renal biopsy. In severe and confusing cases, the renal biopsy will usually enable the correct diagnosis. Of course, there is an understandable reluctance to utilize this invasive procedure in the pregnant patient, and sound clinical judgment is required to decide which patients require a biopsy for optimal management.

As a final point regarding SLE-related hypertension and proteinuria versus preeclampsia, it is the author's experience that in severe cases, the SLE flare and preeclampsia may be either indistinguishable or coexistent as the patient's course advances, tending to render fine points of laboratory distinction between the two conditions moot. Concerns about optimizing the mother's SLE management and avoiding serious complications of preeclampsia, including fetal hypoxemia, often prompt delivery in a relatively short time.

### Renal Disease

Approximately 50% of patients with SLE eventually have clinically obvious renal disease (Schur, 1993). It is generally held that lupus nephropathy (LN) is due to immune complex deposition, with resultant complement activation and inflammatory tissue damage in the kidney. The most common presentation is proteinuria, which occurs at some time in up to 75% of patients. About 40% of patients will have hematuria or aseptic pyuria, and about a third will have urinary casts. Renal biopsy findings are very important to prognosis and treatment and may be grouped into several

basic histologic and clinical categories. Of these, diffuse proliferative glomerulonephritis (DPGN) is the most common as well as the most serious, occurring in about 40% of SLE cases with renal involvement. It typically presents with hypertension, moderate-to-heavy proteinuria and nephrotic syndrome, hematuria, pyuria, casts, hypocomplementemia, and circulating immune complexes. Based on data gathered in the 1980s, the 10-year survival rate is about 60% (Appel, 1987). Focal proliferative glomerulonephritis also presents with proteinuria, but the degree of proteinuria is typically less. Hypertension is less common and also less severe, and serious renal insufficiency is uncommon. Membranous glomerulonephritis typically presents with moderate-to-heavy proteinuria but lacks the active urinary sediment and does not cause renal insufficiency with hypertension. Mesangial nephritis appears as the least severe lesion and carries the best long-term prognosis.

A woman with LN who becomes pregnant faces several special problems. The underlying renal disease probably presages an increased risk for maternal and fetal morbidity and mortality. In addition, those with chronic renal disease resulting in proteinuria are likely to have worsening proteinuria during gestation as the renal blood flow increases. This inevitably poses the question as to whether the increased proteinuria represents an exacerbation of underlying renal disease, preeclampsia, or both.

Early reports suggested that LN was a major contributor to serious maternal morbidity or death (Murray, 1958; Donaldson, 1962; Estes, 1965; Bear, 1976). For example, Estes and Larson (1965) noted progression of renal disease in all 10 pregnant patients with LN, with two of these dying within a year after delivery. Bear (1976) noted worsening of renal disease in five of six patients with LN, and three suffered permanent deterioration. More recent and larger series, however, suggest that the course of renal disease in pregnant women with LN is not so serious (Devoe, 1979; Hayslett, 1980; Fine, 1981; Jungers, 1982; Imbasciati, 1984; Bobrie, 1987; Julkunen, 1993a). All of the studies were retrospective, and patient selection doubtlessly varied from one study to the next. The summary shown in Table 26-4, however, is useful in counseling patients

T A B L E    **26-4**

Deterioration of renal disease during pregnancy in patients with
systemic lupus erythematosus nephropathy

| Author | Pa-tients | Pregnan-cies | No Exacer-bation | Exacer-bation | No Deterio-ration | Deterio-ration | Permanent Deterioration |
|---|---|---|---|---|---|---|---|
| Hayslett, 1980 | | | | | | | |
|    Remission PTC | 23 | 31 | 21/31 (68%) | 10/31 (32%) | 24/31 (77%) | 7/31 (23%) | 2/31 (6%) |
|    Active PTC | 24 | 25 | 13/25 (52%) | 12/25 (48%) | 16/25 (64%) | 9/25 (36%) | 5/25 (20%) |
| Fine, 1981 | 13 | 14 | N/A | N/A | 10/14 (71%) | 4/14 (29%) | 2/14 (14%) |
| Jungers, 1982 | | | | | | | |
|    Remission PTC | 8 | 11 | 9/11 (82%) | 2/11 (18%) | 9/11 (82%) | 2/11 (18%) | 1/11 (9%) |
|    Active PTC | 8 | 15 | 4/15 (27%) | 11/15 (73%) | 13/15 (87%) | 2/15 (13%) | 1/15 (7%) |
| Imbasciati, 1984 | 6 | 18 | 8/18 (44%) | 10/18 (56%) | 14/18 (78%) | 4/18 (22%) | 2/18 (11%) |
| Devoe, 1979 | 14 | 17 | 13/17 (76%) | 4/17 (24%) | 12/17 (71%) | 5/17 (29%) | 2/17 (12%) |
| Bobrie, 1987 | 35 | 53 | 35/53 (66%) | 18/53 (34%) | NA | NA | 4/53 (8%) |
| Julkunen, 1993a | 16 | 23 | 21/23 (91%) | 2/23 (9%) | 23/23 (100%) | 0/23 | 0/23 |
| Median | | | 67% | 33% | 77.5% | 22.5% | 8.5% |
| Range | | | 27%–91% | 9%–73% | 64%–100% | 0%–36% | 0%–20% |

Only patients with LN diagnosed prior to pregnancy are included.

PTC, prior to conception.

with LN. The median rate of SLE exacerbation was 33%, probably no different than that observed in unselected SLE patients. Deterioration of renal status occurred in about a fourth of the patients undertaking pregnancy, and 8.5% of pregnancies were associated with a permanent deterioration in the patient's renal status. Fortunately, the resulting degree of renal impairment was moderate in most cases. Three of the 147 women with LN included in Table 26-4 died of complications related to SLE occurring during a pregnancy or in the postpartum period.

### Pregnancy Loss

It is generally agreed that pregnancy loss is more common among women with SLE than among normal women. Table 26-5 summarizes the pregnancy losses in the more recent series, including four prospective series (Lockshin, 1985a; Mintz, 1986; Wong, 1991; Le Thi Huong, 1994). Overall, the median rate of pregnancy loss is 27%, a figure considerably higher than typically observed in the normal population. The four prospective studies indicate an overall pregnancy loss between 10% and 31%. None of the prospective studies included appropriately matched, prospectively acquired controls. Mintz et al (1986), however, found a statistically higher rate of pregnancy loss among the SLE patients than among more than 100 women followed in a high-risk clinic during the study period.

A large, retrospective case control study by Petri and Allbritton (1993) compared pregnancy outcomes in women with SLE with those of their best friends and relatives. Pregnancy loss was more common in SLE pregnancies (21%) than in pregnancies in friends (14%) or relatives (8%). The investigators also noted that pregnancy loss was greater after the diagnosis of SLE (27%) than before the diagnosis of SLE (19%). Julkunen and colleagues (1993b) published a large, retrospective case control analysis of pregnancy outcomes in women with SLE. The relative risk of pregnancy loss in SLE patients was 2.5 times that of controls.

It appears that a disproportionate number of pregnancy losses in women with SLE occur as fetal deaths in the second or third trimester, with a median rate of 5.45% in the studies listed in Table 26-5. The well-detailed, prospective study of Lockshin et al (1985a) found that more than 20% of the pregnancy losses were second- or

T A B L E    **26-5**

Pregnancy loss in patients with systemic lupus erythematosus

| Author, Year | No. of Patients | No. of Pregnancies | Spontaneous Abortions[a] | Fetal Death[b] | Total Losses |
|---|---|---|---|---|---|
| Fraga, 1974 | 20 | 42 | NA | NA | 17 (40%) |
| Zurier, 1978 | 13 | 25 | 7 (28%) | 2 (8%) | 9 (36%) |
| Zulman, 1979 | 23 | 24 | 0 | 3 (12%) | 3 (12%) |
| Varner, 1983 | 31 | 34 | 3 (9%) | 2 (6%) | 5 (15%) |
| Mor Yosef, 1984 | 40 | 143 | 26 | 13 | — |
| Gimovsky, 1984 | 39 | 65 | 23 (35%) | 7 (11%) | 30 (46%) |
| Lockshin, 1985a | 28 | 32 | 3 (9%) | 7 (22%) | 10 (31%) |
| Yu, 1986 | 28 | 31 | 2 (6.5%) | 0 | 2 (6.5%) |
| Mintz, 1986 | 75 | 92 | 16 (17%)[c] | 4 (4%)[d] | 20 (22%) |
| McHugh, 1989 | NA | 47 | NA | NA | 16 (34%) |
| Nossent, 1990 | 19 | 39 | 4 (10%)[c] | 2 (5%)[d] | 6 (15%) |
| Wong, 1991 | 17 | 19 | 2 (10%) | 0 | 2 (10%) |
| Nicklin, 1991 | 17 | 36 | 9 (25%)[c] | 2 (5.6%)[d] | 11 (31%) |
| Ginsberg, 1992 | 42 | 122 | 30 (25%)[c] | 2 (1.6%)[d] | 32 (26%) |
| Urowitz, 1993 | 46 | 61 | 16 (26%)[c] | 3 (4.9%)[d] | 19 (31%) |
| Petri, 1993 | 42 | 157 | NA | NA | 42 (27%) |
| Le Thi Huong, 1994 | NA | 94 | 13 (14%)[e] | 5 (5.3%)[f] | 18 (19%) |
| Median | | | 15.5% | 5.45% | 27% |
| Range | | | 0%–35% | 0%–22% | 6.5%–40% |

Only pregnancies occurring after the diagnosis of SLE are included. Elective
    pregnancy terminations are excluded.

[a]Whenever possible, losses before 13 completed weeks' gestation are consid-
    ered spontaneous abortions.

[b]Whenever possible, losses ≥ 14 weeks' gestation are considered fetal deaths.

[c]*Spontaneous abortion* is defined as losses < 21 weeks' gestation.

[d]*Fetal death* is defined as losses ≥ 21 weeks' gestation.

[e]*Spontaneous abortions* are defined as losses < 16 weeks' gestation.

[f]*Fetal death* is defined as losses ≥ 16 weeks' gestation.

third-trimester fetal deaths. Unfortunately, neither Mintz et al (1986) nor Petri and Allbritton
(1993) distinguished early pregnancy loss (embryonic loss or first-trimester loss) from fetal
death.

Among SLE patients, fetal deaths are often
associated with the presence of antiphospholipid
antibodies (see the section on Antiphospholipid
Syndrome). In one study of 21 women with SLE,
antiphospholipid antibodies were found to be
the most sensitive indicator of fetal distress or
fetal death (Lockshin, 1985b). In a second study
by the same authors, antiphospholipid antibodies were present in 10 of 11 patients with fetal
death, and the positive predictive value of antiphospholipid antibodies for fetal death was more

than 50% (Lockshin, 1987). The data of Julkunen
et al (1993b) confirm those of Lockshin et al.
They found that women with SLE and lupus anticoagulant were more likely to have a history of
fetal loss than those without (odds ratio, 3.4).
Anticardiolipin antibodies were more sensitive for
fetal loss than lupus anticoagulant (64% vs. 50%),
but the latter was more specific (77% vs. 52%).
Finally, Ginsberg et al (1992) found that SLE patients with prior pregnancy loss were 5 to 20 times
more likely to test positive repeatedly for antiphospholipid antibodies than SLE patients who
had never had pregnancy loss.

Other investigators have emphasized the importance of a history of fetal loss as an independent predictor of fetal loss in women with SLE.

Englert and colleagues (1988) found that the presence of antiphospholipid antibodies *and* a history of fetal loss predicts more than 85% of pregnancy loss in women with SLE. Ramsey-Goldman et al (1993) found a history of fetal loss to be a more powerful predictor of future fetal loss than antiphospholipid antibodies. At present, both antiphospholipid antibodies and a history of prior fetal loss should be considered the most important risk factors for fetal loss in women with SLE.

Three other factors may be associated with pregnancy loss in women with SLE. In a retrospective study of women with SLE and LN, Hayslett and Lynn (1980) suggested that pregnancy loss might be related to the activity of SLE within the several months prior to conception. They found that live births occurred in only 64% of patients with clinically active SLE in the 6 months prior to conception, while 88% of pregnancies were successful if the disease had been quiescent before conception. Other evidence suggests that the onset of SLE during pregnancy may pose a serious threat to the conceptus. Three studies provide enough detail to analyze pregnancy outcome in patients with the onset of SLE during pregnancy (Jungers, 1982; Varner, 1983; Imbasciati, 1984). Of the 21 pregnancies described, five ended in fetal death and one ended in spontaneous abortion, for an overall loss rate of 29%.

Finally, some authors believe that underlying renal disease may have an adverse effect on fetal survival in patients with SLE. An analysis of pregnancy outcomes of women with LN in several major studies (Devoe, 1979; Hayslett, 1980; Jungers, 1982; Imbasciati, 1984; Bobrie, 1987) shows a median spontaneous abortion rate of 13% and a median fetal death rate of 7.5%, figures not remarkably different than those for all patients with SLE shown in Table 26-5. In one study, however, the rate of fetal death was higher after the diagnosis of SLE and LN than before the diagnosis in the same patients (Gimovsky, 1984). Also, the degree of renal impairment is important. Hayslett and Lynn (1980) found that a serum creatinine greater than or equal to 1.5 mg/dL, indicating moderate-to-severe renal insufficiency, was associated with fetal losses in 50% of 10 cases. Fine et al (1981) found fetal loss in 38% and 46%

of pregnancies complicated by proteinuria (>300 mg/25 hr) or a creatinine clearance less than 100 mL/min, respectively. Even without SLE, moderate-to-severe renal insufficiency may be associated with an increased rate of pregnancy loss, especially in patients with chronic hypertension (Katz, 1980; Surian, 1984). Only one small study addresses the important issue of how the renal biopsy findings might influence the pregnancy outcome (Devoe, 1983). Seventeen pregnancies in 14 women with biopsy-proven LN were described. There was no remarkable difference in the pregnancy outcomes of the women with membranous nephropathy compared with those with diffuse or focal proliferative lesions. Although the number of patients studied was quite small, the authors concluded that there was no consistent correlation between renal biopsy findings and pregnancy outcome.

## Preterm Delivery

Preterm delivery is more likely in SLE pregnancies than in normal pregnancies. An analysis of 11 series of pregnant women with SLE, wherein the gestational age of delivery is described, shows that a median of 30% of births occurs before 37 weeks' gestation (range, 3%–73%) (Hayslett, 1980; Houser, 1980; Fine, 1981; Jungers, 1982; Varner, 1983; Imbasciati, 1984; Lockshin, 1985b; Gimovsky, 1984; Mintz, 1986; Englert, 1988; Wong, 1991). There are many confounding variables to consider, not the least of which is the tendency for obstetricians to move to delivery as soon as the fetus is considered mature or the potential for neonatal morbidity is thought to be minimal. In the three studies in which indications for preterm delivery are discussed (Varner, 1983; Gimovsky, 1984; Englert, 1988), 28% to 66% were for preeclampsia and 12% to 33% were for fetal distress. Thus, about one third to one half of preterm deliveries in SLE pregnancies are due to maternal or fetal indications for delivery. Preterm delivery is more common in SLE patients with hypertension (Julkunen, 1993b; Petri, 1993; Le Thi Huong, 1994) if SLE is active at the onset of pregnancy (Le Thi Huong, 1994) or the pregnancy is complicated by SLE flare (Mintz, 1986). Also, preterm birth is probably more common among

SLE patients with antiphospholipid antibodies (Nicklin, 1991; Branch, 1992).

Idiopathic preterm labor is probably not more common among women with SLE than in the general population. Johnson and colleagues (1995), however, found that nearly 44% of preterm deliveries in SLE patients were associated with preterm rupture of the membranes (PROM), statistically higher than the 25% of preterm births associated with PROM in the general obstetric population at the same institution. Fortunately, most of the preterm deliveries associated with PROM occurred after 34 weeks' gestation. Although the authors did not specifically analyze the relationship of PROM to glucocorticoid use, others have found the use of glucocorticoids and PROM to be linked (Cowchock, 1992).

## Pregnancy-Induced Hypertension and Preeclampsia

Interpretation of the literature in terms of pregnancy-induced hypertension (PIH) during SLE pregnancies is difficult due to the varying definitions of the disease, the mix of patients with nephropathy and hypertension in the various studies, and the method of ascertainment. It can be said, however, that PIH is relatively common and potentially serious in SLE pregnancies. Overall, 20% to 30% of SLE pregnancies are complicated by PIH (Lockshin, 1987; Nicklin, 1991; Julkunen, 1993b). A history of renal disease appears to be particularly ominous. In the prospective study of Lockshin et al (1987), eight of 11 (72%) pregnancies in women with LN had PIH, compared with 12 of 53 (22%) in SLE patients without LN.

The reason for the increased frequency of PIH among SLE patients is unknown but may relate to underlying renal disease, a factor recognized to be associated with PIH (Fisher, 1981). Authorities believe that virtually all SLE patients demonstrate some degree of renal abnormality if biopsies are studied by immunofluorescence or electron microscopic methods (Schur, 1993). The use of high doses (>20–30 mg of prednisone daily) of steroids during pregnancy also may predispose to PIH.

## Fetal Growth Impairment

Given the fact that pregnant SLE patients may have PIH, APS, or both, it is not surprising that fetal growth impairment may occur. However, few studies document the occurrence of fetal growth impairment. The best data come from the study of Mintz et al (1986). These investigators found that 20 of 86 (23%) pregnancies progressing beyond 20 weeks' gestation delivered growth-impaired fetuses, including four stillbirths. Only 4% of controls delivered growth-impaired fetuses. Other series indicate that 9.5% to 32% of neonates are growth impaired (Fine, 1981; Varner, 1983; Englert 1988; Nossent, 1990; Nicklin, 1991; Wong, 1991; Julkunen, 1993b; Le Thi Huong, 1994).

## Neonatal Lupus Erythematosus

Neonatal lupus erythematosus is an uncommon condition of the fetus and neonate that is characterized by dermatologic, cardiac, or hematologic abnormalities. The condition results from the transplacental passage of maternal autoantibodies, in particular, antibodies to the Ro/SS-A and La/SS-B antigens. About half of the mothers who deliver an infant with NLE have SLE or another autoimmune disease, but about half have no autoimmune diagnosis. The most common presentation for NLE is probably dermatologic. Cardiac disease is less common but is disproportionately represented in case reports. Hematologic abnormalities, such as autoimmune hemolytic anemia, leukopenia, thrombocytopenia, and hepatosplenomegaly, are the least frequently recognized or reported.

Dermatologic manifestations occur in up to 25% of infants delivered of women with SLE and antibodies (Lockshin, 1988). The typical skin lesions are erythematous, scaling annular or elliptical plaques occurring on the face or scalp. They are analogous to the subacute cutaneous lesions in adults (Lee, 1988) and are probably induced by exposure of the skin to ultraviolet light. The lesions first appear within the first several weeks after delivery and last for up to 6 months. Hypopigmentation may persist for up to 2 years. Skin biopsy shows histopathology and immunofluorescence typical of that of cutaneous lupus.

The cardiac lesions associated with NLE are congenital complete heart block (CCHB) and endocardial fibroelastosis, with the latter being less frequently reported and perhaps uncommon in a severe form. Congenital complete heart block occurs in fewer than 3% of patients with SLE and anti-Ro/SS-A antibodies (Lockshin, 1988). The usual presentation is a fixed fetal bradycardia in the range of 60 to 80 beats per minute detected between the sixteenth and twenty-fifth week of gestation. Ultrasonographic examination of the fetal heart shows a structurally normal heart with atrioventricular dissociation. Hydrops fetalis may develop in utero and is perhaps dependent on the degree of endomyocardial fibrosis rather than the heart rate per se. The histologic lesion is one of fibrosis and interruption of the conduction system, especially in the area of atrioventricular node (Hull, 1966; Lev, 1971). Because the lesion is permanent, a pacemaker is required in at least two thirds of cases for neonatal survival (Waltuck, 1994). The attributable mortality rate is high, with 20% of infants succumbing to cardiac problems within the first month of life and fully 30% of infants dying before age 3 years (Waltuck, 1994).

The diagnosis of NLE is confirmed by testing for autoantibodies associated with the condition. Buyon and colleagues (1993) have shown that CCHB occurs almost exclusively in infants delivered of mothers with antibodies to the 52-kd SS-A antigen and the 48-kd SS-B antigen. Substantial indirect evidence suggests that these maternal autoantibodies are transported across the placenta, where they bind to fetal tissue antigens and cause immunologic damage resulting in NLE. Immunoglobulin has been demonstrated in the heart (Taylor, 1986) and skin (Lee, 1989) of affected infants. Furthermore, intravenously injected affinity-purified anti-Ro/SS-A binds in human skin transplanted onto immunodeficient mice (Lee, 1989).

It is fortunate that the overall frequency of women with SLE having an infant with any manifestation of NLE is low, probably less than 5% (Lockshin, 1988). Of course, patients with antibodies to Ro/SS-A and La/SS-B are at increased risk. If a woman has previously delivered an infant with NLE, the recurrence is approximately 25% for dermatologic manifestations and 10% to 15% for CCHB (Julkunen, 1993c; Waltuck, 1994).

## Management of Systemic Lupus Erythematosus Pregnancy

### Initial Counseling and Assessment

Ideally, a woman with SLE who is contemplating pregnancy will seek preconception counsel. At that time, she should be informed of the potential obstetric problems, including the risk of pregnancy loss, PIH, fetal growth impairment, and preterm delivery. Special concerns related to APS and NLE also should be discussed. Optimally, the patient should be in remission prior to conception. Cytotoxic agents and nonsteroidal antiinflammatory drugs (NSAIDs) should be discontinued prior to conception. She should also be assessed for evidence of anemia or thrombocytopenia, underlying renal disease (urinalysis, serum creatinine, and 24-hr urine for creatinine clearance and total protein), and antiphospholipid antibodies (lupus anticoagulant and anticardiolipin). Some physicians also obtain anti-Ro/SS-A and anti-La/SS-B antibodies on all patients with SLE, but the cost-effectiveness of these tests is somewhat questionable, because one would neither advise avoiding pregnancy nor institute a specific treatment in the absence of a history of an infant with CCHB.

Once pregnant, the patient with SLE may be seen by a physician at least every 2 weeks in the first and second trimesters and every week thereafter. At each visit, the patient should be questioned about signs or symptoms of SLE activity, and her urine should be examined for evidence of blood or protein. Of course, the patient should be urged to notify the physician immediately if she develops symptoms of an SLE flare. There is no evidence that optimal management requires serologic evaluation for hypocomplementemia, circulating immune complexes, or autoantibody levels as long as the patient remains asymptomatic. Some obstetricians obtain urine and hematologic studies from pregnant SLE patients once each trimester.

A primary goal of the antenatal visits after 20 weeks' gestation is the detection of hypertension and/or proteinuria. Because of the risk of uteroplacental insufficiency, fetal ultrasound should be performed every 4 to 6 weeks, starting at 18 to

20 weeks' gestation. In an otherwise uncomplicated SLE patient, fetal surveillance should be started at 30 to 32 weeks' gestation. A program of daily fetal movement counts and once-weekly nonstress tests with amniotic fluid volume determinations are adequate in most cases. More frequent ultrasound and fetal testing is indicated in patients with SLE flare, hypertension, proteinuria, clinical evidence of fetal growth impairment, or APS. In patients with APS, fetal surveillance as early as 24 to 25 weeks may be justified (Druzin, 1987). Appropriate fetal surveillance for fetuses with CCHB would include frequent ultrasonographic evaluation for evidence of hydrops fetalis, biophysical profiles for fetal surveillance, and daily fetal movement counts.

## Antirheumatic Drugs and Pregnancy

**Glucocorticoids** Glucocorticoids are the mainstay of treatment for SLE during pregnancy. In general, the doses of glucocorticoids used in pregnancy are similar to those used in nonpregnant patients. While an increased frequency of cleft palate has been found in the offspring of glucocorticoid-treated laboratory animals, a wealth of human experience and several studies indicate that the risk for human teratogenesis is very low or non-existent (Bongiovanni, 1960; Brooks, 1990). The risk of neonatal adrenal suppression following maternal treatment with hydrocortisone or prednisolone is also low, having been reported only rarely. One reason for the relative safety of these glucocorticoids in the human may be the abundance of 11-β-ol dehydrogenase in the human placenta. This enzyme converts hydrocortisone or prednisolone into the relatively inactive 11-keto forms, leaving no more than 10% of the active drug to reach the fetus (Levitz, 1978). Glucocorticoids with fluorine at the 9α position are considerably less well metabolized by the placenta and should not be administered chronically during pregnancy unless the intent is to treat the fetus with them.

It is imperative that physicians who choose to administer glucocorticoids, especially in higher doses, understand the potential complications that may be caused by these potent immunosuppressives. Minor common side effects include hirsutism, acne, cushingoid appearance, and an increase in the formation and severity of striae. The most important serious, adverse side effect is life-threatening infection, especially bacterial infections such as pneumonia or urinary tract infections. Glucose intolerance is relatively common, especially in pregnant women treated with moderate- to high-dose steroids, and should be sought meticulously and treated aggressively when present. Patients on moderate-to-high doses of glucocorticoids should be screened for gestational diabetes at 24 to 28 weeks' gestation and, if negative, again at 32 to 34 weeks.

Glucocorticoids cause sodium and water retention, and moderate-to-high doses are associated with hypertension. Rapid increases in BP have been observed in patients treated with high-dose pulse therapy (discussion follows). In turn, this may predispose to PIH (Lockshin, 1987) and might be responsible indirectly for the increased frequency of fetal growth impairment in pregnancies treated with glucocorticoids (Rolbin, 1978). Acute psychosis, seizures, and arrhythmias may be induced by glucocorticoids. Finally, some investigators have found that glucocorticoids administered in moderate-to-high doses during pregnancy are associated with premature rupture of the membranes (Cowchock, 1992).

Glucocorticoids are associated with osteonecrosis, a complication that typically involves large, weight-bearing joints (e.g., the femoral head of the hips) and may be permanently disabling. The occurrence of osteonecrosis is correlated positively with the dose and duration of glucocorticoid therapy, but the exact frequency is unknown. In one study of 234 patients with SLE, the estimated frequency of osteonecrosis approached 30% by 15 years of follow-up (Dimant, 1978)! All patients undergoing glucocorticoid treatment should be made aware of this potential complication.

Glucocorticoids also are associated with osteoporosis when used relatively long term. In view of this potential complication, it seems prudent to institute calcium and vitamin D supplementation in all women on glucocorticoids. Weight-bearing exercise also may offset the risk of osteoporosis.

As noted, the routine administration of glucocorticoids to asymptomatic, pregnant SLE patients appears neither prudent nor necessary. Although pregnancy per se is by no means an indication to reduce the dose of glucocorticoids, carefully monitored reduction of the dose of medication during pregnancy is reasonable and safe when the patient's disease appears in remission. So-called stress doses of glucocorticoids should be given during labor or at the time of cesarean section or other obstetric surgery to all patients who have been treated with chronically administered steroids within the year prior to the procedure. Intravenous hydrocortisone sodium succinate, given in doses of 100 mg/8 hr for three doses, is an acceptable regimen.

**Cytotoxic Drugs** Several other immunosuppressives may be encountered in the pregnant woman with SLE. Three of these agents, azathioprine, methotrexate, and cyclophosphamide, are cytotoxic drugs. Limited data suggest that azathioprine, a derivative of 6-mercaptopurine, is not a teratogen in humans. It is associated, however, with fetal growth impairment (Scott, 1977; Armenti, 1994) and evidence of impaired neonatal immunity (Cote, 1974). Azathioprine should be avoided during pregnancy unless the benefits clearly outweigh the risks.

Methotrexate, which is occasionally used in SLE patients, is well known to be embryolethal in early pregnancy. It also is probably a teratogen, being associated with cleft palate, skeletal abnormalities, and hydrocephalus (Thiersch, 1956; Mulinsky, 1968). Also, methotrexate may adversely impact trophoblastic growth or function. Thus, methotrexate should be scrupulously avoided in pregnancy.

Cyclophosphamide is widely used to treat proliferative lupus nephritis. It crosses the placenta and is associated with fetal growth impairment, skeletal abnormalities, and cleft palate in rabbits (Ujhazy, 1993). Although, data in humans are limited, it appears that cyclophosphamide should be avoided in pregnancy except in the unusual case wherein the potential benefits clearly outweigh the risks. One such circumstance for which cyclophosphamide might be indicated is severe, progressive proliferative glomerulonephritis.

**Antimalarials** Antimalarial drugs, such as chloroquine and hydroxychloroquine, cross the placenta and have been associated with several fetal abnormalities. These drugs have an affinity for melanin-containing tissues, such as those in the eye, and case reports suggest that these drugs can cause a dose-related eye damage in the human (Nylander, 1967). Chloroquine also has been associated with ototoxicity in one case report (Hart, 1964). However, most infants born to women taking antimalarials during pregnancy are apparently normal, suggesting that the risks of ocular or ototoxicity are small (Parke, 1988).

**Antiinflammatory Drugs and Analgesics** The most common types of analgesics used in SLE are NSAIDs. Unfortunately, there are serious fetal and neonatal concerns related to the use of these medications in pregnancy. Nonsteroidal antiinflammatory drugs cross the placenta readily and can block prostaglandin synthesis in a wide variety of fetal tissues. They may affect fetoneonatal clotting through the inhibition of platelet aggregation. In the case of aspirin, the inhibition of platelet function lasts the lifespan of the platelet, because aspirin binds irreversibly to the pertinent platelet enzymes. Maternal ingestion of typical adult doses of aspirin in the week prior to delivery has been associated with increased frequency of intracranial hemorrhage in premature infants (Stuart, 1982; Rumack, 1981). Indomethacin, an NSAID, has been associated with constriction of the fetal ductus arteriosus (Moise, 1988), which might result in pulmonary artery thrombosis, hypertrophy of the pulmonary vasculature, impaired oxygenation, and congestive heart failure. Also, NSAIDs have been associated with a decrease in fetal urinary output, and oligohydramnios (Hickok, 1989) and neonatal renal insufficiency (Vanhaesebrouck, 1988) have been described in association with indomethacin. More recently, a retrospective analysis showed that infants delivered after exposure to indomethacin had a lower urine output and higher serum creatinine and higher rates of necrotizing enterocolitis, patent ductus arteriosus, and grades II through

IV intracranial hemorrhage than gestational age-matched controls (Norton, 1993). Given these concerns, high-dose aspirin and NSAIDs should be avoided, if at all possible, during pregnancy.

## Treatment for Specific SLE-Related Problems

**Mild-to-Moderate Exacerbations** Mild-to-moderate exacerbations of symptoms of SLE without CNS or renal involvement may be treated with glucocorticoids or an increase in the dose of glucocorticoids. Relatively small doses of prednisone (e.g., 15–30 mg/day) will result in improvement in most cases. For severe exacerbations without CNS or renal involvement, doses of 1.0–1.5 mg/kg/day of prednisone in divided doses should be used, and a good clinical response can be expected in 5 to 10 days. Thereafter, glucocorticoids may be tapered by several different approaches. The following are two simple and effective methods of tapering:

1. Consolidate to a single morning dose of prednisone. Reduce the daily dose by 10% per week, as tolerated. When a dose of 20 to 30 mg/day is reached, reduce by 2.5-mg increments per week. If the patient remains asymptomatic at a dose of 15 mg/day, reduce the dose by 1-mg increments per week to a dose of 5 to 10 mg/day.
2. Consolidate to a single morning dose of prednisone. Taper to 50 to 60 mg/day by reducing the dose 10% per week. Thereafter eliminate the alternate-day dose by tapering it 10% per week, as tolerated. Thereafter, taper the remaining every other day dose by 10% per week, as tolerated.

**Severe Exacerbations** Severe exacerbations, especially those involving the CNS or kidneys, are treated more aggressively. In recent years, an intravenous pulse glucocorticoid therapy approach has become popular. The initial regimen involves a daily intravenous dose of methylprednisolone at 10 to 30 mg/kg (about 500–1000 mg) for 3 to 6 days. Thereafter, the patient is continued on 1.0 to 1.5 mg/day of prednisone in divided doses and rapidly tapered over the course of 1 month.

One can expect that 75% of patients will respond favorably to this approach (Isenberg, 1982). This regimen may be repeated every 1 to 3 months in severe cases as an alternative to cytotoxic drugs.

In nonpregnant patients, both azathioprine and cyclophosphamide may be used in severe SLE exacerbations to control disease, reduce irreversible tissue damage, and reduce glucocorticoid doses. In particular, severe proliferative lupus nephritis may be treated more effectively with cyclophosphamide, usually in combination with glucocorticoids. The drug may be given either orally or intravenously, but the most effective cyclophosphamide regimen is uncertain. Cyclophosphamide appears to be useful in the treatment of severe cerebral lupus as well. Azathioprine is perhaps less effective than cyclophosphamide, though it is also less toxic. Neither cyclophosphamide nor azathioprine can be recommended in pregnancy, except in unusual or life-threatening cases. In such cases, treatments should be individualized and initiated with the due consideration of and informed consent regarding the potential risks to the mother and fetus.

Plasmapheresis has been used in severe cases of SLE that are unresponsive to high-dose glucocorticoids and cyclophosphamide, although its efficacy is uncertain. It should be considered in life-threatening disease that is unresponsive to other treatments. Because plasmapheresis removes the negative feedback of high levels of autoantibodies, a cytotoxic agent should be administered soon after plasmapheresis is initiated (days 5 through 10 of therapy) if the patient is no longer pregnant.

**Neonatal Lupus** Although some authors have suggested prophylactic treatment of mothers who have previously delivered infants with NLE and CCHB using glucocorticoids and/or plasmapheresis (Barclay, 1987; Buyon, 1988; Kaaja, 1991), the efficacy and safety of this treatment remain unproven. Given that the recurrence risk is fairly low, prophylactic treatment with potentially dangerous therapies does not appear warranted. However, more frequent assessment of the fetal heart rate and serial ultrasounds for development of fetal hydrops would appear reasonable in such cases.

There are several cases wherein fetuses with established CCHB and evidence of cardiac failure or serositis appear to have improved after maternally administered prednisone and betamethasone (Bierman, 1988; Richards, 1990) or maternally administered dexamethasone and plasmapheresis (Buyon, 1987). In all cases, the CCHB persisted, but serous effusions regressed. This suggests that the treatments either improved fetal cardiac function or effectively treated fetal serositis. Others have suggested dexamethasone administered to the mother as a treatment for any infant found to have CCHB, in an effort to avoid further cardiac damage (Rider, 1993; Coppel, 1995). In one series of five cases of heart block discovered in utero, mothers were administered 4 mg of dexamethasone daily (Coppel, 1995). In three cases, hydrops resolved. In two cases, the degree of heart block lessened after treatment. In one, there was improvement from complete heart block to second-degree heart block. In the other, there was improvement from second-degree to first-degree heart block.

Taken together, the currently available data indicate that newly discovered cases of CCHB in utero should be evaluated by sonographic examination of the fetal heart and determination of maternal anti-Ro/SS-A and anti-La/SS-B status. If the diagnosis of CCHB due to neonatal lupus is made, experts are currently recommending administration of a glucocorticoid that crosses the placenta (e.g., dexamethasone, 4 mg/day) to limit further immunologic damage to the fetal heart. This approach is being examined in a registry of cases by Dr. J.P. Buyon at the Hospital for Joint Diseases, in New York City (phone: 212-598-6283).

## Antiphospholipid Syndrome

Antiphospholipid syndrome is an autoimmune condition characterized by certain clinical features associated with the presence of moderate-to-high levels of antiphospholipid (aPLs). The most widely recognized clinical features of APS are thrombotic phenomena (venous or arterial, including stroke), autoimmune thrombocytopenia, and pregnancy loss (Harris, 1986; Asherson, 1989; Alarcon-Segovia, 1989). More debatable clinical features include livedo reticularis, Coombs'-positive hemolytic anemia, cardiac valvular lesions, and others. Antiphospholipid syndrome probably occurs most commonly in patients with other underlying autoimmune diseases, such as SLE. In this setting, the syndrome is known as *secondary* APS. The condition, however, also is diagnosed in women with no other recognizable autoimmune disease. This expression of the syndrome is known as *primary* APS and appears to be what obstetrician-gynecologists encounter most frequently. To be classified as having APS, the patient must have at least one clinical feature of the syndrome along with moderate-to-high levels of aPLs (Table 26-6).

Unfortunately, laboratory testing for aPLs remains somewhat confusing for clinicians. Part of the difficulty is that some laboratories offering aPL testing use assays that are not standardized or operate with inadequate quality control analysis of results (Coulam, 1990; Peaceman, 1992). Underlying this problem is that reliable testing for aPLs is modestly difficult, even in the hands of experienced and interested investigators. Although many of the problems related to aPL testing will be resolved over time, the best advice for the clinician is that he or she identify and use a reliable laboratory with a special interest in aPL testing.

There are two aPLs for which well-established assays are available: (1) lupus anticoagulant and (2) anticardiolipin antibodies (aCLs). Both of these aPLs bind moieties on negatively charged phospholipids or the moieties formed by the interaction of negatively charged phospholipids with other phospholipids or glycoproteins. Lupus anticoagulant is detected in plasma by using phospholipid-dependent clotting assays such as the activated partial thromboplastin time, dilute Russell viper venom time, or kaolin clotting time. Because lupus anticoagulant binds to the phospholipid portion of the clotting tests, the clotting time is prolonged, even though the patients have a thrombotic, not a bleeding, tendency. A sequence of clotting tests is required to determine that the prolonged clotting time is due to lupus anticoagulant, but the clinician needs to know only whether the laboratory detected lupus anticoagulant. Because the sensitivity of the various

T A B L E   **26-6**

Suggested clinical and laboratory criteria for the antiphospholipid syndrome

| Clinical Features | Laboratory Features |
|---|---|
| Pregnancy loss | Lupus anticoagulant |
|   Fetal death | Anticardiolipin antibodies, IgG, medium- |
|   Recurrent pregnancy loss |   or high-positive |
| Thrombosis | Anticardiolipin antibodies, IgM, medium- |
|   Venous |   or high-positive and lupus anticoagulant |
|   Arterial, including stroke | |
| Autoimmune thrombocytopenia | |
| Other | |
|   Coombs'-positive hemolytic anemia | |
|   Livedo reticularis | |

Patients with APS should have at least one clinical and one laboratory feature
    at some time in the course of their disease. Laboratory tests should be
    positive on at least two occasions more than 8 weeks apart.

clotting assays for lupus anticoagulant varies considerably, clinicians should use a laboratory known for performing reliable and sensitive lupus anticoagulant testing.

Anticardiolipin antibodies are detected by conventional immunoassay methods, with serum standards available from the Antiphospholipid Standardization Laboratory in Atlanta, Georgia. Results calibrated against these standards are reported in terms of isotype-specific phospholipid binding units designated as "GPL" (IgG aCL), "MPL" (IgM aCL), or "APL" (IgA aCL) units. Results, however, should be reported and interpreted in semiquantitative terms as either negative, low-positive, medium-positive, or high-positive (Harris, 1990). Low-positive results and isolated IgM aCL results (i.e., IgM-positive, but lupus anticoagulant–negative and IgG aCL–negative) are of questionable clinical significance and should not be regarded as diagnostic of APS (Silver, 1996). Isolated IgA aCL also is of questionable clinical significance, and results must be interpreted carefully in the light of the clinical situation.

At least two groups of investigators find that lupus anticoagulant and aCLs may be separated in the laboratory, suggesting that they are different immunoglobulins (Exner, 1988; Chamley, 1991). Others believe that lupus anticoagulant and aCLs are the same immunoglobulin being detected by different methods. This controversy notwithstanding, lupus anticoagulant and aCLs are associated with the same set of clinical problems and, therefore, seem likely to be members of the same "family" of autoantibodies. The majority of patients with APS have lupus anticoagulant and IgG aCLs. Some patients with APS, however, have either aCLs or lupus anticoagulant but not both. Thus, *both* tests should be obtained when considering the diagnosis of APS.

Tests for aPLs other than lupus anticoagulant and aCL may have merit in the diagnosis of APS, but their status is uncertain. These other aPLs include (1) antibodies binding to phospholipid antigens other than cardiolipin (phosphatidylserine, phosphatidylethanolamine, phosphatidylinositol, phosphatidylglycerol, and phosphatidic acid), (2) antibodies to $\beta$2-glycoprotein I, and (3) antibodies to a complex of cardiolipin and $\beta$2-glycoprotein I. Debate over the importance of these antibodies, independent of lupus anticoagulant and aCLs, continues. For example, some investigators have found that phospholipid-binding antibodies to antigens other than cardiolipin are linked to recurrent pregnancy loss (Kwak, 1992; Aoki, 1993). More recently, other investigators have criticized these studies, and have found that these antibodies are not associated with recurrent pregnancy loss once lupus anticoagulant and aCLs have been excluded (Branch, 1997). Regardless of the debate about recurrent pregnancy loss, aPLs other than lupus anticoagulant and aCLs have not been linked to medically serious complications of APS, such as thrombosis or autoimmune thrombocytopenia, and hence should not be used to make the diagnosis of APS. Antibodies to β2-glycoprotein I or to a complex of cardiolipin and β2-glycoprotein I may be diagnostic of APS, but confirmatory studies are required to be certain.

## Antiphospholipid Syndrome and Pregnancy

### *Thrombosis and Stroke*

Numerous retrospective studies confirm a link between aPLs and thrombosis (Bowie, 1963; Harris, 1983; Lechner, 1985). Venous thrombosis accounts for about 65% to 70% of episodes. The lower extremity is the single most common site of involvement, but no part of the vasculature is spared. In particular, one should entertain the diagnosis of APS in women with venous thrombosis in relatively unusual sites, such as the portal vein, mesenteric vein, splenic vein, and subclavian vein. Antiphospholipid antibodies also are associated with arterial thrombosis and appear to be a predisposing factor in 4% to 46% of cases of stroke in otherwise healthy patients under age 50 (Hart, 1987; Brey, 1990; Ferro, 1993). As with venous thrombosis, one should entertain the diagnosis of APS in individuals with arterial thrombosis in relatively unusual locations, such as the retinal artery, subclavian or brachial artery, and digital arteries. Antiphospholipid antibodies are also associated with transient ischemic attacks and amaurosis fugax (Silver, 1996).

The prospective risk of thrombosis or stroke in women with aPLs is substantial. In a small prospective study, Glueck and colleagues (1985) found that 50% of patients with SLE and lupus anticoagulant had a thrombotic episode during the study period. They estimated that the annual risk of venous thrombosis and arterial thrombosis was 13.7% and 6.7%, respectively, both figures being significantly greater than those among SLE patients without lupus anticoagulant. In a prospective case control study, investigators found that a significant proportion of other-

wise healthy men suffering thrombosis or pulmonary embolism had moderate-to-high titers of aCLs (Ginsburg, 1992). The estimated relative risk for individuals with aCLs developing thrombosis or pulmonary embolism was 5.3. Finally, in an historic cohort study, investigators found that 22% of women with APS had a thromboembolic event, and 6.9% had a cerebrovascular accident over a median follow-up of 60 months (Silver, 1994).

Importantly, a summary of data from women with APS and a history of thrombosis indicates that well over half of thrombotic episodes occurred in relation to pregnancy or the use of combination oral contraceptives (Branch, 1990, 1992). In two prospective studies of pregnancies in women with APS, the rates of thrombosis or stroke were 5% (Branch, 1992) and 12% (Lima, 1996), respectively, with several women having thrombotic events while on prophylactic doses of heparin. These observations suggest that the risk of thrombosis during pregnancy or the postpartum period is substantial enough that relatively aggressive heparin treatment may be required.

### *Postpartum Syndrome*

In a retrospective review of pregnancies in women with APS, three suffered similar postpartum complications, which may represent an autoimmune exacerbation (Kochenour, 1987). None of the women was known to have underlying autoimmune disease, but all developed fever, pulmonary infiltrates, and pleural effusions in the postpartum period. Two of the three also had thrombosis in the postpartum period, and one developed a cardiomyopathy. As reported by others, this syndrome also involves renal insufficiency (Kniaz, 1992) and pulmonary hypertension (Kupferminc, 1994).

### *Catastrophic Antiphospholipid Syndrome*

In 1992, Asherson coined the phrase "catastrophic antiphospholipid syndrome" to describe a case of rapid clinical deterioration associated with accelerated coagulation vasculopathy in a patient with APS (Asherson, 1992a). A number of similar additional cases have been published, although it remains uncertain whether catastrophic APS represents a distinct clinical entity or the superimposition onto APS of another medical problem. Catastrophic APS and the postpartum syndrome mentioned here may be part of the same spectrum.

Patients typically have high titers of aPLs and a rapidly evolving clinical course that may be marked by malignant hypertension, pulmonary hypertension, renal insufficiency, widespread thrombosis (including arterial thrombosis), and disseminated intravascular coagulopathy. In one case report, the patient presented with features suggestive of the HELLP (hemolysis, elevated liver enzymes, and low platelets) syndrome but went on to develop frank coagulopathy and widespread thrombosis (Hochfeld, 1994). The associated mortality rate is quite high, and the condition should be considered a true emergency.

### Pregnancy Loss

Early case reports focused attention on a possible relationship between aPLs and pregnancy loss (Branch, 1987). More recently, several studies have linked aPLs and recurrent pregnancy loss (Petri, 1987; Barbui, 1988; Parazzini, 1991; Parke, 1991; Out, 1991; MacLean, 1994). In these studies, the median frequency of lupus anticoagulant or aCL IgG in women with recurrent pregnancy loss is 12.5% (vs. 2.5% for controls).

Fetal death (death of the conceptus after 10–12 weeks' gestation) appears to be more specific for aPL-related pregnancy loss than embryonic loss. In one summary of data derived from the literature, over 90% of women with APS presenting with pregnancy loss had suffered at least one fetal death (Branch, 1987). A retrospective analysis of women with well-characterized APS showed that 79 of 195 (41%) previous pregnancies were fetal deaths (Branch, 1992). More recently, Oshiro et al (1996) analyzed the obstetric histories of 366 women with two or more consecutive pregnancy losses who were tested for lupus anticoagulant and aCLs. Seventy-six of the patients in this highly selected referral population had

clinically relevant levels of aPLs (lupus anticoagulant or medium-to-high–positive IgG aCLs). Fully 50% of the previous pregnancy losses in this group were fetal deaths, whereas, only 10% of the losses in the 290 women without significant levels of aPLs were fetal deaths. Moreover, over 80% of the women with clinically significant levels of aPLs had suffered at least one fetal death, compared with 24% in women without aPLs. The specificity of one or more fetal deaths for the presence of significant levels of aPLs was 76%. A history of two or more early first-trimester losses without fetal death had a specificity of only 6% for the presence of aPLs.

Most studies linking aPLs to pregnancy loss have found aPLs in highly selected patients with underlying autoimmune disease, a history of fetal death, or a history of thrombosis. Studies of less highly selected populations have led to the emergence of two important facts. First, significant levels of aPLs may be found, albeit infrequently, in otherwise normal women. In the best study, fewer than 2% of over 1000 unselected obstetric patients were found to have IgG aCLs; 4% had IgM aCLs (Harris, 1991). Over 80% of the positive results were in the low-positive range, with only 0.2% of IgG results and 0.7% of IgM results being in the medium- or high-positive range. Other studies have also found a relatively small proportion of positive results in unselected obstetric patients (Pattison, 1988; Lockwood, 1989). It is also clear that sporadic miscarriage or fetal death is infrequently "due to" aPLs (Haddow, 1991; Infante-Rivard, 1991), a finding that is not surprising given the infrequency of APS. Thus, APS is not the "cause" of pregnancy loss in a large proportion of unselected cases, much as parental karyotype abnormalities or uterine malformations are not the "cause" of pregnancy loss in a large proportion of unselected cases. The importance of identifying APS lies not in its prevalence but in its implications for the patient and the fact that it is a potentially treatable cause of pregnancy loss.

### Preeclampsia

An unusually high rate of preeclampsia has been noted in a series of patients with APS (Lockshin, 1985a,b; Branch, 1985, 1992; Caruso, 1993; Lima,

1996), and preeclampsia is a major contributor to the high rate of preterm delivery in this condition. The rate of preeclampsia does not appear to be diminished markedly by treatment with LDA, glucocorticoids, or heparin; in the largest series of treated patients, half developed preeclampsia (Branch, 1992).

Several studies have attempted to determine the rate of aPLs among patients with PIH. In the first, the rate of aPLs was not increased among all patients with PIH, including those near term (Scott, 1987). Three other studies, however, found that 16% to 17% of preeclamptic patients had significant levels of aPLs (Branch, 1990b; Milliez, 1991).

A relationship between aPLs and preeclampsia has been confirmed by a prospective study of unselected obstetric patients (Yasuda, 1995). Of the 60 women who tested positive for IgG aCLs, 12% had preeclampsia, compared with 2% of the 800 women who tested negative.

### Fetal Growth Impairment and Fetal Distress

Several investigators have noted that aPLs are associated with fetal growth impairment (Branch, 1985, 1992; Caruso, 1993; Lima, 1996). Even in treated pregnancies, the rate of fetal growth impairment among live-born infants approaches 30% (Branch, 1992; Lima, 1996), although high-dose immune globulin therapy may reduce the rate (Spinnato, 1995).

Antiphospholipid antibodies may contribute to the overall rate of fetal growth impairment. In one study, nine of 37 mothers (24%) who delivered growth-impaired infants had medium- or high-positive tests for aCLs, significantly more than among controls (Polzin, 1991). In the prospective study of Yasuda and colleagues (1995), 12% of women testing positive for IgG aCLs had small-for-gestational-age infants, compared with 2% of women testing negative.

Fetal distress also appears to be relatively common in APS pregnancy (Lockshin, 1985; Branch, 1985, 1992; Caruso, 1993; Lima, 1996). Here again, treatment does not appear to markedly diminish the rate. Half of all treated, successful pregnancies in 54 women with APS were complicated by fetal distress in one series (Branch, 1992).

### Preterm Birth

Primarily because of the aforementioned complications of aPL pregnancies, preterm delivery is common among patients with APS (Lockshin, 1985b; Branch, 1985, 1992; Caruso, 1993; Lima, 1996). Yasuda and colleagues (1995) found 12% of the 60 women testing positive for IgG aCLs were delivered early, compared with 4% of those testing negative.

The rate of indicated preterm birth remains quite high in spite of treatment during pregnancy with LDA, glucocorticoids, or heparin (Branch, 1992; Lima, 1996), with preterm birth accomplished in at least 30% of cases. Indicated preterm delivery at or before 32 weeks' gestation also is common (Branch, 1992). As with preeclampsia and fetal distress, the rate of indicated preterm birth may be impacted by high-dose immune globulin (Spinnato, 1995).

## Management of Antiphospholipid Syndrome Pregnancy

Patients known to have APS should undergo preconception assessment and counseling. A detailed medical and obstetric history should be obtained, and the presence of significant levels of aPLs should be confirmed. The patient should be informed of the potential maternal and obstetric problems, including the risk of thrombosis or stroke, fetal loss, preeclampsia, fetal growth impairment, and preterm delivery. In those women who also have SLE, issues related to exacerbation of SLE can be discussed. All patients with APS should be assessed for evidence of anemia, thrombocytopenia, and underlying renal disease (urinalysis, a serum creatinine, 24-hr urine for creatinine clearance and total protein).

Once pregnant, the patient with APS may be seen by a physician at least every 2 weeks in the first and second trimesters and every week thereafter. The patient should be instructed to notify the physician immediately if she develops signs or symptoms of thrombosis, thromboembolism, transient ischemic attacks, or amaurosis fugax. Once the diagnosis of APS is made, serial aPL determinations are not useful.

As with SLE, a primary goal of the antenatal visits in APS patients after 20 weeks' gestation is the detection of hypertension and/or proteinuria. Because of the risk of uteroplacental insufficiency, fetal ultrasounds should be performed every 4 to 6 weeks starting at 18 to 20 weeks' gestation. In otherwise uncomplicated APS patients, fetal surveillance should be started at 30 to 32 weeks' gestation. Earlier and more frequent ultrasound and fetal testing is indicated in patients with poor obstetric histories, evidence of PIH, or evidence of fetal growth impairment. In selected cases, fetal surveillance as early as 24 to 25 weeks may be justified (Druzin, 1987).

In women with bona fide APS, the risk of thrombosis in pregnancy is high enough to warrant heparin thromboprophylaxis (Branch, 1992; Lima, 1996). It is important to continue thromboprophylaxis during the postpartum period, probably for about 6 weeks to 2 months. The author prefers to switch from heparin to warfarin for postpartum prophylaxis to limit further risk of heparin osteoporosis. International normalized ratio values of 2.0 to 2.5 would seem a reasonable goal.

### Treatments to Prevent Fetal Loss

Since the early 1980s, clinicians have suggested that women with APS and previous pregnancy loss could be treated during pregnancy to improve the chance of delivering a live infant. Early investigators used prednisone and LDA (Lubbe, 1983; Branch, 1985). This treatment, however, is fraught with minor and major toxic side effects of glucocorticoids, and one group of investigators found the regimen to be ineffective in preventing fetal loss (Lockshin, 1989b).

A regimen of subcutaneous heparin treatment, with or without LDA, is the most widely used treatment for APS pregnancy. The first published series was that of Rosove et al (1990). Using a mean dose of 24,700 units of heparin daily, started in the first trimester, 14 of 15 pregnancies (93%) were successful. In a subsequently published randomized trial, Cowchock and colleagues

(1992) found that treatment of APS pregnancy with heparin and LDA is just as effective as prednisone and LDA in terms of fetal outcome. The mean dose of heparin used was 17,000 units daily. Treatment with heparin and LDA has become the most widely accepted treatment of APS in the United States (Table 26-7).

The experience at the University of Utah now includes in excess of 25 women with APS who were treated with heparin and LDA during pregnancy. Among the first 18 cases (Branch, 1992), the median first-trimester dose of heparin used was 15,000 units/day, and the median second-trimester dose of heparin used was 20,000 units/ day. Sixteen of 18 pregnancies were successful, but two infants delivered prematurely for maternal or fetal indications died of complications of prematurity.

The efficacy of treatment to improve fetal outcome in women with APS is still debated. Recently, Kutteh (1996) completed a prospective trial demonstrating that heparin and LDA are more effective than low-dose aspirin alone in terms of fetal outcome in a selected subset of women with aCLs but no lupus anticoagulant. Doses of heparin were adjusted to maintain the partial thromboplastin time at 1.2 to 1.5 times the control mean. Viable infants were delivered in 80% of women treated with heparin and LDA, compared with only 44% of women treated with aspirin alone.

Heparin treatment is by no means benign. Heparin-induced osteoporosis with fracture occurs in 1% to 2% of women treated during pregnancy (Dahlman, 1993). In an attempt to avoid severe osteoporosis, women treated with heparin should be encouraged to take daily supplemental calcium and vitamin D (e.g., prenatal vitamins). It also seems prudent to encourage daily axial skeleton weight-bearing exercise (e.g., walking). Heparin also is associated with an uncommon idiosyncratic thrombocytopenia, known as heparin-induced thrombocytopenia (HIT). This complication is immune-mediated and usually has its onset 3 to 15 days after initiation of therapy. The frequency is difficult to determine but probably occurs in fewer than 5% of patients treated with heparin, with most cases being relatively mild in nature. A more severe form of HIT, paradoxically involving

T A B L E    26-7

Proposed treatments for pregnant patients with antiphospholipid
antibodies and antiphospholipid syndrome

| Clinical Features | Antiphospholipid Antibodies | Proposed Treatments |
|---|---|---|
| Recurrent embryonic losses, but no fetal deaths, no history of thromboembolic disease, and no history of autoimmune thrombocytopenia | Low-positive IgG aCLs without LA, or IgM or IgA aCLs without IgG aCLs or LA | No treatment or LDA |
| No clinical history suggestive of APS | LA, medium-to-high–positive IgG aCLs | Low-dose aspirin; consider heparin thromboprophylaxis |
| Recurrent embryonic losses, but no fetal deaths, no history of thromboembolic disease, and no history of autoimmune thrombocytopenia | LA, medium-to-high–positive IgG aCLs | Low-dose aspirin; consider heparin thromboprophylaxis |
| Otherwise unexplained fetal death(s), history of thromboembolic disease, history of autoimmune thrombocytopenia, or any combination | LA, medium-to-high–positive IgG aCLs | Heparin, 15,000–20,000 units/day or full anticoagulation doses administered subcutaneously, LDA |

LA, lupus anticoagulant.

---

**CONGENITAL COMPLETE HEART BLOCK IN NEONATAL LUPUS**

I.  *Goal of Therapy*

   A.   To prevent myocardial damage due to ongoing immune-mediated myocarditis

II.  *Management Protocol*

   A.   Once CCHB is suspected, obtain a thorough ultrasonographic evaluation of the fetal heart.
   B.   Start treatment with dexamethasone, 4 mg/day in divided doses, administered to the mother.
   C.   Follow the fetus closely with frequent ultrasonographic assessment.

III.  *Critical Laboratory Tests*

   A.   Anti-SS-A and anti-SS-B antibodies

IV.  *Consultation*

   A.   Jill P. Buyon, M.D. (phone: 212-598-6283)

## SYSTEMIC LUPUS ERYTHEMATOSUS

I. *Goals of Therapy*

   A. Avoidance of maintenance medications that are potentially threatening to the fetus
   B. Timely detection of hypertensive disease in pregnancy and uteroplacental insufficiency
   C. Detection and treatment of exacerbations of SLE in order to modify life-threatening manifestations

II. *Managment Protocol*

   A. Preconception Consultation
      1. Discuss risks and possible outcomes.
      2. If necessary, establish a medical treatment regimen that avoids antirheumatic drugs that are potentially threatening to the fetus.
      3. Assess SLE activity and the presence of nephropathy or aPLs.
   B. Antenatal Care
      1. Frequent prenatal visits to assess SLE disease status.
      2. Frequent assessment for hypertensive disease after 20 weeks' gestation.
      3. Fetal ultrasound every 4 to 6 weeks to detect possible fetal growth restriction or oligohydramnios.
      4. Fetal surveillance testing starting at 30 to 32 weeks' gestation, or sooner if the clinical situation warrants.
   C. Treatment of Exacerbation of SLE
      1. Mild-to-moderate exacerbation
         a. If the patient is currently taking glucocorticoids, increase the dose to at least 20 to 30 mg of oral prednisone per day in divided doses. A higher dose may be required.
         b. If the patient is not currently taking glucocorticoids, start 15 to 20 mg of oral prednisone per day in divided doses.
      2. Severe exacerbation without CNS or renal involvement
         a. Consider hospitalization and rheumatologic consultation.
         b. Start or increase the dose of glucocorticoids at 1.0 to 1.5 mg/kg of oral prednisone per day in divided doses. Expect a clinical response in 5 to 10 days.
         c. Once the patient responds, taper the glucocorticoids as outlined in the text.
      3. Severe exacerbation with CNS or renal involvement
         a. Hospitalize the patient and obtain rheumatologic consultation.
         b. Initiate "pulse" glucocorticoid therapy: daily intravenous methylprednisolone at 10 to 30 mg/kg/day for 3 to 6 days.
         c. Thereafter, maintain 1.0 to 1.5 mg/kg of oral prednisone per day in divided doses until a clinical reponse is established.
         d. Once the patient responds, taper the glucocorticoids as outlined in the text.
         e. In patients unresponsive to this regimen, consider plasmapheresis and cyclophosphamide treatment as outlined in the text.

III. *Critical Laboratory Tests*

   A. Complete blood count, platelet count, urinalysis, ANA, anti-dsDNA, complement levels, electrolytes, creatinine, BUN, and 24-hour urine for total protein and creatinine clearance.

---

## ANTIPHOSPHOLIPID SYNDROME

### I. *Goals of Therapy*

    A.  Fetal survival

    B.  Timely detection of hypertensive disease in pregnancy and uteroplacental insufficiency

    C.  Prevention of maternal morbidity, especially thromboembolic disease

### II. *Management Protocol*

    A.  Uncomplicated Antiphospholipid Syndrome

        1.  Preconceptional consultation

            a.  Evaluate diagnosis; assess for aPLs.

            b.  Discuss risks and possible outcomes.

        2.  Antenatal care

            a.  Frequent prenatal visits to assess maternal and fetal status.

            b.  Start LDA when pregnancy is confirmed.

            c.  Start subcutaneous unfractionated sodium heparin, 15,000 to 20,000 units/day in divided doses, or low-molecular-weight heparin equivalent, when a live embryo is detected (approximately 5.5–6.5 weeks' gestation).

            d.  Calcium supplementation.

            e.  Frequent assessment for hypertensive disease after 20 weeks' gestation.

            f.  Fetal ultrasound every 4 to 6 weeks to detect possible fetal growth restriction or oligohydramnios.

            g.  Fetal surveillance testing starting at 30 to 32 weeks' gestation, or sooner if the clinical situation warrants.

---

venous and arterial thromboses, may occur in up to 0.5% of patients treated with unfractionated sodium heparin. Patients with this complication may have limb ischemia, cerebrovascular accidents, and myocardial infarctions, as well as venous thromboses. It has been shown that low-molecular-weight heparin is much less likely to be associated with HIT (Warkentin, 1995), a major safety feature, compared with unfractionated sodium heparin.

The use of high-dose intravenous immune globulin (IVIG) has generated interest because of anecdotal reports of successful pregnancy outcomes (Scott, 1988; Wapner, 1990; Katz, 1990; Kaaja, 1993). Intravenous immune globulin is particularly attractive because it is associated with relatively few and rare adverse effects. The literature contains nearly a dozen APS pregnancies treated with IVIG, but all but one were also treated with prednisone, heparin, or LDA. For the most

part, the reported cases appear to involve more severe cases of antiphospholipid-related pregnancy loss ("refractory" cases), which had failed other therapies.

A more recently published series of five women with well-characterized APS treated with IVIG during pregnancy is intriguing (Spinnato, 1995). All women received high-dose IVIG as a part of their pregnancy treatment. All also received LDA, and four of the five were additionally treated with heparin (10,000–15,000 units/day). All pregnancies were delivered of live-born infants. In marked contrast to the results summarized earlier, however, none of the patients had preeclampsia, none of the infants were small for gestational age, and no pregnancies required delivery prior to 33 to 34 weeks' gestation. In three of the five cases, IgG anticardiolipin levels were followed through the course of treatment. Intravenous immune

---

## ANTIPHOSPHOLIPID SYNDROME (*cont.*)

   B.  Postpartum Syndrome or Catastrophic APS

      1.  Obtain a thorough cardiovascular and pulmonary evaluation, with appropriate consultations.

      2.  Consider intensive care unit management.

      3.  If the patient is hypertensive, treat with appropriate antihypertensives.

      4.  If there are no contraindications, start heparin anticoagulation.

      5.  If there is evidence of inflammatory conditions, start intravenous methylprednisolone, 10 to 30 mg/kg/day.

      6.  If catastrophic APS is suspected, start plasmapheresis, replacing 40 mL of plasma per kg per exchange. Repeat three times per week for 2 to 6 weeks. Also start cyclophosphamide.

### III. *Diagnostic Tests*

   A.  Pertinent imaging for suspected thrombosis or thromboembolism, chest x-ray for suspected pulmonary infiltrates or pleural effusions, and pelvic imaging to exclude septic focus.

### IV. *Critical Laboratory Tests*

   A.  Complete blood count, platelet count, urinalysis, ANA, anti-dsDNA, aPLs, complement levels, electrolytes, creatinine, BUN, and 24-hour urine for total protein and creatinine clearance.

### V. *Consultations*

   A.  Intensive care, rheumatology, cardiology, pulmonology

---

globulin treatment was associated with marked reductions in the IgG anticardiolipin levels of 76%, 87%, and 96%, respectively. This remarkable suppression of IgG anticardiolipin levels has not been described previously in pregnancy treatment.

As used in these reports, IVIG is extremely expensive. Definitive proof of its efficacy will be necessary before this treatment can be recommended. A prospective, randomized trial is under way (D.W. Branch, University of Utah; phone: 801-581-7647).

*Treatment of Postpartum Syndrome and Catastrophic Antiphospholipid Syndrome*

Early and aggressive treatment of the postpartum syndrome associated with APS and catastrophic APS would appear to be the only hope for survival in many cases. Once either of these conditions is suspected, a thorough cardiovascular and pulmonary evaluation is mandatory. Strong consideration of delivery would seem prudent in pregnant patients with catastrophic APS. Most patients are best managed in an intensive care unit. Medical therapies must be individualized, but certain general principles hold:

1. Control markedly elevated BPs with appropriate antihypertensive medication.
2. If there are no contraindications, start anticoagulation with intravenous heparin. Patients with a prolonged activated partial thromboplastin time (due to lupus anticoagulant) should be monitored using a heparin level assay.
3. If there is evidence of inflammatory conditions, such as serositis or vasculitis, start methylprednisolone (10–30 mg/kg/day).

4. If catastrophic APS is suspected, plasmapheresis should be initiated. A standard regimen involves the replacement of 40 mL of plasma per kilogram of body weight or up to 3 liters per exchange. This should be repeated three times weekly for 2 to 6 weeks. The simultaneous administration of immunosuppressive agents may block potential rebound in production of autoantibodies.

## Variables Influencing Pregnancy Outcomes and Treatments

The diagnosis of APS rests on clinical and laboratory criteria. Women with aPLs but no clinical history compatible with APS pose a difficult dilemma, and it is uncertain as to whether they need treatment during pregnancy. Women with aPLs but no history of fetal loss have a higher rate of delivering a viable infant than women with aPLs and a history of fetal loss (Lockshin, 1989b), and the rate of subsequent fetal loss is correlated positively with the total number of prior losses (Branch, 1992; Out, 1992).

The isotype (class) and level of aPLs have considerable influence on pregnancy outcomes. Lupus anticoagulants are generally not isotyped, but aCLs are usually reported in terms of IgG and IgM. Most authorities agree that IgM aCLs (without IgG aCLs or lupus anticoagulant being present) are of questionable clinical significance (Harris, 1990; Silver, 1996). In contrast, the level of IgG aCLs appears to be one determinant of adverse pregnancy outcome, with high levels of IgG aCLs ($>40$ IgG-binding units [GPL]) associated with a comparatively higher risk of fetal loss (Lockshin, 1989b). In women with aCL levels of 40 GPL units or less, the rate of fetal death is under 20%. The rate of fetal death increases with increasing levels of IgG aCLs, and the presence of more than 80 GPL units predicts nearly a 40% rate of fetal death. The influence of clinical history and IgG aCL levels appear additive. Over 80% of women with a history of prior fetal death and very high levels of anticardiolipin IgG ($>80$ GPL units) will have a fetal death in their next pregnancy.

The apparent risk of maternal thrombosis in women with APS often makes decisions regarding treatment less difficult. Clearly, if the patient has had a thrombotic event in the past, heparin treatment during pregnancy should be strongly considered regardless of prior fetal outcomes. Given that lupus anticoagulant and/or medium-to-high levels of IgG aCLs indicate a thrombotic predisposition, some clinicians would argue that all women with these antibodies are candidates for thromboprophylaxis with heparin during pregnancy.

## REFERENCES

Adelsberg BR. The complement system in pregnancy. Am J Reprod Immunol 1983;4:38.

Alarcon-Segovia D, Deleze M, Oria C, et al. Antiphospholipid antibodies and the antiphospholipid syndrome in systemic lupus erythematosus. A prospective study of 500 consecutive cases. Medicine 1989;68:353.

Aoki K, Hayashi Y, Hirao Y, Yagami Y. Specific antiphospholipid antibodies as a predictive variable in patients with recurrent pregnancy loss. Am J Reprod Immunol 1993;29:82.

Appel GB, Cohen DJ, Pirani CL, et al. Long-term follow-up of patients with lupus nephritis: a study based on the classification of the World Health Organization. Am J Med 1987;83:877.

Armenti VT, Ahlswede KM, Ahlswede BA, et al. National transplantation pregnancy registry: outcomes of 154 pregnancies in cyclosporine-treated female kidney transplant recipients. Transplantation 1994;57:502.

Arnett FC, Reveill JD, Wilson RW, et al. Systemic lupus erythematosus: current state of the genetic hypothesis. Semin Arthritis Rheum 1984; 14:24.

Asherson RA. The catastrophic antiphospholipid syndrome. J Rheumatol 1992a;19:508.

Asherson RA, Cervera R. The antiphospholipid syndrome: a syndrome in evolution. Ann Rheum Dis 1992b;51:147.

Asherson RA, Khamashta MA, Ordi-Ros J, et al. The ''primary'' antiphospholipid syndrome: major clinical and serological features. Medicine 1989;68:366.

Ballegeer V, Spitz B, Kieckens L, et al. Predictive value of increased plasma levels of fibronectin in gestational hypertension. Am J Obstet Gynecol 1989;161:432.

Barbui T, Cortelazzo S, Galli M, et al. Antiphospholipid antibodies in early repeated abortions: a case-controlled study. Fertil Steril 1988;50:589.

Barclay CS, French MAH, Ross LD, Sokol RJ. Successful pregnancy following steroid therapy and plasma exchange in a woman with anti-Ro (SS-A) antibodies. Case report. Br J Obstet Gynaecol 1987;94:369.

Bear R. Pregnancy and lupus nephritis. A detailed report of six cases with a review of the literature. Obstet Gynecol 1976;47:715.

Bierman FZ, Baxi L, Jaffe I, Driscoll J. Fetal hydrops and congenital complete heart block: response to maternal steroid therapy. J Pediatr 1988;112:646.

Block SR, Winfield JB, Lockshin MD, et al. Studies of twins with systemic lupus erythematosus. A review of the literature and presentation of 12 additional sets. Am J Med 1975;59:533.

Bobrie G, Liote F, Houillier P, et al. Pregnancy in lupus nephritis and related disorders. Am J Kidney Dis 1987;9:339.

Bongiovanni AM, McPadden AJ. Steroids during pregnancy and possible fetal consequences. Fertil Steril 1960;11:181.

Bowie EJW, Thompson JH, Pascuzzi CA, Owen CA. Thrombosis in systemic lupus erythematosus despite circulating anticoagulants. J Lab Clin Med 1963;62:416.

Branch DW, Scott JR, Kochenour NK, Hershgold E. Obstetric complications associated with lupus anticoagulant. N Engl J Med 1985;313:1322.

Branch DW. Immunologic disease and fetal death. Clin Obstet Gynecol 1987;30:295.

Branch DW, Scott JR. Clinical implication of antiphospholipid antibodies: the Utah experience. In: Harris EN, Exner T, Hughes GRV, Asherson RA, eds. Phospholipid-binding antibodies. Boca Raton, FL: CRC Press, 1990a:335.

Branch DW, Andres R, Digre KB, et al. The association of antiphospholipid antibodies with severe preeclampsia. Obstet Gynecol 1990b;73:541.

Branch DW, Silver RM, Blackwell JL, et al. Outcome of treated pregnancies in women with antiphospholipid syndrome: an update of the Utah experience. Obstet Gynecol 1992;80:614.

Branch DW, Silver R, Pierangeli S, van Leeuwen I, Harris EN. Antiphospholipid antibodies other than lupus anticoagulant and anticardiolipin antibodies in women with recurrent pregnancy loss, fertile controls, and antiphospholipid syndrome. Obstet Gynecol 1997;89:549–555.

Brey RL, Hart RG, Sherman DG, Tegeler CH. Antiphospholipid antibodies and cerebral ischemia in young people. Neurology 1990;40:1190.

Brooks PM, Needs CJ. Antirheumatic drugs in pregnancy and lactation. Ballieres Clin Rheumatol 1990;4:157.

Burnet FN. The clonal selection theory of acquired immunity. London: Cambridge University Press, 1959.

Buyon JP, Cronstein BN, Morris M, et al. Serum complement values (C3 and C4) to differentiate between systemic lupus activity and preeclampsia. Am J Med 1986;81:194.

Buyon JP, Swersky SH, Fox HE, et al. Intrauterine therapy for presumptive fetal myocarditis with acquired heart block due to systemic lupus erythematosus. Arthritis Rheum 1987;30:44.

Buyon J, Roubey R, Swersky S, et al. Complete congenital heart block: risk of occurrence and therapeutic approach to prevention. J Rheumatol 1988;15:1104.

Buyon JP, Winchester RF, Slade SG, Arnett F, Copel J, Friedman D, Lockshin MD. Identification of mothers at risk for congenital heart block and other neonatal lupus syndromes in their children. Comparison of enzyme-linked immunosorbent assay and immunoblot for measurement of anti-SS-A/Ro and anti-SS-B/La antibodies. Arthritis Rheum 1993;36:1263–1273.

Buyon JP, Tamerius J, Ordorica S, et al. Activation of the alternative complement pathway accompanies disease flares in systemic lupus erythematosus during pregnancy. Arthritis Rheum 1989;35:55.

Caruso A, DeCarolis S, Ferrazzani S, et al. Pregnancy outcome in relation to uterine artery flow velocimetry waveforms and clinical characteristics in women with antiphospholipid syndrome. Obstet Gynecol 1993;82:970.

Chamley LW, Pattison NS, McKay EJ. Separation of lupus anticoagulant from anticardiolipin antibodies by ion-exchange and gel filtration chromatography. Haemostasis 1991;21:25.

Cohen AS, Reynolds WE, Franklin EC, et al. Preliminary criteria for classification of systemic lupus erythematosus. Bull Rheum Dis 1971;21:643.

Coppel JA, Buyon JP, Kleinman CS. Successful in utero therapy of fetal heart block. Am J Obstet Gynecol 1995;173:1384.

Cote CJ, Meuwissen HJ, Pickering RJ. Effects on the neonate of prednisone and azathioprine administered to the mother during pregnancy. J Pediatr 1974;85:324.

Coulam CB, McIntyre JA, Wagenknecht, Rote N. Interlaboratory inconsistencies in detection of anticardiolipin antibodies. Lancet 1990;335:865. Letter.

Cowchock FS, Reece EA, Balaban D, et al. Repeated fetal losses associated with antiphospholipid antibodies: a collaborative randomized trial comparing prednisone to low-dose heparin treatment. Am J Obstet Gynecol 1992;166:1318.

Dahlman TC. Osteoporotic fractures and the recurrence of thromboembolism during pregnancy and the puerperium in 184 women undergoing thromboprophylaxis with heparin. Am J Obstet Gynecol 1993;168:1265.

Deapen DM, Weinrib L, Langholz B, et al. A revised estimate of twin concordance in SLE: a survey of 138 pairs. Arthritis Rheum 1986;29(suppl 4):S26.

Devoe LD, Taylor RL. Systemic lupus erythematosus in pregnancy. Am J Obstet Gynecol 1979; 135:473.

Devoe LD, Loy GL, Spargo BH. Renal histology and pregnancy performance in systemic lupus erythematosus. Clin Exp Hypertens 1983;22: 325.

Devoe LD, Loy GL. Serum complement levels and perinatal outcome in pregnancies complicated by systemic lupus erythematosus. Obstet Gynecol 1984;63:796.

Dimant J, Ginzler EM, Diamond HS, et al. Computer analysis of factors influencing the appearance of aseptic necrosis in patients with systemic lupus erythematosus. J Rheumatol 1978;5:136.

Donaldson BL, Russell BA. Further observations on lupus erythematosus associated with pregnancy. Am J Obstet Gynecol 1962;83:1461.

Druzin ML, Lockshin M, Edersheim TG, et al. Second trimester fetal monitoring and preterm delivery in pregnancies with systemic lupus erythematosus and/or circulating anticoagulant. Am J Obstet Gynecol 1987;157:1503.

Englert HJ, Derue GM, Loizou S, et al. Pregnancy and lupus: prognostic indicators and response to treatment. Q J Med 1988;250:125.

Estes D, Larson DL. Systemic lupus erythematosus and pregnancy. Clin Obstet Gynecol 1965;8:307.

Exner T, Sahan N, Trudinger B. Separation of anticardiolipin antibodies from lupus anticoagulant on a phospholipid-coated polystyrene column. Biochem Biophys Res Commun 1988;155:1001.

Ferro D, Quintarelli C, Rasura M, et al. Lupus anticoagulant and the fibrinolytic system in young patients with stroke. Stroke 1993;24:368.

Fessel WJ. Systemic lupus erythematosus in the community: incidence, prevalence, outcome, and first symptoms; the high prevalence in black women. Arch Intern Med 1974;134:1027.

Fine LG, Barnett EV, Danovitch GM, et al. Systemic lupus erythematosus in pregnancy. Ann Intern Med 1981;94:667.

Fisher KA, Luger A, Spargo BH, et al. Hypertension in pregnancy: clinical-pathologic correlations and remote prognosis. Medicine 1981;60:71.

Fraga A, Mintz G, Orozco J, Orozco JH. Sterility and fertility rates, fetal wastage and maternal morbidity in systemic lupus erythematosus. J Rheumatol 1974;1:293.

Friedman EA, Rutherford JW. Pregnancy in lupus erythematosus. Obstet Gynecol 1956;8:601.

Garenstein M, Pollach VE, Kark RM. Systemic lupus erythematosus and pregnancy. N Engl J Med 1962;267:165.

Gimovsky ML, Montoro M, Paul RH. Pregnancy outcome in women with systemic lupus erythematosus. Obstet Gynecol 1984;63:686.

Ginsberg JS, Brill-Edwards P, Johnston M, et al. Relationship of antiphospholipid antibodies to pregnancy loss in patients with systemic lupus erythematosus: a cross-sectional study. Blood 1992;80:975.

Ginsburg KJ, Liane MH, Newcomer L, et al. Anticardiolipin antibodies and the risk for ischemic stroke and venous thrombosis. Ann Intern Med 1992;117:997.

Glass D, Raum D, Gibson D, et al. Inherited deficiency of the second component of complement. Rheumatic disease associations. J Clin Invest 1976;58:854.

Glueck HI, Kant KS, Weiss MA, et al. Thrombosis in systemic lupus erythematosus. Relation to the presence of circulating anticoagulant. Arch Intern Med 1985;145:1389.

Haddow JE, Rote NS, Dostal-Johnson D, et al. Lack of an association between late fetal death and antiphospholipid antibody measurements in the second trimester. Am J Obstet Gynecol 1991;165:1308.

Haeger M, Unander M, Bengtsson A. Enhanced anaphylatoxin and terminal C5b-9 complement complex formation in patients with the syndrome of hemolysis, elevated liver enzymes, and low platelet count. Obstet Gynecol 1990;76:698.

Haeger M, Bengtsson A, Karlsson K, Heideman M. Complement activation and anaphylatoxin (C3a and C5a) formation in preeclampsia and by amniotic fluid. Obstet Gynecol 1989;73:551.

Hargraves MM, Richmond H, Morton R. Presentation of two bone marrow elements: The "tart" cell and "L.E." cell. Proc Staff Meet Mayo Clin 1948;23:25.

Harris EN, Gharavi AE, Boey ML, et al. Anticardiolipin antibodies: detection by radioimmunoassay and association with thrombosis in systemic lupus erythematosus. Lancet 1983;ii:1211.

Harris EN. Syndrome of the black swan. Br J Rheumatol 1986;26:324.

Harris EN. The second international anti-cardiolipin standardization workshop/The Kingston antiphospholipid antibody study (KAPS) group. Am J Clin Pathol 1990;94:476.

Harris EN, Spinnato JA. Should anticardiolipin tests be performed in otherwise healthy pregnant women? Am J Obstet Gynecol 1991;165:1272.

Hart C, Naughton RF. The ototoxicity of chloroquine phosphate. Arch Otolaryngol 1964;80:407.

Hart RG, Miller VT, Coull BM, et al. Cerebral infarctions associated with lupus anticoagulant. Stroke 1987;18:257.

Hartung K, Fontana A, Klar M, et al. Association of class I, II, and III MHC gene products with systemic lupus erythematosus. Results of a Central European multicenter study. Rheumatol Int 1989;13:18.

Hayslett JP, Lynn RI. Effect of pregnancy in patients with lupus nephropathy. Kidney Int 1980;18:207.

Hickok DE, Hollenbach KA, Reilley SF, et al. The association between decreased amniotic fluid volume and treatment with non-steroidal antiinflammatory agents for preterm labor. Am J Obstet Gynecol 1989;160:1525.

Hochfeld M, Druzin ML, Maia D, et al. Pregnancy complicated by primary antiphospholipid antibody syndrome. Obstet Gynecol 1994;83:804.

Hofmeyer GJ, Wilkins T, Redman CWG. C4 and plasma protein in hypertension during pregnancy with and without proteinuria. Br Med J 1991;302:218.

Hopkins P, Belmont HM, Buyon J, et al. Increased levels of plasma anaphylatoxins in systemic lupus erythematosus predict flares of the disease and may elicit vascular injury in lupus cerebritis. Arthritis Rheum 1984;7:163.

Houser MT, Fish AJ, Tagatz GE, et al. Pregnancy and systemic lupus erythematosus. Am J Obstet Gynecol 1980;138:409.

Howard PF, Hochberg MC, Bias WB, et al. Relationship between C4 null genes, HLA-D region antigens, and genetic susceptibility to SLE in Caucasian and black Americans. Am J Med 1986;81:187.

Hsu C-D, Copel J, Hong S-F, Chan DW. Thrombomodulin levels in preeclampsia, gestational hypertension, and chronic hypertension. Obstet Gynecol 1995;86:897.

Hull D, Binns BAO, Joyce D. Congenital heart block and widespread fibrosis due to maternal lupus erythematosus. Arch Dis Child 1966;41:688.

Imbasciati E, Surian M, Bottino W, et al. Lupus nephropathy and pregnancy. Nephron 1984;36:46.

Imperiale TF, Petrulis AS. A meta-analysis of low-dose aspirin for the prevention of pregnancy-induced hypertensive disease. JAMA 1991;266:260.

Infante-Rivard C, David M, Gauthier R, Rivard G-E. Lupus anticoagulants, anticardiolipin antibodies, and fetal loss. A case control study. N Engl J Med 1991;325:1063.

Isenberg DA, Morrow WJW, Snaith ML. Methylprednisolone pulse therapy in the treatment of systemic lupus erythematosus. Ann Rheum Dis 1982;41:347.

Johnson MJ, Petri M, Witter FR, Repke JT. Evaluation of preterm delivery in a systemic lupus erythematosus pregnancy clinic. Obstet Gynecol 1995;86:396–399.

Julkunen H, Kaaja R, Palosuo T, et al. Pregnancy in lupus nephropathy. Acta Obstet Gynecol Scand 1993a;72:258.

Julkunen H, Jouhikainen T, Kaaja R, et al. Fetal outcome in lupus pregnancy: a retrospective case-control study of 242 pregnancies in 112 patients. Lupus 1993b;2:125.

Julkunen H, Kurki P, Kaaja R, et al. Isolated congenital heart block. Long-term outcome in mothers and characterization of the immune response to SS-A/Ro and SS-B/La. Arthritis Rheum 1993c;36:1588.

Jungers P, Dougados M, Pelissier C, et al. Lupus nephropathy and pregnancy. Arch Intern Med 1982;142:771.

Kaaja R, Julkunen H, Ammala P, et al. Congenital heart block: successful prophylactic treatment with intravenous gamma globulin and corticosteroid therapy. Am J Obstet Gynecol 1991;165:1333.

Kaaja R, Julkunen H, Ammala P, et al. Intravenous immunoglobulin treatment of pregnant patients with recurrent pregnancy losses associated with antiphospholipid antibodies. Acta Obstet Gynecol Scand 1993;72:63–66.

Katz AI, Davison JM, Hayslett JP, et al. Pregnancy in women with kidney disease. Kidney Int 1980;18:192.

Katz VL, Thorp JM, Watson WJ, et al. Human immunoglobulin therapy for preeclampsia associated with lupus anticoagulant and anticardiolipin antibody. Obstet Gynecol 1990;76:986.

Kniaz D, Eisenberg GM, Elard H, et al. Postpartum hemolytic uremic syndrome associated with antiphospholipid antibodies. Am J Nephrol 1992;12:126.

Kochenour NK, Branch DW, Rote NS, et al. A new postpartum syndrome associated with antiphospholipid antibodies. Obstet Gynecol 1987;69:460.

Koffler D, Agnello V, Thoburn R, Kunkel HG. Systemic lupus erythematosus: prototype of immune complex nephritis in man. J Exp Med 1971;134:109.

Kupferminc MJ, Lee M-J, Green D, Peaceman AM. Severe postpartum pulmonary, cardiac, and renal syndrome associated with antiphospholipid antibodies. Obstet Gynecol 1994;83:806.

Kutteh WH. Antiphospholipid antibody-associated recurrent pregnancy loss: treatment with heparin and low-dose aspirin is superior to low-dose aspirin alone. Am J Obstet Gynecol 1996;174:1584–1589.

Kwak JY, Gilman-Sacks A, Beaman KD, Beer AE. Autoantibodies in women with primary recurrent spontaneous abortion of unknown etiology. Am J Reprod Immunol 1992;22:15.

Lahita RG, Bradlow HL, Kunkel HG, Fishman J. Alterations of estrogen metabolism in systemic lupus erythematosus. Arthritis Rheum 1979;22:1195.

Lahita RG, Bradlow HL, Fishman J, Kunkel HG. Abnormal estrogen and androgen metabolism in the human with systemic lupus erythematosus. Am J Kidney Dis 1982;1:206.

Lawrence JS, Martins L, Drake G. A family survey of lupus erythematosus: I. Heritability. J Rheumatol 1987;14:913.

Le Thi Huong D, Wechsler B, Piette J-C, et al. Pregnancy and its outcome in systemic lupus erythematosus. Q J Med 1994;87:721.

Lechner K, Pabinger-Fasching I. Lupus anticoagulants and thrombosis. A study of 25 cases and review of the literature. Haemostasis 1985;15:254.

Lee LA, Gaither KK, Coulter SN, et al. Pattern of cutaneous immunoglobulin G deposition in subacute cutaneous lupus erythematosus is reproduced by infusing purified anti-Ro (SSA) autoantibodies into human skin-grafted mice. J Clin Invest 1989;83:1556.

Lee LA, Weston WL. Neonatal lupus erythematosus. Semin Dermatol 1988;7:66.

Lev M, Silverman J, Fitzmaurice FM, et al. Lack of connection between the atria and the more peripheral conduction system in congenital atrioventricular block. Am J Cardiol 1971;27:481.

Levitz M, Jansen V, Dancis J. The transfer and metabolism of corticosteroids in the perfused human placenta. Am J Obstet Gynecol 1978;132:363.

Lima F, Khamashta MA, Buchanan NM, Kerslake S, Hunt BJ, Hughes GR. A study of sixty pregnancies in patients with the antiphospholipid syndrome. Clin Exp Rheumatol 1996;14:131–136.

Lockshin MD, Reinits E, Druzin ML, et al. Case-control prospective study demonstrating absence of lupus exacerbation during or after pregnancy. Am J Med 1984;77:893.

Lockshin MC, Harpel PC, Druzin ML, et al. Lupus pregnancy II. Unusual pattern of hypocomplementemia and thrombocytopenia in the pregnant patient. Arthritis Rheum 1985a;28:58.

Lockshin MD, Druzin ML, Goei S, et al. Antibody to cardiolipin as a predictor of fetal distress or death in pregnant patients with systemic erythematosus. N Engl J Med 1985b;313:152.

Lockshin MD, Qamar T, Redecha P, et al. Hypocomplementemia with low C1s-C1 inhibitor complex in systemic lupus erythematosus. Arthritis Rheum 1986;29:1467.

Lockshin MD, Qamar T, Druzin ML. Hazards of lupus pregnancy. J Rheumatol 1987;14:214.

Lockshin MD, Bonfa E, Elkon D, Druzin ML. Neonatal lupus risk to newborns of mothers with systemic lupus erythematosus. Arthritis Rheum 1988;31:697.

Lockshin MD. Pregnancy does not cause systemic lupus erythematosus to worsen. Arthritis Rheum 1989a;32:665.

Lockshin MD, Druzin ML, Qamar T. Prednisone does not prevent recurrent pregnancy fetal death in women with antiphospholipid antibody. Am J Obstet Gynecol 1989b;160:439.

Lockwood CJ, Peters JH. Increased plasma levels of $ED1^+$ cellular fibronectin precede the clinical signs of preeclampsia. Am J Obstet Gynecol 1990;162:358.

Lockwood CJ, Romero R, Feinberg RF, et al. The prevalence and biologic significance of lupus anticoagulant and anticardiolipin antibodies in a general obstetric population. Am J Obstet Gynecol 1989;161:369.

Lubbe WF, Butler WS, Palmer SJ, Liggins GC. Fetal survival after prednisone suppression of maternal lupus-anticoagulant. Lancet 1983;i:1361.

Mackworth-Young CG, Parke AL, Morley KD, et al. Sex hormones in male patients with systemic lupus erythematosus: a comparison with other disease groups. Eur J Rheumatol Inflamm 1983;6:228.

MacLean MA, Cumming GP, McCall F, et al. The prevalence of lupus anticoagulant and anticardiolipin antibodies in women with a history of first trimester miscarriages. Br J Obstet Gynaecol 1994;101:103.

McGee CD, Makowski EL. Systemic lupus erythematosus in pregnancy. Am J Obstet Gynecol 1970;107:1008.

McHugh NJ, Reilly PA, McHugh LA. Pregnancy outcome and autoantibodies in connective tissue disease. J Rheumatol 1989;16:42.

Meehan RT, Dorsey JK. Pregnancy among patients with systemic lupus erythematosus receiving immunosuppressive therapy. J Rheumatol 1987;14:252.

Michet CJ, McKenna CH, Elveback LR, et al. Epidemiology of systemic lupus erythematosus and other connective tissue disease in Rochester, Minnesota, 1950 through 1979. Mayo Clin Proc 1985;60:105.

Milliez J, Lelong F, Bayani N, et al. The prevalence of autoantibodies during third-trimester pregnancy complicated by hypertension or idiopathic fetal growth retardation. Am J Obstet Gynecol 1991;165:51.

Mintz R, Niz J, Gutierrez G, et al. Prospective study of pregnancy in systemic lupus erythematosus. Results of a multidisciplinary approach. J Rheumatol 1986;13:732.

Moise KJ, Huhta JC, Sharif DS, et al. Indomethacin in the treatment of premature labor: effects of the fetal ductus arteriosus. N Engl J Med 1988; 319:327.

Mor Yosef S, Navot D, Rabinowitz R, Schenker JG. Collagen diseases in pregnancy. Obstet Gynecol Surv 1984;39:67.

Mulinsky A, Graef JW, Gaynor MF. Methotrexate induced congenital malformations. J Pediatr 1968;72:790.

Murray FA. Lupus erythematosus in pregnancy. J Obstet Gynaecol Br Emp 1958;65:401.

Nicklin JL. Systemic lupus erythematosus and pregnancy at the Royal Women's Hospital, Brisbane 1979–1989. Aust N Z Obstet Gynaecol 1991; 31:128.

Norton ME, Merrill J, Cooper BAB, et al. Neonatal complications after the administration of indomethacin for preterm labor. N Engl J Med 1993;329:1602.

Nossent HC, Swaak TJG. Systemic lupus erythematosus. VI. Analysis of the interrelationship with pregnancy. J Rheumatol 1990;177:771.

Nylander U. Ocular damage in chloroquine therapy. Acta Ophthalmol (Copenh) 1967;45(suppl 92):5.

Oshiro BT, Silver RM, Scott JR, Yu H, Branch DW. Antiphospholipid antibodies and fetal death. Obstet Gynecol 1996;87:489–493.

Out HJ, Bruinse HW, Christiaens GCML, et al. Prevalence of antiphospholipid antibodies in patients with fetal loss. Ann Rheum Dis 1991; 50:553.

Out HJ, Bruinse HW, Christiaens GCML, et al. A prospective, controlled multicenter study on the obstetric risks of pregnant women with antiphospholipid antibodies. Am J Obstet Gynecol 1992;167:26.

Parazzini F, Acaia B, Faden D, et al. Antiphospholipid antibodies and recurrent abortion. Obstet Gynecol 1991;77:854.

Parke A. Antimalarial drugs and pregnancy. Am J Med 1988;85:30.

Parke AL, Wilson D, Maier D. The prevalence of antiphospholipid antibodies in women with recurrent spontaneous abortion, women with successful pregnancies, and women who have never been pregnant. Arthritis Rheum 1991; 34:1231.

Pattison NS, Chamley LW, McKay EJ. Prevalence of antiphospholipid antibodies in a normal pregnant population. Clin Exp Rheumatol 6:210. 1988. Abstract.

Peaceman AM, Silver RK, MacGreger SN, Socol ML. Interlaboratory variation in antiphospholipid antibody testing. Am J Obstet Gynecol 1992; 166:1789.

Petri M, Howard D, Repke J. Frequency of lupus flare in pregnancy; the Hopkins lupus pregnancy center experience. Arthritis Rheum 1991;34:1538.

Petri M, Allbritton J. Fetal outcome of lupus pregnancy: a retrospective case-control study of the Hopkins Lupus Cohort. J Rheumatol 1993; 20:650.

Petri M, Golbus M, Anderson R, et al. Antinuclear antibody, lupus anticoagulant, and anticardiolipin antibody in women with idiopathic habitual abortion: a controlled prospective study of 44 women. Arthritis Rheum 1987;30:601.

Polzin WJ, Kopelman JN, Robinson RD, et al. The association of antiphospholipid antibodies with pregnancy complicated by fetal growth restriction. Obstet Gynecol 1991;78:1108.

Ramsey-Goldman R, Kutzer JE, Kuller LH, et al. Pregnancy outcome and anti-cardiolipin antibody in women with systemic lupus erythematosus. Am J Epidemiol 1993;138:1057.

Reichlin M. Antinuclear antibodies. In: Kelly WN, Harris ED, Ruddy S, Sledge CB, eds. Textbook of rheumatology. 3rd ed. Philadelphia, WB Saunders, 1989:208.

Richards DS, Wagman AJ, Cabaniss ML. Ascites not due to congestive heart failure in a fetus with lupus-induced heart block. Obstet Gynecol 1990;76:957.

Rider LG, Buyon JP, Rutledge J, Sherry DD. Treatment of neonatal lupus: case report and review of the literature. J Rheumatol 1993;20:1208.

Rolbin SH, Levinson G, Shnider SM, et al. Anesthetic considerations for myasthenia gravis and pregnancy. Anesth Analg 1978;57:441.

Rosove MH, Tabsh K, Wasserstrum N, et al. Heparin therapy for pregnant women with lupus anticoagulant or anticardiolipin antibodies. Obstet Gynecol 1990;75:630.

Roubinian JR, Papoian R, Talal N. Androgenic hormones moderate autoantibody responses and improve survival in murine lupus. J Clin Invest 1977;59:1066.

Roubinian JR, Talai N, Greenspan JS, et al. Effect of castration and sex hormone treatment on survival, anti-nucleic acid antibodies, and glomerulonephritis in NZB/NZW mice. J Exp Med 1978;147:1568.

Roubinian JR, Talal N, Siiteri PK, Sadakiam JA. Sex hormone modulation of autoimmunity in NZB/NZW mice. Arthritis Rheum 1979;22:1162.

Rumack CM, Guggenheim MA, Rumack BH. Neonatal intracranial haemorrhage and maternal use of aspirin. Obstet Gynecol 1981;52(suppl):525.

Schur PH, Sandson J. Immunological factors and clinical activity in systemic lupus erythematosus. N Engl J Med 1968;278:533.

Schur PH. Clinical features of SLE. In: Kelly WN, Harris ED, Ruddy S, Sledge CB, eds. Textbook of rheumatology. 4th ed. Philadelphia: WB Saunders, 1993:1017.

Scott JR. Fetal growth retardation associated with maternal administration of immuno-suppressive drugs. Am J Obstet Gynecol 1977;128:668.

Scott RAH. Anti-cardiolipin antibodies and pre-eclampsia. Br J Obstet Gynaecol 1987;94:604.

Scott JR, Branch DW, Kochenour NK, Ward K. Intravenous globulin treatment of pregnant patients with recurrent pregnancy loss due to antiphospholipid antibodies and Rh disease. Am J Obstet Gynecol 1988;159:1055.

Seigel M, Lee SL. The epidemiology of systemic lupus erythematosus. Semin Arthritis Rheum 1973;3:1.

Silver RM, Draper ML, Scott JR, et al. Clinical consequences of antiphospholipid antibodies: an historic cohort study. Obstet Gynecol 1994;83:372.

Silver RM, Porter TR, van Leeuween I, Jeng G, Scott JR, Branch DW. Anticardiolipin antibodies: clinical consequences of "low titers." Obstet Gynecol 1996;87:494–500.

Spinnato JA, Clark AL, Pierangeli SS, Harris EN. Intravenous immunoglobulin therapy for the antiphospholipid syndrome in pregnancy. Am J Obstet Gynecol 1995;172:690.

Steinberg AD, Melez KA, Raveche ES, et al. Approach to the study of the role of sex hormones in autoimmunity. Arthritis Rheum 1979;22:1170.

Stern R, Fishman J, Brusman H, Kunkel HG. Systemic lupus erythematosus associated with Klinefelter's syndrome. Arthritis Rheum 1977;20:18.

Stuart JJ, Gross SJ, Elrad H, et al. Effects of acetylsalicylic acid ingestion on maternal and neonatal hemostasis. N Engl J Med 1982;307:909.

Surian M, Imbasciati E, Cosci P, et al. Glomerular disease and pregnancy. A study of 123 pregnancies in patients with primary and secondary glomerular diseases. Nephron 1984;36:101.

Tan EM, Cohen AS, Fries JF, et al. The 1982 revised criteria for the classification of systemic lupus erythematosus. Arthritis Rheum 1982;25:1271.

Taufield PA, Ales KL, Resnick LM, et al. Hypocalciuria in preeclampsia. N Engl J Med 1987;316:715.

Taylor PV, Scott JS, Gerlis LM, et al. Maternal antibodies against fetal cardiac antigens in congenital complete heart block. N Engl J Med 1986;315:667.

Tedder RS, Nelson M, Eisen V. Effects of serum complement of normal and preeclamptic pregnancy and of oral contraceptives. Br J Exp Pathol 1975;56:389.

Thiersch JB. Early experiences with antimetabolites as abortifacient agents in man. Acta Endocrinol 1956;28:37.

Tozman E, Vrowitz MB, Gladman DD. Systemic lupus erythematosus and pregnancy. J Rheumatol 1980;7:624.

Ujhazy E, Balonova T, Durisova M, et al. Teratogenicity of cyclophosphamide in New Zealand white rabbits. Neoplasma 1993;40:45.

Urowitz MB, Gladman DD, Farewell VT, et al. Lupus and pregnancy studies. Arthritis Rheum 1993; 36:1392.

Vanhaesebrouck P, Thiery M, Leroy JG, et al. Oligohydramnios, renal insufficiency, and ileal perforation in preterm infants after intrauterine exposure to indomethacin. J Pediatr 1988; 113:738.

Varner MW, Meehan RT, Syrop CH, et al. Pregnancy in patients with systemic lupus erythematosus. Am J Obstet Gynecol 1983;145:1025.

Waltuck J, Buyon JP. Autoantibody-associated congenital heart block: outcome in mothers and children. Ann Intern Med 1994;120:544.

Wapner RJ, Cowchock S, Shapiro SS. Successful treatment in two women with antiphospholipid antibodies and refractory pregnancy losses with intravenous immunoglobulin infusions. Am J Obstet Gynecol 1990;162:1271.

Warkentin TE, Levine MN, Hirsh J, et al. Heparin-induced thrombocytopenia in patients treated with low-molecular-weight heparin or unfractionated heparin. N Engl J Med 1995;332:1330.

Weiner CP, Kwaan HC, Xu C, et al. Antithrombin III activity in women with hypertension during pregnancy. Obstet Gynecol 1985;65:301.

Welsh TR, Beischel LS, Balakrishnan K, et al. Major histocompatibility complex extended haplotypes in systemic lupus erythematosus. Dis Markers 1988;247:255.

Wong KL, Chan FY, Lee CP. Outcome of pregnancy in patients with systemic lupus erythematosus. Arch Intern Med 1991;151:269.

Yasuda M, Takakuwa K, Tokunaga A, Tanaka K. Prospective studies of the association between anticardiolipin antibody and outcome of pregnancy. Obstet Gynecol 1995;86:555.

Yu A, Wong VC, Lee AK, et al. Systemic lupus erythematosus in pregnancy in Hong Kong Chinese. Asia Oceania J Obstet Gynaecol 1986;12:321.

Zulman JI, Talal N, Hoffman GS, Epstein WV. Problems associated with the management of pregnancies in patients with systemic lupus erythematosus. J Rheumatol 1979;7:37.

Zurier RB, Argyros TG, Urman JD, et al. System lupus erythematosus. Obstet Gynecol 1978; 51:178.

# CHAPTER 27

# Thrombotic Microangiopathies

The term *thrombotic microangiopathies* defines a fairly uncommon and severe group of syndromes that are associated with multiple etiologies and are distinguished by multiorgan microvascular thromboses. These syndromes can have numerous clinical features, depending on the particular organ system affected. Because of the difficulty in differentiating between some of these disorders, the inclusive term *thrombotic microangiopathy* was first described by Symmers (1952). Terminology in this area is often confusing, as is the relationship of pregnancy to conditions, such as hemolytic-uremic syndrome (HUS), more commonly seen in nonpregnant individuals. This group of conditions is perhaps best conceptualized by considering the terms *hemolytic-uremic syndrome* and *thrombotic thrombocytopenic purpura* (TTP) to refer to different points in the clinical spectrum of a single disorder, thrombotic microangiopathy, which may be initiated by a number of seemingly different antecedent events, including infection, autoimmune disease, and pregnancy. This spectrum also may include the HELLP (hemolysis, elevated liver enzymes, and low platelets) syndrome variant of severe preeclampsia, or, as with other disorders involving renal compromise or abnormal thrombotic tendencies, predispose to this condition.

Various forms of thrombotic microangiopathy can be associated with pregnancy. Some of these are pregnancy-specific, such as preeclamp-sia or its variants (the syndrome of HELLP). Others are uncommon in the nonpregnant adult woman but are noted to occur with greater frequency during gestation, such as TTP and HUS. A few thrombotic microangiopathies are considered only rarely in pregnancy and have distinguishable clinical or laboratory features that may facilitate diagnosis (Evans' syndrome, acute allograft rejection, or thrombotic microangiopathy associated with autoimmune disease) (Martin, 1991).

Except for the spectrum of severe pre-eclampsia-eclampsia, few obstetricians or their consultants have much experience with these pregnancy-associated syndromes, and, thus, the management of affected patients can be a bewildering exercise. Consequently, the aim of this chapter is to describe the differential diagnosis of pregnancy-associated thrombotic microangiopathies, elaborate on the pathophysiologic mechanisms that may underlie the more common forms seen during pregnancy (TTP-HUS), and develop a rational approach to management of the pregnant patient with a thrombotic microangiopathy, focusing in particular on TTP-HUS.

## Historic Considerations

The first case of TTP was described by Moschcowitz (1925), who noted a previously undescribed symptom complex of hemolytic anemia, hemorrhage, neurologic abnormalities, and renal failure, resulting in the death of a 16-year-old girl. Although thrombocytopenia was never documented, autopsy findings were consistent with widespread microvascular thrombosis, which Moschcowitz attributed to a powerful toxin with hemolytic and agglutinative properties. Numerous case reports followed until the 1950s, when the clinical and pathologic features of the disease were established (Barondess, 1952; Gore, 1950).

A similar constellation of signs and symptoms, including hemolytic anemia and thrombocytopenia but associated primarily with acute renal failure, was first described by Gasser and associates (1955). The disturbance was believed to be a distinct entity confined to the kidney and, thus, named "the hemolytic-uremic syndrome." Further investigation has not confirmed Gasser's suspicions (Amorosi, 1966; Eknoyan, 1986), because both TTP and HUS have been associated with multiorgan involvement, including cerebral disturbances (originally thought to be specific to TTP) and acute renal failure. The prevailing opinion is that these disorders represent a spectrum of disease with the common pathologic feature of thrombotic microangiopathy (Byrnes, 1986).

An explosion of various therapies designed to alleviate the devastating effects of these syndromes has occurred during the past 20 years. The list includes corticosteroids, immunosuppressive agents, antiplatelet drugs, plasma exchange (PEX), plasma infusion (PI), and whole blood exchange transfusion. Utilization of a combination of these various modalities has contributed to a dramatic improvement in survival and much speculation concerning the etiology of these disorders (Moake, 1991; Ruggenenti, 1990; Egerman, 1996).

## Thrombotic Thrombocytopenic Purpura–Hemolytic-Uremic Syndrome

### Disease Profile

Thrombotic thrombocytopenic purpura–hemolytic-uremic syndrome is more common in females (10:1, female-male ratio), with no racial predilection. It usually appears in the third decade of life

although certain forms of the syndrome can appear from infancy through the geriatric period. Because TTP-HUS is rare, the true incidence of the disease is difficult to determine. One report from a major teaching institution noted an average of six cases per 50,000 yearly admissions (Bell, 1991).

There is no seasonal variation in the incidence of this syndrome. Although it can occur at any time during pregnancy, the disease is probably most common in the peripartum period (late third trimester, early puerperium) (Bell, 1991a; Egerman, 1996).

## Associated Agents or Conditions

In a significant number of patients with TTP-HUS, it is likely that infectious agents or certain pharmaceuticals may trigger the development of the syndrome. A prodromal illness similar to a viral infection occurs in 40% of patients. Associated agents include coxsackie A and B, mycoplasma pneumonia, or recent vaccinations (Neumann, 1994). A significant relationship between bacterial endotoxins and HUS has been described in numerous reports and will be discussed in detail in the section dealing with pathogenesis (Moake, 1994). A TTP-HUS-like syndrome has been noted in certain patients infected with the human immunodeficiency virus (Ucar, 1994).

There is also a strong association between TTP-HUS and oral contraceptives and antineoplastic and immunosuppressive agents. Triggering chemotherapeutic agents include mitomycin C, bleomycin, mithramycin, cytosine arabinoside, and daunorubicin, while the immunosuppressants cyclosporin A and FK-506 have been associated with a TTP-HUS-like arteriolopathy leading to renal allograft loss. Certain neoplastic conditions also can coexist with the syndrome, including non-Hodgkin's lymphoma, certain forms of leukemia, and particular adenocarcinomas (Kwaan, 1987; Holman, 1993).

There may be familial forms of TTP-HUS. One report described five families with multiple members who contracted TTP, including two sisters who developed the condition during and immediately after pregnancy (Wiznitzer, 1992). Others have noted that the condition may be inherited in an autosomal recessive pattern. In these patients, TTP-HUS is associated with a high mortality rate (70%) and a significant risk of recurrence (Berns, 1992). At present there is no identifiable genetic marker available for TTP-HUS.

There appears to be a significant relationship between the microangiopathic syndromes and underlying connective tissue disease. Thrombotic thrombocytopenic purpura–hemolytic-uremic syndrome has been described in patients with systemic lupus erythematosus (SLE), Sjögren's syndrome, rheumatoid arthritis, and polyarteritis. The most frequent association appears to be between SLE and TTP-HUS, although the incidence varies widely. The postulated mechanism in this situation involves immune-mediated vasculopathy, immune complex deposition, or both (Byrnes, 1986; Stricker, 1992; Meyrier, 1991).

Finally, there is a strong association between TTP-HUS and pregnancy, with most cases occurring in the latter part of gestation and/or the puerperium. The etiologic basis between the two conditions is speculative at present but could include an immune mechanism, vascular endothelial damage, or prostanoid imbalance (Pinette, 1989).

## Clinical Features

Neurologic symptoms often predominate in TTP and may include headache, aphasia, altered consciousness (stupor, confusion, coma), parasthesia, paresis, syncope, cranial nerve palsies, seizures, or stroke (Egerman, 1996). Characteristically, the neurologic symptoms are transient and fluctuating, probably secondary to microvascular platelet aggregation and occlusion of the cerebral arterioles. Patients with HUS can present with neurologic manifestations, but renal involvement is more dramatic, with the majority of patients requiring dialysis, which may help to distinguish between the two syndromes. Other findings elicited during the history and physical examination are listed in Table 27-1. Although fever is not often a notable clinical symptom, it is commonly found on physical examination, as are pallor and hemorrhage.

Thrombotic thrombocytopenic purpura–hemolytic-uremic syndrome is a diagnosis of exclusion. Although there is no single laboratory test that can be used to reliably differentiate it from other disorders, there is a certain group of laboratory findings that should guide the clinician

T A B L E   **27-1**

The spectrum of clinical features in adult thrombotic thrombocytopenic purpura–hemolytic-uremic syndrome

| Presenting Symptoms | Frequency | Presenting Signs |
|---|---|---|
| Neurologic (60%) (often intermittent)<br>  Confusion<br>  Mental status changes<br>  Dizziness<br>  Headache<br>  Focal/central losses | Very common | Fever (98%) |
| | | Hemorrhage (96%)<br>  Petechiae ecchymoses |
| Bleeding (44%) | | Neurologic (92%)<br>  Tremor<br>  Hemiparesis |
| Gastrointestinal (30%)<br>  Abdominal pain (11%)<br>  Nausea/vomiting (24%)<br>  Diarrhea | | Seizures<br>  Coma<br>Pallor (96%)<br>Jaundice (42%) |
| Nonspecific<br>  Fatigue (25%)<br>  Viral prodrome (40%)<br>  Arthralgia (7%) | Least common | Abdominal tenderness (13%) |

Source: Adapted from Bell W. Thrombotic thrombocytopenic purpura. JAMA 1991a;265:91.

to consider the diagnosis (Table 27-2). The test that provides the most immediate clue to TTP-HUS is examination of the peripheral blood smear. Evidence of a fulminant hemolytic process (microangiopathic hemolytic anemia [MHA]), including red-cell fragmentation (burr cells, helmet cells, and schistocytes) and severe thrombocytopenia (platelet count < 50,000), strongly suggests TTP-HUS. Intravascular hemolysis is reflected by a high serum lactic dehydrogenase (LDH), elevated indirect bilirubin, reduced haptoglobin, hemoglobinemia, and occasionally hemoglobinuria. Direct Coombs' testing should be negative.

Both TTP and HUS are commonly associated with renal dysfunction, including proteinuria, hematuria, and azotemia. Histologic confirmation by bone marrow core biopsy (megakaryocytic hyperplasia) or skin biopsy of a petechial spot can sometimes substantiate the diagnosis in confus-

ing cases. The classic clinical pentad associated with TTP-HUS thus consists of fever, thrombocytopenia, MHA, neurologic abnormalities, and renal disease (Amorosi, 1966; Ridolfi, 1981; Bartholomew, 1986).

## Differential Diagnosis

Given the wide range of clinical symptomatology and laboratory findings observed in patients with a thrombotic microangiopathy, the differential diagnosis for TTP-HUS is considerable (Table 27-3). For the obstetrician encountering a pregnant patient with a thrombotic microangiopathy syndrome, the most important disease process in the differential diagnosis to rule out is any form of severe preeclampsia. When adult TTP-HUS is present during the first trimester of pregnancy, the diagnosis is relatively easy to make, and some successful pregnancies after therapy have been reported. Later in gestation, the differential diagnostic problem is more difficult because of striking similarities between the HELLP syndrome and adult TTP-HUS (Thorp, 1991; Vandekerchove, 1984). Both diseases can present with thrombocytopenia and MHA, as well as neurologic and renal dysfunction. Parturients with severe preeclampsia-eclampsia often will manifest

**T A B L E 27-2**

### Laboratory features of TTP

Microangiopathic hemolytic anemia (100%)
  Anemia: often severe (96%)
  Reticulocytosis
  Red-cell fragmentation (100%)
  Nucleated red cells, spherocytes, myelocytes, schistocytes, helmet cells
  High LDH
  Negative direct Coombs' test
  Indirect hyperbilirubinemia (60%)
  Hemoglobinemia (occasional)
  Leukocytosis
  Absent serum haptoglobin
Thrombocytopenia: usually severe (100%)
Azotemia: usually mild to moderate (88%)
Normal coagulation parameters: PT, PTT, fibrinogen, AT III, fibronectin
Abnormal urinary sediment
  Microscopic hematuria
  Proteinuria
  Hemoglobinuria
Bone marrow aspirate: marked megakaryocytic hyperplasia
Gingival/skin biopsy of petechial spot: platelet microthrombi

PT, prothrombin time; PTT, partial thromboplastin time; TT, thrombin time; AT III, antithrombin III.

Source: Adapted from Bell W. Thrombotic thrombocytopenic purpura. JAMA 1991a;265:91.

**T A B L E 27-3**

### Differential diagnoses of adult thrombotic thrombocytopenic purpura–hemolytic-uremic syndrome

Disseminated intravascular coagulopathy
Evans' syndrome (immune-mediated thrombocytopenic purpura + immune-mediated hemolytic anemia)
Vasculitis
  Systemic lupus erythematosus
  Severe glomerulonephritis
Other causes of MHA
  Vascular malformation
  Prosthetic valves
  Metastatic adenocarcinoma
  Malignant hypertension
Adult TTP-HUS-like syndromes
  Acute fatty liver of pregnancy
  Postpartum acute renal failure
  Severe preeclampsia-eclampsia-HELLP

elevation of liver function tests (AST/ALT), and may have hypofibrinogenemia and a depressed antithrombin III (AT III) level (Ceiner, 1987). These findings are infrequent in patients with TTP-HUS, who are also more often febrile and do not initially manifest the acute BP elevations commonly seen in preeclampsia-eclampsia.

It is important to differentiate between the two syndromes, because patients with HELLP/ severe preeclampsia or eclampsia will usually respond dramatically to delivery, while patients with TTP-HUS require other therapy. Because preeclampsia-eclampsia is the more common condition, it should generally be assumed to be present if clinical and pathologic data are not helpful in differentiating these disorders. Generally, it is not in the best interest of the mother or fetus to prolong a gestation beyond 34 weeks in patients with MHA, thrombocytopenia, or elevated liver enzyme levels on the premise that the disease may not actually be severe preeclampsia. If the disease is considered initially to represent severe preeclampsia-eclampsia, yet delivery does not ameliorate the disease process within 48 to 72 hours or AT III activity is not depressed, the patient can be considered to have the less likely diagnosis of adult TTP-HUS and alternate therapy can be undertaken (Martin, 1991).

It is not unusual for TTP-HUS and preeclampsia to be present concomitantly, making it impossible to distinguish between syndromes and forcing the clinician to direct therapy to alleviate both disorders (Ceiner, 1987). A complete listing of the findings common to these disorders and their frequencies is found in Table 27-4. Table 27-5 lists other associated diseases that also may be considered, such as acute fatty liver of pregnancy or autoimmune thrombocytopenic purpura, and their associated differential features (Pinette, 1989).

Disseminated intravascular coagulation (DIC) is not commonly seen in microangiopathic disorders. It is a thrombin-driven disorder characterized by an increased turnover of both platelets and fibrinogen, which is accompanied by a secondary fibrinolytic response. In contrast, the thrombotic microangiopathy disorders are platelet-driven processes in which there is increased platelet consumption, normal fibrinogen turnover, absent local fibrinolysis, and no coagulopathy, although fibrin split products (FSPs) may be increased in some patients with adult HUS (secondary to platelet-fibrinogen degradation).

Evans' syndrome describes the coexistence of immune-mediated idiopathic thrombocytopenic purpura (ITP) and hemolytic anemia and could be confused with adult TTP. In the immune-mediated disorders, platelet or red-cell antibodies should be present and red-cell fragmentation should be absent. As stated before, in TTP, the

TABLE  **27-4**

Distinguishing thrombotic thrombocytopenic purpura–hemolytic-uremic syndrome from preeclampsia

| Feature | TTP-HUS | Preeclampsia |
|---|---|---|
| Microangiopathic hemolytic anemia | Frequent | Only with HELLP |
| Thrombocytopenia | Frequent | Occasional/HELLP |
| Neurologic dysfunction | Frequent/variable | Occasional |
| Fever | Variable | Absent |
| Renal dysfunction | Variable/frequent | Frequent |
| Hypertension | Variable/frequent | Frequent |
| Purpuric skin lesions | Variable | Rare |
| Low fibrinogen | Rare | Variable |
| Elevated FSPs | Infrequent | Variable |
| Antithrombin III | Usually normal | Often decreased |
| 24-hour calcium excretion | Variable | Usually decreased |
| Elevated transaminases | Rare | Frequent/HELLP |

FSPs, fibrin split products.

T A B L E   **27-5**

Comparison table comparing and contrasting TTP-HUS with autoimmune thrombocytopenia (ITP), atypical preeclampsia-eclampsia as HELLP syndrome, and acute fatty liver of pregnancy

| | **TTP** | **ITP** | **HELLP** | **HUS** | **AFLP** |
|---|---|---|---|---|---|
| CNS | + | − | + | − | − |
| Hypertension | − | − | ± | − | ± |
| Fever | + | − | − | − | ± |
| Petechiae | + | + | + | − | − |
| MHA | + | − | + | + | − |
| DIC | − | − | ± | − | + |
| Antibodies | − | + | − | − | − |
| Protein | + | − | + | + | ± |
| LDH | I | N | I | I | I |
| AST/ALT | N | N | I | N | I |
| CR/BUN | I | N | I | I | N/I |

ITP, idiopathic thrombocytopenic purpura; AFLP, acute fatty liver of pregnancy; MHA, microangiopathic hemolytic anemia; DIC, disseminated intravascular coagulopathy; Cr, creatinine; N, no change; I, increased.

Coombs' test should be negative. The distinction between adult TTP and vasculitic disorders is best made on the basis of the composite clinical picture, although biopsy of involved vessels may be useful in making the diagnosis. Other causes of microangiopathy also should be considered and include a connective tissue disorder, vascular malformations, prosthetic heart valves, metastatic adenocarcinoma, and malignant hypertension, all of which are usually easy to distinguish clinically (Martin, 1991; Bell, 1991a).

## Etiology and Pathogenesis

Although HUS and TTP are considered together as thrombotic microangiopathies, certain etiologic agents can be specifically associated with one form of the syndrome.

About 90% of HUS cases are pediatric and occur in late infancy and early childhood and are preceded by the onset of bloody diarrhea (known as D-positive HUS). *Shigella dysenteriae* serotype I and various *E. coli* serotypes have been identified as etiologic agents, and various other organisms have also been implicated, including *Salmonella typhi, Campylobacter jejuni, Streptococcus*, and viruses of the Coxsackie, echo, influenza, and Epstein-Barr varieties (Karmali, 1985).

These organisms produce a powerful protein exotoxin that is detectable in feces.

The prototype of the 70 kDa exotoxin is shiga toxin (ST), encoded in *S. dysenteriae* DNA. The structurally related exotoxins, SLT-1 and SLT-2 (SLT, shiga-like toxin), are encoded in bacteriophage DNA that is incorporated in the genome of specific *E. coli* serotypes. Of these serotypes, the most frequently associated with HUS is *E. coli* 0157:H7 (50% of the cases) (Karmali, 1992; Ashkenazi, 1993). These bacteria may be ingested in contaminated food (beef or poultry) that is insufficiently cooked, then colonize the large intestine and adhere, invade, and destroy colonic mucosal epithelial cells, finally entering the maternal circulation.

Shiga toxin, SLT-1, and SLT-2 are internalized by endocytosis, preferentially in the renal glomerular endothelial cell. By-products of this toxin inhibit protein elongation and lead to an overall suppression of protein synthesis (van de Kar, 1992). Light and electron microscopy studies demonstrate that toxin invasion leads to swelling and detachment of the endothelial cells in capillaries and small arterioles and to eventual necrosis. Exposure of the subendothelial space allows for enhancement of platelet thrombi formation in these areas. In addition, glomerular endothelial cell injury leads to release of various substances, including von Willebrand factor (vWF or factor VIII). Levels of this substance correlate with the degree of microvascular injury associated with HUS. The development of this syndrome following an episode of bloody diarrhea has been termed the *classic* or *postinfectious form* of HUS (Habib, 1992).

Hemolytic-uremic syndrome can develop weeks to months after exposure to various other previously described triggering agents (D-negative HUS), such as oral contraceptive or immunosuppressive medications, or it may appear spontaneously during or after an uncomplicated pregnancy. Exactly why HUS develops remains a mystery, although free radical damage of endothelial cells or enhanced production of antiendothelial cell antibodies have been proposed as theories. In general, HUS that is not associated with diarrhea carries a substantially worse prognosis than the D + form (Moake, 1994).

Thrombotic thrombocytopenic purpura is thought to involve an extreme form of microvascular platelet clumping, a process that can be activated by various substances. These include a 37 kDa (Siddique, 1985) or 59 kDa (Chen, 1989) protein, a calcium-rich enzyme that cleaves vWF multimers into fragments with increased platelet-binding capacity (Moore, 1990), or unusually large vWF multimeric forms (Moake, 1982, 1989).

Von Willebrand factor monomers are naturally linked by disulfide bonds to form large aggregates or multimers (unusually large von Willebrand factor [ULvWF]) of varying sizes that range into the millions of daltons. Multimers are stored inside both endothelial cells and platelets (although the main source of plasma vWF appears to be the endothelial cell) to be degraded by a specific plasma reductase prior to their entrance into the vascular lumen (Frangos, 1989).

Patients who develop TTP are found to have large amounts of circulating plasma ULvWF during the acute episode. This occurs presumably because of endothelial cell injury or intense stimulation of ULvWF release that overwhelms the degradation capability inherent in plasma. Patients who survive the initial episode and have no relapse almost always have absent plasma ULvWF multimer levels. In contrast, those who have persistent plasma ULvWF multimers will most likely have recurrent episodes of TTP secondary to continued endothelial cell pertubation (chronic relapsing TTP). Unusually large von Willebrand factor will then stimulate platelet aggregation to the subendothelial collagen, thus triggering microthrombi formation. Those patients with the chronic relapsing form of TTP may have a congenital defect of the endothelial cell that permits augmented release of ULvWF multimers at frequent and regular intervals (Moake, 1982, 1989).

An alternative theory regarding the genesis of TTP-HUS involves the major vasoactive prostaglandins thromboxane ($TXA_2$) and prostacyclin which are essential for the control of platelet and endothelium interactions (Moncada, 1978). Thromboxane and prostacyclin ($PGI_2$) have agonistic and antagonistic effects, respectively, on platelet aggregation. A number of investigators have associated these syndromes with defective endothelial synthesis of $PGI_2$, leading to relatively greater bioavailability of $TXA_2$, thus stimulating enhanced platelet aggregation and microthrombi formation (Remuzzi, 1978a,b). Although the evidence is indirect, many believe that this same mechanism could explain both the high risk of TTP-HUS in pregnancy and the strong association with preeclampsia. Patients destined to develop severe preeclampsia also may not demonstrate the increase in $PGI_2$ that is observed in normal pregnancies, theoretically leading to a similar clinical presentation of thrombocytopenia and hemolytic anemia (Goodman, 1982; Ylikorkala, 1981).

## Pregnancy

There have been numerous case reports and literature summaries concerning TTP-HUS associated with pregnancy (Permezel, 1992; Helou, 1994; Ambrose, 1985; Kwaan, 1985; Egerman, 1996). The largest summary of cases in the English language noted 40 cases of well-documented TTP in 65 women and 40 cases of HUS in 62 women over a 19-year period (Weiner, 1987). Cases that appear clinically consistent with preeclampsia were rejected, with the author noting a bias toward rejecting mild cases of the syndrome.

The large majority of cases (40/45) of TTP developed during the antepartum period at a mean gestational age of 23.5 weeks ± 10.4 weeks. Fifty-eight percent of the cases presented prior to the twenty-fourth week of pregnancy. The mean maternal age at the time of onset was 23 years. Symptoms and signs consistent with pre-eclampsia were identified in nine of 24 (38%) patients, although only three of these patients were thought to have TTP and preeclampsia simultaneously. Only 25% (10/40) maternal-fetal pairs survived when TTP was diagnosed during the antepartum period, and the fetal mortality rate was 80% (32/40). Maternal mortality was 44% overall in this series but was highly dependent on the treatment modality utilized. For example, if plasma therapy as infusion or exchange was employed, the mortality rate was 0% (0/17). If this form of therapy was not used, however, the mortality rate substantially increased to 68% (19/28).

Hemolytic-uremic syndrome is first recognized in the postpartum period in most patients (58/62, 94%), although symptoms generally precede delivery when viewed retrospectively. In cases presenting during the postpartum period, there is an average symptom-free interval of 26.6 ± 35.0 days (range, 0–180 days). In most cases, the distinction between HUS and severe pre-eclampsia is clear, and in only 15% do both syndromes occur in combination. Maternal mortality was high (55%) and was considered to be an underestimate, because almost half of the survivors were on or nearing dialysis at the time of publication. The overall outcome for patients with HUS was thought to be worse than that of TTP, even though only a small number of women received plasma therapy in one series (3/62), all of whom survived (Weiner, 1987).

## Treatment

A considerable improvement in survival has been recorded in those patients affected with TTP-HUS. In 1964, overall survival was only 10% (Amorosi, 1966). In a series of cases reported from 1964 to 1980, survival had increased to 46% (Ridolfi, 1981). By 1991, the largest reported series of patients treated for TTP-HUS noted a survival rate of 91%

(Bell, 1991b). Undoubtedly, this increase in survival can be attributed to increased availability of improved supportive therapies, including dialysis and antihypertensive regimens and treatment for life-threatening neurologic involvement. In addition, earlier diagnosis has allowed detection and rapid intervention in patients with less fulminant disease. Most authors, however, credit the improved survival of patients with TTP-HUS to the therapeutic effect of PI or PEX therapies, which have become a mainstay of treatment for this disorder (Table 27-6) (Shepard, 1987; Caggiano, 1983; Roberts, 1991; Egerman, 1996).

The goals of therapy in TTP-HUS are three-fold: (1) to improve the patient's renal and/or neurologic status, (2) to control episodes of hypertension, and (3) to reverse the thrombotic microangiopathy.

### Primary Therapy

**Plasma Manipulations** Bukowski and colleagues (1977) suggested the use of plasmapheresis and replacement with fresh-frozen plasma (FFP) as a primary treatment of TTP-HUS.

T A B L E   **27-6**

**Therapeutic approaches to adult thrombotic thrombocytopenic purpura–hemolytic-uremic syndrome**

*Primary Therapy*
  Fresh-frozen plasma infusion
  Plasma exchange
  Hemodialysis (HUS)
*Secondary Therapy*
  Glucocorticoids
  Antiplatelet agents
    Aspirin
    Dipyridamole
    Dextran 70
  Prostacyclin
*Tertiary Therapy*
  Splenectomy
  Immunosuppressants
    Azathioprine
  Chemotherapeutic agents
    Vincristine
    Cyclophosphamide
  High-dose immune globulin

Subsequent reports followed of disease remission following the simple infusion of FFP (PI) (Shepard, 1987; Byrnes, 1977). The beneficial effects of PI were considered to be due to a combination of factors, including increased $PGI_2$ availability, replacement of a deficient $PGI_2$-stimulating factor, or to the normalization of vWF metabolism. Plasma exchange is thought to derive its benefit, at least in part, from the removal of possibly deleterious circulating substances such as immune complexes, antiendothelial antibodies, abnormal vWF multimers, and products of damaged red cells, platelets, and WBCs. Plasma exchange could also supply via FFP putative lacking factors involved in the pathogenesis of disease (Ruggenenti, 1990).

The fundamental principle of PEX is separation of the blood into its components. This is accomplished by a cell separator, which uses centrifugal force to separate the blood components. Essentially, there are two types of these devices: continuous flow and intermittent flow. The continuous flow type is usually favored because it allows simultaneous withdrawal and infusion of blood components and minimizes the amount of blood that is extracorporeal at any given time. Two intravenous (IV) lines of at least 17 to 18 gauge are required in both arms, one to withdraw blood and the other to reinfuse the separated red cells and donor FFP. Complications of PEX include arrhythmia, cardiac arrest, hypovolemia or volume overload (probably accentuated during pregnancy), complications related to vascular access, anaphylaxis, citrate toxicity, or transmission of infectious organisms (Watson, 1990). The estimated risk of posttransfusion hepatitis is 1% per unit of infused FFP, while the risk of HIV is estimated to be between 1 in 40,000 to 1 in 250,000 (Food and Drug Administration, 1989). This is especially important, because a typical adult patient with TTP-HUS who requires multiple PEXs will receive on average more than 200 units of FFP during a disease exacerbation (Bell, 1991b).

In contrast to PI, PEX minimizes volume fluctuations and is thus the treatment of choice for patients with marginal renal function and severe oliguria (Mokrzycki, 1994). During PEX in the undelivered patient with a viable pregnancy, we rec-

ommend continuous electronic fetal monitoring and vigilant monitoring of maternal pulmonary status. Although each patient's therapy is individualized, the usual policy is to exchange 2 to 4 liters of plasma on a daily basis until a platelet count of more than 150,000/$\mu$L is established and then convert to an alternate-day or every-third-day cycle (Martin, 1991).

The goal of PI is to administer the equivalent of one plasma volume (30 mL/kg) over 24 hours, followed by one half to one plasma volume per day until improvement is noted. Risks involved are similar to those of PEX, except that PI is more commonly associated with volume overload.

There is evidence that PEX may be more beneficial than PI for the treatment of TTP-HUS. Rock and co-workers (1991) reported the results of a 7-year multicenter prospective, randomized trial of PI versus PEX in 102 nonpregnant patients with TTP. Patients in the PEX group received FFP and PEX for a minimum of seven procedures over the first 9 hospital days, with 1.5 times the predicted plasma volume exchanged over the first 3 days, followed by 1.0 times the predicted volume thereafter. The other group received PI daily in a cycle of 30 mL/kg body weight over the first 24 hours, followed by 15 mg/kg each day thereafter. In addition to this therapy, all patients received dipyridamole (400 mg/day) and aspirin (325 mg/day) by mouth for at least 2 weeks following entry into the trial.

Plasma exchange proved superior to PI for all clinical endpoints. Overall, more patients on PEX (24/51) had an increase in the platelet count, compared with those on PI (13/51). Only two of 51 patients in the PEX group died during the first treatment cycle, compared with eight of 51 of those randomized to PI. More importantly, after 6 months, patients who received PEX demonstrated a lower rate of relapse and a significantly lower mortality rate. The overall mortality in both groups was 29%. These results are conservative, because a large number of patients in the PI group were classified as treatment failures (31/51) and received PEX as a salvage treatment during the study protocol.

Bell and colleagues (1991b) reported a 91% survival in 108 patients with TTP-HUS who were treated with a combination of corticosteroids and

PEX. Nine percent of the patients in this study were pregnant at the time of the initial episode. The largest series of TTP reported from one institution during pregnancy detailed eight episodes in 16 pregnancies of five patients (Ezra, 1997), with successful disease process reversal in eight of 12 patients treated initially with PEX. In addition to PEX, patients also received corticosteroids (300 mg of hydrocortisone or its equivalent per day), aspirin (100–500 mg/day), and dipyridamole (225 mg/day). In agreement with previous case reports, these authors noted that termination of pregnancy did not affect the course of the disease, although there was a higher incidence of relapse if the patient survived the initial episode and became pregnant again. If therapy were immediate and intensive, the maternal-infant pair could survive.

Based on these reports, we recommend a course of PEX as the initial therapeutic modality in those affected with TTP-HUS during pregnancy. Other therapies (aspirin, steroids, etc.) can be utilized during the primary event or to prevent relapse in accordance with the consulting hematologist's preference.

### Secondary Treatment

While the benefits of plasma infusion, or more often, plasma exchange therapy, appear to be well established, the value of a number of adjunctive therapeutic agents is less certain.

**Corticosteroids**  Corticosteroids were the earliest treatment advocated for TTP-HUS. The rationale for their use was the response seen in occasional patients and the knowledge that platelet survival time is improved with steroid use. Although the efficacy of steroid regimens is debated, nevertheless, most patients affected with the syndrome have been treated with steroids in combination with other drugs, making it difficult to evaluate recommendations for their use in the treatment of TTP (Bell, 1991b; Ridolfi, 1981). Dosages are variable, but an equivalent of 100 to 400 mg of hydrocortisone administered daily for 1 week and tapered thereafter until hematologic parameters improve is a reasonable regimen.

**Antiplatelet Agents**  Although not considered beneficial for those affected primarily with HUS, in noncontrolled studies, therapy inclusive of antiplatelet agents has proven successful in obtaining remissions in patients with TTP (Amorosi, 1977; Bukowski, 1981). As with corticosteroids, the common use of antiplatelet agents in combination with other therapies makes it difficult to evaluate their actual efficacy. Possible modalities include aspirin (325–1500 mg/day), dipyridamole (400–600 mg/day), sulfinpyrazone (400 mg/day), and IV dextran 70 (500 mL every 12 hr).

**Prostacyclin**  The use of prostacyclin infusion in TTP-HUS is consistent with the hypothesis that affected patients may lack a plasma factor required to stimulate prostacyclin production. Unfortunately, experience with this mode of therapy is limited. Some investigators have noted dramatic remissions after failure to respond to PEX as well as $PGI_2$ infusion failures. The authors of a review of this subject noted that most treatment failures were associated with insufficient dosing or duration of therapy (Tardy, 1991). They recommended an initial IV infusion of 4 to 9 ng/kg/min for the first 120 hours of infusion, followed by 48 hours at 9 ng/kg/min. One side effect of prostacyclin infusion is hypotension, which may limit its potential usefulness in pregnancy.

### Tertiary Treatments

The value of these approaches is even less well established and should be considered investigational.

**Splenectomy**  Patients with relapsing disease, especially after PEX, occasionally benefit from splenectomy (Onundarson, 1992; Wells, 1991). Most investigators, however, consider this operation to be ineffective and attribute its purported benefit to blood products and dextran administered during and after the surgery (Ruggenenti, 1990). In the investigation of Bell and associates (1991), six patients underwent splenectomy as a salvage procedure. All of them experienced a rapid deterioration in clinical status, four patients became comatose, and one died abruptly. Thus, splenectomy for TTP-HUS may be ill advised if not contraindicated.

**Immunosuppressive-Chemotherapeutic Agents** These agents include vincristine, azathioprine, and cyclophosphamide. Vincristine may be efficacious because its depolymerizing effect on platelet microtubules produces secondary alterations in the exposure of cell surface receptors. This therapy, however, may be teratogenic and should not be employed in the presence of a live fetus. It is administered IV at an initial dose of 2 mg, followed by 1 mg every 4 days for a period of 4 to 6 weeks (Levin, 1991).

The use of azathioprine (Moake, 1985) and cyclophosphamide (Wallach, 1979) has been associated with the disappearance of very large ULvWF forms and complete recovery in patients with frequently relapsing TTP. These observations suggest that autoantibodies directed against endothelial cells may contribute to the pathogenesis of this disorder.

The effectiveness of all these drugs is unproven at present, although vincristine has been shown to produce remission as a single drug treatment.

**High-Dose Immunoglobulins** Intravenous immunoglobulins in large doses for extended periods (0.5 mg/kg/day for 5 consecutive days) have been advocated as a means to neutralize platelet aggregating factors in patients with TTP. The effectiveness of this therapy needs to be established by controlled trials (Raniele, 1991; Finazzi, 1992).

### Supportive Therapy

In gravidas with adult HUS syndrome, it is critically important to initiate comprehensive supportive therapy to correct fluid and electrolyte imbalance, including, when necessary, dialysis for the control of renal failure. Meticulous attention to salt and water management and correction of hyperkalemia is imperative (Table 27-7). Thereafter, or in concert, PEX is begun as previously described.

Although a significant number of patients with TTP-HUS will be severely thrombocytopenic, with spontaneous bleeding and purpura, the infusion of platelet concentrates should be

T A B L E   **27-7**

Treatment of major electrolyte abnormalities seen in hemolytic-uremic syndrome

| Abnormality | Preferred Treatment | Doses | Comment |
|---|---|---|---|
| Hyponatremia ($<$ 130 mEq/liter) | Fluid restriction Diuretics Dialysis | Furosemide (1–2 mg/kg) Bumetanide (0.1–0.2 mg/kg) | If hypervolemic |
| Hypernatremia ($>$ 150 mEq/liter) | Provide free $H_2O$ ($D_5W$) Dialysis | | If normal GFR |
| Hyperkalemia ($>$ 6.5 mEq/liter) | IV Ca gluconate (10%) IV $NaHco_3$* IV glucose ($D_5W$) IV insulin Cation exchange resin Dialysis | 1-g/kg/dose 1–3 mEq/kg over 3–5 min 500 mg/kg 0.1 units/kg 1-g/kg/dose | If no HTN or hypervolemia If no HTN or hypervolemia over 2 hr  If no HTN or colitis Removes approx. 10 mEq $K^+$/hr |
| Metabolic acidosis (pH $<$ 7.35) ($Hco_3$ $<$ 15 mEq/liter) | $NaHco_3$ Dialysis | 1 mEq/kg | If no HTN or hypervolemia $K^+$ |

*Calcium gluconate and $NaHco_3$ should be given in separate IV lines to avoid calcium carbonate formation and precipitation. Lines must be well flushed between infusions when these substances are given sequentially through the same IV access.

HTN, hypertension; GFR, glomerular filtration rate.

## THROMBOTIC THROMBOCYTOPENIC PURPURA–

### I. *Goals of Therapy*

    A. Impede, arrest, and reverse the abnormal endothelial-platelet interaction causing thrombocytopenia (the thrombotic microangiopathy) and secondary end-organ damage, especially in the kidney and CNS

    B. Relieve symptoms

    C. Protect the pregnancy

    D. Treat any concomitant illness

    E. Control hypertension

### II. *Management Protocol*

    A. *General:* Because there are no pathognomonic tests that are diagnostic of TTP-HUS, more common causations must be excluded (see below). Evaluate closely all possible pertinent signs, symptoms, physical, and laboratory findings.

    B. *Findings:* Once severe thrombocytopenia (usually $<50,000/\mu L$) is detected, assess the patient for the presence of CNS symptoms, fever, petechiae/purpura, evidence of bleeding, malaise/fatigue, nausea/vomiting, jaundice, and areas of pain.

### III. *Critical Tests*

    A. *Laboratory:* Undertake laboratory assessments for evidence of preeclampsia (increased serum uric acid, increased urinary protein, depressed urinary calcium excretion, decreased AT III, elevated BP), HELLP syndrome (increased LDH, transaminases, epigastric pain), ITP (platelet antibodies), DIC (prolongation of PT/PTT, decreased fibrinogen, elevated fibrin degradation products), fatty liver of pregnancy (evidence of liver failure, DIC, elevated bilirubin, hypoglycemia), drugs (cocaine), lupus/connective tissue disorder (ANA, anticardiolipin/lupus anticoagulant antibodies), and renal dysfunction (creatinine, BUN, urinary sediment). Also, assess blood type and screen, HIV and hepatitis screen, complete blood count with differential, and reticulocyte count.

### IV. *Consultation*

    A. If patient appears to have more than preeclampsia/HELLP syndrome and assistance from medical consultants would be beneficial to patient care, request immediate consultation from a maternal-fetal medicine specialist initially and possibly another in hematology. Consider nephrology and neurology consultations or others, as deemed appropriate. Consult neonatology and anesthesia if the patient is pregnant and delivery is imminent.

---

restricted to circumstances of life-threatening hemorrhage or immediately prior to surgery or any invasive procedure in the patient with a platelet count less than $50,000/\mu L$. Administration of platelet concentrates has been associated with worsening of intravascular thrombus formation. Their purported acceleration of the disease process is consistent with the view that intravascular platelet aggregation is probably the initiating event in this disorder (Gordon, 1987).

## HEMOLYTIC-UREMIC SYNDROME

### V. *Pregnancy Surveillance*

A.  Apply continuous electronic fetal monitoring if the fetus is potentially viable, and thoroughly assess with ultrasound. Maintain the mother under close surveillance in the labor and delivery unit or a comparable facility during evaluation and treatment. Biophysical profiles/CST should be used as appropriate, depending on the fetal condition.

### VI. *Other Considerations*

A.  Avoid unnecessary venipunctures and intramuscular injections.

B.  Culture the patient's urine, blood, and other sites if fever is present.

C.  Bone marrow aspiration or biopsy of a skin lesion may be recommended.

D.  If TTP is considered to be present, the leader of the health-care team is generally the hematologist acting in close association with the maternal-fetal specialist; if HUS is the dominant form of the thrombotic microangiopathy, the nephrologist may become the leader of the team. It must be clear to all parties as to who is the primary patient manager.

E.  If TTP is the dominant form of thrombotic microangiopathy, consider initiating prednisone 1 mg/kg/day and initiate a 3-liter plasma exchange procedure; for HUS, consider a similar course of therapy while deciding whether dialysis is indicated as well.

F.  Avoid platelet transfusion; daily plasma exchanges are continued on a daily basis until a response is obtained.

G.  Transfuse red cells at the end of plasma exchange judiciously to sustain a hematocrit minimally acceptable to the providers; minimize red-cell transfusions as much as possible.

H.  Consider initiating LDA (60–80 mg daily), dipyridone (100 mg by mouth every 6 hr), multivitamin with 1.5 g vitamin E daily, 1 mg folic acid daily, control BP, and correct electrolyte (Na, K) imbalances.

I.  Reserve vincristine, high-dose IV gamma globulin, and splenectomy for exceptional circumstances per consultant recommendation. Vincristine should be avoided before delivery.

J.  For the patient well known to have chronic relapsing TTP-HUS and who becomes pregnant, treat prophylactically with daily LDA, dipyridamole (225 mg daily), and prednisone (20 mg daily). Manage in concert with a consulting MFM/hematologist or nephrologist as appropriate to the individual patient.

K.  For the patient with HELLP syndrome, whether of recent onset or complicated by advanced disease, initiate dexamethasone (10 mg IV every 12 hr), support medically, and deliver if appropriate.

Patients with TTP-HUS are best monitored with sequential blood counts, platelet count, serum creatinine, LDH, and indirect bilirubin determinations. Frequent neurologic examinations are indicated. The two most sensitive laboratory indicators of patient recovery are a rising trend in the platelet count and a decreasing serum concentration (Patton, 1994).

## REFERENCES

Ambrose A, Welham RG, Cefalo RC. Thrombotic thrombocytopenic purpura in early pregnancy. Obstet Gynecol 1985;66:267.

Amorosi EL, Karpatkin S. Antiplatelet treatment of thrombotic thrombocytopenic purpura. Ann Intern Med 1977;86:102.

Amorosi EL, Ultman JE. Thrombotic thrombocytopenic purpura: report of 16 cases and review of the literature. Medicine (Baltimore) 1966;45:139.

Ashkenazi S. Role of bacterial cytotoxins in hemolytic uremic syndrome and thrombotic thrombocytopenic purpura. Annu Rev Med 1993;44:11.

Barondess JA. Thrombotic thrombocytopenic purpura: review of the literature and report of three cases. Am J Med 1952;13:294.

Bartholomew JR, Bell WR. Thrombotic thrombocytopenic purpura. J Intensive Care Med 1986;1:341.

Bell W. Thrombotic thrombocytopenic purpura. JAMA 1991a;265:91.

Bell WR, Braine HG, Ness PM, Kickler TS. Improved survival in thrombotic thrombocytopenic purpura–hemolytic uremic syndrome. N Engl J Med 1991b;325:398.

Berns JS, Kaplan BS, Mackow RC, Hefter LG. Inherited hemolytic uremic syndrome in adults. Am J Kidney Dis 1992;19:331.

Bukowski RM, King JW, Hewlett JS. Plasmapheresis in the treatment of thrombotic thrombocytopenic purpura. Blood 1977;50:413.

Bukowski RM, Hewlett JS, Reimer RR, et al. Therapy of thrombotic thrombocytopenic purpura: an overview. Semin Thromb Hemost 1981;7:1.

Byrnes JJ, Khurana M. Treatment of thrombotic thrombocytopenic purpura with plasma. N Engl J Med 1977;297:1386.

Byrnes JJ, Moake JL. Thrombotic thrombocytopenic purpura and the haemolytic-uraemic syndrome: evolving concepts of pathogenesis and therapy. Clin Haematol 1986;15:413.

Caggiano V, Fernando LP, Schneider JM, et al. Thrombotic thrombocytopenic purpura: report of 14 cases—occurrence during pregnancy and response to plasma exchange. J Clin Apheresis 1983;1:71.

Chen SH, Lian EC-Y. Purification and some properties of a 59 kDa platelet-aggregating protein from the plasma of a patient with thrombotic thrombocytopenic purpura. Thromb Haemost 1989;62:568.

Egerman RS, Witlin AG, Friedman SA, Sibai BM. Thrombotic thrombocytopenic purpura and hemolytic uremic syndrome in pregnancy: review of 11 cases. Am J Obstet Gynecol 1996;175:950.

Eknoyan G, Riggs SA. Renal involvement in patients with thrombotic thrombocytopenic purpura. Am J Nephrol 1986;6:117.

Ezra Y, Rose M, Eldor A. Therapy and prevention of thrombotic thrombocytopenic purpura during pregnancy: a clinical study of 16 pregnancies. Am J Hematol (in press) 1997.

Finazzi G, Bellavita P, Falanga A, et al. Inefficacy of intravenous immunoglobulin in patients with low-risk thrombotic thrombocytopenic purpura/hemolytic-uremic syndrome. Am J Hematol 1992;41:165.

Food and Drug Administration. Use of blood components. FDA Drug Bulletin 1989;19:14.

Frangos JA, Moake JL, Nolasco L, et al. Cryosupernatant regulates accumulation of unusually large vWF multimers from endothelial cells. Am J Physiol 1989;256:H1635.

Gasser C, Gautier E, Steck A, et al. Haemolytisch-uramische syndromes bilaterale nierenrindennkrosen bei akuten erworbencheuschr hamolytischen anamien. Schweiz Med Wochenschr 1955;85:905.

Goodman RP, Killam AP, Brash AR, Branch RA. Prostacyclin production during pregnancy: comparison of production during normal pregnancy and pregnancy complicated by hypertension. Am J Obstet Gynecol 1982;142:817.

Gordon LI, Kwaan HC, Rossi EC. Deleterious effects of platelet transfusions and recovery thrombocytosis in patients with thrombotic microangiopathy. Semin Hematol 1987;24:194.

Gore I. Disseminated arteriolar and capillary platelet thrombosis: a morphologic study of its histogenesis. Am J Pathol 1950;26:155.

Habib R. Pathology of the hemolytic uremic syndrome. In: Kaplan BS, Trompeter RS, Moake JL, eds. Hemolytic-uremic syndrome and thrombotic thrombocytopenic purpura. New York: Marcel Dekker, 1992:315.

Helou J, Nakhle S, Shoenfeld S, et al. Postpartum thrombotic thrombocytopenic purpura: report of a case and review of the literature. Obstet Gynecol Surv 1994;49:785.

Holman MJ, Gonwa TA, Cooper B, et al. FK506-associated thrombotic thrombocytopenic purpura. Transplantation 1993;55:205.

Karmali MA. The association of verotoxins and the classical hemolytic uremic syndrome. In: Kaplan BS, Trompeter RS, Moake JL, eds. Hemolytic-uremic syndrome and thrombotic thrombocytopenic purpura. New York: Marcel Dekker, 1992:199.

Karmali MA, Petric M, Lim C, et al. The association between idiopathic hemolytic uremic syndrome and infection by verotoxin-producing *Escherichia coli*. J Infect Dis 1985;151:775.

Kwaan HC. Thrombotic thrombocytopenic purpura and hemolytic uremic syndrome in pregnancy. Clin Obstet Gynecol 1985;28:101.

Kwaan HC. Miscellaneous secondary thrombotic microangiopathy. Semin Hematol 1987;24:141.

Levin M, Grünwald HW. Use of vincristine in refractory thrombotic thrombocytopenic purpura. Acta Haematol 1991;85:37.

Martin JN Jr, Files JC, Morrison JC. Peripartal adult thrombotic thrombocytopenic purpura and hemolytic-uremic syndrome. In: Clark SL, Cotton DB, Hankins GDV, Phelan JP, eds. Critical care obstetrics. 2nd ed. Cambridge: Blackwell Scientific, 1991:464.

Meyrier A, Becquemont L, Weill B, et al. Hemolytic-uremic syndrome with anticardiolipin antibodies revealing paraneoplastic systemic scleroderma. Nephron 1991;59:493.

Moake JL. TTP—desperation, empiricism, progress. N Engl J Med 1991;325:426.

Moake JL. Haemolytic-uraemic syndrome: basic science. Lancet 1994;343:393.

Moake JL, McPherson PD. Abnormalities of von Willebrand factor multimers in thrombotic thrombocytopenic purpura and the hemolytic-uremic syndrome. Am J Med 1989;87:3.

Moake JL, Rudy CK, Troll JH, et al. Unusually large plasma factor VIII: von Willebrand factor multimers in chronic relapsing thrombotic thrombocytopenic purpura. N Engl J Med 1982;307:1432.

Moake JL, Rudy CK, Troll JH, et al. Therapy of chronic relapsing thrombotic thrombocytopenic purpura with prednisone and azathioprine. Am J Hematol 1985;20:73.

Mokrzycki MH, Kaplan AA. Therapeutic plasma exchange: complications and management. Am J Kidney Dis 1994;23:817.

Moncada S, Vane JR. Unstable metabolites of arachidonic acid and their role in haemostasis and thrombosis. Br Med Bull 1978;34:129.

Moore JC, Murphy WG, Kelton JG. Calpain proteolysis of von Willebrand factor enhances its binding to platelet membrane glycoprotein IIb/IIIa: an explanation for platelet aggregation in thrombotic thrombocytopenic purpura. Br J Haematol 1990;74:457.

Moschcowitz E. Acute febrile pleiochromic anemia with hyaline thrombosis of the terminal arterioles and capillaries. An undescribed disease. Arch Intern Med 1925;36:89.

Neumann M, Urizar R. Hemolytic uremic syndrome: current pathophysiology and management. Am Nephrol Nurses Assoc J 1994;21:137.

Onundarson PT, Rowe JM, Heal JM, Francis CW. Response to plasma exchange and splenectomy in thrombotic thrombocytopenic purpura. A 10-year experience at a single institution. Arch Intern Med 1992;152:791.

Patton JF, Manning KR, Case D, Owen J. Serum lactate dehydrogenase and platelet count predict survival in thrombotic thrombocytopenic purpura. Am J Hematol 1994;47:94.

Permezel M, Lee N, Corry J. Thrombotic thrombocytopenic purpura in pregnancy. Aust NZ J Obstet Gynaecol 1992;32:278.

Pinette MG, Vintzileos AM, Ingardia CJ. Thrombotic thrombocytopenic purpura as a cause of thrombocytopenia in pregnancy: literature review. Am J Perinatol 1989;6:55.

Raniele DP, Opsahl JA, Kjellstrand CM. Should intravenous immunoglobulin G be first-line treatment for acute thrombotic thrombocytopenic purpura? Case report and review of the literature. Am J Kidney Dis 1991;28:264.

Remuzzi G, Misiani R, Marchesi D, et al. Haemolytic uraemic syndrome deficiency of plasma factor(s) regulating prostacyclin activity. Lancet 1978a;2:871.

Remuzzi G, Misiani R, Mecca G, et al. Thrombotic thrombocytopenic purpura—a deficiency of plasma factor regulating platelet-vessel wall interaction. N Engl J Med 1978b;299:311.

Ridolfi RL, Bell WR. Thrombotic thrombocytopenic purpura: report of 25 cases and review of the literature. Medicine (Baltimore) 1981;60:413.

Roberts AW, Gillett EA, Fleming SJ. Hemolytic uremic syndrome/thrombotic thrombocytopenic purpura: outcome with plasma exchange. J Clin Apheresis 1991;6:150.

Rock GA, Shumak KH, Buskard NA, et al. Comparison of plasma exchange with plasma infusion in the treatment of thrombotic thrombocytopenic purpura. N Engl J Med 1991;325:393.

Ruggenenti P, Remuzzi G. Thrombotic thrombocytopenic purpura and related disorders. Hematol Oncol Clin North Am 1990;4:219.

Shepard KV, Bukowski RM. The treatment of thrombotic thrombocytopenic purpura with exchange transfusions, plasma infusions, and plasma exchange. Semin Hematol 1987;24:178.

Siddique FA, Lian EC-Y. Novel platelet-agglutinating protein from a thrombotic thrombocytopenic purpura plasma. J Clin Invest 1985;76:1330.

Stricker RB, Davis JA, Gershow J, et al. Thrombotic thrombocytopenic purpura complicating systemic lupus erythematosus. Case report of literature review from the plasmapheresis era. J Rheumatol 1992;19:1469.

Symmers VStC. Thrombotic microangiopathic haemolytic anaemia (thrombotic microangiopathy). Br Med J 1952;2:897.

Tardy B, Page Y, Comtet C, et al. Intravenous prostacyclin in thrombotic thrombocytopenic purpura: case report and review of the literature. J Intern Med 1991;230:279.

Thorp JM Jr, Wells SR, Bowes WA Jr. The obfuscation continues. Severe preeclampsia versus thrombotic thrombocytopenic purpura. N C Med J 1991;52:126.

Ucar A, Fernandez HF, Byrnes JJ, et al. Thrombotic microangiopathy and retroviral infections: a 13-year experience. Am J Hematol 1994;45:304.

van de Kar NCAJ, Monnens LAH, Karmali MA, van Hinsbergh VWM. Tumor necrosis factor and interleukin-1 induce expression of the verocytotoxin receptor globotriaosylceramide on human endothelial cells: implication for the pathogenesis of the hemolytic uremic syndrome. Blood 1992;80:2755.

Vandekerchove F, Noens L, Colardyn F, et al. Thrombotic thrombocytopenic purpura of seven pregnancies mimicking toxemia of pregnancy. Am J Obstet Gynecol 1984;150:320.

Wallach HW, Oren ME, Herskowitz A. Treatment of thrombotic thrombocytopenic purpura with plasma infusion and cyclophosphamide. South Med J 1979;72:1346.

Watson WJ, Katz VL, Bowes WA Jr. Plasmapheresis during pregnancy. Obstet Gynecol 1990;76:451.

Weiner CP. Thrombotic microangiopathy in pregnancy and the postpartum period. Semin Hematol 1987;24:119.

Wells AD, Majumdar G, Slater NGP, Young AE. Role of splenectomy as a salvage procedure in thrombotic thrombocytopenic purpura. Br J Surg 1991;78:1389.

Wiznitzer A, Mazor M, Leigerman JR, et al. Familial occurrence of thrombotic thrombocytopenic purpura in two sisters during pregnancy. Am J Obstet Gynecol 1992;166:20.

Ylikorkala O, Makila UM, Viinikka L. Amniotic fluid prostacyclin and thromboxane in normal, preeclamptic, and some other complicated pregnancies. Am J Obstet Gynecol 1981;141:487.

# CHAPTER 28

# Thyroid and Parathyroid Emergencies

## Maternal and Fetal Thyroid Function

Multiple changes occur in the maternal and fetal thyroid glands during pregnancy. These physiologic changes have been detailed extensively (Fisher, 1981; Burrow, 1994; Millar, 1994; Radunovic, 1991). (The reader is referred to these studies for more detail.) A brief review of changes that affect the interpretation of thyroid tests or thyroid hormone metabolism in relationship to clinical management will follow.

Maternal iodide blood levels fall during gestation, in part due to an increase in glomerular filtration rate, as well as transplacental iodide transport. When iodide intake is mildly decreased (50–75 μg/day), maternal thyroid volume increases by 30%, there is a marked increase in serum thyroglobulin, and 16% of women develop a goiter (Glinoer, 1995). In severely iodide-deficient areas (median iodide intake approximating 25 μg/day), 50% of individuals have a visible goiter, and neonatal hypothyroidism ranges from 2% to 9% (Xue-Yi, 1994). In contrast, in the United States, dietary iodide supplementation is sufficient to maintain normal thyroid function, and neonatal hypothyroidism is also rare, occurring in 1 in 4500 infants. Although some investigators have found that in iodide-replete areas, thyroid volume as measured by ultrasound is unchanged during pregnancy (Berghout, 1994), a

mild increase in thyroid volume of 10% to 20% may be seen (Burrow, 1994). Goiter, therefore, should be investigated and not ascribed to pregnancy changes. Thyroid nodules, particularly solid nodules greater than 2 cm, cystic nodules larger than 4 cm, or enlarging nodules on thyroid suppression, can be evaluated by ultrasound and fine-needle aspiration (Doherty, 1995).

Changes in thyroid hormone levels during pregnancy occur both in the maternal circulation and in the developing fetus. Thyroid-binding globulin (TBG) and total thyroxine blood levels increase in the maternal circulation (Fig 28-1). Prior to the wide availability of free thyroxine measurements, the calculated free thyroxine index was used to adjust for the increase in total thyroxine due to thyroxine-binding globulin and a decrease in the thyroid hormone-binding ratio. More recently, the use of sensitive thyrotropin and free thyroxine assays has largely replaced the free thyroxine index and has improved the diagnosis of thyroid disorders (Surks, 1990). Maternal free T4 and free T3 blood levels remain within the range of normal values but are minimally decreased in the second and third trimesters (Burrow, 1994; Berghout, 1994). One exception to the interpretation of free T4 and thyroid-stimulating hormone (TSH) during pregnancy is the increase in maternal free T4 levels and the decrease in thyrotropin at 8 to 12 weeks of gestation when human chorionic gonadotropin (HCG) levels peak (Glinoer, 1990) (Figs 28-2, 28-3). This is thought to, in part,

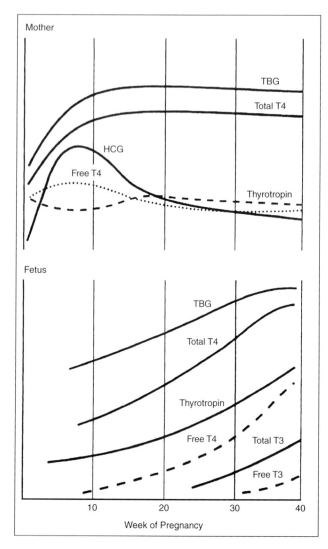

F I G U R E 28-1

**Relative changes in maternal fetal thyroid function during pregnancy**. HCG, human chorionic gonadotropin. (Reproduced by permission from Burrow G, Fisher DA, Larsen PR. Maternal and fetal thyroid function. N Engl J Med 1994;331:1072.)

reflect the weak thyrotropic activity of HCG (Pekary, 1993). Thus, a mild elevation of free T4 and suppressed TSH level in the first trimester, in the absence of clinical signs of thyrotoxicosis, is likely to be physiologic and does not suggest hyperthyroidism. TSH levels may be suppressed in the first trimester and undetectable in as many as 13% of women (Glinoer, 1990).

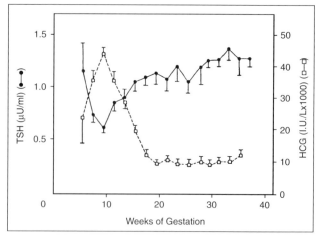

F I G U R E 28-2

**Serum TSH and HCG as a function of gestational age**. (Reproduced by permission from Glinoer D, et al. Regulation of maternal thyroid during pregnancy. J Clin Endocrinol Metab 1990;71:276.)

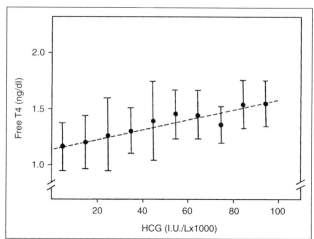

F I G U R E 28-3

**Free T4 in relation to HCG concentrations**. (Reproduced by permission from Glinoer D, et al. Regulation of maternal thyroid during pregnancy. J Clin Endocrinol Metab 1990;71:276.)

Fetal serum total T4, free T4, and thyroxine-binding globulin are detectable at 10 weeks of gestation and increase thereafter, reaching mean maternal values at 36 weeks of gestation (Thorpe-Beeston, 1991). Because fetal thyrotropin levels remain higher than maternal levels despite the increase in T4 levels, this reflects a developmental decrease in sensitivity of the fetal pituitary to negative feedback. An increase in hypothalamic thyrotropin-releasing hormone and thyrotropin also drives the increase in T4. Of particular interest is the success of screening programs in often preventing the neurologic sequelae of congenital hypothyroidism based on replacement after birth (Burrow, 1994). Two factors that are likely important are maternal-fetal transfer of thyroxine and pituitary increases in type II deiodinase regulating conversion of T4 to T3 in hypothyroid states (Burrow, 1994). First, Vulsma et al (1989), studying infants unable to iodinate thyroid proteins and, therefore, unable to make T4, found that maternal-fetal transfer of thyroxine could account for T4 levels in newborns that approximated 50% of normal values. Second, in animal rat models of fetal hypothyroidism induced by maternal administration of methimazole, fetal brain T3 levels can be maintained by maternal T4 supplementation. Thus, increases in type II deiodinase activity may serve to normalize brain T3 concentrations despite peripheral manifestations of hypothyroidism (Ruiz De Ona, 1988).

Much remains to be known of the metabolism of thyroid hormones in pregnancy, but the daily production rate of thyroxine as measured in nonpregnant individuals is roughly 90 $\mu$g/day of thyroxine and 32 $\mu$g/day of triiodothyronine (Degroot, 1984). Virtually 80% of T3 is produced by peripheral conversion of thyroxine to triiodothyronine by 5′-deiodination. Only 0.02% of thyroxine is unbound and in free form, as compared with 0.3% of triiodothyronine. In addition, the half-life of T4 is 8 days (Hermann, 1994) and that of T3, 1 day. Taken together, these data suggest that the relative metabolic potency of triiodothyronine is 3 times that of thyroxine.

The clinical consequences of thyroxine metabolism are threefold. The first is that thyroid replacement in hypothyroid patients usually starts at 100 $\mu$g/day (Toft, 1994; Mandel, 1990). There is some evidence that replacement actually may increase during pregnancy. Mandel et al (1990) found that to normalize thyrotropin levels, the mean thyroxine dose increased from 102 to 147 $\mu$g/day, an increase of 45%. Although the clinical effects of an elevated thyrotropin level and thy-

roxine levels that may be suppressed but are in a normal range are unclear, it is prudent to normalize thyrotropin levels in pregnant women. Second, in the acute setting of thyroid storm, it is logical to use propylthiouracil instead of methimazole, because the former inhibits peripheral conversion of T4 to T3, while the latter does not. Finally, clinical symptomatic improvement in patients with acute hyperthyroidism treated with propylthiouracil (days) precedes normalization of thyroid function tests, which may take 6 to 8 weeks.

## Hyperthyroidism

The evaluation and management of common thyroid disorders in women have been recently discussed by Mazzaferri (1997). Hyperthyroidism during pregnancy is rare, complicating less than 0.2% of all births (Davis, 1989; Wing, 1994). Early treatment and normalization of maternal thyroid function is important because poor metabolic control increases the risk of preterm delivery, fetal wastage, and thyroid crisis (Davis, 1989; Kriplani, 1994). By far, the most common cause of thyrotoxicosis during pregnancy is Graves' disease, accounting for 60% to 90% of cases. Less common causes are listed in Table 28-1 and include thyroid adenomas, thyroiditis, or secondary HCG-dependent disorders (Kendall-Taylor, 1995; Hedberg, 1987).

It is generally accepted that Graves' disease is an autoimmune disorder. Prior to the use of thionamides, it was recognized that some 25% of patients undergo long-term remission without therapy (Volpe, 1991). During pregnancy, the course is variable. As in other autoimmune disorders, some patients appear to improve during pregnancy and relapse postpartum. Amino et al (1982) noted, in women with Graves' disease near remission at the onset of pregnancy, that the free thyroxine index was increased in the first trimester, fell in the second and third trimesters, and was again increased postpartum (Fig 28-4). A fall in antimicrosomal antibodies during pregnancy and an increase postpartum were also measured in patients with Graves' disease or postpartum thyroiditis (Amino, 1978).

## Causes of hyperthyroidism

Autoimmune
    Graves' disease
    Hashimoto's disease
Autonomous
    Toxic multinodular goitre
    Solitary toxic adenoma
Thyroiditis (transient)
    Postpartum thyroiditis
    Subacute thyroiditis
    Painless thyroiditis
Drug-induced
    Iodide-induced (jod basedow)
    Thyroxine (factitious)
Secondary
    TSH-secreting tumor
    HCG-dependent (hyperemesis gravidarum, hy-
        datidiform mole)
Thyroid hormone resistance
Ectopic
    Struma ovarii
    Metastatic follicular carcinoma

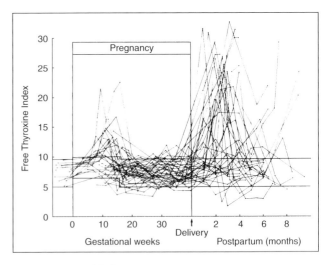

F I G U R E **28-4**

Sequential changes in serum FT4 index during and after pregnancy in patients with Graves' disease in remission or near remission. Horizontal lines indicate the normal range of the FT4 index. (Reproduced by permission from Amino N, Tanizawa O, Mori H, et al. Aggravation of thyrotoxicosis in early pregnancy and after delivery in Graves' disease. J Clin Endocrinol Metab 1982;55:108.)

The diagnosis of Graves' disease is suggested by the presence of thyrotoxicosis, ophthalmopathy, a diffuse goiter, dermopathy, and thyroid receptor antibodies. The diagnosis is clinical and is supported by thyroid function tests; thyroid receptor antibody tests often are not necessary. Pretibial dermopathy, however, is rarely present in pregnant women, and active clinical ophthalmopathy is evident in only half of patients with Graves' disease (Epstein, 1993). The ocular signs of sympathetic overactivity, lid retraction, widening of the palpebral fissure, lid lag, and staring, generally regress with treatment of hyperthyroidism. Exophthalmos, weakness of the extraocular muscles, chemosis, and impairment of convergence are signs of infiltrative ophthalmopathy and may remain despite normalization of thyroid hormone levels.

In pregnancy, the signs and symptoms of hyperthyroidism are slightly more difficult to interpret due to the normal changes that occur during gestation. Heart rate and cardiac output increase, and heat intolerance, nausea, and weight loss are common. Thyrotoxicosis is suggested by clinical findings, which include a pulse rate persistently greater than 100 that fails to decrease with val-

salva in the presence of a tremor, previously mentioned signs, thyroid bruit, thyromegaly, and mild systolic hypertension. The cardiac effects of hyperthyroidism are summarized in Table 28-2. An elevated free thyroxine and low serum thyrotropin by a sensitive assay confirm the diagnosis. Clinical signs of thyrotoxicosis without elevated total or free thyroxine should suggest free T3 thyrotoxicosis or deficient TBG states (Bitton, 1990).

*Thyroid receptor antibodies* is a generalized term that may be used to include both thyroid-stimulating immunoglobulins (TSIs) and thyrotropin-binding inhibitor immunoglobulins (TBIIs) and may be useful as a predictor of neonatal thyroid dysfunction. The nomenclature derives historically from the tests themselves. In 1956, Adams and Purves found a circulating factor in the blood of patients with Graves' disease that was more slowly acting in a guinea pig bioassay model than pituitary TSH. This factor was termed LATS (long-acting thyroid stimulator), identified as an IgG immunoglobulin and standardized using a mouse bioassay. Thyroid-stimulating immunoglobulin assays

T A B L E   **28-2**

Cardiovascular changes in hyperthyroid and hypothyroid states

| | Hyperthyroid | Hypothyroid |
|---|---|---|
| Cardiac output | ↑ | ↓ |
| Heart rate | ↑ | ↓ |
| Stroke volume | ↑ | ↓ |
| Cardiac contractility | ↑ | ↓ |
| Total peripheral resistance | ↓ | ↑ |
| Mean arterial pressure | ↑ | ↑ |
| Blood volume | ↑ | |
| Other | Atrial fibrillation | Ascites |
| | ↓QT ↑PR interval | Pleural effusion |
| | ST elevation | ↑QT interval |
| | | ↑Conduction abnormalities |

Sources: From Easterling TR, Schmucker BC, Carlson KL, et al. Maternal hemodynamics in pregnancies complicated by hyperthyroidism. Obstet Gynecol 1991;78:348; Woeber K. Thyrotoxicosis and the heart. N Engl J Med 1992;327:94; Bent GA. The molecular basis of thyroid hormone action. N Engl J Med 1994;331:847; and Dillman WH. Cardiac function in thyroid disease: clinical features and management considerations. Ann Thorac Surg 1993;56:S9–S15.

are based on the production of cAMP from human thyroid or functioning rat thyroid (FRTL5) cells. Thyrotropin-binding inhibitor immunoglobulin receptor assays measure the inhibition of TSH binding to its receptor by displacement of labeled TSH. As such, the assay does not directly measure receptor activation or thyroid activity; therefore, thyroid stimulating or thyroid inhibiting antibodies may be measured (Mortimer, 1990). Although antimicrosomal antibodies do not cross the placenta, thyroid receptor antibodies do. Consequently, neonatal thyroid effects may occur years after the diagnosis of Graves' disease, when the mother is either euthyroid or hypothyroid after radioactive thyroid ablation (Volpe, 1984).

Neonatal thyroid status may be affected transiently by either thionamide therapy or thyroid receptor antibodies. The incidence of neonatal hyper- or hypothyroidism due to maternal passive transmission of thyroid receptor antibodies appears to be 1% to 3%. Mitsuda et al (1992) reported overt thyrotoxicosis in six neonates of 230 women with Graves' disease. In four of the mothers, TBIIs were elevated. In addition, transient hypothyroidism was found in five neonates with normal TBII levels and thionamide treatment. Mortimer et al (1990) reported a higher incidence of neonatal thyrotoxicosis in four infants of 44 mothers with Graves' disease; in all four cases the mothers had TBII levels greater than 70%. These investigators observed that the neonatal free thyroxine index correlated inversely with maternal thionamide dose. In addition, women who had a free thyroxine index in the lower half of the reference range on thionamides were more likely to deliver a child with an elevated TSH than were women with a free thyroxine index in the upper half of the reference range. Similarly, Momotani et al (1986) studied 43 women maintained on thionamide therapy until delivery and 27 women in whom thionamide therapy was discontinued due to normalization of thyroid function tests prior to delivery. They found that women who took thionamides until delivery had a greater number of fetuses with increased thyrotropin levels, lower thyroxine levels, and higher maternal TBII levels. It is important to note that in both of these studies there was only evidence of mild chemical, not clinical, hypothyroidism. Taken together, however, these data suggest that the minimal dose of thionamide therapy should be used to keep maternal thyroid function at the upper limits of normal. Because TBIIs are positive, although at lower levels in 50% to 70% of women with Graves' disease (Momotani, 1986; Mortimer, 1990), their utility remains to be further demonstrated.

Wing et al (1994) found that only one infant of 185 women treated with propylthiouracil or methimazole had transient hypothyroidism at birth. Similarly, Davis et al (1989) found that one neonate had transient hypothyroidism and a second was euthyroid with an asymptomatic goiter among 43 mothers receiving propylthiouracil. Both women were on high doses of propylthiouracil at the time of delivery. This is consistent with a review of the literature by Mandel et al (1994) in which the incidence of fetal goiter in women exposed to antithyroid medications was 4%. If necessary, when fetal goiter is detected on ultrasound, umbilical cord blood sampling can be used to differentiate between maternal passive transmission of thyroid receptor antibodies or thionamide treatment (Davidson, 1991; Perelman, 1990; Nicolini, 1996). Intra-amniotic injection of thyroxine is effective in treating fetal hypothyroidism.

## Hyperemesis Gravidarum

Hyperemesis gravidarum is an unusual cause of thyrotoxicosis that rarely requires treatment with thionamides because hyperthyroidism is self-limiting (Goodwin, 1992). These investigators found that 66% of patients with hyperemesis had either an increase in free thyroxine index or suppressed TSH, although none had clinical signs of hyperthyroidism requiring therapy. Although HCG appears to stimulate the thyroid, its role in the finding of abnormal thyroid function tests in hyperemesis remains to be defined (Kennedy, 1991). Human chorionic gonadotropin levels are increased in women with hyperemesis, as are free T4 and free T3 blood levels (Kennedy, 1992). Serum from five patients with hyperemesis stimulated cAMP production in human thyroid cells, as did TSH. Sera neutralized with antibodies to HCG, however, also stimulated cAMP production in two of these patients, suggesting that HCG could not completely explain the thyroid stimulation

(Kennedy, 1992). Kimura et al (1993) studied eight patients with hyperemesis and found that HCG levels were not increased compared with controls, but the ratio of thyroid-stimulating activity to HCG was increased in sera from patients with hyperemesis. These studies used a thyroid-stimulating activity assay based on cAMP production in rat thyroid FRTL5. Taken together, these data suggest that thyroid-stimulating activity assays based on human thyroid cell lines may give different results than assays based on rat cell lines. Thus, differences between assays and/or variants in glycosylated HCG may account for thyroid-stimulating activity (Kennedy, 1991; Yoshimura, 1995).

## Thyroid Crisis or Storm

In thyroid crisis or storm, an acute increase in the signs and symptoms of thyrotoxicosis may be life-threatening. The overall incidence of thyroid crisis in women who receive thionamide treatment during pregnancy, some of whom remain thyrotoxic, is about 2% (Davis, 1989). A clinical diagnosis must be established and treatment initiated well before confirmatory thyroid function tests are available. The classic signs of thyroid storm— altered mental status, temperature greater than 41°C, hypertension, and diarrhea—are not always present. Postpartum congestive heart failure, tachycardia, and severe hypertension should suggest the diagnosis and prompt an evaluation for other signs of thyrotoxicosis. Rarely, loss of consciousness following cesarean section (Pugh, 1994) or seizures mimicking eclampsia (Mayer, 1995) may complicate the presentation of thyrotoxicosis.

The risks of thyroid storm appear to be related to metabolic status and to the precipitating cause. Pekonen et al (1978) reported that two of seven untreated thyrotoxic women in labor developed thyroid crisis. Similar results were described in eight untreated women in labor, of whom, five developed heart failure and four had stillbirths (Davis, 1989). In that series, among 16 other women who had received thionamides but were still thyrotoxic at the time of delivery, two had stillbirths and one developed heart failure, whereas there were no complications in 36 women who were euthyroid. Kriplani et al (1994) also reported three patients who developed thyroid storm, including one maternal death, among 32 patients who were hyperthyroid during pregnancy. Although thyroid functions were not detailed specifically, thyroid storm was associated with either emergent operative delivery or infection. Thionamide therapy, even of short duration, is generally effective in preventing storm. Therefore, congestive heart failure that occurs after administration of propylthiouracil should suggest other precipitating events: underlying infection, hypertension, or anemia.

The treatment of thyroid storm is somewhat empiric and consists of thionamides, iodide, and β-blockers (Singer, 1995). Therapy differs from the usual management of hyperthyroidism in the dose and choice of thionamide. Propylthiouracil and methimazole are equally effective in the treatment of hyperthyroidism in pregnancy (Wing, 1994). In the setting of thyroid storm, however, 1 g of propylthiouracil is administered by mouth or by nasogastric tube as a loading dose, and 300 mg are continued three times daily to inhibit peripheral conversion of T4 to T3. Although thyroxine synthesis is also inhibited, this is a long-term goal, because 7 to 8 weeks of therapy are required to deplete thyroid stores and normalize thyroid function tests (Davis, 1989; Wing, 1994). Clinical improvement commonly precedes resolution of the tachycardia due to the long half-life of thyroxine. Iodide, administered as either oral Lugol's solution (20–30 drops in a 24-hr period) or intravenous (IV) sodium iodide (0.5 g/12 hr), inhibits thyroid release rapidly (Tan, 1989; Wartofsky, 1970). Propranolol (1 mg IV/5 min and repeated as necessary) may be used to control autonomic symptoms. Although β-adrenergic blockade may inhibit peripheral thyroxine conversion to triiodothyronine, this does not alter thyroid release and does not prevent thyroid storm (Eriksson, 1977). Because large increases in pulmonary diastolic pressure may be precipitated (Ikram, 1985), and because congestive heart failure may be a common presentation of thyroid crisis in pregnant women, propranolol should be used with caution.

Corticosteroids (dexamethasone, 2 mg/6 hr) have been advocated to inhibit peripheral conversion of thyroxine and prevent adrenal insufficiency, but there are few data to support their use. Fever should be treated with cooling blankets or acetaminophen to decrease cardiovascular demands. Salicylate use is best avoided, because T4 and T3 may be displaced from TBG (Larsen, 1972). A thorough search for underlying infection is necessary, because pyelonephritis, endometritis, or sepsis are common. Because of the increased incidence of atrial arrhythmias and CNS emboli, thromboembolic disease should be considered in patients with altered mental status that does not respond to the aforementioned therapy (Woeber, 1992). If the pregnancy is continued, iodide treatment should be stopped when there is clinical improvement, to avoid the risk of congenital goiter. Propylthiouracil may be continued safely in breastfeeding women if the total dosage does not exceed 300 mg/day (Cooper, 1987). Complications of propylthiouracil or methimazole include chemical hepatitis, rash, or other drug reactions (5%) and agranulocytosis (0.3%) (Cooper, 1983). Because of the seriousness of the latter, patients with fever or sore throat should be instructed to discontinue medication until a WBC count is checked. Agranulocytosis, as defined by a total leukocyte count of less than 1000/μL or a granulocyte count of less than 250/μL, is generally seen in older patients and within 2 months of the onset of therapy (Cooper, 1983).

Thyroid hormones are known to affect both the myocardium and the systemic vasculature; the cause of thyrotoxic heart failure, however, is still controversial. Despite parallels to catecholamine excess, catecholamine levels and secretion rates of norepinephrine are not altered in thyrotoxicosis (Coulombe, 1977; Levey, 1990), and when thyroid hormone concentrations have been measured in thyroid storm, they do not differ from those of thyrotoxic patients (Jacobs, 1973). Exogenous T3 administration in the pig as well as other species does produce eccentric cardiac hypertrophy and an increase in β-adrenergic receptors that is reversible when therapy is discontinued (Hammond, 1987). The increase in β-adrenergic receptors, however, does not necessarily produce an increase in sensitivity of the heart to catecholamines (Woeber, 1992).

Thyroid hormones also increase myocardial myosin isozyme adenosine triphosphatase (ATPase) activity and sarcoplasmic reticulum calcium ATPase, increasing cardiac contractility and heat production (Dillman, 1989). Molecular mechanisms include an increase in cardiac myosin heavy-chain alpha levels and a decrease in myosin heavy-chain beta levels; the myosin heavy-chain alpha form has a greater ATPase activity and velocity of muscle-fiber shortening (Dillman, 1993; Bent, 1994). It has been suggested that because a larger portion of adenosine triphosphate is expended in heat, contractile efficiency is actually decreased (Dillman, 1990). It is also possible that as cardiac work increases due to increases in stroke volume, afterload, and heat production, contractile reserve may be limited (Woeber, 1992). This would help explain the observation that left ventricular ejection fraction is increased at rest in thyrotoxicosis but decreases with exercise (Fofar, 1982). Similarly, in patients with thyrotoxic heart disease, cardiac index falls and systemic vascular resistance increases markedly with exercise. This effect is reversible, because after thionamide therapy, left ventricle ejection fraction again increases in response to exercise (Fofar, 1982). It is important to note that responses of the left ventricle are not normalized with propranolol alone and require normalization of thyroid hormone levels.

The similarities of thyrotoxicosis and pregnancy are striking. Both demonstrate increased blood volume, cardiac output, stroke volume, heart rate, and decreased systemic vascular resistance (Woeber, 1992). Venous compliance in thyrotoxicosis, however, is decreased (Gay, 1987, 1988). Venous constriction superimposed on an increased maternal blood volume might be expected to further increase venous return. Consequently, labor (exercise) as well as the well-known volume shifts that occur with delivery may explain the increased incidence of heart failure seen in pregnant women. Despite this, congestive heart failure, when it presents as thyroid storm, is rapidly reversible when treated with propylthiouracil, iodide, and lasix, as demonstrated in Figure 28-5 (Davis, 1989; Clark, 1985). Gaeza (1995) described

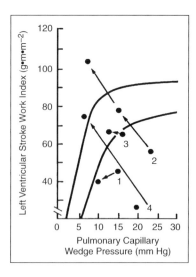

F I G U R E   **28-5**

Data obtained from pulmonary artery catheterization in four pregnant women with thyrotoxicosis and heart failure plotted on a Braunwald ventricular function curve. Values for normal function lie between the two curved lines. Proximal points on the arrows represent initial results, and second points were obtained 24 hours later. (Reproduced by permission from Davis LE, Lucas MJ, Hankins GDV, et al. Thyrotoxicosis complicating pregnancy. Am J Obstet Gynecol 1989;160:63.)

a rapid method of stabilization for hyperthyroid patients requiring surgery.

## Hypothyroidism

Overt hypothyroidism during pregnancy is uncommon because many women are anovulatory. The most common cause is prior surgical thyroidectomy or radioiodine ablation, or autoimmune thyroiditis. Clinical signs and symptoms include delayed deep tendon reflexes, fatigue, weight gain, cold intolerance, hair loss, dry skin, brawny edema, thickened tongue, hoarse voice, hypertension, and bradycardia, some of which are more difficult to ascertain during pregnancy. The hemodynamic changes of hypothyroidism are summarized in Table 28-2. Of note, hyponatremia, ascites, pericardial effusions, or psychosis are not commonly present and may herald myxedema coma. Laboratory confirmation of hypothyroidism can be established by a low free T4 in the presence of an elevated TSH.

Although earlier studies suggested an increase in congenital anomalies, perinatal mortality, and infant neurologic dysfunction, more recently, better outcomes have been obtained (Leung, 1993; Wasserstrum, 1995). Leung et al (1993) studied 23 women with overt hypothyroidism and 45 women with subclinical hypothyroidism (elevated TSH level with a normal thyroxine index). One stillbirth occurred in an untreated, overtly hypothyroid patient who was also eclamptic. Other than one infant with clubfeet, neonatal outcomes were satisfactory. Preeclampsia, pregnancy-induced hypertension, and eclampsia were common in women who were not yet euthyroid at delivery (9/30 subjects). In another study of 16 pregnancies in overtly hypothyroid women and 12 cases of subclinical hypothyroidism, complications were more common in overtly hypothyroid women, including postpartum hemorrhage (3/16), anemia, preeclampsia (7/16), and placental abruption (3/16) (Davis, 1988). In addition, two women had evidence of cardiac dysfunction, one of whom developed congestive heart failure. Prolonged bleeding times in hypothyroid patients are known to normalize with thyroxine replacement (Myrup, 1995). The etiology of the increase in abruption was probably secondary to the higher incidence of chronic hypertension in hypothyroid patients; hypertension is reversible following thyroid replacement in nonpregnant patients (Bing, 1980).

Cardiac dysfunction, although rare, is of particular importance in an acute setting. As discussed earlier, the relationship of thyroid hormones to cardiac function is complex. Indices of cardiac contractility, left ventricular–developed pressure, and the maximal rate of left ventricular–developed pressure, as well as cardiac $Na^+K^+ATPase$ activity are less in a thyroidectomized rat model (Galinanes, 1994). These effects, along with the increase in systemic vascular resistance and afterload in hypothyroidism, as well as volume changes at delivery, may lead to cardiac dysfunction.

As mentioned previously, thyroid replacement doses may increase during pregnancy. Mandel et al (1990) found it necessary to increase the mean thyroxine dose from 102 to 147 μg/day in nine of 12 patients in order to normalize thyrotropin levels. Another group of investigators studied 35 pregnancies, noting that only 20% of women required an increase in thyroxine dosage (Girling, 1992). Because of the advantages of treating subclinical thyroid disease (Toft, 1994), TSH measurements should be used to guide replacement. In acutely hypothyroid patients, pure thyroxine is used for replacement rather than mixtures of T4 and T3 (desiccated thyroid and liotrix) to better control side effects. Caution should be taken in overtly hypothyroid patients with a history of heart disease; replacement is started at 50 μg/day initially and increased progressively to avoid angina.

## Myxedema Coma

Myxedema coma is an extremely rare life-threatening disorder with a mortality of 15% to 20%. The clinical presentation, as reviewed by Jordan (1995), can include coma, respiratory hypoventilation with carbon dioxide retention, hypothermia, bradycardia, hyponatremia, hypoglycemia, and often the presence of an associated infection, most commonly urosepsis. Therapy includes mechanical ventilation to correct hypoxia or hypercarbia, thyroxine replacement in larger doses initially (400 μg IV, followed by 50 μg daily), steroids, passive rewarming to slowly increase body temperature, and correction of hypotension if present. Correction of hyponatremia by fluid restriction or cautious use of hypertonic saline may be necessary. As in thyroid storm, a thorough search for an infectious precipitating event is necessary. Laboratory tests are the same as for hypothyroidism, with the exception that TSH levels may be suppressed (euthyroid sick syndrome). Obtundation in the presence of hypothyroidism suggests the diagnosis.

## Hypoparathyroidism

Hypocalcemia caused by hypoparathyroidism is an extremely rare disorder in pregnancy. The most common cause of hypoparathyroidism is absent parathyroid hormone (PTH) because of excision of the parathyroid gland, usually following thyroidectomy. Although total calcium concentrations decrease in pregnancy, ionized calcium does not (Pitkin, 1985; Seki, 1991). In response to hypocalcemia, PTH normally increases, which in turn augments renal tubular calcium reabsoption and phosphate excretion. Parathyroid hormone also increases 25-hydroxyvitamin D transformation to the active hormone 1,25-dihydroxyvitamin D, which stimulates intestinal calcium and phosphate absorption as well as osteoclastic bone resorption. Apparently, ineffective PTH syndromes may be caused by failure to respond to increased PTH (pseudohypoparathyroidism), deficient vitamin D from malabsorption, or increased vitamin D metabolism seen with phenytoin or other anticonvulsants (Potts, 1991; Zalonga, 1989). Other causes of hypocalcemia include massive citrated blood transfusions (generally transient); alkalosis, with increased ionized calcium binding to albumin; increased phosphate in renal failure; pancreatitis; sepsis; and hypo- or hypermagnesemia (Rebar, 1995). The hypocalcemia of respiratory alkalosis is rarely clinically important, although metabolic alkalosis secondary to bicarbonate administration can be significant. Seriously ill patients often may have depressed total calcium levels; however, the frequency of hypocalcemia when corrected for hypoalbuminemia or when ionized calcium is evaluated is approximately 10% (Potts, 1991).

Chronic candidiasis, alopecia, vitiligo, and multiple endocrinopathies should suggest the autoimmune polyendocrinopathy-candidiasis-ectodermal dystrophy syndrome (Ahonen, 1990). Perioral paresthesias, psychiatric disturbances, and Chvostek's or Trousseau's sign may be present. Trousseau's sign, also known as "the obstetrician's hand," or carpal spasm due to ulnar and median nerve ischemia is elicited by inflating a sphygmomanometer cuff around the arm to 20 mm Hg above systolic pressures (Cain, 1973). The thumb adducts and the fingers are extended, except at the metacarpophalangeal joints, within minutes, indicating latent tetany. Cardiac changes of hypocalcemia are nonspecific but include ECG Q-T prolongation, hypotension, and reversible congestive cardiomyopathy (Csanady, 1990; Zalonga, 1989). Hypopharyngeal tetany may present

as stridor and seizures and may be life-threatening. Magnesium sulfate rarely has been implicated in hypocalcemia and should be used cautiously when preeclampsia is superimposed on hypoparathyroidism (Eisenbud, 1976). If Dilantin is used, it also may increase vitamin D metabolism. In one case, decreased fetal heart rate variability was reported, although there was no evidence of acidosis (Hagay, 1986). Secondary fetal or neonatal hyperparathyroidism, bone demineralization, skeletal and skull fractures have been reported.

Medical treatment of hypocalcemia can be divided into long-term and acute management. Vitamin D (50,000–100,000 units/day) or 1,25-dihydroxyvitamin D (calcitriol 0.5–3.0 μg/day) and 1 to 2 g of elemental calcium daily have been used successfully in pregnancy (Pitkin, 1985). Vitamin D2 is the least expensive form of vitamin D, but several weeks may be needed for its full effect. Calcitriol has a faster onset of action (1–2 days) but requires more frequent monitoring to prevent hypercalcemia. Requirements during pregnancy may increase in the latter half of pregnancy, presumably due to increased vitamin D–binding protein. It is often necessary to reduce replacement doses in the postpartum period to avoid hypercalcemia, even in women who are breastfeeding (Caplan, 1990). The latter require closer monitoring of calcium levels, because it may be difficult to predict calcium needs during lactation. Of interest, in some species (cattle in particular), the onset of lactation can result in hypocalcemia and parturient paresis (Goff, 1989).

Acute hypocalcemia or impending signs of tetany are treated by 10% calcium gluconate (10 mL diluted in 150 mL of D5W over 10 min), followed by continuous infusions of calcium (0.5–2.0 mg/kg/hr). Serial calcium measurements should be measured initially every 2 to 4 hours to assess the adequacy of the administered dose and adjust the infusion rate accordingly (Rebar, 1995). Laboratory evaluation in addition to ionized calcium should include magnesium, phosphorus, and PTH levels. Hypoparathyroidism is diagnosed by a normal serum magnesium, low or inappropriately normal PTH level, and low ionized calcium. High PTH and low phosphorus levels suggest vitamin D deficiency, whereas high

PTH and high phosphorus levels are consistent with the diagnosis of pseudohypoparathyroidism or renal insufficiency.

## Hyperparathyroidism

Approximately 120 cases of primary hyperparathyroidism have been reported during pregnancy. This is less than the expected incidence because primary hyperparathyroidism in women of childbearing age occurs at a rate of eight new cases per 100,000 per year (Carella, 1992). The discrepancy is, in part, due to the asymptomatic nature of most cases of hyperparathyroidism. In one series (Gelister, 1989), 10 of 15 women were diagnosed postpartum following the presentation of neonatal tetany.

The diagnosis of hyperparathyroidism is suggested by fasting hypercalcemia and inappropriately elevated PTH and urinary cAMP levels. Women with primary hyperparathyroidism who are pregnant have biochemical parameters similar to those of women with hyperparathyroidism who are not pregnant (Ammann, 1993). In normal gestation, PTH levels, when measured by newer two-site immunoradiometric assays, are stable or slightly lower in the second trimester, refuting earlier studies of elevated PTH levels (Seki, 1991; Kohlmeier, 1995; Seely, 1997). In addition, the acquisition by the fetus of 25 to 30 g of calcium as well, as the increase in glomerular filtration rate, expanded extracellular fluid volume, and reduced serum albumin levels, results in an overall decrease in total serum calcium levels of 0.5 mg/dL (Pitkin, 1985). Ionized calcium levels are not affected. Thus, repeatedly elevated PTH levels in the presence of increased ionized calcium, or total calcium adjusted for albumin, must be considered significant.

When hyperparathyroidism is diagnosed, a search for multiple endocrine neoplasia is indicated. Most nonparathyroid causes of hypercalcemia are associated with suppression of PTH and urinary cAMP levels. Nonparathyroid causes of hypercalcemia include malignancy (breast, myeloma, lymphoma), hypocalciuric hypercalcemia (familial, thiazides, lithium), granulomatous disease (sarcoidosis, tuberculosis), thyrotoxicosis,

drug-induced causes (hypervitaminosis D or A, calcium, milk-alkali syndrome), adrenal insufficiency, and immobilization. Hypercalcemia secondary to PTH-related protein produced by breast tissue during pregnancy and lactation with normal PTH levels has also been reported (Lepre, 1993). A history should include the use of over-the-counter vitamin preparations and other medications.

Parathyroid adenomas account for 89% of primary hyperparathyroidism, 9% are due to parathyroid hyperplasia, and 2% to parathyroid cancer (Kelly, 1991). The most common signs and symptoms, when present, include nausea or vomiting, fatigue, mental disturbances, nephrolithiasis, pancreatitis, and bone pain (Carella, 1992; Kristoffersson, 1985). Hypercalcemic crisis is characterized by progressive hypercalcemia with hypovolemia, renal insufficiency, altered mentation, and pancreatitis in the most severe cases. Rarely, seizures from hypercalcemia may mimic eclampsia (Whalley, 1963).

There is no satisfactory medical treatment for primary hyperparathyroidism during pregnancy. Mithramycin and bisphosphonates are contraindicated. Asymptomatic patients with mild hypercalcemia can be followed closely through pregnancy, with surgery deferred until after delivery (Croom, 1984; Gelister, 1989; Hill, 1989). Occasionally, patients with significant symptoms from hypercalcemia but are not surgical candidates have been controlled safely and effectively with oral phosphate therapy (1.5 g/day in divided doses) throughout gestation (Montoro, 1980). This therapy is only indicated in patients in whom the initial serum phosphorus level is less than 3 mg/dL; phosphate administration should be adjusted to maintain the serum phosphate below 4 mg/dL. In contrast, patients with progressive symptoms, significant hypercalcemia ($>12$ mg/dL), or deterioration of renal function should be treated surgically by an experienced parathyroid surgeon (Kelly, 1991; Carella, 1992). Neck exploration should not be deferred in the symptomatic woman because of pregnancy, unless delivery is imminent.

Medical management for stabilization in hypercalcemic crisis includes hydration with normal saline (2–3 liters over 3–6 hr); correction of

---

## THYROID STORM

**I. Goals of Therapy**

   A.  Control hyperthyroid state by blocking release of thyroxine and peripheral conversion of thyroxine to triiodothyronine

   B.  Prevent congestive heart failure

**II. Management Protocol**

   A.  One gram of propylthiouracil by mouth or nasogastric tube, followed by 300 mg every 8 hours

   B.  Iodide, oral Lugol's solution 20 to 30 drops in a 24-hr period, or IV sodium iodide, 0.5 g/12 hr

   C.  Dexamethasone, 2 mg/6 hr

   D.  Propranolol 1 mg IV/5 min

   E.  Search for precipitating event and, in particular, infection

   F.  Control temperature if hyperthermic

**III. Critical Laboratory Tests**

   A.  Free T4, TSH, ECG (atrial fibrillation), urine culture, chest x-ray, if indicated. Evaluate for other autoimmune disorders.

**IV. Consultation**

   A.  Endocrinology, internal medicine

---

electrolyte abnormalities; furosemide, which decreases distal tubular calcium reabsorption (10–40 mg IV every 2–4 hr) to maintain urine output at 200 mL/hr, and calcium restriction. Hypercalcemia that is resistant to this regimen may be alleviated with more potent agents, such as calcitonin (100–400 units/day). Although effective initially, tachyphyllaxis to calcitonin generally occurs in 4 to 6 days. Glucocorticocoids can be used to decrease gastrointestinal calcium absorption.

In hyperparathyroid mothers, neonatal hypocalcemia is predictable and can be prevented. Transient neonatal tetany should not be associated with long-term sequelae. Management of maternal hyperparathyroidism diagnosed during pregnancy should be individualized, taking into consideration the patient's symptoms, the gestational age of the fetus, and the severity of the disease.

**REFERENCES**

Adams D, Purves H. Abnormal responses in the assay of thyrotropin. Otago Med School Proc 1956; 34:11.

Ahonen P, Myllarniemi S, Sipila I, et al. Clinical variation of autoimmmune polyendocrinopathy-candidiasis-ectodermal dystrophy (apeced) in a series of 68 patients. N Engl J Med 1990;322: 1829.

Amino N, Kuro R, Tanizawa O, et al. Changes of serum anti-thyroid antibodies during and after pregnancy in autoimmune thyroid diseases. Clin Exp Immunol 1978;31:30.

Amino N, Tanizawa O, Mori H, et al. Aggravation of thyrotoxicosis in early pregnancy and after delivery in Graves' disease. J Clin Endocrinol Metab 1982;55:108.

Amman P, Irion O, Gast J, et al. Alterations of calcium and phosphate metabolism in primary hyperparathyroidism during pregnancy. Acta Obstet Gynecol Scand 1993;72(6):488–492.

Bent GA. The molecular basis of thyroid hormone action. N Engl J Med 1994;331:847.

Berghout A, Endert E, Ross A, et al. Thyroid function and thyroid size in normal pregnant women living in an iodine replete area. Clin Endocrinol (Oxf) 1994;41:375.

Bing RF, Briggs RSJ, Burden AC, et al. Reversible hypertension and hypothyroidism. Clin Endocrinol (Oxf) 1980;13:339.

Bitton RN, Wexler C. Free triiodothyronine toxicosis: a distinct entity. Am J Med 1990;88:531.

Burrow GN. The management of thyrotoxicosis in pregnancy. N Engl J Med 1985;313:562.

Burrow GN, Fisher DA, Larsen PR. Maternal and fetal thyroid function. N Engl J Med 1994;331:1072.

Cain A. The thyroid gland. In: Hamilton Bailey's demonstrations of physical signs in clinical surgery. 15th ed. Bristol: Wright, 1973:164.

Caplan RH, Beguin EA. Hypercalcemia in a calcitriol-treated hypoparathyroid woman during lactation. Obstet Gynecol 1990;76:485.

Carella MJ, Gossain VV. Hyperparathyroidism and pregnancy. J Gen Intern Med 1992;7:448.

Clark SL, Phelan JP, Montoro M, et al. Transient ventricular dysfunction associated with cesarean section in a patient with hyperthyroidism. Am J Obstet Gynecol 1985;151:384.

Cooper DS. Antithyroid drugs: to breast-feed or not to breast-feed. Am J Obstet Gynecol 1987;157:234.

Cooper DS, Goldminz D, Levin A, et al. Agranulocytosis associated with antithyroid drugs. Ann Intern Med 1983;98:26.

Coulombe P, Dussault JH, Walker P. Catecholamine metabolism in thyroid disease: II. Norepinephrine secretion rate in hyperthyroidism and hypothyroidism. J Clin Endocrinol Metab 1977;44:1185.

Croom RD, Thomas CG. Primary hyperparathyroidism during pregnancy. Surgery 1984;96:1109.

Csanady M, Forster T, Julesz J. Reversible impairment of myocardial function in hypoparathyroidism causing hypocalcaemia. Br Heart J 1990;63:58.

Davidson KM, Richards DS, Schatz DA, et al. Successful in utero treatment of fetal goiter and hypothyroidism. N Engl J Med 1991;324:543.

Davis LE, Leveno KJ, Cunningham FG. Hypothyroidism complicating pregnancy. Obstet Gynecol 1988;72:108.

Davis LE, Lucas MJ, Hankins GDV, et al. Thyrotoxicosis complicating pregnancy. Am J Obstet Gynecol 1989;160:63.

DeGroot L, Larsen PR, Refetoff S, Stanbury JB, eds. In: Hormone synthesis, secretion and action. The thyroid and its diseases. New York: Wiley, 1984:76.

Dillman WH. Diabetes and thyroid hormone induced changes in cardiac function and their molecular basis. Annu Rev Med 1989:373.

Dillman WH. Biochemical basis of thyroid hormone action in the heart. Am J Med 1990;88:626.

Dillman WH. Cardiac function in thyroid disease: clinical features and management considerations. Ann Thorac Surg 1993;56:S9–S15.

Doherty CM, Shindo ML, Rice DH, et al. Management of thyroid nodules during pregnancy. Laryngoscope 1995;105:251.

Easterling TR, Schmucker BC, Carlson KL, et al. Maternal hemodynamics in pregnancies complicated by hyperthyroidism. Obstet Gynecol 1991;78:348.

Eisenbud E, BoBue C. Hypocalcemia after therapeutic use of magnesium sulfate. Arch Intern Med 1976;136:688.

Epstein RH. Pathogenesis of Graves' ophthalmopathy. N Engl J Med 1993;329:1468.

Eriksson M, Rubenfeld S, Garber AJ, et al. Propranolol does not prevent thyroid storm. N Engl J Med 1977;296:263.

Fisher DA, Klein AH. Thyroid development and disorders of thyroid function in the newborn. N Engl J Med 1981;304:702.

Fofar JC, Muir AL, Sawers SA, et al. Abnormal left ventricular function in hyperthyroidism. N Engl J Med 1982;307:1165.

Gay R, Lee RW, Appleton C, et al. Control of cardiac function and venous return in thyrotoxic calves. Am J Physiol 1987;252:H467.

Gay RG, Raya TE, Lancaster LD, et al. Effects of thyroid state on venous compliance and left ventricular performance in rats. Am J Physiol 1988; 254:H81.

Gaeza A, Aguayo J, Barria M, et al. Rapid preoperative preparation in hyperthyroidism. Clin Endocrinol (Oxf) 1991;35:439.

Galinanes M, Smolenski R, Haddock P, et al. Early effects of hypothyroidism on the contractile function of the rat heart and its tolerance to hypothermic ischemia. J Thorac Cardiovasc Surg 1994;107:829.

Gelister JSK, Sanderson JD, Chapple CR, et al. Management of hyperparathyroidism in pregnancy. Br J Surg 1989;76:1207.

Girling JC, de Swiet M. Thyroxine dosage during pregnancy in women with primary hypothyroidism. Br J Obstet Gynaecol 1992;99:368.

Glinoer D, De Nayer P, Delange F, et al. A randomized trial for the treatment of mild iodine deficiency during pregnancy: Maternal and fetal effects. J Clin Endocrinol Metab 1995;80:258.

Glinoer D, De Mayer P, Bourdoux P, et al. Regulation of maternal thyroid during pregnancy. J Clin Endocrinol Metab 1990;71:276.

Goff JP, Reinhard TA, Horst RL. Recurring hypocalcemia of bovine parturient paresis is associated with failure to produce 1,25-dihydroxyvitamin D. Endocrinology 1989;125:49.

Goodwin TM, Montoro M, Mestman J. Transient hyperthyroidism and hyperemesis gravidarum: clinical aspects. Am J Obstet Gynecol 1992;167: 648.

Hagay ZJ, Mazor M, Lieberman JR, Piura B. The effect of maternal hypocalcemia on fetal heart rate baseline variability. Acta Obstet Gynecol Scand 1986;65:513.

Hammond HK, White FC, Buxton IL, et al. Increased myocardial B-receptors and adrenergic responses in hyperthyroid pigs. Am J Physiol 1987; 252:H283.

Hedberg CW, Fishbein DB, Janssen RS, et al. An outbreak of thyrotoxicosis caused by the consumption of bovine thyroid gland in ground beef. N Engl J Med 1987;316:993.

Hermann M, Richteer B, Roka R, et al. Thyroid surgery in untreated severe hyperthyroidism: perioperative kinetics of free thyroid hormones in the glandular venous effluent and peripheral blood. Surgery 1994;115:240–245.

Hill NCW, Lloyd-Davies SV, Bishop A, et al. Primary hyperparathyroidism and pregnancy. Int J Gynaecol Obstet 1989;29:253.

Ikram H. The nature and prognosis of thyrotoxic heart disease Q J Med 1985;54:19.

Jacobs HS, Eastman CJ, Ekins RP, et al. Total and free triiodothyronine and thyroxine levels in thyroid storm and recurrent hyperthyroidism. Lancet 1973;2:236.

Jordan RM. Myxedema coma. Med Clin North Am 1995;79:185.

Kelly TR. Primary hyperparathyroidism during pregnancy. Surgery 1991;110:1028.

Kendall-Taylor P. Investigation of thyrotoxicosis. Clin Endocrinol (Oxf) 1995;42:309.

Kennedy R, Darne J, Davies R, Price A. Thyrotoxicosis and hyperemesis gravidarum associated with a serum activity which stimulates human thyroid cells in vitro. Clin Endocrinol (Oxf) 1992; 36:83–89.

Kennedy R, Darne J. The role of hCG in regulation of the thyroid gland in normal and abnormal pregnancy. Obstet Gynecol 1991;78:298.

Kimura M, Amino N, Tamaki H, et al. Gestation thyrotoxicosis and hyperemesis gravidarum: possible role of hCG with higher stimulating activity. Clin Endocrinol (Oxf) 1993;38:343–350.

Kohlmeier L, Marcus R. Calcium disorders of pregnancy. Endocrinol Metab Clin North Am 1995; 24:15.

Kriplani A, Buckshee K, Bhargava VL, et al. Maternal and perinatal outcome in thyrotoxicosis complicating pregnancy. Eur J Obstet Gynecol Reprod Biol 1994;54:159.

Kristoffersson A, Dahlgren S, Lithner F, et al. Primary hyperparathyroidism in pregnancy. Surgery 1985;97:326.

Larsen P. Salicylate-induced increases in free triiodothyronine in human serum. J Clin Invest 1972;51: 1125.

Lepre F, Gril V, Martin TJ, et al. Hypercalcemia in pregnancy and lactation associated with parathyroid hormone-related protein. N Engl J Med 1993;328:666.

Leung AS, Millar LK, Koonings PP, et al. Perinatal outcome in hypothyroid pregnancies. Obstet Gynecol 1993;81:349.

Levey GS. Catecholamine-thyroid hormone interactions and the cardiovascular manifestations of hyperthyroidism. Am J Med 1990;88:642.

Mandel SJ, Larsen RP, Seely EW, et al. Increased need for thyroxine during pregnancy in women with primary hypothyroidism. N Engl J Med 1990;323:91.

Mandel SJ, Brent GA, Larsen PR. Review of antithyroid drug use during pregnancy and report of a case of aplasia cutis. Thyroid 1994;4:129.

Mayer DC, Thorp J, Baucom D, et al. Hyperthyroidism and seizures during pregnancy. Am J Perinatol 1995;12:192.

Mazzaferri EL. Evaluation and management of common thyroid disorders in women. Am J Obstet Gynecol 1997;176:507.

Mestman JH, Manning PR, Hodgman J. Hyperthyroidism and pregnancy. Arch Intern Med 1974; 134:434.

Millar LK, Wing DA, Leung AS, et al. Low birth weight and preeclampsia in pregnancies complicated by hyperthyroidism. Obstet Gynecol 1994;84: 946.

Mitsuda N, Tamaki H, Amino N, et al. Risk factors for developmental disorders in infants born to women with Graves' disease. Obstet Gynecol 1992;80:359–364.

Momotani N, Noh J, Oyanagi H, et al. Antithyroid drug therapy for Graves' disease during pregnancy: Optimal regimen for fetal thyroid status. N Engl J Med 1986;315:24.

Montoro MN, Collear JV, Mestman JH. Management of hyperparathyroidism in pregnancy with oral phosphate therapy. Obstet Gynecol 1980;55:431.

Mortimer RH, Tyuack SA, Galligan JP, et al. Graves' disease in pregnancy: TSH receptor binding inhibiting immunoglobulins and maternal and neonatal thyroid function. Clin Endocrinol 1990; 32:141.

Myrup B, Bregengard C, Faber J. Primary haemostasis in thyroid disease. J Intern Med 1995;238:59–63.

Nicolini V, Venegoni E, Acaia B, et al. Prenatal treatment of fetal hypothyroidism: is there more than one option? Prenatal Diagnosis 1996; 16:443.

Pekary AE, Jackson IM, Goodwin TM, et al. Increased in vitro thyrotropic activity of partially sialated human chorionic gonadotropin extracted from hydatidiform moles of patients with hyperthyroidism. Int J Clin Endocrinol Metab 1993; 76:70.

Pekonen F, Lamberg BA, Ikonen E. Thyrotoxicosis and pregnancy. An analysis of 43 pregnancies in 42 thyrotoxic mothers. Ann Chir Gynaecol 1978;67:1.

Perelman AH, Johnson RL, Clemons RD, et al. Intrauterine diagnosis and treatment of fetal goitrous hypothyroidism. J Clin Endocrinol Metab 1990; 71:618.

Pitkin RM. Calcium metabolism in pregnancy and the perinatal period. A review. Am J Obstet Gynecol 1985;151:99.

Potts JT. Diseases of the parathyroid gland and other hyper- and hypocalcemic disorders. In: Isselbacher KJ, Braunwald E, Wilson JD, et al, eds. Harrison's principles of internal medicine. 12th ed. New York: McGraw-Hill, 1994:2151.

Pugh S, Lalwani K, Awal A. Case report: thyroid storm as a cause of loss of consciousness following anaesthesia for emergency caesarean section. Anaesthesia 1994;49:35–37.

Radunovic N, Dumez Y, Nastic D, et al. Thyroid function in fetus and mother during the second half of normal pregnancy. Biol Neonate 1991;59:139–148.

Rebar PM, Heath H. Hypocalcemic emergencies. Med Clin North Am 1995;79:93–106.

Ruiz De Ona C, Obregon MJ, Escobar Del Rey F, et al. Developmental changes in rat brain 5'-deiodinase and thyroid hormones during the fetal period: the effects of fetal hypothyroidism and maternal thyroid hormones. Pediatr Res 1988;24:588–594.

Seely EW, Brown EM, DeMaggio DM, et al. A prospective study of calcitropic hormones in pregnancy and postpartum: reciprocal changes in serum intact parathyroid hormone and 1,25-dihydroxyvitamin D. Am J Obstet Gynecol 1997;776:214.

Seki K, Makimura N, Mitsui C, et al. Calcium-regulating hormones and osteocalcin levels during pregnancy: a longitudinal study. Am J Obstet Gynecol 1991;164:1248.

Singer PA, Cooper DS, Levy EG, et al. Treatment guidelines for patients with hyperthyroidism and hypothyroidism. JAMA 1995;273:808.

Surks MI, Chopra IJ, Mariash CN, et al. American Thyroid Association guidelines for use of laboratory tests in thyroid disorders. JAMA 1990;263:1529.

Tan TT, Morat P, Ng ML, et al. Effects of Lugol's solution on thyroid function in normals and patients with untreated thyrotoxicosis. Clin Endocrinol (Oxf) 1989;30:645.

Thorpe-Beeston J, Guy, Nicolaides KH, et al. Maturation of the secretion of thyroid hormone and thyroid stimulating hormone in the fetus. N Engl J Med 1991;324:532–536.

Toft AD. Thyroxine therapy. N Engl J Med 1994;331:174.

Volpe R, Ehrlich R, Steiner G, et al. Graves' disease in pregnancy years after hypothyroidism with recurrent passive-transfer neonatal Graves' disease in offspring. Therapeutic considerations. Am J Med 1984;77:572–578.

Volpe R. Graves' disease. In: Braverman LE, Utiger RD, eds. Werner and Ingbar. The thyroid. Philadelphia: Lippincott, 1991:648.

Vulsma T, Gons MH, de Vijlder JM. Maternal-fetal transfer of thyroxine in congenital hypothyroidism due to a total organification defect or thyroid agenesis. N Engl J Med 1989;321:13.

Wartofsky L, Ransil B, Ingbar S. Inhibition by iodine of the release of thyroxine from the thyroid gland of patients with thyrotoxicosis. J Clin Invest 1970;49:78.

Wasserstrum N, Anania CA. Perinatal consequences of maternal hypothyroidism in early pregnancy and inadequate replacement. Clin Endocrinol (Oxf) 1995;42:353.

Whalley PJ. Hyperparathyroidism and pregnancy. Am J Obstet Gynecol 1963;86:517.

Wing DA, Millar LK, Koonings PP, et al. A comparison of propylthiouracil versus methimazole in the treatment of hyperthyroidism in pregnancy. Am J Obstet Gynecol 1994;170:90.

Woeber K. Thyrotoxicosis and the heart. N Engl J Med 1992;327:94.

Xue-Yi C, Xin-Min J, Zhi-Hong D, et al. Timing of vulnerability of the brain to iodine deficiency in endemic cretinism. N Engl J Med 1994;331:1739.

Yoshimura M, Hershman JM. Thyrotropic action of human chorionic gonadotropin. Thyroid 1995;5:425.

Zalonga GP, Eil C. Diseases of the parathyroid glands and nephrolithiasis during pregnancy. In: Brody SA, Ueland K, Kase N, eds. Endocrine disorders in pregnancy. Norwalk, CT: Appleton and Lange, 1989:231.

# CHAPTER 29

# Disseminated Intravascular Coagulation

Disseminated intravascular coagulopathy (DIC) exists whenever intravascular activation of the clotting mechanism results in excess consumption of at least the soluble components of coagulation. Disseminated intravascular coagulopathy is an intermediary manifestation of disease, not a disease in itself. As such, it is usually seen in association with well-defined clinical disorders (Bick, 1994a).

Disseminated intravascular coagulopathy occurs in all areas of medicine and can evoke different connotations to different practitioners due to its varied clinical presentation. It was described as a "consumptive coagulopathy" in the early literature (Rodriquez-Erdman, 1965; Lasch, 1967). Other descriptions have included defibrination syndrome (Mersky, 1967; Dubber, 1967) and defibrinogenation syndrome (Bick, 1994a).

Disseminated intravascular coagulopathy is a thrombohemorrhagic disorder (Marder, 1990) with concurrent activation of the coagulation and fibrinolytic pathways, resulting in simultaneous fibrin clot formation and lysis. Small vessels are occluded by microthrombi, leading directly to tissue ischemia. This is exacerbated further by a concomitant bleeding diathesis from the combination of thrombocytopenia, loss of clotting factors, fibrinolysis, and interference by fibrin degradation products (Gilbert, 1993).

It is imperative to remember that DIC is always a result of an underlying disease process. Table 29-1 lists conditions often associated with DIC. Several disorders are unique to pregnancy: placental abruption, septic abortion, intrauterine fetal demise (IUFD), amniotic fluid embolism (AFE), acute fatty liver of pregnancy, and induced abortion. In this chapter, general concepts, diagnosis, and treatment of DIC are reviewed and the more common causes of DIC in pregnancy are discussed.

## Normal Hemostasis

The successful treatment of DIC requires an understanding of the physiologic mechanisms involved. Figure 29-1 illustrates many of the mechanisms by which a number of unrelated disorders might trigger DIC.

Under normal circumstances, endothelial abnormalities, platelet degranulation, or tissue disruption causes activation of either the intrinsic or extrinsic clotting cascade. Ultimately, thrombin converts fibrinogen to fibrin and activates factor IX, which polymerizes a fibrin monomer to an insoluble dimer (Wessler, 1984).

Activation of coagulation is balanced by the activity of anticlotting mechanisms. Antithrombin III (AT III) is a naturally circulating anticoagulant that forms a complex with heparin, which then neutralizes generated thrombin and blocks factors IXa, Xa, XIa, and XIIa (Savelieva, 1995).

Protein C is a vitamin K–dependent protein that has anticoagulant and fibrinolytic properties.

T A B L E 29-1

Conditions associated with disseminated intravascular coagulopathy

| *Obstetrics* | *Trauma/Tissue Injury* |
|---|---|
| Abruptio placenta | Massive hemorrhage |
| Preeclampsia/eclampsia | Burns |
| Intrauterine fetal demise | *Intravascular Hemolysis* |
| Induced abortion | Hemolytic transfusion reaction |
| Acute fatty liver of pregnancy | Multiple transfusions |
| Amniotic fluid embolism | *Cardiovascular and Pulmonary Disorders* |
| *Infectious* | ARDS |
| Bacterial | Pulmonary embolism |
| Gram-positive and gram-negative | Sickle cell crisis |
| Viral | *Immune Disorders* |
| CMV, hepatitis, varicella | Collagen vascular disease |
| Fungal | Systemic lupus |
| Protozoal | Anaphylaxis |
| Mycobacterial | |

CMV, cytomegalovirus; ARDS, acute repiratory distress syndrome.

Protein C is activated by thrombin, catalyzed by thrombomodulin found in endothelial cells, and, in conjunction with protein S, inactivates factors V and VIII and potentiates the fibrinolytic system (Kisiel, 1979).

Plasmin is activated by tissue plasminogen activator (TPA) from plasminogen. It splits fibrin, removing minute clots from the microcirculation. Plasmin also degrades factors V, VIII, IX, XI, and XII, and other plasma proteins, including ACTH, insulin, and growth hormone (Bick, 1994a).

## Pathophysiology

Disseminated intravascular coagulopathy represents a failure of the normal checks and balances, resulting in systemic, rather than focal, activation and circulation of thrombin and plasmin (Bick, 1988; Mueller-Berghaus, 1989). There may be significant variation in the level of elevation of plasmin and thrombin in different diseases. For example, if the intravascular clotting process dominates and secondary fibrinolysis is minimal, as in sepsis (Takahashi, 1990), the clinical presentation will be thrombosis. If secondary fibrinolysis dominates and fibrin-fibrinogen degradation products circulate at high concentration, the clinical presentation will be hemorrhage. On occasion, thrombosis and hemorrhage occur simul-

taneously. Finally, DIC may exist without being clinically apparent and be detectable only by laboratory evaluation. Figure 29-2 provides a summary of DIC pathophysiology and clinical presentation.

As thrombin circulates systemically, it cleaves fibrinogen, leaving behind a fibrin monomer, which polymerizes into clots, causing vascular thrombosis and restricting blood flow. The resulting tissue hypoxia produces ischemic necrosis within multiple organs. As fibrin is deposited in the microcirculation, platelets become trapped, with resultant thrombocytopenia (Bick, 1992).

The plasmin-induced breakdown products of fibrin and fibrinogen, known as fibrin degradation products (FDPs), bind soluble fibrin monomer and prevent polymerization, resulting in further impairment of hemostasis and hemorrhage. These FDPs are the basis of paracoagulation tests such as protamine sulfate and ethanol gelation (Gurewich, 1971; Breen, 1968). In addition, FDPs inhibit the platelet-mediated primary phase of coagulation and produce profound platelet dysfunction (Kopec, 1968).

Plasmin activates the complement cascade, resulting in red-cell and platelet lysis (Schreiber, 1973). The subsequent release of material from the RBCs propagates the DIC cycle. If the underlying disorder also activates factor XII (as is the case in sepsis), the kinin system will be initiated.

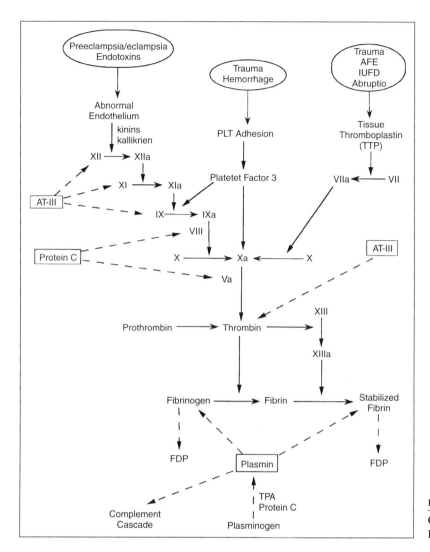

F I G U R E **29-1**
Obstetric disorders that initiate DIC.

Excess bradykinin produces vasodilation, hypotension, increased vascular permeability, and other common clinical manifestations of the DIC syndrome (Mason, 1970; Kaplan, 1976). The cycle of thrombin-induced microvascular thrombosis and plasmin-induced hemorrhage, once established, can become self-perpetuating.

## Diagnosis

### Clinical

Hemorrhage and/or thrombosis associated with one of the clinical conditions listed in Table 29-1

is strongly suggestive of DIC. Laboratory studies are not necessary to make the diagnosis of acute DIC. A patient in acute DIC has multiple hemostatic defects that may present as bleeding from unrelated sites (e.g., venipuncture oozing, epistaxis, hematuria, gingival/mucosal bleeding, purpura, or petechiae). Shock secondary to acute DIC is often out of proportion to the observed blood loss because of bradykinin generation. Renal failure is also common. At other times, DIC may remain subclinical and be manifest only by laboratory abnormalities.

In contrast to acute DIC, the diagnosis of chronic compensated DIC requires laboratory confirmation. Patients with chronic DIC (due to

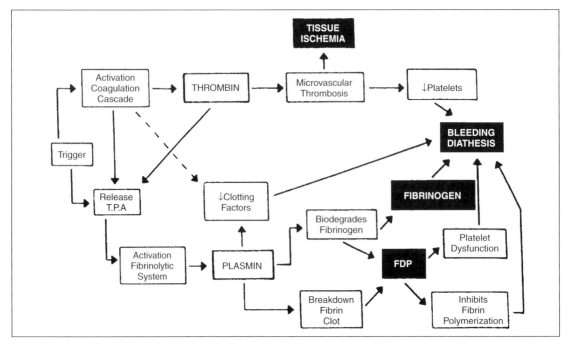

F I G U R E **29-2**

**Summary of DIC pathophysiology.** (Reproduced by permission from Gilbert JA, Scalzi RP. Disseminated intravascular coagulation. Emerg Med Clin North Am 1993;11:465.)

malignancy or IUFD) are well compensated and rarely bleed dramatically. They are more likely to suffer diffuse thrombosis, minor mucosal bleeding, hematuria, epistaxis, or easy bruisability (Bick, 1978). Their clotting mechanism, however, is tenuous and becomes easily deranged if another stress is added.

## Laboratory

Appropriate laboratory tests provide objective criteria for diagnosis and treatment of DIC. Knowledge of the changes in hemostatic components associated with pregnancy is essential for the accurate interpretation of laboratory findings in DIC. These changes are summarized in Table 29-2.

The laboratory abnormalities seen in DIC are listed in Table 29-3. The most specific test for the diagnosis of DIC is the monoclonal assay for the D-dimer, a breakdown product of the cross-linked fibrin polymer (Carr, 1989). It is a rapid (1 hr), widely available test and should, if possible, be used in place of FDP levels.

Over 50% of patients with acute DIC have a prolongation of the prothrombin time (PT) and activated partial thromboplastin time (aPTT). In the remainder, the values are either normal or shortened. Prolongation of the PT and aPTT usually does not occur until factor levels are less than 50% of normal or fibrinogen levels fall below 100 mg/dL (Angelos, 1986). Therefore, while a prolonged PT or an aPTT is strongly suggestive of DIC under appropriate clinical circumstances, a normal PT or aPTT does not rule out the diagnosis of DIC, limiting the usefulness of these tests.

During normal pregnancy, fibrinogen levels normally range between 400 and 700 mg/dL, representing a 74% increase in concentration and a 220% increase in total fibrinogen supply once the increase in vascular volume of pregnancy is considered (Gerbasi, 1990). In pregnancy, therefore, a "normal" fibrinogen level could represent a relative hypofibrinogenemia.

Fifteen percent of patients with acute DIC have normal FDP levels (Myers, 1970), possibly due to incomplete or overdegradation of FDP that result in levels undetectable by commercially available kits. In addition, FDPs as determined by standard tests are elevated in chronic hepatic and renal disease. Despite these difficulties, FDP titers are elevated in most patients.

The platelet count is usually significantly decreased, but the range is quite variable. Most tests of platelet function (bleeding time, platelet aggregation) are abnormal and add little to the diagnosis. Thrombin time (TT) measures the time required to convert fibrinogen to fibrin and is frequently prolonged in DIC. In practice, any prolonged TT not due to heparin administration is suggestive of DIC.

Some of the most specific and reliable tests for DIC are not available on a routine or emergency basis, limiting their clinical usefulness. They may be valuable in the long-term management of a patient with DIC. Antithrombin III levels are a highly sensitive test, because abnormal consumption of this coagulation inhibitor must occur if DIC is present. The conversion of prothrombin to thrombin by factor Xa results in the release of an inactive prothrombin fragment 1 + 2 (PF 1.2), and subsequently, the cleavage of fibrinogen produces fibrinopeptide A. PF 1.2 is a reliable marker

T A B L E   **29-2**

**Changes in hemostatic components associated with normal pregnancy**

Clotting activation
    Fibrinogen
    Factors VII, VIII, IX, X
    Factor V, prothrombin
Anticlotting activation
    Protein C
    Resistance to protein C
    Protein S
    Antithrombin III
    FDP
Platelet count
D-dimer

Sources: From Orlikowski CEP, Rocke DA. Coagulation monitoring in the obstetric patient. In Anesthesiol Clin 1994;32:73; Cumming AM, Tait RC, Fildes S, et al. Development of resistance to activated protein C during pregnancy. Br J Haematol 1995;90:725; and Gerbasi FP, Bottoms S, Farag A, Mammen E. Increased intravascular coagulation associated with pregnancy. Obstet Gynecol 1990;75:385.

T A B L E   **29-3**

**Laboratory tests**

Elevated D-dimer
Abnormal PT
Abnormal aPTT
Decreased fibrinogen
Elevated FDP
Abnormal platelet count
Abnormal thrombin time
AT-III consumption*
Elevated PF 1.2*
Elevated fibrinopeptide A*
Elevated platelet factor 4*

*Usually a 2- to 5-day turnaround time.

PT, prothrombin time; aPTT, activated partial thromboplastin time.

for factor Xa generation, and fibrinopeptide A is a reliable marker for thrombin generation (Sorensen, 1992). Platelet factor 4 levels are markers of general platelet reactivity and are usually elevated in DIC (Matsuda, 1979).

Newer assays that assess other fibrinogen breakdown products (B-beta peptides), including alpha-2-plasmin inhibitor complex, TPA, and tissue plasminogen activator inhibitor, have recently become available. Their role in the diagnosis of DIC remains under investigation (Bick, 1994b).

In summary, the diagnosis of clinically significant DIC is not difficult and involves clinical evidence of hemorrhage and/or thrombosis, the presence of an underlying etiology, and laboratory confirmation. The most reasonable tests to order emergently are complete blood count with platelet count, PT, aPTT, fibrinogen, FDP, D-dimer, and TT. Antithrombin-III levels can be ordered if readily available.

## Therapy

The morbidity and mortality of DIC result from both the coagulopathy and the precipitating illness. The primary therapeutic goal is treatment of the underlying disorder, accompanied by aggressive support of blood volume, BP, and tissue oxygenation. Insufficient volume expansion and fluid resuscitation are the most common therapeutic errors.

An approach applicable to most patients with pregnancy-associated DIC is outlined in Table 29-4. Volume replacement, BP maintenance, and evacuation of the uterus (thus terminating the source of the DIC) constitute adequate therapy in the vast majority of obstetric-related DIC syndromes. In septicemia, appropriate antibiotic therapy is added to the regime.

The next defense is replacement therapy with the deficient clotting factors. The argument that this "adds fuel to the fire" and worsens DIC is unfounded; it may be life-saving. Blood and component therapy is discussed in more detail in Chapter 11.

The third line of therapy is to treat the intravascular thrombosis (Bick, 1994a; Rubin, 1992; Gilbert, 1993). In the obstetric patient, the need for this form of therapy will be rare to nonexistent, except in cases of severe hypofibrinogenemia secondary to IUFD with an intact maternal circulation. Heparin is not recommended in situations associated with vascular disruption and active bleeding. Low-dose subcutaneous heparin

TABLE **29-4**

**Therapy for acute disseminated intravascular coagulopathy**

I. Treatment or Removal of the Triggering Event
  A. Volume replacement and expansion (crystalloid, plasmanate, albumin)
  B. Control of shock, maintenance of BP
  C. Evacuation of uterus (if indicated)
  D. Antibiotics (if indicated)
II. Component Therapy
  A. Fresh-frozen plasma, cryoprecipitate
  B. Prothrombin complex
  C. Platelets
  D. Packed RBCs (in the face of hemorrhage)
III. Anticoagulant Therapy
  A. Heparin, low-modular-weight heparin
  B. AT III concentrates
  C. Antiplatelet drugs (for chronic DIC)
  D. Protein C concentrates
  E. New agents (defibrotide, hirudin, aprotinin, gabexate)
IV. Inhibition of residual fibrinolysis
  A. Epsilon-amino-caproic acid
  B. Tranexamic acid

appears to be as effective and safer than larger doses of intravenous (IV) heparin (Sakuragawa, 1993). If possible, AT III activity should be determined, because heparin is ineffective if AT III levels are insufficient.

Antithrombin III concentrates have been used successfully to treat fulminant DIC. While encouraging, the data are equivocal, and more definitive study is needed to establish a basis for this therapy (Sunder-Plassman, 1991; Fourrier, 1995). Antiplatelet agents are of little clinical use in fulminant DIC. Finally, inhibition of residual fibrinogenolysis has virtually no role in current obstetric practice.

## Obstetric Causes

Pregnancy is one of the most well-documented hypercoaguable conditions (Weiner, 1984; Eby, 1993). Less established is the association of pregnancy with an increased risk of DIC (Gerbasi, 1990). The purpose of this section is not to discuss treatment of the obstetric disorders, but rather to discuss how these clotting abnormalities influence the therapeutic plan.

## Abruptio Placenta

Abruptio is the most common obstetric cause of acute DIC. The incidence varies with the population studied and the diagnostic criteria used, but it ranges from 0.45% to 1.3% (Richey, 1995). Ten percent to 30% of women with a clinically significant abruption will have a gross clotting defect (Creasy, 1994; Finley, 1989).

A large, extravascular clot consuming all available products does not account for the coagulation abnormalities associated with abruptio placenta. Activation of the fibrinolytic system and systemic consumption of soluble components occur out of proportion to blood loss. The degree of thrombocytopenia, AT III consumption, hypofibrinogenemia, and FDP elevation correlates well with the clinical severity of the abruption. Disseminated intravascular coagulopathy occurs most often in the presence of an abruption of magnitude sufficient to cause a fetal demise.

Plasma fibrinolytic activity is similar in the uterine artery and vein when the placenta and fetus are healthy. Following a normal delivery, FDPs increase significantly in the uterine vein. A similar increase occurs after a complete abruption, even when the fetus and placenta remain in utero. Thus, it appears that the process of placental separation contributes to FDP elevation. The FDPs increase throughout labor in the presence of partial abruptio, peak shortly after total separation of the placenta, and then decline, occasionally normalizing by delivery (Basu, 1971; Sher, 1977).

The incidence of postpartum hemorrhage with placental abruption is not increased in the absence of a clotting abnormality. Of any single laboratory parameter, FDP elevation has the greatest correlation with postpartum hemorrhage. Uterine inertia is uncommon unless the FDPs are in excess of 330 mg/mL. In vitro, a concentration of FDPs higher than that usually found in the peripheral circulation inhibits myometrial contractility (Basu, 1971). Therefore, inhibition of myometrial contractions by FDPs would seem a possible mechanism for postpartum hemorrhage if the myometrial concentration of FDPs is considerably higher than that in the peripheral blood. This is likely in light of the uterine arterial-venous differences in fibrinolytic activity after placental separation. Further, the concentration of FDP in the lochia of women who have had an abruption is markedly higher than concentrations in normal controls (Basu, 1971). The IV infusion of an antifibrinolytic agent has been reported to promptly overcome uterine inertia secondary to abruptio unresponsive to amniotomy and oxytocin (Sher, 1977). These data support a direct, pathophysiologic relationship between elevated FDPs and postpartum hemorrhage after placental abruption.

The management of acute placental abruption is well established. Recommendations follow the outline of Table 29-4, empty the uterus, and in the interim, vigorously support the intravascular volume. This action effectively terminates consumption, although component therapy may be required to correct deficiencies. (ACOG, 1994; National Blood Resource Education Program Expert Panel, 1993). In this circumstance, heparin could cause bleeding, especially if surgery were required, and should be avoided.

## The Preeclampsia-Eclampsia Syndrome

The inability of many investigators to consistently demonstrate alterations in commonly measured clotting parameters led to the logical dismissal of DIC as an etiology of preeclampsia. Rather, it is considered a manifestation of disease severity (Pritchard, 1976). While the causal relationship between preeclampsia-eclampsia and overt DIC is fiercely debated, there is substantial clinical evidence that the majority of women with preeclampsia have a subclinical, consumptive coagulopathy.

Fibrin or a fibrin-like substance has been identified as a variable constituent of the renal lesion termed *glomerular endotheliosis* (Kincaid-Smith, 1975; Morris, 1964). The activation of coagulation may cause fibrin deposition in both the kidney and lung (Birmingham Eclampsia Study Group, 1971). Fibrin is consistently detected in liver biopsy specimens obtained from women with preeclampsia (Anas, 1976). There is an increased incidence of fibrin deposition in placental perivillous spaces (McKay, 1981) and in placental microvessels (Lebarrere, 1992). Also, blood levels of D-dimer are elevated in women with preeclampsia (Trofatter, 1989). Kanfer and colleagues (1996) demonstrated increased fibrin deposition and increased antifibrinolytic potential in preeclamptic placentas.

There is increasing evidence that endothelial cell injury and altered endothelial cell function plays an important role in the pathogenesis of preeclampsia and eclampsia. Blood-borne products from the diseased placenta injure endothelial cells, with subsequent increases in the level of factor VIII-related antigen, endothelin, and fibronectin, and loss of normal antithrombogenic function (Zeeman, 1992; Koh, 1993; Saleh, 1987).

Elevated plasma thrombin-antithrombin complexes and a significant decrease in plasma AT III activity occur in women with preeclampsia and eclampsia (Terao, 1991; Halim, 1995; Savelieva, 1995). A characteristic fall in the platelet counts occurs (Redman, 1978), coupled with platelet damage and dysfunction (Halim, 1996). Additionally, the concentration of fibrinopeptide A is significantly higher in the preeclamptic pregnancy (Douglas, 1982).

Although a subtle, subclinical consumptive state may be demonstrated in preeclampsia by using sophisticated labortory tests, frank DIC or alterations in clinically measured clotting parameters (other than thrombocytopenia) are virtually never seen in severe preeclampsia or eclampsia in the absence of placental abruption. Usually, no treatment is necessary beyond delivery. Transfusion of packed RBCs may be necessary if there is significant hemorrhage at delivery, and platelet transfusion may be required in women with platelet counts below 50,000 per mL who require cesarean delivery. It is usually not necessary to replace other components.

### Intrauterine Fetal Demise

The association between IUFD and subsequent coagulopathy is well established. Coagulopathy can occur after the death of a singleton or of one fetus of a multiple gestation. The development of coagulopathy is gradual, occurring 3 to 4 weeks after the demise is diagnosed (Pritchard, 1959), and consists of varying degrees of hypofibrinogenemia, decreased plasminogen, decreased AT III activity, generation of fibrinopeptide A and FDP, and thrombocytopenia (Jimenez, 1968). The etiology of the DIC is most likely via release of tissue thromboplastin from the necrotic fetus into the maternal circulation, with activation of the procoagulant system (Bick, 1994a). Although controversial, neither primary nor secondary fibrinolysis appears to have a significant role in the coagulopathy (Jimenez, 1968).

Heparin is the treatment of choice for the chronic DIC associated with IUFD if delivery is required. Although full anticoagulation was used in the past, low-dose heparin (5000–10,000 units) given subcutaneously twice daily should be adequate in most patients. Treatment should be continued until there is correction of the hypofibrinogenemia, after which delivery may be effected.

Romero and colleagues (1984) reported the long-term use of heparin in a single twin demise

to reverse coagulopathy, but because the hypofibrinogenemia tends to be transitory, this may not be necessary (Chescheir, 1988). Management of the demise of one fetus in a multiple gestation must be individualized for each pregnancy.

At a very early gestational age (approximately 26–28 wk), if the surviving fetus is healthy and there is no overt maternal coagulopathy, appropriate treatment includes either expectant management, allowing spontaneous resolution of the hypofibrinogenemia, or the administration of low-dose heparin (Romero, 1984).

In the presence of severe DIC with clinical bleeding, immediate delivery may be required. To assure survival of the remaining twin or the mother, the associated DIC should be treated as outlined in Table 29-4. Once volume replacement and expansion and component therapy stabilize the patient, delivery can be initiated. Aggressive treatment should continue until normalization of laboratory parameters has been achieved.

At more advanced gestational ages, delivery may be warranted, even for subclinical DIC, but is generally not an emergent problem. Low-dose heparin therapy can be instituted and continued for 48 to 96 hours or until normalization of fibrinogen levels occurs. Delivery can then be accomplished safely.

### Abortion

Coagulopathy may occur as a result of septic abortion, massive hemorrhage with shock, or instillation of hypertonic saline. With the development of safer, easier methods of pregnancy termination, saline abortion has been relegated largely to historic status. If DIC does occur, the management is the same as outlined in Table 29-4: evacuation of the uterus, restoration of volume status, maintenance of BP, and component therapy as needed.

### Acute Fatty Liver

Acute fatty liver is a rare, potentially fatal disorder of the third trimester of pregnancy. Holzbach

(1974) proposed that the coagulopathy associated with acute fatty liver was the result of DIC initiated by severe hepatic dysfunction. Later studies demonstrated markedly decreased levels of AT III (Liebman, 1983; Hellgren, 1983). Castro and colleagues (1996) found evidence of DIC and profoundly depressed AT III levels in 100% of patients with acute fatty liver. Transfusion of AT III transiently increased plasma levels but did not affect clinical outcome. Treatment consists of delivery, aggressive fluid resuscitation and volume expansion, and transfusion of necessary blood components (see Chapter 11).

## Sepsis

Severe infections, such as septic abortion, pyelonephritis, chorioamnionitis, or endomyometritis, can be associated with shock and DIC. Gram-negative organisms are responsible for the majority of cases, but gram-positive organisms and viral, fungal, protozoan, and mycobacterial etiologies must be considered. Bacterial endotoxin (bacterial coat lipopolysaccharide) or exotoxin provides the initiating event. Endotoxin activates factor XII, induces a platelet-release reaction, triggers endothelial sloughing, releases granulocyte procoagulants, and ultimately liberates histamines, kinins, and serotonin. Any of these events might trigger DIC. What more commonly occurs is a summation of several or all of these events (Table 29-5).

At least some of the clinical findings in septic shock are secondary to the DIC. Kinin activation occurs early in the clotting cascade. The quantity of kallikrein that is generated correlates directly with the severity of the shock (Mason, 1970). While the kidney is almost always affected in the early stages of shock, death is most often secondary to pulmonary complications (Beller, 1974; Duff, 1980).

Treatment of DIC secondary to sepsis follows the plan outlined in Table 29-4. The major controversy involves the use of anticoagulants. Sepsis is associated with the widespread activation of the clotting cascade, and fibrin thrombi within the microvasculature exacerbates the syndrome. Heparin administration could alleviate this complication but would not effect kinin activation or platelet aggregation. Further, the coagulopathy generally resolves rapidly after removal of the septic focus and antibiotic administration. Thus, the use of heparin is controversial. Some investigators recommend the administration of low-dose heparin (Bick, 1994a; Rubin, 1992) in patients with septic-related DIC, while others find its use contraindicated (Richey, 1995). A more thorough review of septic shock in pregnancy is found in Chapter 22.

T A B L E    **29-5**

Summary of some pathophysiologic effects of endotoxin

| Direct Endotoxic Effects Related to Endotoxic Shock | Secondary Effects Not Necessarily Related to Toxic Effects of Endotoxin |
|---|---|
| Release of biogenic hormones (catecholamines, serotonin, histamine, kinins, etc.) | Hemoconcentration, hypovolemia |
| Thrombocytopenia, platelet aggregation | DIC |
| Leukopenia-leukocytosis | Ischemia-necrosis-renal cortical necrosis |
| Vascular hyperreactivity | Increase in lactate |
| Interference with reticuloendothelial system function | Interstitial pulmonary edema |
| Cardiogenic shock | Microangiopathic anemia |
| Lysosomal breakdown | |
| Tolerance phenomenon | |
| Abortion | |
| Pyrogens | |

---

### DISSEMINATED INTRAVASCULAR COAGULOPATHY

**I. *Goals of Therapy***

  A. Treat/remove underlying etiology.
  B. Maintain blood volume and oxygenation.
  C. Stop intravascular clotting/inhibit fibrinolysis.

**II. *Management Protocol***

  A. Aggressive maintenance of blood volume (crystalloid, plasma expanders, or albumin)
  B. Maintenance of BP (pressors if necessary)
  C. Maintenance of oxygenation (oxygen administration or mechanical ventilation)
  D. Additional supportive therapy as required
  E. Treatment of underlying etiology of DIC
   1. Evacuation of uterus, if indicated
   2. Antibiotics for sepsis
  F. Component therapy (aggressive replacement with packed RBCs; choose coagulation components based on deficiencies)
  G. Anticoagulant therapy (only if an intact circulatory system; rarely required in obstetric causes of DIC)
  H. Fibrinolysis inhibition (rarely indicated)

**III. *Critical Laboratory Tests***

  A. Complete blood count with platelet count, PT, aPTT, fibrinogen, FDP, D-dimer, TT, and AT III

**IV. *Consultation***

  A. Hematology, anesthesia

---

### Amniotic Fluid Embolism

Amniotic fluid embolism is rare, but it is associated with a maternal mortality rate of up to 80% (Clark, 1990). If the initial cardiovascular insult is not fatal, DIC can follow in 45% or more of the cases. Amniotic fluid extraction and massive placental abruption are the only two obstetric causes of clinically significant, acute DIC. The hemorrhage of AFE is treated by volume and component replacement, often in massive quantities. The clinician is advised to continue replacement therapy until normalization of laboratory parameters. A complete discussion of AFE can be found in Chapter 20.

**REFERENCES**

American College of Obstetricians and Gynecologists. Blood component therapy. Am Coll Obstetricians Gynecologists Technical Bulletin, November 1994; No. 199.

Anas F, Mancilla-Jimenez R. Hepatic fibrinogen deposits in preeclampsia-immunofluorescent evidence. N Engl J Med 1976;295:578.

Angelos MG, Hamilton GC. Coagulation studies: prothrombin time, partial thromboplastin time, bleeding time. Emerg Med Clin North Am 1986; 4:95.

Basu HK. Fibrinolysis and abruptio placenta. Br J Obstet Gynaecol 1971;109:604.

Beller FK, Uszynski M. Disseminated intravascular coagulation in pregnancy. Clin Obstet Gynecol 1974;17:250.

Bick RL, Baker WF. Disseminated intravascular coagulation. Hematol Pathol 1992;6:1.

Bick RL. Disseminated intravascular coagulation and related syndromes: a clinical review. Semin Thromb Hemost 1988;14:299.

Bick RL. Disseminated intravascular coagulation: objective criteria for diagnosis and management. Med Clin North Am 1994a;78:511.

Bick RL. Disseminated intravascular coagulation: objective laboratory diagnostic criteria and guidelines for management. Clin Lab Med 1994b;14: 729.

Bick RL. Disseminated intravascular coagulation and related syndromes: etiology, pathophysiology, diagnosis, and management. Am J Hematol 1978;5:265.

Birmingham Eclampsia Study Group. Intravascular coagulation and abnormal lung-scans in preeclampsia and eclampsia. Lancet 1971;2:889.

Breen FA, Tullis JZ. Ethanol gelation, a rapid screening test for intravascular coagulation. Ann Intern Med 1968;69:111.

Carr JM, McKinney M, McDonagh J. Diagnosis of disseminated intravascular coagulation role of d-dimer. Am J Clin Pathol 1989;91:280.

Castro MA, Goodwin TM, Shaw KJ, et al. Disseminated intravascular coagulation and antithrombin III depression in acute fatty liver of pregnancy. Am J Obstet Gynecol 1996;174:211.

Chescheir NC, Seeds JW. Spontaneous resolution of hypofibrinogenemia associated with death of a twin in utero: a case report. Am J Obstet Gynecol 1988;159:1183.

Clark SL. New concepts of amniotic fluid embolism: a review. Obstet Gynecol Surv 1990;45:360.

Creasy RK, Resnik R, eds. Placenta previa and abruptio placentae. In: Maternal-fetal medicine: principles and practice. 3rd ed. Philadelphia: WB Saunders, 1994:615.

Cumming AM, Tait RC, Fildes S, et al. Development of resistance to activated protein C during pregnancy. Br J Haematol 1995;90:725.

Douglas JT, Shaw M, Lowe GDO, et al. Fibrinopeptide A and beta thromboglobulin levels in preeclampsia and hypertensive pregnancy. Thromb Haemost 1982;47:54.

Dubber AHC, McNicol GP, Douglas AS. Acquired hypofibrinoo-genemia: the "defibrination syndrome." A study of seven patients. Scott Med J 1967;12:138.

Duff P. Pathophysiology and management of septic shock. J Reprod Med 1980;24:109.

Eby CS. A review of the hypercoagulable state. Hematol Oncol Clin North Am 1993;7:1121.

Finley BE. Acute coagulopathy in pregnancy. Med Clin North Am 1989;73:723.

Fourrier F, Jourdain M, Tournois A, et al. Coagulation inhibitor substitution during sepsis. Intensive Care Med 1995;21(suppl 2):S264.

Gerbasi FP, Bottoms S, Farag A, Mammen E. Increased intravascular coagulation associated with pregnancy. Obstet Gynecol 1990;75:385.

Gilbert JA, Scalzi RP. Disseminated intravascular coagulation. Emerg Med Clin North Am 1993;11: 465.

Gurewich V, Hutchinson E. Detection of intravascular coagulation by a serial dilution protamine sulfate test. Ann Intern Med 1971;75:895.

Halim A, Bhuiyan AB, Azim FA, et al. Blood coagulation and fibrinolysis in eclamptic patients and their correlation with the clinical signs. Gynecol Obstet Invest 1995;39:97.

Halim A, Kanayama N, Maradny E, et al. Plasmin P selectin (GMP-140) and glycocalicin are elevated in preeclampsia and eclampsia: their significance. Am J Obstet Gynecol 1996;174:272.

Hellgren M, Hagenevik K, Robbe H, et al. Severe acquired anti-thrombin III deficiency in relation to hepatic and renal insufficiency and intrauterine fetal death in late pregnancy. Gynecol Obstet Invest 1983;16:107.

Holzbach R. Acute fatty liver of pregnancy with disseminated intravascular coagulation. Obstet Gynecol 1974;43:740.

Jimenez JM, Pritchard JA. Pathogenesis and treatment of coagulation defects resulting from fetal death. Obstet Gynecol 1968;32:449.

Kanfer A, Bruch JF, Nguyen G, et al. Increased placental antifibrinolytic potential and fibrin deposits in pregnancy-induced hypertension and preeclampsia. Lab Invest 1996;74:253.

Kaplan A, Meier H, Handle R. The Hageman factor: dependent pathways of coagulation, fibrinolysis, and kinin generation. Semin Thromb Hemost 1976;3:6.

Kincaid-Smith P. Participation of intravascular coagulation in the pathogenesis of glomerular and vascular lesion. Kidney Int 1975;7:242.

Kisiel W. Human plasma protein C: isolation, characterization, and mechanism of activation and alpha-thrombin. J Clin Invest 1979;64:761.

Koh SCL, Anandakumar C, Montan S, Ratnam SS. Plasminogen activators, plasminogen activator inhibitors and markers of intravascular coagulation in pre-eclampsia. Gynecol Obstet Invest 1993;35:214.

Kopec M, Wegrzynowiczy Z, Budzynski A, et al. Interaction of fibrinogen degradation products with platelets. Exp Biol Med 1968;3:73.

Labarrere CA, Faulk WP. Microvascular perturbations in human allografts: analogies in preeclamptic placentae. Am J Reprod Immunol 1992;27:109.

Lasch HG, Henne DL, Huth K, Sandruitter W. Pathophysiology, clinical manifestations, and therapy of consumptive coagulopathy. Am J Cardiol 1967;20:381.

Liebman H, McGehee W, Patch J, Feinstein I. Severe depression of AT-III with disseminated intravascular coagulopathy in women with fatty liver of pregnancy. Ann Intern Med 1983;98:330.

Marder VJ. Consumptive thrombohemorrhagic disorders. In: Williams WJ, Beutler E, Ersleu AJ, et al, eds. Hematology. 4th ed. New York: McGraw-Hill, 1990:1522.

Mason JW, Kleeberg U, Dolan P, et al. Plasma kallikrein and Hageman factor in gram negative bacteremia. Ann Intern Med 1970;1973:545.

Matsuda T, Seki T, Ogawara M, et al. Comparison between plasma levels of b-thromboglobulin and platelet factor 4 in various diseases. Thromb Haemost 1979;42:288.

McKay DC. Chronic intravascular coagulation in normal pregnancy and preeclampsia. Contrib Nephrol 1981;25:108.

Mersky C, Johnson AJ, Kleiner GJ, Wohl H. The defibrination syndrome: clinical features and laboratory diagnosis. Br J Haematol 1967;13:528.

Morris RH, Vassalli P, Beler FK, et al. Immunofluorescent studies of renal biopsies in the diagnosis of toxemia of pregnancy. Obstet Gynecol 1964;24:32.

Muller-Berghaus G. Pathophysiologic and biochemical events in disseminated intravascular coagulation: dysregulation of procoagulant and anticoagulant pathways. Semin Thromb Hemost 1989;15:58.

Myers AR, Bloch KJ, Coleman RW. A comparative study of four methods for detecting fibrinogen degradation products in patients with various diseases. N Engl J Med 1970;283:663.

National Blood Resource Education Program Exper Panel. Indications for the use of red blood cells, platelets, and fresh frozen plasma. National Institutes of Health National Heart, Lung, and Blood Institute, August 1993; No. 93-2974a.

Orlikowski CEP, Rocke DA. Coagulation monitoring in the obstetric patient. Int Anesthesiol Clin 1994;32:73.

Pritchard JA, Cunningham FG, Mason RA. Coagulation changes in eclampsia: their frequency and pathogenesis. Am J Obstet Gynecol 1976;124:855.

Pritchard JA. Fetal death in utero. Obstet Gynecol 1959;15:48.

Redman CWG, Bonnar J, Berlin L. Early platelet consumption in preeclampsia. Br Med J 1978;1:467.

Richey ME, Gilstrap LC, Ramin SM. Management of disseminated intravascular coagulopathy. Clin Obstet Gynecol 1995;38:514.

Rodriquez-Erdman F. Bleeding due to increased intravascular blood coagulation: hemorrhagic syndromes caused by consumption of blood-clotting factors (consumption coagulopathies). N Engl J Med 1965;273:1370.

Romero R, Duffy TP, Berkowitz RL, et al. Prolongation of a preterm pregnancy complicated by death of a single twin in utero and disseminated intravascular coagulation: effects of treatment with heparin. N Engl J Med 1984;310:772.

Rubin RN, Colman RW. Disseminated intravascular coagulation: Approach to treatment. Drugs 1992;44:963.

Sakuragawa N, Hasegawa H, Maki M, et al. Clinical evaluation of low-molecular-weight-heparin (FR-860) on disseminated intravascular coagulation (DIC): a multicentric cooperative double-blind trial in comparison with heparin. Thromb Res 1993;72:475.

Saleh AA, Bottoms SF, Welch RA, et al. Preeclampsia, delivery, and the hemostatic system. Am J Obstet Gynecol 1987;157:331.

Savelieva GM, Efimov VS, Grishin VL, et al. Blood coagulation changes in pregnant women at risk of developing preeclampsia. Int J Gynaecol Obstet 1995;48:3.

Schreiber AD, Austen KF. Interrelationships of the fibrinolytic, coagulation, kinin generation, and complement systems. Semin Hematol 1973;6: 593.

Sher G. Pathogenesis and management of uterine inertia complicating abruptio placenta with consumption coagulopathy. Am J Obstet Gynecol 1977;129:164.

Sorensen JV, Jensen HP, Rahr HR, et al. F 1 + 2 and FPA in urine from patients with multiple trauma and healthy individuals: a pilot study. Thromb Res 1992;67:429.

Sunder-Plassman G, Speiser W, Korninger C, et al. Disseminated intravascular coagulation and decrease in fibrinogen levels induced by vincristine/prednisolone therapy of lymphoid blast crisis of chronic myeloid leukemia. Ann Hematol 1991;62:169.

Takahashi H, Tatewaki W, Wada K, et al. Thrombin vs. plasma generation in disseminated intravascular coagulation associated with various underlying disorders. Am J Hematol 1990;32:90.

Terao T, Maki M, Ikenoue T, et al. The relationship between clinical signs and hypercoagulable state in toxemia of pregnancy. Gynecol Obstet Invest 1991;31:74.

Trofatter KF, Howell MC, Greenberg CS, Hage ML. Use of the fibrin D-dimer in screening for coagulation abnormalities in preeclampsia. Obstet Gynecol 1989;73:435.

Weiner C, Kwaan H, Hauck WW, et al. Fibrin generation in normal pregnancy. Obstet Gynecol 1984;64:46.

Wessler S, Gitel SN. Warfarin: from bedside to bench. N Engl J Med 1984;311:645.

Zeeman GG, Dekker GA. Pathogenesis of preeclampsia: a hypothesis. Clin Obstet Gynecol 1992;35:317.

# CHAPTER *30*

# Sickle Cell Crisis

*S*ickle cell diseases represent a spectrum of heritable disorders of hemoglobin synthesis that includes homozygous S disease (HbSS), the double heterozygous variants of sickle cell disease (HbSC), and sickle β-thalassemia (HbS β-thal) (Table 30-1). These disorders are characterized by chronic hemolytic anemia, acute, episodic vaso-occlusive crises that can cause organ failure, and heightened susceptibility to infection. Pregnancies complicated by sickle hemoglobinopathies are associated with significant maternal and perinatal morbidity and mortality. The incidence of preeclampsia, preterm labor, spontaneous abortion, stillbirth, and maternal death is increased in women with sickle cell disease (Seoud, 1994). A better understanding of the pathogenesis of these diseases has led to improvements in prenatal care and obstetric outcomes (Milner, 1980; Powars, 1986).

## Pathogenesis

The genes that code for sickle hemoglobinopathies are inherited as autosomal recessive traits. Hemoglobin S is caused by a molecular mutation that results in the single substitution of the neutral amino acid valine for the negatively charged glutamic acid at the sixth position of the beta hemoglobin chain. Hemoglobin C results from lysine substitution for glutamic acid at the number six position. These seemingly minor amino

acid substitutions have profound physiologic and clinical consequences.

In contrast to the qualitative defect in hemoglobin structure produced by sickle genes, the inheritance of thalassemia genes results in a quantitative defect in globulin chain production. The peripheral blood film reflects this reduction in globulin synthesis by the presence of target red cells, which represent the mismatch between intracellular hemoglobin and cell membrane constituents.

The definitive diagnosis of sickle cell anemia and the classification of the compound hemoglobinopathies requires a quantitative measurement of cellular hemoglobins. Clinical laboratories routinely perform hemoglobin electrophoresis to identify the common sickle cell diseases. Quantitation also assists the therapeutic management of sickle cell crises.

Hemoglobin S retains its normal form and function under oxygenated conditions. Once deoxygenated, the neutral charge of valine allows hydrophobic bonds to form between adjacent amino acids within the polypeptide structure of hemoglobin. These bonds lead to the formation of deoxyhemoglobin tetramers that aggregate to form strands of polymerized hemoglobin within the erythrocyte. These aggregates go through a process of gelation, organizing into structures that distort the red cell into the classic sickle cell shape (Dean, 1978). Gelation is enhanced by reductions in the oxygen concentration or pH or

T A B L E   **30-1**

Approximate frequency of common hemoglobinopathies in North Americans of African descent

| Hemoglobinopathy | Frequency |
|---|---|
| Hemoglobin C trait | 1:40 |
| Sickle hemoglobin trait | 1:120 |
| Sickle cell anemia | 1:700 |
| Sickle cell–hemoglobin C disease | 1:750 |
| Hemoglobin S β-thalassemia disease | 1:1700 |
| Hemoglobin C disease | 1:4800 |

by increases in the concentrations of 2-3 diphosphoglycerate or hemoglobin S. Initially, oxygen can restore the erythrocyte to normal, but with repetitive cycles of deoxygenation, the red-cell membrane becomes rigid and irreversibly sickled in shape.

Because of its abnormal shape, the life span of a sickled erythrocyte is usually 10 to 20 days, compared with 120 days for a normal erythrocyte. These permanently damaged red cells are prematurely cleared by the reticuloendothelial system. A third of this hemolysis occurs intravascularly, which accounts for the depression of serum haptoglobin and the loss of iron in the urine, as well as the elevation in the serum level of indirect, unconjugated bilirubin and the appearance of icterus. Bone marrow and extramedullary erythropoiesis leads to a chronic, compensated anemia.

This heightened clearance of abnormally sickled red cells is postulated to account for the persistence of the sickle gene (Pasrol, 1978). Malarial parasitization of the red cell enhances the rate of erythrocyte sickling, which prompts the removal of infected cells from the circulation. Sickle heterozygosity thus conferred a survival advantage in geographic regions of endemic falciparum malaria prior to the advent of antimicrobial therapy.

The presence of fetal hemoglobin (HbF) protects against hemoglobin aggregation by altering the contact sites involved in deoxyhemoglobin S polymer formation. The hereditary persistence of more than 20% HbF appears to be highly pro-

tective against the development of crises in sickle cell patients (Noguchi, 1988).

Factors other than the disordered structure of hemoglobin S play a role in the clinical expression of sickle cell disease. Sickle erythrocytes display an increased adhesiveness to vascular endothelium, and the degree of adhesiveness correlates with the severity of vaso-occlusive crises (Hebbel, 1985). In the presence of plasma proteins liberated from damaged endothelial cells, young, light, deformable sickle cells adhere to the lining of the venular capillaries. By narrowing the capillary lumen, these erythrocytes may impede the flow of older, denser, less deformable sickle cells, leading to vessel occlusion.

This cascade of events explains the clinical observation that concurrent infection and recent sickle crisis predispose to the development of vaso-occlusive crisis. Infectious agents can disrupt the endothelium and lead to the release of von Willebrand's factor multimers, which will enhance sickle cell adhesion. Vaso-occlusive crisis leads to reticulocytosis and the production of youthful cohorts of deformable erythrocytes, whose increased vascular adhesiveness can beget subsequent crises (Bookchin, 1991).

The alteration of the microvasculature during vaso-occlusive episodes feeds back on gelation kinetics. Obstruction to blood flow shortens the delay time to deoxyhemoglobin S polymerization, thus propagating vascular occlusion.

Repetitive deformation of the red-cell membrane by sickle polymerization also leads to disordered salt and water homeostasis. Disruption of the cation barriers leads to cellular dehydration and red cells with high mean corpuscular hemoglobin concentrations (MCHCs). These dense, rigid cells are likely derived from subpopulations of erythrocytes low in hemoglobin F and are prone to occlude the capillary beds, leading to distal hypoxia.

In situ thrombosis also has also been postulated to play a role in sickle occlusion. Serial measurements of biochemical markers indicative of ongoing thrombosis and thrombolysis have been exploited in the diagnosis of vaso-occlusive events.

The clinical manifestations of sickle cell disease intensify in the presence of conditions that promote deoxyhemoglobin S polymerization (e.g., hypoxemia, acidosis, and red cell dehydration), that produce inflammation of the vascular endothelium, and that alter blood viscosity and the rheology of blood flow.

## Clinical Presentation

In contrast to the steady state chronic hemolytic anemia, the sickle crisis is a potentially life-threatening complication of sickle cell disease. The term *crisis* encompasses a number of clinical events seen in sickle cell disease. Crises can be divided into two major categories: hematologic and vaso-occlusive.

## Hematologic Crisis

Hematologic crises occur infrequently in pregnancy and are characterized by a sudden worsening of anemia. Affected patients present with weakness and exertional dyspnea and may show signs of high-output cardiac failure. Icterus is not remarkable because intravascular hemolysis is not a prominent feature.

The most common type of hematologic crisis is an aplastic crisis caused by parvovirus B-19 infection (Rao, 1992). Infection by human parvovirus destroys erythropoietic precursors and leads to a dramatic decrease in circulating hemoglobin. A diagnostic hallmark of parvovirus infection is the appearance of giant pronormoblasts on bone marrow examination. Marrow aplasia resolves spontaneously within 2 weeks of the onset of infection. Although the infection is self-limiting, transfusion support may be necessary prior to marrow recovery.

Megaloblastic crisis occasioned by folic acid deficiency is induced by the chronic hemolysis and compensatory reticulocytosis of stable sickle anemia. The peripheral blood smear shows macro-ovalocytes and hypersegmented neutrophils. The bone marrow reveals megaloblastic erythroid hyperplasia. Depression of red cell folate levels reflects tissue deprivation. Although now rare in pregnant women due to the current emphasis on prophylactic folate supplementation, folate depletion can be seen in sickle cell patients with multiple gestation or in adolescent mothers

with frequent and closely spaced pregnancies (Alperin, 1967). In most patients, a hematologic response is seen with the oral administration of 1 mg of folic acid daily.

Splenic sequestration syndrome is due to the acute intrasplenic trapping of blood, leading to severe anemia (Emond, 1985). This hematologic crisis occurs predominantly in children with sickle cell anemia whose spleens have not undergone autoinfarction and fibrosis. Sequestration crisis is more common in adults with HbSC disease as a consequence of persisting splenic function beyond childhood (Orringer, 1991). The syndrome is characterized by abdominal pain, sudden splenic enlargement, and a precipitous drop in hemoglobin level, resulting in hypovolemic shock. Red blood cell transfusions during the acute event have been shown to reverse splenic sequestration (Rao, 1985). Recurrent sequestration crises are common and may be treated by a chronic transfusion program or splenectomy (Kinney, 1990). Splenic hypofunction is a normal consequence of sickle cell disease, thus the risk of infectious complications postsplenectomy is not increased (Pegelow, 1980).

Although uncommon, hepatic sequestration crises have been observed, as evidenced by rapid enlargement of the liver and an accompanying drop in hemoglobin level (Hernandez, 1989). Acute management is similar to that for splenic sequestration.

Whether hyperhemolytic crises, defined as accelerated hemolysis, associated with elevated levels of serum bilirubin occur in sickle cell disease is a matter of debate (Diggs, 1973). It is more likely that these episodes represent mild transient hepatic dysfunction.

Sickle cell anemia is generally associated with increased total body iron stores due to transfusion therapy. Anemia worsened by iron deficiency is rare, except in those patients living in low socioeconomic environments with poor access to medical care.

## Vaso-occlusive Crisis

The majority of sickle crises during pregnancy are vaso-occlusive. These sickle crises are painful and dramatic expressions of vascular occlusion and may lead to organ dysfunction. The pain of sickle crisis is usually caused by avascular necrosis of the bone marrow. The pain is usually stereotypical for each particular patient. The frequency of past pain crises may be predictive of the frequency of crisis during pregnancy. The rheologic changes induced by pregnancy, however, may predispose to increased vascular occlusive events, especially during the third trimester and the postpartum period.

Painful crisis is precipitated by the rigidity of the sickle erythrocyte caused by deoxyhemoglobin S polymerization and cellular dehydration with the attendant rise in the MCHC. In the presence of a microcirculation impaired by the adherence of sickle erythrocytes to the endothelium, the transit of rigid sickle cells may be arrested, leading to vascular occlusion and ischemic infarction. The amplifying effect of stasis-induced hypoxemia leads to progressive sickle crisis.

Often, the initiating event in vaso-occlusive crisis is elusive. Risk factors predisposing to painful crises include a rise in hematocrit that increases blood viscosity, an elevated reticulocyte count that leads to the production of adhesive erythrocytes, inflammatory states that lead to the increased production of acute-phase plasma proteins, low oxygen tension, cold weather, low concentrations of fetal hemoglobin, and pregnancy (Baum, 1987).

The clinical manifestations of vaso-occlusive crisis relate to the site of the capillary bed involved. Portal circulations in which oxygen tension is low, as in the liver and kidney, are at significant risk for occlusion. Hepatopathy is caused by impaired blood flow as a result of sickling in the hepatic sinusoids and Kupffer-cell erythrophagocytosis (Mills, 1988). During painful crises, the liver is enlarged and tender, and liver-associated enzymes are elevated, representing intrahepatic cholestasis. Elevated alkaline phosphatase is common in asymptomatic sickle cell patients but is usually bone derived. Gamma-glutamyl transferase, which is not found in bone, is helpful in distinguishing hepatic from other causes of elevated alkaline phosphatase. Serum total bilirubin levels may be markedly elevated, and coagulation abnormalities may lead to hemorrhagic complications. Frank hepatic failure is

quite unusual during pregnancy, although most cases are fatal.

Congestive hepatopathy secondary to heart failure; viral hepatitis, which may develop as a result of blood product transfusions; and cocaine abuse should be considered in the differential diagnosis of the etiology of hepatotoxicity in sickle cell patients (Saltzman, 1992).

Hepatic crisis accompanied by right upper quadrant pain, fever, and leukocytosis must be differentiated from acute cholecystitis. Cholelithiasis is a common complication of sickle disease that occurs in 30% to 70% of patients (Rennels, 1984). The frequency of gallstones in the sickle hemoglobinopathies is related to the severity and chronicity of the hemolytic process. In contrast to the general population, there is no gender difference in the incidence of gallstones in sickle cell patients. The majority are pigmented stones produced by the accelerated metabolism of heme. Pigmented gallstones are predominantly calcium bilirubinate and are usually radiopaque, although the majority of those found in sickle disease are radiolucent because they are not heavily calcified (Billa, 1991). Abdominal sonography assists in the differentiation of intrahepatic cholestasis from extrahepatic obstruction. Although prophylactic cholecystectomy has been advocated to avoid confusion between acute cholecystitis and hepatic pain crises, there are no randomized trials to guide decision making (Ware, 1992).

The extremely hypertonic milieu of the renal medulla dehydrates sickle red cells, inducing severe vaso-occlusion and destruction of the vasa recta. Water loss as a result of an inability to concentrate urine enhances the sickling process in the kidney and elsewhere (de Jong, 1985). Ischemic disruption of the nephron leads to hematuria and papillary necrosis. Renal tubular clearance of hydrogen and potassium ions is impaired in most patients with sickle cell disease, and in a minority of patients may lead to frank renal tubular acidosis and hyperkalemia (De Fronzo, 1979). Renal insufficiency is a rare complication and is marked by proteinuria (Falk, 1992). Transfusion has no effect on the restoration of maximum urinary concentrating ability or correction of other renal disturbances.

Pulmonary complications are the most common cause of death in adult sickle cell patients (Platt, 1994; Kirkpatrick, 1989). Acute pulmonary complications include local infection and vascular occlusion in the pulmonary artery bed. Differentiation between the two, which may be causally related, is difficult. The clinical features of this acute chest syndrome include fever, nonproductive cough, chest pain of a pleuritic quality, and tachypnea. Hypoxemia is usually apparent, and progressive worsening may herald the development of the acute respiratory distress syndrome. Elevation of pulmonary-derived lactic dehydrogenase (LDH) and leukocytosis are associated laboratory abnormalities. The syndrome is radiographically characterized by the development of patchy pulmonary infiltrates that predominantly involve lower lobes. The infrequent confirmation of an infectious etiology in the acute chest syndrome suggests that vaso-occlusive processes count for much of the clinical picture (Kirkpatrick, 1991). The differential diagnosis includes pulmonary embolism due to deep venous thrombosis, fat embolus due to bone marrow infarction, and amniotic fluid embolus. Chronic pulmonary abnormalities due to recurrent episodes of acute chest syndrome may compromise interpretation of the otherwise diagnostic ventilation-perfusion scan.

Therapy for acute pulmonary crisis is directed toward maintenance of adequate oxygenation, treatment of any underlying infection, relief of pain, repletion of intravascular volume, and reduction of HbS concentration. Arterial blood gas analysis should be obtained and supplemental oxygen provided to maintain an arterial oxygen tension greater than 70 mm Hg. Incentive spirometry can be helpful to minimize atelectasis and infiltrates (Bellet, 1995). Data characterizing the spectrum of bacterial infectious organisms in the acute chest syndrome are limited, but empiric antibiotic coverage for both encapsulated and atypical organisms commonly causing community-acquired pneumonia is recommended (De Ceulaer, 1985). Chest pain secondary to pulmonary infarction may cause hypoventilation and exacerbation of the syndrome. Likewise, pain control through the use of narcotic analgesics must be employed cautiously because respiratory depression and deoxygenation may be precipitated. Transfusion to an HbA concentration of 30% to 50% without exceeding a hematocrit of 30% is the only therapeutic modality demonstrated to reverse the acute respiratory distress seen in this syndrome, independent of its etiology (Mallouh, 1988). Prospective data on chronic transfusion therapy to decrease the frequency of the acute chest syndrome are not available.

Central nervous system (CNS) involvement, including cerebral infarct, may also be seen in sickle crisis (Adams, 1988). Neurological changes must be differentiated from preeclampsia or meningitis. Computed tomography or lumbar puncture may be indicated. Blood transfusion has been demonstrated to ameliorate acute ischemic stroke syndromes (Rothman, 1986). Vaso-occlusive pain crisis without major organ involvement is the most common crisis seen in uncomplicated pregnancies. Approximately one third of patients with sickle cell disease will experience at least one pain crisis during pregnancy (Koshy, 1987). Musculoskeletal pain, tenderness, and limitation of motion may occur without signs of local inflammation. The exact location, intensity, and duration of pain are variable among sickle cell patients, although most patients have similar manifestations with each crisis. The presence of pain in the patient with sickle cell disease is not always due to vaso-occlusive crisis. A detailed history and physical examination are required to differentiate medical, surgical, and obstetric conditions that can present with similar clinical scenarios. Obstetric complications that should be considered in the differential diagnosis include placental abruption, preterm labor, uterine rupture, threatened abortion, and ectopic pregnancy. Narcotic-seeking behavior also should be assessed.

## Diagnosis

The lack of objective physical or laboratory findings makes the diagnosis of sickle cell vaso-occlusive pain crisis problematic. Clinical acumen is necessary to render an accurate diagnosis and to provide optimal treatment to these patients. Data from recent investigations suggest that signs of vaso-occlusion can be demonstrated in the majority of patients if reliable steady-state values have been established and are available for comparison.

Alterations in the vital signs occur in approximately 50% of adult patients suffering from a sickle pain crisis (Ballas, 1988). These include fever, BP elevation, tachypnea, and tachycardia. Fever can be due to the crisis itself, the result of tissue ischemia, and the release of endogenous pyrogens, or due to an underlying infection. Whenever fever is encountered, a thorough search for an infectious etiology is advised.

A moderate leukocytosis is seen in steady-state sickle cell anemia. Marked increases in leukocyte counts can be seen in patients with sickle cell crisis in the absence of infection. However, an increase in nonsegmented leukocytes and an elevation in the leukocyte alkaline phosphatase activity are not observed during an uncomplicated sickle crisis and should suggest concurrent infection.

Serum lactate dehydrogenase values, especially isoenzymes 1 and 2, are elevated in sickle cell crisis. These levels tend to rise in proportion to the severity of vaso-occlusion. The increase in LDH is likely due to bone marrow infarction.

Ischemic tissue damage induces an acute-phase inflammatory response that is mediated by cytokines released from local monocytes and macrophages. In a vaso-occlusive crisis, ischemia generates interleukins, which induce hepatic synthesis and release of acute-phase proteins. Elevations of C-reactive protein (CRP) and fibrinogen levels lead to a rapid erythrocyte sedimentation rate (ESR). C-reactive protein concentrations increase within 1 to 2 days of crisis onset, while other acute-phase reactants show a more delayed rise, with a peak around 6 to 7 days (Akinola, 1992). The more severe and protracted the course of the pain crisis, the higher the concentration of acute-phase reactants. Unfortunately, the acute-phase response to tissue injury is nonspecific and is not demonstrably different between vaso-occlusive infarction and infection.

Thrombosis is believed to play a pathogenic role in the development of vaso-occlusive crisis. Fibrin D-dimer levels are elevated in sickle cell patients at baseline and rise to high levels with vaso-occlusion (Francis, 1989). D-dimer is produced by plasma degradation of cross-linked fi-brin. Increased amounts of D-dimer indicate increased degradation of fibrin and indirectly indicate increased thrombin activity and fibrin formation. A documented rise in D-dimer levels may be useful in differentiating vaso-occlusive crisis from infection.

Nuclear medicine and magnetic resonance imaging studies have demonstrated changes in the bone marrow during painful crisis (Rao, 1989). Although these studies are able to detect areas of tissue damage, they cannot distinguish reliably between newly infarcted areas and those altered by previous necrosis and fibrosis (van Zanten, 1989). The prior studies needed for comparative judgments are unlikely to be available for review. Imaging studies deemed "negative" may allow for expedited discharge planning or confirm suspicions of narcotic-seeking behavior (Feldman, 1993).

Reports suggest that the typical painful crisis in adults evolves in two distinct phases, with corresponding hematologic markers (Ballas, 1988, 1992). The first phase in which the pain escalates is associated with decreased red-cell deformability and increased numbers of dense sickle cells. An increase in measures of cell heterogeneity, such as the red-cell distribution width (RDW), is also noted. Anemia worsens due to preferential occlusion and destruction of dense cells. Resolution of the pain crisis is accompanied by an increase in red-cell deformability, a fall in the percentage of dense cells, a return in hemoglobin to precrisis level, and a decrease in the RDW as reticulocytosis abates. The charting of these changes in the degree of anemia and RDW has been proposed as a method to diagnose and track the progression of painful crises (Lande, 1988).

Ischemia, infarction, and inflammation may be responsible for initiating vaso-occlusive events, yet no simple laboratory test that gauges the presence and extent of painful crises is available. Fluctuations in leukocyte differential counts, biochemical values, acute-phase reactants, measurements of fibrinolysis, and erythrocyte subpopulations suggest that serial assessments of these markers may assist in objective judgments regarding painful crisis. The subjective nature of pain itself, however, often clashes with objectively based assessments.

## Management

The standard conservative management of sickle pain crisis consists of appropriate examination followed by rest, hydration, and analgesia. Advances in the understanding of the molecular and cellular pathophysiology of sickle hemoglobinopathies and the precipitates of painful, vaso-occlusive crises provide the rationale for current therapy. Overall, the therapy of sickle cell crisis is supportive and symptomatic.

In most cases of sickle crisis, the pregnant patient should be admitted to the obstetric unit, preferably to a warm, quiet, comfortable area where her family can provide support and necessary medical needs can be met. Major characteristics of acute pain include fear and anxiety, which are especially pronounced when associated with fear of death. A vicious cycle of pain, anxiety, fear, helplessness, and sleep deprivation accompanies acute painful crisis (Ballas, 1990). Bed rest and relaxation should be encouraged.

## Hydration

Because the majority of patients will be dehydrated, rehydration constitutes a cornerstone of supportive therapy. The kidney in sickle cell disease manifests an inability to concentrate urine, and thus, hypotonic solutions should be employed in intravenous fluid maintenance after initial isotonic fluid resuscitation. It is unlikely that fluid therapy can produce a positive impact on dehydrated, dense sickle cells themselves, due to the irreversible nature of cell membrane impairment. Blood viscosity can be lowered with maintenance of a euvolemic state, which can decrease the predisposition to ongoing vaso-occlusive crisis. Intravenous hydration should be prudently monitored because pulmonary edema is a commonly recognized complication of the acute chest syndrome. Intake and output should be recorded, although urinary catheterization should be avoided, if possible, to decrease the risk of ascending infection.

## Oxygen

The benefit of oxygen therapy in nonhypoxic patients is uncertain. Although oxygen has been shown to reduce the number of reversibly sickled cells in vitro, clinical trials of such therapy have not produced a reduction in the duration of pain, analgesic administration, or length of hospitalization (Zipursky, 1992). Oxygen therapy inhibits erythropoiesis, which may account for these contradictory findings (Embory, 1984). It is possible that the number of reticulocytes prone to vascular adhesion could rebound after the cessation of oxygen therapy and predispose to recurrent vaso-occlusive crisis. Therefore, oxygen supplementation should be reserved for those patients with a documented $Pao_2$ of less than 70 mm Hg or those with evidence of pulmonary infection or infarction or labor. The therapeutic goal is to maintain a normal $Pao_2$, thus minimizing microvascular occlusion and exaggeration of any underlying pulmonary hypertension. There is no proven benefit to increasing the $Pao_2$ above the normal 100 mm Hg. Incentive spirometry every 2 hours during the waking hours is recommended for any patient with acute chest or back pain above the diaphragm.

If oxygen therapy is needed, 3 liters supplied by nasal cannula is usually sufficient. In severe oxygenation failure refractory to supplemental oxygen, the use of continuous positive airway pressure or positive end-expiratory pressure may be necessary. Arterial blood gases should be obtained as clinically indicated.

As many as one third of adult vaso-occlusive crises are associated with apparent or occult infection. The most frequently encountered infections in pregnant sickle cell patients are pneumonia, urinary tract infection, osteomyelitis, and puerperal endomyometritis. Whereas the pneumococcus predominates in childhood, gram-negative organisms and salmonella are more commonly recovered as the major offending infectious organisms during pregnancy and the reproductive years. Atypical agents such as mycoplasma and chlamydia can also cause pneumonia in these patients. The striking susceptibility to infection in gravidas with sickle hemoglobinopathies is considered to be multifactorial and related to defective activation of the complement system, decreased serum immunoglobulin levels, impaired serum opsonizing capacity, inhibited neutrophil migration, defective granulocyte phagocytosis, and hyposplenism (Boghossian, 1991; Hand, 1978; Johnston, 1973; Pearson, 1969). A thorough search for infection is mandatory. Empiric broad-spectrum antibiotic coverage should be administered prior to the isolation of a causative organism if infection is suspected.

## Pain Control

Avascular necrosis of the bone marrow produces excruciating pain that can last up to 1 week. For mild pain, peripherally acting analgesics such as acetaminophen may suffice for pharmacologic management. Oral narcotics are commonly used for outpatient therapy of mild-to-moderate pain, with codeine being the most widely used. For maximal effect, oral narcotics should be given with a peripherally acting analgesic. Stronger oral narcotics, such as hydrocodone or immediate- and sustained-release morphine, are reserved for patients with moderate-to-severe vaso-occlusive crisis. Narcotics can cause nausea and emesis, which should be controlled by antiemetic suppositories. Inpatient withdrawal of patients who require extended narcotic treatment may be necessary to appropriately prevent or manage chemical dependency.

Caution should be exercised in the use of nonsteroidal antiinflammatory drugs (NSAIDs) to enhance the efficacy of narcotic analgesia in pregnant women. These agents are contraindicated after 32 weeks of gestation due to the high risk of premature closure of the ductus arteriosus and the development of oligohydramnios. If NSAIDs are used prior to this date, serial fetal echocardiograms and ultrasounds may be necessary to assess ductal closure and amniotic fluid volume.

For the relief of severe pain, meperidine is often given by the intramuscular or intravenous route. Meperidine has a long-acting metabolite, normeperidine, which has poor analgesic activity but has been associated with dysphoria, CNS excitability, and even seizures. Risk factors for normeperidine seizures include renal failure, high drug doses, and coadministration of hepatic enzyme-inducing medicines such as phenothiazines. To avoid this adverse effect, some consultants recommend morphine as the parenteral analgesic of choice. Morphine also has its share of unwanted side effects, such as nausea, vomiting, pruritus, and possible respiratory depression. Development of the latter should be avoided because it has been hypothesized that narcotic-induced respiratory depression may predispose the patient to develop the acute chest syndrome.

Sickle cell patients who are provided patient-controlled analgesic (PCA) pumps use less medication, develop less respiratory depression, and report better pain control than those patients receiving intermittent bolus injections on demand (Shapiro, 1993). Because dosing meperidine through PCA pumps increases the risk of normeperidine-related seizures, morphine or other synthetic narcotics should be employed (Hagmeyer, 1993).

Epidural analgesia with local anesthetics alone or in combination with narcotic analgesics has been shown to effectively and safely treat the pain of sickle cell crisis (Yaster, 1994). More importantly, it does so without causing sedation, respiratory depression, or significant ambulatory limitation, which may worsen oxygenation.

Transcutaneous electric nerve stimulation (TENS) devices have been used in patients with sickle cell disease. At least one group of investigators has reported that TENS was helpful, although a large placebo effect was noted (Wang, 1988). The role of nonpharmacologic analgesic technologies in debilitating painful crises likely is limited.

In a double-blinded randomized study, a short course of high-dose intravenous methylprednisolone decreased the duration of severe pain in children and adolescents with sickle cell–associated vaso-occlusive pain crisis (Griffin, 1994). Unfortunately, these patients tended to have more rebound attacks. The potential benefit of this modality of therapy has not yet been studied in pregnancy.

The role of hydroxyurea in decreasing the frequency of painful sickle crises has been investigated (Charache, 1995). Due to its mutagenic and teratogenic effects, this medication is contraindicated in women contemplating pregnancy or who are pregnant.

## Exchange Transfusion

Although controversial, several clinicians support the use of prophylactic hypertransfusion or partial exchange transfusion during pregnancy (Cunningham, 1983; Morrison, 1989). The potential benefits of an infusion of erythrocytes is mediated by increases in oxygen-carrying capacity, decreases in the percentage of hemoglobin S, and temporary decreases in disordered erythropoiesis. Through these mechanisms, the incidence of red cell deoxygenation and subsequent polymerization can be prevented and vaso-occlusive crises avoided.

The goal of a program of transfusion therapy is to maintain a hematocrit less than 30% with a hemoglobin A concentration of 30% to 50% documented by electrophoresis. Although the use of prophylactic transfusions has been shown to reduce the incidence of vaso-occlusive crisis during pregnancy, debate continues regarding the issue of whether the practice actually has a beneficial impact on maternal and perinatal outcomes (Koshy, 1988). The major disadvantages of transfusion therapy include the risks of transfusion reactions, alloimmunization complicating later transfusion therapy, and the acquisition of blood-rne infectious diseases.

One of the most important therapeutic mea-·es for treating an established sickle cell crisis, especially one that has not responded to conservative management, is partial exchange transfusion (Morrison, 1976). The older manual methods have been replaced at most comprehensive sickle cell disease centers with automated erythrocytopheresis. The advantage of the newer method is the controlled rate of red-cell withdrawal and return, which protects the patient from hypovolemia or overload and the fetus from uteroplacental insufficiency (Morrison, 1991). Simple transfusion alone is helpful when the hemoglobin level is less than 6 g/dL.

Whenever transfusion is deemed necessary, blood donors should be family members or African-American, if possible, to reduce the risk of alloimmunization. The use of buffy coat poor, washed red cells also may help to reduce the risk of alloimmunization and allergic reactions. Intensive screening of donated blood to detect the human immunodeficiency virus, cytomegalovirus, and hepatitis B and C is critically important.

## Fetal Evaluation

Fetal loss is a major concern in pregnant patients with sickle cell disease. It can occur during or immediately after a crisis. Continuous electronic monitoring should be undertaken for patients during crisis if the fetus is potentially viable. Caution is necessary in interpreting tracings as nonreassuring. A nonreactive fetal heart rate pattern is common during vaso-occlusive episodes, and one third of patients will have a biophysical profile of 6 or less (Anyaegbunum, 1991). However, fetal assessments tend to normalize as the crisis improves. In utero resuscitation should be initiated prior to consideration of emergent operative delivery.

## Operative Considerations

Anesthesia may enhance sickling due to hypoxemia and vascular stasis and may lead to sickle cell crisis in the postoperative period. Opinions are divided on the risks of regional and general anesthesia in pregnant patients with sickle cell anemia. Although specific intraoperative goals of maintaining a normal pH, avoiding circulatory stasis or sludging, and maintaining optimal oxygenation and body temperature are agreed on, the issue of prophylactic or exchange transfusions prior to vaginal or cesarean delivery remains controversial. The transfusion of 1 unit of packed red cells per week for 4 weeks prior to planned surgical procedures in asymptomatic sickle cell patients has been advocated (Rawstron, 1976). Because sickled red cells have a shorter half-life than normal transfused cells and because transfusion dampens erythropoietic response and suppresses bone marrow production of new sickle erythrocytes, this degree of supplementation should produce a level of approximately 50% hemoglobin A at the time of surgery (Schmalzer, 1982). Nevertheless, a mix of 50% normal cells and 50% sickle cells does not reduce anesthetic and surgical risk to the minimal levels experienced by heterozygous sickle trait patients whose red cells contain approximately 50% hemoglobin A and 50% hemoglobin S. Unlike the red cells of the patient

**SICKLE CELL CRISIS**

I. *Goals of Therapy*

  A.  To relieve symptoms.
  B.  To treat any concomitant illness.

II. *Management Protocol*

  A.  Admit the patient to a warm quiet area in an obstetric unit.
  B.  Place the patient at bed rest.
  C.  Apply continuous electronic fetal monitoring if the fetus is potentially viable.
  D.  Rehydrate the patient with warm fluids.
  E.  Strictly record intake and output.
  F.  Avoid unnecessary urinary catheters and central venous lines.
  G.  Administer acetaminophen for mild pain, oral opioids for moderate pain, and parenteral opioids for severe pain.
  H.  Obtain appropriate cultures and empirically administer antibiotics if infection is suspected.
  I.  Administer oxygen at 3 to 6 liters by nasal cannula if the patient is in labor or is hypoxic ($Pao_2$ <70 mm Hg).
  J.  Initiate incentive spirometry every 2 hours in the presence of acute chest pain or back pain above the diaphragm.
  K.  Employ automated partial exchange transfusion (erythrocytopheresis) if the patient does not respond to initial conservative management or if the hemoglobin A concentration is less than 30%. Use warmed, washed, leukocyte-poor, screened blood to minimize complications.
  L.  Monitor postpartum febrile morbidity.
  M.  Encourage early ambulation.
  N.  Discuss genetic counseling and contraceptive methods with the patient.

III. *Critical Laboratory Tests*

  A.  Complete blood count with differential
  B.  Reticulocyte count
  C.  Hemoglobin electropheresis
  D.  Chemistry panel, including LDH fractionation, CRP, ESR
  E.  Blood type and screen
  F.  Human immunodeficiency virus and hepatitis screen
  G.  Urinalysis
  H.  Urine, sputum, and blood cultures as clinically indicated
  I.  Chest x-ray, ECG, and arterial blood gas as clinically indicated
  J.  Crossmatch 6 units of buffy coat poor, washed packed RBCs if erythrocytopheresis is planned.

IV. *Consultation*

  A.  Medicine (hematology and critical care)
  B.  Newborn medicine (if delivery is contemplated)
  C.  Anesthesia (if delivery is contemplated)

with sickle trait, sickle cells in the transfused patient will still sickle on deoxygenation and exposure to other stressors and a vaso-occlusive crisis may be precipitated.

Studies support withholding prophylactic transfusions in routine, elective procedures, although transfusion or exchange transfusion is advocated in preparation for emergent or prolonged surgery under general anesthesia (Homi, 1979). These studies have been conducted in general surgery patients, and the applicability of these recommendations to the obstetric population is unknown. The choice of anesthetic technique or agent for general anesthesia does not seem to be a major factor in obstetric morbidity in sickle cell patients if proper monitoring standards are maintained (Gross, 1993).

## REFERENCES

Adams RJ, Nichols RG, McKie V. Cerebral infarction in sickle cell anemia: mechanism based on CT and MRI. Neurology 1988;38:1012.

Akinola NO, Stevens SME, Franklin IM, et al. Rheological changes in the prodromal and established phases of sickle cell vaso-occlusive crisis. Br J Haematol 1992;81:598.

Alperin JB. Folic acid deficiency complicating sickle cell anemia. Arch Intern Med 1967;120:298.

Anyaegbunum A, Morel M, Merkatz IR. Antepartum fetal surveillance tests during sickle cell crisis. Am J Obstet Gynecol 1991;165:1081.

Ballas SK. Treatment of pain in adults with sickle cell disease. Am J Hematol 1990;34:49.

Ballas SK, Larner J, Smith ED, et al. Rheologic predictors of the painful sickle cell crisis. Blood 1988;72:1216.

Ballas SK, Smith ED. Red blood cell changes during the evolution of the sickle cell painful crisis. Blood 1992;79:2154.

Baum KF, Dunn DT, Maude GH, Serjeant GR. The painful crisis of homozygous sickle cell disease: a study of risk factors. Arch Intern Med 1987;147:1231.

Bellet PS, Kalinyak KA, Shukla R, et al. Incentive spirometry to prevent acute pulmonary complications in sickle cell diseases. N Engl J Med 1995;333:699.

Billa RF, Biwole MS, Juimo AG, et al. Gallstone disease in African patients with sickle cell anaemia: a preliminary report from Yaounde, Cameroon. Gut 1991;31:539.

Boghossian SH, Nash G, Dormandy J, Bearan DH. Abnormal neutrophil adhesion in sickle cell anaemia and crisis: relationship to blood rheology. Br J Haematol 1991;78:437.

Bookchin RM, Ortiz OE, Lew VL. Evidence for a direct reticulocyte origin of dense red cells in sickle cell anemia. J Clin Invest 1991;87:113.

Charache S, Terrin ML, Moore RD, et al. Effect of hydroxyurea on the frequency of painful crises in sickle cell anemia. N Engl J Med 1995;332:1317.

Cunningham F, Pritchard JA, Mason R, Chase G. Pregnancy and sickle cell hemoglobinopathies: results with and without prophylactic transfusions. Obstet Gynecol 1983;62:419.

De Ceulaer K, McMullen KW, Maude GH, et al. Pneumonia in young children with homozygous sickle cell disease: risk and clinical features. Eur J Pediatr 1985;144:255.

De Fronzo RA, Taufield PA, Black H. Impaired renal tubular potassium secretion in sickle cell disease. Ann Intern Med 1979;90:310.

de Jong PE, Statius van Eps LW. Sickle cell nephropathy: new insights into its pathophysiology. Kidney Int 1985;27:711.

Dean J, Schechter AN. Sickle-cell anemia: molecular and cellular bases of therapeutic approaches (pts 1, 2, and 3). N Engl J Med 1978;299:752, 804, 863.

Diggs LW. Anatomic lesions in sickle cell disease. In: Abramson H, Bertles JF, Wethers DL, eds. Sickle cell disease: diagnosis, management, education and research. St. Louis: Mosby, 1973:189.

Embory SH, Garcia JF, Mohandas N, et al. Effects of oxygen inhalation on endogenous erythropoietin kinetics, erythropoiesis, and properties of blood cells in sickle cell anemia. N Engl J Med 1984;311:291.

Emond AM, Collis R, Darrill D, et al. Acute splenic sequestration in homozygous sickle cell disease: natural history and management. J Pediatr 1985;107:201.

Falk RJ, Scheinman J, Phillips G, et al. Prevalence and pathologic features of sickle cell nephropathy and response to inhibition of angiotensin-converting enzyme. N Engl J Med 1992;326:910.

Feldman F, Zwass A, Staron RB, Haramati N. MRI of soft tissue abnormalities: a primary cause of sickle cell crisis. Skeletal Radiol 1993;22:501.

Francis RB Jr. Elevated fibrin D-dimer fragment in sickle cell anemia: evidence for activation of coagulation during the steady state as well as in painful crisis. Haemostasis 1989;19:105.

Griffin TC, McIntire D, Buchanan GR. High-dose intravenous methylprednisolone therapy for pain in children and adolescents with sickle cell disease. N Engl J Med 1994;330:733.

Gross ML, Schwedler M, Bischoff RJ, Kerstein MD. Impact of anesthetic agents on patients with sickle cell disease. Am Surg 1993;59:261.

Hagmeyer KO, Mauro LS, Mauro VF. Meperidine-related seizures associated with patient-controlled analgesia pumps. Ann Pharmacother 1993;27:29.

Hand WL, King NL. Serum opsonization of salmonella in sickle cell anemia. Am J Med 1978; 64:388.

Hebbel RP, Schwartz RS, Mohanda SN. The adhesive sickle erythrocyte: cause and sequence of abnormal interactions with endothelium, monocytes/macrophages and model membranes. Clin Haematol 1985;14:141.

Hernandez P, Dorticos E, Espinoza E, et al. Clinical features of hepatic sequestration in sickle cell anaemia. Haematologia 1989;22:169.

Homi J, Reynolds J, Skinner A, et al. General anesthesia in sickle cell disease. Br Med J 1979;1: 1599.

Johnston RB, Newman SL, Struth AG. An abnormality of the alternate pathway of complement activation in sickle cell disease. N Engl J Med 1973;288:803.

Kinney TR, Ware RE, Schultz WH. Long-term management of splenic sequestration in children with sickle cell disease. J Pediatr 1990;117:194.

Kirkpatrick MB, Bass JB. Pulmonary complications in adults with sickle cell disease. Pulm Perspect 1989;6:6.

Kirkpatrick MB, Haynes J, Bass JB. Results of bronchoscopically obtained lower airway cultures from adult sickle cell disease patients with the acute chest syndrome. Am J Med 1991;90:206.

Koshy M, Burd L, Dorn L, Hoff G. Frequency of pain crisis during pregnancy. Prog Clin Biol Res 1987;240:305.

Koshy M, Burd L, Wallace D, et al. Prophylactic red cell transfusion in pregnant patients with sickle cell disease. A randomized cooperative study. N Engl J Med 1988;319:1447.

Lande WM, Andrews DL, Clark MR. The incidence of painful crisis in homozygous sickle cell disease: correlation with red cell deformability. Blood 1988;72:2056.

Mallouh AA, Asha MA. Beneficial effect of blood transfusion in children with sickle cell chest syndrome. Am J Dis Child 1988;142:178.

Mills LR, Marakyusa D, Milner P. Histopathologic features of liver biopsy specimens in sickle cell disease. Arch Pathol Lab Med 1988;112:290.

Milner PF, Jones BR, Dobler J. Outcome of pregnancy in sickle cell anemia and sickle cell hemoglobin C disease. Am J Obstet Gynecol 1980; 138:239.

Morrison JC, Morrison FS. Prophylactic transfusions in pregnant patients with sickle cell disease. N Engl J Med 1989;320:1286.

Morrison JC, Morrison FS, Floyd RC, et al. Use of continuous flow erythrocytopheresis in pregnant patients with sickle cell disease. J Clin Apheresis 1991;6:224.

Morrison JC, Wiser WL. The use of prophylactic partial exchange transfusion in pregnancies associated with sickle cell hemoglobinopathies. Obstet Gynecol 1976;48:516.

Noguchi CT, Rodgers GP, Serjeant RG, Schechter AN. Levels of fetal hemoglobin necessary for treatment of sickle cell disease. N Engl J Med 1988;318:96.

Orringer EP, Fowler VG, Owens CM, et al. Case report: splenic infarction and acute splenic sequestration in adults with hemoglobin SC disease. Am J Med Sci 1991;302:374.

Pasrol G, Weatherall DJ. Cellular mechanism for the protective effect of haemoglobin S against *P. falciparum* malaria. Nature 1978;274:701.

Pearson HA, Spence RP, Cornelius EA. Functional asplenia in sickle cell anemia. N Engl J Med 1969;281:923.

Pegelow CH, Wilson B, Overturf GD. Infection in splenectomized sickle cell disease patients. Clin Pediatr 1980;19:102.

Platt OS, Brambilla DJ, Wendell RF, et al. Mortality in sickle cell disease: life expectancy and risk factors for early death. N Engl J Med 1994;330:1639.

Powars DR, Meeno S, Niland-Weiss J, et al. Pregnancy in sickle cell disease. Obstet Gynecol 1986;67:217.

Rao S, Gooden S. Splenic sequestration in sickle cell disease: role of transfusion therapy. Am J Pediatr Hematol Oncol 1985;7:298.

Rao SP, Miller ST, Cohen BJ. Transient aplastic crisis in patients with sickle cell disease: B1 parvovirus studies during a 7-year period. Am J Dis Child 1992;146:1328.

Rao VM, Mitchell DG, Rifkin MD, et al. Marrow infarction in sickle cell anemia: correlation with marrow type and distribution by MRI. Magn Reson Imaging 1989;7:39.

Rawstron RE. Preoperative haemoglobin levels. Anaesth Intensive Care 1976;4:176.

Rennels MB, Dunne MG, Grossman NJ, Schwartz AD. Cholelithiasis in patients with major sickle hemoglobinopathies. Am J Dis Child 1984;138:66.

Rothman SM, Fulling KH, Nelson JS. Sickle cell anemia and central nervous system infarction: a neuropathological study. Ann Neurol 1986;20:684.

Saltzman JR, Johnston DE. Sickle cell crisis and cocaine hepatotoxicity. Am J Gastroenterol 1992;87:1661.

Schmalzer EH, Lee JO, Brown AF. Viscosity of mixtures of sickle and normal red cells in varying hematocrit levels: implications for transfusion. Transfusion 1982;22:17.

Seoud MAF, Cantwell C, Nobles G, Lery DL. Outcome of pregnancies complicated by sickle cell and sickle-C hemoglobinopathies. Am J Perinatol 1994;11:187.

Shapiro BS, Cohen DE, Howe CJ. Patient-controlled analgesia for sickle-cell-related pain. J Pain Symptom Manage 1993;8:22.

van Zanten TEG, Van Eps LW, Golding RP, Valk J. Imaging the bone marrow with magnetic resonance during a crisis and in chronic forms of sickle cell disease. Clin Radiol 1989;40:486.

Wang WC, George SL, Wilimas JA. Transcutaneous electrical nerve stimulation treatment of sickle cell pain crises. Acta Haematol 1988;80:99.

Ware RE, Kinney TR, Casey JR, et al. Laparoscopic cholecystectomy in young patients with sickle hemoglobinopathies. J Pediatr 1992;120:58.

Yaster M, Tobin JR, Billett C, et al. Epidural analgesia in the management of severe vaso-occlusive sickle cell crisis. Pediatrics 1994;93:3310.

Zipursky A, Robieux I, Brown EJ, et al. Oxygen therapy in sickle cell disease. Am J Pediatr Hematol Oncol 1992;14:222.

# CHAPTER 31

# Intracranial Hemorrhage

*I*ntracranial hemorrhage (ICH) is a rare but often catastrophic event that can occur in the gravid population. Anatomically, intracranial bleeds can be classified as intracerebral hemorrhage or subarachnoid hemorrhage (SAH), with the latter being most common (Dias, 1990). Although there is some etiologic overlap, SAH during pregnancy is primarily the result of ruptured cerebral aneurysms or arteriovenous malformations (AVM). Intracerebral hemorrhage, on the other hand, is associated primarily with pregnancy-induced hypertension. The pathophysiology and management of ICH due to cerebral aneurysm, AVM, and eclampsia are discussed in this chapter. Less common etiologies include moyamoya disease, dural venous sinus thrombosis, mycotic aneurysm, choriocarcinoma, vasculitides, brain tumors, and coagulopathies (Enomoto, 1987; Isla, 1997). Cocaine and phenylpropanolamine also have been associated with ICH in pregnant patients (Henderson, 1988; Iriye, 1995; Maher, 1987).

## Regulation of Cerebral Blood Flow

Human cerebral blood flow averages approximately 50 mL/min/100 g of brain tissue and is normally regulated to maintain constant flow over a wide range of systemic BPs (Kety, 1948; Lassen, 1959). In addition, cerebral blood flow is markedly affected by levels of systemic oxygen and carbon dioxide; elevation of $pco_2$ by as little as 15

mm Hg results in a 75% increase in cerebral blood flow (Kety, 1948). Similarly, a reduction in arterial $po_2$ to 50 mm Hg results in a 100% increase in cerebral blood flow. On the other hand, elevation of the normal arterial $po_2$ by the inhalation of pure oxygen results in a 15% decrease in cerebral blood flow, and hyperventilation with a decrease in $pco_2$ by 15 mm Hg results in a 33% decrease (Kety, 1948). In the previously normotensive patient, the process of cerebral blood flow autoregulation is not reliably maintained at levels of mean arterial pressure in excess of 140 mm Hg; this level is somewhat higher for patients with long-standing chronic hypertension. Pressures in excess of these levels can result in SAH, even in the absence of underlying vascular defects.

## Subarachnoid Hemorrhage

### Pathophysiology

Aneurysms and AVMs are believed to develop secondary to congenital defects in cerebral vasculature formation. Aneurysms generally are located at an angle of vessel bifurcation in or near the circle of Willis. Arteriovenous malformations, on the other hand, can be located anywhere between the frontal region and the brain stem, but they occur with a higher frequency in the frontoparietal and temporal regions. The anatomic

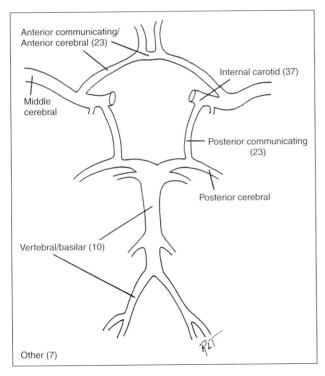

F I G U R E **31-1**

Location of cerebral aneurysms in pregnancy (%).

distribution of both lesions is similar to that in the nongravid population (Dias, 1990). Figure 31-1 displays the most common locations of aneurysms in the pregnant patient.

The natural history of intracranial aneurysms in the nonpregnant patient varies, depending on several clinical factors. Asymptomatic lesions account for 95% of intracranial aneurysms and are typically identified incidentally. They rupture at a rate of 1% to 2% per year (Barrow, 1993). Activities reported to precede aneurysmal rupture include emotional strain, heavy lifting, coughing, coitus, urination, and defecation. All may increase intracranial pressure (ICP) and alter hemodynamics. Symptomatic aneurysms present a greater risk. Their annual risk of rupture is 6.25%. Once bleeding has occurred, the patient's course is altered significantly. Untreated, half of all patients will die as a result of the initial event, with another 25% to 35% succumbing to a subsequent bleed. Other factors affecting the patient's ultimate out-

come are neurologic grade, the development of secondary vasospasm, and BP (Barrow, 1993).

Outcomes of patients with AVMs are influenced by the presenting symptoms and subsequent treatment. Most present with spontaneous bleeding, and these patients have the worst prognosis. Other presenting symptoms in order of frequency include seizures, headache, and neurologic deficit. If left untreated, there is an annual hemorrhage rate of 4%, with a mortality rate of 1% per year (Barrow, 1993).

During pregnancy, the incidence of SAH is one to five per 10,000 pregnancies. Maternal mortality is 30% to 40%, but rates as high as 80% have been reported (Dias, 1990; Wilterdink, 1994). Kitner (1996) recently presented evidence that the risks of cerebral infarction and intracerebral hemorrhage are increased in the first six weeks postpartum, but not during pregnancy itself. Fetal outcome parallels that of the mother and reflects the maternal condition as well as gestational age at delivery (Dias, 1990). Because the condition is rare, pregnancy's effect on cerebral aneurysms or AVMs continues to be controversial. Most episodes of SAH occur later in pregnancy (Wilterdink, 1994; Reichman, 1995). The timing of SAH during pregnancy is shown in Figure 31-2. Several physiologic changes occurring during pregnancy

F I G U R E **31-2**

**Gestational age distribution of aneurysmal SAH.**

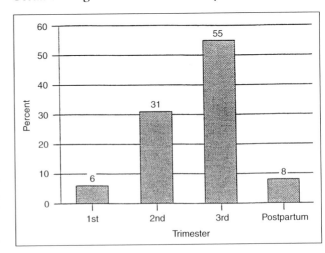

may theoretically predispose these cerebrovascular abnormalities to bleed. These factors include increases in blood volume, stroke volume, and cardiac output. Estrogen levels also are increased and may result in vasodilation of already abnormal vessels (Pritchard, 1985). The hemodynamic fluctuations occurring during labor and delivery would seem to make this a particularly high risk time.

Despite the associated physiologic changes, pregnancy does not appear to increase the incidence of SAH and, surprisingly, bleeding during the time of labor and delivery is infrequent (Dias, 1990; Weibers, 1985; Cannell, 1956; Amias, 1970; Copelan, 1962; Robinson, 1972, 1974; Forster, 1993; Weibers, 1988). Most pregnancies complicated by SAH are preceded by unaffected gestations. In a review of 154 patients prepared by Dias and Sekhar (1990), only 25% were nulliparous, and the mean parity of patients with aneurysmal and AVM ruptures was 2.0 and 1.4, respectively ($p > .05$). Barno and Freeman (1976) reviewed 24 years of maternal mortality in Minnesota resulting from SAH. The mean parity among the 37 deaths was 2.9. Forster et al (1993) reported their experience with AVMs in reproductive-age women. Although the annual hemorrhage rate was higher when these women were pregnant than when not (9.3% vs. 4.5%), it was no different than the 9.6% annual rate in reproductive-age women who never became pregnant. Compared with the above study, Horton et al (1990) identified a lower annual rate of hemorrhage in both their pregnant and nonpregnant patients with AVMs (3.5% vs. 3.1%). They concluded that pregnancy was not a risk factor for bleeding.

The maternal mortality associated with aneurysmal bleeding is not increased due to pregnancy (Dias, 1990; Cannell, 1956; Amias, 1970; Pedowitz, 1957). Conversely, AVM-associated mortality appears to be increased in gravid compared with nongravid patients. This likely is related to the poor neurologic condition of these patients at presentation.

Major complications associated with SAH include vasospasm, recurrent hemorrhage, and hydrocephalus. Vasospasm is a serious problem seen in 30% to 40% of aneurysm patients but less commonly in those with AVMs (Wilterdink, 1994; Kas-

sel, 1985). This complication is caused, at least in part, by the release of several vasoactive products of hemoglobin breakdown in the subarachnoid space; the degree of vasospasm appears to correlate with the amount and distribution of subarachnoid blood (Grolimund, 1988; Heros, 1983; Fisher, 1980; Hijdra, 1988; Adams, 1987; Giannotta, 1977). The resultant ischemia is a major cause of permanent disability and death (Giannotta, 1986). Angiographically, vasospasm appears as cerebral arterial narrowing, sometimes with a beaded pattern. Vasospasm is associated with decreased cerebral blood flow as measured by radioactive tracers such as xenon 133 and by transcranial Doppler (Kassel, 1985).

Recurrent hemorrhage is a particularly morbid complication and is especially likely in patients with ruptured aneurysm. In the untreated patient, the risk of rebleeding is 6% during the first 48 hours. Rebleeding continues to occur at a rate of 1.5% per day for the remainder of the first 2 weeks. By the end of 6 months, 30% to 40% will have had a subsequent hemorrhage (Barrow, 1993). Mortality increases with each successive bleed, with a rate of 64% and 80% after the first and second rebleed, respectively (Adams, 1976). Although few data are available that specifically address the pregnant patient, the risk of recurrent bleeding appears to be similar in this population (Wilterdink, 1994).

Acute hydrocephalus is a very poor prognostic factor in SAH. It has received relatively little attention in pregnant and nonpregnant patients alike. In a large prospective series of nonobstetric patients reported by van Gijn et al (1985), the incidence of acute hydrocephalus was 20%. The accompanying mortality rate was significantly higher when ventricular dilation was present. Ventricular drainage did not decrease overall mortality despite an initial clinical improvement.

## Clinical Presentation

Pregnancy does not significantly alter the clinical presentation of SAH. Signs and symptoms of aneurysmal or AVM bleeding are indistinguishable. Intracerebral bleeding associated with severe preeclampsia may also have similar findings. A sudden-onset "bursting" headache is generally the initial symptom. Frequently, other signs and symptoms accompany the headache. These may include nausea and vomiting, meningeal signs, decreased level of consciousness, hypertension, focal neurologic signs, and seizures (Giannotta, 1986). Specific findings are dependent on the size, location, and rapidity of the bleed. When the hemorrhage is massive, the patient may be moribund at presentation.

The most important prognostic indicator of outcome is the patient's condition at presentation. Grading scales have been developed to categorize the severity of the clinical condition in order to guide management and determine prognosis. The Hunt and Botterell scales combine the level of consciousness and the presence of neurologic deficit to describe the patient as follows (Grenvik, 1981):

Grade I: Alert with or without nuchal rigidity

Grade II: Drowsy or severe headache with no neurologic deficits other than those of the cranial nerves

Grade III: Focal neurologic deficit such as mild hemiparesis

Grade IV: Stupor with severe neurologic deficits

Grade V: Moribund

Figure 31-3 displays maternal mortality as it relates to the initial clinical grade of aneurysmal hemorrhage.

## Diagnosis

It is imperative that the clinician maintain a high index of suspicion due to the rarity and life-threatening nature of the condition. Occasionally, SAH is confused with eclampsia, resulting in diagnostic delays and a worse outcome (Giannotta, 1986). Table 31-1 compares clinical findings of SAH and eclampsia. All abnormal neurologic signs and symptoms in the gravida should be evaluated thoroughly. A team approach, with appropriate maternal-fetal medicine, neurology, and neurosurgery consultation should be sought

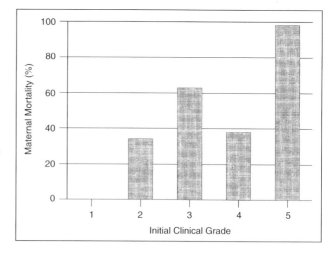

F I G U R E   **31-3**

**Maternal mortality and initial clinical grade after aneurysmal hemorrhage.**

to guide the diagnostic work-up. A computed tomography (CT) scan of the brain, lumbar puncture (if necessary), and cerebral angiography is the common sequence of testing. The CT scan can predict, with a high degree of accuracy, the type of hemorrhage and its site of origin. In addition, cerebral CT can be useful in determining the presence of life-threatening hematomas that require surgical evacuation, as well as the development of hydrocephalus. If the CT scan is normal, the CSF should be examined for blood or xanthochromia. Nonclearing bloody CSF found at lumbar puncture supports the diagnosis of SAH, but it also may be seen occasionally with other conditions, such as preeclampsia. Cerebral angiography, including magnetic resonance angiography, remains the best diagnostic tool for identifying any vascular abnormality. In addition, important anatomic (and therefore prognostic) information usually is obtained with this invasive technique. Angiography may fail to visualize the cause of SAH in 20% of patients, however (Giannotta, 1986). In these cases, a repeat angiogram may be necessary to rule out false-negative results secondary to vasospasm or clot filling of the aneurysm. A magnetic resonance imaging (MRI) scan also may be helpful in situations in which the initial angiogram fails to identify the lesion. This technique also can identify vascular lesions in the spinal cord (Wilterdink, 1994). Abdominal shielding should be considered during any radiologic examination of the gravid patient.

## Management

Pregnancy alters the standard management of SAH only slightly, because the clinical goals remain prevention and treatment of neurologic complications. Neurosurgical principles should guide therapy. In all patients thought to be viable, immediate management involves evacuation of any life-threatening hematoma (Sadasivan, 1990; Giannotta, 1979). A number of considerations have led neurosurgeons to perform early aneurysm clipping in the post-SAH period (<4 days) for patients with grades I through III. These considerations include the disastrous consequences of rebleeding and the decreased vasospasm with early removal of cisternal blood. Advances in neurosurgery and neuroanesthesia have aided the early surgical approach (Giannotta, 1979, 1986; Kassell, 1981, 1984; Taneda, 1982; Ljunggren, 1982, 1984). Early operation also allows for therapies such as induced hypertension and volume expansion to be instituted to combat vasospasm

T A B L E  **31-1**

Comparison of subarachnoid hemorrhage and eclampsia

|  | SAH | Eclampsia |
|---|---|---|
| Headache | Explosive-severe | Insidious-dull |
| Nausea and vomiting | Common | Uncommon |
| Loss of consciousness | 2/3 | All (seizure) |
| Nuchal rigidity | 90% | Uncommon |
| Seizures | 15% | All |
| Hypertension | 30% to 50% | All |
| Proteinuria | Uncommon | Common |
| Focal motor weakness | 20% | Rare |

Adapted with permission from Giannotta SL, Daniels J, Golde SH, et al. Ruptured intracranial aneurysms during pregnancy: a report of four cases. J Reprod Med 1986;31:139.

without increasing the risk of rebleeding (Kassell, 1981, 1982, 1985; Giannotta, 1979; Buckland, 1988). Improved outcomes for both the mother and the fetus have been realized with early surgical intervention in pregnant patients (Dias, 1990). Patients with significant neurologic deficits (grades IV and V) are less likely to undergo early aneurysm clipping due to an extremely high operative mortality. Rather, such patients receive medical therapy until their condition improves. The proper timing for resection of AVMs is more controversial due to the smaller number of cases reported. No clear benefit to surgery in these patients has been found, with some surgeons advocating operative intervention in AVMs only to remove clinically significant hematomas (Dias, 1990; Grenvik, 1981). One alternative is embolization of the AVM under angiographic control prior to surgical excision (Aminoff, 1994).

Adjunctive medical therapy for SAH is directed toward reducing the risks of rebleeding and cerebral ischemia due to vasospasm. Patients are generally confined to bed rest in a dark, quiet room. They are administered stool softeners, sedatives, and analgesics. Because of the presumed benefits of volume expansion, colloid solutions are frequently administered. Vasospasm is often combated by induced hypertension using vasopressors or inotropic agents, and systolic BP is maintained between 150 and 200 mm Hg (Awad, 1987; Soloman, 1988; Levy, 1990). Nimodipine, a dihydropyridone calcium channel blocker, is often given because it has been shown to improve neurologic outcome by combating vasospasm following SAH (Allen, 1983; Ljunggren, 1984). Caution is advised in using this drug in pregnancy because the fetal effects have not been completely defined. Belfort et al (1994) have reported on the use of nimodipine for seizure prophylaxis in a small number of preeclamptic patients with no apparent adverse fetal outcomes. On the other hand, Ducsay et al (1987) reported that nicardipine, another dihydropyridine calcium channel blocker, may be poorly tolerated by the fetus and may result in the development of fetal acidosis and hypoxemia in an animal model. The clinician also must be alert for the development of respiratory depression in patients with SAH;

prompt intubation is essential in such cases. Hyperthermia also may contribute to increases in cerebral blood flow and elevated ICP and should be treated aggressively when present.

In surviving patients, most aneurysm ruptures have initially bled only a few milliliters before a platelet plug sealed the leak. This tenuous hemostasis is strengthened over several days by a process of fibrosis. Interference of early physiologic fibrinolysis, therefore, theoretically improves the patient's chances of avoiding rebleed. Epsilon-aminocaproic acid and tranexamic acid block the activation of plasminogen, a precursor of plasmin, a major fibrinolytic protein. Clinical trials initially found a reduction in the incidence of rebleeding with these agents; however, later work failed to demonstrate significant improvement in outcome (Sengupta, 1976; Van Rossum, 1977).

A complete discussion of the neurosurgical and anesthetic principles of craniotomy for aneurysm clipping is beyond the scope of this chapter. However, there are two intraoperative therapies—hypotension and hypothermia—commonly instituted to reduce complications, which raise special concerns in the pregnant patient. Hypotension is sometimes instituted to reduce the risk of rupture of the aneurysm during dissection. Although maternal hypotension may pose a threat to fetal well-being, it has been successfully induced with sodium nitroprusside or isoflurane in a number of cases (Rigg, 1981; Donchin, 1978; Willoughby, 1984; Newman, 1986). Based on experimental evidence, administration of sodium nitroprusside in pregnant patients has raised concerns regarding potential fetal cyanide toxicity. Thus, if surgery is to be preformed during pregnancy, it is recommended that infusion rates not exceed 10 µg/kg/min (Willoughby, 1984). The fetal effects of maternal hypotension should be evaluated throughout the perianesthetic period with electronic fetal heart rate monitoring. Adverse changes in fetal cardiac activity suggest the need for elevation in maternal BP if safe and feasible from the maternal standpoint. Many of the drugs used in anesthesia may decrease fetal heart rate variability, thereby complicating fetal heart rate monitor interpretation (van Buul, 1993). Excessive hyperventilation has been

shown to further decrease uterine blood flow during sodium nitroprusside administration and should be avoided (Levinson, 1974). Because of the potential fetal risks of maternal hypotension, some authors recommend cesarean delivery immediately prior to intracranial surgery in term or near-term gestation (Kassell, 1981).

Hypothermia is instituted during cerebral aneurysm clipping as a means of cerebral protection from potential ischemia due to aneurysm rupture, retractor injury, or hypotension. Stange and Hallidin (1983) have suggested that hypothermia is well tolerated by the mother and fetus, provided that other confounding variables (e.g., respiratory exchange, acidosis, and electrolyte balance) are controlled. The majority of experience with hypothermia and hypotension in pregnancy, however, is anecdotal. Regardless of the neurosurgical technique employed, maternal outcome remains the most important predictor of eventual fetal outcome.

After a successful repair of an aneurysm or AVM, the most frequent obstetric concern relates to mode of delivery. Earlier authors routinely recommended elective cesarean section for these patients. This was particularly true along with consideration of sterilization if an AVM was responsible for the SAH (Robinson, 1974). More recent data and reanalysis of some older studies suggest that labor and vaginal delivery pose no additional risk to mother or fetus (Dias, 1990; Copelan, 1962; Forster, 1993; Horton, 1990; Minielly, 1979; Robinson, 1972; Parkinson, 1980; Fliegner, 1969). It has been suggested that these recommendations probably also hold true for the patient who begins labor before surgical correction is attempted or in the case in which the intracranial lesion is inaccessible to surgical intervention (Dias, 1990; Young, 1983). The number of cases on which such recommendations are based, however, is small. In the review by Dias and Sekhar (1990), involving 53 patients with uncorrected AVM or aneurysm, those delivering vaginally had almost twice the mortality rate of those undergoing cesarean section. Nevertheless, this difference did not reach statistical significance, possibly due to small sample size. Moreover, even those authors suggesting vaginal delivery for such women generally hedge their bets by recommending shortening of the second stage of labor with forceps delivery, recommendations not entirely consistent with the presumed safety of the labor and delivery process. Given the long-standing recognition that ICH is often preceded by activities involving Valsalva, it seems unreasonable at this time to conclude that vaginal delivery is as safe as cesarean for women with uncorrected lesions that have resulted in ICH. We suggest that the available data be discussed with the patient in planning route of delivery. Ultimate management decisions should be based primarily on the maternal condition, with modifications for fetal intervention based on gestational age. Figure 31-4 summarizes the management of the pregnant patient with SAH.

## Preeclampsia-Associated Intracerebral Hemorrhage

### Pathophysiology

Intracerebral hemorrhage is the most common cause of death in the eclamptic patient; it is identified in up to 60% of all deaths associated with this condition (Table 31-2). Intracerebral hemorrhage is more likely to occur in the older parturient and is correlated better with advancing maternal age and hypertension than with seizure activity. When hemorrhage does occur, it often does not coincide with the onset of seizures but rather may be manifested as long as 6 hours or

F I G U R E   **31-4**

**Management scheme for SAH due to cerebral aneurysm or AVM during pregnancy.** C/S, cesarean section.

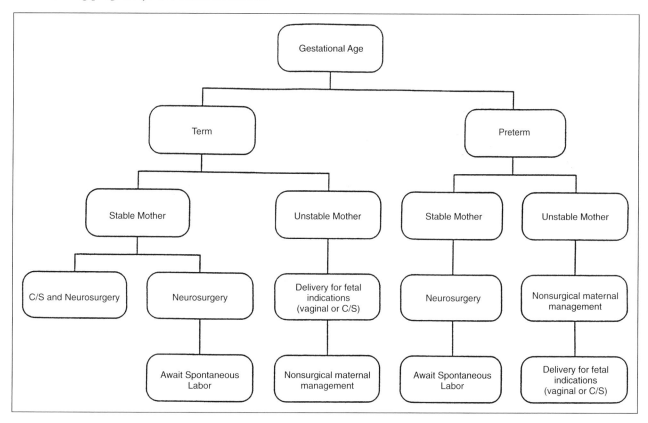

T A B L E   **31-2**

Causes of death in patients with preeclampsia/eclampsia

|  | Donnelly (1954) | Hibbard (1973) | Lopez-Llera (1982) | Evan (1983) |
|---|---|---|---|---|
| Cerebral |  |  |  |  |
|   Hemorrhage | 180 | 21 | 62 | 14 |
|   Edema | — | 13 | — | 6 |
| Pulmonary |  |  |  |  |
|   Edema | 133 | 3 | — | 3 |
|   Insufficiency | 29 | 4 | 10 | — |
| Hepatic |  |  |  |  |
|   Rupture | 30 | — | 1 | 3 |
|   Necrosis | — | 10 | — | 2 |
| Renal |  |  |  |  |
|   Failure | — | 2 | — | 7 |
|   Necrosis | — | 5 | 1 | — |
| Coagulopathy | 39 | 6 | 7 | 6 |
| Anesthesia | 12 | — | — | — |
| Sepsis | 18 | — | 2 | — |
| Drug overdose | — | 2 | — | — |
| Undetermined | 92 | 1 | 3 | 8 |
| Total | 533 | 67 | 86 | 49 |

Modified from Evan S, Frigoletto FD, Jewett JF. Mortality of eclampsia: a case
   report and the experience of the Massachusetts Maternal Mortality Study.
   N Engl J Med 1983;309:1644.

more after the onset of convulsions (Sheehan, 1973). The pathology of preeclampsia-related intracerebral hemorrhage has been described by Sheehan and Lynch (1973). They described five categories of pathologic findings and speculated on the mechanisms involved:

1. Cortical petechiae arranged radially, possibly as a result of transient vasoconstriction severe enough to result in ischemia
2. Multiple areas of ischemic softening found throughout the brain, similar in character and perhaps in etiology to the cortical petechiae
3. Multiple capillary hemorrhages in the subcortical region, with no evidence of thrombosis
4. Multiple medium-sized (1–3 cm in diameter) hemorrhages in white matter
5. Single large hemorrhage arising from deep in the white matter, in proximity to large vessels

Beck and Menezes (1981) added a sixth category:

6. Periventricular subependymal hemorrhage found in preeclamptic patients with disseminated intravascular coagulopathy or hyperemesis gravidarum

The clinical report of flashes of light and other fluctuating neurologic signs and symptoms in these patients supports the concept of intermittent ischemia, although the definitive pathologic events involved still remain to be elucidated.

## Clinical Presentation

A detailed presentation on the clinical aspects of eclampsia has been presented elsewhere in this text. In brief, the eclamptic patient traditionally presents with hypertension and tonic-clonic convulsions. The occurrence of seizure activity, however, does not necessarily result in the subsequent development of intracerebral hemorrhage, even if a transient neurologic deficit is identified in the postictal period. When small intracerebral hemorrhages do occur, the patient may present initially with only drowsiness or complaints of flashes of light. If the disease progresses, stupor and focal neurologic deficits worsen. Hemiplegia or rapidly progressive coma and cerebral death may be identified when a more massive cerebral bleed occurs (Donnelly, 1954; Hibbard, 1973; Lopoez-Llera, 1982; Evan, 1983). When assessing the timing of intracerebral hemorrhage in these patients, it is important to consider the fact that a sudden increase in blood pressure may be a sign of, rather than a cause of, intracranial bleeding.

## Diagnosis

The diagnosis of preeclampsia is well engrained in the practicing obstetrician's mind. The clinician, however, may not always be alert to the fact that a variety of subtle neurologic abnormalities, such as lethargy, visual disturbances, and even acute psychosis, can herald the onset of an intracerebral hemorrhage. With newer-generation CT scanners, there is an increased incidence of abnormal radiologic findings that correlate with the pathologic findings described by Sheehan and Lynch (Brown, 1988; Milliez, 1990). Despite these findings, CT and MRI scans are not recommended as a routine part of the evaluation for uncomplicated eclamptic patients, because management is rarely altered. These diagnostic tools should be reserved for atypical presentations, focal neurologic signs, or prolonged coma (Brown, 1988; Milliez, 1990; Digre, 1993).

## Management

Acute surgical intervention, even for the removal of a large intracerebral hematoma, is rarely of benefit. Control of seizure activity and severe hypertension, however, is always indicated. Thrombocytopenia is not an uncommon complication of preeclampsia and may aggravate the intracerebral bleeding process. Appropriate management requires monitoring of coagulation indices and replacement therapy as indicated. If the patient's outcome appears to be grave, consideration of perimortem cesarean delivery should be made.

## Adjunctive Approaches

Potent glucocorticoids such as dexamethasone have been used widely for the treatment of cerebral edema and ischemia. Support for this use comes not only from laboratory evidence of steroid-induced membrane stabilization but also from the often dramatic clinical improvement of patients with brain tumors (Fishman, 1982). Little clinical evidence exists, however, for the efficacy of steroids, in any dose, in altering the progress and outcome in the presence of ICP (Dearden, 1986).

Cerebral edema can result in elevated ICP. The neurosurgeon may wish to invasively monitor this variable in some patients to avoid severe intracranial hypertension. In patients with SAH, monitoring usually is done with a ventriculostomy so that CSF can be drained if hydrocephalus is present. The ventriculostomy may be connected to a transducer for continuous monitoring. Intracranial pressure elevations resulting from cerebral edema may be treated with mannitol, an osmotic diuretic. The mechanism of action for mannitol is felt to be primarily an extraction of both intracellular and extracellular fluid from brain tissue (Nath, 1986). However, mannitol also may produce vasoconstriction, alter blood viscosity, and effect local oxygen delivery (Muizelaar, 1984). Mannitol is a nonmetabolized sugar that is available in 20% and 25% solutions. Typically, 12.5 to 50.0 g are administered intravenously, as needed, to keep the ICP below 20 mm Hg. The development of hyperosmolality is a potential hazard of mannitol therapy and can be monitored by serum osmolality determinations. Normal values are 280 to 300 mosm/liter; the drug should be withheld when a level of 315 to 320 mosm/liter or a serum sodium of 150 mEq/dL is reached. Evidence exists to suggest that the combination of mannitol and furosemide may result in a greater and more sustained reduction in ICP than either agent given alone (Wilkinson, 1983; Pollay, 1983). Care must be taken to prevent hypovolemia resulting from the accompanying diuresis, which could aggravate placental and cerebral hypoperfusion. Barbiturate therapy also may be useful in otherwise refractory intracranial hypertension. Pentobarbital is administered slowly in a dose of

---

## INTRACRANIAL HEMORRHAGE

### I. *Goals of Therapy*

    A.  To prevent vasospasm and cerebral ischemia
    B.  To minimize cerebral edema and reduce ICP
    C.  To support respiration
    D.  To support or reduce BP, as necessary
    E.  To surgically correct lesions when appropriate

### II. *Management Protocol*

    A.  Ruptured Aneurysm
       1.  Grades I, II, and III: Early surgical intervention
       2.  Grades IV and V: Stabilization and conservative management
          a.  Bed rest, quiet environment
          b.  Sedative, analgesic support, supplemented by a stool softener
          c.  Surgery after stabilization
    B.  Arteriovenous Malformation: Early surgical intervention versus embolization
    C.  Labor and Delivery After Repair
       1.  Cesarean for obstetric indications only
       2.  Labor with epidural anesthesia
       3.  Outlet forceps to shorten second stage of labor
    D.  Cerebral Edema: Mannitol 12.5 to 50.0 g intravenously (serum osmolality not to exceed 315 mosm/liter). Furosamide and barbiturates as necessary if adjunctive measures are needed.

### III. *Critical Laboratory Tests*

    A.  Computed tomography scan of head, cerebral angiography, complete blood count, platelets, prothrombin time, partial thromboplastin time, fibrinogen

### IV. *Consultation*

    A.  Neurosurgery, neurology, intensivist

---

5 to 10 mg/kg actual body weight and may be continued in doses of 2 to 4 mg/kg/hr. Patients who do not respond to these pharmacologic measures require intubation and hyperventilation to a $pco_2$ of 25 to 30 mm Hg to reduce ICP.

In the presence of either ICH or cerebral edema, rapid initiation of diagnostic procedures and therapy is essential. Although pregnancy may complicate the diagnosis, once this life-threatening condition is recognized, pregnancy should not slow or alter the mode of therapy.

**REFERENCES**

Adams EBT, Loach AB, O'Laoire SA. Intracranial aneurysms: analysis of results of microneurosurgery. Br Med J 1976;2:607.

Adams HP, Kassell NF, Torner JC, et al. Predicting cerebral ischemia after aneurysmal subarachnoid hemorrhage: influences of clinical condition, CT results, and antifibrinolytic therapy. Neurology 1987;37:1586.

Allen GS, Ahn HS, Preziosi TJ, et al. Cerebral arterial spasm: a controlled trial of nimodipine in patients with subarachnoid hemorrhage. N Engl J Med 1983;308:619.

Amias AG. Cerebral vascular disease in pregnancy. I. Haemorrhage. J Obstet Gynaecol Br Cwlth 1970; 77:100.

Aminoff MJ. Maternal neurologic disorders. In: Creasy RK, Resnik R, eds. Maternal-fetal medicine. Philadelphia: WB Saunders, 1994.

Awad IA, Carter LP, Spetzler RF, et al. Clinical vasospasm after subarachnoid hemorrhage: response to hypervolemic hemodilution and arterial hypertension. Stroke 1987;18:365.

Barno A, Freeman DW. Maternal deaths due to spontaneous subarachnoid hemorrhage. Am J Obstet Gynecol 1976;125:384–392.

Barrow DL, Reisner A. Natural history of intracranial aneurysms and vascular malformations. Clin Neurosurg 1993;40:3.

Beck DW, Menezes AH. Intracerebral hemorrhage in a patient with eclampsia. JAMA 1981;246: 1442.

Belfort MA, Saade GR, Moise, KJ Jr, et al. Nimodipine in the management of preeclampsia: maternal and fetal effects. Am J Obstet Gynecol 1994;171:417–424.

Brown CEL, Purdy P, Cunningham FG. Head computed tomographic scans in women with eclampsia. Am J Obstet Gynecol 1988;159:915–920.

Buckland MR, Batjer HH, Giesecke AH. Anesthesia for cerebral aneurysm surgery: use of induced hypertension in patients with symptomatic vasospasm. Anesthesiology 1988;69:116.

Cannell DE, Botterell EH. Subarachnoid hemorrhage and pregnancy. Am J Obstet Gynecol 1956;72: 844.

Copelan EL, Mabon RF. Spontaneous intracranial bleeding in pregnancy. Obstet Gynecol 1962;20: 373.

Dearden NM, Gibson JS, McDowall DG, et al. Effect of high-dose dexamethasone on outcome from severe head injury. J Neurosurg 1986;64:81–88.

Dias M, Sekhar L. Intracranial hemorrhage from aneurysms and arteriovenous malformations during pregnancy and the puerperium. Neurosurg 1990;27:855–866.

Digre KB, Varner MW, Osborn AG, Crawford S. Cranial magnetic resonance imaging in severe preeclampsia vs eclampsia. Arch Neurol 1993;50: 399–406.

Donchin Y, Amirav B, Yarkoni S. Sodium nitroprusside for aneurysm surgery in pregnancy. Br J Anaesth 1978;50:849.

Donnelly JF, Lock FR. Causes of death in five hundred thirty-three fatal cases of toxemia of pregnancy. Am J Obstet Gynecol 1954;68:184.

Ducsay CA, Thompson JS, Wu AT, et al. Effects of calcium entry blocker (nicardipine) tocolysis in rhesus macaques: fetal plasma concentrations and cardiorespiratory changes. Am J Obstet Gynecol 1987;157:1482.

Enomoto H, Got H. Moyamoya disease presenting as intracerebral hemorrhage during pregnancy: case report and review of the literature. Neurosurgery 1987;20:33.

Evan S, Frigoletto FD, Jewett JF. Mortality of eclampsia: a case report and the experience of the Massachusetts Maternal Mortality Study. N Engl J Med 1983;309:1644.

Fisher CM, Kistler JP, Davis JM. Relation of cerebral vasospasm to subarachnoid hemorrhage visualized by computerized tomographic scanning. Neurosurgery 1980;6:1.

Fishman RA. Steroids in the treatment of brain edema. N Engl J Med 1982;306:359.

Fleigner JR, Hooper RS, Kloss M. Subarachnoid hemorrhage and pregnancy. J Obstet Gynaecol Br Cwlth 1969;76:912.

Forster DMC, Kunkler IH, Hartland P. Risk of cerebral bleeding from arteriovenous malformations in pregnancy: the Sheffield experience. Stereotact Funct Neurosurg 1993;61(suppl 1):20–22.

Giannotta SL, McGillicuddy JE, Kindt GW. Diagnosis and treatment of postoperative cerebral vasospasm. Surg Neurol 1977;8:286.

Giannotta SL, Daniels J, Golde SH, et al. Ruptured intracranial aneurysms during pregnancy: a report of four cases. J Reprod Med 1986;31:139.

Giannotta SL, Kindt GW. Total morbidity and mortality rates of patients with surgically treated intracranial aneurysms. Neurosurgery 1979;4:125.

Grenvik A, Safar P. Brain failure and resuscitation. New York: Churchill Livingstone, 1981.

Grolimund P, Weber M, Seiler RW, et al. Time course of cerebral vasospasm after severe head injury. Lancet 1988;ii:1173.

Henderson CE, Torbey M. Rupture of intracranial aneurysm associated with cocaine use during pregnancy. Am J Perinatol 1988;5:142.

Heros RC, Zervas NT, Varsos V. Cerebral vasospasm after subarachnoid hemorrhage: an update. Ann Neurol 1983;14:599.

Hibbard LT. Maternal mortality due to acute toxemia. Obstet Gynecol 1973;42:263.

Hijdra A, van Gijn J, Nagelkerke NJD, et al. Prediction of delayed cerebral ischemia, rebleeding, and outcome after aneurysmal subarachnoid hemorrhage. Stroke 1988;19:1250.

Horton JC, Chambers WA, Lyons SL, et al. Pregnancy and the risk of hemorrhage from cerebral arteriovenous malformations. Neurosurgery 1990;27:867–871.

Iriye BK, Asrat T, Adashek JA, Carr MH. Intraventricular haemorrhage and maternal brain death associated with antepartum cocaine abuse. Br J Obstet Gynaecol 1995;102:68–69.

Isla A, Alvarez F, Gonzalez A, et al. Brain tumor and pregnancy. Obstet Gynecol 1997;89:19.

Kassel NF, Sasaki T, Colohan ART, et al. Cerebral vasospasm following aneurysmal subarachnoid hemorrhage. Stroke 1985;16:562.

Kassell NF, Boarini DJ, Adams HP, et al. Overall management of ruptured aneurysm: comparison of early and later operation. Neurosurgery 1981;9:120.

Kassell NF, Torner JC. The International Cooperative Study on Timing Aneurysm Surgery: an update. Stroke 1984;15:566.

Kassel NF, Peerless SJ, Durward QJ, et al. Treatment of ischemic deficits from vasospasm with intravascular volume expansion and induced arterial hypertension. Neurosurg 1982;11:337.

Kety SS, Schmidt CF. The nitrous oxide method for the quantitative determination of cerebral blood flow in man: theory, procedure and normal values. J Clin Invest 1948;27:476.

Kitner SJ, Stern BJ, Feeser BR, et al. Pregnancy and the risk of stroke. N Engl J Med 1996;335:768.

Lassen NA. Cerebral blood flow and oxygen consumption in man. Physiol Rev 1959;39:183.

Levinson G, Shnider SM, DeLorimier AA, et al. Effects of maternal hyperventilation on uterine blood flow and fetal oxygenation and acid-base balance. Anesthesiology 1974;40:340.

Levy ML, Giannotta SL. Induced hypertension and hypervolemia for treatment of cerebral vasospasm. Neurosurg Clin North Am 1990;1:357.

Ljunggren B, Brandt L, Sunbarg G, et al. Early management of aneurysmal subarachnoid hemorrhage. Neurosurgery 1982;11:412.

Ljunggren B, Brandt L, Saveland H, et al. Outcome in 60 consecutive patients treated with early aneurysm operation and intravenous nimodipine. J Neurosurg 1984;61:864.

Lopez-Llera M. Complicated eclampsia: fifteen years' experience in a referral medical center. Am J Obstet Gynecol 1982;142:28.

Maher LM. Postpartum intracranial hemorrhage and phenylpropanolamine use. Neurology 1987;37:1686.

Milliez J, Dahoun A, Boudraa M. Computed tomography of the brain in eclampsia. Obstet Gynecol 1990;75:975.

Minielly R, Yuzpe AA, Drake CG. Subarachnoid hemorrhage secondary to ruptured cerebral aneurysm in pregnancy. Obstet Gynecol 1979;53:64.

Muizelaar JP, Lutz HA, Becker DP. Effect of mannitol on ICP and CBF and correlation with pressure autoregulation in severely head-injured patients. J Neurosurg 1984;61:700.

Nath F, Galbraith S. The effect of mannitol on cerebral white matter content. J Neurosurg 1986;65:41.

Newman B, Lam AM. Induced hypotension for clipping of a cerebral aneurysm during pregnancy: a case report and brief review. Anesth Analg 1986;65:675.

Parkinson D, Bachers G. Arteriovenous malformations: summary of 100 consecutive supratentorial cases. J Neurosurg 1980;53:285.

Pedowitz P, Perrell A. Aneurysm complicated by pregnancy. Am J Obstet Gynecol 1957;73:736.

Pollay M, Fullenwider C, Roberts PA, et al. Effect of mannitol and furosemide on blood-brain osmotic gradient and intracranial pressure. J Neurosurg 1983;59:945.

Pritchard JA, MacDonald PC, Gant NF, eds. Maternal adaptation to pregnancy. In: Williams obstetrics. 17th ed. Norwalk, CT: Appleton-Century-Crofts, 1985.

Reichman OH, Karlman RL. Berry aneurysm. Surg Clin North Am 1995;75:115–121.

Rigg D, McDonogh P. Use of sodium nitroprusside in deliberate hypotension during pregnancy. Br J Anaesth 1981;53:985.

Robinson JL, Hall CS, Sedzimir CB. AV malformations, aneurysms, and pregnancy. J Neurosurg 1974;41:63.

Robinson JL, Hall CJ, Sedzimir CB. Subarachnoid hemorrhage in pregnancy. J Neurosurg 1972;36:27.

Sadasivan B, Malik G, Lee C, Ausman J. Vascular malformations and pregnancy. Surg Neurol 1990;33:305–313.

Sengupta RP, So SC, Villarejo-Orteja FJ. Use of epsilon aminocaproic acid (EACA) in the preoperative management of ruptured intracranial aneurysms. J Neurosurg 1976;44:479.

Sheehan HL, Lynch JB. Pathology of toxemia of pregnancy. Baltimore: Williams and Wilkins, 1973.

Solomon RA, Fink ME, Lennihan L. Early aneurysm surgery and prophylactic hypervolemic hypertensive therapy for the treatment of aneurysmal subarachnoid hemorrhage. Neurosurgery 1988;23:699.

Stange K, Hallidin M. Hypothermia in pregnancy. Anesthesiology 1983;58:460.

Taneda M. Effect of early operation for ruptured aneurysms on prevention of delayed ischemic symptoms. J Neurosurg 1982;57:622.

van Buul BJA, Nijhuis JG, Slappendel R, et al. General anesthesia for surgical repair of intracranial aneurysm in pregnancy: effects on fetal heart rate. Am J Perinatol 1993;10:183–186.

van Gijn J, Hijdra A, Wijdicks EFM, et al. Acute hydrocephalus after aneurysmal subarachnoid hemorrhage. J Neurosurg 1985;63:355–362.

Van Rossum J, Wintzen AR, Endtz LJ, et al. Effect of tranexamic acid on rebleeding after subarachnoid hemorrhage: a double blind controlled clinical trial. Ann Neurol 1977;2:242.

Weibers D, Whisnant J. The incidence of stroke among pregnant women in Rochester, Minn., 1955 through 1979. JAMA 1985;254:2055–2057.

Wiebers DO. Subarachnoid hemorrhage in pregnancy. Semin Neurol 1988;8:226–229.

Wilkinson HA, Rosenfeld S. Furosemide and mannitol in the treatment of acute experimental intracranial hypertension. Neurosurgery 1983;12:405.

Willoughby JS. Sodium nitroprusside, pregnancy and multiple intracranial aneurysms. Anaesth Intensive Care 1984;12:358.

Wilterdink JL, Feldmann E. Cerebral hemorrhage. In: Devinsky O, Feldman E, Hainline B, eds. Neurological complications of pregnancy. New York: Raven, 1994:13–23.

Young DC, Leveno KJ, Whalley PS. Induced delivery prior to surgery for ruptured cerebral aneurysm. Obstet Gynecol 1983;61:749.

# CHAPTER *32*

# Acute Spinal Cord Injury

*B*ecause of both acute and long-term effects, spinal fracture with cord damage can be one of the most devastating injuries a person can incur. Approximately 11,000 new spinal cord injuries (SCIs) occur annually in the United States, more than 50% in persons younger than 30 years of age. The most prevalent age range at injury is 15 to 34 years. About 3000 women of childbearing age suffer SCI each year (Griffin, 1985).

There are a number of important issues concerning the care of the pregnant patient who has sustained an acute SCI (ASCI). Serious acute maternal morbidity, especially due to cardiopulmonary dysfunction, can develop in the ASCI pregnant patient. Therefore, it must be anticipated and properly managed in addition to any other trauma the patient may have sustained at the time of her accident (Patterson, 1984). General management principles for patients with acute spinal injury have recently been renewed by Chiles (1996).

## Immediate Considerations

The obstetric caregiver should be involved early in the emergency stabilization of the pregnant ASCI patient. The patient's neck must be stabilized until the extent of SCI has been determined and transfer to a tertiary care center has been accomplished. Initial airway management includes the jaw thrust maneuver (American Heart Association, 1994) rather than the head tilt/chin lift measure (Fig 32-1). Nasal intubation of the trachea may be required if the need for assisted ventilation arises (Committee on Trauma, 1993). An anesthesiologist skilled in this technique is preferred although not always available. Circulatory system assessment includes efforts to rule out occult internal hemorrhage secondary to other injuries sustained during the patient's accident that could lead to hypovolemic shock. The usual signs of intraperitoneal bleeding may be obscured not only by the pregnancy but also by the sensory and motor deficits caused by the ASCI. Peritoneal lavage is often an appropriate early diagnostic maneuver. A high epigastric entry point and an open technique in late pregnancy are usually advisable in order to avoid injury to the enlarged uterus. Ultrasound (vaginal or abdominal) might be helpful to quickly indicate the presence of free peritoneal fluid and thereby obviate the need for peritoneal lavage. A grading scale for evaluating motor function has been developed by Chiles, and is detailed in Table 32-1.

Fetal monitoring provides an excellent additional vital sign to indirectly assess overall maternal hemodynamic status. Use of this tool can provide reassurance of fetal well-being and may be used even in the nonviable fetus as an internal oximeter (Gilson, 1995). One of the first signs of maternal and uterine hypovolemia is a fetal heart rate stress pattern of tachycardia, followed eventually by bradycardia.

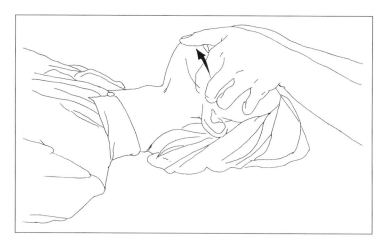

F I G U R E   **32-1**

Jaw thrust maneuver for establishing an airway in a woman with
suspected spinal cord injury.

T A B L E    **32-1**

Innervation of spinal segments and muscles and grading scale
for evaluation of motor function

| Spinal Segment* | Muscle | Action |
|---|---|---|
| **C5**, C6 | Deltoid | Arm abduction |
| C5, **C6** | Biceps | Elbow flexion |
| **C6**, C7 | Extensor carpi radialis | Wrist extension |
| **C7**, C8 | Triceps | Elbow extension |
| **C8**, T1 | Flexor digitorum profundus | Hand grasp |
| C8, **T1** | Hand intrinsics | Finger abduction |
| L1, **L2**, **L3** | Iliopsoas | Hip flexion |
| L2, **L3**, **L4** | Quadriceps | Knee extension |
| L4, **L5**, **S1**, S2 | Hamstrings | Knee flexion |
| L4, **L5** | Tibialis anterior | Ankle dorsiflexion |
| **L5**, S1 | Extensor hallucis longus | Great-toe extension |
| **S1**, S2 | Gastrocnemius | Ankle plantar flexion |
| S2, S3, S4 | Bladder, anal sphincter | Voluntary rectal tone |

| Grade | **Muscle Strength** |
|---|---|
| 5 | Normal strength |
| 4 | Active power against both resistance and gravity |
| 3 | Active power against gravity but not resistance |
| 2 | Active movement only with gravity eliminated |
| 1 | Flicker or trace of contraction |
| 0 | No movement or contraction |

*The predominant segments of innervation are shown in boldface type.

Reprinted with permission from Chiles (1996).

Acute use of methylprednisolone after ASCI has been associated with significant improvement in motor and sensory function 6 months after the insult in treated patients, compared with those who received naloxone or placebo (Bracken, 1990). Methylprednisolone is given as an intravenous bolus dose of 30 mg/kg, followed by infusion at 5.4 mg/kg/hr for 23 hours. It should be initiated within 8 hours of the ASCI injury.

## Neurogenic Shock

Neurogenic shock is a severe early complication of ASCI with significant maternal and fetal implications. The typical signs of hypovolemic shock, such as tachycardia and cool clammy skin, are obscured. Patients in neurogenic shock are usually hypotensive and bradycardic, with warm dry skin reflecting the dominance of parasympathetic effects, which develop when sympathetic autonomic function is blocked by the cord lesion. As vasomotor tone is lost, systemic arteriolar resistance decreases profoundly, and venous capacitance increases. Thus, decreased afterload and preload develop, with a subsequent drop in cardiac output. Unopposed vagal tone produces significant bradycardia. The loss of sympathetic tone also results in an inability to shunt blood from the periphery to the core. Thus, heat loss through the skin becomes excessive, and hypothermia develops. Hypothermia itself can cause an even more profound bradycardia, which may be reflected by fetal bradycardia in the pregnant patient. The period of potential neurogenic shock can be anticipated to last from 1 to 3 weeks.

Initial treatment of the patient in neurogenic shock includes judicious fluid replacement, often best guided by the use of a pulmonary artery flow-directed catheter. In the absence of this surveillance tool, pulmonary edema can result from overzealous volume replacement. The use of inotropic pressor agents, such as dopamine and dobutamine, at the lower dosage levels (1–5 µg/kg/min) are very helpful for enhancing cardiac output, raising perfusion pressure, and improving renal hemodynamics. Despite animal evidence to the contrary, adverse fetal effects from long-term use of these inotropes have not been observed in humans (Rolbin, 1979).

Surgery can be performed without anesthesia in a patient in neurogenic shock if the lesion is above T-10. If the patient is receiving a dopamine infusion, uterine atony could result from the betamimetic effects of the drug on uterine smooth muscle. After delivery of the fetus, phenylephrine can be useful for maintaining pressure support without the side effect of uterine relaxation (Lucas, 1965).

Although conduction anesthesia in the obstetric patient has been reported to cause spinal hypotension, study of the effects of neurogenic shock on uteroplacental perfusion is limited (American Society of Anesthesiologists, 1991). In experiments on near-term pregnant ewes in which spinal hypotension (50% drop in maternal mean arterial pressure) was induced via the progressive subarachnoid administration of 1% lidocaine, a 35% decrease in maternal heart rate and a 65% decrease in uterine blood flow were recorded (Shnider, 1968). Despite the induction of relative uterine ischemia due to spinal hypotension, adverse fetal effects, including hypoxemia, hypercapnia, or metabolic acidosis, did not ensue. Because there was a greater decrease in uterine arterial flow than pressure, uterine vascular resistance increased. These experiments suggested that intrinsic control of uterine vasoconstrictor tone may be partially independent of autonomic control. Decreased uterine and fetoplacental unit blood supply in this situation could induce a compensatory enhancement of oxygen extraction, producing a larger arteriovenous oxygen content difference while sustaining oxygen consumption at a near-normal level. Although these findings suggest that some fetuses can tolerate short periods of decreased placental perfusion, others with baseline uteroplacental insufficiency may not tolerate any amount of hypotension or uterine vasoconstriction (Shnider, 1968, 1970).

## Later Considerations

There are important long-term considerations for the patient with acute or chronic SCI. These include urinary tract infections, respiratory infections, decubitus ulcers, muscle spasms, preterm labor, anemia, unrecognized labor, and autonomic hyperreflexia.

Urinary tract infections are reported in all retrospective analyses of pregnant patients with SCIs. As a major infectious complication, it is encountered frequently in relation to the status of urine bladder management with progressively decreasing frequency from the retention catheter and ileal conduit to intermittent catheterization, the Crede method, and normal voiding (Cross, 1992).

Urinary incontinence and increased urinary frequency are almost universal and pose problems in changing clothes, transfer, and bathroom accessibility. Urinary incontinence often persists after delivery, with difficulty returning to prepregnancy urinary programs (Greenspoon, 1986; Baker, 1992). To avoid the complications involved with urinary tract infection, including autonomic hyperreflexia associated with pyelonephritis, the performance of frequent urine cultures is recommended, with prophylactic antibiotics given for persistent or recurrent urinary tract infections (American College of Obstetricians and Gynecologists, 1993).

When the level of the spinal cord lesion is above T-5, voluntary use of abdominal muscles is absent (Fig 32-2). This may impair reflex cough ability and thereby increase the potential for respiratory complications. In pregnant tetraplegic women, abdominal distention can further compromise essential ventilatory diaphragmatic function (Hughes, 1991).

F I G U R E **32-2**

Radiographic demonstration of C5–6 cervical spine dislocation.

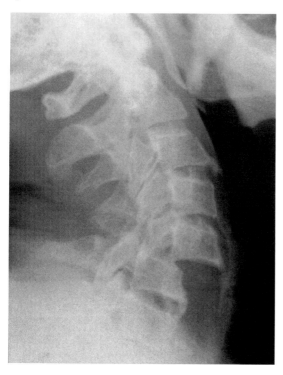

Pregnant spinal cord injured women must take proactive measures to prevent pressure sores. These include wearing loose-fitting clothing, frequent position changes, and frequent skin inspections. While pressure sores are not a frequent complication, they can have serious sequelae, such as cellulitis, soft-tissue necrosis, sepsis, and even loss of an extremity related to infection (Cross, 1992).

All pregnant SCI patients are at increased risk for unexpected, unattended delivery. This is especially true in the patient with spinal cord transection above the T-10 segment, because her labor is painless. In the patient with total transection at a lower thoracic level, labor pain can be so minimal that there is no perception of uterine contractions. Other symptoms that are under sympathetic nervous system control, such as abdominal or leg spasms or shortness of breath, might be concurrent with labor contractions and could trigger patient awareness of labor.

Patients should be instructed in uterine palpation techniques in order to detect contractions at home. Otherwise, the use of a home uterine activity monitor could be considered. Regular, gentle cervical examinations, which are initiated in the late second or early third trimester, may be helpful, with gentle care and precautions taken in any patient at risk for autonomic hyperreflexia. With good monitoring techniques, early and prolonged hospitalization is not necessary but should be considered in patients remote from the hospital or with transportation problems.

Preterm labor is a risk in the SCI patient who has had a prior preterm delivery or recurrent urinary tract infections. Hospitalization should be considered in any patient with signs of preterm labor. Otherwise, traditional therapy can be utilized, with transfer to a tertiary care center when appropriate (American College of Obstetricians and Gynecologists, 1993).

Muscle spasms can be treated with frequent position changes and muscle relaxers, but they are difficult to control (Hughes, 1991). They can be localized either to segments of sensory input or may involve a more generalized response, with increased tone and spasms of the abdominal and leg muscles.

Anemia represents a minor problem in this group of women and should be managed cautiously when it does occur. Iron supplements may have the compounding effects of constipation and difficulty with bowel evacuation.

Patients with SCI at or above the T-6 segment are subject to autonomic hyperreflexia syndrome. This serious and potentially life-threatening complication is attributed to a loss of hypothalamic control over sympathetic spinal reflexes. It occurs in patients with complete and incomplete lesions in the upper thoracic or cervical region with viable cord segments distal to the level of injury. In susceptible patients, afferent stimuli from either a hollow viscous (the bladder, bowel, or uterus), the genital area, or an area of skin below the level of the lesion ascend in the spinothalamic tracts and posterior columns. This causes reflex sympathetic activation that is unmodified by the supraspinal centers. Catecholamine release and vasoconstriction leads to hypertension associated with headache, bradycardia, cardiac arrhythmia, sweating, flushing, tingling, nasal congestion, and occasionally, respiratory distress. Uteroplacental vasoconstriction may produce fetal hypoxemia (Gilson, 1995).

Autonomic hyperreflexia can be caused by distention of the vagina, bladder, or bowel. It could be provoked by a simple manipulation, such as changing a urinary catheter or a cervical examination during labor. Any unnecessary stimuli should be avoided in these patients. Constipation should be treated with increased dietary fiber and stool softeners. During labor, the symptoms of autonomic hyperreflexia are commonly synchronous with uterine contractions and abate with uterine relaxation, ceasing after placental expulsion. The severity of the syndrome during labor ranges from annoying symptoms to serious conditions including hypertensive encephalopathy, cerebrovascular accidents, intraventricular and retinal hemorrhages, and death. Continuous monitoring of cardiac rhythm and BP during labor is mandatory in all patients at risk for autonomic hyperreflexia so that serious sequelae can be averted (Wanner, 1987).

Although patients with SCI may perceive no pain in labor, anesthesia should be used to prevent autonomic hyperreflexia. A rapidly induced subarachnoid block is recommended for emergency cesarean section. Labor and nonurgent cesarean delivery are best managed with epidural anesthesia. Both methods of anesthesia prevent hyperreflexia by blocking stimuli that arise from the pelvic organs. If the spine is not stable, the patient can be "log-rolled" onto her side with the guidance of a neurosurgeon. Antepartum consultation with an anesthesiologist and the establishment of a plan for induction of epidural or spinal anesthesia at the onset of labor are highly desirable in susceptible patients. If autonomic hyperreflexia occurs before a regional anesthetic is available or occurs despite regional anesthesia, hypertension is treated with antihypertensive agents that have a rapid onset and offset. Suggested agents to use include sodium nitroprusside or nitroglycerin, ganglionic blocking agents (trimethaphan), adrenergic blocking agents (guanethidine), or a direct vasodilator (hydralazine) (Gilson, 1995; Wanner, 1987).

If there is evidence of autonomic hyperreflexia during the second stage of labor, delivery can be expedited by operative forceps or vacuum extraction. If symptoms cannot be controlled by any means, cesarean delivery may be indicated. Adequate anesthesia is needed for cesarean delivery in all patients with SCIs (American Society of Anesthesiologists, 1991).

Most physicians skilled at managing trauma and specifically SCI often are less familiar with the special needs of the obstetric patient; thus, the obstetrician needs to be involved very early in the care of the pregnant SCI patient. The ABCs (airway, breathing, and circulation) of resuscitation are important. Until the possibility of injury is excluded, stabilization of the airway and immobilization of the cervical spine are important concepts. Placement of the patient in the left lateral tilt position with oxygen supplementation is advocated for fetal well-being. If necessary, support the circulation and initiate acute cardiac life support. The uterus may need to be emptied to facilitate maternal resuscitation. Assess SCIs, neurologic status, and any associated injuries. Evaluate the extent of the patient's injuries including the use of x-rays, computed tomography scan, and magnetic resonance imaging, if necessary, and the abdomen should be shielded when possible.

---

## ACUTE SPINAL CORD INJURY

### I. *Goals of Therapy*

A. To stabilize the patient
B. To control the spine in an attempt to prevent further injuries
C. To evaluate and treat other injuries
D. To achieve early recognition, prevention, and management of frequently encountered complications

### II. *Management Protocol*

A. Initial stabilization should be achieved, including stabilization of the patient's neck, airway management, circulatory system assessment, and fetal monitoring.
B. Methylprednisolone should be initiated within 8 hours of the SCI and given as a bolus dose of 30 mg/kg, followed by infusion at 5.4 mg/kg/hr for 23 hours.
C. Central hemodynamic monitoring may be required for optimum fluid management of neurogenic shock.
D. Adequate fluid and pressor support may be necessary during the period of neurogenic shock.
E. Delivery may be indicated for obstetric indications, to facilitate maternal resuscitation, or in conjunction with surgery for other injuries.

---

Begin high-dose steroids in accordance with the recommendations. Recognize the indications for immediate surgery, which may need to be coordinated with cesarean section for the following findings: (1) acute anterior cord syndrome, (2) cephalad progression of an earlier determined level of function, (3) compound fractures requiring surgical debridement, (4) foreign body within the spinal canal, and (5) pedicle fracture associated with nerve root compression at that level.

Because most women continue to enjoy an active lifestyle during their pregnancy, SCIs will continue to occur. Seat belts with a shoulder harness in accordance with American College of Obstetricians and Gynecologists recommendations will prevent many of these injuries and should be encouraged (American College of Obstetricians and Gynecologists, 1991).

---

**REFERENCES**

American College of Obstetricians and Gynecologists. Automobile passenger restraints for children and pregnant women. Technical Bulletin No. 151, January 1991.

American College of Obstetricians and Gynecologists. Obstetric management of patients with spinal cord injury. Technical Bulletin No. 121, April 1993.

American Heart Association. Textbook of basic life support for health care providers. American Heart Association, 1994.

American Society of Anesthesiologists. Standards for basic intra-operative monitoring. In: ASA standards, guidelines and statements. Park Ridge, IL: American Society of Anesthesiologists, 1991:6

Baker ER, Cardenas DD, Benedetti TJ. Risks associated with pregnancy in spinal cord-injured women. Obstet Gynecol 1992;80:425.

Bracken MB, Shepard MJ, Collins WR, et al. A randomized, controlled trial of methylprednisolone or naloxone in the treatment of acute spinal cord injury. N Engl J Med 1990;322:1405.

Chiles BW III, Cooper PR. Acute spinal injury. N Engl J Med 1996;334:514.

Committee on Trauma. Advanced trauma life support course for physician-student manual. Chicago: American College of Surgeons, 1993.

Cross LL, Meythaler JM, Tuel SM, Cross AL. Pregnancy, labor, and delivery post spinal cord injury. Paraplegia 1992;30:890.

Gilson GJ, Miller AC, Clevenger FE, Curet LB. Acute spinal cord injury and neurogenic shock in pregnancy. Obstet Gynecol Surv 1995;50:556.

Greenspoon JS, Paul HP. Paraplegia and quadriplegia. Special considerations during pregnancy and labor and delivery. Am J Obstet Gynecol 1986;155:738.

Griffin JP. Anesthesia for acute and chronic spinal cord injuries. In: Barash PG, ed. American Society of Anesthesiologists review course, vol. 13. 1985:69.

Hughes SJ, Short DJ, Userwood MM, Tebbitt H. Management of the pregnant woman with spinal cord injuries. Br J Obstet Gynaecol 1991;98:513.

Lucas W, Kirschbaum T, Assali NS. Spinal shock and fetal oxygenation. Am J Obstet Gynecol 1965;93:583.

Patterson RM. Trauma in pregnancy. Clin Obstet Gynecol 1984;27:32.

Rolbin SH, Levinson G, Shnider SM, et al. Dopamine treatment of spinal hypotension decreases uterine blood flow in the pregnant ewe. Anesthesiology 1979;51:36.

Shnider SM, de Lorimier AA, Holl AW, et al. Vasopressors in obstetrics. I. Correction of fetal acidosis with ephedrine during spinal hypotension. Am J Obstet Gynecol 1968;102:911.

Shnider SM, de Lorimier AA, Asling JH, et al. Vasopressors in obstetrics. II. Fetal hazards of methoxamine during obstetric spinal anesthesia. Am J Obstet Gynecol 1970;106:680.

Wanner MG, Rageth CJ, Zach GA. Pregnancy and autonomic hyperreflexia in patients with spinal cord lesions. Paraplegia 1987;25:482.

CHAPTER **33**

# Trauma and Envenomation

**M**ajor trauma affects up to 8% of pregnant patients, with life-threatening maternal injuries complicating three to four per 1000 deliveries (Laverly, 1995). Trauma is the leading cause of non-obstetric maternal death (Varner, 1989). The maternal death rate secondary to trauma is 1.9 in 1000 live births (Sachs, 1987). Trauma caused by battering or abuse occurs in up to 10% of pregnant women (Helton, 1987). Thus, trauma is a significant cause of both maternal and fetal mortality and morbidity. The appropriate multidisciplinary treatment of trauma during pregnancy is of great importance for any provider who cares for pregnant women. The aim of this chapter is to discuss principles of general trauma management and to examine the specific aspects of trauma care that affect or are affected by the state of pregnancy. While minor trauma only rarely produces morbid sequelae during pregnancy, optimal maternal and perinatal outcome can come only through a thorough understanding of both trauma and pregnancy.

## Maternal Physiologic Adaptations Applicable to Trauma During Pregnancy

The physiologic changes the woman's body undergoes during pregnancy have a significant influence on the pathophysiologic responses the mother and her fetus manifest as a result of trauma. Furthermore, the physiologic changes of pregnancy may alter the clinician's ability to accurately diagnose trauma and may either favorably or adversely influence maternal outcome. The most important physiologic changes, as applicable to the pregnant trauma victim, are summarized in Table 33-1.

## Cardiovascular Alterations

One of the most extensive and important physiologic adaptations to pregnancy that affects trauma care and pregnancy outcome is the associated increase in blood and plasma volume. While some plasma volume expansion is evident by the end of the first trimester, by 28 to 32 weeks, it is expanded by 45% to 50% (Scott, 1972). Red-cell mass, also expanded during pregnancy, increases relatively less than plasma volume. The result is a dilutional anemia of pregnancy with a small decrease in hematocrit (Pritchard, 1965). Consequently, normal pregnancy imparts a natural buffer to the expected 500- to 1000-mL blood loss of normal vaginal or cesarean delivery (Cunningham, 1993a). Additionally, during blood loss associated with trauma, the pregnant woman is apt to display relative physiologic stability until massive blood loss ensues (Kuhlman, 1994).

Table 33-2 categorizes hemorrhage according to the amount of blood loss and related manifestations (Collicott, 1985). In pregnancy, due to the described blood volume changes plus the

597

T A B L E   33-1

Trauma-related maternal adaptations to pregnancy

| Parameter | Change | Implications |
|---|---|---|
| Plasma volume | Increases by 45%–50% | Relative maternal resistance to limited blood loss |
| Red-cell mass | Increases by 30% | Dilutional anemia |
| Cardiac output | Increases by 30%–50% | Relative maternal resistance to limited blood loss |
| Uteroplacenta blood flow | 20%–30% shunt | Uterine injury may predispose to increased blood loss |
| | | Increased uterine vascularity |
| Uterine size | Dramatic increase | Increased incidence of uterine injury with abdominal trauma |
| | | Change in position of abdominal contents |
| | | Supine hypotension |
| Minute ventilation | Increases by 25%–30% | Diminished $Paco_2$ |
| | | Diminished buffering capacity |
| Functional residual volume | Decreased | Predisposition to atelectasis and hypoxemia |
| Gastric emptying | Delayed | Predisposition to aspiration |

See text for sources of data.

fact that most pregnant patients are young and otherwise healthy, signs and symptoms of profound blood loss are usually attenuated and the diagnosis of ongoing blood loss may be missed or delayed until profound hemodynamic collapse occurs. Conversely, providers who do not normally care for pregnant women could be oppositely misled by the normal dilutional anemia of pregnancy if they compare hematocrit values with normal nonpregnant values. Recognition of the volume changes evident during pregnancy *must*

be considered during evaluation of the pregnant trauma patient.

In addition to the blood volume changes, BP and cardiac output also change during normal pregnancy. Systolic and diastolic BPs decrease to nadir values by approximately 28 weeks of gestation (Wilson, 1980). Heart rate increases by approximately 15% to 20% over nonpregnancy levels. Cardiac output increases by 30% to 50% over control values by the late second trimester, secondary to increases in both heart rate and stroke

T A B L E   33-2

Categorization of acute hemorrhage

| | Class 1 | Class 2 | Class 3 | Class 4 |
|---|---|---|---|---|
| Blood loss (% blood volume) | 15% | 15%–30% | 30%–40% | >40% |
| Pulse rate | <100 | >100 | >120 | >140 |
| Pulse pressure | Normal | Decreased | Decreased | Decreased |
| Blood pressure | Normal or increased | Decreased | Decreased | Decreased |

Source: Adapted from Ramenofsky ML, Alexander RH, Ali J, et al, eds. Advanced trauma life support—1993 instructor manual. American College of Surgeons. Chicago: First Impressions, 1993.

volume (Clark, 1989). The etiology of the increase in cardiac output may be hormonal, volume related, or secondary to the functional 20% to 30% arteriovenous shunt produced by the low-resistance placental circuit. Despite an increase in stroke volume, left ventricular filling pressures are not increased during pregnancy. Systemic vascular resistance decreases during gestation, with a partial return toward prepregnancy values by late pregnancy. An often unrecognized pregnancy-associated cardiovascular effect is the profound hypotension that can occur with supine positioning of the pregnant woman. Supine hypotension results from aortocaval compression by the enlarged gravid uterus and can have profound effects on both normal and hemodynamically compromised patients (Lees, 1967). Avoidance of supine hypotension often can be accomplished by proper patient positioning (Vaizey, 1994), using a wedge placed under the right hip or by placing the operating room table on a tilt.

Labor itself imposes additional cardiovascular demands on the pregnant patient. In healthy pregnant subjects, cardiac output increases by an additional 40% over basal third-trimester values. This increase is attenuated partially by pain relief and the provision of conduction anesthesia (Ueland, 1969a,b). Immediately after delivery, cardiac output is often at its peak. Cardiac output and stroke volume may increase by nearly 60% and more than 70%, respectively. Ventricular filling pressure and pulmonary artery pressure also increase immediately postpartum (Ueland, 1975). Progressive diuresis and resolution of hormonal changes produce normalization of hemodynamic parameters by about 6 weeks postpartum (Chesley, 1959).

## Pulmonary and Respiratory Changes

Several mechanical and metabolic changes in respiratory physiology occur during pregnancy. Minute ventilation increases by some 40%, predominantly secondary to an increase in tidal volume, but also with a much smaller increase in respiratory rate. As a consequence of increased minute volume, the arterial partial pressure of carbon dioxide ($Paco_2$) diminishes to approxi-

mately 30 mm Hg (de Swiet, 1991; Prowse, 1965). The resulting compensated respiratory alkalosis causes pH to trend to the alkalemic range of normal. Concomitantly, serum bicarbonate ($Hco_3$) decreases to 18 to 22 mEq/liter, and serum-buffering capacity is thereby reduced (Hankins, 1995). Finally, it is important to remember that other derangements, such as hypoxia, sepsis, ketoacidosis, and so on, exert an additive effect on underlying blood gas changes of pregnancy. Hyperventilation from moderately high altitude has been shown to reduce $Paco_2$ in the third-trimester gravida to values as low as 25 to 26 mm Hg (Hankins, 1996). Therefore, any pathophysiologic acid-base derangement in pregnancy should be interpreted in light of the fact that a primary acid-base disturbance exists normally.

Functional residual volume (FRV) is decreased during pregnancy (Alaily, 1978). Tidal breathing may be at or near critical closing volume, potentially predisposing the pregnant patient to hypoxemia, particularly in situations that normally reduce FRV anyway (e.g., supine positioning, intrinsic pulmonary disease, chest wall trauma) (Hankins, 1995; Gerrard, 1978). The diaphragm is elevated by about 4 cm during pregnancy, making injury during thoracostomy tube placement potentially more likely (Laverly, 1995).

## Gastrointestinal Changes

The mechanical effect of the enlarged uterus as pregnancy progresses causes displacement of the small bowel into the upper abdomen (Kuhlman, 1994). As will be discussed in the section on abdominal trauma, the change in position of the abdominal viscera has an impact on mechanisms, diagnosis, and treatment of abdominal trauma. Hormonal and metabolic factors result in delayed gastric emptying and increased gastrointestinal transit time. Consequently, pulmonary aspiration of stomach contents is more likely during pregnancy (Mendelson, 1946; Davison, 1977).

## Genitourinary Changes

The progestational effect of smooth muscle relaxation, along with mechanical compression from the gravid uterus, cause dilation of the ureters and the renal pelvises. Consequently, radiographic imaging of the genitourinary system may show some degree of "physiologic" hydronephrosis (Kuhlman, 1994; Lindheimer, 1970; Bellina, 1976). Ureteropelvical dilation also may predispose the urinary collecting system to stasis. Bacteriuria and pyelonephritis are more common during pregnancy (Cunningham, 1993). Creatinine clearance is increased in normal pregnancy. Simplistically, the increase in creatinine clearance is due to a cardiac output–mediated increase in renal blood flow. Therefore, in pregnancy, a serum creatinine at the upper limit of what is considered normal when not pregnant may reflect diminished renal function (Lindheimer, 1970; Cunningham, 1993b). The urinary bladder is "abdominalized" after the first trimester of pregnancy, increasing the propensity for the female bladder to become injured during abdominal trauma.

## Hematologic Changes

As discussed previously, normal pregnancy is associated with a relative dilutional anemia despite an increase in overall red-cell mass. A mild leukocytosis also is noted during pregnancy (Taylor, 1981). Factors VII, VIII, IX, X, and fibrinogen are elevated during pregnancy. Factors IX and XIII and platelet count are unchanged or minimally decreased during pregnancy (Cunningham, 1993a; Burrows, 1988). Despite these somewhat conflicting changes, pregnancy is a hypercoagu-

lable state. Consequently, pregnancy accentuates other predisposing factors, leading to the development of deep venous thrombosis (Rutherford, 1991). Coagulation factor changes in pregnancy are summarized in Table 33-3.

## Uterus

By 12 weeks of gestation, the uterus becomes an abdominal organ. Prior to 12 weeks' gestation, the small size and the pelvic location of the uterus make it resistant to injury (Crosby, 1971). Conversely, late in pregnancy, the abdominal location of the uterus predisposes it to injury from blunt or penetrating abdominal trauma (Kuhlman, 1994). Perhaps even more important is the dramatic increase in uteropelvic blood flow during pregnancy. By late pregnancy, a volume equivalent to the mother's entire circulating blood volume passes through the uterus at least every 10 minutes (Vaizey, 1994). This dramatic increase in uterine blood flow, coupled with the abdominalization of the dramatically larger gravid organ, pose a synergistic propensity for hemorrhage in the face of uterine trauma (Esposito, 1994). Fortunately, uterine rupture is an infrequent complication of multiorgan trauma during pregnancy. Rupture of the uterus is found in less than 1% of pregnant trauma victims (Hankins, 1995). Uterine rupture is most usually associated with direct and substantial abdominal impact or other predisposing obstetric factors, such as gestational age or previous uterine surgery (Williams, 1990). Fetal death usually occurs with uterine rupture.

T A B L E   **33-3**
Hemostatic changes during pregnancy

| Factor | Change | Normal in Late Pregnancy |
|---|---|---|
| Fibrinogen | 50% increase | 300–600 mg/dL |
| Factor II | Slight increase | Variable |
| Factor VII | Increased | Variable |
| Factor IX | Increased | Variable |
| Factor X | Increased | Variable |
| Factor IX | Minimal decrease | Variable |
| Factor XIII | Minimal decrease | Variable |
| Platelet count | Normal or slightly lower | Variable |

See text for source of data.

Maternal death from uterine rupture is reported to occur in 10% of cases with traumatic uterine rupture (Pearlman, 1991). Often, however, death is from other severe injuries that tend to occur in patients with uterine rupture.

## Management of Trauma

The American College of Surgeons, through their Advanced Trauma Life Support program, has advocated standardized initial trauma management (Ramenofsky, 1993). Resuscitation is based on a systematic survey and intervention method. Some review of this philosophy as it relates to pregnant patients is justified. A modified basic algorithm for initial resuscitation of the pregnant trauma patient is provided in Figure 33-1.

## Primary Survey

The primary survey encompasses the immediate evaluation of the pregnant or nonpregnant trauma patient. The letters A-B-C-D-E are used to de-

scribe the steps of the primary survey (see Fig 33-1) (Ramenofsky, 1993; Moore, 1990; Trunkey, 1991; Vaizey, 1994; Laverly, 1995). Little is different in performing the primary survey during pregnancy, as compared with the nonpregnant individual. Foremost in the primary survey is stabilization of a proper airway (A). If an adequate functioning airway is not present, chin lift (with a stabilized neck and cervical spine) and oral or nasal airway insertion may be necessary. Early endotracheal intubation by qualified personnel must be performed if the just-described measures fail. Because of a potential for aspiration, intubation should be pursued more aggressively in the pregnant trauma victim than in her nonpregnant counterpart (Kuhlman, 1994). After airway stabilization, adequate respiration (B) must be established. Supplemental oxygen is given as necessary and its adequacy assessed via pulse oximetry. Arterial blood gas determination, if obtained, must be interpreted in reference to what is found normally during pregnancy. A decreased serum bicarbonate level may be indicative of significant risk for fetal loss. One series

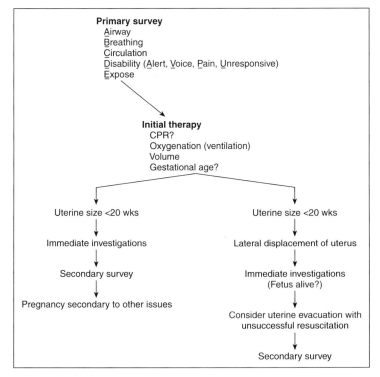

**F I G U R E   33-1**

**Initial resuscitation of the pregnant trauma patient.** CPR, cardiopulmonary resuscitation. (See text for sources of data.)

reported that initial serum bicarbonate levels were significantly lower (16.4 ± 3.0 mEq/liter vs. 20.3 ± 2.2 mEq/liter) in pregnant major trauma victims in which fetal loss was noted (Scorpio, 1992).

C refers to circulation. Pulse quality, BP, and capillary refill are basic clinical determinants of the adequacy of perfusion. As mentioned earlier, clinical evaluation of maternal intravascular homeostasis is altered by the underlying physiologic changes of pregnancy. Also, fetal effects from maternal hypovolemia are not addressed by basic hemodynamic physical diagnosis (Scorpio, 1992; Hoff, 1991; Dilts, 1967; Greiss, 1966). In any case, because of the ongoing hemorrhage often present in any severely injured trauma patient, immediate assessment and treatment of hypovolemia must be provided. In nearly all trauma cases, a large-bore (14- or 16-gauge) intravenous (IV) access should be established. In the multiple trauma patient, it is our custom to insert a large-bore IV in both an upper and lower extremity. Central venous access is not immediately indicated, provided adequate peripheral access can be established. An appropriately sized peripheral IV (14- or 16-guage) will provide the ability to rapidly instill large amounts of volume. Hypotension in the trauma patient is assumed to be hypovolemia until proven otherwise. Because of the blood volume changes described previously, it is not uncommon for pregnant patients to seemingly "tolerate" 1500 to 2000 mL of blood loss with only subtle hemodynamic changes (Laverly, 1995). Splanchnic and uterine blood flow is nonetheless compromised (Dilts, 1967; Greiss, 1966), and deterioration of the patient can develop rapidly with any further blood loss. *Initial* therapy for hypotension found during the primary survey is rapid infusion of up to 2000 mL of crystalloid solution and preparation for blood transfusion as necessary. Cardiopulmonary resuscitation, discussed in subsequent sections of this chapter, is begun if pulses are not palpated.

Up to this point in the primary survey, obstetric and non-obstetric management is very similar. At this stage of the resuscitation process, however, attention to great vessel compression by the gravid uterus must be addressed in pregnancies beyond 20 weeks' gestation. In multiple trauma, because of potential vertebral injury, pa-

tients are generally placed on a rigid spinal board, and usual methods for avoiding aortocaval compression (e.g., lateral roll, lateral tilt, etc.) are not possible. Manual lateral displacement of the uterus is therefore performed. Alternatively, if the gravid trauma patient is on a trauma backboard, the entire board can be tilted 15 degrees, providing stabilization of the vertebral column is maintained (Hankins, 1995; Ramenofsky, 1993).

The letter D in the sequence stands for "disability." With any trauma, early neurologic evaluation is undertaken. A rapid assessment is by the A-V-P-U method (*Alert, Voice, Pain, Unresponsive*) (Ramenofsky, 1993). The Glasgow Coma Scale (GCS) also can be used (Table 33-4) (Tessdale, 1974). A GCS of 8 or less may be indicative of significant ongoing neurologic pathology (Baxt, 1987; Rutherford, 1995).

T A B L E **33-4**

Glasgow Coma Scale

| | Points |
|---|---|
| ***Eye-opening Response (E-score)*** | |
| Spontaneous (already open and blinking) | 4 |
| Opens in response to speech | 3 |
| Opens in response to pain (not to face) | 2 |
| No response | 1 |
| ***Verbal Response (V-score)*** | |
| Oriented and appropriate response | 5 |
| Confused response | 4 |
| Inappropriate wording | 3 |
| Incomprehensible words | 2 |
| No response | 1 |
| ***Motor Response (M-score)*** | |
| Obeys command | 6 |
| Localizes pain | 5 |
| Withdraws to pain | 4 |
| Flexion response to pain | 3 |
| Extension response to pain | 2 |
| No response | 1 |

Glasgow Coma Scale score is the sum of scores in the three areas listed. A GCS score ≤ 8 is consistent with coma. Caregivers need to consider intubated patients' inability to speak.

Source: From Tessdale G, Jennett B. Assessment of coma and impaired consciousness: a practical scale. Lancet 1974;1:81.

Assessment of the patient with trauma in the fashion just described will immediately identify significant cardiovascular or CNS dysfunction. The next step in the evaluation is to expose (E) the patient. *Expose* means completely undressing the patient and examining her from head to toe. The back is examined for entrance or exit wounds, the extremities are briefly palpated, and any obvious visible injuries are noted. At this stage, the pregnant patient must undergo some preliminary determination of gestational age, the presence or absence of labor, and attempted measurement of fetal heart rate. Because of both the potential for fetal viability and for the supine hypotension effects described previously, pregnancies greater than 20 to 24 weeks' gestation evoke different management concerns than do gestations at less than the midpoint of pregnancy. For the patient undergoing cardiopulmonary resuscitation (CPR), perimortum cesarean section may be necessary. It should be emphasized, however, that *initial* management of the pregnant patient should be the same as for the nonpregnant individual. Maternal resuscitation *initially* takes precedence over fetal evaluation. Always remember that the leading cause of fetal mortality in trauma is maternal mortality, and rapid recognition and resuscitation reduces maternal mortality.

Inflatable military antishock trousers (MAST) have enjoyed some past popularity in the resuscitation or transport of the hypotensive trauma patient. These trousers are less frequently used in general adult trauma, with the device's most compelling indication being stabilization of the severely fractured pelvis. Conventional wisdom holds that if used in pregnancy, only the lower (leg) compartments should be inflated. The abdominal compartment should probably not be inflated in any patient with a potentially salvageable gestation, because uteroplacental blood flow is not preserved (Esposito, 1994; Pearlman, 1990a,b). Other potential obstetric-gynecologic indications for MAST include temporary stabilization of unremitting vaginal bleeding from uterine inversion, advanced reproductive tract malignancy, and recalcitrant uterine atony remote from a medical facility. Generally speaking, however, MAST should not be used in the pregnant *trauma* patient except under special circumstances.

## Investigations

At the conclusion of the primary survey, critical resuscitation is under way, major injuries are identified, and a general idea about the status of the pregnancy itself is known. At this juncture in management, diagnostic testing is ordered. *Immediate investigations* include necessary imaging studies, laboratory evaluation, and ancillary examination. Particular attention should be paid to the maternal bladder. Catheterization is undertaken, and if gross hematuria is noted on the perineum, consideration of bladder, urethral, ureteral, renal, or uterine trauma is essential. Evaluation for ruptured fetal membranes, cervical dilatation, vaginal bleeding, and fetal malpresentation is accomplished at this time. Cervical spine and other necessary radiographs are not contraindicated in the pregnant trauma victim. Nearly all pregnant trauma patients with multiple injuries should be considered candidates for chest and cervical vertebral radiographs. Other immediate investigations may include blood gas analysis, complete blood count, coagulation studies, serum electrolytes, and serum glucose determinations.

Measurement of fetomaternal hemorrhage (FMH) is indicated during the immediate investigation stage (Neufield, 1993). The Kleihauer-Betke citric acid elution stain can identify as little as 0.1 mL of fetal cells in the maternal circulation (Fig 33-2). The incidence of FMH is four- to fivefold higher in pregnant women who have experienced trauma than in uninjured controls (Pearlman, 1990b; Goodwin, 1990). Rh-negative gravidas who may be carrying Rh-positive fetuses need Rh-immune globulin (RIG). To calculate the appropriate dose of RIG in the Rh-negative patient with evidence of FMH, Rose et al describe the following formula (Rose, 1985; Laverly, 1995):

(Number of fetal cells/Number of adult cells)
× Maternal red-cell volume
= Fetal cells in maternal circulation

One milliliter of RIG (300 μg) is used for each 15 mL of fetal cells or 30 mL of fetal blood detected. The mean volume of FMH is usually less than 15 mL of blood, and over 90% of patients exhibit less than 30 mL of FMH. Therefore, in the majority of

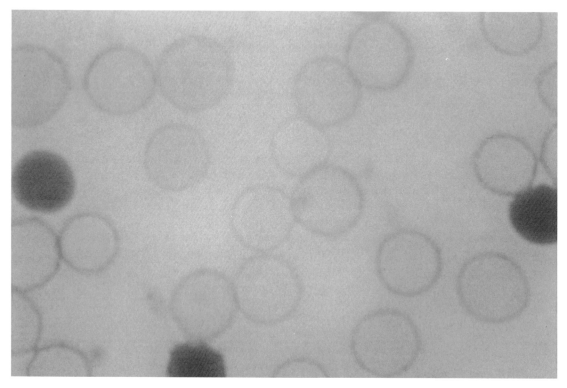

F I G U R E   **33-2**

Positive Kleihauer-Betke stain indicative of FMH. Fetal cells stain darkly with acid elucidation. (Photograph courtesy of Dr. Thomas F. Rowe.)

such patients, 300 μg of RIG will suffice. Measurement of RIG in the maternal circulation on the day following administration via indirect Coombs' assay should be weakly positive, thereby reflecting some residual "unused" RIG. If the follow-upindirect Coombs' assay is negative, additional RIG may be needed (Bowman, 1994, 1978a,b). Finally, even in the absence of detectable fetal cells in the Rh-negative and previously nonimmunized trauma victim, administration of a 300-μg dose of RIG should be considered anyway, given the significant risk of FMH in the presence of trauma coupled with the relatively small amount of fetal blood required to sensitize the Rh-negative mother (Hankins, 1995). Fetomaternal hemorrhage also may be a marker for occult or active placental abruption or uterine

rupture, albeit less reliably than fetal heart rate monitoring or clinical signs (Pearlman, 1990a,b; Goodwin, 1990).

## Secondary Survey and Treatment

At the conclusion of the primary survey, a second top-to-bottom physical assessment is made. This point in the resuscitation is ideal for a more extensive fetal evaluation. Earlier efforts were aimed at (1) general evaluation of fetal age and presence of life, (2) ascertainment of the appropriateness of perimortem cesarean section during unsuccessful CPR, (3) minimizing the effects of uterine compression on maternal resuscitation, and (4) indirect fetal resuscitation through successful maternal hemodynamic resuscitation.

During the secondary survey, however, specific fetal investigations are indicated. Identification of vaginal bleeding, ruptured fetal membranes, preterm labor, placental abruption, direct uterine or fetal injury, and/or fetal distress is accomplished.

## Fetal Evaluation

Fetal injury or death from maternal trauma occurs by several mechanisms. Pearlman and Tintinalli (1991) noted a 41% fetal loss rate with life-threatening maternal injuries and a 1.6% fetal loss rate with non-life-threatening maternal injuries. Generally, fetal loss is correlated with the severity of maternal injury; unfortunately, however, lethal fetal injury can occur readily in the absence of significant maternal injury (Fries, 1989).

Placental abruption complicates up to 5% of otherwise minor injuries and up to 50% of major injuries during pregnancy (Hankins, 1995; Esposito, 1994; Pearlman, 1991; Neufield, 1993; Pearlman, 1990a,b; Vaizey, 1994). Placental abruption is a frequent cause of fetal death from trauma. The relatively inelastic placenta is thought to shear secondary to deformation of the much more elastic myometrium. The placental abruption is worsened by bleeding-perpetuated worsening of placental separation. Uterine tenderness, uterine contractions, vaginal bleeding, and fetal heart rate abnormalities are clinical hallmarks of placental abruption. The association of contractions with placental abruption is a significant one. Williams et al (1990) studied pregnant trauma patients with electronic fetal monitoring. Placental abruption did not occur in women who did not have uterine contractions, or who had contractions at a frequency of less than one every 10 minutes after 4 hours of fetal monitoring. In patients with more frequent contractions, nearly 20% had placental abruption. Other fetal heart rate abnormalities, such as bradycardia, late decelerations, and tachycardia, also were seen frequently in patients who had experienced abruption (Fig 33-3). Continuous fetal monitoring is therefore usually indicated

F I G U R E   **33-3**

Fetal heart rate monitor strip in a 28-week fetus exhibiting FMH from traumatic abruption. Uterine activity was not recorded, but a characteristic sinusoidal fetal heart rate pattern is evident. (Courtesy of Carol Harvey, RNC, MS.)

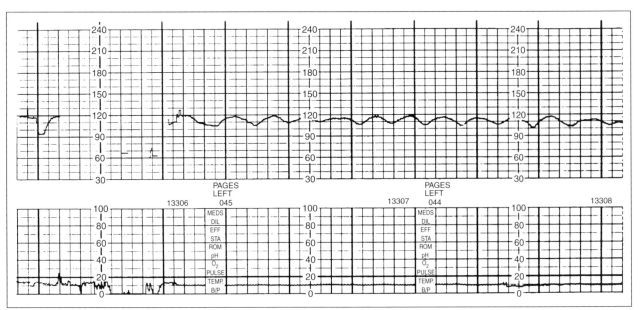

in the 22–24+-week pregnant trauma patient (Williams, 1990; ACOG, 1991; Hankins, 1995). Finally, placental abruption may be associated with a consumptive coagulopathy, and, if so, it will be additive to other trauma-associated coagulopathies (Pritchard, 1967).

The duration of electronic fetal heart rate monitoring after maternal trauma is problematic. Delayed manifestation of catastrophic abruption has been reported more than 48 hours after trauma (Higgins, 1984). Fortunately, the majority of catastrophic events occur much sooner. Patients with regular uterine contractions or fetal heart rate abnormalities should be monitored until resolution of such findings. In patients without uterine contractions, or fetal heart rate abnormalities, or other objective signs or symptoms of abruption, it is suggested that a period of 2 to 6 hours of monitoring will suffice (ACOG, 1991). Electronic fetal monitoring is probably the best tool for detection of abruption in the trauma patient. In one large series, no abruption was identified unless uterine activity was noted within the first 4 hours of monitoring (Pearlman, 1990b).

In the woman actively undergoing resuscitation, continuous electronic fetal monitoring of the potentially viable fetus is a useful indicator of fetal response to and adequacy of resuscitation. Fetal heart rate monitoring is a proven sensitive indicator of maternal hypovolemia (Katz, 1976). Given the relatively large uteroplacental perfusion requirements during pregnancy, coupled with the poor placental autoregulation in the face of hypotension, fetoplacental blood flow often will undergo pathophysiologic alterations in the absence of any obvious maternal manifestations of hypovolemia. The risk of fetal loss is related directly to the degree of maternal hemorrhagic shock (Scorpio, 1992). Hence, aggressive volume replacement and shock treatment, coupled with continuous electronic fetal monitoring, are indicated in the gravid trauma victim who is otherwise a candidate for fetal monitoring.

## The Fetal Patient

Direct fetal injury is infrequent, albeit the reported incidence is uncertain (Hankins, 1995). Fetal injury is uncommon in early pregnancy unless severe pelvic fractures are found. The uterus of the early-pregnant and nonpregnant patient is well protected by the bony pelvis. Direct fetal injury from blunt abdominal trauma most often involves the fetal skull and head and is seen in the third trimester in patients with pelvic fractures (Esposito, 1994).

Very few diagnostic or therapeutic interventions are *absolutely* contraindicated in the pregnant trauma victim with life-threatening injuries. While the effects of high doses of ionizing radiation on the fetus may be pronounced, the degree and amount of fetal exposure from routinely obtained conventional or computerized tomography (CT) radiography is considerably less. Animal and human data show little or no risk to the fetus from up to 0.1 Gy or more of ionizing radiation (Briss, 1994; Shepard, 1992). A single pelvic film delivers less than 0.01 Gy to the fetus. Although fetal exposure is higher with CT scans or pyelography, they should not be avoided if they are needed to evaluate and treat the mother (Esposito, 1994). Despite the requirement to use fluoroscopy in conjunction with the technique, angiography may also be relatively beneficial to the pregnant trauma victim because of its ability to produce hemostasis (Ben-Menachem, 1985).

Few medications produce harmful fetal effects, and most teratogens have an impact only in early pregnancy. With the supposition that fetal survival and well-being is related directly to maternal survival and well-being, most medically necessary interventions applied to the pregnant trauma victim are indicated for both maternal and fetal well-being. Tetanus toxoid administration and tetanus immune globulin are not contraindicated in the gravid trauma victim. Administration should be identical to that in the nonpregnant trauma patient. Most obstetricians are familiar with the benefits and limitations of ultrasound. Diagnostic ultrasound is not as sensitive as electronic fetal monitoring in the diagnosis of abruption (Pearlman, 1990a). Ultrasound use for obstetric anthropometric parameters and as a screening modality for direct fetal injury, hematoma formation, and free fluid should be encouraged (Bode, 1993; Nyberg, 1987). A recent review that analyzed the accuracy of ultrasound in the initial evaluation of the blunt trauma victim underscored ultrasound's usefulness in trauma evaluation (McKenney, 1996).

## Volume Resuscitation

Volume replacement in pregnancy merits special consideration. By virtue of young age and the volume changes inherent in normal pregnancy, the pregnant woman may not exhibit clinically significant symptomatology of blood loss until 1500 to 2000 mL are lost. Blood loss greater than 2000 mL often produces rapid maternal deterioration. Because fetal status is a sensitive indicator of maternal hemodynamic homeostasis, fetal compromise may occur at maternal blood losses significantly less than 2000 mL. Fetal heart rate changes may be an early indicator of maternal hypovolemia. Initial treatment of suspected hypovolemia should consist of rapid infusion of isotonic crystalloid solution (normal saline or lactated Ringer's solution). Blood products should be considered in trauma with hemorrhage greater than 1000 mL (Esposito, 1994; Mighty, 1994). Theoretic concerns about hyperchloremia from excessive normal saline make lactated Ringer's solution more ideal for volume resuscitation (Crosby, 1987). Fetal oxygen delivery is also better when lactated Ringer's solution is used instead of normal saline in volume resuscitation (Boba, 1966). Type- and Rh-specific blood should be available as soon as possible. Until blood is available, isotonic crystalloid solutions are replaced at a rate of 3 mL for each milliliter of estimated blood loss. While whole blood may be preferable to packed RBCs, it is generally not available. Component therapy should not be given empirically, except perhaps in the case of massive exsanguination. Initial resuscitation goals include restoration of maternal vital signs, normalization of fetal heart rate, and resumption of normal urine output. It should be reemphasized that up to a 20% reduction in uteroplacental blood flow can occur without changes in maternal BP. Maternal resuscitation should be taken in the context of fetal resuscitation during pregnancy (Greiss, 1966; Boba, 1966).

## Perimortem Cesarean Section

Under normal circumstances, cesarean section in the trauma victim is reserved for the usual obstetric indications and is performed at gestational ages consistent with fetal viability. Unique clinical circumstances may alter these guidelines somewhat when perimortem cesarean section is considered during unsuccessful maternal CPR. Uterine evacuation may be indicated for either maternal or fetal reasons, or both. Due to the inefficiency of CPR in the provision of adequate cerebral and coronary blood flow, prolonged CPR in the nonpregnant individual is rarely successful. Because of aortocaval compression from the uterus after 20 to 24 weeks' gestation, the significant circulatory shunt produced by the uteroplacental circuit, and the force vector–mediated degradation of chest compression effectiveness in the laterally tilted pregnant patient, CPR is likely to be even less effective in the patient who has been pregnant longer than 20 weeks (Kuhlman, 1994). Therefore, during CPR of this gravid female, uterine evacuation after 5 to 10 minutes of unsuccessful resuscitation may be therapeutic for the mother. In Katz's (1986) review of fetal outcome from perimortem cesarean section, intact fetal survival is excellent if delivery is accomplished within 5 minutes of arrest. Survival and *intact* survival decrease profoundly after the 10-minute interval. Therefore, when there is a living fetus at a potentially viable gestational age, perimortem cesarean section should be strongly considered within 4 to 5 minutes of seemingly unsuccessful CPR (Fig 33-4). This would potentially allow delivery to occur within the 5- to 10-minute window, affording perhaps the best overall balance of risk and benefit to the fetus and mother (see Chapter 12). Bedside laparotomy and delivery should always be considered during the CPR of any advanced-gestation-age trauma patient. Little equipment beyond gloves and a scalpel is needed. The hypotension from the arrest often results in minimal blood loss from the surgery. Perimortem cesarean section should not be delayed to take the patient to an operating room, although a qualified physician should perform the surgery.

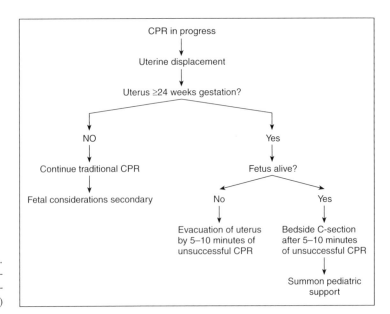

CPR in progress

Uterine displacement

Uterus ≥24 weeks gestation?

NO — Yes

NO: Continue traditional CPR → Fetal considerations secondary

Yes: Fetus alive?

No → Evacuation of uterus by 5–10 minutes of unsuccessful CPR

Yes → Bedside C-section after 5–10 minutes of unsuccessful CPR → Summon pediatric support

FIGURE **33-4**

**Perimortem cesarean section.** (From Katz VL, Dotters DJ, Droege-mueller W. Perimortem cesarean delivery. Obstet Gynecol 1986;68:571.)

## Manifestations of Trauma

### Blunt Abdominal Trauma

Motor vehicle accidents account for a large portion of severe, blunt obstetric trauma. Other causes of blunt abdominal trauma include accidental falls and intentional trauma (violence) (Goodwin, 1990; Pearlman, 1990a,b; Rothenberger, 1978; Esposito, 1989).

Motor vehicle accidents produce blunt abdominal trauma in addition to other forms of maternal injury. In motor vehicle accidents, the most common cause of fetal death is maternal death (Crosby, 1971). Expulsion from the vehicle and the presence of coexisting head trauma portend poor maternal and fetal outcomes. The value of automobile passenger restraint systems is evident from both fetal and maternal trauma data. Crosby and Costiloe (1971) noted a 33% mortality in unrestrained gravid automobile accident victims, compared with a 5% mortality in those pregnant victims using two-point restraints (traditional lap belt). The fetal death rate also was lower in the restraint group. The three-point restraint system (lap and shoulder belt) limits "jackknifing" of the gravid abdomen during sudden deceleration. The mechanism of fetal loss may be

different since the introduction and more widespread use of three-point restraints and the arguably better crash engineering of most modern automobiles. The impact of air bags is expected to be positive on both maternal and fetal outcomes, but thus far, there are no data to address this. The majority of fetal deaths occur in conjunction with relatively minor maternal injury, and most are due to placental abruption (Fries , 1989; Agran, 1987; Lane, 1989; Stafford, 1988; Pearlman, 1995). Lap belts should be positioned low across the bony pelvis instead of over the mid or upper uterine fundus. Shoulder belts should be adjusted for comfort and lie across the gravid uterus. Although fetal injury and death have been attributed to lap belts, restraint systems are still recommended and in most states are mandatory (Griffiths, 1991; Pearce, 1992; Crosby, 1971; Pearlman, 1996a,b).

Up to 40% of severe blunt abdominal trauma is associated with placental abruption, but a 2.6% rate of abruption is seen with otherwise "minor" abdominal trauma (Fries, 1989; Agran, 1987; Lane, 1989; Hankins, 1995). Preterm labor is seen de novo in approximately 1% of non-life-threatening abdominal trauma and is probably more frequent in severe abdominal trauma. As stated earlier in this chapter, contractions are associated frequently with the eventual manifestation of placental abruption. Most patients without clinical evidence of abruption eventually cease to contract (Pearlman, 1995).

Evaluation of the pregnant patient with blunt abdominal trauma generally is similar to evaluation in the nonpregnant patient. Up to 25% of severe blunt trauma victims suffer hemodynamically significant hepatic and/or splenic injuries (Kuhlman, 1994). Upper abdominal pain, referred shoulder pain, sudden onset of pain, and elevated transaminases are consistent with injuries to the liver or spleen. Computerized tomographic scanning may aid diagnosis in less obvious cases. Embolization or hepatic lobe resection, coupled with packing and local control may ameliorate hepatic hemorrhage. Splenectomy is generally the preferred treatment for splenic rupture. Other indications for exploratory laparotomy in the pregnant patient with blunt abdominal trauma include hemodynamic instability with suspected active bleeding, viscus perforation, infection, and fetal distress in the viable gestation. In less severe cases, diagnostic peritoneal lavage (DPL) is as useful in pregnant as in nonpregnant abdominal trauma patients. During pregnancy, an open technique (analogous to open laparoscopy), in which the lavage catheter is placed in the abdomen to

help the operator avoid the enlarged uterus, is recommended. Guidelines for a positive DPL are included in Table 33-5. Fetal outcome is not adversely affected by the performance of a DPL during pregnancy.

An important caveat does exist in the evaluation of the pregnant patient with blunt abdominal trauma. Because of maternal volume changes and pregnancy-associated intra-abdominal anatomic alterations, many pregnant patients who ultimately require a laparotomy for intra-abdominal injuries present without significant abdominal signs or symptoms! In one series, 44% of those patients who eventually required laparotomy for intra-abdominal pathology were initially asymptomatic. Rib or pelvic fractures in the pregnant trauma victim should heighten one's suspicion for hepatic, splenic, genitourinary, uterine or other abdominal injury (Laverly, 1995; Davis, 1976).

Blunt abdominal trauma is one of the more common results of physical abuse during pregnancy. As many as 10% of pregnant women will experience physical or sexual abuse during pregnancy. In addition to blunt abdominal trauma, other injuries commonly occur on the face, neck, and proximal extremities. Providers must maintain an index of suspicion for physical or sexual abuse during pregnancy (Newberger, 1992; Parker, 1994).

T A B L E   **33-5**

Diagnostic peritoneal lavage[a]

|  | **Positive** | **Equivocal** | **Negative**[b] |
|---|---|---|---|
| *Aspirate* | | | |
| Blood | > 10 mL | > 5 mL but < 10 mL | < 5 mL |
| Fluid | Enteric fluid | — | — |
| *Lavage* | | | |
| RBCs | > 100,000/μL | > 50,000/μL | < 50,000/μL |
| WBCs | > 500/μL | > 200/μL but < 500/μL | < 200/μL |
| Amylase | > 20 IU/liter | — | — |
| Bile | Present | — | — |

Ten milliliters per kilogram (approx 1 liter) of warmed Ringer's lactate or isotonic normal saline infused and allowed to return to IV base.

[a]"Negative" findings must be interpreted in clinical context.

[b]Open technique recommended during pregnancy.

Sources: McAnena OJ, Moore EE, Marx JA. Initial evaluation of the patient with blunt abdominal trauma. Surg Clin North Am 1990;70:495, and Esposito TJ, Gens DR, Smith CG, Scorpio R. Evaluation of blunt abdominal trauma occurring during pregnancy. J Trauma 1989;29:1628.

## Penetrating Abdominal Trauma

The two most common types of penetrating abdominal injury are stab and gunshot wounds. Pregnancy often changes the usual manifestations of penetrating abdominal injury. The gravid uterus displaces lower abdominal organs cephalad. Maternal mortality is lower from abdominal gunshot wounds than it is in nonpregnant adults (3.9% vs. 12.5%). Fetal mortality (71%), however, is high (Sandy, 1989). Reported data from abdominal stab wounds were similar in that fetal mortality was high (42%) and maternal mortality was not seen (Sakala, 1988). The reduced maternal mortality, yet high fetal loss, from penetrating abdominal injury are probably due to the gravid uterus shielding other abdominal contents from the force of the penetrating projectile when the impact of the shell or penetrating object is below the uterine fundus (Sandy, 1989; Sakala, 1988; Laverly, 1995; Esposito, 1994). Contrawise, upper abdominal penetrating injuries are more likely to produce small bowel injury in the advanced gravida than would occur in nonpregnant victims.

Management of gunshot wounds to the pregnant abdomen include the general resuscitation measures outlined previously. Particular attention should be paid to the pathway of the projectile. Both entry and exit wounds must be identified. If the missile has not exited the abdomen, radiographic localization aids bullet location and injury prognostication. Gunshot projectiles that enter into the uterus often will remain in utero. Fetal death may be direct or indirect. Most authors recommend abdominal exploration for all extrauterine intra-abdominal gunshot wounds and most intrauterine wounds. Experience from the Middle East conflict and other reports suggest an individualized approach to intrauterine injuries (Kuhlman, 1994; Del Rossi, 1990; Awwad, 1994). We generally advocate surgical exploration of the pregnant intra-abdominal gunshot wound victim (Grubb, 1992).

Abdominal stab wounds generally are less serious than gunshot wounds. Because of less likelihood for "collateral damage," many pregnant stab wound victims will not have abdominal organ damage that requires surgical repair. Because of the compartmentalization that occurs with advanced pregnancy, the mechanism of injury changes with abdominal stab wounds during pregnancy. Small bowel involvement is more frequent with upper abdominal stab wounds during pregnancy. Also, the upper abdomen is the most frequent site of abdominal stab wounds during pregnancy, comprising some two out of three anterior abdominal penetrating wounds (Kuhlman, 1994). Because of the propensity for small intestine injury and the potentially catastrophic effects of diaphragmatic involvement, with up to a 66% mortality with thoracic herniation and strangulation of small intestine, most authors recommend exploration of upper abdominal stab wounds during pregnancy.

Lower abdominal stab wounds during pregnancy may involve the uterus, fetus, uteropelvic vessels, or urinary bladder. An individualized approach to management is suggested. Diagnostic peritoneal lavage is useful for evaluating intra-abdominal bleeding (Esposito, 1994). Amniocentesis and ultrasound help in the evaluation of intrauterine bleeding (Kuhlman, 1994). Urinary bladder involvement may be determined by radiographic evaluation (retrograde cystogram). Actual abdominal cavity entry can be determined through direct exploration of the wound or the performance of a wound fistulogram (Cornell, 1976). While not all lower abdominal stab wounds need to be explored, a very high index of suspicion for the need to explore the abdomen should be maintained.

During exploratory laparotomy for penetrating abdominal trauma, the uterus must be carefully inspected for injury. If direct uterine perforation is noted in the presence of a living term fetus, abdominal delivery is probably warranted. Less extensive uterine or adnexal injury or the presence of intrauterine fetal death does not necessarily dictate emptying of the uterus (Franger, 1989). Likewise, the uterus should not necessarily be emptied via cesarean section or hysterectomy during surgery for nonuterine injuries. In cases in which direct uterine injury is found and the fetus is alive, premature, but potentially viable, cesarean section may be obvious for fetal or maternal hemorrhage or intrauterine infection (Laverly, 1995; Kuhlman, 1994). These are incredibly difficult cases and will require an assessment of the risk-benefit ratio of expectant management versus delivery by cesarean section specific to the best estimate of gestational age, of fetal injury, and of both the maternal and fetal prognosis if left undelivered.

Other obstetric considerations for delivery also apply in that direct uterine injury to the active uterine segment probably necessitates eventual cesarean section as the preferred route of delivery. Injury to the lower uterine segment with delayed delivery probably needs to be approached on an individual case-by-case basis.

In cases of direct uterine injury, preterm labor may be treated with tocolytics, although betasympathomimetics and nonsteroidal antiinflammatory agents generally should be avoided because of their effects on maternal hemodynamics and platelet function, respectively (Hankins, 1991; Caritis, 1992). Magnesium sulfate is probably the drug of choice for treatment of preterm labor in the circumstance of maternal trauma. The usual precautions for administration of magnesium sulfate are to be considered with its use in trauma.

### Chest Trauma

Thoracic trauma represents a particular challenge to the clinician caring for the pregnant trauma victim. There is a paucity of information regarding thoracic trauma (or its management) during pregnancy. In the United States, chest trauma accounts for one in four trauma deaths annually. Recognition and stabilization of chest trauma is vital, because fewer than 10% of blunt chest trauma and fewer than 30% of penetrating chest injuries require immediate thoracotomy (Ramenofsky, 1993). Most cases of thoracic trauma initially respond to nonsurgical stabilization. Effective stabilization ultimately results in improved operative outcome if surgery is required. A basic understanding of the types of chest trauma will help the obstetric member of the trauma team function more effectively in the overall resuscitation of the injured gravida.

Chest trauma can be classified functionally or mechanistically. Mechanistically, thoracic trauma is subdivided into blunt and penetrating injuries (much like abdominal trauma). Of pri-

mary importance is the recognition of immediately life-threatening chest trauma, with differentiation of life-threatening trauma from potentially serious but less immediately life-threatening subtypes of chest trauma. In this discussion we generally divide chest trauma into immediately life-threatening and non-life-threatening subtypes (Ramenofsky, 1993; Del Rossi, 1990).

The primary survey of a trauma patient will identify several types of life-threatening thoracic trauma. When identified, life-threatening injuries require expedient management. Fortunately, many immediately life-threatening injuries can be managed initially by oxygen administration, mechanical ventilation, needle pneumothoracocentesis, or tube thoracostomy (chest tube) placement. Life-threatening chest injuries include airway obstruction, open pneumothorax, massive hemothorax, tension pneumothorax, flail chest, cardiac tamponade and trauma-mediated severe myocardial dysfunction (Table 33-6) (Ramenofsky, 1993).

Airway obstruction should be managed initially as described in Chapter 12 (CPR), and then systematically with early intubation or cricothyroidotomy, if required. Cervical spine protection

T A B L E **33-6**

**Life-threatening chest injuries**

| Immediately Life-Threatening | Initial Treatment* |
|---|---|
| Airway obstruction | Airway control |
| Open pneumothorax | Injury site control and thoracotomy tube |
| Tension pneumothorax | Needle thoracostomy |
| Flail chest | Supportive (± intubation) |
| Cardiac tamponade | Volume therapy and pericardiocentesis |
| Severe myocardial damage | Inotropic support and treatment of dysrhythmias |

*Qualified consultants should be involved in the care of any chest trauma patient. These treatment recommendations are guidelines. Each case should be individualized.

Source: Ramenofsky ML, Alexander RH, Ali J, et al, eds. Advanced trauma life support—1993 instructor manual. American College of Surgeons. Chicago: First Impressions, 1993.

by neck stabilization and jaw thrust is vital during intubation of any patient with an unevaluated cervical spine. In pregnancy, the additional increased risk of aspiration of gastric contents may necessitate the more aggressive use of endotracheal intubation or surgical airway control. The requirement for oxygenation and effective pulmonary gas exchange precedes all other aspects of resuscitation (Rutherford, 1995; Barone, 1986).

Tension pneumothorax develops when a one-way flow of gas collects in the pleural space. Intrapleural pressure increases progressively with each inspiration. When intrapleural pressure increases to a level higher than great vessel pressures, hemodynamic instability results. The clinical diagnosis of tension pneumothorax is made by a combination of respiratory distress, hypotension, tachycardia, diminished or absent breath sounds, possible jugular venous distention, and tracheal deviation. The differential diagnosis of tension pneumothorax includes massive hemothorax (similar thoracic pathophysiology and treatment) and pericardial tamponade (much less common) (Wilson, 1995). Radiographic confirmation of a suspected tension pneumothorax is usually useful only for postmortem correlation (Weaver, 1986)!

In addition to trauma, other causes of tension pneumothorax include central line placement, bullous emphysema, and mechanical ventilation. Regardless of its etiology, immediate recognition and treatment of a tension pneumothorax or massive hemothorax is vital. Needle thoracostomy, performed in the second intercostal space–midclavicular line, will convert a tension pneumothorax to a simple pneumothorax. Definitive treatment is by insertion of a thoracostomy tube in the affected hemithorax. For this indication, a thoracostomy tube is usually placed in the fifth intercostal space (nipple level), anterior to the midaxillary line (Feliciano, 1992). Additional care during pregnancy must be taken because of the normally elevated diaphragm (Laverly, 1995). Inadvertent abdominal insertion of a chest tube with the resultant diaphragmatic, hepatic, or splenic injury is potentially more likely during pregnancy. Particular attention to this potentially catastrophic complication must be heeded if additional thoracostomy tubes are placed in locations other than the anterior midaxillary fifth intercostal space, and especially if such tubes are placed in lower intercostal spaces. To reduce the chance of abdominal placement, consideration should be taken to place the thoracostomy tube at least one interspace higher than usual.

Massive hemothorax is treated initially by thoracostomy tube placement, as described. To facilitate drainage of thoracic blood, the chest tube should be directed inferiorly (after its insertion in the midaxillary fifth intercostal space). Once again, care should be taken to avoid abdominal entry. A large chest tube (i.e., no. 38 Fr) is usually recommended. If the initial volume of blood drained from the tube is greater than or equal to 1500 mL, early thoracotomy is probably necessary. Continued loss of 300 mL or more per hour from the chest tube also may indicate the need of a thoracotomy. Other temporizing measures, such as volume replacement, transfusion, and potential use of cell-saving autotransfusion, should be initiated until the patient is evaluated by a qualified thoracic trauma surgeon (Wilson, 1995; Mattox, 1989; Mansour, 1992).

Open pneumothorax is often referred to as a sucking chest wound. If the size of the opening to the hemothorax is near to or greater than the size of the tracheal diameter, physics dictates that air will enter the chest preferentially through the chest wall rather than through the trachea during inspiratory attempts. Consequently, to restore effective ventilation temporarily, a large occlusive dressing is placed on the open injury. Ultimately, thoracostomy tube placement at a site distal to the thoracic entry wound and surgical repair are required (Ramenofsky, 1993).

Cardiac tamponade was mentioned previously in the discussion of tension pneumothorax. Tamponade usually occurs with penetrating injuries and is less common than tension pneumothorax. Catastrophic hypotension and, ultimately, pulseless electrical activity (electromechanical disassociation) result from cardiac tamponade. Because of noncompliance of the pericardial sac, a relatively small amount of rapidly collected blood will cause hemodynamic compromise. Diagnosis is possible from clinical features (Becks' triad: venous pressure elevation, decreased arterial pressure, and muffled heart tones), radiographic examination (enlarged cardiac silhouette), or echocardiography. Unfortunately, as with tension pneumothorax, time is often not available to diagnose cardiac tamponade definitively. Pericardiocentesis by a qualified operator is a life-saving temporizing measure. Rapid volume infusion also will often temporarily alleviate the problem. As with thoracostomy tube placement, pericardiocentesis should be undertaken with recognition of the fact that the pregnant patient's diaphragm is normally elevated. Definitive treatment of pericardiocentesis is usually by the opening of the pericardium by a qualified thoracic trauma surgeon (Shoemaker, 1970, 1975).

Flail chest happens secondary to trauma-mediated separation of a part of the bony chest wall from the remaining thorax. Hypoxemia from severe atelectasis and underlying pulmonary contusion is produced by flail chest. Paradoxical movement of part of the chest during respiration, direct physical examination of the chest, and radiographic evaluation lead to the diagnosis of this condition. Intubation and mechanical ventilation may be required in the flail chest victim with intractable hypoxemia or other injuries (Trinkle, 1975; Sankaran, 1976).

Massive chest trauma can produce intrinsic myocardial damage. Myocardial contusion, myocardial ischemia from hypoperfusion, or underlying substance abuse all may cause or contribute to myocardial injury. Although usually diagnosed during the secondary survey, potentially lethal dysrhythmias also can be noted during the primary survey. These dysrhythmias may be produced by the initial injury or from reperfusion of injured myocardium. Standard treatment of such dysrhythmias is recommended to reduce the likelihood of malignant degeneration of the rhythm or cardiac arrest (Paone, 1993; Mattox, 1992; Fiazee, 1986).

The secondary survey also may uncover evolving life-threatening thoracic injuries, albeit *usually* the progression of such injuries is less fulminant than when they are diagnosed during the primary survey. Potentially lethal secondary survey injuries include pulmonary contusion, myocardial contusion, aortic disruption, esophageal disruption, tracheal or bronchial rupture, and traumatic diaphragmatic rupture (Ramenofsky, 1993).

Pulmonary contusion is the most common potentially lethal chest injury seen in North America (Fig 33-5) (Ramenofsky, 1993). Progressive hypoxemia results from the secondary effects of the contusion. Typically, respiratory failure from pulmonary contusion progresses insidiously and often is not present immediately. A diffuse radiographic injury pattern is characteristic of pulmonary contusion. Careful clinical monitoring, frequent blood gas analysis, and a low threshold for intubation and mechanical ventilation in the patient with a severe pulmonary contusion help reduce mortality (Ramenofsky, 1993; Stellin, 1981).

Myocardial contusion may initiate malignant dysrhythmias as a delayed event. Ischemia, new-onset bundle branch block, presence of ventricular or supraventricular dysrhythmias, and pure myocardial pump failure in the victim of severe thoracic trauma should heighten the suspicion for myocardial contusion (Paone, 1993; Mattox, 1992). Continuous ECG monitoring is suggested in any patient felt to be predisposed to the sequelae of myocardial contusion (Wilson, 1995). Prompt recognition and treatment may prevent hemodynamic deterioration. Diagnosis is by ECG or echocardiography.

The increased frequency of traumatic diaphragmatic rupture in association with upper abdominal injury during pregnancy needs to be considered in any pregnant chest or upper abdominal trauma victim (Ramenofsky, 1993).

Traumatic aortic rupture occurs frequently in conjunction with motor vehicle accidents or falls from great heights (Ramenofsky, 1993; Wilson, 1995). Aortic rupture mechanistically occurs from the relative fixation of the aorta, thereby reducing its ability to move or flex with sudden deceleration. Tearing of one or more of the layers of the vessel is produced. Aortic rupture is often associated initially with only modest hypotension, especially with lesions near the ligamentum arteriosum. With aortic rupture, those patients with unconfined lesions or transection usually exsanguinate before or shortly after arrival to the hospital, while patients with contained hematomas are more frequently alive at hospital presentation. Diagnosis of the contained aortic rupture may be difficult. Mediastinal widening, obliteration of the aortic knob, or first or second

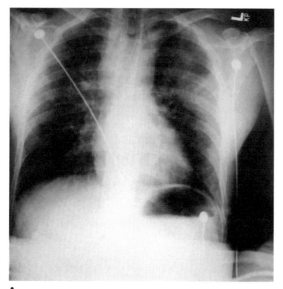

**A**

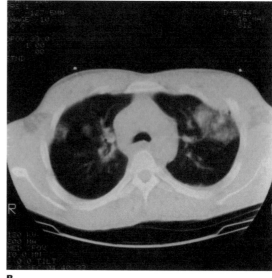

**B**

FIGURE **33-5**

Trauma victim with bilateral pulmonary contusions as evident on (A) chest x-ray and (B) CT-scan. Fluffy contusion infiltrate is more apparent and larger in the left lung field. (Images courtesy of Dr. Sanford Rubin.)

rib fractures suggest an increased probability of aortic rupture (Mattox, 1989). Ultrasound, magnetic resonance imaging, or CT may assist in the diagnosis of aortic rupture, but angiography is the penultimate diagnostic procedure for traumatic aortic rupture (Ramenofsky, 1993). Once again, any needed radiographic studies are not to be deferred in the severely ill pregnant trauma victim.

Tracheobronchial tree injuries (TBIs) may produce sudden airway obstruction. A high clinical index of suspicion, especially in cases of refractory pneumothorax, subcutaneous emphysema, or blast injuries, is necessary for timely diagnosis. Operative intervention is frequently necessary in patients with TBIs (Scorpio, 1992; Wilson, 1995; Taskinen, 1989).

Esophageal trauma often is an insidious feature of chest trauma. It is usually, but not always, associated with penetrating chest trauma. Esophageal rupture is suspected in any patient with severe epigastric injury, substernal trauma, and pneumothorax without chest wall injury, and/or

in patients with continued particulate material in their thoracostomy tube drainage. Esophagoscopy or contrast studies confirm the diagnosis. Death may result directly from hemorrhage or from unrelenting mediastinitis (Jones, 1992; Tilanus, 1991).

While thoracic trauma should be evaluated by a thoracic specialist familiar with chest trauma management, an understanding of the ramifications of potentially lethal chest trauma often will allow the obstetrician to recognize and stabilize the chest trauma victim.

### Head Trauma

Approximately 50% of all trauma deaths are associated with head injury. More than 60% of motor vehicle–associated trauma deaths occur as a result of head trauma (Scorpio, 1992). In a review of pregnant trauma deaths in Cook County (Illinois), approximately 10% of maternal trauma deaths were due directly to head injury (Fildes, 1992).

Several aspects of cranial and cerebral physiology and pathophysiology are very important in head trauma victims. The brain is one of the most carefully protected organs of the body; the calvarium and CSF cushion the brain from minor trauma. In severe trauma, however, these two otherwise protective features may contribute to or precipitate brain injury. The brain has poor tolerance of diminished perfusion, with little or no metabolic reserve in brain tissues. Global cerebral oxygen consumption of at least 1.5 mL/100 g/min must be maintained to prevent injury. Oxygen delivery to the brain is determined by BP, blood oxygen content, blood flow distribution, and relative perfusion pressure. Because the closed space of the calvarium is occupied by blood, CSF, and brain volume, intracranial pressure (ICP) is a function of all three components (the Monro-Kellie doctrine). Cerebral edema results in increased brain volume, thereby producing elevated ICP. Traumatic collections of blood in the cranial vault will similarly increase ICP. Often, both of these mechanisms are present in the head trauma victim (Hayek, 1991).

Cerebroautoregulation is normally maintained over a wide range of BP. Extremes of BP, such as hypotension found in the multiple trauma victim, tax the brain's ability to autoregulate. When coupled with cerebral edema and/or intracranial bleeding, hypotension further aggravates the inability of the brain to autoregulate. Furthermore, the injured brain may lose its ability to autoregulate, yet another mechanism for self-perpetuation of brain injury. Finally, because the cranium is a closed system, propagation of elevated extravascular cerebral pressure transmurally causes the driving pressure in the cerebral circulation to be decreased significantly. If that flow is directly determined by a change in pressure, diminished cerebral perfusion pressure (mean arterial BP − ICP) causes decreased effective cerebral blood flow. Cerebral mass lesions will, therefore, diminish cerebral perfusion pressure in proportion to their size, even in the face of normal BP. Thus, it should be obvious that acute brain injury is often a self-perpetuating, dynamic process which is poorly tolerated by the fastidious neuronal cells. Cell death and permanent injury may result. The therapeutic goal of acute cerebral resuscitation is to limit cell death by regulated reperfusion to nonfunctioning but still viable brain tissue (ischemic penumbra). The clinician's ability to accomplish this goal is often limited (Hayek, 1991; Robertsen, 1992; Maset, 1987).

Another feature of brain injury is the concept of secondary, or reperfusion, injury. An initial insult produces the loss of autoregulation, as described. Unfortunately, reperfusion of the injured area may occur in the presence of absent or diminished autoregulation. Injury is produced either mechanically (through edema) or metabolically (through inappropriate substrate production) through reperfusion (Hayek, 1991; Bruce, 1973; Smith, 1990).

To avoid or limit permanent cerebral injury, specific cerebral resuscitation must be performed. The sooner resuscitation is begun, the greater the chance that injured but living neuronal tissue will survive.

Penetrating head injuries produce injury by obvious mechanisms. With blunt head trauma, especially in deceleration events, movement of the brain occurs first in one direction with a secondary rebound movement in the opposite direction, producing a *coup-countercoup* effect. Closed head injuries can occur without significant injury of the cutaneous tissues and calvarium through bruising or contusion of the brain at coup or countercoup sites. Intracerebral hemorrhage from traumatic brain injury often results from severe contusion. Subdural or epidural hematomas are produced by direct laceration or tearing of subdural or epidural vessels, respectively (Scorpio, 1992).

Initial management of suspected brain injury starts with the basic ABCs discussed previously. Profound hypotension, defined as systolic BP less than 60 mm Hg in nonpregnant individuals, may cause or contribute to altered consciousness. Correction of hypotension is important. Although possible, hypotension as a result of the neurologic insult is uncommon. Until proven otherwise, hypotension in the presence of head injury is from other causes. Severe hypertension in the comatose trauma victim may be centrally mediated. This Cushing response is also characterized by bradycardia and a diminished respiratory rate (Hayek, 1991). Altered levels of consciousness also may be produced by alcohol or drug ingestion. Toxicologic assessment is recommended in most trauma patients with altered levels of consciousness. Conversely, an altered level of consciousness should never be attributed totally to alcohol or other drug ingestion alone, unless confirmed. Finally, other medical conditions, such as hypoglycemia, occasionally may be coincidental with trauma.

A baseline and ongoing mental assessment is necessary as a frame of reference for all trauma patients (Scorpio, 1992). The A-V-P-U mini-exam (see Fig 33-1) is a brief primary survey tool. In the secondary survey, more extensive evaluation, such as by the GCS, is recommended (see Table 33-4) (Tessdale, 1974). As mentioned previously, a score of 8 or less is indicative of the diagnosis of coma and is classified as severe head injury (Baxt, 1987; Rutherford, 1995). If the GCS is from 9 to 12, the injury is classified as moderate. Glasgow Coma Scale scores greater than 12 are classified as minor head injuries (Jordan, 1994). Once again, the GCS and other neurologic examinations need to be performed frequently so that trends in neurologic response can be identified. A decrease in the GCS score of 2 or more points is indicative of deterioration (Kuhlman, 1994; Scorpio, 1992). Irrespective of the GCS score, unequal pupils, unequal motor findings, open head injury with leaking CSF or exposed brain tissue, and/or the presence of a depressed skull fracture also indicate severe head injury. Finally, if headache severity increases dramatically, pupillary size increases unilaterally, or lateralizing weakness is noted to develop, particular concern is warranted.

Appropriate immediate investigations of the head trauma victim may include roentgenograms (x-ray), CT, and neurologic or neurosurgical consultation. Sedation and/or paralysis is delayed until the consultant examines the patient, if possible. Generally, all patients with moderate or severe head injury should be evaluated radiographically for cervical spine fracture. Conversely, skull roentgenograms often are not helpful (Scorpio, 1992), because physical examination or CT imaging provides higher quality data. Computed tomographic imaging is a vital tool in the evaluation of head injuries and, except for women with minor injuries, all head-injured patients require CT imaging. Severe injury dictates imaging as soon as possible. It is important, however, to adequately monitor the victim while she undergoes imaging. Once C-spine fractures are ruled out, the 20 + -week gestation pregnant patient is placed on a left lateral tilt during the scanning (Kuhlman, 1994). Head injuries can be classified simply into the categories of diffuse brain injury, focal brain injury, and skull fractures (Table 33-7) (Scorpio, 1992).

Diffuse brain injury can be classified as a concussion or diffuse axonal injury. Concussion is produced from widespread brief interruption of global brain function. Although confusion, headache, dizziness, and so on, are often present in the recovering concussion victim, any persistent neurologic abnormalities in the patient with a presumed concussion must be investigated for other etiologies. Many authors feel that the patient with 5 minutes or more of lost consciousness should be observed in the hospital for at least 24 hours (Scorpio, 1992; Jordan, 1994). Diffuse axonal injury (DAI), more commonly known as closed head injury, is produced by widespread global brain injury or the cerebral edema resulting from diffuse brain injury (Adams, 1982). Prolonged coma is the hallmark of DAI. Computed tomographic imaging will show cerebral edema

T A B L E   **33-7**

**Classification of acute head trauma**

I.  Diffuse Brain Injury
    A. Concussion
    B. Diffuse Axonal Injury
II. Focal Brain Injury
    A. Contusion
    B. Hemorrhage/Hematoma
       1. Parenchymal Hemorrhage
       2. Meningeal Hemorrhage/Hematoma
          a. Acute Epidural Hemorrhage/ Hematoma
          b. Subarachnoid Hemorrhage/ Hematoma
          c. Subdural Hematoma
III. Skull Fractures
    A. Simple Fracture
    B. Basilar Skull Fracture
    C. Depressed Skull Fracture

without focal lesions. Nearly 50% of coma-producing brain injuries are caused by DAI. Diffuse axonal injury is classified clinically into mild, moderate, and severe categories (Jordan, 1994). Severe DAI carries a 50% mortality. Long-term supportive care and control of intracranial hypertension are the only treatments for the condition. Partial or complete recovery is possible, but permanent coma (chronic vegetative state) often is an inexorable consequence of severe DAI (Scorpio, 1992).

Focal brain injuries are those in which damage occurs in a relatively local area. Types of focal brain injury include contusions, hemorrhages, and hematomas. Because focal injuries may produce a mass effect and damage underlying normal brain tissue, rapid diagnosis and treatment of focal brain injuries may improve outcome and recovery.

Contusions are usually caused by deceleration coup-countercoup trauma, as previously described. Although contusions can occur anywhere, they are found most commonly in the tips of the frontal and temporal lobes. In addition to producing deficits from focal injury, delayed bleeding and edema can produce injury from mass effects (Kuhlman, 1994). Prolonged observation is recommended. If neurologic deterioration is detected and is thought to be from a mass effect, surgery may be indicated.

Hemorrhages and hematomas can be classified functionally into those occurring in the meningeal or parenchymal regions of the brain. Parenchymal hemorrhage includes intracerebral hematomas, impalement injuries, and missile (bullet) wounds. Meningeal hemorrhage is classified further as acute epidural hemorrhage (AEH), acute subdural hematoma (SDH), or subarachnoid hemorrhage (SAH).

Acute epidural hemorrhage usually occurs from tears in the middle meningeal artery. Although found in 1% or less of coma-producing acute brain injuries, AEH can be rapidly progressive and fatal. Figure 33-6 describes the usual sequence of events associated with AEH. It is important to note that the patient with AEH may display an intervening period of lucidity prior to a rapid deterioration from massive rebleeding of the lesion (Adams, 1972). If surgically treated

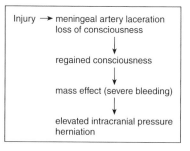

FIGURE **33-6**

Sequence of events associated with acute epidural hemorrhage.

early, the prognosis is good (91% survival) (Scorpio, 1992). If not evacuated until hemiparesis and pupil fixation, the prognosis is poor. Acute epidural hemorrhage is, in effect, the vasa previa of acute brain injury. Rapid recognition and treatment yields markedly improved results.

Subarachnoid hemorrhage produces bleeding in the subarachnoid space. Meningeal irritation occurs, with the resulting symptoms of headache and/or photophobia. Because the subarachnoid space is much larger than the epidural space, bleeding does not usually progress rapidly to death. Although bloody spinal fluid is a hallmark of SAH, CT scanning has basically replaced lumbar puncture in the diagnosis of SAH. Evacuation is rarely required; treatment is supportive. Meningeal irritation can produce unwanted cerebral artery vasospasm. Therefore, neuroselective calcium channel blocking agents such as nimodipine often are used in patients with SAH (American Nimodipine Study Group, 1992).

Acute subdural hematoma is one of the more common causes of serious brain hemorrhage. This hematoma commonly occurs from rupture of bridging veins between the cerebral cortex and dura. Direct laceration of the brain or cortical arteries also can produce SDH (Gennarelli, 1982). The clinical presentation of SDH often depends on the rapidity of expansion of the hematoma. Rapidly expanding hematomas carry a poorer prognosis than do stable, chronic SDHs. Early evacuation of rapidly growing SDHs may favorably impact the 60% mortality that SDH carries (Scorpio, 1992).

Intracerebral hematomas can occur anywhere in the brain. Symptoms and outcome depend on the size and location. Intraventricular and intracerebellar hemorrhages portend poor outcome. With impalement injuries, the missile or projectile should be left in place until neurosurgical evaluation is obtained. Bullet wounds should be mapped as to entrance and potential exit. Skull films may help the localization process of any remaining missile fragments. Nonpenetrating bullet wounds may result in significant blunt trauma (Bullock, 1990)!

Skull fractures are relatively common and may or may not be associated with severe brain injury. Because skull fractures may be an indicator that significant energy dispersal occurred on the cranial vault, most patients with seemingly uncomplicated skull fractures should be hospitalized for serial neurosurgical evaluations.

Different types of skull fractures have different considerations. Linear nondepressed skull fractures that traverse suture lines or vascular arterial grooves may be associated with epidural hemorrhage. Depressed skull fractures may require operative elevation of the bony fragment. Open skull fractures nearly always require early operative intervention. Basilar skull fractures may not be apparent immediately. Anterior basilar skull fractures may predispose to inadvertent placement of a nasogastric tube into the intracranial space (Scorpio, 1992).

Skull fractures need to be evaluated initially with cranial CT scanning and physical examination. Skull x-rays may be subsequently useful. Attempt at precise delineation of skull fractures should not delay recognition and treatment of other head injuries.

Mainstays in the treatment of head trauma include maintenance of brain perfusion, reduction of cerebral edema, elimination or reduction of hemorrhage, and prevention of infection. Patients with evolving symptomatology or unremitting coma need to be evaluated immediately for potential neurosurgical intervention. Maintenance of normal arterial BP will aid the often impaired cerebral autoregulation seen with head trauma. Normalization of blood glucose will help supply cerebral metabolic needs. However, hyperglycemia is as undesirable as hypoglycemia and is to be avoided (Bullock, 1995).

Figure 33-7 outlines a general scheme for severe head injury triage and features of high-, moderate-, and low-risk lesions. It should be noted that a lateralizing defect and a GCS score of 8 or less require immediate evaluation for surgical treatment. Generally, all comatose patients should receive ICP monitoring. Abnormal ICP is treated medically with controlled hyperventilation, mannitol administration, loop diuretics, volume restriction, and head-up positioning (Scorpio, 1992; Bullock, 1995).

Hyperventilation works to decrease ICP by reducing cerebral blood flow. Hyperventilation should be undertaken to a $Paco_2$ endpoint of 26 to 28 mm Hg (Enevoldsen, 1978), although the appropriate level for pregnancy is not established. Hyperventilation is most effective within the first 48 hours of acute injury. It is *not* effective in "prophylaxis" against elevated ICP (Muizelear, 1991). If hyperventilation is discontinued abruptly, ICP may rise rapidly. The effects of normal pregnancy (compensated respiratory alkalosis) on carbon dioxide–mediated regulation of cerebral blood flow are not known. In the absence of conclusive data, we recommend a 26- to 28-mm Hg endpoint in pregnant women who require hyperventilation.

Mannitol functions as a hyperosmotic diuretic. Doses of 0.5 to 1.0 g/kg body weight are typically used (Muizelear, 1983). Frequent monitoring of serum osmolality is needed, and mannitol should be withheld if osmolality is greater than 315 to 320 mosm/liter. Theoretically, mannitol can affect uteroplacental perfusion and/or fetal volume homeostasis. Given the grave circumstances for which mannitol is used in severe head trauma, however, the benefits of its administration far outweigh these risks (Kuhlman, 1994). Diuresis with furosemide or other loop diuretics also may be used. Overhydration, especially with hypotonic solutions, should be avoided. Head-up positioning at 20 degrees may marginally reduce hydrostatic pressure (Bullock, 1995).

It is emphasized that prompt neurosurgical consultation should be undertaken in patients requiring ICP therapy. Continuous monitoring via a transcranial transducer is generally indicated when ICP therapy is used (Bullock, 1995). Medical therapy is more successful when it is a temporizing measure until definitive surgical therapy is

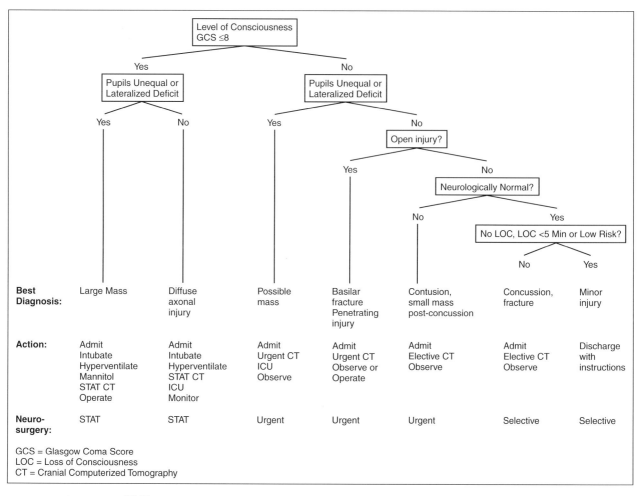

F I G U R E  **33-7**

**Head injury triage scheme.** (Reproduced by permission from Ra-menofsky ML, Alexander RH, Ali J, et al, eds. Advanced trauma life support—1993 instructor manual. American College of Surgeons. Chicago: First Impressions, 1993:176.)

undertaken. In patients with refractory ICPs greater than 25 mm Hg, a midventricular shift on CT scan of greater than 5 mm, or rapid deterioration, prompt surgical intervention may be necessary. In patients who are not surgical candidates but who have intractably elevated ICP, other medical therapies have only limited success. Barbiturate coma and hypothermia are generally last-ditch efforts. Both techniques probably work by reducing cerebral oxygen consumption (Bullock, 1995). Corticosteroids are not indicated for ther-

apy of cerebral edema from trauma (Dearden, 1986; Rutherford, 1995).

The best route of delivery in the patient with acute brain injury is controversial. The only large series of data germane to the delivery of the pregnant head trauma patient without surgical correction of a specific bleeding site is Hunt et al's series involving uncorrected ruptured cerebral aneurysms. Their investigation of 142 cases of *non-traumatic* SAH led them to conclude that vaginal delivery was not contraindicated. Importantly, stable, *nontraumatic* lesions leading to cerebral hemorrhage may behave quite differently than acute brain injuries (Hunt, 1974). We favor ICP monitoring in any at-risk head trauma patient undergoing labor and vaginal or cesarean-section delivery. We also use cesarean section liberally in such patients, with team management by obstetricians, neurosurgeons, and obstetric anesthesiologists.

Rapid diagnosis, early neurosurgical intervention, and meticulous attention to support measures offer the best hope for a good outcome in patients with severe brain injuries. Comanagement with consultants, appropriate and timely use of cranial CT scans, and serial neurologic examination may reduce mortality and morbidity in brain trauma. Improvement in maternal outcome offers the best hope for improved fetal outcome.

## Thermal Injury

In the United States, approximately 4% of patients seeking care for burns are pregnant (Laverly, 1995). Irrespective of pregnancy, the management of burns depends on their extent, thickness, and location. Burns are classified as partial thickness and full thickness. Full-thickness burns involve complete destruction of the dermal layers of the skin, and regeneration of skin does not occur. Minor burns are partial thickness and involve less than 10% of body surface area (BSA). Major burns involve greater than 10% BSA and can be partial or full thickness. Major burns are subdivided into moderate (10%–19% BSA), severe (20%–39% BSA), and critical (>39% BSA). Estimation of BSA involvement is performed quickly by using the "rule of nines" (Fig 33-8). Body surface area is altered by the pregnant body habitus. Although the rule of nines is often still used in its uncorrected form (Kuhlman, 1994), correction for the changed BSA of pregnancy would probably be appropriate.

Burn mortality is correlated directly with the size of the burn. Maternal mortality of 50% to 90% is expected when total BSA exceeds 70% to 80%. Pregnancy does not appear to have any direct effect on maternal survival (Laverly, 1995; Kuhlman, 1994). Fetal survival, however, is affected. In burns of less than 30% total BSA, fetal

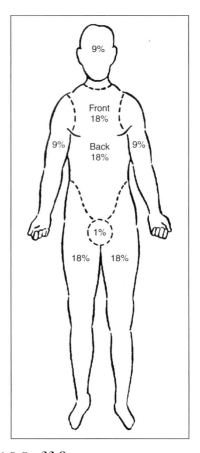

F I G U R E  **33-8**

Estimation of burn size (rule of nines). The accuracy of this system in pregnancy may be altered.

outcome is generally good, with a 70% or greater survival. Conversely, in burns of greater than 30%, Rayburn et al (1984) showed only a 6% fetal survival. Fetal survival may be diminished because of inadequate volume resuscitation, maternal demise, maternal infection, and/or preterm labor. Preterm labor is thought to occur through the mechanisms of dehydration, and hypoxemia from inhalation injuries and by mediator release from burned tissues. Some recommend immediate delivery of pregnant patients who have greater than 50% BSA burns and fetuses of viable gestational ages (Rayburn, 1984; Mathews, 1982). We favor individualization of care. Betasympathomimetics are not recommended for preterm labor treatment in the burn patient (Kuhlman, 1994). Magnesium sulfate can be used, but with great caution, in patients with concomitant renal failure.

Resuscitation of the pregnant burn patient includes oxygenation, pain relief, and volume resuscitation. Many authorities recommend 4 mL/kg body weight per percent burn of isotonic crystalloid infusion during the first 24 hours following a thermal injury (Demling, 1983). Constant vigilance regarding electrolyte disturbances, urinary output, and follow-up volume requirements is necessary. Fetal monitoring is used in the patient with a potentially viable fetus. Sterile monitoring can be used on the burned abdomen through use of a plastic sleeve. Topical and systemic antibiotics and topical silver sulfadiazine cream are applied to the burn. Split-thickness skin grafts or cadaveric grafts are eventually placed after necessary debridement. Timing of delivery is determined by obstetric considerations and fetal condition. The delivery route is determined by obstetric considerations and by burn location, if a large abdominal burn is present (Srivastava, 1988). Even remote from the acute burn, delivery through the severely scarred abdominal wall can be quite taxing.

## Electrical Injury

Limited data exist on maternal or fetal outcome from electrical accidents. Available studies imply that maternal outcome is variable and probably not affected by the presence of pregnancy. Fetal

outcome is either "all or none"—fetal death occurs in conjunction with the electrical insult or intact survival is noted. Similar data from lightning strikes also are noted (Strong, 1987; Pierce, 1986).

## Snakebite

Snakebite during pregnancy is an uncommon event. The majority of snakebites during pregnancy cases reported worldwide arise from envenomation by snakes in the Crotalidae or pit viper family. Common pit vipers in the United States include cottonmouths (water moccasins, *Agkistrodon*), copperheads (*Agkistrodon*), and rattlesnakes (*Sistrusus* and *Crotalus*). In their review of English language cases, Dunnihoo et al (1992) reported an overall fetal wastage of 43% and a maternal mortality of 10%. Bleeding diathesis results from pit viper envenomation. Fetal and placental effects from the anticoagulation are postulated to produce the fetal wastage. We are unable to find any English-language reports of Elapidae (e.g., coral snake) envenomation during pregnancy. Elapidae venom functions as a neurotoxin. Snakes of the Elapidae family are much less efficient in injecting venom into their prey; thus, their poor efficiency at envenomation, coupled with their relatively small size and retiring nature, may play a role in the paucity of information concerning coral snake bites during pregnancy.

Snakebite poisoning is graded according to severity (Table 33-8) (Dunnihoo, 1992; Wood,

TABLE  **33-8**
Grading of snakebite poisoning

| Grade | Skin Effects | Envenomation | Symptoms |
|---|---|---|---|
| 0 | < 1 in of edema or erythema | None | None |
| I | 1–5 in of edema or erythema within first 12 hr | Minimal | None |
| II | 6–12 in of edema or erythema in first 12 hr | Moderate | Minimal (nausea, vomiting, paresthesias) |
| III | > 12 in of edema or erythema in first 12 hr | Severe | System involvement |
| IV | Rapidly progressing symptoms | Severe | Severe |

Sources: Adapted from Wood et al, 1995 and Dunnihoo et al, 1992.

1955). Local measures include positive identification of the type of snake and rapid transport to definitive medical care. Because venom may be transported, a *loose* constriction bandage may be used to delay spread of the venom. If care is available within 60 minutes, wound incision and suctioning is not recommended. With pit viper poisoning, antivenin is usually recommended for grade III or IV bites. Because copperheads carry a less potent venom, their bites usually do not require antivenin. Hypersensitivity reactions are common with antivenin use. Skin testing and careful monitoring must be available and used when antivenin is given.

Coral snake bites often show little local reaction. Systemic effects may be delayed for several hours. Because of the neurotoxicity of coral snake venom, coral snake antivenin is usually recommended for victims of Elapidae bites.

Local and supportive measures for poisonous snakebite include careful cleaning of the wound, supportive care, potential use of antibiotics, and tetanus prophylaxis (Pennell, 1987). Tetanus prophylaxis is not contraindicated in any pregnant snakebite or trauma victim who otherwise would be a candidate for the toxoid booster or antiglobulin.

Occasionally, a victim will present with the bite of a rare, exotic snake. Most zoos or poison control centers have specific information on unusual breeds of snakes. Timely consultation is highly recommended.

## Poisonous Spider Bite

Two main types of poisonous spider bites are of concern in the United States. The *Latrodectus*

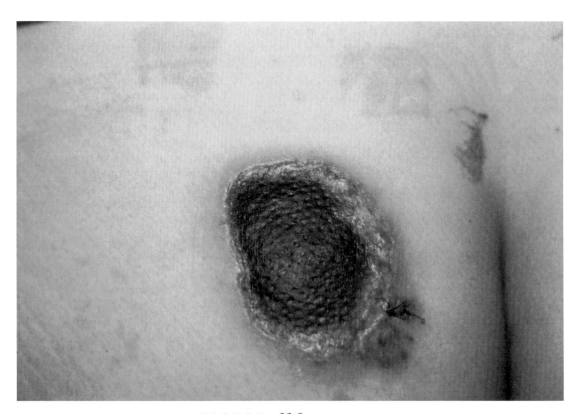

FIGURE **33-9**

Effects of *Loxosceles reclusa* bite. (Photograph courtsey of Dr. Ramon L. Sanchez.)

(black widow) spider occasionally has been reported to envenomate a pregnant victim. The venom of the black widow is a neurotoxin. Therefore, much like the coral snake, little local irritation results from the bite of a female *Latrodectus* (Pennell, 1987). While maternal mortality is postulated to be as high as 5%, care is generally supportive only. Limited evidence suggests no adverse fetal effects from the black widow spider bite if the mother does well (Scalzone, 1994).

*Loxosceles reclusa*, also known as the brown recluse spider, enjoys a nationwide distribution. The usual habitat of the brown recluse is in dark closet corners and the sides of cardboard boxes. Although not aggressive, the spider will bite when trapped. The venom of *Loxoscelis reclusa* produces tissue necrosis. Severe cases of brown recluse poisoning cause systemic hemolysis. Children appear more susceptible to this severe complication. Although large areas of necrosis require debridement and skin grafting, most cases of loxoscelism cause self-limited wounds that require only local care (Fig 33-9) (Pennell, 1987). Anderson (1991) reported five cases of loxoscelism in pregnant patients. He surmised that no special risks or complications resulted from being bitten by the brown recluse during pregnancy. He recommended conservative management and low doses of systemic corticosteroids.

## Conclusion

Trauma during pregnancy poses a special and immediate challenge to the obstetrician and to the emergency room provider. Generally speaking, most diagnostic and therapeutic modalities relating to trauma care should not be avoided or modified during pregnancy. Comanagement, with input from obstetric and non-obstetric services, functions to ensure appropriate care of the pregnant trauma victim and her fetus.

**REFERENCES**

Adams H, Graham DI. The pathology of blunt head injuries. In: Critchley M, O'Leary JL, Jennet B, eds. Scientific foundations of neurology. Philadelphia: Davis, 1972:478–491.

Adams J, Graham D, Murray L, et al. Diffuse axonal injury due to non-missile head injury in humans: an analysis of 45 cases. Ann Neurol 1982;12:557.

Agran PF, Dunkle DE, Winn DG, Kent D. Fetal death in motor vehicle accidents. Ann Emerg Med 1987;16:1355.

Alaily AB, Carrol KB. Pulmonary ventilation in pregnancy. Br J Obstet Gynaecol 1978;85:518.

American College of Obstetricians and Gynecologists. Trauma during pregnancy. Technical Bulletin No. 161; 1991.

American Nimodipine Study Group. Clinical trial of nimodipine in acute ischemic stroke. Stroke 1992;23:3.

Anderson PC. Loxoscelism threatening pregnancy: five cases. Am J Obstet Gynecol 1991;165:1454.

Awwad JT, Azar GB, Seoud MA, et al. High-velocity penetrating wounds of the gravid uterus: review of 16 years of civil war. Obstet Gynecol 1994;83:259.

Barone JE, Pizzi WS, Nealon TF Jr, et al. Indications for intubation in blunt chest trauma. J Trauma 1986;26:334.

Baxt WG, Moody P. The differential survival of trauma patients. J Trauma 1987;27:602.

Bellina JA, Dougherty CM, Mickal A. Pyeloureteral dilatation and pregnancy. Am J Obstet Gynecol 1976;108:356.

Ben-Menachem Y, Handel SF, Ray RD, et al. Embolization procedures in trauma, a matter of urgency. Semin Intervent Radiol 1985;2:107.

Boba A, Linkie DM, Plotz EJ. Effects of vasopressor administration and fluid replacement on fetal bradycardia and hypoxia induced by maternal hemorrhage. Obstet Gynecol 1966;27:408.

Bode PJ, Niezen RA, van Vost AB, et al. Abdominal ultrasound as a reliable indicator for conclusive laparotomy in blunt abdominal trauma. J Trauma 1993;34:27.

Bowman JM. Hemolytic disease (erythroblastosis fetalis). In: Creasy RK, Resnik R, eds. Maternal fetal medicine—principles and practice. 3rd ed. Philadelphia. WB Saunders, 1994:711–743.

Bowman JM. Management of Rh-isoimmunization. Obstet Gynecol 1978a;52:1.

Bowman JM, Chown B, Lewis M, et al. Rh-isoimmunization during pregnancy: antenatal prophylaxis. Can Med Assoc J 1978b;118:623.

Briss GG, Freeman RK, Jaffe SJ. A reference guide to fetal and neonatal risk—drugs in pregnancy and lactation. 4th ed. Baltimore: Williams and Wilkins, 1994.

Bruce DA, Lansfitt TW, Miller JD, et al. Regional cerebral blood flow, intracranial pressure, and brain metabolism in comatose patients. J Neurosurg 1973;38:131.

Bullock R, Teasdale GM. Surgical management of traumatic intracranial hematomas. In: Breakman R, ed. Handbook of clinical neurology—head injury. Amsterdam: Elsevier, 1990:259–297.

Bullock R, Ward JD. Management of head trauma. In: Ayres SM, Granuik A, Holbrook PR, Shoemaker WC, eds. Textbook of critical care. Philadelphia: WB Saunders, 1995:1449–1457.

Burrows RF, Kelton JG. Incidentally detached thrombocytopenia in healthy mothers and their infants. N Engl J Med 1988;319:142.

Caritis SN, Kuller JA, Watt-Morse ML. Pharmacologic options for treating preterm labor. In: Rayburn WF, Zuspan FP, eds. Drug therapy in obstetrics and gynecology. 3rd ed. St Louis: Mosby Year Book, 1992:74–89.

Chesley LC, Valenti C, Uichano L. Alterations in body fluid compartments and exchangeable sodium in early puerperium. Am J Obstet Gynecol 1959;77:1054.

Clark SL, Cotton DB, Lee W, et al. Central hemodynamic assessment of normal term pregnancy. Am J Obstet Gynecol 1989;161:1439.

Collicott PE, et al, eds. Advanced trauma life support course for physicians. American College of Surgeons, Committee on Trauma, Subcommittee on Advanced Trauma Life Support. Chicago: American College of Surgeons, 1985:48–50.

Cornell WP, Ebert PA, Zvidma GD. X-ray diagnosis of penetrating wounds of the abdomen. J Surg Res 1976;5:142.

Crosby WM, Costiloe JP. Safety of lap belt restraints for pregnant victims of automobile collisions. N Engl J Med 1971;284:632.

Crosby WM, Haycock CE, Carbac SS, eds. An emergency care protocol for trauma in pregnancy. Emerg Med Rep 1987;8:73.

Cunningham FG, McDonald PG, Leveno KJ, et al. Maternal adaptations to pregnancy. In: Williams obstetrics. 19th ed. Norwalk, CT: Appleton and Lange, 1993a:209–246.

Cunningham FG, MacDonald PG, Leveno KJ, et al. Renal and urinary tract diseases. In: Williams Obstetrics. 19th ed. Norwalk, CT: Appleton and Lange, 1993b:1127–1144.

Davis JJ, Cohn I, Nance FC. Diagnosis and management of blunt abdominal trauma. Ann Surg 1976;83:672.

Davison JS, Davison MC, Hay DM. Gastric emptying time in late pregnancy and labor. J Obstet Gynaecol Br Comwlth 1977;77:37.

Dearden NM, Gibson JS, McDowell DG, et al. Effect of high dose dexamethasone on outcome from severe head injury. J Neurosurg 1986;64:81.

Del Rossi AJ, ed. Blunt thoracic trauma. Trauma Q 1990;6:1.

Demling RH. Fluid resuscitation after major burns. JAMA 1983;250:1438.

de Swiet M. The respiratory system. In: Hytten F, Chamberlain G, eds. Clinical physiology in obstetrics. 2nd ed. London: Blackwell Scientific, 1991:83–100.

Dilts PV, Brintzman CR, Kirschbaum TH, et al. Uterine and systemic hemodynamic interrelationships and their response to hypoxia. Am J Obstet Gynecol 1967;103:38.

Dunnihoo DR, Rush BM, Wise RB, et al. Snake bite poisoning in pregnancy: a review of the literature. J Reprod Med 1992;37:653.

Enevoldsen EM, Jensen FT. Autoresolution and $CO_2$ responses of cerebral blood flow in patients with acute head injury. J Neurosurg 1978;48:689.

Esposito TJ. Trauma during pregnancy. Emerg Med Clin North Am 1994;12:167.

Feliciano DV. Tube thoracostomy. In: Benumof JL, ed. Clinical procedures in anesthesia and intensive care. Philadelphia: JB Lippincott, 1992:305–314.

Fiazee RC, Mucha P, Fainell MB, et al. Objective evidence of blunt cardiac trauma. J Trauma 1986;26:510.

Fildes J, Reed L, Jones N, et al. Trauma: the leading cause of maternal death. J Trauma 1992;32:643.

Franger AL, Buschbaum HJ, Peaceman AM. Abdominal gunshot wounds in pregnancy. Am J Obstet Gynecol 1989;29:1628.

Fries MH, Hankins GDV. Motor vehicle accident associated with minimal maternal trauma, but subsequent fetal demise. Ann Emerg Med 1989;18:301.

Gennarelli TA, Thibault LE. Biomechanics of acute subdural hematoma. J Trauma 1982;22:680.

Gerrard BS, Littler WA, Redman CWG. Closing volume during pregnancy. Thorax 1978;33:488.

Goodwin TM, Breen MT. Pregnancy outcome and fetomaternal hemorrhage after noncatastrophic trauma. Am J Obstet Gynecol 1990;162:665.

Greiss F. Uterine vascular response to hemorrhage during pregnancy. Obstet Gynecol 1966;27:408.

Griffiths M, Hillman G, Usherwood M. Seat belt injury in pregnancy resulting in fetal death. A need for education? Case reports. Br J Obstet Gynaecol 1991;98:320.

Grubb DK. Non-surgical management of penetrating uterine trauma in pregnancy—a case report. Am J Obstet Gynecol 1992;166:583.

Hankins GDV. Complications of beta-sympathomimetic tocolytic agents. In: Clark SL, Cotton DB, Hankins GDV, Phelan JP, eds. Critical care obstetrics. 2nd ed. Boston: Blackwell Scientific, 1991:223–250.

Hankins GDV, Barth WH, Satin AJ. Critical care medicine and the obstetric patient. In: Ayres SM, Grenuik A, Holbrook PR, Shoemaker WC, eds. Textbook of critical care. 3rd ed. Philadelphia: WB Saunders, 1995:50–64.

Hankins GDV, Clark S, Uckan E, et al. Arterial blood gas analysis during normal third-trimester pregnancy and the effects of position changes. Am J Obstet Gynecol 1996;174(Part 2):376. Abstract.

Hayek DA, Veremakis C. Intracranial pathophysiology of brain injury. Probl Crit Care 1991;5:135.

Helton AS, McFarlane J, Anderson ET. Battered and pregnant: a prevalence study. Am J Public Health 1987;77:1337.

Higgins SD, Garite TJ. Late abruptio placentae in trauma patients: implications for monitoring. Obstet Gynecol 1987;63(suppl):510.

Hoff WS, D'Amelio LF, Tinkhoff GH, et al. Maternal predictors of fetal demise during pregnancy. Surg Gynecol Obstet 1991;172:175.

Hunt HB, Schifrin BS, Suzuki K. Ruptured berry aneurysms and pregnancy. Obstet Gynecol 1974;43:827.

Jones WG, Ginsberg RJ. Esophageal perforation: a continuing challenge. Ann Thorac Surg 1992;53:534.

Jordan BD. Maternal head trauma during pregnancy. In: Devinsky O, Feldman E, Hainlinc B, eds. Neurologic complications of pregnancy. New York: Raven, 1994:131–138.

Katz JD, Hook R, Baragh PG. Fetal heart rate monitoring in pregnant patients undergoing surgery. Am J Obstet Gynecol 1976;125:267.

Katz DL, Dotters DJ, Droegemueller W. Perimortem cesarean delivery. Obstet Gynecol 1986;68:571.

Kuhlman RS, Cruikshank DP. Maternal trauma during pregnancy. Clin Obstet Gynecol 1994;37:274.

Lane PL. Traumatic fetal death. J Emerg Med 1989;7:433.

Laverly JP, Staten-McCormick M. Management of moderate to severe trauma in pregnancy. Obstet Gynecol Clin North Am 1995;22:69.

Lees M, Scott D, Carr MG, et al. Circulatory effects of recumbent postural changes in late pregnancy. Clin Sci 1967;32:453.

Lindheimer M, Katz H. The kidney and pregnancy. N Engl J Med 1970;283:1095.

Mansour MA, Moore EE, Moore FA, et al. Exigent post-injury thoracotomy. Analysis of blunt versus penetrating trauma. Surg Gynecol Obstet 1992;175:97.

Maset AL, Marmarou A, Ward JD, et al. Pressure-volume index in head injury. J Neurosurg 1987; 67:832.

Mathews RN. Obstetric implications of burns in pregnancy. Br J Obstet Gynaecol 1982;89:603.

Mattox KL. Approaches to trauma involving the major vessels of the thorax. Surg Clin North Am 1989;69:77.

Mattox KL, Flint LM, Carrico CJ. Blunt cardiac injury (formerly termed "myocardiac contusion"). J Trauma 1992;33:649. Editorial.

McKenney MG, Martin L, Lentz K, et al. 1000 consecutive ultrasounds for blunt abdominal trauma. J Trauma Inj Infect Crit Care 1996;40:607.

Mendelson CL. The aspiration of stomach contents into the lungs during obstetric anesthesia. Am J Obstet Gynecol 1946;52:191.

Mighty H. Trauma in pregnancy. Crit Care Clin 1994; 10:623.

Moore EE, ed. Early care of the injured patient. 4th ed. Philadelphia: Decker, 1990.

Muizelear JP, Maramou A, Ward JD, et al. Adverse effects of prolonged hyperventilation in patients with severe head injury: a randomized clinical trial. J Neurosurg 1991;75:731.

Muizelear JP, Wei EP, Kontos HA, et al. Mannitol causes compensatory cerebral vasoconstriction and vasodilation on response to blood viscosity changes. J Neurosurg 1983;59:822.

Neufield JDG. Trauma in pregnancy, what if . . .? Emerg Med Clin North Am 1993;11:207.

Newberger EH, Barkan SE, Lieberman ES, et al. Abuse of pregnant women and adverse birth outcomes. Current knowledge and implications for practice. JAMA 1992;267:2370.

Nyberg DA, Cyr DR, Mack LA, et al. Sonographic spectrum of placental abruption. Am J Radiol 1987;148:161.

Paone RF, Peacock JB, Smith DLT. Diagnosis of myocardiac contusion. South Med J 1993;86:867.

Parker B, McFarlane J, Soeken K. Abuse during pregnancy: effects on maternal complications and birth weight in adult and teenage women. Obstet Gynecol 1994;84:323.

Pearce M. Seat belts in pregnancy. Br Med J 1992; 304:586.

Pearlman MD, Tintinalli JE, Lorenz RP. Blunt trauma during pregnancy. N Engl J Med 1990a;323:1609.

Pearlman MD, Tintinalli JE, Lorenz RP. A prospective controlled study of outcome after trauma during pregnancy. Am J Obstet Gynecol 1990b; 162:1502.

Pearlman MD, Tintinalli JE. Evaluation and treatment of the gravida and fetus following trauma during pregnancy. Obstet Gynecol Clin North Am 1991;18:371.

Pearlman MD. Trauma. In: Hankins GDV, Clark SL, Cunningham FG, Gilstrap LC, eds. Operative obstetrics. Norwalk, CT: Appleton and Lange, 1995:651–666.

Pearlman MD, Viano D. Automobile crash stimulation with the first pregnant crash test dummy. Am J Obstet Gynecol 1996a;175:977.

Pearlman MD, Phillips ME. Safety belt use during pregnancy. Obstet Gynecol 1996b;88:1026.

Pennell TC, Babu SS, Meredith JW. The management of snake and spider bites in the southeastern United States. Am Surg 1987;53:198.

Pierce MR, Henderson RA, Mitchell JM. Cardiopulmonary arrest secondary to lightning injury in a pregnant woman. Ann Emerg Med 1986;15:597.

Pritchard JA. Changes in blood volume during pregnancy and delivery. Anesthesiology 1965;26:393.

Pritchard JA, Brekken AL. Clinical and laboratory studies on severe abruptio placentae. Am J Obstet Gynecol 1967;97:681.

Prowse CM, Gaensler EA. Respiratory and acid base changes during pregnancy. Anesthesiology 1965;26:381.

Ramenofsky ML, Alexander RH, Ali J, et al, eds. Advanced trauma life support—1993 instructor manual. American College of Surgeons. Chicago: First Impressions, 1993.

Rayburn W, Smith B, Feller J, et al. Major burns during pregnancy: Effect on fetal well-being. Obstet Gynecol 1984;63:392.

Robertson CS, Contant CF, Gokaslan ZL, et al. Cerebral blood flow, arteriovenous oxygen difference and outcome in head injured patients. J Neurol Neurosurg Psychiatry 1992;55:594.

Rose PG, Strohm PL, Zuspan FP. Fetomaternal hemorrhage following trauma. Am J Obstet Gynecol 1985;153:844.

Rothenberger D, Quattlebaum FW, Perry JF Jr, et al. Blunt maternal trauma: a review of 103 cases. J Trauma 1978;18:173.

Rutherford SE, Phelan JP. Deep venous thrombosis and pulmonary embolus. In: Clark SL, Cotton DB, Hankins GDV, Phelan JP, eds. Critical care obstetrics. 2nd ed. Boston: Blackwell Scientific, 1991:150–179.

Rutherford EJ, Nelson LD. Initial assessment of the multiple trauma patient. In: Ayres SM, Grenvitz A, Holbrook PR, Shoemaker WC, eds. Textbook of critical care. 3rd ed. Philadelphia: WB Saunders, 1995:1382–1389.

Sachs BP, Brown DAT, Driscoll SG, et al. Maternal mortality in Massachusetts: trends and prevention. N Engl J Med 1987;316:667.

Sakala EP, Kost DD. Management of stab wounds to the pregnant uterus. A case report and review of the literature. Obstet Gynecol Surv 1988;43:319.

Sandy EA, Koerner M. Self-inflicted gunshot wound to the pregnant abdomen: report of a case and review of the literature. Am J Perinatol 1989;6:30.

Sankaran S, Wilson RF. Factors affecting prognosis in patients with flail chest. J Thorac Cardiovasc Surg 1976;60:402.

Scalzone JM, Wells SL. *Latrodectus mactans* (black widow spider) envenomation: an unusual cause for abdominal pain in pregnancy. Obstet Gynecol 1994;83:830.

Scorpio RJ, Esposito TJ, Smith LG, Gens DR. Blunt trauma during pregnancy: factors affecting fetal outcome. J Trauma 1992;32:213.

Scott DE. Anesthesia during pregnancy. Obstet Gynecol Annu 1972;1:219.

Shepard TH. Catalog of teratogenic agents. 7th ed. Baltimore: Johns Hopkins, 1992.

Shoemaker WC, Carey JS, Yao ST, et al. Hemodynamic alterations in acute cardiac tamponade after penetrating injuries of the heart. Surgery 1970;67:754.

Shoemaker WC. Algorithm for early recognition and management of cardiac tamponade. Crit Care Med 1975;3:59.

Smith DS, Levy W, Maris M, et al. Reperfusion hyperoxia in brain after circulatory arrest in humans. Anesthesiology 1990;73:12.

Srivastava S, Bang RL. Burns during pregnancy. Burns 1988;14:228.

Stafford PA, Biddinger PW, Zumwalt RE. Lethal intrauterine fetal trauma. Am J Obstet Gynecol 1988;159:485.

Stellin G. Survival in trauma victims with pulmonary contusion. Am Surg 1981;57:780.

Strong TH, Gocke SE, Levy AV, et al. Electrical shock in pregnancy: a case report. J Emerg Med 1987;5:381.

Taskinen SO, Salo JA, Halttunen PEA, et al. Tracheobronchial rupture due to blunt chest trauma: a follow-up study. Ann Thorac Surg 1989;48:846.

Taylor DJ, Phillips P, Lind T. Puerperal hematological indices. Br J Obstet Gynaecol 1981;88:601.

Tessdale G, Jennett B. Assessment of coma and impaired consciousness: a practical scale. Lancet 1974;1:81.

Tilanus HW, Bossuyt P, Schattenkeck ME, et al. Treatment of oesophageal perforation: a multivariate analysis. Br J Surg 1991;78:582.

Trinkle JK, Richardson JD, Franz JL, et al. Management of flail chest without mechanical ventilation. Ann Thorac Surg 1975;19:355.

Trunkey DD, Lewis FR Jr, ed. Current therapy of trauma. 3rd ed. Philadelphia: Decker, 1991.

Ueland K, Hansen JM. Maternal cardiovascular dynamics, III. Labor and delivery under local and caudal anesthesia. Am J Obstet Gynecol 1969a;103:8.

Ueland K, Hansen JM. Maternal cardiovascular dynamics, II. Posture and uterine contractions. Am J Obstet Gynecol 1969b;103:1.

Ueland K, Metcalfe J. Circulatory changes in pregnancy. Clin Obstet Gynecol 1975;18:41.

Vaizey CJ, Jacobson MJ, Cross FW. Trauma in pregnancy. Br J Surg 1994;81:1406.

Varner MW. Maternal mortality in Iowa from 1952 to 1986. Surg Obstet Gynecol 1989;168:555.

Weaver WD, Cobb LA, Hallstrom AP, et al. Factors influencing survival after out of hospital cardiac arrest. J Am Coll Cardiol 1986;7:752.

Williams JK, McClain L, Rosemursy AS, Colorado NM. Evaluation of blunt abdominal trauma in the third trimester of pregnancy. Obstet Gynecol 1990;75:33.

Wilson M, Morganti AA, Zervodakis I, et al. Blood pressure, the renin-aldosterone system, and sex steroids throughout normal pregnancy. Am J Med 1980;68:97.

Wilson RF. Thoracic injuries. In: Ayres SM, Grenvik A, Holbrook PR, Shoemaker WC, eds. Textbook of critical care. Philadelphia: WB Saunders, 1995: 1429–1438.

Wood JT, Hoback WW, Green TW. Poisonous snakebites resulting in lack of venom poisoning. Va Med Monthly 1955;82:130.

# CHAPTER 34

# Thermal and Electrical Injury

$\mathcal{E}$ xposure to a thermal, electrical, or chemical source causes most common types of burns. While some studies estimate the incidence of thermal burns during pregnancy at approximately one in 250, the actual incidence of burns during pregnancy is unknown, due in part to the underreporting of minor burn injuries (Kuhlmann, 1994). In the nonpregnant population, the highest incidence is reported in the 18 to 30 age group (Demling, 1991). Pregnancy does not appear to alter the incidence or etiology of burns when compared with the nonpregnant state.

Burns are classified by degree based on the depth of the burn into the skin and also by the amount of surface area involved. Partial-thickness injury includes first- and second-degree burns; full-thickness includes third-degree burns. A first-degree, or superficial, burn involves the epidermis. The skin appears red and is painful to touch. A typical example of this type of burn is sunburn.

Second-degree burns are divided into two categories. A superficial partial-thickness burn involves the epidermis and part of the corium or dermis. This type of burn is typically characterized by fluid-filled blisters. A deep partial-thickness burn includes the majority of the corium. While blisters may or may not be present, eschar formation is common. On initial evaluation, it may be difficult to assess the depth of injury. Regardless of the type of second-degree burn, such injuries are extremely painful.

Third-degree, or full-thickness, burns involve the epidermis and the corium (dermis), extending into the fat layer or further. The skin has a thick layer of eschar and may or may not be painful depending on the amount of damage to the surrounding nerves (Caine, 1993; Krob, 1992; Demling, 1991).

Estimation of the total body surface area (TBSA) involved in the burn can be determined in two ways, the "rule of nines" or the Lund-Browder chart. The rule of nines divides the body into sections, which allows for quick estimation of the burn area, and is especially useful in emergency situations (Table 34-1). The Lund-Browder chart also divides the body into sections but is more accurate because it takes into account changes in BSA related to patient age. In both methods, only second- and third-degree burns are estimated. A chart specific to pregnancy has not been developed.

## Classification

### Thermal Burns

Burns are most commonly associated with thermal injury. This injury may result from exposure to heat, flame, or hot materials (e.g., scalding). This type of burn also commonly involves smoke inhalation injury. The burn involves only the area of the body that has been in direct contact with

T A B L E  **34-1**

The rule of nines chart for estimation of burns

| Anatomic Area | % BSA |
|---|---|
| Head | 9 |
| Upper extremities | 9 (each) |
| Lower extremities | 9 (each) |
| Anterior trunk | 18 |
| Posterior trunk | 18 |
| Neck | 1 |

Small burns are classified as less than 20% of the TBSA.

the cause of injury. Thermal burns are described based on the degree of injury, as described previously (Caine, 1993 ).

## Chemical Burns

The amount of injury to the skin from a chemical burn is dependent on several factors: (1) the concentration of the chemical, (2) the length of exposure to the chemical, (3) the amount of chemical involved, (4) the type of chemical, and (5) the effect of the chemical on the skin or exposed area. Unlike thermal burns, the degree of injury is related directly to the length of exposure. Flushing of the skin or exposed area should be accomplished as soon as possible after exposure. While water is usually the flushing medium of choice, a careful history should be taken, because water actually may potentiate the injury when used with certain chemicals.

## Electrical Burns

The passage of high-voltage electrical energy through tissues results in its conversion to thermal energy (Holliman, 1982). This results in a burn that involves not only the skin and subcutaneous tissues, but also additional tissue in the path of the current. The amount of damage to the tissues depends on the characteristics of the electrical current.

The most obvious burn areas usually involve an entry and an exit site. The amount of additional underlying tissue, muscle, and nerve damage can be extremely difficult to assess. Electrical current may be delivered in a wave or alternating

pattern, called AC, or in DC. Current is created when the flow of electricity (which is measured by voltage) meets resistance, generating a current (measured by amperage). The higher the current, the more severe the injury.

Alternating current is more dangerous than DC because it can cause tonic muscle contractions, and the victim may be unable to release the source of electrical energy. Because different parts of the body provide varying degrees of resistance, the current, and thus the damage caused by electricity, can vary from tissue to tissue. In addition, the same current can generate varying amounts of heat in difficult tissues (Caine, 1993).

Electrical injury can occur through four mechanisms. Direct contact with the electrical source results in injury to the skin in contact with the source and the surrounding subcutaneous tissues. Arcing of electricity usually occurs across joint areas as electrical charge is transferred. This results in cutaneous burns in areas not involved with entry or the exit site. Conduction burns occur when the current is conducted through another medium, such as water, to the body area. Secondary ignition burns occur when the electrical source ignites a flammable material. The most common causes of electrical burns include occupational hazards, household appliances, and lightning. In a review of 31 women exposed to nonfatal accidental electric shock in pregnancy, the incidence of adverse pregnancy outcome was not increased, compared to matched controls. Thus, for the most part, electric shock during pregnancy does not pose major fetal risk (Einarson, 1997).

## Maternal Concerns

A number of physiologic changes occur during pregnancy, making the management of the pregnant burn patient especially challenging. This section addresses these changes and their relationship to maternal complications of burns.

## Cardiovascular System

During pregnancy, cardiac output and plasma volume are increased. Systemic vascular resistance is decreased to compensate the increased circulatory volume. Colloid osmotic pressure is decreased in the vascular spaces. This high-flow, low-resistance state is essential for maintaining perfusion to the uterus and for increasing oxygen delivery to the fetus. The loss of the integrity of the skin results in a loss of body water. This loss is more exaggerated in pregnancy due to the decreased colloid osmotic pressure. Therefore, the pregnant burn patient is at increased risk for losing circulatory volume, compared with her nonpregnant counterpart.

## Pulmonary System

Increased oxygen delivery and consumption are the hallmark changes in the pulmonary system during pregnancy. Respiratory rate, tidal volume, and minute ventilation are increased. Arterial blood gases in pregnancy reflect a higher resting oxygen tension and a resting carbon dioxide tension below 30 mm Hg.

Oxygen delivery also is facilitated by the increased cardiac output and circulating red-cell volume. Oxygen needs of the placenta and fetus increase oxygen consumption, making the patient especially susceptible to hypoxemia if oxygen delivery decreases.

Because many thermal and chemical inhalation injuries involve the pulmonary system, early evaluation is warranted. Burns involving the face, neck, or chest also may involve damage to the respiratory passages, leading to a loss of a patent airway. Because the trachea tends to be more edematous, especially during the third trimester of pregnancy, consideration should be given to early intubation in order to protect the airway.

## Integumentary System

The skin is the organ system most often involved in burns. The skin serves as a barrier to infection and a regulator of fluid, electrolyte, and thermal balance. During pregnancy, the skin also adapts to changes in body habitus. Severe burns involving the trunk of the patient before or during early pregnancy may lead to problems with skin expansion, especially during the second and third

trimesters when the abdomen must expand to accommodate the growing fetus (Widgerow, 1991). A longitudinal study of seven patients with circumferential truncal burns sustained during childhood revealed one case of scar tissue breakdown in the third trimester. Burn treatment of all seven patients included excision and split-thickness skin grafts (McCauley, 1991). Cultured epidermal autograft has also been used successfully in pregnancy in the case of severe burns over a large surface area when the patient has a shortage of skin suitable for grafting (Barillo, 1992).

## Management Strategies

Management of burns in the nonpregnant patient can be divided into four periods: the resuscitation period (0–36 hr postinjury), the postresuscitation period (2–5 days postinjury), the inflammation-infection period (from 6 days to postwound closure), and rehabilitation (Demling, 1995). The initial management of the burn victim was recently reviewed by Monafo (1996).

## Resuscitation Period

The primary treatment goal of the patient suffering a large burn is the avoidance of complications related to fluid and electrolyte deficits in the immediate postburn period. Cardiovascular and pulmonary support is crucial.

Estimation of the TBSA and the severity of the burns is the first step toward management. While there are many formulas for calculating fluid replacement based on TBSA, the modified Brooke or Parkland formulas are two of the most frequently used. A Foley catheter should be placed to monitor renal perfusion. In patients with a history of cardiac or pulmonary disease, patients with combined cutaneous and pulmonary injury, or patients who are unresponsive to initial resuscitative efforts, a pulmonary artery catheter should be considered.

Early intubation is recommended in those patients with suspected inhalation injury, because intubation after inflammation and the formation of tissue edema may prove difficult. Exposure of the respiratory passages to certain chemicals may require intubation to provide the adequate pulmonary toilet necessary for healing. Serial serum chemistry and electrolyte studies should be performed. Care should be taken to monitor glucose carefully, because hypoglycemia can occur as the patient attempts to regulate body temperature. Arterial blood gases should be obtained immediately, as should a complete blood count and coagulation panel. A chest radiograph can be performed, remembering that morphologic changes may lag behind clinical presentation.

Crystalloid is given in the form of lactated Ringer's at a rate of 4 mL/kg per percent of body burn during the first 24 hours. For example, in a 65-kg patient with a TBSA burn of 50%, 13,000 mL of fluid would be required. One half of the volume should be given over the first 8 hours, the remaining one half is given over the next 16 hours in divided increments (Georgiade, 1987). Red-cell replacement may be required and assist in volume expansion as well as increasing oxygen-carrying capacity. The hematocrit may be falsely elevated in the face of volume depletion. Urinary output should be maintained at 100 mL/hr. Hypoproteinemia secondary to losses from the burn area and the decreased colloid osmotic pressure of pregnancy may be associated with massive tissue edema during the resuscitation period.

The wound should be treated daily with debridement, cleansing, and topical antibacterial creams. External fetal monitoring should be instituted at a viable gestational age, usually around 24 to 26 weeks (Kuhlmann, 1994).

## Postresuscitation Period

This period typically begins 2 to 5 days after the injury has occurred. If the patient is hemodynamically stable and oxygen delivery is adequate, operative management of the wound can begin. It is important to accomplish excision of the burn tissue and skin closure at this time, before inflammation and infection occur. This is achieved in a series of short surgical procedures to decrease hypothermia. To combat infection, topical antibiotic administration and cultures to determine specific bacteria colonization are done. Intravenous antibiotics are targeted to organisms identified in culture. A consumptive coagulopathy may occur

during this period, requiring component replacement therapy. It should be remembered that fibrinogen levels are increased above normal during pregnancy and that a fibrinogen in the normal nonpregnant range may be a sign of an early coagulopathy.

## Inflammation-Infection Period

The hypermetabolic response to injury begins at about 4 to 5 days after injury and peaks at about 7 to 10 days ( Alexander, 1987). Cardiac output is often more than doubled in order to supply the necessary increase in oxygen demands. Carbon dioxide production also is increased, which can lead to a rapid deterioration of respiratory status because the injured lung may be unable to exchange gases satisfactorily.

The inability to differentiate the hypermetabolic process from sepsis can make care during this period extremely difficult. The injured lung also is at an increased risk for pneumonia secondary to hypoxia, atelectasis, mucous plugging, and increased tissue edema. The decreased colloid osmotic pressure of pregnancy also contributes to the development of acute respiratory distress syndrome (ARDS).

Adequate nutritional support is crucial during this period. Supplementation through the gastrointestinal route is optimal. Parenteral nutrition also may be needed to meet caloric demands. It is important to remember the metabolic demands of pregnancy when calculating nutritional needs. A true assessment of caloric needs can be obtained from indirect calorimetry.

The burn wound is best managed by the use of topical antibiotics. Silver sulfadiazine is used most commonly and is not contraindicated in pregnancy. *Staphylococcus aureus* is the most common wound infection; however, gram-negative organisms, especially *Pseudomonas aeruginosa,* also may be cultured (Boss, 1985). Skin-grafting usually takes place 2 to 3 weeks after injury if needed.

## Rehabilitation

Active range of motion exercises in the burn patient should be instituted as soon as possible to prevent loss of muscle and joint functions. In the parturient, movement of the lower extremities and early ambulation can prevent the formation of deep venous thrombosis. The route of delivery should be based on obstetric considerations.

## Maternal Complications

### Acute Renal Failure

Acute renal failure presenting as oliguria or anuria is not uncommon in the burn patient. Prerenal azotemia occurs frequently, because underestimation of the extent of injury may lead to an underestimation of fluid requirements. In the pregnant patient, assessment of vital signs alone may be insufficient as a marker of volume status, because the increased cardiac output and intravascular volume associated with pregnancy may mask early signs of hemodynamic compromise. Treatment should be aimed at maintaining adequate intravascular volume and urine output. In the patient whose oliguria is unresponsive to reasonable fluid replacement, hemodynamic monitoring should be instituted to assist in providing appropriate fluid replacement.

In the electrical burn patient, deep tissue injury may not be readily apparent. Massive muscle injury, common in the electrical burn patient, may lead to the production of myoglobin. Myoglobin, a breakdown product of necrotic muscle, is directly toxic to the renal tubule. Hypovolemia may potentiate renal injury in patients with myoglobinuria. Hyperkalemia can accompany myoglobinuria and be life-threatening. The diagnosis of myoglobinuria can be performed easily at the bedside. The presence of reddish-brown urine and a negative urine dipstick for heme confirms the presence of myoglobin. Treatment should be undertaken to maintain urine output through volume replacement. Mannitol also may be used to aid in increasing urinary output. Bicarbonate should be placed into all intravenous fluids in order to alkalize the urine and assist in the excretion of myoglobin.

## Sepsis and Acute Respiratory Distress Syndrome

Multisystem end-organ failure in the burn patient has a mortality rare of nearly 100%. The immunosuppressive effects of pregnancy, as well as host compromise secondary to injury, may make the parturient especially susceptible to the developing septic complications. Recognition and appropriate treatment are crucial. In interpreting pulmonary artery catheter values, the hyperdynamic state of pregnancy must be considered (Clark, 1989). Appropriate cultures should be obtained and antibiotic therapy tailored to culture results.

During pregnancy, the development of sepsis leads frequently to the development of ARDS (see Chapter 18). As mentioned, changes in the respiratory system during pregnancy may make the lung especially susceptible to injury. Smoke inhalation injury associated with some thermal burns, as well as massive fluid shifts during the postresuscitation period, also may predispose the patient to bacterial colonization and the development of pneumonia. Because respiratory failure is the leading cause of death in the burn patient, early recognition of respiratory compromise is imperative. Early intubation and the use of positive end-expiratory pressure may prevent further injury. While parameters for intubation have not been formally established for the pregnant burn patient, intubation should be considered strongly in patients with a respiratory rate greater than 40, a $Pao_2$ less than 80 mm Hg, or a $Paco_2$ greater than 35.

## Fractures

Evaluation for skeletal trauma should occur early in the assessment in patients experiencing electrical injury. Increased tetany of the muscles during electrocution may result in long bone fractures as well as fractures of the vertebral column.

## Mortality

Maternal mortality following burn injury is related to the severity of the initial injury and the development of later complications. When less than

50% of the total BSA is involved, maternal mortality is less than 5%. When greater than 80% of the total BSA is involved, mortality is 100%.

## Fetal Complications

### Preterm Labor

Prostaglandin levels are increased uniformly in the burn patient. Inadequate volume resuscitation may also lead to a decrease in uteroplacental perfusion and tissue hypoxia. These factors combine to lead to a high incidence of labor and delivery within a few days of a massive burn injury. Because burn patients are at great risk for complications from tocolytic therapy, care should be taken with the use of these agents. Because betamimetics and magnesium sulfate may be associated with increased capillary permeability and electrolyte imbalances, it has been suggested that the safest tocolytic agent in these patients may be indomethacin. In the patient beyond 32 to 34 weeks' gestation, tocolysis would generally not be indicated.

### Abortions

Several authors have noted an increase in the spontaneous abortion rate in patients who experience burns during the first trimester. In one study, four of six patients who were injured during this period miscarried (Jain, 1993). Some authors have advocated therapeutic terminations in patients with severe burns in the first trimester, but there are no data to associate this procedure with an improved maternal outcome.

### Fetal Distress and Stillbirths

Fetal distress secondary to hypoxia and uteroplacental insufficiency may necessitate the need for emergent delivery. For this reason, all parturients with a viable fetus should have fetal monitoring instituted. Perinatal morbidity is related directly to the severity of the burn. When less than 40% of the BSA is involved, the perinatal mortality rate is approximately 25%; when 50% of the BSA is involved, 50%; and when greater than 80% of the BSA is involved, 100%.

Because of the technical difficulties involved with external fetal heart rate monitoring in the patient with truncal burns and the extremely high rate of preterm labor and fetal demise, Matthews (1982) has recommended cesarean delivery of the viable fetus if the maternal burn involves more than 50% of the BSA. Depending on the ability to utilize external fetal heart rate monitoring, delivery also should be considered in late third-trimester fetuses with lesser degrees of maternal burn injury. Additional considerations in this regard are discussed in Chapter 36.

**REFERENCES**

Alexander J. The role of infection in the burn patient. In: Boswick J, ed. The art and science of burn care. Rockville, MD: Aspen, 1987:103–112.

Barillo DJ, Nangle NE, Farrell K. Preliminary experience with cultured epidermal autograft in a community hospital burn unit. J Burn Care Rehabil 1992;13:158.

Boss WK, Brand DA, Acampora D. Effectiveness of prophylactic antibiotics in the outpatient treatment of burns. J Trauma 1985;25:244.

Caine R, Lefcourt N. Patients with burns. In: Clochesy J, Breu C, Cardin S, et al, eds. Critical care nursing. Philadelphia, WB Saunders, 1993.

Clark SL, Cotton DB, Lee W, et al. Central hemodynamic assessment of normal term pregnancy. Am J Obstet Gynecol 1989;161:1439.

Demling RH. Management of the burn patient. In: Grenvik A, Holbrook PR, Shoemaker WC, eds. Textbook of critical care. 3rd ed. Philadelphia: WB Saunders, 1995.

Demling RH. Burn management. In: Wilmore D, ed. Pre- and postoperative care. New York: Scientific American, 1991.

Einarson A, Bailey B, Inocencion G, et al. Accidental electric shock in pregnancy: a prospective cohort study. Am J Obstet Gynecol 1997;176:678.

Georgiade G, Pederson C. Burns. In: Sabiston DC, ed. Essentials of surgery. Philadelphia: WB Saunders, 1987:122–131.

Holliman CJ, Saffle JR, Kravitz M, et al. Early surgical decompression in the management of electrical injuries. Am J Surg 1982;144:733.

Jain ML, Gang AK. Burns with pregnancy: a review of 25 cases. Burns 1993;19:166.

Krob M, Deppe S, Thompson DC. Burn injury. In: Civetta J, Taylor R, Kirby R, eds. Critical care. 2nd ed. Philadelphia, JB Lippincott, 1992.

Kuhlman RS, Cruikshank DP. Maternal trauma during pregnancy. Clin Obstet Gynecol 1994;37:274.

Lippin Y, Shvoron A, Tsur H. Therapeutic abortion in a severely burned woman. J Burn Care Rehabil 1993;14:398.

McCauley RL, Sternberg BA, Phillips LG, et al. Long-term assessment of the effects of circumferential truncal burns in pediatric patients on subsequent pregnancies. J Burn Care Rehabil 1991;12:51.

Matthews RN. Obstetric implications of burns in pregnancy. Br J Obstet Gynaecol 1982;89:603.

Monafo WW. Initial management of burns. New Engl J Med 1996;335:1581.

Widgerow AD, Ford TD, Botha M. Burn contracture preventing uterine expansion. Ann Plast Surg 1991;27:269.

# CHAPTER 35

# Overdose and Poisoning

All substances are poisons.

*Paracelsus (1493–1541)*

**S**everal factors modify the intake of drugs during pregnancy. Pregnancy, in and of itself, is a symptom-producing condition with the potential to increase the intake of medications in otherwise healthy women. Despite an increased awareness of the dangers of taking medications other than iron and vitamins during pregnancy, the natural hesitance to take prescription drugs and chemicals does not always apply to the use of recreational and illicit drugs. There are many pregnant women using such drugs and chemicals. The aim of this chapter is to provide a general approach to the problem of overdose and poisoning in pregnancy, with some practical and specific considerations for management of the most common causes of poisoning and toxicity.

## Definitions

*Poisoning* is a morbid state produced by exposure to a toxic agent that by its chemical action causes damage to structure or disturbance of function (Stine, 1983). *Drug overdosage* refers to the state produced by an excess or abuse of a drug or substance. *Poisoning* connotes clinical symptomatology and generally implies that the toxic exposure was unintentional or unknown to the recipient (Litovitz, 1995). In contrast, *drug overdose* generally infers an intentional drug exposure. For the purposes of this chapter, the terms will be used in a similar way.

## Drug Ingestion

According to a multinational survey by the World Health Organization in 1992, 86% of pregnant women took medications during pregnancy (Noji, 1989). The average number of prescriptions filled during pregnancy was 2.9, with a range of 15. These figures do not take into account over-the-counter prescriptions or intrapartum medications. Almost three fourths of the prescriptions were given by an obstetrician.

The American Association of Poison Control Centers Toxic Exposure Surveillance System noted that almost 2 million people reported a toxic exposure in 1994, yielding a rate of exposure of approximately 8.9 per thousand population (Litovitz, 1989). The majority of these exposures were unintentional, but suicidal intent was present in 7.7% of the cases. A single substance was implicated in 93.2%, with ingestion being the most common exposure route, followed by dermal and inhalational routes. Of these exposures, 0.03% were lethal and 77% of the deaths were the result of intentional exposure. Overall, a female-to-male preponderance was found in the reproductive age group, as well as in the category of intentional exposures and adverse reactions.

TABLE  **35-1**

Substances most frequently involved in human exposures

| Substance | % | Substance | % |
|---|---|---|---|
| Cleaning substances | 10.6 | Foreign bodies | 3.7 |
| Analgesics | 9.4 | Food products/food poisoning | 3.5 |
| Cosmetics/personal care products | 8.5 | Hydrocarbons | 3.4 |
| Plants | 5.4 | Antimicrobials | 3.2 |
| Cough/cold preparations | 5.2 | Sedatives/hypnotics/antipsychotics | 3.1 |
| Bites/envenomations | 4.3 | Alcohols | 2.6 |
| Pesticides (including rodenticides) | 4.1 | Antidepressants | 2.6 |
| Topicals | 3.7 | Chemicals | 2.5 |
| | | Vitamins | 2.3 |

Sources: Litovitz TL, Felberg L, Soloway RA, et al. 1994 Annual report of the American Association of Poison Control Centers Toxic Exposure Surveillance System. Am J Emerg Med 1995;13:551–597.

Little is known about the specific prevalence of toxic exposures, overdoses, and poisonings during pregnancy, and the available data are either incomplete or directed to specific toxic substances, usually illicit drugs or alcohol. It is known, however, that at least 0.3% of the toxic exposures reported in 1994 in the United States were in pregnant women (Litovitz, 1989). Of those for which gestational age was known, 31% occurred in the first trimester, 38% in the second trimester, and 31% in the third trimester. There are, unfortunately, no reported data on the outcome of these pregnancies. The National Poison Control Center in Washington, DC, does not maintain data specifically on poisoning in pregnancy.

During pregnancy, drug overdose frequently is part of a suicide gesture (Gilstrap, 1992; Rogers, 1988). Less often, it is the result of an attempt to induce abortion. In one series of 162 pregnant women who were evaluated for poisoning, 86% had intended to overdose, with 78% attempting suicide and 8% attempting to induce an abortion (Haddad, 1990). Approximately 1% of suicide gestures in a gravid woman will result in a maternal death (Bayer, 1983). More than 95% of suicide gestures involve ingestion of a combination of drugs.

## Toxic Agents and Poisons

Most commonly, information regarding the history of the exposure and the agent responsible can be obtained from the patient, her relatives,

or paramedical personnel at the patient's home; during transport to the hospital; or in the emergency room. Particular care should be taken with patients who exhibit suspicious behavior, who have a history of psychiatric illnesses, or a history of a previous suicide attempt, because they may be intentionally or unintentionally misleading.

More than 250,000 drugs and commercial products are available for ingestion (Olson, 1994; Weisman, 1990). Tables 35-1 and 35-2 (Litovitz,

TABLE  **35-2**

Thirteen most common causes of death from acute poisoning per group of medications

| Category | No. | % of All Exposures |
|---|---|---|
| Analgesics | 205 | 0.113 |
| Antidepressants | 175 | 0.353 |
| Sedative/hypnotics/psychotics | 99 | 0.166 |
| Stimulants/street drugs | 91 | 0.312 |
| Cardiovascular drugs | 90 | 0.307 |
| Alcohols | 76 | 0.150 |
| Gases/fumes | 56 | 0.154 |
| Asthma therapies | 36 | 0.204 |
| Automotive products | 33 | 0.250 |
| Chemicals | 26 | 0.055 |
| Hydrocarbons | 26 | 0.040 |
| Antihistamines | 23 | 0.060 |
| Cleaning substances | 22 | 0.011 |

Sources: Litovitz TL, Felberg L, Soloway RA, et al. 1994 Annual report of the American Association of Poison Control Centers Toxic Exposure Surveillance System. Am J Emerg Med 1995;13:551–597.

1995) list the most frequent causes of morbidity and mortality from poisoning in the United States. Table 35-3 (Rayburn, 1984) details the most frequently seen classes of drugs used in suicide or suicide gestures among 111 pregnant women.

Some groups of agents produce a complex of signs and symptoms that can be recognized as a typical syndrome (toxidrome) (Noji, 1989; Briggs, 1994). A knowledge of such toxidromes is particularly useful when information about the substance is not available. A list of the most common toxidromes is shown in Table 35-4 (Briggs, 1994; Doyon, 1994). Other physical findings that are useful in the recognition of a toxic exposure are outlined in Table 35-5.

Urine and serum samples may be analyzed and the concentration of the ingested toxic substances measured to confirm the diagnosis and manage the overdose. Some groups of agents will produce characteristic laboratory findings that can be helpful in the diagnosis and management

of overdose and poisoning. Toxicologic analysis is useful in confirming the toxic substance(s) ingested (Tables 35-6, 35-7). Serum drug levels of the agent are important to determine the severity of the intoxication and should be used selectively in serious and potentially life-threatening poisonings (e.g., acetaminophen, methanol, ethylene glycol, paraquat) (Stine, 1983). In general, when solid substances have been ingested, a quantitative serum level should be measured within 4 hours of ingestion. Different agents have different pharmokinetics and metabolism. As such, Tables 35-6 (Thorpe, 1995) and 35-7 (Mowry, 1995) list the different types of specimens needed (serum, whole blood), time required to check the level after ingestion, whether a repeat level is needed, and which other tests may be useful in diagnosis and treatment. In general, specimens sent to the laboratory should include the following: 10 to 15 mL of serum (whole blood for certain toxic substances), 50 to 100 mL of urine, and 100 mL of initial gastric aspirate or emesis (Shannon, 1995).

To assist with patient management, the anion gap should be calculated as follows:

$$(Na^+) - (HCO_3 + Cl)$$

The normal anion gap is 12 to 14 mEq/liter. Causes of an increased or decreased anion gap are presented in Table 35-8. As part of the differential diagnosis, common causes of acidosis, such as hypoxia and ischemia, will need to be excluded. Of note, false depression of carbon dioxide and sodium bicarbonate can result from inadequate filling of blood collection tubes and from heparin-containing syringes.

Additionally, and depending on the clinical circumstances, the osmolal gap (Bolgiano, 1994; Thorpe, 1995) will need to be measured. For accuracy, the freezing-point method (Bolgiano, 1994) should be used. Then, the difference between calculated osmolality (2 × Na$^+$ (mEq/liter) + glucose (mg/dL)/18 + BUN (mg/dL)/2.8 + ethanol (mg/dL)/4.3) and measured osmolality is determined. This is normally less than 10. The causes of increased osmolal gap are illustrated in Table 35-9. In cases of severe hyperlipidemia, the osmolal gap can be falsely elevated.

T A B L E    **35-3**

**Ten most frequently seen drug classes used in suicide gestures among 111 pregnant women**

| Drug Class | % |
|---|---|
| Nonnarcotic analgesics (acetaminophen, aspirin, ibuprofen) | 26 |
| Nutritional supplements (prenatal vitamins, iron) | 12 |
| Antianxiolytics (diazepam, hydroxyzine, other benzodiazepines) | 11 |
| Hypnotics and sedatives (phenobarbital, flurazepam, others) | 10 |
| Narcotic analgesics (codeine, propoxyphene, others | 8 |
| Antibiotics (cephalexin, amoxicillin, trimethoprim-sulfamethoxazole) | 7 |
| Antihistamines (diphenhydramine, others) | 6 |
| Antipsychotics (thioridazine, trifluoperazine) | 3 |
| Anorectics (sympathomimetics, phenylpropanolamine) | 2 |
| Hormonal agents (corticosteroids, oral contraceptives) | 2 |

Sources: Bayer MJ, Romack BH. Poisoning and overdose. Aspen Systems, 1983: and modified from Rayburn W, Anonow R, Delay B, Hogan MJ. Drug overdose during pregnancy: an overview from a metropolitan poison control center. Obstet Gynecol 1984;64:611.

T A B L E   **35-4**

The most common toxic syndromes

| Class of Drug | Common Signs | Common Causes |
|---|---|---|
| Anticholinergic | Dementia with mumbling speech<br>Tachycardia<br>Dry flushed skin<br>Dilated pupils (mydriasis)<br>Myoclonus<br>Temperature slightly elevated<br>Urinary retention<br>Decreased bowel sounds<br>Seizures/dysrhythmias (severe cases) | Antihistamines<br>Antiparkinsonian medications<br>Atropine<br>Scopolamine<br>Amantadine<br>Antipsychotics<br>Antidepressants<br>Antispasmodics<br>Mydriatics<br>Skeletal muscle relaxants<br>Some plants (i.e., jimson weed) |
| Sympathomimetics | Delusions<br>Paranoia<br>Tachycardia<br>Hypertension<br>Hyperpyrexia<br>Diaphoresis<br>Piloerection<br>Mydriasis<br>Hyperreflexia<br>Seizures/dysrhythmias (severe cases) | Cocaine<br>Amphetamines<br>Methamphetamines and derivatives<br>Over-the-counter decongestants (phenylpropanolamine, ephedrine, pseudoephedrine)<br>NB: Caffeine and theophylline overdoses have similar findings, except for organic psychiatric signs. |
| Opiates/sedatives | Coma<br>Respiratory depression<br>Constricted pupils (miosis)<br>Hypotension<br>Bradycardia<br>Hypothermia<br>Pulmonary edema<br>Decreased bowel sounds<br>Hyporeflexia<br>Needle marks | Narcotics<br>Barbiturates<br>Benzodiazepines<br>Ethchlorvynol<br>Glutethimide<br>Methyprylon<br>Methaqualone<br>Meprobamate |
| Cholinergics | Confusion/CNS depression<br>Weakness<br>Salivation<br>Lacrimation<br>Urinary and fecal incontinence<br>Gastrointestinal cramping<br>Emesis<br>Diarrhea<br>Diaphoresis<br>Muscle fasciculations<br>Bronchospasm<br>Pulmonary edema<br>Miosis<br>Bradycardia (or tachycardia)<br>Seizures | Organophosphate and carbamate insecticides<br>Physostigmine<br>Edrophonium<br>Some mushrooms (*Amanita muscaria; Amanita pantherina, Inocybe* sp, *Clitocybe* sp) |

Sources: Briggs GG, Freeman RK, eds. Drugs in pregnancy and lactation. 4th ed. Baltimore: Williams and Wilkins, 1994; and Doyon S, Roberts J. Reappraisal of the "coma cocktail." Emerg Med Clin North Am 1994;12.

T A B L E   **35-5**

**Physical findings in poisoning**

*Pupils*
Dilation
    Alkaloids
    Aminophylline
    Anticholinergics
    Antihistaminics
    Barbiturates
    Carbon monoxide
    Cocaine
    Cyanide
    Ergot
    Ethanol

    Ethylene glycol
    Glutethimide
    LSD
    Methaqualone
    Mushrooms
    Phenothiazines
    Phenytoin
    Quinine
    Reserpine
    Sympathomimetics

    Toluene
    Tricyclics
    Withdrawal states

Constriction
    Acetone
    Barbiturates
    Benzodiazepines
    Caffeine
    Chloral hydrate
    Cholinergics
    Cholinesterase inhibitors
    Clonidine
    Codeine

    Ethanol
    Meprobamate
    Opiates (except meperidine)
    Organophosphates
    Phencyclidine
    Phenothiazines
    Propoxyphene
    Sympatholytics

*Breath Odor*
    Acetone
    Acrid or pear-like
    Bitter almonds
    Carrots
    Garlic
    Mothballs
    Pungent aromatic
    Violets
    Wintergreen

    Acetone, chloroform, ethanol, isopropyl alcohol, salicylates
    Chloral hydrate, paraldehyde
    Cyanide
    Cicutoxin (water hemlock)
    Arsenic, organophosphates, phosphorus, selenium, thallium
    Camphor, naphthalene, paradichlorobenzene
    Ethchlorvynol (Placidyl)
    Turpentine
    Methyl salicylate

*Reflexes*
Depressed
    Antidepressants
    Barbiturates
    Benzodiazepines
    Chloral hydrate
    Clonidine
    Ethanol

    Ethchlorvynol
    Glutethimide
    Meprobamate
    Narcotics
    Phenothiazines
    Tricyclic antidepressants
    Valproic acid

Hyperreflexia
    Amphetamines
    Carbamazepine
    Carbon monoxide
    Cocaine
    Cyanide
    Haloperidol
    Methaqualone

    Phencyclidine
    Phenothiazines
    Phenytoin
    Propoxyphene
    Propranolol
    Strychnine
    Tricyclic antidepressants

Source: Data for "Breath Odor" from Olson K. Poisoning and drug overdose.
    2nd ed. Norwalk, CT: Appleton and Lange, 1994:__ – __.

T A B L E    **35-6**

Time intervals for detecting drugs in urine after use

| Drug | Detectable After Use | Drug | Detectable After Use |
|---|---|---|---|
| Alcohol | < 24 hr | Benzodiazepines | < 72 hr |
| Amphetamines | < 48 hr | Cocaine | < 72 hr |
| Barbiturates | | Marijuana | |
|   Short-acting | < 48 hr |   Single use | < 72 hr |
|   Long-acting | < 7 days |   Chronic use | < 30 days |

Source: Thorp J. Management of drug dependency, overdose, and withdrawal
    in the obstetric patient. Obstet Gynecol Clin North Am 1995;22.

Finally, an approximation of the concentration of the drug in the blood can be obtained from the following formula:

$$(\text{Osmolar gap} - 10) \times \text{mol wt}/10 = \text{Serum concentration (mg/dL)}$$

Diagnostic studies such as ECGs and x-rays (see Table 35-9) also can assist in determining the cause of the overdose.

## Advanced Poisoning Treatment and Life Support

Noji and Kelen (1989) developed the concept of Advanced Poisoning Treatment and Life Support (APTLS), which is equivalent to the approach used in trauma victims (ATLS) or advanced cardiac life support (ACLS), to evaluate the poisoned patient in a systematic and relatively simple way. A modification of such approach is presented here. The APTLS has five phases of evaluation and management.

In the first two phases, the objective is to identify immediate life-threatening problems and to initiate resuscitative measures as needed. The standard ABCs of patient management are implemented. First, establish and maintain an airway. If necessary, cervical spine control in patients with trauma or altered mental status is necessary. Then, assess breathing and smell the breath. Next, evaluate the circulation. This will include an estimation of rate, rhythm, and BP by feeling for pulses. (Radial pulse implies a systolic BP of at least 80 mm Hg, a femoral BP of 70 mm Hg, and a carotid BP of 60 mm Hg).

Once the patient has been initially assessed, the level of consciousness using the AVPU (*a*lert, *v*erbal stimuli response, *p*ainful stimuli response, *u*nresponsive) is evaluated. As part of that evaluation, pupil size and reactivity should be assessed.

After completing the initial assessment, fully expose the body by completely undressing the patient. Preserve all clothing. Then, look for identifications, Medic-Alert types of tags, bracelets, or collars, even if soiled with blood, vomit, or mud, and begin the search for toxic or toxics responsible for the exposure.

The patient should undergo ECG monitoring and, in general, should receive oxygen by mask. Intravenous (IV) access should be established in all but trivial toxic exposures. Blood should be obtained for immediate blood glucose determination and basic laboratory work (10–15 mL of serum). Patients with altered mental status should receive 50% dextrose solution, naloxone, and thiamine. Obtain arterial blood gases if appropriate. Antidotes should be given for specific symptomatic exposures if the diagnosis is certain or very likely. Wash or irrigate exposed areas such as eyes and skin.

Next, a complete history and physical examination are obtained and documented, and diagnostic laboratory and radiographic studies are then obtained. As part of the history, include circumstances of the toxic exposure, such as what, when, how, how much, and why? Then, a full examination should be completed, and fetal heart tones should be sought and documented. Additional laboratory or radiographic tests may be ordered as indicated.

T A B L E    **35-7**

Quantitative toxicology testing

| Test | Time to Sample Postingestion | Repeat Sample | Implication Positive Test |
|------|------------------------------|---------------|---------------------------|
| Acetaminophen | 4 hr | None | Blood level<br>Nomogram and N-acetylcysteine |
| Carbamazepine | 2–4 hr | 2–4 hr | Repetitive doses of activated charcoal/hemoperfusion |
| Carboxyhemoglobin | Immediate | 2–4 hr | 100% oxygen |
| Cholinesterase blood RBC | Immediate | 12–24 hr | Confirm exposure to insecticide |
| Digoxin | 2–4 hr | 2–4 hr | Digoxin antibody fragments (Fab) |
| Ethanol | 0.5–1 hr | Not necessary | If negative, not ethanol intoxication; if positive, inconclusive (tolerance) |
| Ethylene glycol | 0.5–1 hr | 2 hr | Ethanol therapy, hemodialysis, sodium bicarbonate |
| Heavy metals | First 24 hr | 2–4 hr | Chelation therapy, dialysis |
| Iron | 2–4 hr (chewable/liquid preparation absorbed faster) | 2–4 hr | Serum iron >350 µg use deferoxamine |
| Isopropanol | 0.5–1 hr | 2 hr | Supportive-care hemodialysis |
| Lithium | 2–4 hr | 4 hr | Hemodialysis |
| Methanol | 0.5–1 hr | 2 hr | Ethanol therapy folinic acid, $NaHCO_3$, hemodialysis |
| Methemoglobin | Immediate | 1–2 hr | Methylene blue |
| Phenobarbital | 1–2 hr | 4–6 hr | Alkaline diuresis<br>Repeated activated charcoal; hemoperfusion |
| Phenytoin | 1–2 hr | 4–6 hr | Supportive care<br>Repeated activated charcoal |
| Salicylates | 2–4 hr | 2–4 hr | Serum & urine alkalinization<br>Repeated activated charcoal, hemodialysis |
| Theophylline | 1-hr peak at 12–36 hr | 1–2 hr | Repeat activated charcoal, hemoperfusion |

PT, prothrombin time; PTT, partial thromboplastin time; ABGs, arterial blood gases; Fab, fragment antigen-binding; 2-PAM, pralidoxime.

Sources: Mowry JB, Furbee RB, Chyka PA. Poisoning. In: Chernow B, Borater DC, Holaday JW, et al, eds. The pharmacological approach to the critically ill patient. 3rd ed. Baltimore: Williams and Wilkins, 1995.

During the definitive phase, the less immediately life-threatening problems or injuries and social and psychological issues are addressed and managed. Continuous reevaluation and monitoring of the patient, especially airway and mental status, should be carried out in the appropriate setting. As part of the process, the medical team should initiate general and specific treatment measures directed at the underlying toxin. A member of the team may communicate with the regional agency or poison control center (Table 35-10). Evaluate each patient for suicide potential and document the information. Patients at heightened risk for suicide may require constant

| Supportive Tests | Interference | Specimen |
|---|---|---|
| Liver function bilirubin, PT, PTT | Increased bilirubin | Serum |
| — | — | Serum |
| Cyanide, ECG, ABGs | — | Whole blood (EDTA or sodium fluoride) |
| ABGs | 2-PAM Normalize RBC cholinesterase | Whole blood (heparin) |
| ECG, K | Fab fragments | Serum |
| Serum osmolarity | Alcohol dehydrogenase | Serum |
| BUN, electrolytes, calcium, serum osmolarity gap, anion gap, ABGs, ethanol, urine oxalate crystals, hippurate crystals | Propylene glycol | Serum |
| 24-hr urine collection | — | Whole blood (heparin) |
| Deferoxamine challenge test | Deferoxamine interferes with subsequent tests | Serum |
| Urine/serum ketones, serum acetone, osmolarity | — | Serum |
| Renal function test, ECG, lytes | — | Serum |
| BUN, lytes, osmolarity gap, ABGs, anion gap | Same as ethanol | Serum |
| Chocolate color blood | Sulfhemoglobin | Whole blood |
| ABGs, urine pH | Phenobarbital vs total barbiturates | Serum |
| — | — | Serum |
| BUN, lytes, ABGs, urine pH, urine ferric chloride | — | Serum |
| ECG, $K^+$, ABGs | — | Serum |

observation and special precautions. Once the evaluation is complete, decisions with respect to consultation and disposition (e.g., admission, observation, or discharge) are made. If the patient is admitted, the team leader should decide if the condition or toxin warrants admission to an intensive care unit (Table 35-11).

## Labor and Delivery Admission

Pregnant women at greater than 20 weeks' gestation should be admitted to the labor and delivery suite once they are resuscitated and stable. Remember, there may be a delayed effect on the fetus, placenta, or uterus that may compromise

T A B L E    **35-8**

Causes for an increased or decreased anion gap

| Increased Anion Gap | | Decreased Anion Gap |
|---|---|---|
| Lactic acidosis | Other | Bromates |
|   Beta-adrenergic drugs |   Benzyl alcohol | Lithium |
|   Caffeine |   Ethanol | Nitrites |
|   Carbon monoxide |     (ketoacidosis) | |
|   Cyanide |   Ethylene glycol | |
|   Hydrogen sulfide |   Exogenous organic | |
|   Ibuprofen |     and mineral acids | |
|   Iron |   Formaldehyde | |
|   Isoniazid |   Methaldehyde | |
|   Phenformin |   Methanol | |
|   Salicylates |   Toluene | |
|   Seizures | | |
|   Theophylline | | |

T A B L E    **35-9**

Causes of increased osmolal gap

Methanol (mol wt = 32)
Ethanol (mol wt = 46)
Acetone (mol wt = 58)
Isopropyl alcohol (mol wt = 60)
Ethylene glycol (mol wt = 62)
Propylene glycol (mol wt = 76)
Mannitol (mol wt = 182)
Ethyl ether
Magnesium
Renal failure without dialysis
Severe alcoholic or lactic ketoacidosis

the pregnancy. Thus, the patient should be admitted for a period of observation to monitor the fetus and uterine activity. At the time of admission, a blood type and antibody screening test should be sent, preparations for urgent delivery should be made (if appropriate), and the pediatric service should be notified if there is potential for urgent delivery.

## General Detoxification Measures

### Decontamination

The immediate therapy for poison victims should include local or systemic decontamination (Table 35-12). Decontamination often requires the use of special equipment and methodologies to enhance elimination of poisons.

### Skin Decontamination

Absorption of toxins such as organic chemicals and industrial compounds through the skin is common. Substances such as organophosphate insecticides, organochlorines, nitrates, and industrial aromatic hydrocarbons can produce significant systemic toxicity through transdermal absorption. Organophosphates, in particular, can pass through intact skin very rapidly without causing any specific skin sensation or reaction. This would predispose the pregnant woman to a greater risk of toxicity due to the normal physiologic increase in skin perfusion during pregnancy.

In the exposed pregnant woman, the entire skin surface should be cleaned. This will require rapid removal of all clothing, including footware. When removed, the clothes should be handled with gloves and placed in a labeled plastic bag for sampling later. Do not permit the patient to re-dress in the same clothes if there is history of exposure to any of the aforementioned substances, particularly organophosphates and carbamates, or if the clothes have a distinct chemical odor. Once the clothes are removed completely, the skin should be flushed thoroughly with a large volume of soapy water administered at a relatively high velocity. A rare exception to immediate decontamination with water is exposure

T A B L E **35-10**

Certified regional poison control centers in the United States

| State | Poison Center | Phone Number |
|---|---|---|
| Alabama | Children's Hospital of Alabama, Birmingham | 800/292-6678 (AL only) 205/939-9201 |
| Arizona | Arizona Poison and Drug Information Center, Tucson | 800/362-0101 (AZ only) 602/626-6016 |
| | Samaritan Regional Poison Center, Phoenix | 602/253-3334 |
| California | Fresno Regional Poison Control Center, Fresno | 800/346-5922 (CA only) 209/445-1222 |
| | San Diego Regional Poison Center, UC-San Diego | 800/876-4766 (CA only) 619/543-6000 |
| | San Francisco Bay Area Regional Poison Center, San Francisco | 800/523-2222 (CA only) |
| | Santa Clara Valley Regional Poison Center, San Jose | 800/662-9886 (CA only) 408/299-5112 |
| | UC Davis Medical Center Regional Poison Center, Sacramento | 800/342-9293 (CA only) 916/734-3692 |
| Colorado and Montana | Rocky Mountain Poison Center, Denver | 303/629-1123 |
| Florida | Florida Poison Information Center, Tampa | 800/282-3171 (FL only) 813/253-4444 |
| Georgia | Georgia Poison Center, Atlanta | 800/282-5846 (GA only) 404/589-4400 |
| Indiana | Indiana Poison Center, Indianapolis | 800/382-9097 (IN only) 317/929-2323 |
| Maryland | Maryland Poison Center, Baltimore | 800/492-2414 (MD only) 410/528-7701 |
| Massachusetts | Massachusetts Poison Control System, Boston | 800/682-9211 (MA only) 617/232-2120 |
| Michigan | Blodgett Regional Poison Center, Grand Rapids | 800/632-2727 (MI only) |
| | Poison Control Center, Children's Hospital, Detroit | 313/745-5711 |
| Minnesota | Hennepin Regional Poison Center, Minneapolis | 612/347-3141 |
| | Minnesota Regional Poison Center, St. Paul | 612/221-2113 |
| Missouri | Cardinal Glennon Children's Hospital Regional Poison Center, St. Louis | 800/366-8888 (MO only) 314/772-5200 |
| Nebraska and Wyoming | Mid-Plains Poison Center, Omaha | 800/955-9119 (NE only) 402/390-5555 |
| New Jersey | New Jersey Poison Information and Education System, Newark | 800/962-1253 (NJ only) |
| New Mexico | New Mexico Poison and Drug Information Center, Albuquerque | 800/432-6866 (NM only) 505/843-2551 |
| New York | Hudson Valley Poison Center, Nyack | 800/336-6997 914/353-1000 |
| | Long Island Regional Poison Control Center, East Meadow | 516/542-2323 |
| | New York City Poison Center, New York City | 212/340-4494 212/764-7667 |
| Ohio | Central Ohio Poison Center, Columbus | 800/682-7625 (OH only) 614/228-1323 |
| | Cincinnati Drug and Poison Information Center | 800/872-5111 513/558-5111 |

T A B L E 35-10

*Continued*

| State | Poison Center | Phone Number |
|-------|---------------|--------------|
| Oregon | Oregon Poison Center, Portland | 800/452-7165 (OR only)<br>503/494-8968 |
| Pennsylvania | Central Pennsylvania Poison Center, Hershey | 800/521-6110 |
| | Pittsburgh Poison Center | 412/681-6669 |
| | The Poison Center, Philadelphia | 215/386-2100 |
| Rhode Island | Rhode Island Poison Center, Providence | 401/277-5727 |
| Texas | North Texas Poison Center, Dallas | 800/441-0040 (TX only)<br>214/590-5000 |
| | Texas State Poison Center, Galveston, Houston | 409/765-1420<br>713/654-1701 |
| Utah | Intermountain Regional Poison Center, Salt Lake City | 800/456-7707 (UT only)<br>801/581-2151 |
| Virginia | Blue Ridge Poison Center, Charlottesville | 800/451-1428<br>804/924-5543 |
| Washington, DC | National Capitol Poison Center, Washington, DC | 202/625-3333 |
| West Virginia | West Virginia Poison Center, Charleston | 800/642-3625 (WV only)<br>304/348-4211 |

T A B L E 35-11

**Criteria for consideration of admission to the intensive care unit**

Mechanical ventilation required
Vasopressor support necessary
Arrhythmia management or need for hemodialysis
Signs of severe poisoning
Worsening signs of toxicity
Predisposing underlying medical conditions
Potential for prolonged absorption of toxin
Potential for delayed onset of toxicity
Invasive procedures or monitoring needed
Antidotes with potential for serious side effects
Suicidal patients requiring observations

T A B L E 35-12

**Decontamination issues in poison victims**

Skin, mucous membrane, and eye decontamination
Gastrointestinal decontamination
    Dilution
    Emesis
    Lavage
    Adsorption
    Cathartics and bowel irrigation
Enhanced elimination
    Diuresis
    Hemofiltration
    Hemoperfusion
    Hemodialysis
    Exchange transfusion/plasmapheresis
    Immunotherapy

to agents such as chlorosulfonic acid, titanium tetrachloride, calcium oxide, and phosphorus, which react violently with water.

If the eyes are involved, the foreign material should be removed immediately after exposure. Preferably, this should occur at the site of the incident, with copious amounts (4–6 liters) of saline solution (or water). After 20 minutes of irrigation, verify neutrality with pH strip paper. In the case of alkalis, the eyes should be irrigated continuously for 1 to 2 hours, because this kind of injury is associated with rapid and deep penetration. The irrigation should be done from the nasal side to the temporal side of the eye to avoid contamination to the contralateral eye. After the immediate treatment, the minimum examination should include a visual acuity evaluation, a slit lamp evaluation, funduscopy, and tonometry. An ophthalmologic consult is strongly recommended.

## Gastrointestinal Decontamination

To decontaminate the gastrointestinal tract, various approaches have been suggested (Table 35-13). Not all of these methods are clinically acceptable in each instance. *Dilution* is generally not an appropriate therapy for gastrointestinal decontamination. Not only has it been shown not to be effective, but it may also increase the absorption of many drugs and induce emesis. As a result, the upper gastrointestinal (GI) tract is reexposed to the caustic agent. In circumstances of caustic ingestion (acids or alkalis), however, dilution with the oral administration of 200 to 300 mL of milk may be appropriate.

The induction of *emesis* has been questioned as the first-line therapy of an overdose for a number of reasons. First, emesis is not immediately effective. Second, the effect of syrup of ipecac may persist for 2 hours, and the administration of adsorbents is delayed. This is important, because the ability to prevent absorption requires its administration within 1 to 2 hours after ingestion of a poison. Finally, emesis has not proven to be better than lavage. Moreover, the use of emesis has several contraindications, such as caustic ingestion, altered level of consciousness, unprotected airway, seizures or seizure potential, hemorrhagic diatheses, hematemesis, and ingestion of drugs that lead to rapid change in the patient's condition, such as tricyclics, β-blockers, phencyclidine, or isoniazid. Emesis has no value in cases of ethanol intoxication and poisoning with certain hydrocarbons. Importantly, where there is failure to induce emesis (5% of patients), the stomach should be evacuated by other means, because ipecac can be cardiotoxic.

The usual adult dose of ipecac is 30 mL with water and can be repeated after 15 to 30 minutes if vomiting is not induced. The primary indications for the use of syrup of ipecac are listed in Table 35-14. The most common side effects of ipecac are drowsiness and diarrhea. Persistent vomiting can be controlled with the use of antiemetics or $H_2$-blockers. In pregnant women, emesis is second-line therapy and should be employed only after lavage has failed because of the greater risk for aspiration during pregnancy.

*Gastric lavage* is employed when gastric emptying is indicated and emesis is inappropriate or contraindicated. These circumstances include comatose patients, those with altered mentation, and when the ingested substance has the potential for seizures, is lethal, and/or is rapidly absorbed and delay could result in death. Gastric lavage is contraindicated following the ingestion of caustics and in hemorrhagic diatheses. The advantages of lavage are that it can be performed immediately on arrival of the patient, that it takes only 15 to 20 minutes to complete, and that it facilitates the administration of charcoal.

A large gastric tube (Ewald, Lavaculator, and others), size 36 to 40 Fr, should be passed orally with lubricant. Concominant endotracheal intubation should be considered for patients with depressed mental status, an altered gag reflex, and/or seizures or seizure potential. The patient needs to be placed in a Trendelenburg or sitting position, and aspiration should be performed

T A B L E **35-13**

Clinical approaches to
gastrointestinal decontamination

Dilution
Emesis
Gastric lavage
Adsorption
Cathartics
Whole bowel irrigation

T A B L E **35-14**

For induction of emesis, syrup of ipecac is
indicated in the following drug circumstances

Gastric concretion formation
   Salicylates
   Meprobamate
   Barbiturates
   Glutethimide
Gastric emptying delay
   Tricyclics
   Narcotics
   Salicylates
Conditions producing adynamic ileus

prior to lavage to collect samples for analysis and to confirm placement of the tube. Lavage is performed with normal saline or water in boluses of 1.5 mL/kg (up to 200 mL) until clear. Once clear lavage fluid is seen, an additional 1 to 2 liters is indicated. In selected circumstances, positional changes of the patient to dislodge potential residues or undissolved pills may be necessary. Possible complications of gastric lavage include esophageal rupture or perforation, pharyngeal perforation, nasopharyngeal trauma, pneumothorax, and tracheal intubation.

Activated charcoal use for *adsorption* is a fine powder made from pyrolysis of carbonaceous material. It consists of small particles with an internal network of pores that absorb substances. It is indicated after gastric emptying procedures and should also be given in repeated doses (every 2 to 4 hr) for drugs with an enterohepatic circulation (theophylline, digoxin, nor- and amitriptyline, salicylates, benzodiazepines, phenytoin, and phenobarbital). Activated charcoal may be used immediately after ipecac and N-acetylcysteine. It is contraindicated in caustic ingestion and ineffective after ingestion of elemental metals (iron), some pesticides (malathion, DDT), cyanide, ethanol, and methanol.

The dose is 30 to 100 g in adults, and it is usually given with a cathartic (50 mL of 70% sorbitol or 30 g of magnesium sulfate) to accelerate the transit time of the toxin-charcoal complex. Charcoal can generate an empyema if aspirated or create a charcoal impaction in patients with atonic bowel. In some poisonings, a specific neutralizing agent is preferable to charcoal for instillation (Table 35-15).

*Cathartics* are used as adjunctive treatment with activated charcoal and are contraindicated in the presence of diarrhea, dehydration, electrolyte imbalance, abdominal trauma, intestinal obstruction, and adynamic ileus. Sorbitol is the most frequently used agent in the treatment of poisoning because of its short onset of action (< 1 hr), duration of effect (8–12 hr), and lack of interaction with charcoal. Oil cathartics are contraindicated because they can be aspirated and can increase the absorption of hydrocarbons. Of note, overaggressive use of cathartics can lead to fluid and electrolyte imbalances (see Chapter 4).

T A B L E   **35-15**

**Poisoning in which a specific neutralizing agent is preferable to activated charcoal**

| | |
|---|---|
| Mercury | Sodium formaldehyde (20 g) converts HgCl to less soluble metallic mercury |
| Iron | Iodium bicarbonate (200–300 mL) converts ferrous iron to ferrous carbonate |
| Iodine | Starch solution (75 g of starch in 1 liter of water; continue until aspirate is no longer blue) |
| Strychnine, nicotine, quinine, physostigmine | Potassium permanganate (1:10,000) |

*Whole bowel irrigation* with polyethylene glycol is given at a rate of 2 liters/hr orally or via a nasogastric tube to flush the bowel of whole or undissolved pills. This procedure may be helpful in clearing the GI tract of iron or delayed-release formulations not adsorbed by activated charcoal, or in cases in which there is a very delayed onset of treatment. The procedure takes 3 to 5 hours and may be complicated by bowel perforation or obstruction, ileus, or GI hemorrhage.

## Enhanced Elimination

A number of toxic agents can be eliminated by diuresis, dialysis, or hemoperfusion. The facility with which an agent can be actively eliminated is dependent on its *volume of distribution* (Vd). Volume of distribution (liters per kilogram) is the hypothetical volume of water required to produce the same concentration as that seen in the serum for a given amount of drug. Substances with a large Vd are highly tissue soluble. Substances with a small Vd remain confined within the vascular compartment and are, thus, more amenable to enhanced elimination by processes such as diuresis, dialysis, or hemoperfusion.

The Vd also can be used to estimate the amount of drug ingested:

Serum level (Cp) = Amount ingested (A)/Vd
Amount ingested (A) = Body weight × Vd × Cp

There are a number of clinical situations in which enhanced elimination of toxic compounds would hasten recovery of the patients (Pond, 1990). These include cases of severe poisoning and progressive deterioration, and when the normal route of elimination is impaired.

### Diuresis

*Forced neutral diuresis* (FND) can be used to enhance the elimination of a drug if it is a renal-excreted polar substance with small Vd and poor protein binding, such as isoniazid, bromide, and ethanol (Stine, 1983; Haddad, 1990). Here, the aim is to maintain a urinary flow rate of 5 to 7 mL/kg/hr using IV solute (0.45% normal saline) and repeated doses of furosemide (20 mg IV). A mannitol infusion of 20 to 100 g also may be used to enhance diuresis. In the presence of hypotension, pulmonary edema, and cerebral edema, FND is contraindicated. During FND, patient monitoring will include an assessment of vital signs (ECG, BP, heart rate, respiratory rate, body temperature), blood chemistries (hyponatremia, hypokalemia), blood gases (acid-base disturbances), and hemodynamic parameters.

In the pregnant patient, fetal condition (nonstress test, biophysical profile) (Roberts, 1994) should be monitored, not only for the effect of the poison, but also because of the potential for hemodynamic perturbations during this type of therapy. Furosemide crosses the placenta readily and reaches peak levels in fetal serum in 9 hours. By 8 hours, fetal serum levels are equivalent to maternal levels. Exposure to furosemide prior to delivery may result in increased diuresis and increased excretion of sodium and potassium in the neonate.

*Forced acid diuresis* (FAD) is used for many toxic compounds that are weak acids or bases. When these agents are exposed to a solution with a pH that is equivalent to their pKa, they become 50% ionized and 50% non-ionized. In a weak acid solution, compounds that are weak bases become more ionized. The cell membrane is relatively impermeable to ionized molecules; this principle can be applied in the kidney to reduce reabsorption of toxic substances and enhance renal excretion. The acidification of the urine will ionize weak bases, preventing reabsorption and enhancing elim-

ination. Substances with a small Vd, poor protein binding, and preferential renal excretion, such as amphetamines, phencyclidine, quinidine/quinine, and fenfluramine, may be eliminated this way. Of note, some toxicologists believe that urinary acidification is no longer appropriate therapy, because it does not significantly enhance removal of toxic compounds and has the potential for causing severe metabolic acidosis (Pond, 1990).

The most common approach to FAD is to prescribe ascorbic acid, 500 mg to 1 g, orally or IV, every 6 hours to maintain a urinary pH of 5.5 to 6.5. Furosemide and supplemental fluids are given to maintain a urine output of 5 to 7 mL/kg/hr. Alternately, ammonium chloride (4 g every 2 hr) via nasogastric tube or 1% to 2% solution of ammonium chloride in normal saline can be infused to maintain the urinary pH in the required range. During therapy, maternal serum electrolytes and urinary pH will need to be monitored. Forced acid diuresis is contraindicated in the presence of myoglobinuria. Ascorbic acid poses no threat to the fetus in doses up to 2 g/day (Korner, 1972). Close fetal monitoring, however, is needed due to the potential hemodynamic disturbances that may accompany volume expansion and repeated doses of diuretics.

Following the same principles with FAD, *forced alkaline diuresis*, or alkalization of the urine in the kidney, will ionize weak acids, such as long-acting barbiturates (phenobarbital, mephobarbital, pyrimidine), salicylates, lithium, isoniazid, and 2,4-dichlorophenoxy acetic acid, and prevent their renal reabsorption (Stine, 1983; Rayburn, 1984). Here, sodium bicarbonate ($NaHCO_3$) is given as a constant infusion (1 to 2 ampules $NaHCO_3$/liter of 0.25%–0.45% normal saline) to maintain a urinary pH of 7.3 to 8.5 (1–2 mEq/kg every 3–4 hr). Furosemide is given along with supplemental 0.45% normal saline to maintain the urinary output at 5 to 7 mL/kg/hr. For example, salicylate has a pKa of 3.0, and by increasing the urine pH from 6.5 to 7.5, the renal clearance of salicylate increases fourfold. During therapy, the patient will need to be monitored with blood gases (metabolic alkalosis), blood chemistry (hypernatremia), serum osmolality (hyperosmolality), and fluid retention. In pregnancy, toxic exposure to sodium bicarbonate may lead to maternal metabolic anomalies such as hypernatremia, hypokalemia, hypochloremia, alkalosis, and hypocalcemia (Poisindex, 1975–1995). In adults with normal renal function, alkalosis is rare. Nonetheless, close fetal monitoring is needed in the event of hemodynamic disturbances that may accompany volume expansion and repeated doses of diuretics.

## Hemodialysis

Hemodialysis has a very important but limited role in the elimination of toxic agents. One specific advantage of hemodialysis is that it can be used to correct metabolic acidemia (Pond, 1990). Compounds with the highest hemodialysis clearance potential will have the following properties: molecular weight (mol wt) less than 500 daltons, water soluble, small volume of distribution, minimal protein binding, and a concentration gradient that ensures that the compound remains in the dialysate.

Peritoneal dialysis also can be utilized, but it is only 10% to 25% as effective as hemodialysis (Shannon, 1995; Pond, 1990). Compounds with a mol wt less than 500 daltons have the highest peritoneal dialysis clearance. The effectiveness of peritoneal dialysis is decreased when there is hypotension, which is commonly seen in overdose patients. In addition to the compounds enumerated in Table 35-16 (Stine, 1983; Reynolds, 1990), dialysis also may be appropriate when severe intoxication is associated with progressive deterioration despite intensive supportive therapy or in patients with impaired excretory function.

The primary complications of hemodialysis include an increased risk of acute bleeding or thrombosis at the access site, as well as electrolyte disturbances. Thus, patients undergoing dialysis should have their electrolytes monitored for possible hypo- and hypernatremia, hypo- and hyperkalemia, hypercalcemia, and hypermagnesemia (Blagg, 1981).

TABLE **35-16**

Compounds for which dialysis is an appropriate consideration

| | | | |
|---|---|---|---|
| Acetaminophen | Chloride | Gallamine | Nitrofurantoin |
| Aluminum | Chromate | Gentamicin | Ouabain |
| Amanita toxin | Cimetidine | Glutethimide | Paraquat |
| Amikacin | Cisplatin | Hydrogen ions | Penicillin |
| Ammonia | Citrate | Iodide | Phenobarbital |
| Amobarbital | Colistin | Iron desferrioxamine | Phosphate |
| Amoxicillin | Creatinine | Isoniazid | Potassium |
| Amphetamines | Cyclobarbital | Isopropyl alcohol | Primidone |
| Ampicillin | Cyclophosphamide | Kanamycin | Procainamide |
| Aniline | Cycloserine | Lactate | Quinidine |
| Arsenic | Demeton | Lead edetate | Quinine |
| Azathioprine | Diazoxide | Lithium | Salicylates |
| Barbital | Dimethoate | Magnesium | Sodium |
| Borate | Diquat | Mannitol | Streptomycin |
| Bromide | Diisopyramide | Meprobamate | Strontium |
| Butabarbital | Ethambutol | Methanol | Sulfonamides |
| Calcium | Ethanol | Methaqualone | Theophylline |
| Camphor | Ethchlorvynol | Methotrexate | Thiocyanate |
| Carbenicillin | Ethionamide | Methyldopa | Ticarcillin |
| Carbon tetrachloride | Ethylene glycol | Methylprednisolone | Tobramycin |
| Cephalosporins | Flucytosine | Methyprylon | Trichloroethylene |
| Chloral hydrate | Fluoride | Metronidazole | Urea |
| Chloramphenicol | 5-Fluorouracil | MAO inhibitors | Uric acid |
| Chlorate | Fosfomycin | Neomycin | Water |

In the pregnant patient, preterm contractions and labor occur in up to 41% of patients in association with hemodialysis (Hou, 1985; Unzelman, 1973; Johnson, 1979). Additionally, maternal hypotension and fetal distress may be encountered in 20% to 30% of patients (Sanchez-Casajus, 1978; Kurtz, 1966). Thus, continuous electronic fetal monitoring during dialysis may be helpful in the fetus beyond 24 weeks' gestation. Additional complications of dialysis include disequilibrium syndrome (headache, nausea, muscle twitching, disorientation, seizures, and rarely, coma), cerebral and pulmonary edema (Hou, 1985; Unzelman, 1973; Johnson, 1979; Sanchez-Casajus, 1978; Posner, 1977), hemorrhage and placental abruption, and hypertension (Hou, 1994; Yasin, 1988; Elliott, 1991).

### Hemoperfusion

Hemoperfusion has limitations similar to those seen in hemodialysis. These include the low affinity of the absorbent for many of the toxins, the slow rate of blood flow through the absorbent, the volume of distribution, and the slow rate of equilibration between peripheral tissue and blood. However, this method can better circumvent the lipid solubility, plasma protein binding, and molecular weight issues that may complicate hemodialysis (Shannon, 1995; Pond, 1990). A distinct advantage of hemoperfusion is that both antidepressants and their metabolites are removed by this method (Pond, 1990). The primary indications for this procedure involve removal of the compounds listed in Table 35-17 (Stine, 1983; Reynolds, 1990).

With hemoperfusion, heparinized blood is pumped through a column of activated charcoal or resin via a single- or double-lumen catheter that is usually placed in the femoral vein. The cartridge should be changed every 4 to 6 hours to ensure optimal affinity of the absorbent and to maintain a high rate of blood flow through the system (Pond, 1990). Potential complications are hematologic and electrolyte disturbances. For example, platelet depletion is common. Patients with liver failure secondary to acetaminophen overdose do not tolerate hemoperfusion and develop severe thrombocytopenia. In addition, reductions in serum calcium, glucose, and fibrinogen, and a transient leukopenia have been observed. As a result, patients undergoing hemoperfusion should have frequent monitoring of complete blood count, electrolytes and glucose, prothrombin and activated partial thromboplastin times, and fibrinogen.

In the pregnant woman, complications are similar to those experienced with hemodialysis. These include sudden blood volume shifts that can lead to hypotension, fetal distress, and possible preterm contractions.

### Hemofiltration

Hemofiltration is indicated in circumstances of severe intoxication and intoxication by so-called middle molecules with a molecular weight of 500 daltons (e.g., aminogylcosides). Because the

T A B L E  **35-17**

**Compounds for which hemoperfusion is appropriate**

| | | | |
|---|---|---|---|
| Acetaminophen | Chloroquine | Heptabarbital | Procainamide |
| *Amanita* toxins | Creatinine | Meprobamate | Quinalbital |
| Ammonia | Cyclobarbital | Methaqualone | Quinidine |
| Amobarbital | Demeton | Methotrexate | Salicylates |
| Barbital | Digoxin | Methyprylon | Secobarbital |
| Bromide | Dimethoate | Nitrostigmine | Theophylline |
| Butabarbital | Diquat | Paraquat | Thyroxine |
| Camphor | Diisopyramide | Parathion | Tricyclic antidepressant |
| Carbon Tetrachloride | Ethanol | Pentobarbital | Triiodothyronine |
| Carbamazepine | Ethchlorvynol | Phenobarbital | Uric acid |
| Chloral hydrate | Glutethimide | Phenytoin | |

complications are similar to those of hemodialysis, the monitoring of the pregnant patient is also the same.

With hemofiltration, a catheter is placed in a peripheral artery and blood is filtered through a continuous arteriovenous hemofiltration system (CAVH) using arterial pressure (if it is high enough) or a pump in the presence of hypotension. The blood is then drained into a peripheral vein. Heparin is infused into the arterial side of the hemofilter, which is a hollow fiber filter composed of polysulfone or polyamide (mol wt < 10,000 daltons). This extracorporeal system can be used only when the volume of blood in the system does not exceed 10% of the patient's blood volume. A particular advantage of this method is that by using the patient's own arterial pressure to pump the blood, hemofiltration can be continued 24 hours per day. Some clinicians recommend that hemofiltration be used after hemodialysis or hemoperfusion in order to minimize rebound in blood levels of toxic compounds once they are released from tissue-binding sites (Pond, 1990).

### Exchange Transfusion and Plasmapheresis

Plasmapheresis and exchange transfusion are distinctly different methods for the treatment of poisonings. *Plasmapheresis* is the removal of the patient's plasma and the transfusion of fresh plasma. The benefit of this method is the enhancement of the elimination of drugs with strong plasma-protein binding. In contrast, *exchange transfusion* is the removal of the patient's blood and the transfusion of donor blood in situations such as severe poisoning that may lead to hemolysis and methemoglobinemia (Roberts, 1994). Because these techniques involve the use of blood products, complications from these procedures are blood reactions, hemodynamic instability, and sequelae such as hepatitis and HIV. During therapy, patient monitoring is similar to that for hemodialysis. In pregnancy, exchange transfusion will need to be carried out more slowly and with close monitoring of the fetus. Of note, excessive reduction of the patient's circulating blood volume may lead to fetal distress.

### Immunotherapy

Immunotherapy has limited usefulness, although the use of digoxin-specific antibody fragments has been successful in treating patients with severe digoxin toxicity.

### Additional Considerations during Pregnancy

The presence of a fetus in utero presents some additional concerns to the management team. As a result, clinical management will involve consideration of the items listed in Table 35-18 when handling the pregnant poison victim. Clinical indications for enhanced elimination of toxic compounds are listed in Table 35-19 (Pond, 1990).

## Specific Agents

### Acetaminophen

#### Background

Acetaminophen (paracetamol, N-acetyl-para-aminophenol) is one of the most commonly used medications in pregnancy, and it is also the most commonly used substance in suicide attempts by

T A B L E   **35-18**

**Factors to consider in the clinical management of the pregnant poison victim**

Supine hypotensive syndrome
Lower potential to resist acidosis in pregnancy
Need for preservation of a maternal $Pao_2$ of at least 60 to 70 mm Hg for fetal oxygenation
Increased maternal cardiac output and oxygen consumption
Increased renal clearance of antidotes and therapeutic drugs
Different "normal" values of blood tests such as BUN and creatinine
Effects of various resuscitative drugs on the uteroplacental circulation and myometrium
Increased potential for gastric aspiration in pregnant women and heightened need for airway protection
Additional physiologic changes in circulatory, respiratory, and metabolic systems

T A B L E  **35-19**

Clinical indications for enhanced elimination of toxic compounds

Patients with signs of severe poisoning, such as hypotension, uncontrolled seizures or arrhythmias, and severe depression of the CNS. In deeply comatose patients, the mortality rate is approximately 13% to 35%, despite intensive supportive care.

Progressively deteriorating condition despite full supportive care. Prolonged coma is associated with a number of acute hazards (aspiration pneumonia, infection, and ARDS) that can be decreased with shortening of the toxin-induced coma time.

The amount of the toxic compound ingested/absorbed or its plasma concentration indicates the likelihood of serious morbidity/mortality. Such substances include acetaminophen, arsenic trioxide, ethylene glycol, lithium, mercuric chloride, methanol, paraquat, salicylates, and theophylline.

The normal route of elimination of the toxic compound is impaired, secondary to coexisting chronic disease or acute injury, acute tubular necrosis, hypotension, or low-output cardiac failure.

Compound produces delayed but serious toxic effects (e.g., arsenic trioxide, ethylene glycol, lithium, mercuric chloride, methanol, or paraquat).

Concurrent disease state or age group that places the patient at an increased risk of morbidity or mortality.

ARDS, acute respiratory distress syndrome.

pregnant women (Rayburn, 1984). It is found in many analgesic, antipyretic, and antiinflammatory preparations. In 1994, a total of 102,619 cases of acetaminophen overdose were reported in the United States, of which 29,682 were in adults and 100 resulted in death (Litovitz, 1995). The serum half-life of acetaminophen in pregnancy is 3.7 hours, and the pharmacokinetics (absorption, metabolism, and renal clearance) are similar in the pregnant and nonpregnant states (Reynolds, 1990; Rayburn, 1986).

The lethal dosage is in excess of 140 mg/kg and primarily involves hepatotoxicity (Peterson, 1978). The lethality of acetaminophen is not related directly to the dose, and other factors such

as age, nutritional status, and other compounds ingested may affect the amount of cytochrome P-450 present and, thus, its toxicity. Renal failure, myocardial depression, and pancreatitis also have been observed in acute overdoses.

Acetaminophen is metabolized in the liver to nontoxic sulfate (52%) and glucuronide (42%) forms and then excreted by the kidneys. Approximately 4% is metabolized by the hepatic cytochrome oxidase P-450 system, resulting in a toxic reactive intermediate. This toxic metabolite is conjugated with glutathione and excreted in the urine as nontoxic mercaptourate. Two percent of acetaminophen is excreted unchanged. In an overdose, the hepatic glutathione stores are depleted and the toxic intermediates become covalently bound to hepatic cellular proteins, resulting in hepatocellular necrosis (Peterson, 1978).

The symptoms of acetaminophen toxicity have been divided into four stages (Table 35-20). Plasma acetaminophen level (obtained 4 or more hours after ingestion) can be plotted on the Rumack-Matthew (1975) nomogram (Fig 35-1). A level drawn less than 4 hours after ingestion may reflect a partially absorbed and falsely low level. N-acetylcysteine (Mucomyst) is indicated for plasma levels in the hepatic toxicity range (usually regarded as > 120 mg/mL) or for any patient with a documented ingested dose of 7.5 g or greater of acetaminophen.

T A B L E  **35-20**

Stages of acetaminophen toxicity

| Phase | Time | Symptoms |
|-------|------|----------|
| I | 0–24 hr | Gastrointestinal symptoms (anorexia, nausea, vomiting), malaise, diaphoresis |
| II | 24–48 hr | Clinical improvement, but abnormal liver function tests |
| III | 72–96 hr | Peak hepatotoxicity with encephalopathy, coagulopathy, and hypoglycemia |
| IV | 7–8 days | Death, or recovery from hepatic failure (begins within 5 days and usually progresses to complete resolution within 3 mo) |

In general, the primary short-term problem of acetaminophen overdose is hepatocellular necrosis, which peaks at 72 to 96 hours. Cardiac, renal, and pancreatic complications rarely occur, but appropriate monitoring should be instituted. Perhaps the most serious long-term consequence is residual liver damage. Acetaminophen is considered a class B agent (Briggs, 1994). Although it crosses the placenta, none of the reported studies has shown an increase in fetal anomalies after an overdose (Rumack, 1975).

In cases of maternal overdose, fetal distress, premature labor, premature delivery, and fetal demise have been described. In one case, fetal death occurred at 27 weeks of gestation after the mother ingested 29.5 g of acetaminophen. Autopsy revealed extensive lysis of the fetal liver and kidneys (Levy, 1975). There have been case reports of newborns with normal liver function who were born 6 to 20 weeks after maternal ingestion of a toxic dose of acetaminophen. In each of these cases, prompt administration of IV N-acetylcysteine (Haibach, 1984; Byer, 1982; Stokes, 1984) had been performed. There is a relationship between pregnancy outcome and the interval between drug exposure and administration of N-acetylcysteine, with an increase in the incidence of spontaneous abortion and stillbirth as the interval increases (Lumir, 1986; Riggs, 1989). In cases in which there was prompt treatment with N-acetylcysteine, hypoglycemia and mild jaundice were reported in the newborn, although liver function appeared to remain normal (Haibach, 1984; Byer, 1982; Stokes, 1984).

### Clinical Management

With acetaminophen overdose, the therapeutic goal is to prevent, if possible, hepatic toxicity and maternal and/or fetal death. Thus, the first step is immediate gastric lavage or induced emesis with ipecac. With acetaminophen, activated charcoal or cathartics should be avoided because they impair absorption of the antidote.

*N-acetylcysteine (Mucomyst)*, a glutathione substitute or precursor, is used as an effective antidote to acetaminophen toxicity. The earlier Mucomyst therapy is initiated, the more effective it is. The best results are obtained when therapy

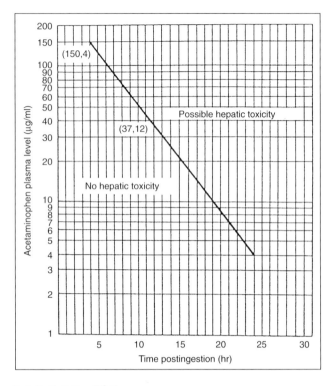

F I G U R E **35-1**

**Nomogram for acetaminophen toxicity.** (From Rumack RH, Matthew H. Acetaminophen poisoning and toxicity. Pediatric 1975;55:871. Reproduced by permission of Pediatrics.)

is started within 16 hours of the overdose, but N-acetylcysteine is still indicated up to 24 hours after ingestion of the overdose (Rumack, 1981). If an acetaminophen level cannot be readily obtained, therapy should be initiated anyway. If the plasma level is within the toxic range, N-acetylcysteine must be continued for the full 18-dose course of treatment. The initial loading dose is 140 mg/kg, followed by 17 doses of 70 mg/kg/4 hr given orally or via a gastric tube (Table 35-21). In selected circumstances, hemoperfusion and hemodialysis have been found to be effective, but these techniques are not usually indicated.

As part of the clinical management of these patients, the serum acetaminophen level should be plotted on the Rumack-Matthew nomogram (see Fig 35-1). In addition, renal and hepatic function will need to be monitored with liver function tests, ammonia levels if indicated, electrolyte and

T A B L E   **35-21**

Antidotes

| Poison | Antidote | Dosage |
|---|---|---|
| Acetaminophen | N-Acetylcysteine | 140 mg/kg PO, followed by 70 mg/kg/4 hr × 17 doses |
| Anticholinergics (atropine) | Physostigmine salicylate | 0.5–2.0 mg IV (IM) over 2 min every 30–60 min prn |
| Anticholinesterases (organophosphates) | Atropine sulfate | 1–5 mg IV (IM, SQ) every 15 min prn |
| | Pralidoxime (2-PAM) chloride | 1 g IV (PO) over 15–30 min every 8–12 hr × 3 doses prn |
| Benzodiazepines | Flumazenil (British data) | 1–2 mg IV (for respiratory arrest) |
| Carbon monoxide | Oxygen | 100%, hyperbaric |
| Cyanide | Amyl nitrite | Inhalation pearls for 15–30 sec every minute |
| | Sodium nitrite | 300 mg (10 mL of 3% solution) IV over 3 min, repeated in half dosage in 2 hr if persistent toxicity |
| | Sodium thiosulfate | 12.5 g (50 mL of 25% solution) IV over 10 min, repeated in half dosage in 2 hr if persistent toxicity |
| Digoxin | Antidigoxin Fab fragments | — |
| Ethylene glycol | Ethanol | 0.6 g/kg ethanol in D5W IV (PO) over 30–45 min, followed initially by 110 mg/kg/hr to maintain blood level of 100–150 mg/dL |
| Extrapyramidal signs | Diphenhydramine HCl | 25–50 mg IV (IM, PO) prn |
| | Benztropine mesylate | 1–2 mg IV (IM, PO) prn |
| Heavy metals (arsenic, copper, gold, lead, mercury) | Chelator | — |
| | Calcium disodium edetate (EDTA) | 1 g IV (IM) over 1 hr every 12 hr |
| | Dimercaprol (BAL) | 2.5–5.0 mg/kg IM every 4–6 hr |
| | Penicillamine | 250–500 mg PO every 6 hr |
| Heparin | Protamine | 1 mg/100 units heparin and for every 60 min after heparin, halved dose |
| Iron | Desferrioxamine mesylate | 1 g IM (IV at a rate of ≤ 15 mg/kg/hr if hypotension) every 8 hr prn (maximum 80 mg/kg in 24 hr) |
| Isoniazid | Pyridoxine | Gram per gram ingested; 5 g, if INH dose unknown |
| Magnesium sulfate | Calcium glutamate | 2–3 g IV over 5 min (in 30-mL D10) |
| Methanol | Ethanol | See Ethylene glycol |
| Methemoglobinemia (nitrites) | Methylene blue | 1–2 mg/kg (0.1–0.2 mL/kg 1% solution) IV over 5 min, repeated in 1 hr prn |
| Opiates/narcotics | Naloxone HCl | 0.4–2.0 mg IV (IM, SQ, ET) prn |
| Warfarin | Phytonadione/vitamin K$_1$ | 0.5 mg/min IV (in NS or D5W) |

PO, by mouth; IM, intramuscularly; prn, as circumstances may require; SQ, subcutaneously; z-PAM, pralidoxime; INH, isoniazid; ET, endotracheal; NS, normal saline.

Sources: Thorp J. Management of drug dependency, overdose, and withdrawal in the obstetric patient. Obstet Gynecol Clin North Am 1995;22:222–228; and Roberts JM. Pregnancy related hypertension. In: Creasy RK, Resnick R, eds. Maternal-fetal medicine: principles and practice. 3rd ed. Philadelphia: WB Saunders, 1994:804–843.

renal function tests, amylase, and ECG. When the patient is ready to be discharged, she should undergo a psychiatric evaluation as well as a determination of the extent of her hepatic disease. Clinical follow-up may include a social worker, obstetrician, hepatologist, and psychiatrist. Depending on the proximity of the overdose to the delivery date, the pediatric service should be informed of the exposure and possible fetal liver damage.

## Amphetamines

### Background

Amphetamines (amphetamine sulfate [Benzedrine] [Briggs, 1994], dextroamphetamine [Dexedrine], methamphetamine [Methedrine]) are a group of sympathomimetic drugs used to stimulate the CNS via norepinephrine- and dopamine-mediated pathways. Although the precise mechanism of action is unknown, proposed mechanisms have included presynaptic release of catecholamines, direct postsynaptic stimulation, and inhibition of monoamine oxidase. These drugs are used frequently for appetite suppression, to treat narcolepsy, or for illicit recreational reasons.

In 1994, there were 10,180 reported cases of amphetamine overdose. Of these, 2791 were in adults, and 16 fatalities were reported (Litovitz, 1995). In one study, the prevalence of amphetamine use in pregnancy was 13% in an inner city, indigent population and 11% in a private practice population (Matera, 1990). The lethal dose in adults is 20 to 25 mg/kg. Smaller doses, however, have been known to be fatal (Haddad, 1990).

Amphetamines are weak bases with a pKa of 9.9 and are metabolized in the liver. Both active metabolites and free amphetamines are excreted in the urine. Chronic abusers develop tolerance to amphetamines and may ingest lethal doses without effect. Thus, most cases of fatal intoxication seen are people who are not chronic abusers.

The signs and symptoms of amphetamine overdose (Stine, 1983; Shannon, 1995) are listed in Table 35-22. Blood levels correlate partly with both clinical status and mortality risk secondary to the development of tolerance (Tables 35-6, 35-22).

Short-term problems are manifested by cardiovascular changes such as severe hypertension, tachyarrhythmias, and cardiovascular collapse. There have been reports of maternal anemia and fetal meconium passage in women who abuse amphetamines. Paradoxically, the incidence of fetal distress, preterm labor, and premature rupture of membrane is reduced in these women (Matera, 1990; Gillogley, 1990). The potential long-term consequence of chronic abuse is psychosis.

The teratogenic potential of amphetamines depends on the type and teratogenic category (Briggs, 1994). Presently, there is no evidence that these drugs are associated with an increase in the frequency of major and/or minor congenital malformations (Little, 1989; Biggs, 1975). Correcting for confounding factors (tobacco, alcohol), however, babies of amphetamine abusers have significantly decreased birth weight, length, and head circumference (Little, 1989). Infants exposed to methamphetamine and/or cocaine have significantly greater frequency of prematurity, intrauterine growth retardation, placental hemorrhage, and anemia (Rayburn, 1984; Oro, 1987).

T A B L E    **35-22**

**Signs and symptoms of amphetamine overdose**

*Mild Toxicity*
 Respiratory (tachypnea)
 Cardiovascular (tachycardia, mild hypertension, chest pain, palpitations)
 Gastrointestinal (abdominal cramping, nausea, vomiting, diarrhea)
 Sympathetic stimulation (mild hyperpyrexia, dry mouth, mydriasis, diaphoresis, hyperreflexia)
 Central nervous system symptoms (dizziness, hyperactivity, irritability, confusion, and panic)

*Severe Toxicity*
 Cardiovascular (severe hypertension with intracranial hemorrhage, tachyarrhythmias, ventricular tachycardia or fibrillation, hypotension, and cardiovascular collapse)
 Severe hyperthermia (associated with coagulopathies, rhabdomyolysis, and renal failure)
 Metabolic (systemic acidosis)
 Central nervous system (convulsions, delirium, psychosis, usually in chronic abusers with paranoia, delusions, and hallucinations, coma)

Neonatal amphetamine and methamphetamine withdrawal syndromes have been described (Oro, 1987; Sussman, 1965; Newberg, 1970).

## Clinical Management

With amphetamine overdose, the therapeutic goal is to provide primarily supportive care until the patient is stabilized. Then, the patient should be placed in a cool, quiet environment to diminish external stimulation. There, the first step is gastric emptying, followed by charcoal instillation and cathartic administration for oral overdoses. Forced acid diuresis is indicated in severe toxicity to enhance renal excretion. In addition, symptomatic therapy for psychosis and agitation can best be treated with haloperidol (chlorpromazine may increase the half-life of amphetamines and cause greater respiratory depression) or diazepam. Along with these complications, seizures may be terminated with diazepam, and recurrent seizures may be treated with phenytoin.

Cardiovascular complications such as arrhythmias and hypertension can be managed with propranolol and haloperidol or chlorpromazine, respectively. Severe or refractory hypertension may require phentolamine or nitroprusside. Hypotension may be treated initially with IV fluids. Refractory hypotension may be due to catecholamine depletion and may require a direct-acting agent such as norepinephrine.

Hyperthermia is an ominous sign. Haloperidol or chlorpromazine and active cooling should be used to manage temperatures in excess of 102°F. Finally, hemodialysis may be useful for life-threatening cases that are unresponsive to supportive care or in patients with renal compromise.

As part of patient management, appropriate patient monitoring is essential. This includes ECG, BP, respiratory rate and blood gases, electrolytes, temperature, urine myoglobin levels, and fetal heart rate and uterine activity, when applicable.

When the patient is considered ready for discharge, she should be considered for drug rehabilitation. Clinical follow-up may include a social worker, obstetrician, and psychiatrist. Subsequently, she should be monitored for evidence of preterm labor, placental hemorrhage, and intrauterine growth restriction.

## Antidepressant Agents

### Background

Antidepressant drugs (imipramine, amitriptyline, Doxepin, trimipramine, trazadone, fluoxetine) may produce three major toxidromes: anticholinergic crisis, cardiovascular failure, or seizure activity. A patient may experience one or all three of these toxic effects, depending on the dose and the drug taken. Patients who initially are awake may abruptly lose consciousness and/or develop seizures without warning. The signs and symptoms associated with antidepressant overdose are illustrated in Table 35-23. In patients with an overdose, an ECG is a most helpful diagnostic test. Here, the clinician is looking for a sinus tachycardia with prolonged PR, QRS, and QT intervals. Prolongation of the QRS segment greater than 0.12 is a reliable indicator of serious cardiovascular and neurologic toxicity (with the exception of amoxapine). In addition, bradyarrhythmias carry a bad prognosis. Additional ECG changes include atrioventricular block and ventricular tachycardia. Although drug levels can be obtained, these are not generally useful in the acute management of an overdose. Arterial blood gases, electrolytes, glucose, and complete blood count also are helpful laboratory tests.

T A B L E   **35-23**

**Signs and symptoms of antidepressant overdose**

| Signs | Symptoms |
|---|---|
| Tachycardia | Blurred vision |
| Dry skin and mucous membranes | Dysarthria |
| Blisters | Visual hallucinations |
| Mydriasis | Sedation |
| Divergent strabismus | Delirium |
| Decreased bowel sounds | Coma |
| Urinary retention | |
| Increased muscular tone | |
| Hyperreflexia | |
| Myoclonic activity | |
| Rapid loss of consciousness | |
| Seizures | |
| Cardiac dysrhythmias | |
| Hypotension | |
| Pulmonary edema | |

Short-term problems include cardiac dysrhythmias, seizures, urinary retention, GI hypomotility, aspiration pneumonitis, and acute respiratory distress syndrome (ARDS). Long-term problems include rhabdomyolysis, brain damage, and multisystem failure.

The effects of antidepressants on the fetus are variable. The teratogenic potential appears to involve an increased risk of cardiovascular defects in exposed fetuses. While the potential for fetal distress exists due to maternal seizures, hypotension, or dysrhythmias, cesarean delivery is reserved for the usual obstetric indications. Postnatally, the neonate may be predisposed to tachypnea, cyanosis, irritability, urinary retention, and paralytic ileus.

## Clinical Management

With antidepressant overdose, the therapeutic goal is to prevent complications in the first 24 hours after a significant ingestion. The first step is decontamination with activated charcoal and a cathartic. A gastric lavage also should be performed. Because of the risk of sudden onset of seizures, emesis should not be induced. Forced diuresis, dialyses, and hemoperfusion are generally ineffective.

Once decontamination has been initiated, supportive therapy is warranted to maintain the airway, and, if necessary, mechanical ventilation should be instituted. Agitation, seizures, hyperthermia, hypotension, and arrhythmias should be treated. Because painful interventions and patient movement can precipitate seizures, such stimuli should be avoided.

If the patient manifests coma, seizures, QRS greater than 0.1 second, ventricular arrhythmias, or hypotension, alkalinization therapy with IV sodium bicarbonate is indicated. To alkalinize the patient, one ampule (44–50 mEq) of sodium bicarbonate should be given IV slowly over 1 to 5 minutes. This is followed by an infusion at 0.5 mEq/kg/hr to maintain an arterial pH of 7.45–7.55. If perfusion is compromised or there is hypotension despite bicarbonate therapy, phenytoin, 100 mg over 3 minutes, should be considered. Antiarrhythmics are used to control dysrhythmia.

If seizures are not immediately controlled with anticonvulsants, muscle relaxation with a nondepolarizing long-acting agent (pancuronium, norcuronium) should be instituted to avoid hyperthermia and lactic acidosis. An EEG may be required to evaluate the effectiveness of the anticonvulsant therapy.

Controversy exists regarding the use of physostigmine salicylate (usually given as a 2-mg bolus over 2 min) because it may precipitate convulsions or ventricular tachycardia. In situations in which there is doubt as to the cause of the coma, or in patients with altered mental status and serious respiratory compromise, physostigmine may be considered.

During therapy, 12 hours of maternal and fetal cardiac monitoring is recommended in asymptomatic pregnant patients. If there are signs of significant maternal toxicity, 24 hours in an intensive care setting appears warranted.

Prior to the discharge of the patient, a final dose of charcoal should be considered. In addition, the patients will need to be evaluated for suicide potential. Observe (or make arrangements for outpatient monitoring) for 72 hours, because deaths from the original overdose have been reported up to 3 days after ingestion. Clinical follow-up may include a social worker, obstetrician, and a psychiatrist.

## Barbiturates

### Background

Barbiturate abuse in therapeutic and illicit settings is high. In 1994, there were 4684 reported overdose cases in the United States. Of these 2111 were in adults, and 16 were fatal cases (Litovitz, 1995).

Barbiturates (Table 35-24) (Winchester, 1977) are weak acids with pKa values ranging between 7.2 and 8.0. The more lipid-soluble drugs have a faster onset but shorter duration of action. Barbiturates cause CNS depression and in toxic doses depress other excitable tissues (skeletal, cardiac, and smooth muscle) (Stine, 1983). The short-acting agents cause more potent CNS depression, are more toxic, and are more commonly abused. The quantity of drug ingested and the

T A B L E   **35-24**

Barbiturates commonly associated with overdose*

| Type | Duration of Action | Drug |
|---|---|---|
| Ultra-short-acting (methohexital) | 20 min | Thiopental, thiamylal |
| Short-acting | 3 hr | Pentobarbital, secobarbital, hexobarbital |
| Intermediate-acting | 3–6 hr | Amobarbital, butabarbital, aprobarbital |
| Long-acting | 6–12 hr | Barbital, phenobarbital, mephobarbital, primidone |

*Lethal dosage: Short-acting, ingestion of 3 g (lethal level, 3.5 mg/dL); long-acting, ingestion of 5 g (lethal level, 8 mg/dL) (Winchester, 1977).

blood level may not correlate with the clinical status, because chronic abusers develop tolerance (Stine, 1983). The patient's clinical condition is the best predictor of morbidity and mortality in cases of barbiturate toxicity. Death occurs from cardiopulmonary depression and is seen only in deeply comatose patients.

Maternal complications arise from either acute intoxication or chronic addiction of mother and fetus. Signs and symptoms are illustrated in Table 35-25. Barbiturate withdrawal is characterized by insomnia, excitement, delirium, hallucinations, toxic psychosis, tremors, nausea and vomiting, orthostatic hypotension, and seizures. This condition may not present until 48 to 72 hours after the last dose but must be considered whenever managing a chronic abuser, because deaths have been reported with severe withdrawal reactions (Victor, 1980).

In cases of suspected barbiturate overdose, blood levels may be useful for confirming the identity of the drug, although the quantitative level may not reflect the clinical status of the patient. Regardless, maternal ECG, respiratory rate, and peripheral oxygen saturation, as well as fetal heart rate monitoring, are suggested (see Tables 35-6, 35-7).

Because barbiturates cross the placenta, the teratogenic potential depends on the agent and the category (B/C/D/Y) (Briggs, 1994). Epileptic pregnant women taking phenobarbital in combination with other anticonvulsants have a two- to threefold greater risk of minor congenital defects in the fetus (Briggs, 1994).

The potential for fetal distress depends on maternal clinical status. In severe intoxication, cardiopulmonary depression may lead to fetal compromise. Cesarean delivery is reserved for the usual obstetric indications. Fetal and neonatal addiction have been reported (Shubert, 1994). Neonatal withdrawal complications may occur 3 to 14 days after delivery and may require

T A B L E   **35-25**

Signs and symptoms of barbiturate overdose

*Central Nervous System*
Mild intoxication: drowsiness
Moderate intoxication: CNS depression, slurred speech, ataxia, nystagmus, and miosis
Severe intoxication: extraocular motor palsies, absent corneal reflexes, sluggish pupillary reaction, mydriasis, absent deep tendon reflexes, absent Babinski sign, and coma. A flatline EEG has been reported.

*Respiratory System*
Respiratory depression (typically 3 times the hypnotic dose) (Stine, 1983; Roberts, 1994)
Aspiration pneumonia, atelectasis, pulmonary edema, and bronchopneumonia also have been reported.

*Cardiovascular System*
Hypotension, low cardiac output, and direct myocardial depression (Stine, 1983; Roberts, 1994)

*Other*
Hypothermia due to depressed thermal regulation in the brainstem
Cutaneous bullae (barb-burns) over pressure points (Roberts, 1994)
Decreased GI motility
Renal failure due to cardiovascular shock or rhabdomyolysis

treatment (Desmond, 1972). Phenobarbital and other anticonvulsant agents also have been associated with early hemorrhagic disease of the newborn (Bleyer, 1982).

### Clinical Management

With barbiturate overdose, the initial therapeutic goal is stabilization of maternal cardiopulmonary status. Gradual detoxification is then instituted to prevent abrupt withdrawal complications. Gastric emptying should be followed by the administration of charcoal (Bleyer, 1982) (every 4 hr) and cathartic agents. Lavage should continue for 8 hours because there may be delayed gastric emptying. Because phenobarbital may form gastric concretions, endoscopic removal (Shannon, 1995) may be surgically necessary. Hypotension may be supported by oxygen and IV fluids. With severe hypotension, dopamine or norepinephrine may be required. Alkaline diuresis may be indicated in stage III or IV coma induced by long-acting barbiturates (Stine, 1983). Charcoal hemoperfusion is indicated for life-threatening overdoses of short- and long-acting barbiturates that are refractory to supportive care (Berg, 1982). Hemodialysis is useful in long-acting barbiturate overdose.

Because there are no specific antidotes, the focus is on gradual withdrawal. Thus, a decremental dosage regimen, beginning with 200 mg of phenobarbital every 6 hours should be used to prevent withdrawal complications in both mother and fetus (Shannon, 1995; Shubert, 1994). During therapy, there should be close monitoring of the maternal CNS, respiratory, and cardiovascular status. Severe toxicity requires management in an intensive care unit (Stine, 1983). Clinical follow-up with a social worker, obstetrician, and psychiatrist is warranted. As part of the patient's ongoing care, drug rehabilitation should be considered.

## Benzodiazepines

### Background

Benzodiazepines (Table 35-26) are CNS depressants and are widely prescribed for their anxi-

T A B L E **35-26**

**Benzodiazepines commonly associated with overdose and their teratogenic classification**

| | |
|---|---|
| Alprazolam ($D_M$) | Chlordiazepoxide (D) |
| Chlorazepate (D) | Diazepam (D) |
| Flurazepam (Y) | Flunitrazepam (D) |
| Lorazepam ($D_M$) | Midazolam ($D_M$) |
| Oxazepam (D) | Triazolam ($X_M$) |
| Temazepam ($X_M$) | |

olytic, muscle relaxant, anticonvulsant, and hypnotic effects. In 1994, there were 34,940 reported overdoses in the United States. Of these, 8672 were in adults, and 47 were fatalities (Litovitz, 1995).

Benzodiazepines are metabolized in the liver by desmethylation (active metabolites) and/or conjugation (inactive metabolites) and are excreted in the urine (predominantly) and in the bile (Hardman, 1996). Gastrointestinal absorption is rapid and complete, while intramuscular absorption is erratic (Shannon, 1995). Benzodiazepines have a wide therapeutic index (Shannon, 1995) and are relatively safe when taken orally and as a single agent (Stine, 1983). Intravenous administration, however, has been associated with a 2% mortality from respiratory or cardiac arrest (Shannon, 1995).

Mild overdose is manifested by drowsiness, nystagmus, dysarthria, ataxia, dizziness, weakness, and confusion. Occasionally, paradoxical irritability, excitation, or delirium may occur (MacGregor, 1992). Coma is the manifestation of severe overdose. Uncommonly, respiratory and/or circulatory depression may be present. A qualitative drug screen confirms diagnosis for all the benzodiazapines except clonazepam. Of note, drug levels do not correlate with clinical status. If severe toxicity is present, respiratory and cardiovascular support may be required. Seizures have been reported up to 12 days after withdrawal in chronic users (MacGregor, 1992).

The teratogenic potential of these agents is illustrated in Table 35-26 and generally falls in category C/D/Y (Briggs, 1994). In one study, chlordiazepoxide (category D) was associated with a fourfold increase in congenital anomalies (mental deficiency, diplegia and deafness, duodenal atresia, and Meckel's diverticulum) (Milkovich, 1974). However, there was no such association noted in the Collaborative Perinatal Project with first-trimester exposure (Hartz, 1975). Diazepam (category D) has been reported to be associated with oral clefts (Saxen, 1975; Safra, 1975). This association, however, has not been confirmed (Shiono, 1984; Rosenberg, 1983). Laegreid et al (1987) reported on seven children who were prenatally exposed to benzodiazepines and developed minor anomalies, growth deficiency, and CNS abnormalities, including mental retardation. Thus, there is some evidence that a cause-and-effect relationship exists between benzodiazepines and congenital fetal anomalies. High-dose or recent use prior to delivery has been associated with birth depression and withdrawal stigmata in neonates, the latter occurring up to 6 days after delivery (Athinarayanan, 1976).

## Clinical Management

With benzodiazepine overdose, the therapeutic goal is supportive care and gradual withdrawal of the benzodiazepines in long-term abusers. The first step is gastric emptying with the administration of charcoal and cathartics. Occasionally, respiratory and cardiovascular support will be needed.

If the patient develops seizures, IV injection of benzodiazepine may be required to terminate withdrawal seizures, followed by a gradual withdrawal of the agent (MacGregor, 1992). An alternative treatment is phenobarbital for seizure control (Table 35-27). During therapy, maternal vital signs should be monitored for evidence of respiratory or cardiovascular compromise. Fetal heart rate monitoring is indicated in appropriate cases. Clinical follow-up with a social worker, obstetrician, and psychiatrist is warranted. As part of the

T A B L E   **35-27**

Therapy for maternal drug withdrawal

| Drugs | Therapy |
|---|---|
| Alcohol | Barbiturates |
| | Pentobarbital sodium (short-acting) followed by phenobarbital (longer-acting) |
| | Benzodiazepines (cleared slowly by fetus) |
| Amphetamines | Tricyclic antidepressants (severe depression) |
| Barbiturates | Barbiturates: 200 mg pentobarbital sodium IV or by mouth to test for physical dependence (short-acting), followed by phenobarbital (withdrawal equivalent, 30 mg phenobarbital/100 mg of short-acting). Estimated dose of phenobarbital is administered by mouth every 8 hr (maximum daily dose, 500 mg; if toxicity, daily dose is halved; if withdrawal symptoms, 200 mg phenobarbital intramuscularly). Once stable, decrease daily dose by 30 mg. |
| Benzodiazepine | Benzodiazepine: slow tapering over a 1- to 2-week period |
| | Barbiturates (see Barbiturates) |
| | Withdrawal equivalents: 30 mg phenobarbital/100 mg chlordiazepoxide or 50 mg diazepam |
| Opiates | Librium 10–25 mg by mouth every 8 hr ± compazine, as warranted, for nausea/vomiting |
| | Methadone 10–20 mg intramuscularly |
| | Refractory withdrawal may require short-acting narcotics (morphine, meperidine, hydromorphine). |

Sources: Stine RJ, Marcus RH. Toxicologic emergencies. In: Haddad LM, Winchester JF, eds. Clinical management of poisoning and drug overdose. Philadelphia: WB Saunders, 1983:297–342; and Thorp J. Management of drug dependency, overdose, and withdrawal in the obstetric patient. Obstet Gynecol Clin North Am 1995;22:131.

patient's ongoing care, drug rehabilitation should be considered.

## Carbon Monoxide

### Background

Carbon monoxide is a colorless, odorless gas. It is a by-product of cigarette smoking (the most common source of carbon monoxide exposure), automobile exhaust, faulty heating systems, and fire (Balaskas, 1992). It is absorbed rapidly through the respiratory tract. Hemoglobin's affinity for carbon monoxide is 250 to 300 times greater than for oxygen.

Maternal signs and symptoms relate to the reduction of the oxygen carrying capacity of hemoglobin as it is bound by carbon monoxide (Table 35-28). Thus, diagnostic tests focus on oxygen-sensitive structures such as the heart, lungs, kidneys, and brain. Cardiac evaluation will include an ECG; sinus tachycardia, ST depression, atrial fibrillation, and prolonged PR and QT intervals, and atrioventricular or bundle branch block can be seen. Additionally, arterial blood gases and a COHb level are helpful. The latter correlates with the patient's signs and symptoms. Finally, a complete blood count, transaminases, electrolytes and creatinine, and urinalysis are recommended.

Short-term concerns with carbon monoxide poisoning include myocardial ischemia or infarction, rhabdomyolysis, renal failure, pulmonary

T A B L E   **35-28**

Signs and symptoms of carbon monoxide overdose

| Signs | Symptoms |
|---|---|
| Vasodilation | Headache |
| Disturbed judgment | Shortness of breath |
| Collapse | Nausea |
| Coma | Dizziness |
| Convulsions | Visual disturbances |
| Cheyne Stokes respiration | Weakness |

Signs and symptoms will vary depending on the concentration of carboxyhemoglobin.

edema, blindness, and hearing loss. Delayed problems include CNS toxicity due to perivascular infarction and demyelination of basal ganglia. This is usually seen in patients who are comatose or acidotic on arrival to the hospital.

Carbon monoxide crosses the placenta and has a higher affinity for fetal than adult hemoglobin. As a result, fetal concentrations of carbon monoxide are 10% to 15% higher than those in the mother (Athinarayanan, 1976). Although the teratogenic potential is unclear, fetal brain damage and subsequent developmental delays may be seen.

### Clinical Management

With carbon monoxide poisoning, the therapeutic goal is to obtain a carbon monoxide level less than 5% and an asymptomatic patient. Initial therapy is directed at reducing the carbon monoxide concentration by removing the patient from the contaminated environment and instituting complete rest to decrease oxygen consumption. Oxygen (100%) is administered via a tight-fitting non-rebreathing mask. The oxygen should be continued for a period equal to 5 times the duration that it took for the maternal carbon monoxide levels to normalize. If the COHb level is more than 20% (as opposed to >40% in the nonpregnant state), hyperbaric oxygen is indicated (see Table 35-21).

During therapy, any pregnant woman who is exposed to carbon monoxide and has a potentially viable fetus should be monitored for a minimum of 12 hours. If cardiovascular complications are present, she should be admitted to the intensive care unit. Such complications are expected in nonpregnant patients with a COHb greater than 15%. This level is lower in pregnant women (COHb >10%). Additionally, each patient's mental state and acid-base status should be monitored.

Prior to discharge, the identification and avoidance of the source of exposure should be done. If clinically necessary, a suicide evaluation should be conducted. Clinical follow-up should include ultrasound assessment for possible intrauterine growth evaluation.

# Cocaine

## Background

Cocaine is a naturally occurring agent that is legally available for use as a topical anesthetic. It is more commonly used illegally as a CNS stimulant with a street-sample purity of 15% to 60% (Gay, 1982). It is principally used in one of two forms: either as the hydrochloride salt ("snorted" intranasally or IV) or as an alkaloid ("crack," "free base"). Illegally produced cocaine is frequently adulterated with foreign substances such as lactose, mannitol, lidocaine, and/or procaine (Gay, 1982).

Prevalence rates as high as 10% to 18% have been reported in indigent pregnant women seen in an inner-city hospital population. The cocaine abuse rate among fee-for-service patients is reported to be in the range of 1.4% (Riggs, 1989; Zuckerman, 1989).

The lethal dosage of cocaine is approximately 1400 mg taken orally or 750 mg taken parenterally or inhaled (Gay, 1982). Lethal overdoses can be taken via any route but are more likely with parenteral use or "freebasing" (smoking purified cocaine).

Cocaine is absorbed through mucous membranes and can be inhaled; smoked; swallowed; injected IV, intramuscularly, or subcutaneously; or placed in the vagina or rectum (Grinspoon, 1981). It is a sympathomimetic with direct cardiovascular stimulant activity that causes hypertension and vasoconstriction. Cocaine has both direct and indirect cardiotoxic effects (sensitizing the myocardium to epinephrine and norepinephrine) (Zuckerman, 1989). It is detoxified by liver and plasma cholinesterase. The fetus, infant, and pregnant woman experience slower metabolism and elimination (Bingol, 1987; Moore, 1989). The peak effects of cocaine in nonpregnant women occur within 3 to 5 minutes IV or at 60 to 90 minutes orally. The plasma half-life is 1 hour.

Symptoms and signs are secondary to adrenergic stimulation and depend on the severity of the toxicity. Mild-to-moderate toxicity is manifested by nausea, vomiting, abdominal pain, pallor, headache, hyperreflexia, apprehension, dysphoria, confusion, and hallucinations (Stine,

1983). Additionally, one may see increased respiratory rate, tachycardia, increased BP, and diaphoresis.

Severe toxicity is manifested by psychotic behavior, seizures, coma, ventricular arrhythmias (myocardial ischemia/infarction), hypertension (severe), circulatory collapse, pulmonary edema and respiratory depression, ARDS ("crack lung"), pneumomediastinum, rhabdomyolysis, hyperthermia, and hepatic infarction (Poisindex, 1975–1995). Death may occur rapidly from respiratory depression and/or circulatory collapse (Balaskas, 1992). Cerebral infarction is more common among alkaloidal cocaine users, and hemorrhagic stroke is seen more frequently in IV cocaine hydrochloride use. Cerebral catastrophes can occur within minutes of the use of cocaine (Levine, 1991).

Cocaine is detectable in blood within 24 hours of ingestion and in urine for several days. In addition to a drug screen, an ECG, blood gases, and liver and renal function tests should be obtained in patients suspected of cocaine use.

In pregnancy, there is a significant increase in the incidence of preterm labor (25% to 30% vs. 12% to 17%) and anemia (57% vs. 39%) (Matera, 1990; Gillogley, 1990). There is also a higher incidence of pregnancy-induced hypertension (25% vs. 4%) (Gillogley, 1990) and abruptio placentae (Chasnoff, 1987a). Meconium aspiration, preeclampsia, premature rupture of membrane, and fetal distress are all increased (Matera, 1990; Gillogley, 1990). Long-term problems include the aftermath of intracranial hemorrhage or infarction and rhabdomyolysis.

Cocaine has high water and lipid solubility, a low molecular weight, and a low degree of ionization, all of which facilitate its passage across the placenta and into the fetus (Bingol, 1987). Cocaine metabolites are found in the urine of neonates who were exposed in utero. In the sheep model, the fetal plasma level is approximately 14% of the maternal level at 5 and 30 minutes after administration. Cocaine infusion is associated with a decrease in uterine blood flow, leading to fetal hypoxic damage in the short term and to intrauterine growth retardation over time (Zuckerman, 1989; Neerhof, 1989).

The teratogenic potential for cocaine falls into category C. For nonmedicinal use, cocaine is classified as category X (Briggs, 1994). Urinary tract malformations (hydronephrosis, hypospadias, prune-belly syndrome), congenital heart defects (transposition of the great vessels, hypoplastic right-heart, ventricular septal defect, patent ductus arteriosus), and skull defects (exencephaly, encephalocele) (Briggs, 1994) are associated with cocaine use in pregnancy.

When compared with non-drug-using patients, cocaine-exposed women demonstrate shorter pregnancies (2 weeks) (Levine, 1991). After controlling for other factors, using multivariate analysis, however, Zuckerman et al (1989) could not show that cocaine exposure was the only factor responsible for the shortened gestation. The incidence of abruptio placentae–related stillbirths in cocaine users was 8%, as compared with 0.8% among drug-free control women (Bingol, 1987). Up to 13% of women who used cocaine during pregnancy develop an abruption, which may be sudden, unpredictable, and catastrophic (Chasnoff, 1987a, 1989). Cocaine has been shown to be associated with significantly increased perinatal distress hypotonia and significantly lower 5-minute Apgar scores (Chasnoff, 1987a).

Obstetric indications for delivery will depend on the maturity of the fetus and the degree of growth retardation. Postnatally, perinatal or newborn cerebrovascular accidents may be found in neonates with a positive cocaine screening test (Chasnoff, 1987a,b). The pathology of such cocaine-induced injury may include, in addition to hypoxic ischemic encephalopathy, hemorrhagic infarction, cystic lesions, posterior fossa hemorrhage, absent septum pellucidum, atrophy, and brain edema (Dixon, 1988). Necrotizing enterocolitis also has been described in neonates exposed to cocaine (Tesley, 1988).

### Clinical Management

With cocaine overdose, the initial therapeutic goal is to stabilize and support the patient for 24 hours. In addition, most patients require symptomatic management of specific problems (Stine, 1983). In selected circumstances, overdose victims or

users will suffer from seizures, arrhythmias, hyperthermia, hypertension, hypotension, behavioral problems, and rhabdomyolysis. When seizures occur, diazepam can be used to abort them. If the patient has recurrent seizures, phenytoin is used. Status epilepticus may require paralysis and ventilation.

For the treatment of ventricular arrhythmias and transient hypertension, propranolol or esmolol may be used to block adrenergic stimulation. In severe cases of hypertension, nitroprusside or phentolamine may be needed for control. Hyperthermia is managed with external cooling. This is especially important in pregnancy to protect the fetus. In cases of hypotension, treatment with IV fluids should be initiated. For refractory hypotension, dopamine or norepinephrine may be required.

Rhabdomyolysis is treated with maintenance and alkalinization of urine flow with IV fluids and sodium bicarbonate infusion. For behavioral problems, diazepam is used. During therapy, close monitoring of the fetus is essential. Evaluation may include ECG, BP, temperature, blood gases, chest x-ray, renal and liver function tests, prothrombin and partial thromboplastin times and platelets, hemoglobin/hematocrit, and urinalysis for myoglobin.

On discharge, the patient will need clinical follow-up with a social worker, obstetrician, or psychiatric service. Fetal follow-up will require ultrasound evaluations to monitor fetal growth and anatomy. Once the fetus is potentially viable, assessment of fetal well-being is warranted. In addition, evaluation of the newborn for cerebral, urologic, and gastrointestinal sequelae is indicated.

## Ethanol

### Background

According to the National Natality Survey, 39% of women admitted to alcohol use during their pregnancies. The prevalence of heavy or problem drinkers has been estimated to be 6% to 11% (Andres, 1994). Clinical presentation may vary with acute and/or chronic ethanol abuse or withdrawal. Only acute overdosage is considered here. With acute alcohol overdosage, the signs and symptoms vary depending on the severity of intoxication and may include euphoria, incoordination, impaired judgment, abnormal reflexes, ataxia, nystagmus, altered mental status, constricted pupils, and a characteristic smell on the breath. At the same time, social inhibitions are loosened. As such, aggressive or boisterous behavior is commonly seen. In severe overdose, hypothermia, bradycardia, hypotension, respiratory depression, hypoglycemia, respiratory distress, and coma are seen. To assess the patient with an acute ethanol overdose, blood glucose, electrolytes, BUN, creatinine, transaminases, prothrombin time, magnesium, arterial blood gases, or noninvasive oximetry are obtained (see Tables 35-6, 35-7). If aspiration is suspected, a chest x-ray should be obtained.

The most important short-term problems of a severe overdose are respiratory depression, pulmonary aspiration, hypoglycemia, and coma. Less frequently, gastrointestinal bleeding or rhabdomyolysis are encountered. Long-term problems are both organic and social. Organic problems include pancreatitis, hepatitis, cirrhosis, hepatic encephalopathy, portal hypertension, gastrointestinal bleeding, anemia, thiamine deficiency, alcoholic ketoacidosis, decreased resistance to infection, hypomagnesemia, hypokalemia, and hypophosphatemia. Social problems are manifested by malnutrition, isolation, depression, or suicide attempts.

The fetal signs of acute maternal alcohol ingestion are a decrease in fetal heart rate accelerations and variability, suppression of fetal breathing movements, and lower fetal weight. In the neonate, suppression of neonatal electrocorticographic activity and electrooculographic activity (Brien, 1991) is seen. The clinician should allow metabolism of the ethanol load before acting on a nonreassuring fetal heart rate pattern.

The major teratogenic potential of alcohol involves fetal alcohol syndrome (FAS), characterized by craniofacial dysmorphology (short palpebral fissures, ptosis, strabismus, epicanthal folds, myopia, microphthalmia, hypoplastic philtrum and maxilla, short upturned nose, posterior rotation of ears, poorly formed concha), prenatal growth deficiencies (body length more than weight), and CNS dysfunction (mild-to-moderate retardation, hypotonia, poor coordination, microcephaly). Other abnormalities, mainly cardiac, renogenital, and hemangiomas, are seen in at least 30% to 40% of exposed infants. Of note, the neonatal diagnosis of FAS may be delayed until 9 to 12 months of age.

Postnatally, the potential for withdrawal syndrome in neonates should be considered and the infant carefully monitored. Because ethanol passes freely into breast milk, there is the potential for sedation and dose-related psychomotor and developmental delay in breast-fed infants. In infants with FAS, the literature suggests an increased risk for the development of acute nonlymphocytic leukemia (Van Duija, 1994) and possibly other neoplasias.

### Clinical Management

With ethanol overdose, the therapeutic goal is to prevent acute complications in the first 6 to 8 hours following admission. Although the first step in ethanol overdose is decontamination, its use will depend on the proximity to the ingestion. Emesis is not indicated unless a substantial ingestion has occurred within minutes of presentation or other drug ingestion is suspected. Similarly, gastric lavage is indicated if there has been an intake of large amounts within 30 to 45 minutes of presentation. Of note, charcoal does not adsorb ethanol efficiently but may be useful if other drugs also were ingested. Respiratory depression and seizures may require treatment, and the airway should be protected because of the possibility of gastric aspiration.

While there is no specific antidote, flumazenil and naloxone may alleviate respiratory depression. There is anecdotal evidence for improved level of consciousness after the use of naloxone. Glucose and thiamine should be given routinely to ethanol overdose patients. During therapy, continuous pulse oximetry should be used if the patient is asleep or if the initial reading is abnormal. On discharge, clinical follow-up may involve a social worker, drug counselor, or obstetrician, and/or psychiatrist. Fetal follow-up will require ultrasound evaluations to monitor fetal growth.

## Opiates

### Background

Opiates are naturally occurring substances that are isolated from the *Papaver somniferum* poppy with the potential for addiction and overdose. In 1994, for example, there was a total of 6173 exposures. Of these, 3376 were adults, and 52 were fatal. The overdose rate in pregnancy was 0.9% (clinical patients, 1.1%; private patients, 0.7%) (Jones, 1994).

Maternal signs and symptoms of opiate overdose are variable and depend on the level of toxicity. Clinical signs of opiate overdose may include symmetrical miosis, altered level of consciousness, delirium, seizures, depressed respiration, pulmonary edema, cardiac arrhythmias, and coma. Of note, miosis may not be noted if anticholinergic drugs or meperidine have been coingested or if head trauma or hypoxia are involved. Maternal symptoms include nausea, vomiting, constipation, jitteriness, tremors, and involuntary muscle contractions.

Diagnostic tests should focus on confirmation of the opiate via urine and blood screens. In addition, maternal ECG, blood gases, and renal and liver function should generally be evaluated (see Table 35-6).

Short-term problems of opiate overdose relate primarily to maternal signs and symptoms. There is no increase in pregnancy complications such as preterm labor, premature rupture of the membranes, intrauterine fetal demise, or fetal distress (Gillogley, 1990; Sussman, 1965). Long-term problems relate to addiction and injuries sustained during the acute event.

In general, opiates are not considered to be clinically significant teratogens. In neonates, however, respiratory depression and other cardiovascular features seen in adult overdosage may be encountered. As with barbiturate use, withdrawal is a concern during the neonatal period.

### Clinical Management

With opiate overdose, the therapeutic goal is to maintain cardiovascular and respiratory function.

To do so, basic life support measures usually are necessary. Subsequent measures to reduce the opiate load are variable and depend on the circumstance. Dialysis and diuresis are not useful in eliminating opiates. In patients who have swallowed a large number of opiate-containing condoms ("body packers"), activated charcoal and cathartics or whole bowel irrigation may be indicated. In cases in which CNS depression is evident, surgical removal of the drug load may be life-saving.

Naloxone, a direct opiate receptor antagonist, is effective in reversing the respiratory depression, coma, miosis, analgesia, delayed gastric emptying, and cardiovascular depression that results from opiate overdose (see Table 35-21). For respiratory depression, a dose of 2 mg IV (adult or child) can be used initially. If there is no response in 2 to 3 minutes, the dose can be repeated up to a total of 10 mg before it should be regarded as ineffective. Naloxone may be given repeatedly due to its short duration of action (20–60 min). If repeated dosage is required, an hourly infusion of two thirds of the bolus dose that initially resulted in reversal of symptoms may be used and titrated to symptoms. Although IV administration is preferred, naloxone may be given intramuscularly, intralingually, intratracheally, or intraosseously. In a small number of cases, rapid naloxone administration has been associated with pulmonary edema, hypertension, dysrhythmias, and cardiac arrest. During the management of opiate overdose, maternal and fetal vital signs will need to be monitored, and an ECG and blood gases may be helpful.

On discharge, clinical follow-up with a social worker, obstetrician, and psychiatrist would be warranted. Frequent ultrasound evaluations are indicated to monitor for fetal growth problems. Once the fetus is potentially viable, antenatal assessment of fetal well-being may be warranted.

**REFERENCES**

Andres RL, Jones KL. Social and elicit drug use in pregnancy. In: Creasy RK, Resnik R, eds. Maternal-fetal medicine: principles and practice. 3rd ed. Philadelphia: WB Saunders, 1994:182.

Athinarayanan P, Pieroy SH, Nigan SK, Glass L. Chlordiazepoxide withdrawal in the neonate. Am J Obstet Gynecol 1976;124:212–213.

Balaskas TN. Common poisons. In: Gleicher N, Elkayam U, Galgraith RM, et al, eds. Principles and practice of medical therapy in pregnancy. 2nd ed. Norwalk, CT: Appleton and Lange, 1992: 236.

Bayer MJ, Rumack BH. Poisoning and overdose. Aspen Systems, 1983.

Berg MJ, Berlinger WG, Goldberg MJ, et al. Acceleration of the body clearance of phenobarbital by oral activated charcoal. N Engl J Med 1982; 507:642.

Biggs GG, Samaon JH, Crawford DJ. Lack of abnormalities in a newborn exposed to amphetamine during gestation. Am J Dis Child 1975;129:249–250.

Bingol N, Fuchs M, Diaz V. Teratogenicity of cocaine in humans. J Pediatr 1987;110:93–96.

Blagg CH. Acute complications associated with hemodialysis. In: Druker N, Parsons F, eds. Replacement of renal functions by dialysis. 2nd ed. Boston: Martinus-Njhoff, 1981:611–629.

Bleyer WA, Skinner AL. Fatal neonatal hemorrhage after maternal anticonvulsant therapy. JAMA 1976;235:826–827.

Bolgiano EB, Barish RA. Use of new and established antidotes. In: Emerg Med Clin North Am 1994;12:22–27.

Brien JF, Smith GN. Effects of alcohol (ethanol) on the fetus. J Dev Physiol 1991;15:21.

Briggs GG, Freeman RK, eds. Drugs in pregnancy and lactation. 4th ed. Baltimore: Williams and Wilkins, 1994.

Byer AJ, Taylor TR, Semmer JR. Acetaminophen overdose in the third trimester of pregnancy. JAMA 1982;247:3114–3115.

Chasnoff IJ, Burns KA, Burns WJ. Cocaine use in pregnancy: perinatal morbidity and mortality. Neurotoxicol Teratol 1987a;9:291–293.

Chasnoff IJ, MacGregor S. Maternal cocaine use and neonatal morbidity. Pediatr Res 1987b;21:356.

Chasnoff IJ, Griffith DR, MacGregor S, et al. Temporal patterns of cocaine use in pregnancy: perinatal outcome. JAMA 1989;261:1741–1744.

Desmond MM, Schwanecke PP, Wilson GS, et al. Maternal barbiturate utilization and neonatal withdrawal symptomatology. J Pediatr 1972;80: 190–197.

Dixon SD, Bejar R. Brain lesions in cocaine and methamphetamine exposed neonates. Pediatr Res 1988;23:405.

Doyon S, Roberts J. Reappraisal of the "coma cocktail." Emerg Med Clin North Am 1994;12:55–61.

Elliott JP, O'Keeffe DF, Schon DA, Cheron LB. Dialysis in pregnancy: a critical review. Obstet Gynecol Survey 1991;46:319–324.

Gay GR. Clinical management of acute and chronic cocaine poisoning. Ann Emerg Med 1982;11: 562.

Gillogley KM, Evans AT, Hansen RL, et al. The perinatal impact of cocaine, amphetamine and opiate use detected by universal intrapartum screening. Am J Obstet Gynecol 1990;163:1535–1542.

Gilstrap L III, Little BB. Drugs and pregnancy. New York: Elsevier, 1992.

Grinspoon L, Bakalan JB. Adverse effects of cocaine: selected issues. Ann NY Acad Sci 1981; 326:125.

Haddad LM, Winchester JF, eds. Clinical management of poisoning and drug overdose. 2nd ed. Philadelphia: WB Saunders, 1990.

Haibach H, Akhter JE, Muscato MS. Acetaminophen overdose with fetal demise. Am J Clin Pathol 1984;82:240–242.

Hardman JG, Limbird LE, eds. Goodman & Gilman's the pharmacological basis of therapeutic. 9th ed. New York: McGraw-Hill, 1996.

Hartz SC, Heinonen OP, Shapiro S, et al. Antenatal exposure to meprobamate and chlordiazepoxide in relation to malformations, mental development and childhood mortality. N Engl J Med 1975;292:726–728.

Hou S. Pregnancy in women on hemodialysis and peritoneal dialysis. Baillieres Clin Obstet Gynaecol 1994:481–500.

Hou S, Grossman SZ, Malius N. Pregnancy in women with renal disease and moderate renal insufficiency. Am J Med 1985;78:185–194.

Johnson T, Lorenz R, Menor KMJ, et al. Successful outcome of pregnancy requiring dialysis: effects on serum progesterone and estrogen. J Reprod Med 1979;22:217.

Jones KL. Effects of therapeutic, diagnostic and environmental agents. In: Creasy RK, Resnik R, eds. Maternal-fetal medicine: principles and practice. 3rd ed. Philadelphia: WB Saunders, 1994:171–181.

Korner WF, Weber F. Zur tolerenz hohr ascobinsauredosen. Int J Vitam Nutr Res 1972;42:528–544.

Kurtz GG, Michael OF, Morosi HJ, et al. Hemodialysis during pregnancy: report of a case of glutethamide poisoning complicated by acute renal failure. Arch Intern Med 1996;118:30.

Laegreid L, Olegard R, Wahlstrom J, et al. Abnormalities in children exposed to benzodiazepines in utero. Lancet 1987;1:108.

Levine SR, Brust JC, Futrell W, et al. A comparative study of the cerebrovascular complications of cocaine: alkaloid versus hydrochloride—a review. Neurology 1991;41:1173.

Levy G, Garretson LK, Socha DM. Evidence of placental transfer of acetaminophen. Pediatrics 1975;55:895.

Litovitz TL, Felberg L, Soloway RA, et al. 1994 Annual report of the American Association of Poison Control Centers Toxic Exposure Surveillance System. Am J Emerg Med 1995;13:551–597.

Little BB, Snell LM, Klein VR, Gilstrap LC. Cocaine abuse during pregnancy: maternal and fetal implication. Obstet Gynecol 1989;72:157–160.

Lumir J, Main DM, Landon MB, Gabbe SG. Maternal acetaminophen overdose at 15 weeks of gestation. Obstet Gynecol 1986;67:750–751.

MacGregor SN, Keith LG. Drug abuse during pregnancy. In: Rayburn RF, Zuspan FP, eds. Drug therapy in obstetrics and gynecology. 3rd ed. St. Louis: Mosby Year Book, 1992:164–189.

Marchand LL. Trends in birth defects for a Hawaiian population exposed to heptachlor and for the United States. Arch Environ Health 1986;41:145.

Matera C, Warren WB, Moomjy M, et al. Prevalence of use of cocaine and other substances in an obstetric population. Am J Obstet Gynecol 1990;163:797–801.

Milkovich L, van den Berg BJ. Effects of prenatal meprobamate and chlordiazepoxide, hydrochloride in human embryonic and fetal development. N Engl J Med 1974;291:1268–1271.

Moore TR, Sorg J, Miller L. Hemodynamic effects of intravenous cocaine on the pregnant ewe and fetus. Am J Obstet Gynecol 1989;155:883–888.

Mowry JB, Furbee RB, Chyka PA. Poisoning. In: Chernow B, Borater DC, Holaday JW, et al, eds. The pharmacological approach to the critically ill patient. 3rd ed. Baltimore: Williams and Wilkins, 1995.

Neerhof MG, MacGregor SN, Retzky SS, Sullivan JP. Cocaine abuse during pregnancy: peripartum prevalence and perinatal outcome. Am J Obstet Gynecol 1989;161:633–638.

Neuberg R. Drug dependence and pregnancy: a review of the problems and their management. J Obstet Gynaecol Br Cmwlth 1970;66:1117–1122.

Noji E, Kelen G. Manual of toxicologic emergencies. St. Louis: Year Book Medical, 1989.

Olson K. Poisoning and drug overdose. 2nd ed. Norwalk, CT: Appleton and Lange, 1994.

Oro AS, Dixon SD. Perinatal cocaine and methamphetamine exposure: maternal and neonatal correlates. J Pediatr 1987;111:571–578.

Peterson RG, Rumack BH. Toxicity of acetaminophen overdose. JACEP 1978;7:202.

Poisindex® toxicologic management. Micromedex. 1975–1995;84.

Pond SM. Principles of techniques used to enhance elimination of toxic compounds. In: Goldfrank LR, Flomenbaum NE, Lewin NA, et al, eds. Goldfrank's toxicologic emergencies, 4th ed. Norwalk, CT: Appleton and Lange, 1990:21–28.

Posner JB, Posner P. Spinal fluid pH and neurologic symptoms in systemic acidosis. N Engl J Med 1977;277:605.

Rayburn W, Anonow R, Delay B, Hogan MJ. Drug overdose during pregnancy: an overview from a metropolitan poison control center. Obstet Gynecol 1984;64:611.

Rayburn W, Shukla U, Stetson P, et al. Acetaminophen pharmacokinetics: comparison between pregnant and nonpregnant women. Am J Obstet Gynecol 1986;155:1353–1356.

Reynolds JR, Howland MA, Weisman RS. Pharmacokinetic and toxicokinetic principles. In: Goldfrank LR, Flomenbaum NE, Lewin NA, et al, eds. Goldfrank's toxicologic emergencies, 4th ed. Norwalk, CT: Appleton and Lange, 1990:29–38.

Riggs BS, Bronstein AC, Kuling K, et al. Acute acetaminophen overdose during pregnancy. Obstet Gynecol 1989;74:247–253.

Roberts JM. Pregnancy related hypertension. In: Creasy RK, Resnik R, eds. Maternal-fetal medicine: principles and practice. 3rd ed. Philadelphia: WB Saunders, 1994:804–843.

Rogers BD, Lee RV. Drugs abuse. In: Burrow GN, Ferris TF, eds. Medical complications during pregnancy. 3rd ed. Philadelphia: WB Saunders, 1988:570–581.

Rosenberg L, Mitchell AA, Parsells JL, et al. Lack of relation of oral clefts to diazepam use during pregnancy. N Engl J Med 1983;309:1282.

Rumack BH, Peterson RC, Koch GG, Amara IA. Acetaminophen overdose: 662 cases with evaluation of oral acetylcysteine treatment. Arch Intern Med 1981;141:380.

Rumack BH, Matthew H. Acetaminophen poisoning and toxicity. Pediatrics 1975;55:871.

Safra MJ, Oakley JP. Association between cleft lip with and without cleft palate and prenatal exposure to diazepam. Lancet 1975;2:478.

Sanchez-Casajus, Ramos I, Sanchez M. Hemodialysis durante el embrarrazo. Rev Clin Esp 1978;149:187–188.

Saxen I, Saxen L. Association between maternal intake of diazepam and oral clefts. Lancet 1975; 2:498.

Shannon BE, Jenkins JL, Loscalzo J. Poisoning and ingestion. In: Jenkins JL, Loscalzo J, eds. Manual of emergency medicine—diagnosis and treatment. 2nd ed. 1995:417–469.

Shiono PH, Mills JL. Oral clefts and diazepam use during pregnancy. N Engl J Med 1984;311:920.

Shubert PJ, Savage B. Smoking, alcohol and drug abuse. In: James DK, Stein RJ, Weiner CP, Gonik B, eds. High risk pregnancy management options. Philadelphia: WB Saunders, 1994:51–66.

Stine RJ, Marcus RH. Toxicologic emergencies. In: Haddad LM, Winchester JF, eds. Clinical management of poisoning and drug overdose. Philadelphia: WB Saunders, 1983:297–342.

Stokes IM. Paracetamol overdose in the second trimester of pregnancy—case report. Br J Obstet Gynaecol 1984;91:286–288.

Sussman S. Narcotic and methamphetamine use during pregnancy: effect on newborn and infants. Am J Dis Child 1965;106:325–330.

Telsey AM, Merrit TA, Dixon SD. Cocaine exposure in a term neonate: necrotizing enterocolitis as a complication. Clin Pediatr 1988;27:547–550.

Thorp J. Management of drug dependency, overdose, and withdrawal in the obstetric patient. Obstet Gynecol Clin North Am 1995;22.

Unzelman RF, Alderfer GR, Chojnacki RE. Pregnancy and chronic hemodialysis. Trans Am Soc Artif Intern Organs 1973;129:141.

VanDuija CM, vanSteensel-Moll HA, Coebergh JW, et al. Risk factors for childhood acute non-lymphocytic leukemia association with maternal alcohol consumption during pregnancy. Cancer Epidemiol Biomarkers Prev 1994;3:457.

Victor M, Adams RD. Barbiturates. In: Isselbacher KS, Adams RD, Braunswald E, et al, eds. Principles of internal medicine. 9th ed. New York: McGraw-Hill, 1980:982–985.

Weisman RS, Howland MA, Flomenbaum NE. The toxicology laboratory. In: Goldfrank LR, Flomenbaum NE, Lewin NA, et al. Goldfrank's toxicologic emergencies. 4th ed. Norwalk, CT: Appleton and Lange, 1990:45–46.

Winchester JF, Gelfand MC, Knepshield JH, Schreiner GE. Dialysis and hemoperfusion of poisons and drugs update. Trans Am Soc Artif Intern Organs 1977;23:762.

Yasin SY, BeyDoun SW. Hemodialysis in pregnancy. Obstet Gynecol Survey 1988;43:655–668.

Zuckerman B, Frank DA, Hingson R, et al. Effects of maternal marijuana and cocaine use on fetal growth. N Engl J Med 1989;320:762–768.

# $\mathcal{P}$ART **IV**

# Fetal Consideration

# CHAPTER 36

# Fetal Considerations in the Critically Ill Gravida

*U*nlike any other medical or surgical specialty, obstetrics deals with the simultaneous management of two—and sometimes more—individuals. Under all circumstances, the obstetrician must delicately balance the effects of each treatment decision on the pregnant woman and her fetus, seeking always to minimize the risks of harm to each. Throughout this text, the primary focus has been on the critically ill obstetric patient and, secondarily, her fetus. Although the fetal effects of those illnesses were reviewed in part, the goal of this chapter is to highlight, especially for the non-obstetric clinician, the important clinical fetal considerations encountered when caring for these high-risk mothers. To achieve that objective, this chapter reviews (1) current techniques for assessing fetal well-being, (2) fetal considerations in several maternal medical and surgical conditions, and (3) the role of perimortem cesarean delivery in modern obstetrics.

## Detection of Fetal Distress in the Critically Ill Obstetric Patient

More than two decades ago, Hon and Quilligan (1968a) demonstrated the relationship between certain fetal heart rate (FHR) patterns and fetal condition by using continuous electronic FHR monitoring. Since then, continuous electronic FHR monitoring has remained a universally ac-

cepted method of assessing fetal well-being (Paul, 1980; Shenker, 1990), which permits the clinician to promptly identify fetuses at a greater likelihood of fetal death and to intervene when certain FHR abnormalities are present.

Although the presence of a reassuring FHR tracing is virtually always associated with a well-perfused and oxygenated fetus, an abnormal tracing is not necessarily predictive of an adverse fetal outcome. While it was anticipated that the detection of abnormal FHR patterns during labor and expeditious delivery of such fetuses might impact the subsequent development of cerebral palsy, this expectation has clearly not been fulfilled. Despite the ubiquitous use of electronic FHR monitoring during labor and a rise in the cesarean section rate from 5% to over 20% in the past two decades, a corresponding decline in the rate of cerebral palsy has not been seen. Indeed, a recent report documented a 99.8% false-positive rate of ominous FHR patterns for the subsequent development of cerebral palsy (Nelson, 1996).

Although it is now generally accepted that the specific entity of cerebral palsy is, in almost all cases, related to prenatal developmental events or complications of prematurity, the basic physiologic observations relating hypoxia and acidemia to specific FHR patterns remain, for the most part, valid. Because the critically ill mother will shunt blood from the splanchnic bed (including the uterus) in response to shock, and because the fetus operates on the steep portion of the oxyhemoglobin dissociation curve, any degree of hypoxia or hypoperfusion in the mother may first be manifest as an abnormality of the FHR. In this sense, the late second- and third-trimester fetus acts as a physiologic oximeter and cardiac output computer. Observation of FHR changes, thus, may assist the clinician in managing the mother, as well as alerting him or her to subtle degrees of physiologic instability, which would be unimportant in a nonpregnant adult but may have detrimental effects on the fetus (Clark, 1990).

The next few pages present an overview of FHR patterns pertinent to the critically ill patient; certain of these observations may not generally apply to the laboring but otherwise well mother. For a more detailed description of antepartum and intrapartum FHR tracings, the reader is referred to the classic descriptions by Hon (1968b).

## Baseline Fetal Heart Rate

The baseline FHR is the intrinsic heart rate of the fetus. A normal baseline FHR is between 110 beats per minute (bpm) and 160 bpm. A baseline FHR less than 100 bpm is termed a *bradycardia,* and 160 bpm or higher is considered a tachycardia.

### Bradycardia

*Bradycardia* is defined as the intrinsic heart rate of the fetus of less than 110 bpm and is subclassified as follows: mild (100–110 bpm) and marked (< 100 bpm). An FHR bradycardia is associated with an underlying congenital fetal abnormality, such as a structural defect of the fetal heart. In addition, congenital bradyarrhythmias may involve fetal heart block secondary to a prior maternal infection, a structural defect of the fetal heart, or a systemic lupus erythematosus (Lee, 1984). In these circumstances, an FHR bradycardia is not an indicator of hypoxia, and alternative methods of fetal assessment, such as the fetal biophysical profile (FBP) (Manning, 1990), may be necessary to assure fetal well-being.

## Prolonged Fetal Heart Rate Deceleration

Prolonged FHR deceleration is distinctly different from a bradycardia. In the latter circumstance, the baseline FHR was previously normal (110–160 bpm), but due to acute events, such as a uterine rupture, the FHR has dropped and remains at a lower level. In the critically ill obstetric patient with hypertension, preeclampsia, or trauma, a common cause of a prolonged FHR deceleration is an abruption of the placenta. Intrapartum, a prolonged FHR deceleration also may be associated with fetal conditions that cause umbilical cord compression, such as cord prolapse, nuchal cord, oligohydramnios, or uterine hypertonus. Investigators also have described the presence of a prolonged FHR deceleration in association with the overaggressive lowering of maternal BP with antihypertensive agents (Rigg, 1981). In addition, an acute, prolonged FHR deceleration may herald sudden maternal hypoxia in conditions such as amniotic fluid embolus syndrome, acute respiratory insufficiency, or eclamptic seizure (Paul, 1978). Prolonged FHR decelerations have been described in patients undergoing cardiopulmonary bypass (Koh, 1975). It is believed that this pattern is the result of inadequate maternal flow rates during cardiopulmonary bypass and may be alleviated with higher flow rates (Koh, 1975). In addition, fetuses whose mothers are undergoing neurosurgical procedures with hypothermia also may exhibit a slowing of the heart rate (Strange, 1983).

In a patient with a prior normal baseline FHR, the abrupt occurrence and persistence of a fetal heart rate of less than 110 bpm for an extended period generally constitute an obstetric emergency and require either prompt correction of the precipitating cause or immediate delivery.

### Tachycardia

*Fetal tachycardia* is defined as a baseline FHR of 160 bpm or greater and is subclassified as follows: mild (160–180 bpm) and marked (> 180 bpm). Most commonly, this type of baseline FHR abnormality is associated with prematurity, maternal pyrexia, or chorioamnionitis (Fig 36-1). In addition, beta-mimetic administration, hyperthyroidism, or fetal cardiac arrhythmias may produce an FHR tachycardia. The clinical observation of an FHR tachycardia, in and of itself, is not an ominous finding but probably reflects a normal physiologic adjustment to an underlying maternal or fetal condition. Although operative intervention is rarely required, a search for the underlying basis for the tachycardia may be necessary.

The patient with a previously normal FHR pattern (Fig 36-2) who develops an FHR tachycardia (Figs 36-3, 36-4) in the absence of maternal pyrexia and in association with a loss of accelerations, repetitive FHR decelerations, and diminished FHR variability is at risk for hypoxic ischemic injury (Phelan, 1994a). As before, assessment of the usual causes of FHR tachycardia should be undertaken. If none is identified, the patient should undergo assessment of fetal acid-base status or delivery as soon as it is practical.

## Fetal Heart Rate Variability

*Fetal heart rate variability* is defined as the beat-to-beat variation in the FHR resulting from the continuous interaction of the parasympathetic and sympathetic nervous systems on the fetal heart. For clinical purposes, normal FHR variability may be viewed as a beat-to-beat variation of the FHR of 6 bpm or more above and below the baseline FHR.

Decreased FHRV, in and of itself, is not an ominous observation. In most cases, the diminished FHRV represents normal fetal physiologic adjustments to a number of medications or simply behavioral state changes such as IF and IV F (Smith, 1994). For example, narcotic administration (Petrie, 1978) or magnesium sulfate infusion (Babakania, 1978) can decrease FHRV by inducing a sleep state or behavioral state IF. Clinically, diminished FHRV has meaning in apparently only one selected circumstance (Phelan, 1994a). Here (see Figs 36-2, 36-3, 36-4), the diminished FHRV should be associated with a loss of FHR reactivity, a substantial change in the baseline FHR, an FHR tachycardia, and repetitive FHR decelerations (Phelan, 1994a). Under these circumstances, the potential for fetal asphyxia appears to be increased.

## Sinusoidal Fetal Heart Rate Pattern

A *sinusoidal FHR pattern* is defined as a regular sine wave variation of the baseline FHR that has a frequency of 3 to 6 cycles per minute (Clark, 1984a). The degree of oscillation correlates with fetal outcome (Katz, 1984). For instance, infants with oscillations of 25 bpm or more have a significantly greater perinatal mortality rate than do

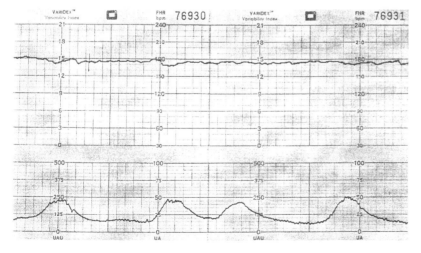

F I G U R E  **36-1**

Baseline FHR tachycardia in a pregnancy complicated by maternal fever due to chorioamnionitis.

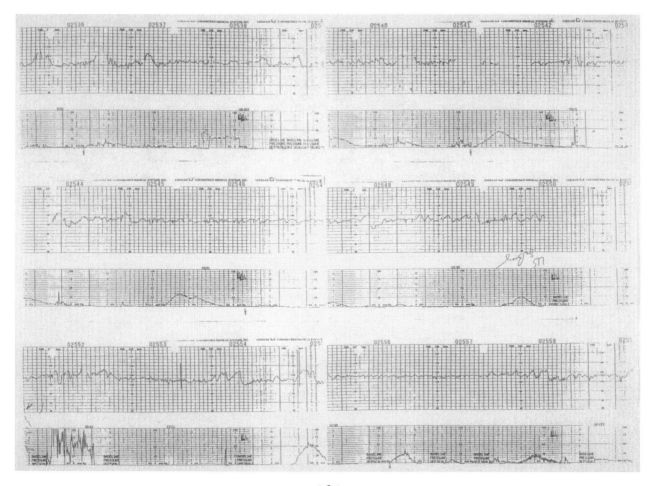

F I G U R E    **36-2**

The admission FHR of a term pregnancy exhibits numerous FHR accelerations or a reactive FHR pattern.

infants whose oscillations are less than 25 bpm (67% vs. 1%). A favorable fetal outcome also is associated with the presence of FHR accelerations and/or a nonpersistent sinusoidal FHR pattern.

Regardless, the key to the management of a persistent sinusoidal FHR pattern is recognition. Once this FHR pattern is identified, a search for the underlying cause should be undertaken. One common cause for intermittent sinusoidal FHR pattern is maternal narcotic administration, such as alphaprodine or meperidine (Epstein, 1982; Modanlou, 1982). In the absence of maternal narcotic administration, the presence of a persistent sinusoidal FHR pattern suggests fetal anemia.

Fetal anemia may be associated with placental abruption or previa, fetomaternal hemorrhage, vasa previa, Rh sensitization, and nonimmune hydrops (Modanlou, 1982). If, for example, a persistent sinusoidal FHR pattern is observed in a patient who recently has been involved in a motor vehicle accident, the diagnosis of placental abruption would be one consideration. Evidence of an abruption or other forms of fetal hemorrhage may also be suggested by a positive Kleihauer-Betke test for fetal RBCs in the maternal circulation. Finally, as suggested by Katz and associates (1984), a persistent sinusoidal FHR pattern in the absence of accelerations is a sign of potential

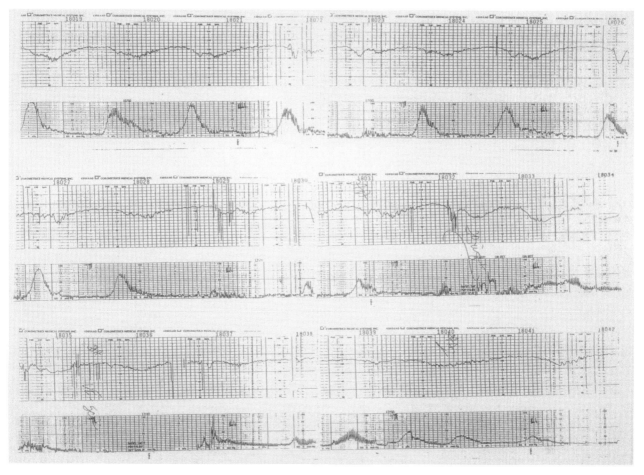

F I G U R E   **36-3**
Sometime later, the fetus exhibits an FHR tachycardia of 160 to
170 bpm, repetitive FHR decelerations, and diminished FHR variability.

fetal hypoxia with acidemia. In this latter circumstance, either delivery or some form of fetal acid-
base assessment can be considered (Theard,
1984). Often, patients with a persistent sinusoidal FHR pattern will have a history of reduced
fetal activity and, occasionally, an abnormal
Kleihauer-Betke test.

## Periodic Changes

Fetal heart rate decelerations are usually benign
and frequently reflect changes in the intrauterine
environment. The focus of this section is on FHR
accelerations, as well as variable and late decelerations. Fetal heart rate decelerations, in and of
themselves, are not associated necessarily with
an increased perinatal morbidity and mortality
(Phelan, 1994a).

## Accelerations

An *FHR acceleration* is defined as an abrupt increase in the FHR above baseline, spontaneously
or in relation to uterine activity (Fig 36-5), fetal
body movement (Fig 36-6), or fetal breathing.
Criteria for FHR accelerations (i.e., a ''reactive''

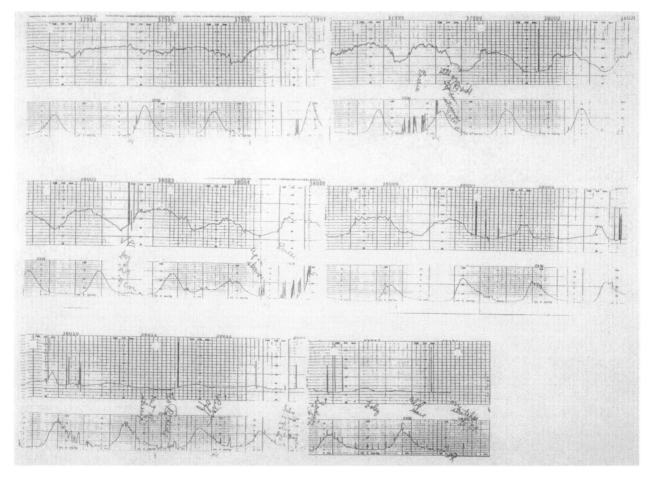

FIGURE 36-4

Later in the labor, the FHR pattern has continued, but near the end, the FHR shows a progressive bradycardia or what this author terms a *stair steps to death pattern.* This fetus was born with hypoxic ischemic encephalopathy and later died.

tracing) include a rise in the FHR of at least 15 bpm from baseline, lasting at least 15 seconds from the time it leaves baseline until it returns (Phelan, 1982a, 1988a, 1994b). Whenever spontaneous or induced FHR accelerations are present, significant fetal metabolic acidosis is absent. This is true, regardless of whether otherwise worrisome features of the FHR tracing are present (Lee, 1975; Clark, 1982, 1984b; Smith, 1986; Shaw, 1988). The presence of FHR accelerations is the basis for the nonstress test (NST) as a primary form of fetal surveillance to assess fetal well-being (Phelan, 1982a, 1988a, 1994b).

In the pregnant patient, the presence of FHR accelerations has been shown to be a sign of fetal well-being with a low probability of fetal compromise (Phelan, 1982a) or death within several days to a week (Phelan, 1982b). This observation persists irrespective of the method used to generate the acceleration, for example, mechanical (Druzin, 1985) or sound stimulation (Smith, 1985, 1986a,b; Phelan, 1993a; Clark, 1989), scalp sampling (Clark, 1982), or scalp stimulation (Clark, 1984b). In contrast, the fetus with a persistent nonreactive FHR pattern lasting longer than 120 minutes has significantly greater

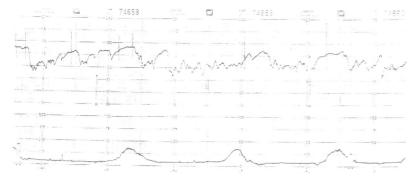

F I G U R E   **36-5**

Intrapartum FHR tracing with a normal baseline FHR and FHR accelerations.

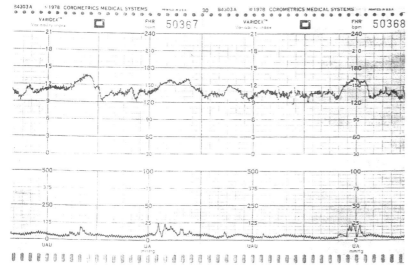

F I G U R E   **36-6**

Antepartum FHR pattern illustrating FHR accelerations in response to apparent fetal movement.

probability of an adverse fetal outcome (Phelan, 1994a; Leveno, 1983; Brown, 1981). Often, a persistent nonreactive FHR pattern with a fixed or wandering baseline heart rate may represent underlying chronic fetal brain injury (Phelan, 1994a), a structurally abnormal fetus (Garite, 1979), or a fetus with a chromosomal anomaly (Slomka, 1981).

To assist in the assessment of fetal health, acoustic stimulation of the fetus has been developed and permits prompt and immediate assessment of fetal status (Smith, 1985, 1986a,b; Phelan, 1993a; Clark, 1989). A transabdominal vibroacoustic stimulus can be applied with an electronic artificial larynx (EAL), a Model 5C (American Telephone Telegraph, New York), or a Corometrics Acoustic Stimulator (Wallingford,

CT). The EAL emits a fundamental frequency of 80 Hz and a sound pressure level averaging 82 decibels (dB) at 1 m through air.

Briefly, the clinical approach to antepartum fetal assessment begins with monitoring the baseline FHR for a reasonable period to determine the presence of fetal reactivity. If the test is nonreactive, a sound stimulus is applied for 3 seconds or less. If no response is observed, the stimulus may be repeated. With this approach, the incidence of nonreactive test results were reduced 50% when compared with historical controls (Smith, 1985), and overall testing time declined (Smith, 1986b). Most important, the predictive reliability of the reactive test was unchanged (Smith, 1986b). If, after acoustic stimulation, the fetus has a persistent nonreactive pattern, the contraction stress test (Phelan, 1989a) or the FBP (Manning, 1980, 1990; Phelan, 1988a) are two options that can be used to evaluate fetal status.

The performance of an FBP (Table 36-1) requires real-time ultrasound. Since the introduction of the FBP, this technique has been modified to include the four-quadrant technique (amniotic fluid index) to estimate the amniotic fluid volume (Fig 36-7). Using this approach, the clinician divides the uterus into four quadrants. The linea nigra divides the uterus into right and left halves, while the umbilicus divides it into upper and lower halves. The vertical diameter of the largest pocket in each of these quadrants is determined with the transducer perpendicular to the floor. The summation of these four values provides a single number known as the amniotic fluid index (AFI). From the prior work of Phelan and associates (1987, 1993b), an AFI ≤5.0 cm is considered oligohydramnios. Consequently, if a patient has an AFI ≤5.0 cm, her FBP score for that component will be 0. Additional components of the FBP include fetal breathing movements, fetal limb movements, fetal tone, and reactivity on an NST. Based on the presence or absence of each component, the patient receives 0 or 2 points.

An FBP score of 8 or 10 is considered normal (see Table 36-1). In patients whose score is 6, the

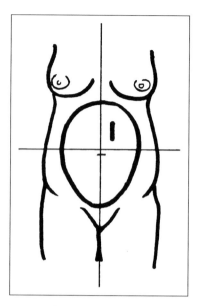

F I G U R E   **36-7**
**The technique for the performance of the amniotic fluid index.** (Reproduced from Phelan, 1993b, with permission from the author.)

test is considered equivocal or suspicious. In such patients, repeat FBP is performed within 12 to 24 hours. If the patient is considered to be term, she should be evaluated for delivery (Phelan, 1988a). The patient with a biophysical profile score of 0, 2, or 4 is considered for delivery.

T A B L E   **36-1**

Fetal biophysical profile components required over a 30-minute period*

| Components | Normal Result | Score |
|---|---|---|
| Nonstress test | Reactive | 2 |
| Fetal breathing movements | Duration ≥ 1 min | 2 |
| Fetal movement | ≥3 movements | 2 |
| Fetal tone | Flexion and extension of limb | 2 |
| Amniotic fluid volume | Amniotic fluid index >5.0 cm | 2 |
| | Maximum score   =  | 10 |

Components of the FBP (Phelan, 1981), which includes the modification for determining the amniotic fluid volume using the amniotic fluid index (Phelan, 1987, 1993b).

*This represents one approach to the fetal biophysical profile.

## Variable Decelerations

As implied by the name, *variable FHR decelerations* have a variable or non-uniform shape and bear no consistent relationship to a uterine contraction. The decline in rate is rapid and is followed by a quick recovery. Umbilical cord compression leading to an increased fetal BP and baroreceptor response is felt to be the most likely etiology. Umbilical cord compression is more likely to occur in circumstances of an abnormal cord position, such as nuchal cords, knots, prolapse (Phelan, 1981), or a diminished amniotic fluid volume (Gabbe, 1976; Phelan, 1989b).

To simplify labor management, investigators such as Kubli et al (1969) and Krebs et al (1983) have attempted to classify variable decelerations.

For example, Kubli and associates have correlated fetal outcome with mild, moderate, or severe variable decelerations. Kubli's criteria, however, are cumbersome and do not lend themselves to easy clinical use. In contrast, Krebs et al (1983) have advocated a method of interpretation that relies on the visual characteristics of the variable decelerations rather than on the degree or amplitude of the FHR deceleration. These investigators have shown that when repetitive, atypical variable decelerations are present over a prolonged period in a patient with a previously normal FHR tracing, the risk of fetal acidosis is increased. These atypical features (Fig 36-8) include (1) loss of the initial FHR acceleration and loss of the secondary FHR acceleration, (2) prolonged acceleration after the deceleration, (3) decreased FHR variability within the deceleration, (4) baseline rate continuation at a level lower than that preceding the deceleration, (5) a biphasic deceleration, and (6) delayed return of the FHR to baseline. The potential for an adverse fetal outcome, such as a low Apgar, is greater with persistent atypical variable FHR decelerations than is seen in patients with

FIGURE   **36-8**

**Atypical variable FHR decelerations.** (From Krebs HB, Petres RE, Dunn LH. Intrapartum fetal heart rate monitoring. VII. Atypical variable decelerations. Am J Obstet Gynecol 1983;145:305–310. Reproduced with permission from CV Mosby Co, St. Louis, MO.)

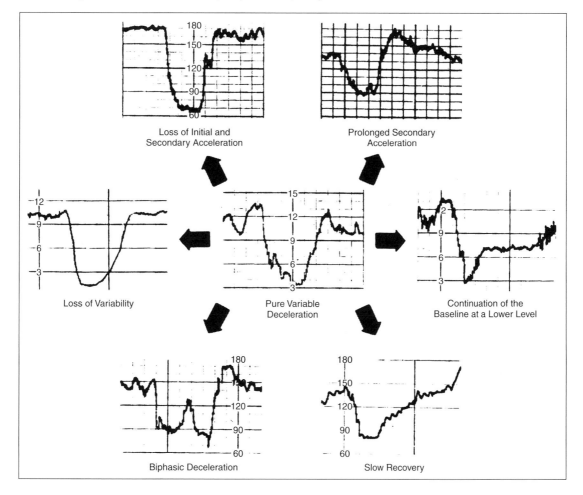

"typical" variable decelerations. Consequently, whenever persistent, atypical variable FHR decelerations are present in association with a substantial rise in baseline FHR, an absence of accelerations, and a loss of FHRV (see Figs 36-2, 36-3, 36-4), the patient should be considered for fetal acid-base assessment and/or delivery.

## Late Decelerations

*Late decelerations* are a uniform deceleration pattern with onset at or beyond the peak of the uterine contraction, the nadir in heart rate at the offset of the uterine contraction, and a subsequent return to baseline (Fig 36-9). To be signif-

icant clinically, late decelerations must be repetitive (i.e., occur with each contraction of similar magnitude and be associated with a substantial rise in baseline FHR, a loss of reactivity, and a diminished FHRV) (Phelan, 1994a). The mechanism for this FHR pattern is fetal hypoxia.

In any patient who presents with this FHR pattern, a search for the underlying etiology is helpful. A review of her history may give some clue as to the basis of this abnormality. For instance, trauma victims with placental abruption or patients in hypovolemic shock may manifest repetitive late decelerations on the fetal monitor. In addition, patients with underlying vascular disease resulting from diabetes mellitus, sickle cell

F I G U R E   **36-9**

Two late decelerations of the fetal heart rate during labor.

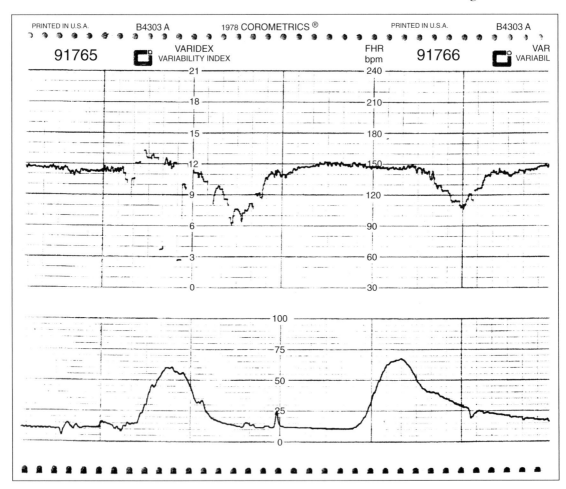

crisis, hypertensive disease, or systemic lupus erythematosus may have fetuses that manifest this FHR pattern.

Whenever repetitive late decelerations are observed, the pregnant woman should be positioned on her side, oxygen should be administered, intravenous fluids should be increased, and a search should be made for a correctable underlying cause (e.g., hypotension). If this repetitive pattern persists in the presence of nonreactivity, a substantial rise of the baseline FHR, and absent or diminished FHRV, fetal acid-base assessment and/or delivery should be considered.

Treatable causes of late decelerations can occasionally be seen, especially in women with diabetic ketoacidosis (LoBue, 1978; Rhodes, 1984), sickle cell crisis (Cruz, 1979), or anaphylaxis (Klein, 1984; Witter, 1983). With correction of the underlying maternal metabolic abnormality, the FHR abnormality may resolve, and operative intervention is often unnecessary. Persistence of the FHR pattern after maternal metabolic recovery, however, may suggest an underlying fetal diabetic cardiomyopathy (Sheehan, 1986) or preexisting fetal compromise and should, when accompanied by the aforementioned additional signs of fetal compromise, lead to fetal acid-base assessment or delivery.

## Fetal Acid-Base Assessment

In the past, fetal acid-base status was thought to be an integral part of labor management. Fetal scalp blood sampling was first described by Saling (1964). He found that infants with a pH less than 7.2 were more likely to be delivered physiologically depressed. Conversely, a normal fetal outcome was more likely to be associated with a nonacidotic fetus (pH > 7.20) (Saling, 1967). Even at the peak of its popularity, fetal scalp blood sampling was used in a limited number of pregnancies (~3%) (Clark, 1985a).

In many institutions, fetal scalp sampling is technically not feasible because of the lack of readily available equipment. Additionally, the technique is cumbersome and time consuming. Fetal scalp sampling also requires a dilated cervix. Nevertheless, clinical circumstances today

may dictate in a rare patient the need to know precise fetal acid-base status. Rather than employ scalp sampling techniques, alternative noninvasive methods have been developed (Smith, 1986a, 1994; Phelan, 1994b; Clark, 1982, 1984b).

A historical review of noninvasive techniques to assess fetal acid-base status reveals that the presence of FHR accelerations (Table 36-2), spontaneous or evoked, is associated with normal fetal acid-base status (Clark, 1982, 1984b; Smith, 1986a). In key studies, Clark et al (1982, 1984a) and Smith et al (1986a), using scalp and acoustic stimulation, demonstrated that a loss of reactivity was associated with a significantly greater likelihood of fetal acid-base abnormality.

Therefore, as part of the management of the critically ill obstetric patient with an abnormal FHR pattern, either scalp or acoustic stimulation of the fetus appears to be a reasonable alternative to scalp blood sampling, and the latter technique is rarely used outside of select teaching institutions today.

## Maternal and Surgical Conditions

### Anaphylaxis

*Anaphylaxis* is an acute allergic reaction to food ingestion or drugs. It is generally associated with rapid onset of pruritus and urticaria and may result in respiratory distress, vascular collapse, and shock. Medicines, primarily penicillins; food substances, such as shellfish; exercise; and contrast dyes are common causes of anaphylaxis (Van Arsdel, 1981; Reisman, 1989).

TABLE  36-2

The likelihood of fetal acid-base abnormality in patients with or without a spontaneous or evoked FHR acceleration

| | **Fetal pH** | |
|---|---|---|
| FHR pattern | < 7.20 | ≥ 7.20 |
| Reactive | 1 (0.3%) | 278 (99.7%) |
| Nonreactive | 65 (46%) | 76 (54%) |

Reproduced by permission from Phelan JP. Labor admission test. Clin Perinatol 1994b;21:879–885.

When an anaphylactic reaction occurs during pregnancy, the accompanying maternal physiologic changes may result in fetal distress. In a case described by Klein and associates (1984), a woman at 29 weeks' gestation presented with an acute allergic reaction after eating shellfish. On admission, she had evidence of regular uterine contractions and repetitive, severe late decelerations. The fetal distress was believed to be the result of maternal hypotension and relative hypovolemia, which accompanied the allergic reaction. Prompt treatment of the patient with intravenous fluids and ephedrine corrected the fetal distress. Subsequently, the patient delivered a healthy male infant at term with normal Apgar scores.

As suggested by these investigators and by Witter and Niebyl (1983), while acute maternal allergic reactions do pose a threat to the fetus, treatment directed at the underlying cause often remedies the accompanying fetal distress. To afford the fetus a wider margin of safety, efforts should be directed at maintaining maternal systolic BP above 90 mm Hg. In addition, oxygen should be administered to correct maternal hypoxia; in the absence of maternal hypervolemia, a maternal $Pao_2$ in excess of 60 to 70 mm Hg will assure adequate fetal oxygenation (Klein, 1984; Witter, 1983). A persistent fetal tachycardia or other abnormal FHR patterns suggest the need for additional maternal hemodynamic support or oxygenation, even in the nominally "stable" mother.

## Eclampsia

Maternal seizures are a well-known but infrequent sequel of preeclampsia. Although the maternal hemodynamic findings in patients with eclampsia are similar to those with severe preeclampsia (Clark, 1985b), maternal convulsions require prompt attention to prevent harm to both mother and fetus (Naidu, 1996; Lucas, 1995). During a seizure, the fetal response usually is manifested as an abrupt, prolonged FHR deceleration (Paul, 1978; Boehm, 1974). The theoretical underpinnings for the observed FHR changes are illustrated in Figure 36-10. During the seizure, which generally lasts less than 1.5 minutes (Paul, 1978), transient maternal hypoxia and uterine artery

vasospasm occur and combine to produce a decline in uterine blood flow. In addition, uterine activity increases secondary to the release of norepinephrine, resulting in additional reduction in uteroplacental perfusion. Ultimately, the reduction of uteroplacental perfusion causes the FHR deceleration. Such a deceleration may last up to 9 minutes (Paul, 1978). Following the seizure and recovery from the FHR deceleration, a loss of FHRV and a compensatory rise in baseline FHR are characteristically seen. Transient late decelerations are not uncommon but resolve once maternal metabolic recovery is complete.

The cornerstone of patient management during an eclamptic seizure is to maintain adequate maternal oxygenation and to administer appropriate anticonvulsants. After a convulsion occurs, an adequate airway should be maintained and oxygen administered. To optimize uteroplacental perfusion, the mother is repositioned onto her side. Anticonvulsant therapy with intravenous magnesium sulfate (Naidu, 1996; Lucas, 1995; Pritchard, 1984) to prevent seizure recurrence is recommended. In spite of adequate magnesium sulfate therapy, adjunctive anticonvulsant therapy

F I G U R E **36-10**

**The theoretical basis for the observed FHR changes associated with eclampsia.**

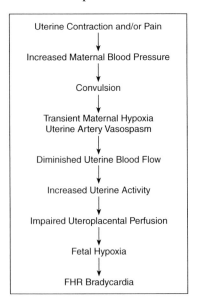

occasionally may be necessary (Paul, 1978; Pritchard, 1984). In the event of a persistent FHR deceleration, intrauterine resuscitation with a betamimetic (Barrett, 1984) or additional magnesium sulfate (Reece, 1984) may be helpful in relieving eclampsia-induced uterine hypertonus. Continuous electronic fetal monitoring should be used to follow the fetal condition. After the mother has been stabilized, and if the fetus continues to show signs of distress after a reasonable recovery period, assessment of fetal acid-base status (Phelan, 1993a) and/or delivery would be indicated.

## Disseminated Intravascular Coagulopathy

Disseminated intravascular coagulopathy (DIC) occurs in a variety of obstetric conditions, such as abruptio placenta, amniotic fluid embolus syndrome, and the dead fetus syndrome. The pathophysiology of this condition is discussed in greater detail in Chapter 29.

Infrequently, DIC may be advanced to a point of overt bleeding (Porter, 1996). Under these circumstances, laboratory abnormalities accompany the clinical evidence of consumptive coagulopathy. In the rare circumstance of overt fetal distress and a clinically apparent maternal coagulopathy, obstetric management requires prompt replacement of deficient coagulation components before attempting to deliver the distressed fetus. This frequently requires balancing the interests of the pregnant woman with those of her unborn child.

For example, a 34-year-old woman presented to the hospital at 33 weeks' gestation with the FHR tracing illustrated in Figure 36-11. Real-time sonography demonstrated asymmetrical intrauterine growth retardation. Oxygen was administered, and the patient was repositioned on her left side. Appropriate laboratory studies were drawn, and informed consent for a cesarean was obtained. When a Foley catheter was inserted, grossly bloody urine was observed. The previously drawn blood did not clot, and she was observed to be bleeding from the site of her intravenous line. The abnormal FHR pattern persisted.

In this circumstance, the interests of the mother and fetus are at odds with one another,

and a difficult clinical decision must now be made. Whose interest does the obstetrician protect in this instance? Immediate surgical intervention without blood products would lessen the mother's chances of survival. If the clinician waits for fresh-frozen plasma and platelets infusion before undertaking surgery, however, the fetus will be exposed to a significant risk of death or permanent neurologic impairment. Ideally, the mother and/or her family should participate in such decisions. In reality, because of the unpredictable nature of these dilemmas and the need for rapid decision making, family involvement often is not possible. Under such circumstances, it is axiomatic that maternal interests take precedence over those of the fetus, especially given the poor predictive value of an abnormal FHR tracing (Nelson, 1996).

Because blood products were not readily available, the decision was made to move the patient to the operating room. Once she was in the operating room, the clinical management should be to oxygenate the mother; maintain her in the left lateral recumbent position; have an anesthesiologist, operating room personnel, and surgeons present; and be prepared to operate. As soon as the blood products were available, she was infused with fresh-frozen plasma, platelets, and packed cells, and the cesarean was begun under general anesthesia. Maternal and fetal outcomes for this case were ultimately favorable.

In summary, the cornerstone of management of the patient with full-blown DIC and clinically apparent fetal distress is to correct the maternal clotting abnormality before initiating surgery. While waiting for the blood products to be infused, the patient should be prepared and ready for immediate cesarean delivery. If the fetus dies in the interim, the cesarean should not be performed; and, the patient should be given the opportunity to deliver vaginally.

## The Burn Victim

Although burn victims are uncommonly encountered in high-risk obstetric units, the pregnant burn patient is sufficiently complex to require a team approach to enhance maternal and perinatal survival (Smith, 1983; Matthews, 1982; Daw,

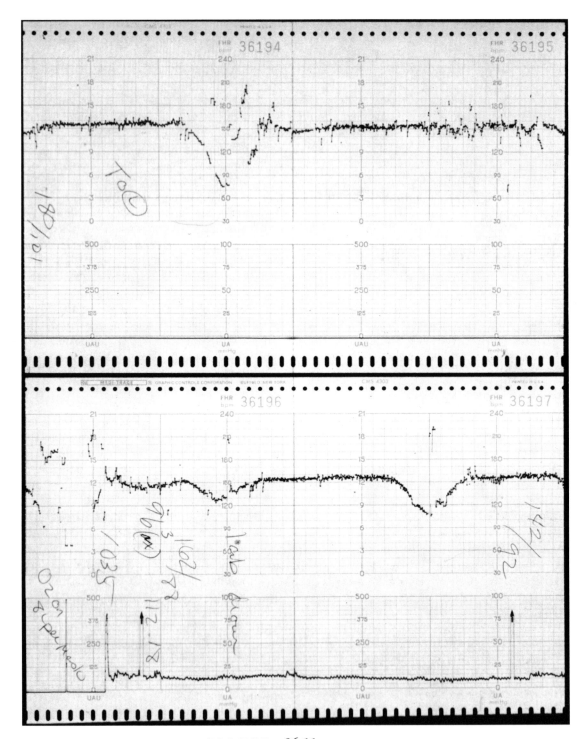

F I G U R E    **36-11**

The FHR pattern from a 33-week fetus with asymmetrical intrauterine growth retardation whose mother presented with clinical DIC.

1983; Rayburn, 1984). In most cases, this will require maternal-fetal transfer to a facility skilled to handle burn patients. Transfer will depend primarily on the severity of the burn and the stability of the pregnant woman and her fetus.

The first step in the management of the pregnant burn victim is to determine the depth and size of the burn. The depth of a burn may be partial or full thickness. A full-thickness burn, formerly called a third-degree burn, is the most severe and involves total destruction of the skin. As a result, regeneration of the epithelial surface is not possible.

The second element of burn management is the percent of body surface area involved (Table 36-3). The percentage of maternal body surface area covered by the burn is linked to maternal and perinatal outcome (Fig 36-12); the more severe the maternal burn, the higher is the maternal and perinatal mortality (Smith, 1983; Matthews, 1982; Daw, 1983; Rayburn, 1984).

The subsequent clinical management of the pregnant burn patient will depend on the patient's burn phase (e.g., acute, convalescent, or remote). Each phase has unique problems. For example, the acute phase is characterized by premature labor, electrolyte and fluid disturbances, maternal cardiopulmonary instability, and the potential for fetal compromise. In contrast, the convalescent and remote periods are unique for their problems of sepsis and abdominal scarring, re-

T A B L E    **36-3**

Classification of burn patients based on the percent of body surface area involved

| Classification | Body Surface Area (%) |
| --- | --- |
| Minor | < 10 |
| Major | |
| Moderate | 10–19 |
| Severe | 20–39 |
| Critical | ≥ 40 |

spectively. Because the potential for fetal compromise is greatest during the window of time immediately following the burn, the focus here is on acute-phase burn patients.

In the acute phase of a severe burn, the primary maternal focus centers on stabilization. Here, electrolyte disturbances due to transudation of fluid and altered renal function mandate close attention to the maternal intravascular volume. At the same time, these patients are also potentially compromised from airway injury and/or smoke inhalation, and ventilator support may be necessary to maintain cardiopulmonary stability. Given the complexities of these patients, invasive hemodynamic monitoring may be necessary. Because most of these patients will be in an intensive care unit (ICU), appropriate medical consultation and intensive nursing care for the mother and fetus are essential.

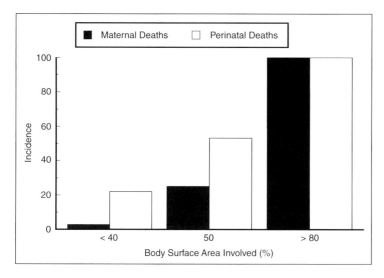

F I G U R E    **36-12**

Estimated maternal and perinatal mortality rates following maternal burn injuries separated by the amount of body surface area involved. (Smith, 1983; Matthews, 1982; Daw, 1983; Rayburn, 1984.)

Assessing fetal well-being in the burn patient may be difficult. The ability to determine fetal status with ultrasound or fetal monitoring will depend on the size and location of the burn. If, for example, the burn involves the maternal abdominal wall, alternative methods of fetal assessment, such as fetal kick counts (alone or in response to acoustic stimulation) (Clark, 1990; Smith, 1994) or a modified FBP (Manning, 1980, 1990; Phelan, 1988a) using vaginal ultrasound, may be necessary. In the absence of a maternal abdominal burn, continuous electronic fetal monitoring can generally be used. Because of such monitoring difficulties and the direct relationship between the size of the maternal burn and perinatal outcome (see Fig 36-12), Matthews (1982) has recommended immediate cesarean delivery (assuming maternal stability) in any pregnant burn patient with a potentially viable fetus and a burn that involves 50% or more of the maternal body surface area. As a reminder, burn patients with electrolyte disturbances may exhibit alterations in fetal status similar to those of a patient in sickle cell crisis (Cruz, 1979) or diabetic ketoacidosis (LoBue, 1978; Rhodes, 1984). Once the maternal electrolyte disturbance is corrected, fetal status may return to normal and intervention often can be avoided.

Fetal considerations specific to cardiac bypass procedures and electrical shock are discussed in previous chapters.

## Maternal Brain Death

With the advent of artificial life-support systems, prolonged viability of the brain-dead pregnant woman is now a reality (Dillon, 1982). As a consequence, an increasing number of obstetric patients on artificial life support will be encountered in the medical community. Maternal brain death poses an array of medical, legal, and ethical dilemmas for the obstetric health-care provider (Black, 1978; Bernat, 1982; Field, 1988). Should extraordinary care for the brain-dead mother be initiated to preserve the life of her unborn child, and if so, at what gestational age? If artificial life support is elected, how should the pregnancy be managed? When should the fetus be delivered? When should maternal life support be terminated? Is consent required to maintain the pregnancy? If so, from whom should it be obtained? Such questions illustrate the complexities of these cases.

It is not within the scope of this chapter to deal with the ethical, moral, and legal issues related to the obstetric care of the brain-dead gravida. Rather, the emphasis is on the clinical management of these patients when a decision has been made to maintain artificial life support of the brain-dead gravida for the benefit of her unborn child.

To date, three cases of maternal brain death during pregnancy have been reported (Table 36-4).

T A B L E  **36-4**

Perinatal outcome in reported cases of maternal brain death during pregnancy

| | Gestational Age (wk) | | Indication for Delivery | Mode of Delivery | Apgar Scores (5 min) | Weight (g) |
|---|---|---|---|---|---|---|
| | **Brain Death** | **Delivery** | | | | |
| Dillon (1982) | | | | | | |
| Case I | 25 | 26 | Fetal distress | Cesarean | 8 | 390 |
| Case II | 18 | Life support terminated at 19 weeks | | | | |
| Field (1988) | 22 | 31 | Growth retardation, septicemia | Cesarean | 8 | 1440 |

In one, life support was terminated after a discussion between the patient's physician and family at 19 weeks' gestation. In the other cases, the pregnancies were maintained for 1 and 9 weeks (Dillon, 1982; Field, 1988). Infants were delivered by classical cesarean and ultimately had favorable outcomes. For optimal care of such patients and fetuses, a cooperative effort among various healthcare providers is essential. The goal is to maintain maternal somatic survival until the fetus is viable and reasonably mature. To achieve this goal, a number of maternal and fetal considerations must be addressed (Field, 1988) (Table 36-5).

As pointed out by Field and associates (1988), maternal medical considerations involve the regulation of most, if not all, maternal bodily functions. For example, the loss of the pneumotaxic center in the pons, which is responsible for cyclic respirations, and the medullary center, which is responsible for spontaneous respirations, make mechanical ventilation mandatory. Ventilation, under these circumstances, is similar to that for the nonpregnant patient. In contrast to the nonpregnant patient, however, the maternal $Paco_2$ should be kept between 28 mm Hg and 32 mm Hg and the maternal $Paco_2$ greater than 60 to 70 mm Hg, to avoid deleterious effects on uteroplacental perfusion.

Maternal hypotension occurs frequently in these patients and may be due to a combination of factors, including hypothermia, hypoxia, and panhypopituitarism. Maintenance of maternal BP can often be achieved with the infusion of low-dose dopamine, which elevates BP without affecting renal or splanchnic blood flow.

With maternal brain death, the thermoregulatory center located in the ventromedian nucleus of the hypothalamus does not function, and maternal body temperature cannot be maintained normally. As a result, maternal hypothermia is the rule. Maintenance of maternal euthermia is important and usually can be accomplished through the use of warming blankets and the administration of warm, inspired, humidified air.

Maternal pyrexia suggests an infectious process and the need for a thorough septic work-up. If the maternal temperature remains elevated for a protracted period, cooling blankets may be necessary to avoid potentially deleterious effects on the fetus (Edwards, 1977).

Nutritional support, usually in the form of enteral or parenteral hyperalimentation, is required for maternal maintenance and fetal growth and development (see Chapter 10). Because of poor maternal gastric motility, parenteral rather than enteral hyperalimentation is often preferred (Field, 1988). The use of hyperalimentation during pregnancy does not appear to have deleterious effects on the fetus (Smith, 1981). As a rule, the amount of hyperalimentation should be in keeping with the caloric requirements of pregnancy.

In such patients, panhypopituitarism frequently occurs. As a result, a variety of hypoendocrinopathies, such as diabetes insipidus, secondary adrenal insufficiency, and hypothyroidism, may develop, each mandating therapy to maintain the pregnancy. Treatment of these conditions requires the use of vasopressin, corticosteroids, and thyroid replacement, respectively.

Because of the hypercoagulable state of pregnancy and the immobility of the brain-dead gravida, these patients also are at an increased risk for thromboembolism. Therefore, to minimize the potential for deep venous thrombosis or pulmonary embolus, heparin prophylaxis (5000–7500 units twice or three times a day) and/or intermittent pneumatic calf compression are recommended (Clark-Pearson, 1993).

By artificially supporting the maternal physiologic system, the intrauterine environment can

T A B L E  **36-5**

**Medical and obstetrical considerations in providing artificial life support to the brain-dead gravida**

*Maternal Considerations*
Mechanical ventilation
Cardiovascular support
Temperature lability
Hyperalimentation
Panhypopituitarism
Infection surveillance
Prophylactic anticoagulation

*Fetal Considerations*
Fetal surveillance
Ultrasonography
Steroids
Timing of delivery

be theoretically maintained to allow for adequate fetal growth and development (see Table 36-5). Obstetric management should focus on monitoring fetal growth with frequent ultrasound evaluations, antepartum FHR assessment, and the administration of corticosteroids between 24 and 34 weeks' gestation to enhance fetal lung maturation (Field, 1988; NIH, 1995). For stimulation of fetal maturity, the National Institutes of Health (1995) recommends betamethasone, 12 mg, initially and then a second dose 24 hours later. Though not specifically recommended by the NIH consensus conference, a weekly injection of betamethasone, 12 mg, is commonly administered.

The timing of delivery is based on the deterioration of maternal or fetal status or the presence of fetal lung maturity. Classical cesarean is the procedure of choice (Field, 1988) and is the least traumatic procedure for the fetus (Phelan, 1988b). To assure immediate cesarean capability, a cesarean pack and neonatal resuscitation equipment should be immediately available in the intensive care unit.

## Perimortem Cesarean Delivery

For centuries, postmortem cesarean delivery has been described as an attempt to preserve the life of the unborn child (Weber, 1971). In 237 B.C., Pliny the Elder described the first successful postmortem cesarean delivery, that of Scipio Africanus. Subsequently, in 1280, the Catholic Church at the Council of Cologne decreed that postmortem cesarean delivery must be performed to permit the unborn child to be baptized and to undergo a proper burial. Failure to perform the delivery was considered a punishable offense. This law mandated postmortem cesarean delivery only in women whose pregnancies were advanced beyond 6 months. To date, there have been 269 cases of postmortem cesarean delivery reported in the English literature, with 188 (70%) surviving infants (Katz, 1986).

Since Weber's monumental review of the subject in 1971, the causes of maternal death leading to a postmortem cesarean delivery have not changed substantially (Katz, 1988). These include hypertension, hemorrhage, and sepsis. With unanticipated or sudden death, such as amniotic fluid embolus syndrome, pulmonary embolus, or acute respiratory failure, the timing of cesarean delivery becomes an especially critical issue.

If a pregnant woman does sustain a cardiopulmonary arrest, cardiopulmonary resuscitation (CPR) should be initiated immediately (see Chapter 12). Optimal performance of CPR results in a cardiac output of 30% to 40% of normal in the nonpregnant patient. For best efficiency, the patient should be placed in the supine position. In this position, however, dextrorotation of the uterus may impede venous return and may further reduce maternal cardiac output, thus compromising cardiac output. Lateral uterine displacement may help to remedy this problem.

If maternal and fetal outcomes are to be optimized, the timing of the cesarean delivery is critical. Katz and associates (1986) have suggested that "cesarean delivery should be begun within 4 minutes, and the baby delivered within 5 minutes of maternal cardiac arrest." Care must be taken to continue maternal CPR, not only until the birth of fetus, but also after the delivery. Similar results were presented in a series of patients undergoing cardiac arrest in association with amniotic fluid embolism; if delivery occurred within 15 minutes, most fetuses survived and were neurologically intact. However, poor neonatal outcome was seen occasionally, even with delivery within 5 minutes of maternal cardiac arrest (Clark, 1995).

As demonstrated in Table 36-6, fetal outcome is linked closely to the interval between maternal arrest and delivery. Although the probability of a surviving, normal infant diminishes the longer the time interval from maternal death, the potential exists for a favorable fetal outcome even beyond 20 minutes of maternal cardiac arrest (Katz, 1988). Although delivery within 5 minutes of maternal cardiac arrest is ideal, in reality this rarely can be accomplished in a clinical setting, even with optimal care. Perhaps the most realistic guideline would be to perform cesarean section as soon as possible following maternal cardiac arrest; in late second- or third-trimester pregnant patients, the standard ABCs of cardiopulmonary resuscitation (airway, breathing, circulation) should be expanded to include D (delivery).

While the timing of cesarean delivery is a major determinant of subsequent fetal outcome,

T A B L E   **36-6**

Perimortem cesarean delivery with the outcome of surviving infants from the time of maternal death until delivery

| Time Interval (min) | Surviving Infants (no.) | Intact Neurologic Status of Survivors (%) |
|---|---|---|
| 0–5 | 45 | 98 |
| 6–15 | 18 | 83 |
| 16–25 | 9 | 33 |
| 26–35 | 4 | 25 |
| 36 + | 1 | 0 |

Sources: Katz VL, Dotters DJ, Droegemueller W. Perimortem cesarean delivery. Obstet Gynecol 1986;68:571–576; and Clark SL, Hankins GD, Dudley DA, et al. Amniotic fluid embolism: analysis of the National Registry. Am J Obstet Gynecol 1995;172:1158.

the gestational age of the fetus also is an important consideration. The probability of survival is related directly to the neonatal birth weight or gestational age (Copper, 1993; Robertson, 1992; Ferrara, 1989, 1994). At what gestational age should a postmortem cesarean delivery be considered? Is there a lower limit? It becomes obvious immediately that there are no clear answers to these questions. As a general rule, intervention appears prudent whenever the fetus is potentially viable or is "capable of a meaningful existence outside the mother's womb" (*Roe v. Wade,* 1973). Ideally, criteria for intervention in such circumstances would be formulated with the aid of an institution's current neonatal survival statistics and guidance from its bioethics committee. In light of the continual technologic advances in neonatology, care must be taken to periodically review these criteria because the gestational age and weight criteria may be lowered in the future (Copper, 1993; Robertson, 1992; Ferrara, 1989, 1994; *Roe v. Wade,* 1973).

When maternal death is not an unforeseeable event, is informed consent necessary? For instance, patients hospitalized with terminal cancer, class IV cardiac disease, pulmonary hypertension, or previous myocardial infarction are at an increased risk of death during pregnancy. Although these cases are infrequent, it seems reasonable to prepare for such an eventuality. Decisions regarding intervention should be made in advance with the patient and family. When intervention has been agreed to, one consideration is to have a cesarean delivery pack and neonatal resuscitation equipment immediately available in the ICU.

In the unforeseeable, sudden, unexpected maternal death, consent to deliver the potentially viable fetus does not appear to be required (Katz, 1986). When maternal death is foreseeable, however, maternal consent for cesarean delivery in the event of death is desirable.

**REFERENCES**

Babakania A, Niebyl R. The effect of magnesium sulfate on fetal heart rate variability. Obstet Gynecol 1978;51(suppl):2S–4S.

Barrett JM. Fetal resuscitation with terbutaline during eclampsia-induced uterine hypertonus. Am J Obstet Gynecol 1984;150:895.

Benedetti TJ, Hargrove JC, Rosene KA. Maternal pulmonary edema during premature labor inhibition. Obstet Gynecol 1982;59(suppl):33S–37S.

Benedetti TJ, Kates R, Williams V. Hemodynamic observations in severe preeclampsia complicated by pulmonary edema. Am J Obstet Gynecol 1985;152:330–334.

Bernal JM, Growdon JH. Cardiac surgery with cardiopulmonary bypass during pregnancy. Am J Obstet Gynecol Surv 1986;41:1–6.

Bernat JL, Culver CM, Gert B. On the definition and criterion of death. Ann Intern Med 1982;94:389.

Black PM. Brain death. N Engl J Med 1978;229:338–344, 393–401.

Boehm FH, Growdon JH. The effect of eclamptic convulsions of the fetal heart rate. Am J Obstet Gynecol 1974;120:851–853.

Brown R, Patrick J. The nonstress test: how long is enough? Am J Obstet Gynecol 1981;141:646–651.

Clark SL. Shock in the pregnant patient. Semin Perinatol 1990;14:52.

Clark SL, Gimovsky ML, Miller FD. Fetal heart rate response to scalp blood sampling. Am J Obstet Gynecol 1982;144:706–708.

Clark SL, Hawkins GD, Dudley DA, et al. Amniotic fluid embolism: analysis of the National Registry. Am J Obstet Gynecol 1995;172:1158.

Clark SL, Miller FC. Sinusoidal fetal heart rate pattern associated with massive fetomaternal transfusion. Am J Obstet Gynecol 1984a;149:97–99.

Clark SL, Gimovsky ML, Miller FC. The scalp stimulation test: a clinical alternative to fetal scalp blood sampling. Am J Obstet Gynecol 1984b;148:274–277.

Clark SL, Paul RH. Intrapartum fetal surveillance; the role of fetal scalp sampling. Am J Obstet Gynecol 1985a;153:717–720.

Clark SL, Divon M, Phelan JP. Preeclampsia/eclampsia: hemodynamic and neurologic correlations. Obstet Gynecol 1985b;66:337–340.

Clark SL, Sabey P, Jolley K. Non-stress testing with acoustic stimulation: 5960 tests without a fetal demise. Am J Obstet Gynecol 1989;160:694–697.

Clark-Pearson DL, Synan IS, Dodge R, et al. A randomized trial of low-dose heparin and intermittent pneumatic calf compression for the prevention of deep venous thrombosis after gynecologic oncology surgery. Am J Obstet Gynecol 1993;168:1146–1154.

Copper RL, Goldenberg RL, Creasy RK, et al. A multicenter study of preterm birth weight and gestational age specific neonatal mortality. Am J Obstet Gynecol 1993;168:78–84.

Cruz AC, Spellacy WN, Jarrell M. Fetal heart rate tracing during sickle cell crisis: a cause for transient late decelerations. Obstet Gynecol 1979;54:647–649.

Daw E, Mohandas I. Pregnancy in patients after severe abdominal burns. Br J Obstet Gynaecol 1983;90:69–72.

Dillon WP, Lee RV, Tronolone MJ, et al. Life support and maternal brain death during pregnancy. JAMA 1982;248:1089–1091.

Druzin ML, Gratacos J, Paul RH, et al. Antepartum fetal heat rate testing. XII. The effect of manual manipulation of the fetus on the nonstress test. Am J Obstet Gynecol 1985;151:61–64.

Edwards MJ, Wanner RA. Extremes of temperature. In: Wilson JG, Graser FC, eds. Handbook of teratology. vol. 1. New York: Plenum, 1977:421.

Epstein H, Waxman A, Fleicher N, et al. Meperidine-induced sinusoidal fetal heart rate pattern and its reversal with naloxone. Obstet Gynecol 1982;59(suppl):22–25.

Ferrara TB, Hoekstra RE, Couser RJ, et al. Survival and follow-up of infants born at 23–26 weeks of gestational age: effects of surfactant therapy. J Pediatr 1994;124:119.

Ferrara TB, Hoekstra RE, Gaziano E, et al. Changing outcome of extremely premature infants (<26 weeks gestation and <750 gm): survival and follow-up at a tertiary center. Am J Obstet Gynecol 1989;161:1114–1118.

Field DR, Gates EA, Creasy RK, et al. Maternal brain death during pregnancy: medical and ethical issues. JAMA 1988;260:816–822.

Gabbe SG, Ettinger RB, Freeman RK, et al. Umbilical cord compression with amniotomy: laboratory observations. Am J Obstet Gynecol 1976;126:353–355.

Garite TJ, Linzey EM, Freeman RK, et al. Fetal heart rate patterns and fetal distress in fetuses with congenital anomalies. Obstet Gynecol 1979;53:716–720.

Hon EH, Quilligan EJ. Electronic evaluation of the fetal heart rate. Clin Obstet Gynecol 1968a;11:145–155.

Hon EH, ed. An atlas of fetal heart rate patterns. New Haven, CT: Hardy, 1968b.

Katz M, Meizner I, Shani N, et al. Clinical significance of sinusoidal fetal heart rate pattern. Br J Obstet Gynaecol 1984;149:97–100.

Katz M, Robertson PA, Creasy RK. Cardiovascular complications associated with terbutaline treatment for preterm labor. Am J Obstet Gynecol 1981;139:605–608.

Katz VL, Cefalo RC. The history and the evolution of cesarean delivery. In: Phelan JP, Clark SL, eds. Cesarean delivery. New York: Elsevier, 1988:1–18.

Katz VL, Dotters DJ, Droegemueller W. Perimortem cesarean delivery. Obstet Gynecol 1986;68:571–576.

Klein VR, Harris AP, Abraham RA, Niebyl JR. Fetal distress during a maternal systemic allergic reaction. Obstet Gynecol 1984;64(suppl):15S–17S.

Koh KD, Friesen RM, Livingstone RA, et al. Fetal monitoring during maternal cardiac surgery with cardiopulmonary bypass. Can Med Assoc J 1975;112:1102–1106.

Krebs HB, Petres RE, Dunn LH. Intrapartum fetal heart rate monitoring. VII. Atypical variable decelerations. Am J Obstet Gynecol 1983;145:297–305.

Kubli FW, Hon EH, Hhazin AF, et al. Observations in heart rate and pH in the human fetus during labor. Am J Obstet Gynecol 1969;104:1190–1206.

Lamp MP, Ross K, Johnstone AM, et al. Fetal heart rate monitoring during open heart surgery: two case reports. Br J Obstet Gynaecol 1981;88:669–673.

Lee CY, Diloreto RC, O'Lane JM. A study of fetal heart rate acceleration patterns. Obstet Gynecol 1975;45:142–146.

Lee LA, Weston WL. New findings in neonatal lupus syndrome. Am J Dis Child 1984;138:233–238.

Leveno KJ, Williams ML, DePalma RT, et al. Perinatal outcome in the absence of antepartum fetal heart rate acceleration. Obstet Gynecol 1983;61:347.

Levy DL, Warriner RA, Burgess GE. Fetal response to cardiopulmonary bypass. Obstet Gynecol 1980;56:112–115.

Lieberman JR, Mazar M, Molcho J, et al. Electrical accidents during pregnancy. Obstet Gynecol 1986;67:861–863.

LoBue C, Goodlin RC. Treatment of fetal distress during diabetic ketoacidosis. J Reprod Med 1978;20:101–104.

Lucas MJ, Leveno KJ, Cunningham FG. A comparison of magnesium sulfate with phenytoin for the prevention of eclampsia. N Engl J Med 1995;333:201–205.

Manning FA, Morrison I, Harman CR, Menticoglou SM. The abnormal fetal biophysical profile score V: predictive accuracy according to score composition. Am J Obstet Gynecol 1990;162:918–927.

Manning FA, Platt LD, Sipos L. Antepartum fetal evaluation: development of a fetal biophysical profile. Am J Obstet Gynecol 1980;136:787–795.

Martin MC, Pernoll ML, Boruszak AM, et al. Cesarean section while on cardiac bypass: report of a case. Obstet Gynecol 1981;57(suppl):41S–45S.

Matthews RN. Obstetric implications of burns in pregnancy. Br J Obstet Gynaecol 1982;89:603–609.

Meffert WB, Stansel HC. Open heart surgery during pregnancy. Am J Obstet Gynecol 1968;102:1116.

Modanlou HD, Freeman RK. Sinusoidal fetal heart rate pattern: its definition and clinical significance. Am J Obstet Gynecol 1982;142:1033–1038.

Naidu S, Payne AJ, Moodley J, et al. Randomised study assessing the effect of phenytoin and magnesium sulfate on maternal cerebral circulation in eclampsia using transcranial doppler ultrasound. Br J Obstet Gynaecol 1996;103:111–116.

Nelson KB, Dambrosia JM, Ting TY, Grether JK. Uncertain value of electronic fetal monitoring in predicting cerebral palsy. N Engl J Med 1996;334:613–618.

Nielsen JL, Hankins GDV. Pulmonary edema in pregnancy. Female Patient 1990;15:66–72.

NIH Consensus Conference on Effect of Corticosteroids for Fetal Maturation on Perinatal Outcomes. JAMA 1995;273:413–418.

Paul RH, Gauthier RJ, Quilligan EJ. Clinical fetal monitoring: the usage and relationship to trends in cesarean delivery and perinatal mortality. Acta Obstet Gynecol Scand 1980;59:289.

Paul RH, Koh KS, Bernstein SG. Changes in fetal heart rate: uterine contraction patterns associated with eclampsia. Am J Obstet Gynecol 1978;130:165–169.

Petrie RH, Yeh SY, Maurata Y, et al. Effect of drugs on fetal heart rate variability. Am J Obstet Gynecol 1978;130:294–299.

Phelan JP. The non-stress test: a review of 3000 tests. Am J Obstet Gynecol 1982a;139:7–10.

Phelan JP, Cromartie AP, Smith CV. The nonstress test: the false negative test. Am J Obstet Gynecol 1982b;142:293–296.

Phelan JP. Pulmonary edema in obstetrics. Obstet Gynecol Clin North Am 1991;18:319–331.

Phelan JP, Ahn MO. Fetal acoustic stimulation. In: Chervenak FA, Isaacson G, Campbell S, eds. Textbook of ultrasound in obstetrics and gynecology. Vol. 1. Boston: Little, Brown, 1993a:507–516.

Phelan JP. The amniotic fluid index. In: Chervenak FA, Isaacson G, Campbell S, eds. Textbook of ultrasound in obstetrics and gynecology. Vol. 1. Boston: Little, Brown, 1993b:565–568.

Phelan JP, Ahn MO. Perinatal observations in forty-eight neurologically impaired term infants. Am J Obstet Gynecol 1994a;171:424–431.

Phelan JP. Labor admission test. Clin Perinatol 1994b;21:879–885.

Phelan JP. Antepartum fetal assessment—newer techniques. Semin Perinatol 1988a;12:57–65.

Phelan JP, Clark SL. Cesarean delivery: transperitoneal approach. In: Phelan JP, Clark SL, eds. Cesarean delivery. New York: Elsevier, 1988b:201–218.

Phelan JP, Lewis PE. Fetal heart rate decelerations during a nonstress test. Obstet Gynecol 1981; 57:228–232.

Phelan JP, Smith CV. Antepartum fetal assessment: the contraction stress test, In: Hill A, Volpe JJ, eds. Fetal neurology. New York: Raven, 1989a: 75–90.

Phelan JP. The postdate pregnancy: an overview. Clin Obstet Gynecol 1989b;32:221–227.

Phelan JP, Smith CV, Broussard P, et al. Amniotic fluid volume assessment using the four-quadrant technique in the pregnancy between 36 and 42 weeks gestation. J Reprod Med 1987; 32:540–543.

Porter TF, Clark SL, Dildy GA, et al. Isolated disseminated intravascular coagulation and amniotic fluid embolism. Am J Obstet Gynecol 1996; 174:486.

Pritchard JA, Cunningham FG, Pritchard SA. The Parkland Memorial Hospital protocol for treatment of eclampsia: evaluation of 245 cases. Am J Obstet Gynecol 1984;148:951–963.

Rayburn W, Smith B, Feller I, et al. Major burns during pregnancy: effects on fetal well-being. Obstet Gynecol 1984;63:392–395.

Reece E, Chervenak F, Romero R, Hobbins J. Magnesium sulfate in the management of acute intrapartum fetal distress. Am J Obstet Gynecol 1984;148:104–106.

Reisman RE. Responding to acute anaphylaxis. Contemp Obstet Gynecol 1989;33:45–57.

Rhodes RW, Ogburn PL. Treatment of severe diabetic ketoacidosis in the early third trimester in a patient with fetal distress. J Reprod Med 1984;29:621–625.

Rigg D, McDonough J. Use of sodium nitroprusside in deliberate hypotension during pregnancy. Br J Anaesth 1981;53:985.

Robertson PA, Sniderman SH, Laros RK, et al. Neonatal morbidity according to gestational age and birth weight from five tertiary care centers in the United States. 1983 through 1986. Am J Obstet Gynecol 1992;166:1629–1645.

*Roe v. Wade.* 410 US 113, 93 Sct 705, 35 Led 2d 147 (1973).

Saling E. Technik der endoskopischen microbluentnahme am feten. Geburtshilfe Frauenheilkd 1964;24:464–467.

Saling E, Schneider D. Biochemical supervision of the fetus during labor. J Obstet Gynaecol Br Cwlth 1967;74:799–803.

Shaw K, Clark SL. Reliability of intrapartum fetal heart rate monitoring in the postterm fetus with meconium passage. Obstet Gynecol 1988;72: 886–889.

Sheehan PQ, Rowland TW, Shah BL, et al. Maternal diabetic control and hypertrophic cardiomyopathy in infants of diabetic mothers. Clin Pediatr 1986;25:226–230.

Shenker L, Post RC, Seiler JS. Routine electronic monitoring of fetal heart rate and uterine activity during labor. Obstet Gynecol 1980;46:185–189.

Slomka C, Phelan JP. Pregnancy outcome in the gravida with a nonreactive nonstress test and positive contraction stress test. Am J Obstet Gynecol 1981;139:11–15.

Smith BK, Rayburn WF, Feller I. Burns and pregnancy. Clin Perinatol 1983;10:383–398.

Smith CV. Vibroacoustic stimulation for risk assessment. Clin Perinatol 1994;21:797–808.

Smith CV, Nguyen HM, Phelan JP, et al. Intrapartum assessment of fetal well-being: a comparison of fetal acoustic stimulation with acid-base determination. Am J Obstet Gynecol 1986a;155:726–728.

Smith CV, Phelan JP, Platt LD, et al. Fetal acoustic stimulation testing (the "FASTEST"). II. A randomized clinical comparison with the nonstress test. Am J Obstet Gynecol 1986b;155:131–134.

Smith CV, Phelan JP, Paul RH, et al. Fetal acoustic stimulation testing: a retrospective experience with the fetal acoustic stimulation test. Am J Obstet Gynecol 1985;153:567–568.

Smith CV, Rufleth P, Phelan JP, et al. Longterm enteral hyperalimentation in the pregnant woman with insulin dependent diabetes. Am J Obstet Gynecol 1981;141:180–183.

Strange K, Halldin M. Hypothermia in pregnancy. Anesthesiology 1983;58:460–465.

Strong TH, Gocke SE, Levy AV, Newel GJ. Electrical shock in pregnancy: a case report. J Emerg Med 1987;5:381–383.

Szekely P, Turner R, Snaith L. Pregnancy and the changing pattern of rheumatic heart disease. Br Heart J 1973;35:1293–1298.

Theard FC, Penny LL, Otterson WN. Sinusoidal fetal heart rate: ominous or benign? J Reprod Med 1984;29:265–268.

Van Arsdel PP. Drug allergy update. Med Clin North Am 1981;65:1089–1092.

Weber CE. Postmortem cesarean section: review of the literature and case reports. Am J Obstet Gynecol 1971;110:158.

Werch A, Lamberg HM. Fetal monitoring and maternal open heart surgery. South Med J 1977;70:1024–1027.

Witter FR, Niebyl JR. Drug intoxication and anaphylactic shock in the obstetric patient. In: Berkowitz RL, ed. Critical care of the obstetric patient. New York: Churchill Livingstone, 1983:527–543.

Yoong AFE. Electrical shock in pregnancy followed by placental abruption. Postgrad Med J 1990;66:563–564.

# CHAPTER *37*
# Fetal Effects of Drugs Commonly Used in Critical Care

*I*nformation regarding fetal and sub-sequent neonatal effects of drugs given to the mother in critical care situations is limited by a number of factors. Generally, such situations arise infrequently and, therefore, the number of cases available for analysis is limited. Critical care events are, by definition, crises; therefore, they usually are unanticipated, and the major concern is usually for the mother. When these crises arise, the effects of drugs on the fetus may be overlooked. The fact that multiple drugs are usually used makes any adverse effect difficult to ascribe to a given agent. Moreover, in the critically ill patient, altered placental blood flow, fetal oxygenation, and other maternal conditions affecting fetal well-being make such analyses even more complex. Depending on the interval between drug administration and delivery, neonatal effects may vary significantly. Therefore, much of the available data on the effects of such drugs comes from situations in which these drugs were used chronically or in less critical situations, as with propranolol for chronic hypertension or epinephrine for asthmatic episodes.

The drugs listed in Table 37-1 are described with respect to their effects on the fetus and neonate. (The reader is referred to the work by Briggs et al (1994a) for a more extensive review of the drugs in Table 37-1.)

## Adenosine

Adenosine (Briggs, 1994a; Podolsky, 1991; Harrison, 1992; Mason, 1992; Afridi, 1992; Matfin, 1993; Hagley, 1994, 1995; Elkayam, 1995; Kohl, 1995; Page, 1995), a rapid acting, very short half-life (<10 sec), antiarrhythmic agent, is used for the treatment of paroxysmal supraventricular tachycardia. Adenosine is not an animal teratogen. The drug has been used in a number of pregnant women during the second and third trimesters, sometimes immediately prior to delivery, without observable adverse effects in the fetus or newborn. Treatment of the mother with adenosine apparently has no effect on fetal heart rate (FHR). In one case, adenosine was administered directly to a 28-week-old fetus to successfully terminate a tachycardia secondary to severe hydrops.

## Amiodarone

The antiarrhythmic, amiodarone (Page, 1995; Briggs, 1994b; Sloskey, 1983; De Wolf, 1988; Laurent, 1987), is embryotoxic (increased fetal resorption and growth retardation) in rats and in one strain of mice. Following chronic administration, amiodarone has an elimination half-life of 14 to 58 days. Because the drug contains about 75 mg of iodine per 200-mg dose, its use during pregnancy may result in congenital hypothyroidism in the newborn. Hypothyroidism with

T A B L E   **37-1**

Effects of drugs on the fetus and neonate

| Generic Name | Trade Name[a] | Class/Action | Fetal Risk[b] |
| --- | --- | --- | --- |
| Adenosine | Adenocard | Antiarrhythmic | Low |
| Amiodarone | Cordarone | Antiarrhythmic | High |
| Amrinone | Inocor | +Inotropic/vasodilator | Unknown |
| Atenolol | Tenormin | β-Blocker | High |
| Atropine | — | Anticholinergic | Low |
| Bretylium | — | Antiarrhythmic | Moderate |
| Bumetanide | Bumex | Loop diuretic | Low |
| Cardioversion | — | Antiarrhythmic | Low |
| Diazepam | Valium | Sedative/anticonvulsant | High |
| Diazoxide | Hyperstat | Antihypertensive | High |
| Digoxin | Lanoxin | Cardiac glycoside | Low |
| Diltiazem | Cardizem | Calcium channel blocker | Unknown |
| Dobutamine | — | Vasopressor | Low |
| Dopamine | — | Vasopressor | Low |
| Enalapril | Vasotec | Antihypertensive | High |
| Ephedrine | — | Vasopressor | Low |
| Epinephrine | — | Vasopressor | Moderate |
| Esmolol | Brevibloc | β-Blocker | High |
| Flecainide | Tambocor | Antiarrhythmic | Low |
| Furosemide | Lasix | Loop diuretic | Low |
| Glycopyrrolate | Robinul | Anticholinergic | Low |
| Hydralazine | Apresoline | Peripheral vasodilator | High |
| Isoproterenol | Isuprel | Vasopressor | Low |
| Labetalol | Normodyne | α/β-Blocker | Moderate |
| Lidocaine | — | Antiarrhythmic | Moderate |
| Magnesium sulfate | — | Anticonvulsant | Moderate |
| Mephentermine | Wyamine | Vasopressor | Moderate |
| Metaraminol | Aramine | Vasopressor | Moderate |
| Methoxamine | Vasoxyl | Vasopressor | High |
| Metoprolol | Lopressor | β-Blocker | Moderate |
| Mexiletine | Mexitil | Antiarrhythmic | Low |
| Midazolam | Versed | Sedative | High |
| Milrinone | Primacor | +Inotropic/vasodilator | Unknown |
| Moricizine | Ethmozine | Antiarrhythmic | Unknown |
| Naloxone | Narcan | Narcotic antagonist | Low |

[a]Only one trade name is shown, even though some older drugs may have multiple commercial sources. No trade name is shown when the generic name is commonly used.

[b]Estimates of fetal risk include both the potential for teratogenic and toxic effects. Toxic effects may be direct (e.g., β-blockade, neuromuscular toxicity) or indirect (e.g., high potential for maternal hypotension with resulting decreased placental perfusion).

*Low:* Fetal risk cannot be excluded, but the absence or low frequency of adverse effects indicates that the risk is probably minimal.

*Moderate:* Fetal and/or neonatal adverse effects have been reported, but the benefits of therapy appear to outweigh the risks. Safer alternatives should be considered if available.

*High:* The reported (or potential based on the pharmacology of the drug) incidence of fetal and/or neonatal severe adverse effects is high. The drug should be used only if safer alternatives are unavailable.

*Unknown:* There are inadequate human data to determine the risk the drug represents to the fetus and/or neonate. The drug should be used only if safer alternatives are unavailable.

TABLE 37-1
*Continued*

| Generic Name | Trade Name[a] | Class/Action | Fetal Risk[b] |
|---|---|---|---|
| Nicardipine | Cardene | Calcium channel blocker | Low |
| Nifedipine | Procardia | Calcium channel blocker | Low |
| Nimodipine | Nimotop | Calcium channel blocker | Low |
| Nitroglycerin | — | Vasodilator | Low |
| Nitroprusside | — | Antihypertensive | Low |
| Norepinephrine | Levophed | Vasopressor | High |
| Phentolamine | Regitine | Antihypertensive | Low |
| Phenylephrine | NeoSynephrine | Vasopressor | High |
| Phenytoin | Dilantin | Anticonvulsant | High |
| Procainamide | Pronestyl | Antiarrhythmic | Low |
| Propafenone | Rythmol | Antiarrhythmic | Unknown |
| Propranolol | Inderal | β-Blocker | High |
| Quinidine | — | Antiarrhythmic | Low |
| Sotalol | Betapace | β-Blocker | Low |
| Streptokinase | Streptase | Thrombolytic | Moderate |
| Tissue plasminogen activator | Activase | Thrombolytic | Unknown |
| Tocainide | Tonocard | Antiarrhythmic | Unknown |
| Torsemide | Demadex | Loop diuretic | Low |
| Urokinase | Abbokinase | Thrombolytic | Unknown |
| Verapamil | Calan | Calcium channel blocker | Low |

goiter was observed in two newborns, one of whom was growth retarded, following chronic use of amiodarone during gestation. Intrauterine growth retardation is a frequent finding following chronic exposure to the antiarrhythmic, but a causal relationship to the drug has not been proven. However, the transient bradycardia and prolonged QT intervals that have been observed in some newborns is probably attributable directly to amiodarone.

## Amrinone

Amrinone (Briggs, 1994a; Fishburne, 1988; Jelsema, 1991) is a positive inotropic agent with vasodilator activity. The drug is unrelated to cardiac glycosides or catecholamines. The principal indication for amrinone is for the short-term management of congestive heart failure. Amrinone is teratogenic in rabbits (skeletal and gross external malformations). In pregnant baboons, amrinone infusion did not significantly effect uterine artery blood flow. A woman at 18 weeks' gestation was treated with a continuous intravenous (IV) infusion of amrinone. No fetal adverse effects attributable to the drug were observed, but the fetus died 11 days later due to the deteriorating medical condition of the mother.

## Atenolol

Atenolol (Briggs, 1994a) is a cardioselective $\beta_1$-adrenergic blocking agent used for the treatment of hypertension. An unpublished surveillance study observed 12 (11.4%) major birth defects (four expected) in 105 newborns exposed to atenolol during the first trimester, but a causal relationship cannot be determined without confirming studies. Most published studies described use of the drug after the first trimester. Intrauterine growth retardation has been noted in several studies and appears to be related to increased vascular resistance in the mother and fetus. Persistent β-blockade in the newborn may occur when the drug is administered close to delivery.

## Atropine

Atropine (Briggs, 1994a; Kivalo, 1977; Hellman, 1965; Heinonen, 1977; Diaz, 1980; Abboud, 1983), a parasympatholytic agent, rapidly crosses the placenta. The Collaborative Perinatal Project observed 401 mother-child pairs who received the drug in the first trimester. For use anytime in pregnancy, 1198 exposures were recorded. In neither case was evidence found for an association with malformations. When the group of parasympatholytics was taken as a whole, however, a possible association was found. Atropine has been used prior to cesarean section without producing apparent fetal or neonatal effects. One study analyzed the effect of IV atropine, 0.01 mg/kg, on FHR and found no significant change in rate or variability nor any effect on uterine activity. In contrast, the ability of atropine to produce a fetal tachycardia was used in the past as a test of placental function in complicated pregnancies.

## Bretylium

Bretylium (Briggs, 1994a; Page, 1995), a quaternary ammonium compound, is an adrenergic blocker used as an antiarrhythmic agent. No information on its use in pregnancy has been located. Hypotension has been observed in 50% of patients who have been administered bretylium. Although reports are lacking, reduced uterine blood flow with fetal hypoxia and associated bradycardia or late decelerations are potential risks.

## Bumetanide

Bumetanide (Briggs, 1994a) is a potent loop diuretic similar in action to furosemide. The drug is not teratogenic in animals, but doses 3 to 10 times the maximum therapeutic human dose resulted in an increased incidence of embryocidal effect in rabbits. Limited human data following exposure during the first trimester were not suggestive of a fetal risk.

## Cardioversion

Direct-current cardioversion (Briggs, 1994a; Vogel, 1965; Sussman, 1966; Schroeder, 1971; McKenna, 1983; Brown, 1989; Rotmensch, 1987), with energies of 10 to 50 joules, has been used in all trimesters and is considered to be a safe and usually effective procedure for arrhythmias during pregnancy.

## Diazepam

The relationship between human congenital malformations and diazepam (Briggs, 1994a), a sedative and emergency anticonvulsant, is controversial. Associations between the drug and oral clefts, inguinal hernia, congenital heart defects, and multiple other malformations have been reported, but, in most cases, a causal relationship could not be proven. Moreover, other studies found no association with birth defects. On the other hand, fetal and newborn toxicity directly attributable to diazepam includes loss of beat-to-beat variability in the FHR, decreased fetal movements, altered neonatal thermogenesis, newborn "floppy infant" syndrome (hypotonia, lethargy, sucking difficulties), and neonatal withdrawal (after chronic maternal therapy). Based on this toxicity and the uncertain relationship with birth defects, diazepam administration is best avoided during organogenesis and immediately prior to delivery.

## Diazoxide

A number of maternal and fetal adverse effects have been associated with the use of diazoxide (Briggs, 1994a; Newman, 1979; Paulissian, 1978; Milsap, 1980), including dose-related severe maternal hypotension with resulting fetal bradycardia, a tocolytic action during labor, and marked hyperglycemia. Because of these toxicities, the drug should not be considered as primary therapy during pregnancy.

## Digoxin

Because of increased elimination and increased volume of distribution in pregnancy, a significant increase in the dose of digoxin (Briggs, 1994a; Page, 1995; Rotmensch, 1987; Shepard, 1992; Rogers, 1972; Pladetti, 1979; Sherman, 1960; Weaver, 1973; Ho, 1980) is required to maintain adequate therapeutic maternal serum levels. No reports linking digoxin or the other various digitalis glycosides with congenital defects have been located. These agents have been used in all stages of pregnancy without causing fetal harm. Animal studies also have failed to show any teratogenic effect. Rapid passage of digoxin to the fetus occurs with the amount of drug in fetal serum dependent on the length of gestation.

Fetal toxicity resulting in neonatal death has been reported following a maternal overdose. The mother, in her eighth month of pregnancy, took an estimated 9 mg of digitoxin as a single dose. Delivery occurred 4 days later. The newborn exhibited toxic digitalis cardiac effect until death at 3 days of age.

There has been controversy regarding the effect of digitalis on the onset and duration of labor. Some data suggest earlier onset and shorter labors, and other data show no apparent effect.

## Diltiazem

The calcium channel blocker, diltiazem (Briggs, 1994a; Page, 1995; Lubbe, 1987), is embryo- and fetotoxic and teratogenic in some animal species, but published human first-trimester experience is limited to a single case. A woman was treated throughout most of pregnancy with diltiazem and isosorbide dinitrate for symptomatic myocardial ischemia and delivered normal twins at 37 weeks' gestation. In an unpublished surveillance study, 27 newborns were exposed to diltiazem during the first trimester. Four (14.8%) of the newborns had major congenital defects (one expected), two of which were cardiovascular defects (0.3 expected). A causal relationship cannot be determined without confirming studies.

## Dobutamine

Dobutamine (Briggs, 1994a; Stokes, 1984) is a sympathomimetic agent structurally related to dopamine. It has not been studied in human pregnancy. Short-term use in one patient with a myocardial infarction at 18 weeks' gestation was not associated with any known fetal adverse effects.

## Dopamine

Experience with dopamine (Briggs, 1994a; Fishburne, 1988; Gerstner, 1980; Clark, 1980; Kirshon, 1988) in human pregnancy is limited. Dopamine has been used to prevent renal failure in nine oliguric eclamptic patients. In another study of six women with severe preeclampsia and oliguria, low-dose dopamine (1–5 μg/kg/min) infusion produced a significant rise in urine and cardiac output. No significant changes in BP, central venous pressure, or pulmonary capillary wedge pressure occurred. Dopamine also has been used in patients undergoing cesarean section to treat hypotension. No adverse effects attributable to dopamine were observed in the fetuses or newborns of the mothers in these studies. Animal studies have found both increases and decreases in uterine blood flow with dopamine. This effect of the drug may be dose and plasma volume dependent, as is its effect on renal blood flow.

## Enalapril

Enalapril (Briggs, 1994a; Scott, 1989; Rosa, 1989; Cunniff, 1990; Piper, 1992; Barr, 1991; Brent, 1991; Martin, 1992) is a member of a class of agents that are competitive inhibitors of angiotensin I–converting enzyme, the enzyme that catalyses the conversion of angiotensin I to angiotensin II. Because fetal renal perfusion and glomerular plasma flow are low during gestation, high levels of angiotensin II appear to be physiologically required to maintain glomerular filtration at low perfusion pressures. In pregnant rats, fetal growth retardation and incomplete skull ossification have been observed.

In humans, chronic enalapril therapy is teratogenic and fetal/neonatal toxic when used during the second and third trimesters. Teratogenicity, represented by fetal hypocalvaria, is most likely a mechanical defect due to fetal hypotension and has been observed in a number of cases. Congenital renal malformations also may be related to in utero exposure to these agents. Fetal/neonatal toxicity is characterized by in utero renal failure, at times accompanied by oligohydramnios, and marked neonatal hypotension resistant to volume expansion and pressor agents. Severe and at times fatal, anuria may occur both in the fetus and newborn.

## Ephedrine

Ephedrine (Briggs, 1994a; Matfin, 1993; Nishimura, 1976; Wright, 1981; Hughes, 1985) is used for the treatment of bronchospasm and hypotension. Ephedrine is often used to treat hypotension in the pregnant patient that is caused by spinal or epidural anesthesia, because it causes peripheral vasoconstriction without reducing uterine blood flow. Ephedrine-like drugs are teratogenic in some animal species, but clear-cut human teratogenicity has not been demonstrated. There is a suggestion of minor malformations, including inguinal hernia and clubfoot, associated with first trimester administration. Adverse effects associated with near-term use have not been observed. Increases in FHR and decreases in beat-to-beat variability have been seen following IV administration, but these effects may have been the result of normal reflexes following hypotension-associated bradycardia. One study, however, has demonstrated the placental passage of ephedrine with fetal levels at delivery approximately 70% of the maternal concentration. The presence of ephedrine in the fetal circulation is probably a major cause of the FHR changes.

## Epinephrine

Epinephrine (Briggs, 1994a; Heinonen, 1977; Nishimura, 1976; Morgan, 1972; Beermann, 1978; Entman, 1984) is a drug widely used for the treatment of conditions such as shock, cardiac conditions, allergic reactions, and bronchospasm. This drug readily crosses the placenta. Epinephrine is teratogenic in some animal species, but human teratogenicity has not been clearly demonstrated. The findings of one surveillance study did suggest an increased incidence of major and minor birth defects; however, the only specific anomaly associated with epinephrine was inguinal hernia. Theoretically, epinephrine's α-adrenergic properties might lead to a decrease in uterine blood flow. A large IV dose of epinephrine, 1.5 mL of a 1:1000 solution over 1 hour to reverse severe hypotension secondary to an allergic reaction, may have contributed to intrauterine anoxic insult to a 28-week-old fetus. Decreased fetal movements occurred after treatment and the infant, delivered at 34 weeks' gestation, had evidence of intracranial hemorrhage at birth and died 4 days later. In hypotensive situations, therefore, use of ephedrine is a better choice. In bronchial asthma, use of subcutaneous epinephrine is apparently safe, but the β-adrenergics, such as terbutaline, offer a useful alternative.

## Esmolol

Esmolol (Briggs, 1994a; Losasso, 1991; Ducey, 1992) is a short-acting cardioselective β-adrenergic blocking agent that is structurally related to atenolol and metoprolol. The drug is used for the rapid, temporary treatment of supraventricular tachyarrhythmia, such as atrial flutter and/or fibrillation, and sinus tachycardia, and for hypertension occurring during surgery. Use of esmolol in two pregnant women, at 22 and 38 weeks' gestation, respectively, has been described. In the first case, the FHR decreased from 139 to 144 beats per minute (bpm) to 131 to 137 bpm, but no loss in FHR variability was observed. In the second case, however, an emergency cesarean section was required when persistent bradycardia (70–80 bpm) occurred despite discontinuance of the drug. The severe fetal bradycardia was thought to have been due to an esmolol-induced decrease in placental blood flow or interference with fetal compensation for a marginal placental perfusion. Because hypotension may occur with the use of esmolol—up to 50% in some trials—the potential for decreased uterine blood flow and resulting fetal hypoxia must be considered.

## Flecainide

Flecainide (Briggs, 1994a; Page, 1995; Wren, 1988; Macphail, 1988; Wagner, 1990; Kofinas, 1991; Allan, 1991; van Engelen, 1994) is an antiarrhythmic agent that is structurally related to encainide and procainamide. Structural defects have been observed in one breed of rabbits but not in a second breed of rabbits or in mice or rats. Use of flecainide has been described in a limited number of human pregnancies, both for maternal and fetal indications. Pregnancy outcomes were normal in all of these cases except for a single case of intrauterine death that occurred after 3 days of flecainide therapy. Therapy had been initiated in 14 women at a mean gestational age of 31 weeks (range, 23–36 wk) to treat fetal hydrops and ascites secondary to supraventricular tachycardia or atrial flutter. The death of the fetuses was attributed to either a flecainide-induced arrhythmia or to fetal blood sampling. A 1994 study involving 51 fetuses with tachycardia concluded that digoxin and flecainide were drugs of first choice for this condition because of their efficacy and safety.

## Furosemide

Furosemide (Briggs, 1994a; Beermann, 1984; Wladimiroff, 1975; Percorari, 1969; Votts, 1975; Sibai, 1984) is a potent diuretic and one of the most commonly used medications in critical care obstetrics. Furosemide readily crosses the placenta. Peak fetal serum concentrations are reached at about 9 hours; by 8 hours, fetal serum levels are roughly equal to maternal levels. Transiently increased fetal urine production following maternal administration has been documented, but chronic therapy does not result in significant alterations in amniotic fluid volumes. Newborns exposed to furosemide shortly before birth have been found to have increased diuresis and increased sodium and potassium excretion. Fetal and neonatal hypokalemia is a theoretical com-

plication. No teratogenic effects have been described, but the use of this agent in the first trimester is uncommon. The greatest concern regarding the use of potent diuretics is maternal plasma volume reduction, especially in preeclamptics, which could result in decreased placental perfusion, hypoxia, acidosis, and resulting complications. Unlike thiazide diuretics, neonatal thrombocytopenia has not been reported with furosemide.

## Glycopyrrolate

Glycopyrrolate (Briggs, 1994a) is an anticholinergic agent commonly used prior to surgery, including cesarean section, to decrease gastric secretions. Because it is a quaternary ammonium compound, its placental transfer is markedly less than that of atropine, and, thus, significant effects on FHR and variability have not been observed.

## Hydralazine

No reports linking the use of the antihypertensive hydralazine (Briggs, 1994a; Widerlov, 1980; Liedholm, 1982; Heinrich, 1977; Mabie, 1987; Lodeiro, 1989; Yemini, 1989) with congenital malformations have been located. Neonatal thrombocytopenia and secondary bleeding have been associated with the use of hydralazine. Because this toxicity has also been reported with pregnancy-induced hypertension, however, it may have been related to the maternal disease rather than to the drug. Hydralazine readily crosses the placenta; fetal serum concentrations are equal to or greater than those in the mother.

Fetal premature atrial contractions, but without tachyarrhythmia, were observed in a 36-week-old fetus whose mother was treated with hydralazine. The arrhythmia resolved 24 hours after the drug was stopped. A lupus-like syndrome developed in a mother and her fetus following treatment with IV hydralazine at 28 weeks' gestation. The infant was delivered at 29 weeks' gestation because of fetal distress but expired 36 hours after birth secondary to cardiac tamponade induced by 7 mL of clear sterile transudate in the pericardial space. Because hydralazine is a potent antihypertensive agent, excessive doses may result in too rapid and too profound a reduction in BP, causing decreased uteroplacental blood flow and reduced oxygen delivery to the fetus. Frequent, small incremental doses (5–10 mg IV every 20 min) are probably preferable to avoid such problems.

## Isoproterenol

Isoproterenol (Briggs, 1994a; Tamari, 1982) is a $\beta_1/\beta_2$-adrenergic agent that is teratogenic in some animal species, but human teratogenicity has not been shown. Although no specific evidence links this drug to birth defects, the number of reported exposures is small. There has been a reported association with the sympathomimetic class of drugs and minor birth defects, including inguinal hernia and club foot. Isoproterenol has been used during pregnancy to increase heart rate in the presence of high-grade atrioventricular block, to treat ventricular arrhythmias associated with a prolonged QT interval, and in cases of primary pulmonary hypertension. As a $\beta$-adrenergic agent, isoproterenol will also inhibit uterine contractions.

## Labetalol

Labetalol (Briggs, 1994a; Mabie, 1987) is a combined $\alpha/\beta$-adrenergic blocking agent used for the treatment of hypertension. Fetal concentrations of the drug average 40% to 80% of maternal levels. No congenital malformations have been reported in published studies after the use of labetalol in human pregnancy, but first-trimester experience is very limited. In an unpublished surveillance study, 29 newborns had been exposed to labetalol during the first trimester. Four (13.8%) of the newborns had major, unspecified, congenital defects (one expected), but a causal relationship cannot be determined without confirming studies. Labetalol apparently does not effect uteroplacental blood flow despite a reduction in BP. The lack of effect is probably due to reduced peripheral resistance. $\beta$-blockade, as evidenced by persistent, marked bradycardia (< 100 bpm), and hypotension, has been observed in some newborns exposed to labetalol close to delivery.

Because of the potential for birth defects, labetalol should not be used during the first trimester unless other alternatives are unavailable.

## Lidocaine

Lidocaine (Briggs, 1994a; Page, 1995; Heinonen, 1977; Stokes, 1984; Shnider, 1968; Blankenbaker, 1975; Abboud, 1982; Scanlon, 1974) is a local anesthetic that is also used for the treatment of cardiac ventricular arrhythmias. The majority of information on the use of this drug in pregnancy derives from its use as a local or regional anesthetic during labor and delivery. The drug rapidly crosses the placenta and appears in the fetal circulation within a few minutes of injection. Ratios of fetal cord to maternal serum range from 0.5 to 0.7 after IV injection or epidural anesthesia. Both the fetus and newborn are capable of metabolizing and eliminating lidocaine. Following epidural anesthesia, the elimination half-life in the newborn averages 3 hours, but levels may be detectable for 48 hours or longer after birth.

Several studies have evaluated lidocaine's effect on the newborn. Serum levels in excess of 2.5 $\mu$g/mL have been associated with significant neonatal depression. Lower levels more commonly found following regional or local anesthesia have been associated with neonatal muscular weakness, decreased tone, and altered neurobehavior. Other studies, however, have been unable to show these effects with similar serum levels. Fetuses born following maternal lidocaine administration both for anesthesia and as an antiarrhythmic agent have shown no teratogenic or development abnormalities.

## Magnesium Sulfate

Magnesium sulfate (Briggs, 1994a; Lamm, 1988; Dudley, 1989; Waisman, 1988; Snyder, 1989; Rodis, 1987; Ben-Ami, 1994) (MgSO$_4$) is an anticonvulsant used frequently to prevent or treat seizures in obstetric patients with preeclampsia or eclampsia and as a tocolytic agent in patients with premature labor. This agent also is used to prevent early mortality in patients with acute myocardial infarction and in asthmatic patients as adjunctive treatment of acute exacerbations of moderate to severe asthma. Although magnesium sulfate is not teratogenic, it can produce significant toxicity in the fetus and newborn. Long-term use of magnesium sulfate during pregnancy is associated with sustained hypocalcemia in the fetus, resulting in congenital rickets. When used close to delivery, neonatal neurologic depression may occur, with respiratory depression, muscle weakness, and loss of reflexes. This toxicity is not usually correlated with cord serum magnesium levels. Other toxicities observed with magnesium sulfate include maternal hypothermia and fetal bradycardia. Two clinically significant drug interactions have been described between magnesium sulfate and nifedipine. In one report, severe hypotension occurred in two hypertensive women being treated with oral methyldopa and magnesium sulfate when oral nifedipine was added, resulting in the death of one of the fetuses. In another woman, maintained on nifedipine for tocolysis, the addition of magnesium sulfate resulted in maternal neuromuscular blockade. Symptoms included pronounced muscle weakness, jerky movements of the extremities, difficulty in swallowing, paradoxical respirations, and an inability to lift her head from the pillow. The symptoms resolved 25 minutes after magnesium sulfate was stopped. Neuromuscular blockade was also observed in a woman with preeclampsia treated concurrently with magnesium sulfate and nifedipine. Because of these toxicities, newborns of mothers treated with magnesium sulfate near delivery should be observed closely for signs of toxicity during the first 24 to 48 hours after birth.

## Mephentermine

Mephentermine (Briggs, 1994a) is a sympathomimetic used in emergency situations to treat hypotension. Experience in pregnancy with this agent is very limited. The pharmacologic effect of mephentermine is to increase cardiac output by enhancing cardiac contraction and, to a lesser extent, from peripheral vasoconstriction. Its effect on uterine blood flow should be minimal.

## Metaraminol

Metaraminol (Briggs, 1994a; Smith, 1970) is an agent used to treat hypotension in critical care situations. Because of this limited indication, experience in pregnancy is minimal. The drug has predominantly α-adrenergic properties; vasoconstriction of the uterine vessels with fetal hypoxia is, therefore, a probable effect. Metaraminol also may interact with oxytocics or ergot preparations to produce significant maternal hypertension with the potential for rupture of a cerebral vessel. If a pressor agent is required, other drugs, such as ephedrine, should be used.

## Methoxamine

Methoxamine (Briggs, 1994a; Smith, 1970) is a predominate α-adrenergic sympathomimetic used in emergency situations for the treatment of hypotension. Vasoconstriction of the uterine vessels may occur, thereby producing fetal hypoxia. As with other agents in this class, an interaction with oxytocics or ergot preparations may occur, resulting in severe persistent maternal hypertension with the potential for rupture of a cerebral vessel. If a pressor agent is required, other drugs, such as ephedrine, should be used.

## Metoprolol

Metoprolol (Briggs, 1994a; Jannet, 1994) is a cardioselective β-adrenergic blocking agent that has been used during pregnancy for the treatment of maternal hypertension and tachycardia. The drug rapidly enters the fetal circulation, and fetal and maternal concentrations are approximately equal. No reports linking the use of metoprolol with congenital defects have been located, but experience during the first trimester is minimal. Use during the second and third trimesters has not been associated with adverse effects in the fetus or newborn. However, persistent β-blockade in the newborn may occur if the drug has been used near delivery.

## Mexiletine

Mexiletine (Briggs, 1994a; Page, 1995; Rotmensch, 1987; Lownes, 1987; Lewis, 1981; Timmis, 1980) is a local anesthetic, structurally similar to lidocaine, that is used as an antiarrhythmic. This drug is not teratogenic in animals. Limited human pregnancy experience includes three cases. In one of these cases, mexiletine was used throughout gestation. No adverse effects in the fetuses or newborns were observed.

## Midazolam

Midazolam (Briggs, 1994a; Crawford, 1989; Ravlo, 1989) is a short-acting benzodiazepine used for anesthetic induction. The drug is not teratogenic in animals, and no reports associating the use of this agent with birth defects in humans have been located. However, published human pregnancy experience is limited to the third trimester. Midazolam crosses the placenta to the fetus and, when used immediately prior to delivery, results in neurobehavioral and respiratory depression in some newborns. These adverse effects are similar to the "floppy infant" syndrome observed with diazepam and are greater than those observed with thiopental.

## Milrinone

Milrinone (Briggs, 1994a) is a positive inotropic and vasodilator agent with phosphodiesterase inhibitor activity used for the short-term treatment of congestive heart failure. The drug is embryotoxic (increased resorption rate) but not teratogenic in rabbits. No reports describing the use of milrinone in human pregnancy have been located.

## Moricizine

Moricizine (Briggs, 1994a; Page, 1995) is an orally active agent used in the treatment of ventricular arrhythmias. No fetotoxicity or teratogenicity was observed in pregnant rats and rabbits administered doses above the maximum recommended

human dose. No reports describing the use of moricizine in human pregnancy have been located.

## Naloxone

Naloxone (Briggs, 1994a; Goodlin, 1981) is a narcotic antagonist normally used in emergency situations to reverse the effects of narcotic overdose. The drug rapidly crosses the placenta and will reverse toxic narcotic effects in the fetus. In one study, naloxone was used at term to treat FHR baselines with low beat-to-beat variability that was thought to be due to elevated endogenous fetal endorphins. However, naloxone may have enhanced fetal asphyxia in one case, resulting in fatal respiratory failure in the newborn.

## Nicardipine

The calcium channel blocker, nicardipine (Briggs, 1994a; Jannet, 1994; Holbrook, 1989; Carbonne, 1993; Walker, 1992), is used for the treatment of angina and hypertension. This drug is not teratogenic in animals or in humans, but published human pregnancy experience is limited to the second and third trimesters. Nicardipine has been used as a tocolytic in pregnant rabbits and monkeys but, although it was successful in stopping uterine contractions, it caused significant acidemia and hypoxemia in the fetuses. Decreased uteroplacental blood flow, however, has not been observed in humans.

## Nifedipine

Nifedipine (Briggs, 1994a; Childress, 1994), a calcium channel blocker, appears to be a safe and effective agent during pregnancy for the treatment of hypertension and as a tocolytic agent. Nifedipine is teratogenic and embryotoxic in animals, but these toxicities have not been observed in humans. Severe hypotension has been reported infrequently and is a potential concern. Interactions between nifedipine and magnesium sulfate, resulting in severe hypotension or neuromuscular blockade, have been observed and are described in the section on magnesium sulfate.

## Nimodipine

Nimodipine (Briggs, 1994a; Belfort, 1994) is a calcium channel blocking agent used to reduce the incidence and severity of ischemic deficits in patients with subarachnoid hemorrhage after rupture of congenital aneurysms. One study has described the safe use of nimodipine in the management of preeclampsia, concluding that the drug had significant maternal and fetal cerebral vasodilator activity. Nimodipine is teratogenic and embryotoxic in animals. Based on the experience with other calcium channel blockers of the same class (e.g., nicardipine, nifedipine), these toxic effects in humans are not expected, but human experience with nimodipine during the first trimester is lacking.

## Nitroglycerin

The rapid-onset, short-acting vasodilator, nitroglycerin (Heinonen, 1977; Briggs, 1995; Cotton, 1986a,b), is used for the treatment or prevention of angina pectoris and for the control of severe hypertension. Nitroglycerin also has been used as an emergency tocolytic agent to relax the uterus, allowing delivery of entrapped infants, and during external and internal versions. In addition, nitroglycerin transdermal patches have been used for long-term tocolysis. Although experience is limited, use of nitroglycerin for any of these indications has not resulted in fetal harm. In one report of nitroglycerin administration for severe preeclampsia, an association with reduced short-term FHR variability, without change in fetal acid-base status, was reported. In another study, nitroglycerin infusion was effective in rapidly correcting the hemodynamic disturbances in pregnancy-induced hypertension complicated by hydrostatic pulmonary edema, but a rapid improvement in arterial oxygenation did not occur. Despite a very small sample size, a surveillance study noted an unusually high incidence of malformed children of women exposed in the first trimester to vasodilators, including nitroglycerin. Unfortunately, the effects of this drug alone could not be separated from the other drugs in the class.

## Nitroprusside

No reports linking the use of sodium nitroprusside (Briggs, 1994a) with congenital defects have been found. Nitroprusside has been used in pregnancy to produce deliberate hypotension during aneurysm surgery and to treat severe hypertension. Transient fetal bradycardia was the only adverse effect noted. Nitroprusside crosses the placenta and produces fetal cyanide concentrations higher than maternal levels in animals, but this has not been studied in humans. Avoidance of prolonged use and monitoring of serum pH, plasma cyanide, red-cell cyanide, and methemoglobin levels in the mother have been recommended. Standard recommended doses of nitroprusside apparently do not pose a major risk of excessive accumulation of cyanide in the fetal liver.

## Norepinephrine

Norepinephrine (Shepard, 1992; Schardein, 1993) is a potent arterial and venous vasoconstrictor ($\alpha$-adrenergic) and cardiac inotropic stimulant ($\beta_1$-adrenergic) used for the treatment of severe hypotension and cardiac arrest. The drug is teratogenic in some animal species. No reports describing the use of norepinephrine in human pregnancy have been located. Due to the $\alpha$-adrenergic activity, use of this agent during pregnancy could compromise placental perfusion, resulting in fetal bradycardia and hypoxia.

## Phentolamine

Phentolamine (Briggs, 1994a) is a short-acting $\alpha$-adrenergic blocker used for the treatment of severe hypertension secondary to maternal pheochromocytoma. This agent is neither teratogenic nor embryotoxic in animals. Phentolamine has been used in a small number of human pregnancies for the treatment of hypertension due to pheochromocytoma, apparently without causing drug-induced toxicity. Use during the first trimester, however, has not been reported.

## Phenylephrine

Phenylephrine (Briggs, 1994a) is a predominately α-adrenergic sympathomimetic used in the emergency treatment of hypotension. As such, the possibility of reduced uterine blood flow and fetal hypoxia is a major concern if this agent is used in pregnancy. Phenylephrine also may interact with oxytocics and ergot preparations to produce severe persistent maternal hypertension. A surveillance study found an association between phenylephrine and minor malformations, but confirming studies have not been reported. If a pressor agent is indicated, other drugs, such as ephedrine, should be used.

## Phenytoin

Phenytoin (Briggs, 1994a; Page, 1995; Tamari, 1982) is an anticonvulsant that has been used in the treatment of cardiac arrhythmias, such as those caused by digitalis intoxication (considered by some to be the treatment of choice for this indication), ventricular tachycardia, and paroxysmal atrial tachycardia. This drug is teratogenic when administered to pregnant epileptic women, producing, in some cases, a recognizable pattern of malformations termed the *fetal hydantoin syndrome.* Moreover, numerous other congenital defects have resulted from chronic exposure to phenytoin. Multiple mechanisms have been proposed for this teratogenicity, including genetic factors, induction of folic acid deficiency, and the disease itself. Early hemorrhagic disease of the newborn is a potential complication of maternal phenytoin therapy but probably only after sustained use. Although the exact mechanism is unknown, the induction of fetal liver microsomal enzymes resulting in the depletion of already low reserves of vitamin K is the most likely cause. The fetal risk from short-term use, such as might be used in a critical care setting, is unknown but is probably less than when used chronically in epileptic women.

## Procainamide

Procainamide (Briggs, 1994a; Page, 1995; Rotmensch, 1987; Tamari, 1982) is an antiarrhythmic agent that is most commonly used for ventricular arrhythmias. The experience with the use of this drug in human pregnancy is small. Limited data suggest that fetal levels are approximately 25% of maternal concentrations. In a case in which digitalis and propranolol both failed, maternal administration of procainamide was used for successful fetal cardioversion. There was no evidence of teratogenicity when this drug was given in the first trimester, nor are there any reports of adverse fetal or neonatal effects from maternal administration.

## Propafenone

Propafenone (Briggs, 1994a; Page, 1995; Gembruch, 1989) is an orally active antiarrhythmic drug used in the treatment of ventricular tachycardia. The agent is embryotoxic but not teratogenic in animals. Propafenone, in combination with a digitalis glycoside, was used in an unsuccessful attempt to treat refractory fetal supraventricular tachycardia and hydrops fetalis during the second trimester.

## Propranolol

The β-adrenergic blocking agent, propranolol (Briggs, 1994a; Page, 1995; Calderoney, 1982; Rubin, 1981; Redmond, 1982), has been used for many indications in pregnancy, such as hypertension, hyperthyroidism, prevention of arrhythmias, and other cardiac problems, and for fetal supraventricular tachycardia. This drug readily crosses the placenta. Cord serum levels have varied between 19% and 127% of maternal levels. Oxytocic properties also have been demonstrated.

A number of fetal/neonatal adverse effects have been reported following the use of propranolol in pregnancy. These adverse effects include intrauterine growth retardation, hypoglycemia, bradycardia, neonatal respiratory depression, and coagulation defects. Whether all of these effects result from the drug, the maternal disease, or other drugs consumed concurrently is not always clear. Daily doses of 160 mg or higher have produced the most serious effects, but toxicity also has occurred with lower doses. Large doses have been related to the loss of FHR accelerations associated with fetal movement. Respiratory depression and bradycardia have been described in newborns delivered shortly after IV use of propranolol, but no lasting effects were seen. Newborn infants of women consuming this drug near delivery should be observed closely for bradycardia, hypoglycemia, and other signs and symptoms of β-blockade during the first 24 to 48 hours after birth.

## Quinidine

No reports linking the use of the antiarrhythmic, quinidine (Briggs, 1994a; Page, 1995; Rotmensch, 1987; Hill, 1979) with congenital defects have been found. Although eighth nerve damage has been observed with quinine, the optical isomer of quinidine, this effect is apparently not a problem with quinidine. The drug crosses the placenta and achieves levels similar to maternal concentrations. No apparent deleterious effects on the fetus or newborn have been reported. Caution, however, should be used with high doses because of the potential oxytocic properties of quinidine.

## Sotalol

Sotalol (Briggs, 1994a) is a β-blocker used for the treatment of ventricular arrhythmias and hypertension. This drug is not teratogenic in animals or humans. A few reports have described the use of sotalol during human gestation either for the treatment of maternal hypertension or ventricular tachycardia or, in one case, in an unsuccessful attempt to treat a hydropic fetus with supraventricular tachycardia. No adverse effects, other than bradycardia, have been observed in exposed newborns. Newborns should be monitored closely for 24 to 48 hours after birth for signs and symptoms of β-blockade, as in all cases in which drugs of this category have been used close to delivery.

## Streptokinase

The thrombolytic agent, streptokinase (Briggs, 1994a; Fagher, 1990; Ramamurthy, 1994; Turrentine, 1995), has been used at various times during all trimesters in fewer than 200 human pregnancy cases. Two fetal deaths (1.2%), in which a direct relationship between the drug and the fetal death could not be excluded, have been observed from a total of 172 patients. An increased risk of intrapartum and/or immediate postpartum hemorrhage exists if therapy is given at the time of delivery. Other potential drug-induced complications include uterine bleeding not related to delivery, spontaneous abortion, and the onset of premature labor. Streptokinase does not appear to cause preterm rupture of membranes or delivery. Although only minimal amounts of the drug cross the placenta, streptokinase antibodies are transferred to the fetus. The resulting passive sensitization would have clinical significance only if the neonate required streptokinase therapy.

## Tissue Plasminogen Activator

The use of tissue plasminogen activator (Turrentine, 1995) (also known as Alteplase, recombinant), a thrombolytic agent, has been described in only four human pregnancies, one of which also included the use of urokinase. No fetal adverse effects were observed in these cases, but as with streptokinase and urokinase, the potential exists for both fetal and maternal morbidity.

## Tocainide

Tocainide (Briggs, 1994a) is an antiarrhythmic used in the treatment of ventricular arrhythmias. This drug also has been used in the treatment of myotonic dystrophy and trigeminal neuralgia. Tocainide is not teratogenic or embryotoxic in animals. No reports describing its use during human pregnancy have been located.

## Torsemide

Torsemide (Boehringer Mannheim Pharmaceuticals) is a loop diuretic, in the same class as bumetamide and furosemide, that is used in the treatment of congestive heart failure and hypertension. This drug is not teratogenic or embryotoxic in animals. No reports describing its use during human pregnancy have been located.

## Urokinase

The thrombolytic agent, urokinase (Briggs, 1994a; Turrentine, 1995), is not teratogenic in animals. Reports on the use of urokinase during human pregnancy are limited to four cases. One woman was treated at 3 and 6 months, and the others were treated between 14 and 32 weeks' gestation. In two of the women, another thrombolytic agent was used: streptokinase in one and tissue plasminogen activator in another. Although no adverse fetal effects were described, uterine bleeding occurred in one patient.

## Verapamil

Verapamil (Briggs, 1994a; Page, 1995; Rotmensch, 1987; Goodnick, 1993; Magee, 1994) is a calcium channel blocker used as an antiarrhythmic, antihypertensive, and tocolytic agent. Maternal administration has been used to treat fetal supraventricular tachycardia. In one report, moreover, verapamil was prescribed during the first trimester as an alternative to lithium for the treatment or prevention of bipolar disorder (mania). No reports linking the use of verapamil with congenital malformations have been located. In one case, however, coadministration of verapamil and digoxin for the treatment of fetal supraventricular tachycardia may have resulted in complete heart block and fetal death. After IV administration, hypotension has been observed in 5% to 10% of patients. Because of this effect, reduced uterine blood flow with fetal hypoxia is a potential risk.

### REFERENCES

Abboud T, Raya J, Sadri S, et al. Fetal and maternal cardiovascular effects of atropine and glycopyrrolate. Anesth Analg 1983;62:426.

Abboud TK, Sarkis F, Blikian A, et al. Lack of adverse neurobehavioral effects of lidocaine. Anesthesiology 1982;57(suppl):A404.

Afridi J, Moise KJ Jr, Rokey R. Termination of supraventricular tachycardia with intravenous adenosine in a pregnant woman with Wolff-Parkinson-White syndrome. Obstet Gynecol 1992;80:481.

Allan LD, Chita SK, Sharland GK, et al. Flecainide in the treatment of fetal tachycardias. Br Heart J 1991;65:46.

Barr M Jr, Cohen MM Jr. ACE inhibitor fetopathy and hypocalvaria: the kidney-skull connection. Teratology 1991;44:485.

Beermann B, Groschinsky-Grind M, Fahraens L, et al. Placental transfer of furosemide. Clin Pharmacol Ther 1978;24:560.

Belfort MA, Saade GR, Moise KJ Jr, et al. Nimodipine in the management of preeclampsia: maternal and fetal effects. Am J Obstet Gynecol 1994;171:417.

Ben-Ami M, Giladi Y, Shalev E. The combination of magnesium sulphate and nifedipine: a cause of neuromuscular blockade. Br J Obstet Gynaecol 1994;101:262.

Blankenbaker WL, DiFazio CA, Berry FA Jr. Lidocaine and its metabolites in the newborn. Anesthesiology 1975;42:325.

Boehringer Mannheim Pharmaceuticals. Product information. Demadex: Gaithersburg, MD, 1995.

Brent RL, Beckman DA. Angiotensin-converting enzyme inhibitors, an embryopathic class of drugs with unique properties: information for clinical teratology counselors. Teratology 1991;43:543.

Briggs GG, Freeman RK, Yaffe SJ. Drugs in pregnancy and lactation. A reference guide to fetal and neonatal risk. 4th ed. Baltimore: Williams and Wilkins, 1994a.

Briggs GG, Freeman RK, Yaffe SJ. Amiodarone. UPDATE 1994b;7:1.

Briggs GG, Freeman RK, Yaffe SJ. Nitroglycerin. UP-DATE 1995;8:4.

Brown CEL, Wendel GD. Cardiac arrhythmias during pregnancy. Clin Obstet Gynecol 1989;32:89.

Calderoney RD. Beta blockers in pregnancy. N Engl J Med 1982;306:810.

Carbonne B, Jannet D, Touboul C, et al. Nicardipine treatment of hypertension during pregnancy. Obstet Gynecol 1993;81:908.

Childress CH, Katz VL. Nifedipine and its indications in obstetrics and gynecology. Obstet Gynecol 1994;83:616.

Clark RB, Brunner JA III. Dopamine for the treatment of spinal hypotension during cesarean section. Anesthesiology 1980;53:514.

Cotton DB, Longmire S, Jones MM, et al. Cardiovascular alterations in severe pregnancy-induced hypertension: effects of nitroglycerin coupled with volume expansion. Am J Obstet Gynecol 1986a;154:1053.

Cotton DB, Jones MM, Longmire S, et al. Role of intravenous nitroglycerin in the treatment of severe pregnancy-induced hypertension complicated by pulmonary edema. Am J Obstet Gynecol 1986b;154:91.

Crawford ME, Carl P, Bach V, et al. A randomized comparison between midazolam and thiopental for elective cesarean section anesthesia. I. Mothers. Anesth Analg 1989;68:229.

Cunniff C, Jones KL, Phillipson J, et al. Oligohydramnios sequence and renal tubular malformation associated with maternal enalapril use. Am J Obstet Gynecol 1990;162:187.

De Wolf D, De Schepper J, Verhaaren H, et al. Congenital hypothyroid goiter and amiodarone. Acta Paediatr Scand 1988;77:616.

Diaz DM, Diaz SF, Marx GF. Cardiovascular effects of glycopyrrolate and belladonna derivatives in obstetric patients. Bull NY Acad Med 1980;56:245.

Ducey JP, Knape KG. Maternal esmolol administration resulting in fetal distress and cesarean section in a term pregnancy. Anesthesiology 1992;77:829.

Dudley D, Gagnon D, Varner M. Long-term tocolysis with intravenous magnesium sulfate. Obstet Gynecol 1989;73:373.

Elkayam U, Goodwin TM. Adenosine therapy for supraventricular tachycardia during pregnancy. Am J Cardiol 1995;75:521.

Entman SS, Moise KJ. Anaphylaxis in pregnancy. South Med J 1984;77:402.

Fagher B, Ahlgren M, Astedt B. Acute massive pulmonary embolism treated with streptokinase during labor and the early puerperium. Acta Obstet Gynecol Scand 1990;69:659.

Fishburne JI Jr, Dormer KJ, Payne GG, et al. Effects of amrinone and dopamine on uterine blood flow and vascular responses in the gravid baboon. Am J Obstet Gynecol 1988;158:829.

Gembruch U, Manz M, Bald R, et al. Repeated intravascular treatment with amiodarone in a fetus with refractory supraventricular tachycardia and hydrops fetalis. Am Heart J 1989;118:1335.

Gerstner G, Grunberger W. Dopamine treatment for prevention of renal failure in patients with severe eclampsia. Clin Exp Obstet Gynecol 1980;7:219.

Goodlin RC. Naloxone and its possible relationship to fetal endorphin levels and fetal distress. Am J Obstet Gynecol 1981;139:16.

Goodnick PJ. Verapamil prophylaxis in pregnant women with bipolar disorder. Am J Psychiatry 1993;150:1560.

Hagley MT, Cole PL. Adenosine use in pregnant women with supraventricular tachycardia. Ann Pharmacother 1994;28:1241.

Hagley MT, Haraden B, Cole PL. Adenosine use in a pregnant patient with supraventricular tachycardia. Ann Pharmacother 1995;29:938.

Harrison JK, Greenfield RA, Wharton JM. Acute termination of supraventricular tachycardia by adenosine during pregnancy. Am Heart J 1992;123:1386.

Heinonen OP, Sloan D, Shapiro S. Birth defects and drugs in pregnancy. Littleton, MA: Publishing Sciences Group, 1977.

Heinrich WL, Cronin R, Miller PD, et al. Hypotensive sequelae of diazoxide and hydralazine therapy. JAMA 1977;237:264.

Hellman LM, Fillisti LP. Analysis of the atropine test for placental transfer in gravidas with toxemia and diabetes. Am J Obstet Gynecol 1965;91:797.

Hill LM, Malkasian GD Jr. The use of quinidine sulfate throughout pregnancy. Obstet Gynecol 1979;54:366.

Ho PC, Chen TY, Wong V. The effect of maternal cardiac disease and digoxin administration on labour, fetal weight and maturity at birth. Aust NZ J Obstet Gynaecol 1980;20:24.

Holbrook RH, Voss EM, Gibson RN. Ovine fetal cardiorespiratory response to nicardipine. Am J Obstet Gynecol 1989;161:718.

Hughes SC, Ward MG, Levinson G, et al. Placental transfer of ephedrine does not affect neonatal outcome. Anesthesiology 1985;63:217.

Jannet D, Carbonne B, Sebban E, et al. Nicardipine versus metoprolol in the treatment of hypertension during pregnancy: a randomized comparative trial. Obstet Gynecol 1994;84:354.

Jelsema RD, Bhatia RK, Ganguly S. Use of intravenous amrinone in the short-term management of refractory heart failure in pregnancy. Obstet Gynecol 1991;78:935.

Kirshon B, Lee W, Mauer MB, et al. Effects of low-dose dopamine therapy in the oliguric patient with preeclampsia. Am J Obstet Gynecol 1988; 159:604–607.

Kivalo I, Saarikasi S. Placental transmission of atropine at full-term pregnancy. Br J Anaesth 1977; 49:1017.

Kofinas AD, Simon NV, Sagel H, et al. Treatment of fetal supraventricular tachycardia with flecainide acetate after digoxin failure. Am J Obstet Gynecol 1991;165:630.

Kohl T, Tercanli S, Kececioglu D, Holzgreve W. Direct fetal administration of adenosine for the termination of incessant supraventricular tachycardia. Obstet Gynecol 1995;85:873.

Lamm CI, Norton KI, Murphy RJC, et al. Congenital rickets associated with magnesium sulfate infusion for tocolysis. J Pediatr 1988;113:1078.

Laurent M, Betremieux P, Biron Y, LeHelloco A. Neonatal hypothyroidism after treatment by amiodarone during pregnancy. Am J Cardiol 1987; 60:942.

Lewis AM, Patel L, Johnson A. Mexiletine in human blood and breast milk. Postgrad Med J 1981;57: 546.

Liedholm H, Wahlin-Boll E, Ingemarsson I, et al. Transplacental passage and breast milk concentration of hydralazine. Eur J Clin Pharmacol 1982;21:417.

Lodeiro JG, Feinstein SJ, Lodeiro SB. Fetal premature atrial contractions associated with hydralazine. Am J Obstet Gynecol 1989;160:105.

Losasso TJ, Muzzi DA, Cucchiara RF. Response of fetal heart rate to maternal administration of esmolol. Anesthesiology 1991;74:782.

Lownes HE, Ives TJ. Mexiletine use in pregnancy and lactation. Am J Obstet Gynecol 1987;157: 446.

Lubbe WF. Use of diltiazem during pregnancy. NZ Med J 1987;100:121.

Mabie WC, Gonzalez AR, Sibai BM, et al. A comparative trial of labetalol and hydralazine in the acute management of severe hypertension complicating pregnancy. Obstet Gynecol 1987;70: 328.

Macphail S, Walkinshaw SA. Fetal supraventricular tachycardia: detection by routine auscultation and successful in-utero management: case report. Br J Obstet Gynaecol 1988;95:1073.

Magee LA, Conover B, Schick B, et al. Exposure to calcium channel blockers in human pregnancy. A prospective, controlled, multicentre cohort study. Teratology 1994;49:372. Abstract.

Martin RA, Jones KL, Mendoza A, et al. Effect of ACE inhibition on the fetal kidney: decreased renal blood flow. Teratology 1992;46:317.

Mason BA, Ricci-Goodman J, Koos BJ. Adenosine in the treatment of maternal paroxysmal supraventricular tachycardia. Obstet Gynecol 1992;80: 478.

Matfin G, Baylis P, Adams P. Maternal paroxysmal supraventricular tachycardia treated with adenosine. Postgrad Med J 1993;69:661.

McKenna WJ, Harris L, Rowland E, et al. Amiodarone therapy during pregnancy. Am J Cardiol 1983; 51:1231.

Milsap RL, Auld PAM. Neonatal hyperglycemia following maternal dioxide administration. JAMA 1980;243:144.

Morgan CD, Sandler M, Panigel M. Placental transfer of catecholamines in vitro and in vivo. Am J Obstet Gynecol 1972;112:1068.

Neuman J, Weiss B, Rabello Y, et al. Diazoxide for the acute control of severe hypertension complicating pregnancy: a pilot study. Obstet Gynecol 1979;53(suppl):50S.

Nishimura H, Tanimura T. Clinical aspects of the teratogenicity of drugs. Amsterdam: Excerpta Medica, 1976:231.

Page RL. Treatment of arrhythmias during pregnancy. Am Heart J 1995;130:871.

Paulissian R. Diazoxide. Int Anesthesiol Clin 1978; 16:201.

Percorari D, Ragni N, Autera C. Administration of furosemide to women during confinement, and its action on newborn infants. Acta Biomed (Italy) 1969;40:2.

Piper JM, Ray WA, Rosa FW. Pregnancy outcome following exposure to angiotensin-converting enzyme inhibitors. Obstet Gynecol 1992;80:429.

Pladetti L, Porciani MC, Scimone G. Placental transfer of digoxin in man. Int J Clin Pharmacol Biopharm 1979;17:82.

Podolsky SM, Varon J. Adenosine use during pregnancy. Ann Emerg Med 1991;20:1027.

Ramamurthy S, Talwar KK, Saxena A, et al. Prosthetic mitral valve thrombosis in pregnancy successfully treated with streptokinase. Am Heart J 1994;127:446.

Ravlo O, Carl P, Crawford ME, et al. A randomized comparison between midazolam and thiopental for elective cesarean section anesthesia. II. Neonates. Anesth Analg 1989;68:234.

Redmond GP. Propranolol and fetal growth retardation. Semin Perinatol 1982;6:142.

Rodis JF, Vintzileos AM, Campbell WA, et al. Maternal hypothermia: an unusual complication of magnesium sulfate therapy. Am J Obstet Gynecol 1987;156:435.

Rogers MC, Willserson JT, Goldblatt A, et al. Serum digoxin concentrations in the human fetus, neonate and infant. N Engl J Med 1972;287:1010.

Rosa FW, Bosco LA, Graham CF, et al. Neonatal anuria with maternal angiotensin-converting enzyme inhibition. Obstet Gynecol 1989;74:371.

Rotmensch HH, Rotmensch S, Elkayam U. Management of cardiac arrhythmias during pregnancy. Current concepts. Drugs 1987;33:623.

Rubin PC. Beta blockers in pregnancy. N Engl J Med 1981;305:1323.

Scanlon JW, Brown WU Jr, Weiss B, et al. Neurobehavioral responses of newborn infants after maternal epidural anesthesia. Anesthesiology 1974; 40:121.

Schardein JL. Chemically induced birth defects. 2nd ed. New York: Marcel Dekker, 1993:341, 343.

Schroeder JS, Harrison DC. Repeated cardioversion during pregnancy; treatment of refractory paroxysmal atrial tachycardia during 3 successive pregnancies. Am J Cardiol 1971;27:445.

Scott AA, Purohit DM. Neonatal renal failure: a complication of maternal antihypertensive therapy. Am J Obstet Gynecol 1989;160:1223.

Shepard TH. Catalog of teratogenic agents. 7th ed. Baltimore: Johns Hopkins University, 1992:140.

Shepard TH. Catalog of teratogenic agents. 7th ed. Baltimore: Johns Hopkins University, 1992:289.

Sherman JL Jr, Locke RV. Transplacental neonatal digitalis intoxication. Am J Cardiol 1960;6:834.

Shnider SM, Way EL. The kinetics of transfer of lidocaine across the human placenta. Anesthesiology 1968;29:944.

Sibai BM, Grossman RA, Grossman HG. Effects of diuretics on plasma volume in pregnancies with long term hypertension. Am J Obstet Gynecol 1984;150:831.

Sloskey GE. Amiodarone: a unique antiarrhythmic agent. Clin Pharm 1983;2:330.

Smith NT, Corbascio AN. The use and misuse of pressor agents. Anesthesiology 1970;33:58.

Snyder SW, Cardwell MS. Neuromuscular blockade with magnesium sulfate and nifedipine. Am J Obstet Gynecol 1989;161:35.

Stokes IM, Evans J, Stone M. Myocardial infarction and cardiac arrest in the second trimester followed by assisted vaginal delivery under epidural analgesia at 38 weeks' gestation: case report. Br J Obstet Gynaecol 1984;91:197.

Sussman HF, Duque D, Lesser ME. Atrial flutter with 1:1 A-V conduction; report of a case in a pregnant woman successfully treated with DC countershock. Dis Chest 1966;49:99.

Tamari I, Edgar M, Rabinowitz B, et al. Medical treatment of cardiovascular disorders during pregnancy. Am Heart J 1982;104:1357.

Timmis AD, Jackson G, Holt DW. Mexiletine for control of ventricular dysrhythmias in pregnancy. Lancet 1980;2:647.

Turrentine MA, Braems G, Ramirez MM. Use of thrombolytics for the treatment of thromboembolic disease during pregnancy. Obstet Gynecol Surv 1995;50:534.

van Engelen AD, Weijtens O, Brenner JI, et al. Management outcome and follow-up of fetal tachycardia. J Am Coll Cardiol 1994;24:1371.

Vogel JHK, Pryor R, Blount SG Jr. Direct-current defibrillation during pregnancy. JAMA 1965;193: 970.

Votts RA, Parada OH, Windgrad RH, et al. Furosemide action on the creatinine concentration of amniotic fluid. Am J Obstet Gynecol 1975; 123:621.

Wagner X, Jouglard J, Moulin M, et al. Coadministration of flecainide acetate and sotalol during pregnancy: lack of teratogenic effects, passage across the placenta, and excretion in human breast milk. Am Heart J 1990;119:700.

Waisman GD, Mayorga LM, Camera MI, et al. Magnesium plus nifedipine: potentiation of hypotensive effect in preeclampsia? Am J Obstet Gynecol 1988;159:308.

Walker JJ, Mathers A, Bjornsson S, et al. The effect of acute and chronic antihypertensive therapy on maternal and fetoplacental Doppler velocimetry. Eur J Obstet Gynecol Reprod Biol 1992;43: 193.

Weaver JB, Pearson JF. Influence of digitalis on time of onset and duration of labour in women with cardiac disease. Br Med J 1973;3:519.

Widerlov E, Karlman I, Storsater J. Hydralazine induced neonatal thrombocytopenia. N Engl J Med 1980;303:1235.

Wladimiroff JW. Effect of furosemide on fetal urine production. Br J Obstet Gynaecol 1975;82:221.

Wren C, Hunter S. Maternal administration of flecainide to terminate and suppress fetal tachycardia. Br Med J 1988;296:249.

Wright RG, Shnider SM, Levinson G, et al. The effect of maternal administration of ephedrine on fetal heart rate and variability. Obstet Gynecol 1981;57:734.

Yemini M, Shoham (Schwartz) Z, Dgani R, et al. Lupus-like syndrome in a mother and newborn following administration of hydralazine: a case report. Eur J Obstet Gynecol Reprod Biol 1989; 30:193.

# Physiologic Tables and Formulas

## Normal third-trimester physiologic values

| Hemodynamics Abbreviation | Definition | Normal Value/Units |
|---|---|---|
| BSA | Body surface area | $m^2$ |
| MAP | Mean systemic arterial pressure | 84–96 mm Hg |
| CVP | Central venous pressure | 4–10 mm Hg |
| PA | Mean pulmonary artery pressure | 10–17 mm Hg |
| PCWP | Mean pulmonary capillary wedge pressure | 6–12 mm Hg |
| CO | Cardiac output | 5.5–7.5 L/min |
| SVR | Systemic vascular resistance | 1000–1400 dynes/sec/cm$^{-5}$ |
| PVR | Pulmonary vascular resistance | 55–100 dynes/sec/cm$^{-5}$ |
| HR | Heart rate | 75–95 beats/min |
| SV | Stroke volume | 60–100 mL/beat |
| LVSWI | Left ventricular stroke work index | 40–55 gmM/m$^2$ |
| EF | Ejection fraction | 0.67 |
| EDV | End-diastolic volume | 70–75 mL/m$^2$ |
| COP | Colloid oncotic pressure | 16–19 mm Hg |
| COP-PCWP | Colloid oncotic pressure-wedge pressure gradient | 8–14 mm Hg |
| $PAo_2$ | Mean partial pressure of oxygen in the alveolus | 104 mm Hg |
| $Pao_2$ | Partial pressure of oxygen in arterial blood | 106–108 mm Hg (first trimester); 101–104 mm Hg (third trimester) |
| $P(A-a)o_2$ | Alveolar-arterial, gradient | 25–65 mm Hg with $Fio_2 = 1.0$ |
| $PAco_2$ | Partial pressure of carbon dioxide in the alveolus | 40 mm Hg |
| $Paco_2$ | Partial pressure of carbon dioxide in arterial blood | 35 mm Hg |
| $P\bar{v}o_2$ | Partial pressure of oxygen in mixed venous blood | Varies, dependent upon cardiac output, $Fio_2$ and oxygen consumption from approximately 35–40 mm Hg |
| $P\bar{v}co_2$ | Partial pressure of carbon dioxide in mixed venous blood | 40–50 mm Hg |
| $Sao_2$ | Oxyhemoglobin saturation of arterial blood | 98% (room air) |
| $S\bar{v}o_2$ | Oxyhemoglobin saturation of mixed venous blood | 75% (room air) |
| $Cao_2$ | Arterial oxygen content | 18–22 mL/dL |
| $C\bar{v}o_2$ | Mixed venous oxygen content | 14–17 mL/dL |
| $C(a-v)o_2$ | Arteriovenous oxygen content difference | 4–6 mL/100 mL |
| $O_2$ extraction ratio | | 0.25 |
| $Vo_2$ | Oxygen consumption | 270–320 mL/min |
| $Vco_2$ | Carbon dioxide production | 240–280 mL/min |
| R | Respiratory quotient | 0.8 |

*(continued)*

# Normal third-trimester physiologic values *(continued)*

| Hemodynamics Abbreviation | Definition | Normal Value/Units |
|---|---|---|
| FRC | Functional residual capacity | 2000 mL |
| VC | Vital capacity | 65–75 mL/kg |
| Ventilation | | 11–13 L/min |
| IF | Inspiratory force | 75–100 cm $H_2O$ |
| EDC | Effective compliance | 35–45 mL/cm $H_2O$ |
| $V_D$ | Dead space | 150 mL |
| $V_T$ | Tidal volume | 500 mL |
| $V_D/V_T$ | Dead space to tidal volume ratio | 0.30–0.35 |
| $\dot{Q}_s/\dot{Q}_t$ | Right-to-left shunt (percent of cardiac output flowing past nonventilated alveoli or the equivalent) | 3.3% |
| Flow volume loops (mean) | | |
| $\dot{V}_{50}$ | Instantaneous flow at 50% VC | 3.5 L/sec |
| $\dot{V}_{25}$ | Instantaneous flow at 25% VC | 1.5 L/sec |
| $\dot{V}_{50R}$ | Expiratory/inspiratory flow at 50% VC | 1.0 |
| $\dot{V}_{25R}$ | Expiratory/inspiratory flow at 25% VC | 0.5 |
| $V_{50/25}$ | Ratio of exp. flow at 50% VC to exp. flow at 25% VC | 2.3 |

## Useful formulas

$$MAP = 2 \cdot (\text{diastolic pressure}) + (\text{systolic pressure})/3$$

$$CI \ (\text{L/min/m}^2) = \frac{\text{Cardiac output (L/min)}}{\text{Body surface area (m}^2)}$$

$$SVR \ (\text{dynes} \cdot \text{sec} \cdot \text{cm}^{-5}) = \frac{\text{MAP[mm Hg]} - \text{CVP[mm Hg]} \times 79.9}{(\text{Cardiac output[L/min]})}$$

$$PVR \ (\text{dynes} \cdot \text{sec} \cdot \text{cm}^{-5}) = \frac{\text{MPAP[mm Hg]} - \text{PCWP[mm Hg]} \times 79.9}{\text{Cardiac output(L/min)}}$$

$$SV \ (\text{mL/beat}) = \frac{\text{Cardiac output}}{\text{Heart rate}}$$

$$SVI \ (\text{mL/min/m}^2) = \frac{\text{Stroke volume}}{\text{Body surface area}}$$

$$RVSWI \ (\text{gmM/m}^2) = SVI \times MPAP \ (\text{mm Hg}) \times 0.0136$$

$$LVSWI \ (\text{gmM/m}^2) = SI \times MAP \ (\text{mm Hg}) \times 0.0136$$

$$C(a-v)o_2 \ (\text{mL/100 mL or vol\%}) = Cao_2 - Cvo_2$$

$$\dot{V}o_2 \ (\text{mL/min/m}^2) = CI \times C(a-v)o_2 \times 10$$

$$RQ = \frac{Vco_2}{Vo_2}$$

$$O_2 \ \text{avail} \ (\text{mL/min/m}^2) = CI \times Cao_2 \times 10$$

$$\dot{Q}s/\dot{Q}t \ (\%) = \frac{Cco_2 - Cao_2}{Cco_2 - Cvo_2} \times 100$$

$$\dot{Q}s/\dot{Q}t \ (\%) = \frac{0.0031 \times P(A-a)o_2}{[C(a-v)o_2 + (0.0031 \times P(A-a)o_2)]} \times 100$$

$$EDC \ (\text{mL/cm H}_2O) = \frac{\text{Tidal volume (mL)}}{\text{Peak airway pressure (cm H}_2O)}$$

$$VD/VT = \frac{Paco_2 - P\bar{E}co_2}{Paco_2}$$

$$P(A-a)o_2 \ (\text{mm Hg}) = PAo_2 - Pao_2$$

$$Cao_2 = (\text{Hgb}) \ (1.34) \ Sao_2 + (Pao_2 \times 0.0031)$$

$$(Sao_2 = \text{Arterial saturation})$$

$$C\bar{v}o_2 = (\text{Hgb}) \ (1.34) \ S\bar{v}o_2 + (Pv\bar{o}_2 \times 0.0031)$$

$$S\bar{v}o_2 = \text{Percent saturation of mixed venous blood}$$

$$\frac{\dot{Q}s}{\dot{Q}t} = \frac{Cc'o_2 - Cao_2}{Cc'o_2 - C\bar{v}o_2}$$

$$C\dot{c}o_2 = (1.34) \ (\text{Hgb}) \ 100\% \ \text{saturation} + 0.0031 \ Pao_2$$

$$PAo_2 = (P_B - P_{H_2O}) \ Fio_2 - P_{CO_2}/0.8$$

$$(P_{H_2O} = \text{Water vapor pressure})$$

$$(P_B = \text{Barometric pressure})$$

## Body surface area calculation

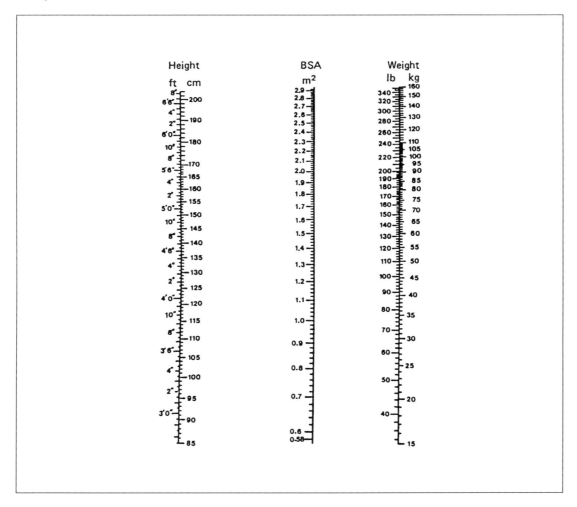

DuBois nomogram for calculating the body surface area of adults. To find body surface of a patient, locate height in inches (or centimeters) on scale 1 and weight in pounds (or kilograms) on scale 3 and place straight edge (ruler) between these two points.

## Serum osmolality calculation

$$\text{Osmolality (mosm/kg)} = 2[\text{Na(mEq/L)} + \text{K(mEq/L)} + \frac{\text{Urea(mg/dL)}}{2.8} + \frac{\text{Glucose (mg/dL)}}{18}$$

## EKG changes in pregnancy

|  | 1TM | 2TM | 3TM | D | PP |
|---|---|---|---|---|---|
| Heart rate (bpm) | 77 | 79 | 87 | 80 | 66 |
| QT interval(s) | 0.378 | 0.375 | 0.361 | 0.362 | 0.406 |
| QT$_c$ interval(s) | 0.424 | 0.427 | 0.431 | 0.414 | 0.423 |
| PR interval(s) | 0.160 | 0.160 | 0.155 | 0.155 | 0.160 |
| P wave |  |  |  |  |  |
| Duration (s) | 0.092 | 0.092 | 0.091 | 0.091 | 0.096 |
| Amplitude (mm) | 1.9 | 1.9 | 2.0 | 2.0 | 1.9 |
| Axis (degrees) | 40 | 38 | 38 | 41 | 35 |
| QRS complex |  |  |  |  |  |
| Duration (s) | 0.074 | 0.074 | 0.074 | 0.076 | 0.077 |
| Amplitude (mm) | 11.5 | 11.5 | 12.4 | 12.2 | 11.2 |
| Axis (degrees) | 49 | 46 | 40 | 44 | 44 |
| T wave |  |  |  |  |  |
| Duration (s) | 0.168 | 0.171 | 0.165 | 0.166 | 0.176 |
| Amplitude (mm) | 3.4 | 3.5 | 3.4 | 3.6 | 3.5 |
| Axis (degrees) | 27 | 25 | 22 | 33 | 34 |

1TM = first trimester; 2TM = second trimester; 3TM = third trimester; D = 1–3 days after delivery; PP = 6–8 weeks postpartum.

Mean EKG measurements during normal pregnancy, delivery, and postpartum in 102 patients

(Reprinted with permission from Carruth JE, Mirvis SB, Brogan DR, et al. The electrocardiogram in normal pregnancy. Am Heart J 1981;6:1075.)

## Thyroid function in pregnancy

| | Total T$_4$ | Free T$_4$ | Total T$_3$ | Free T$_3$ | T$_3$ resin uptake | Free thyroxine index (T$_7$) |
|---|---|---|---|---|---|---|
| Normal nonpregnant | 5–13 μg/100 ml | 2.70 μg/100 ml | 70–150 μg/100 ml | 1.5 μg/100 ml | 0.8–1.15 | 4.5–12 |
| Normal pregnant | ↑ | ↔ | ↑ | ↔ | ↓ | 4.5–12 |
| Pregnant hyperthyroid | ↑ ↑ to ↑ ↑ ↑ | ↑ ↑ to ↑ ↑ ↑ | ↑ ↑ to ↑ ↑ ↑ | Not measured | Normal to ↑ ↑ | ↑ ↑ ↑ |
| Pregnant hypothyroid | ↔ to ↓ | ↓ | ↓ | Not measured | ↓ to ↓ ↓ | Low |

T$_4$ = thyroxine; T$_3$ = triiodothyronine; ↔ = stays the same.

(Reproduced with permission from Komins JI, et al. Hyperthyroidism in pregnancy. Obstet Gynecol Sur Baltimore: Williams & Wilkins, 1975;30: 527.)

## Modified Glasgow Coma Score (GCS)*

| Sign | Evaluation | Score |
|---|---|---|
| Eye opening | Spontaneous | 4 |
| | To speech | 3 |
| | To pain | 2 |
| | None | 1 |
| Best verbal response | Oriented | 5 |
| | Confused | 4 |
| | Inappropriate | 3 |
| | Incomprehensible | 2 |
| | None | 1 |
| Best motor response | Obeys commands | 6 |
| | Localizes pain | 5 |
| | Withdrawal to pain | 4 |
| | Flexion to pain | 3 |
| | Extension to pain | 2 |
| | None | 1 |

*GCS < 8 = severe brain injury; GCS < 7 = immediate intubation.

(Modified from Jennett B. Assessment of severity of head injury. J Neurol Neurosurg Psychiatry 1976;39:647.)

## Coagulation factor requirements for hemostasis

| Coagulation factor | Requirement (% of normal) |
|---|---|
| Prothrombin | 40 |
| Factor V | 10–15 |
| Factor VII | 5–10 |
| Factor VIII | 10–40 |
| Factor IX | 10–40 |
| Factor X | 10–15 |
| Factor XI | 20–30 |
| Factor XII | 0 |
| Prekallikrein | 0 |
| High-molecular-weight kininogen | 0 |
| Factor XIII | 1–5 |

(Reproduced with permission from Orland MJ, Saltmaur J, eds. Manual of medical therapeutics, 25th ed. Boston: Little, Brown, 1986: 277.)

## Plasma coagulation factors in pregnancy

| Factor | Name | Change in pregnancy |
|---|---|---|
| I | Fibrinogen | 4.0–6.5 g/L |
| II | Prothrombin | 100%–125% |
| IV | $Ca^H$ | |
| V | Proaccelerin | 100%–150% |
| VII | Proconvertin | 150%–250% |
| VIII | Antihemophilic factor A (AHF) | 200%–500% |
| IX | Antihemophilic B (Christmas factor) | 100%–150% |
| X | Stuart Prower factor | 150%–250% |
| XI | Antihemophilic factor C | 50%–100% |
| XII | Hageman factor | 100%–200% |
| XIII | Fibrin-stabilizing factor | 35%–75% |
| | Antithrombin III | 75%–100% |
| | Antifactor Xa | 75%–100% |

(Modified from Romero R. The management of acquired hemolytic failure in pregnancy. In: Berkowtiz RL, ed. Critical care of the obstetric patient. New York: Churchill Livingstone, 1983.)

# The coagulation cascade

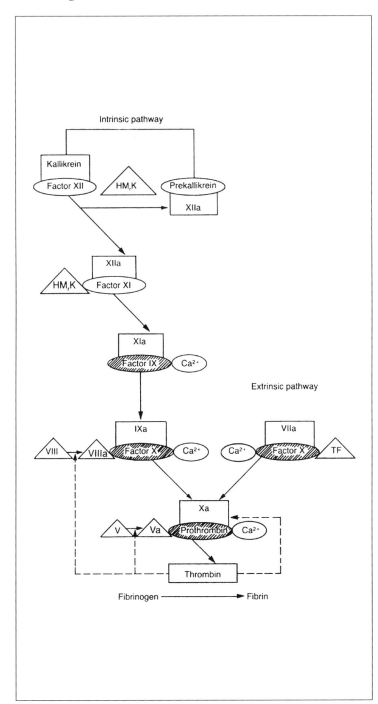

Ovals represent inactive protease precursors. Rectangles represent active proteases. Nonenzymatic protein cofactors are represented by triangles. Hatched ovals represent factors which are felt to be activated on a tissue phospholipid surface. The feedback reactions accelerate the coagulation process. (Reproduced with permission from Orland MJ, Saltmaur J, eds. Manual of medical therapeutics, 25th ed. Boston: Little, Brown, 1986: 272.)

## Anemia: differential diagnosis

| Anemia Type | Peripheral Smear |
| --- | --- |
| Iron deficiency | Hypochromic microcytic |
| Anemia of chronic disease | Microcytic/normocytic |
| Thalassemia | Target cells, anisocytosis, microcytic |
| B$_{12}$/folate deficient | Macrocytic, hypersegmented PMNs |
| Microangiopathic hemolysis anemia | Normocytic schistocytes, helmet cells |
| Sickling disorders | Normocytic sickled cells |

## Pulmonary function in pregnancy

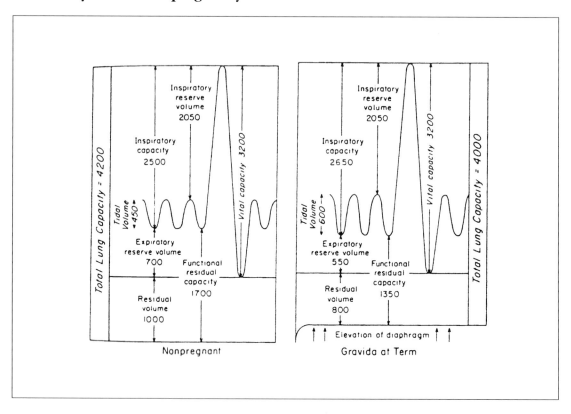

Pulmonary volumes and capacities in the nonpregnant state and in the gravida at term. (Courtesy of Bonica J J. Principles and practice of obstetric analgesia and anesthesia. Philadelphia: F.A. Davis Company, 1967.)

## Oxygenation throughout pregnancy

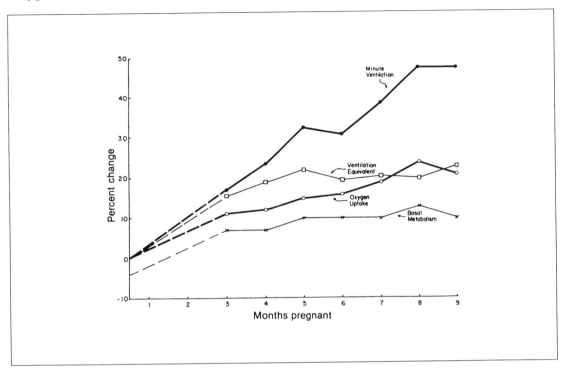

Percentage changes of minute volume, oxygen uptake, basal metabolism, and the ventilation equivalent for oxygen at monthly intervals throughtout pregnancy. (Reproduced by permission from Prowse CM, Gaensler EA. Respiratory and acid-base changes during pregnancy. Anesthesiology 1965;26:381.)

## Postpartum hematocrit and blood volume changes

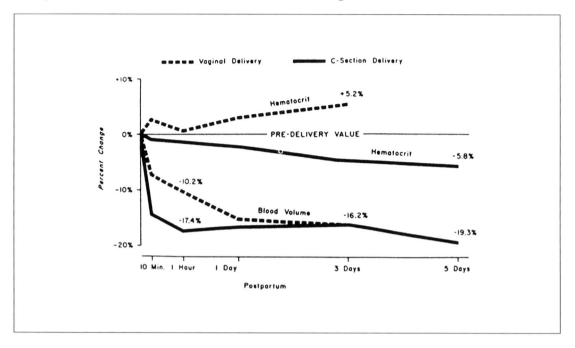

Percentage changes in blood volume and venous hematocrit following vaginal delivery or cesarean section. (Reproduced by permission from Metcalfe J, Ueland K. Heart disease and pregnancy. In: Fowler NO, ed. Cardiac diagnosis and treatment, 3rd ed. Hagerstown, MD: Harper & Row, 1980:1153–1170.)

## Body water distribution

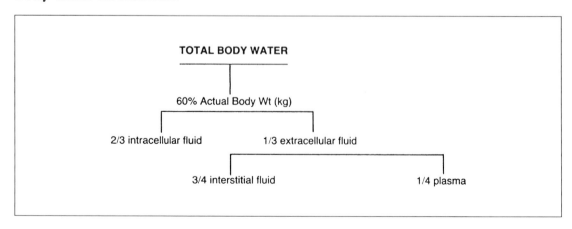

# Electrolyte content of body fluids

| Sweat or gastrointestinal secretion | Electrolyte concentration (mEq/L) | | | | | Replacement amount for each liter lost | | | |
|---|---|---|---|---|---|---|---|---|---|
| | $Na^-$ | $K^-$ | $H^-$ | $Cl^-$ | $HCO_3^-$ | Isotonic saline (mL) | 5% D/W (mL) | KCl* (mEq) | $NaHCO_3$[†] (mEq) |
| Sweat | 30–50 | 5 | | 45–55 | | 300 | 700 | 5 | |
| Gastric secretions | 40–65 | 10 | 90[‡] | 100–140 | | 300 | 700 | 20[§] | |
| Pancreatic fistula | 135–155 | 5 | | 55–75 | 70–90 | 250 | 750 | 5 | 90 |
| Biliary fistula | 135–155 | 5 | | 80–110 | 35–50 | 750 | 250 | 5 | 45 |
| Ileostomy fluid | 120–130 | 10 | | 50–60 | 50–70 | 300 | 700 | 10 | 67.6 |
| Diarrhea fluid | 25–50 | 35–60 | | 20–40 | 30–45 | | 1000 | 35 | 45 |

*Caution should be used in administering potassium faster than 10 mEq/hour.

[†]One ampule of 7.5% NaHCO₃ contains 45 mEq $HCO_3^-$.

[‡]Variable (e.g., achlorhydria).

[§]Administration of more than the observed gastric loss of potassium is often required because of enhanced urinary potassium excretion in alkalosis. (Reproduced with permission from Orland MJ, Saltmaur J, eds. Manual of medical therapeutics, 25th ed. Boston: Little, Brown, 1986: 43).

APPENDIX *2*

# Drugs, Devices, and Fluid Therapy

## Guidelines for the institution and discontinuation of mechanical ventilation

| Parameter | Normal range | Indication for ventilatory assistance | Indication for weaning |
|---|---|---|---|
| Mechanics | | | |
| Respiratory rate | 12–20 | >35 | <30 |
| Vital capacity (mL/kg of body weight) | 65–75 | <15 | 12–15 |
| FEV$_1$ (mL/kg of body weight) | 50–60 | <10 | >10 |
| Inspiratory force | 75–100 | <25 | >25 |
| Oxygenation | | | |
| Pao$_2$ (mm Hg) | 100–75 (room air) | <70 (on mask O$_2$) | — |
| P(A−a)o$_2$ (Fio$_2$ = 1.0) | 25–65 | 450 | <400 |
| Ventilation | | | |
| Paco$_2$ (mm Hg) | 35–45 | >55 | — |
| V$_D$/V$_T$ | 0.25–0.40 | >0.60 | <0.58 |

## Oxygen delivery systems

| Delivery | Common flow (L/min) | Inspired O$_2$ concentration (%) | Comments |
|---|---|---|---|
| Nasal cannula | 1–6 | 24–44 | Inspired O$_2$ concentration increases by approximately 4% for each 1 L/min flow; exact FIo$_2$ is uncertain. |
| Face mask | 8–10 | 40–60 | Oxygen flow should be higher than 5 L/min to avoid accumulatioin of exhaled air. |
| Face mask with oxygen reservoir | 6–10 | 60–100 | Inspired O$_2$ concentration increases by 10% for each 1 L/min flow. |
| Venturi mask | — | 24, 28, 31, 35, 40, 50 | Provides constant controlled FIo$_2$. |
| Mouth-to-mouth | — | 17 | — |
| Mouth-to-mask | 10–15 | 50–80 | — |

## Vitamin requirements in pregnancy (compared with standard intravenous vitamin preparation)

| Vitamin | RDA | MVI-12 |
|---------|-----|--------|
| A | 800 μg RE | 3300 USP (retinol)* |
| D | 400 IU (10 μg cholecalciferol) | 200 USP units[†] |
| E (de-alpha-tocopherol acetate) | 10 mg a-TE | 10 USP units* |
| Ascorbic acid | 70 mg | 100 mg |
| Thiamine (B$_1$) | 1.5 mg | 3.0 mg |
| Riboflavin (B$_2$) | 1.6 mg | 3.6 mg |
| Pyridoxine (B$_6$) | 2.2 mg | 4.0 mg |
| Niacin | 17 mg | 40.0 mg |
| Pantothenic acid | 4–7 mg[‡] | 15.0 mg |
| Biotin | 30–100 μg[‡] | 60 μg |
| Folic Acid | 400 μg | 400 μg |
| B$_{12}$ | 2.2 μg | 5 μg |
| K | 0.03–1.5 μg/kg (RDA) | —[§] |

*Equivalent to RDA.

[†]May require additional supplementation for women with a history of poor intake.

[‡]Estimated safe and adequate daily dietary intakes in nonpregnant adults (RDA).

[§]Must be added to vitamin regimens.

(Reproduced with permission from Nutrition Support Dietetics, 2nd ed. American Society for Parenteral and Enteral Care, Silver Springs, MD, 1993.)

## Mineral and trace element requirements in pregnancy

| Mineral | Enteral Nutrition | Parenteral Nutrition |
|---------|-------------------|----------------------|
| Calcium | 1200 mg | 200–250 mg (9.6–12.5 mEq) |
| Phosphorus | 1200 mg (38 mm) | 30–45 mm |
| Magnesium | 450 mg (37.5 mEq) | 10–15 mEq |
| Zinc | 15 mg | 2.55–3.0 mg |
| Copper | 1.5–3.0 mg* | 0.5–1.5 mg |
| Manganese | 2.0–5.0 mg* | 0.15–0.8 mg |
| Iodine | 175 μg | 50 μg[†] |
| Selenium | 65 μg | 20–40 μg[‡] |
| Iron | 10 + 30–60 mg supplemental iron | 3–6 mg |
| Chromium | 0.05–0.2 mg* | 10–15 μg |

*Estimated safe and adequate daily intakes in nonpregnant adults.

[†]Assuming 80% absorption.

[‡]Recommended intravenous dose for stable adults.

(Reproduced with permission from Nutrition Support Dietetics, 2nd ed. American Society for Parenteral and Enteral Nutrition, Silver Springs, MD, 1993.)

## Insulin preparations and properties

| Type | Action (Hours)* | | |
|------|------|------|------|
|      | Onset | Peak | Duration |
| Rapid |  |  |  |
| Regular (crystalline) | 0.3–1 | 2–4 | 6–8 |
| Semilente | 0.5–1.0 | 2–6 | 10–12 |
| Intermediate |  |  |  |
| NPH | 1–2 | 6–12 | 18–24 |
| Lente | 1–2 | 6–12 | 18–24 |
| Slow |  |  |  |
| Ultralente | 3–8 | 18–24 | 36 |
| Protamine zinc | 3–8 | 14–24 | 36 |

*These are approximate figures. There is significant variation from patient to patient and from dose to dose in the same patient.

## Topical corticosteroid preparations

Low potency
Hydrocortisone 0.5%
Hydrocortisone 1%
Desonide 0.05%

Medium potency
Triamcinolone acetonide 0.1%
Betamethasone dipropionate 0.05%
Betamethasone valerate 0.1%
Fluocinolone acetonide 0.025%
Flurandrenolide 0.05%

High potency
Fluocinonide 0.05%
Halcinonide 0.1%
Desoximetasone 0.25%

## Glucocorticoids

| Steroid action | Available tablet size (mg) | Relative anti-inflammatory effect | Relative mineralo-corticoid effect | Duration |
|---|---|---|---|---|
| Hydrocortisone | 5, 10, 20 | 1.0 | 1.0 | S |
| Prednisone | 1, 2.5, 5, 10, 20, 50 | 4.0 | 0.8 | I |
| Prednisolone | 5 | 4.0 | 0.8 | I |
| Methyl-prednisolone | 2, 4, 8, 16, 24, 32 | 5.0 | 0.5 | I |
| Dexamethasone | 0.25, 0.5, 0.75, 1.5, 4, 6 | 25.0 | 0.0 | L |
| Betamethasone | 0.6 | 25.0 | 0.0 | L |

S = short; I = intermediate; L = long.

## Narcotics: relative potency

| Drug | Potency Relative to Morphine | Oral-Parenteral Potency |
|---|---|---|
| Hydromorphone | 6.0 | 1:5 |
| Morphine | 1.0 | 1:6 |
| Oxycodone | 1.0 | 1:2 |
| Pentazocine (Talwin) | 0.25 | 1:3 |
| Meperidine (Demerol) | 0.15 | 1:3 |
| Codeine | 0.1 | 2:3 |

## Commonly used antihypertensive agents

| Drug | Indication | Oral Dose | Parenteral Dose |
|------|-----------|-----------|-----------------|
| Alphamethyldopa | Chronic hypertension | 250–500 mg b.i.d.–q.i.d. | |
| Hydralazine hydrochloride | Acute control of hypertensive crisis (IV) chronic hypertension (p.o.) | 25–50 mg b.i.d.–q.i.d. | 5–10 mg IV q 20 minutes |
| Atenolol | Chronic hypertension | 50–100 mg p.o. q.i.d. | |
| Propranolol | Chronic hypertension | 40–160 mg b.i.d.–q.i.d. | |
| Labetolol | | 200–400 mg b.i.d. | 20–80 mg IV q 10 minutes |
| Nifedipine | | 10–20 mg q 6–8 h | |

## Commonly used agents for hemodynamic manipulation

| Drug | Method of Preparation | Microdrop Concentration[†] µg/µgtt | Begin at Low Dosage[†] µg/kg/min | Progress to High Dosage[†] µg/kg/min | Comments |
|---|---|---|---|---|---|
| Dopamine (Inotropin) (Single Strength) | 1 amp (200 mg) in 250 mL | 13.3 | 5 (26)[‡] | 20 (105)[‡] | Renal 0–3; Mixed renal/beta 3–7; Renal/beta/alpha >7 µg/kg/min |
| Dopamine (Inotropin) (Double Strength) | 2 amps (400 mg) in 250 mL | 26.6 | 5 (13)[‡] | 20 (52)[‡] | NEJM 1979;300:17. |
| Dobutamine (Dobutrex) | 1 amp (250 mg) in 250 mL | 16.6 | 5 (21)[‡] | — | |
| Epinephrine | 2 amps (2 mg) in 250 mL | 0.13 | 0.01 (5)[‡] | 0.20 (100)[‡] | Beta 0.01–0.03; mixed 0.03; alpha >0.15; µg/kg/min |
| Isoproterenol (Isuprel) | 1 large amp (1 mg) in 250 mL (or 5 small amps in 250 mL) | 0.066 | 0.01 (10)[‡] | 0.30 (300)[‡] | |
| Phenylophrine (Neosynephrine) | 1 amp (10 mg) in 250 mL | 0.66 | 0.1 (11)[‡] | 0.7 (74)[‡] | Practically, pure alpha |
| Norepinephrine (Levophed) | 2 amps (8 mg) in 250 mL | 0.53 | 0.05 (7)[‡] | 1 (132)[‡] | |
| Phentolamine (Regitine) | 1.5 amps (7.5 mg) in 250 mL | 0.5 | 0.5 (70)[‡] | 20 (2800)[‡] | |
| Nitroprusside (Nipride) | 1 bottle (50 mg) in 250 mL | 3.3 | 0.4 (8)[‡] | 5 (106)[‡] | Toxic 8 µg/kg/min; or acute toxicity 1.5 mg/kg over 3 h period |
| Nitroglycerin | 50 mg in 250 mL via millipore filter | 3.3 | 0.4 (8)[‡] | 1.5; may up to 5 in awake patients (106)[‡] | No known metabolic toxicity as yet |

[†]Microdrop (µgtt) is provided by an infusion apparatus giving 60 drops per mL.

[‡]Microdrops per minute for a 70 kg patient

Some guidelines are approximate and modulated by clinical response and indications

## Blood component therapy

| Product | Volume (mL) | Content | Life |
|---|---|---|---|
| Whole blood | 450 | All blood components | 35 d No granulocytes or platelets after 24 hours. Decreased but functionally adequate levels of factors V and VIII for 1–2 weeks |
| Packed red blood cells | 250 | Red cells only | 35 d |
| Fresh-frozen plasma | 200–250 | All stable and labile clotting factors | 1 y |
| Cryoprecipitate | 50 | Factors V, VIII:c, VIII: Von Willibrand, XIII, fibronectin fibrinogen | 1 y |
| Platelets | 50 (per pack) | Platelets | 5 d |

## Electrolyte equivalencies

| | mg/mEq |
|---|---|
| NaCl | 58 |
| NaHCO$_3$ | 84 |
| KCl | 75 |
| KHCO$_3$ | 100 |
| MgSO$_4 \cdot$ 7 H$_2$O | 123 |
| CaCO$_3$ | 50 |
| CaCl$_2 \cdot$ 2 H$_2$O | 73 |
| Ca gluconate$_2 \cdot$ 1 H$_2$O | 224 |

## Intravenous fluids

| | Osmolality (mosm/kg | Glucose concentration (g/L) | Na (mEq/L) | Cl (mEq/L |
|---|---|---|---|---|
| 5% dextrose/water | 252 | 50 | — | — |
| 10% dextrose/water | 505 | 100 | — | — |
| 50% dextrose/water | 2520 | 500 | — | — |
| 0.45% NaCl | 154 | — | 77 | 77 |
| 0.9% NaCl | 308 | — | 154 | 154 |
| Lactated Ringer's solution | 272 | — | 130 | 109 |

*Also contains K (4 mEq/L), Ca (3 mEq/L), and lactate (28 mEq/L)

## Solution for total parenteral nutrition in pregnancy

### Pharmacy Orders

| | |
|---|---|
| Aminosyn 2, 8.5% | 454.0 mL |
| Dextrose, 50% | 516.0 mL |
| Lypholyte II | 20.0 mL |
| Sodium phosphate (4.0 mEq/mL) | 4.0 mL |
| MVI | 5.5 mL |
| Trace elements* | 0.7 mL |

Make 2 bottles, send 500 mL of lipid emulsion 10%.

### Nursing Orders

1. Run TPN bottles at 80 mL per hour.
2. Run lipid 10% emulsion at 125 mL per hour until 500 mL of lipid have been infused.
3. Routine monitoring (Weight, I&O, and Urinary Glucose q 6 h).

Each bottle of TPN (total volume 1000 mL) supplies the following:

| | |
|---|---|
| Aminosyn 2, 8.5% | 454 cc (38.6 gm protein) |
| Dextrose, 50% | 516 cc (end concentration 25.8%) |
| | 1.03 cal/mL TPN |
| Sodium | 51.0 mEq |
| Potassium | 20.0 mEq |
| Calcium | 4.5 mEq |
| Magnesium | 5.0 mEq |
| Zinc | 3.5 mg |
| Copper | 0.7 mg |
| Manganese | 0.4 mg |
| Chromium | 7.0 mcg |
| Chloride | 35.0 mEq |
| Acetate | 29.5 mEq |
| Phosphate | 24.0 mEq |

*Add 800 μg folic acid and 6 mg iron to one bottle daily.

Sample TPN Solution in Pregnancy for 63-kg woman, height 168 cm, age 23.

## Solution for total parenteral nutrition in pregnancy (*continued*)

MVI-12                          5.5 cc
Folic acid                      800 mg
Iron                            6 mg

### Calories

Using the Harris-Benedict equation, these factors calculate a basal energy expenditure (BEE) of 1461 kcal/d. Since calorie and protein requirements parenterally are the same as for a pregnant woman being fed orally or enterally, we used the factor of 1.5 × BEE to calculate caloric need.

Pt's BEE (1461) × 1.5 − 2192 + additional kcals for 2nd + 3rd trimester (300 kcals/d) − 2500 kcals/d.

### Protein

The current recommended dietary allowance (RDA) for protein has been reduced to an additional 10 g/d.

Feeding 1 g/kg/d would provide 63 g of protein for this patient on her ideal weight. An additional 10 g were added to her TPN for a total of 73 g or 1.2 g/kg/d.

### Fats

The requirement for essential fatty acids (EFA) is slightly increased in pregnancy to 4.5% of total calories. It is important to use a fat emulsion that contains both linoleic and linolenic acids. Liposyn is the brand of fat emulsion used in this TPN order and it is composed of 60% essential fatty acids.

### Electrolytes, trace elements

Most standard packs provide adequate amounts except for folate and iron. The iron can be safely infused intravenously, dependent upon rate and dosage.

# Index